KEY TO ESSENTIAL TERMINOLOGY

Client Assessment Database

Provides an overview of the more commonly occurring etiology and coexisting factors associated with a specific medical and/or surgical diagnosis as well as the signs and symptoms and corresponding diagnostic findings.

Nursing Priorities

Establishes a general ranking of needs and concerns on which the Nursing Diagnoses are ordered in constructing the plan of care. This ranking would be altered according to the individual client situation.

Discharge Goals

Identifies generalized statements that could be developed into short-term and intermediate goals to be achieved by the client before being "discharged" from nursing care. They may also provide guidance for creating long-term goals for the client to work on after discharge.

Nursing Diagnosis

The general need or problem (diagnosis) is stated without the distinct cause and signs and symptoms, which would be added to create a client diagnostic statement when specific client information is available. For example, when a client displays increased tension, apprehension, quivering voice, and focus on self, the nursing diagnosis of Anxiety might be stated: severe Anxiety related to unconscious conflict, threat to self-concept as evidenced by statements of increased tension, apprehension; observations of quivering voice, focus on self.

In addition, diagnoses identified within these guides for planning care as actual or risk can be changed or deleted and new diagnoses added, depending entirely on the specific client information.

May Be Related to/Possibly Evidenced by

These lists provide the usual or common reasons (etiology) why a particular need or problem may occur with probable signs and symptoms, which would be used to create the "related to" and "evidenced by" portions of the *client diagnostic statement* when the specific situation is known.

When a risk diagnosis has been identified, signs and symptoms have not yet developed and therefore are not included in the nursing diagnosis statement. However, interventions are provided to prevent progression to an actual problem. The exception to this occurs in the nursing diagnosis risk for Violence, which has possible indicators that reflect the client's risk status.

Desired Outcomes/Evaluation Criteria—Client Will

These give direction to client care as they identify what the client or nurse hopes to achieve. They are stated in general terms to permit the practitioner to modify or individualize them by adding time lines and specific client criteria so they become "measurable." For example, "Client will appear relaxed and report anxiety is reduced to a manageable level within 24 hours."

Nursing Outcomes Classification (NOC) labels are also included. The outcome label is selected from a standardized nursing language and serves as a general header for the outcome indicators that follow.

Actions/Interventions

Nursing Interventions Classification (NIC) labels are drawn from a standardized nursing language and serve as a general header for the nursing actions that follow.

Nursing actions are divided into independent—those actions that the nurse performs autonomously; and collaborative—those actions that the nurse performs in conjunction with others, such as implementing physician orders. The interventions in this book are generally ranked from most to least common. When creating the individual plan of care, interventions would normally be ranked to reflect the client's specific needs and situation. In addition, the division of independent and collaborative is arbitrary and is actually dependent on the individual nurse's capabilities and hospital and community standards.

Rationale

Although not commonly appearing in client plans of care, rationale has been included here to provide a pathophysiological basis to assist the nurse in deciding about the relevance of a specific intervention for an individual client situation.

Clinical Pathway

This abbreviated plan of care or care map is event- or task-oriented and provides outcome-based guidelines for goal achievement within a designated length of stay. Several samples have been included to demonstrate alternative planning formats.

NURSING DIAGNOSES ACCEPTED FOR USE AND RESEARCH FOR 2009–2011

Activity Intolerance [specify level]
Activity Intolerance, risk for
Activity Planning, ineffective
Airway Clearance, ineffective
Allergy Response, latex
Allergy Response, risk for latex
Anxiety [specify level]
Anxiety, death
Aspiration, risk for
Attachment, risk for impaired
Autonomic Dysreflexia
Autonomic Dysreflexia, risk for
Behavior, risk-prone health
Bleeding, risk for
Body Image, disturbed
Body Temperature, risk for imbalanced
Bowel Incontinence
Breastfeeding, effective
Breastfeeding, ineffective
Breastfeeding, interrupted
Breathing Pattern, ineffective
Cardiac Output, decreased
Caregiver Role Strain
Caregiver Role Strain, risk for
Childbearing Process, readiness for enhanced
Comfort, impaired
Comfort, readiness for enhanced
Communication, impaired verbal
Communication, readiness for enhanced
Conflict, decisional
Conflict, parental role
Confusion, acute
Confusion, risk for acute
Confusion, chronic
Constipation
Constipation, perceived
Constipation, risk for
Contamination
Contamination, risk for
Coping, defensive
Coping, ineffective
Coping, readiness for enhanced
Coping, ineffective community
Coping, readiness for enhanced community
Coping, compromised family
Coping, disabled family
Coping, readiness for enhanced family
Death Syndrome, risk for sudden infant
Decision-Making, readiness for enhanced
Denial, ineffective
Dentition, impaired
Development, risk for delayed
Diarrhea
Dignity, risk for compromised human
Distress, moral
Disuse Syndrome, risk for
Diversional Activity, deficient
Electrolyte Imbalance, risk for
Energy Field, disturbed
Environmental Interpretation Syndrome, impaired
Failure to Thrive, adult
Falls, risk for
Family Processes, dysfunctional
Family Processes, interrupted
Family Processes, readiness for enhanced
Fatigue
Fear
Feeding Pattern, ineffective infant
Fluid Balance, readiness for enhanced
[Fluid Volume, deficient hyper/hypotonic]
Fluid Volume, deficient [isotonic]
Fluid Volume, excess
Fluid Volume, risk for deficient

Fluid Volume, risk for imbalanced
Gas Exchange, impaired
Glucose Level, risk for unstable blood
Grieving
Grieving, complicated
Grieving, risk for complicated
Growth, risk for disproportionate
Growth and Development, delayed
Health Maintenance, ineffective
Health Management, ineffective self [formerly
    Therapeutic Regimen Management, ineffective]
Health Management, readiness for enhanced self
    [formerly Therapeutic Regimen Management,
    readiness for enhanced]
Home Maintenance, impaired
Hope, readiness for enhanced
Hopelessness
Hyperthermia
Hypothermia
Identity, disturbed personal
Immunization Status, readiness for enhanced
Infant Behavior, disorganized
Infant Behavior, readiness for enhanced organized
Infant Behavior, risk for disorganized
Infection, risk for
Injury, risk for
Injury, risk for perioperative positioning
Insomnia
Intracranial Adaptive Capacity, decreased
Jaundice, neonatal
Knowledge, deficient [Learning Need] [specify]
Knowledge [specify], readiness for enhanced
Lifestyle, sedentary
Liver Function, risk for impaired
Loneliness, risk for
Maternal/Fetal Dyad, risk for disturbed
Memory, impaired
Mobility, impaired bed
Mobility, impaired physical
Mobility, impaired wheelchair
Motility, dysfunctional gastrointestinal
Motility, risk for dysfunctional gastrointestinal
Nausea
Neglect, self
Neglect, unilateral
Noncompliance [Adherence, ineffective] [specify]
Nutrition: less than body requirements, imbalanced
Nutrition: more than body requirements, imbalanced
Nutrition: more than body requirements, risk for
    imbalanced
Nutrition, readiness for enhanced
Oral Mucous Membrane, impaired
Pain, acute
Pain, chronic
Parenting, impaired
Parenting, readiness for enhanced
Parenting, risk for impaired
Perfusion, ineffective peripheral tissue
Perfusion, risk for decreased cardiac tissue
Perfusion, risk for ineffective cerebral tisse
Perfusion, risk for ineffective gastrointestinal
Perfusion, risk for ineffective renal
Peripheral Neurovascular Dysfunction, risk for
Poisoning, risk for
Post-Trauma Syndrome [specify stage]
Post-Trauma Syndrome, risk for
Power, readiness for enhanced
Powerlessness [specify level]
Powerlessness, risk for
Protection, ineffective
Rape-Trauma Syndrome
(Rape-Trauma Syndrome: compound reaction—
    retired 2009)

(Rape-Trauma Syndrome: silent reaction—retired
    2009)
Relationship, readiness for enhanced
Religiosity, impaired
Religiosity, risk for impaired
Religiosity, readiness for enhanced
Relocation Stress Syndrome
Relocation Stress Syndrome, risk for
Resilience, impaired individual
Resilience, readiness for enhanced
Resilience, risk for compromised
Role Performance, ineffective
Self-Care, readiness for enhanced
Self-Care Deficit: bathing
Self-Care Deficit: dressing
Self-Care Deficit: feeding
Self-Care Deficit: toileting
Self-Concept, readiness for enhanced
Self-Esteem, chronic low
Self-Esteem, situational low
Self-Esteem, risk for situational low
Self-Mutilation
Self-Mutilation, risk for
Sensory Perception, disturbed (specify: visual,
    auditory, kinesthetic, gustatory, tactile, olfactory)
Sexual Dysfunction
Sexuality Pattern, ineffective
Shock, risk for
Skin Integrity, impaired
Skin Integrity, risk for impaired
Sleep, readiness for enhanced
Sleep Deprivation
Sleep Pattern, disturbed
Social Interaction, impaired
Social Isolation
Sorrow, chronic
Spiritual Distress
Spiritual Distress, risk for
Spiritual Well-Being, readiness for enhanced
Stress Overload
Suffocation, risk for
Suicide, risk for
Surgical Recovery, delayed
Swallowing, impaired
(Therapeutic Regimen Management, effective—
    retired 2009)
(Therapeutic Regimen Management, ineffective
    community—retired 2009)
Therapeutic Regimen Management, ineffective
    family
Thermoregulation, ineffective
(Thought Processes, disturbed—retired 2009)
Tissue Integrity, impaired
Transfer Ability, impaired
Trauma, risk for
Trauma, risk for vascular
Urinary Elimination, impaired
Urinary Elimination, readiness for enhanced
Urinary Incontinence, functional
Urinary Incontinence, overflow
Urinary Incontinence, reflex
Urinary Incontinence, stress
(Urinary Incontinence, total—retired 2009)
Urinary Incontinence, urge
Urinary Incontinence, risk for urge
Urinary Retention [acute/chronic]
Ventilation, impaired spontaneous
Ventilatory Weaning Response, dysfunctional
Violence, [actual/]risk for other-directed
Violence, [actual/]risk for self-directed
Walking, impaired
Wandering [specify sporadic or continual]
[ ] author recommendations

Nursing Care Plans

Guidelines for Individualizing Client Care Across the Life Span

EDITION 8

Nursing Care Plans

Guidelines for Individualizing Client Care Across the Life Span

Marilynn E. Doenges, APRN, BC-Retired
Clinical Specialist, Adult Psychiatric/Mental Health Nursing, Retired
Adjunct Faculty
Beth-El College of Nursing and Health Sciences, UCCS
Colorado Springs, Colorado

Mary Frances Moorhouse, RN, MSN, CRRN, LNC
Adjunct Faculty/Clinical Instructor
Pikes Peak Community College
Nurse Consultant/TNT-RN Enterprises
Colorado Springs, Colorado

Alice C. Murr, RN, BSN, LNC
Legal Nurse Consultant
Telephone Triage Nurse
Macon, Mississippi

EDITION 8

F.A. Davis Company • Philadelphia

F. A. Davis Company
1915 Arch Street
Philadelphia, PA 19103
www.fadavis.com

Printed in the United States of America

Last digit indicates print number: 10 9 8 7 6 5 4 3 2 1

Publisher, Nursing: Joanne Patzek DaCunha, RN, MSN
Director of Content Development: Darlene Pederson, MSN, APRN, BC
Project Editor: Kim DePaul Mackey
Design and Illustrations Manager: Carolyn O'Brien

As new scientific information becomes available through basic and clinical research, recommended treatments and drug therapies undergo changes. The author(s) and publisher have done everything possible to make this book accurate, up to date, and in accord with accepted standards at the time of publication. The author(s), editors, and publisher are not responsible for errors or omissions or for consequences from application of the book, and make no warranty, expressed or implied, in regard to the contents of the book. Any practice described in this book should be applied by the reader in accordance with professional standards of care used in regard to the unique circumstances that may apply in each situation. The reader is advised always to check product information (package inserts) for changes and new information regarding dose and contraindications before administering any drug. Caution is especially urged when using new or infrequently ordered drugs.

Library of Congress Cataloging-in-Publication Data

Doenges, Marilynn E., 1922–
  Nursing care plans : guidelines for individualizing client care across the life span / Marilynn E. Doenges, Mary Frances Moorhouse, Alice C. Murr.—Ed. 8.
    p. ; cm.
  Includes bibliographical references and index.
  ISBN-13: 978-0-8036-2210-4
  ISBN-10: 0-8036-2210-4
  1. Nursing care plans—Handbooks, manuals, etc. I. Moorhouse, Mary Frances, 1947– II. Murr, Alice C., 1946– III. Title.
  [DNLM: 1. Patient Care Planning—Handbooks. 2. Nursing Process—Handbooks. WY 49 D651na 2010]
  RT49.D64 2010
  610.73—dc22

2009014629

*To our spouses, children, parents, and friends, who much of the time
have had to manage without us while we work as well as having to
cope with our struggles and frustrations.*

*The Doenges families: the late Dean, whose support and
encouragement is sorely missed; Jim; Barbara and Bob Lanza;
David, Monita, Matthew, and Tyler; John, Holly, Nicole, and
Kelsey; and the Daigle families, Nancy, Jim, Jennifer, Brandon,
Anna, Will, and Henry Smith-Daigle, and Jonathan, Kim,
and Mandalyn JoAn.*

*The Moorhouse family: Jan, Paul; Jason, Thenderlyn, Alexa,
and Mary Isabella.*

*To Mary and Marilynn, I couldn't have done it without you.
In loving memory of my parents, who were my biggest promoters
in my early days of writing. To my children and grandchildren
with love. You have expanded my horizons so wonderfully!—Alice*

*To our F. A. Davis family, especially Bob Martone and Bob Butler,
whose support is so vital to the completion of a project of
this magnitude. And to Joanne DaCunha, who is not just our
acquisitions editor, but also a colleague and friend who has seen
the project from both sides now. Thank you for your support
and understanding. We are fourtunate to have you working
with us.*

*To the nurses we are writing for, who daily face the challenge of caring
for the acutely ill client and are looking for a practical way to organize
and document this care. We believe that nursing diagnosis and these
guides will help.*

*To NANDA and to the international nurses who are developing
and using nursing diagnoses—here we come!*

*Finally, to the late Mary Lisk Jeffries, who initiated the
original project. The memory of our early friendship and struggles
remains with us. We miss her and wish she were here to see the
growth of the profession and how nursing diagnosis has contributed
to the process.*

Mope T. Adeola, RN, MSN, CNS, OCN

Clinical Assistant Professor
Purdue University School of Nursing
West Lafayette, Indiana

Jane V. Arndt, MS, RN, CWOCN

Clinical Nurse Specialist
Poudre Valley Hospital
Fort Collins, Colorado

Nancy Buttry, MSN, RN

Associate Dean of Nursing and Allied Health
Illinois Eastern Community Colleges
Olney, Illinois

Kathleen A. Curtis, RN, MSN

Instructor, Course Coordinator
Mount Carmel College of Nursing
Columbus, Ohio

Rosemary Fliszar, PhD, RN, CNE

Assistant Professor Nursing
Kutztown University
Kutztown, Pennsylvania

Brenda Hicks, RN, OCN

Memorial Cancer Medicine Specialists
Memorial Hospital
Colorado Springs, Colorado

Christie A. Hinds, MSN, APRN-BC

Primary Care Nurse Practitioner
Health Essentials
Chattanooga, Tennessee

Jennifer Limongiello, MSN, ARNP

Associate Professor
NHTI-Concord Community College
Concord, New Hamshire

Bill Loughmiller, CRT

Respiratory Therapist
St. Francis Medical Center
Colorado Springs, Colorado

Larry Manalo, RN, MSN

Nursing Instructor
Allan Hancock College
Santa Maria, California

Julie Matheny, RRT

ICU Specialist
Penrose Hospital
Colorado Springs, Colorado

Kathleen Molden, RN, MSN, CNE

Nurse Educator
St. Francis Medical Center School of Nursing
Trenton, New Jersey

Kimberly Tucker Pfennigs, MA, BAN, RN

Case Manager, Warrior Transition Unit
Fort Carson, Colorado

Gilda Rolls-Dellinger, RN

Staff Nurse, Skin, Wound, and Burn Team
Penrose-St. Francis Health Services
Colorado Springs, Colorado

Rochelle Salmore, MSN, RN, CGRN, NE, BC

Clincal Manager, GI Lab, Wound Clinic
Penrose/Centura Hospital
Colorado Springs, Colorado

April Sheker, RN, MSN(c), CMSRN

Clinical Instructor
Pennsylvania State University
College of Nursing
Allentown, Pennsylvania

Geri L. Tierney, RN, BSN, ONC

Nursing Simulation Lab Coordinator
Pikes Peak Community College
Past-President National Association of Orthopaedic
 Nurses
Colorado Springs, Colorado

Kathleen H. Winder, RN, BSN

Clinical Manager, Pediatric Specialty Clinic
Memorial Hospital
Colorado Springs, Colorado

Anne Zobec, MS, RN, CS, NP, AOCN

Oncology Nurse Practitioner
Rocky Mountain Cancer Center
Colorado Springs, Colorado

Jennie C. Denker, RN, MSN, EdDc

Director Year I
Galen College of Nursing
Goshen, Kentucky

Dianne Marie Johnson, MA, APRN-BC, AHN-BC

Assistant Professor, School of Nursing
College of St. Scholastica
Duluth, Minnesota

Carol A. Kincaid, RN, MS, CNS, ANP

Full-time faculty
Chair of Fundamentals Level
Crouse Hospital School of Nursing
Syracuse, New York

Priscilla A. Lee, MN, NP

Nurse Practitioner
Assistant Clinical Professor
UCLA Gonda Vascular Center
Los Angeles, California

Pamela Y. Mahon, PhD, RN, CNAA

Associate Professor
Hunter College/CUNY
New York, New York

Mary Tan, AAS/ADN, BSN, MSN, PhD, RN

Assistant Director and Allied Health
Holmes Community College
Ridgeland, Missouri

ACKNOWLEDGMENTS

Joe Ruskin, RPH
Colorado Springs, Colorado

James I. Burns, BS
Disaster Science
Aurora, Colorado

The late Nancy Lea Carter, RN, MA
Clinical Nurse, Orthopedics
Albuquerque, New Mexico

We are often asked how we came to write the Care Plan books. In the late 1970s we were involved with some publishing efforts that did not come to fruition. In this work we had included care plans, so ensuing discussions revolved around the need for a Care Plan book. We spent a year struggling to write care plans before we realized our major difficulty was the lack of standardized labels for client problems. At that time, we were given a list of nursing diagnoses from the Clearinghouse for Nursing Diagnosis, which became the North American Nursing Diagnosis Association (NANDA), and is now NANDA International (NANDA-I). This work answered our need by providing concise titles that could be used in various plans of care and followed across the spectrum of client care. We believed these nursing diagnosis labels would both define and focus nursing care.

Because we had long been involved in direct client care in our nursing careers, we knew there was a need for guidelines to assist nurses in planning care. As we began to write, our focus was the nurse in a small rural community who at 2 a.m. needed the answer to a burning question for her client and had few resources available. We believed the book would give definition and direction to the development and use of individualized nursing care. Thus, in the first edition, the theory of nursing process, diagnosis, and intervention was brought to the clinical setting for implementation by the nurse. We also anticipated that nursing students would appreciate having access to these guidelines as they struggled to learn how to provide nursing care. Therefore, we did not consider the book to be an end in itself, but rather a vehicle for the continuing growth and development of the profession. Obviously we struck a chord and met a need because the first edition was an immediate success.

In becoming involved with NANDA, we acknowledged that maintaining a strict adherence to their wording, while adding our own clearly identified recommendations, would help develop this neophyte standardized language and would promote the growth of nursing as a profession. We have continued our involvement with NANDA-I, promoting the use of the language by practicing nurses in the United States and around the world and encouraging them to participate in updating and refining the diagnoses. The wide use of our books within the student population has supported and fostered the acceptance of both the activity of diagnosing client problems or needs and the use of standardized language.

Nursing instructors initially expressed concern that students would simply copy the plans of care and thus limit their learning. However, as students used the plans to individualize care and to develop practice priorities and client care outcomes, the book met with more acceptance. Instructors began not only to recommend the book, but also to adopt it as an adjunct text. Today, it remains the best-selling nursing care plan book recognized as an important adjunct for student learning.

In writing the second edition, we recognized the need for an assessment tool with a nursing focus instead of a medical focus. Not finding one that met our needs, we constructed our own. To facilitate problem identification, we categorized the nursing diagnosis labels and the information obtained in the client assessment database into a framework entitled "Diagnostic Divisions." Our philosophy is to provide a way in which to gather information and to intervene beneficially, while thinking about the rationale for every action we take and the standardized language that best expresses it. When nurses do this they are defining their practice and are able to identify it with a code and charge for it. By doing this, we promote client protection (quality of care issue), provide for the definition and protection of nursing practice, and the protection of the individual (legal implications). The latter is important because we live in a litigation-minded society and the nurse's license and livelihood are at stake.

One of the most significant achievements in the healthcare field over the past 20 or more years has been the emergence of the nurse as an active coordinator and initiator of client care. Although the transition from physician's helpmate to healthcare professional has been painfully slow and is not yet complete, the importance of the nurse within the system can no longer be denied or ignored. Today's nurse designs nursing care interventions that move the total client toward improved health and maximum independence.

Professional care standards and healthcare providers and consumers will continue to increase the expectations for nurses' performance. Each day brings new challenges in client care and the struggle to understand the human responses to actual and potential health problems. To meet these challenges competently, the nurse must have up-to-date assessment skills and a working knowledge of pathophysiological concepts concerning the common diseases and conditions presented. We believe that this book is a tool, providing a means of attaining that competency.

In the past, plans of care were viewed principally as learning tools for students and seemed to have little relevance after graduation. However, the need for a written format to communicate and document client care has been recognized in all care settings. In addition, healthcare policy, governmental regulations, and third-party payor requirements have created the need to validate many things, including appropriateness of care provided, staffing patterns, and monetary charges. Thus, although the student's "case studies" are too cumbersome to be practical in the clinical setting, it has long been recognized that the client plan of care meets certain needs and therefore its appropriate use was validated.

The practicing nurse, as well as the nursing student, can welcome this text as a ready reference in clinical practice. It is designed for use in the acute care, community, and home-care settings. It is organized by systems for easy reference.

Chapter 1 examines current issues and trends and their implications for the nursing profession. An overview of cultural, community, sociological, and ethical concepts affecting the nurse is included. The importance of the nurse's role in collaboration and coordination with other healthcare professionals is integrated throughout the plans of care.

Chapter 2 reviews the historical use of the nursing process in formulating plans of care and the nurse's role in the delivery of that care. Nursing diagnoses, outcomes, and interventions are discussed to assist the nurse in understanding her or his role in the nursing process. In this book, we have also linked NANDA-I diagnoses with Nursing Interventions Classification (NIC) and Nursing Outcomes Classification (NOC) languages.

Chapter 3 discusses care plan construction and describes the use and adaptation of the guides presented in this book. A nursing-based assessment tool is provided to assist the nurse in identifying appropriate nursing diagnoses. A sample client situation with individual database and a corresponding plan of care is included to demonstrate how critical thinking is used to adapt nursing process theory to practice. Finally, a dynamic and creative approach for developing and documenting the planning of care is also included. Mind Mapping is a new technique or learning tool provided to assist you in achieving a holistic view of your client, enhance your critical thinking skills, and facilitate the creative process of planning client care.

Chapters 4 through 15 present plans of care that include information from multiple disciplines to assist the nurse in providing holistic care. Each plan includes a Client Assessment Database presented in a nursing format, and associated Diagnostic Studies. After the database is collected, Nursing Priorities are sifted from the information to help focus and structure the care. Discharge Goals are created to identify what should be generally accomplished by the time of discharge from the care setting.

Nursing diagnosis labels are then chosen and combined with possible related factors disignated by "may be related to," and the signs and symptoms or defining characteristics as "possibly evidenced by" if present to create Client Diagnostic Statements that provide a clear picture of the client's needs. Next, Desired Client Outcomes are stated in measurable behavioral terms to evaluate both the client's progress and the effectiveness of care provided.

Corresponding actions/interventions are designed to promote resolution of the identified client needs. The nurse acting independently or collaboratively within the health team then uses a decision-making model to organize and prioritize nursing interventions. No attempt is made in this book to indicate whether independent or collaborative actions come first because this must be dictated by the individual situation. We do, however, believe that every collaborative action has a component that the nurse must identify and for which nursing has responsibility and accountability.

Rationales for the nursing actions, which are not required in the customary plan of care, are included to assist the nurse in deciding whether the interventions are appropriate for an individual client. Additional information is provided to further assist the nurse in identifying and planning for rehabilitation as the client progresses toward discharge and across all care settings. A bibliography is provided as a reference and to allow further research as desired.

This book is designed for students who will find the plans of care helpful as they learn and develop skills in applying the nursing process and using nursing diagnoses. It will complement their classroom work and support the critical thinking process. The book also provides a ready reference for the practicing nurse as a catalyst for thought in planning, evaluating, and documenting care.

As a final note, this book is not intended to be a procedure manual, and efforts have been made to avoid detailed descriptions of techniques or protocols that might be viewed as individual or regional in nature. Instead, the reader is referred to a procedure manual or text covering Standards of Care if detailed direction is desired.

As we always say when we sign a book, "Use and enjoy."

MD, MM, and AM

CONTENTS IN BRIEF

INDEX OF NURSING
DIAGNOSES APPEARS
ON PAGES   958–961

INTRODUCTION   xv

CHAPTER 1
Issues and Trends in Nursing
    and Healthcare Delivery   1

CHAPTER 2
The Nursing Process: Planning Care
    Using Nursing Diagnoses   7

CHAPTER 3
Critical Thinking: Adaptation
    of Theory to Practice   14

CHAPTER 4
Cardiovascular   37
    Hypertension: Severe   37
    Heart Failure: Chronic   48
    Angina (Coronary Artery Disease, Acute
        Coronary Syndrome)   64
    Myocardial Infarction   74
    Dysrhythmias   88
    Cardiac Surgery: Postoperative
        Care—Coronary Artery Bypass Graft
        (CABG), Minimally Invasive Direct
        Coronary Artery Bypass (MIDCAB),
        Cardiomyoplasty, Valve Replacement 100
    Thrombophlebitis: Deep Vein Thrombosis
        (Including Pulmonary Emboli
        Considerations)   111

CHAPTER 5
Respiratory   120
    Chronic Obstructive Pulmonary Disease
        (COPD) and Asthma   120
    Pneumonia   131
    Lung Cancer: Postoperative Care 144
    Pneumothorax/Hemothorax   154
    Radical Neck Surgery: Laryngectomy
        (Postoperative Care)   160
    Ventilatory Assistance (Mechanical) 173
    Pulmonary Tuberculosis (TB)   186
    Respiratory Acid-Base
        Imbalances   195

Respiratory Acidosis (Primary Carbonic
    Acid Excess)   195
Respiratory Alkalosis (Primary Carbonic
    Acid Deficit)   200

CHAPTER 6
Neurological/Sensory Disorders   204
    Glaucoma   204
    Seizure Disorders   210
    Craniocerebral Trauma—Acute
        Rehabilitative Phase   220
    Cerebrovascular Accident (CVA)/Stroke 238
    Herniated Nucleus Pulposus (Ruptured
        Intervertebral Disc)   254
    Disc Surgery   262
    Spinal Cord Injury (Acute Rehabilitative
        Phase)   271
    Multiple Sclerosis (MS)   290

CHAPTER 7
Gastrointestinal Disorders   306
    Upper Gastrointestinal/
        Esophageal Bleeding   306
    Gastrectomy/Gastric Resection   317
    Inflammatory Bowel Disease (IBD):
        Ulcerative Colitis, Crohn's Disease 321
    Fecal Diversions: Postoperative Care
        of Ileostomy and Colostomy   334
    Appendectomy   344
    Peritonitis   349
    Cholecystitis With Cholelithiasis 357
    Cholecystectomy   364

CHAPTER 8
Metabolic and Endocrine Disorders   369
    Eating Disorders: Anorexia
        Nervosa/Bulimia Nervosa   369
    Eating Disorders: Obesity   387
    Obesity: Bariatric Surgery—Gastric
        Partitioning/Gastroplasty, Gastric
        Bypass   396
    Diabetes Mellitus/Diabetic Ketoacidosis 405
    Hyperthyroidism (Graves' Disease,
        Thyrotoxicosis)   419
    Thyroidectomy   429
    Hepatitis   434
    Cirrhosis of the Liver   445
    Pancreatitis   458

Total Nutritional Support: Parenteral/Enteral
   Feeding   469
Metabolic Acid-Base Imbalances   483
Metabolic Acidosis—Primary Base
   Bicarbonate (HCO$_3$-) Deficiency   483
Metabolic Alkalosis—Primary Base
   Bicarbonate Excess   488

CHAPTER 9
Diseases of the Blood/
Blood-Forming Organs   **493**
Anemias—Iron Deficiency, Anemia
   of Chronic Disease, Pernicious,
   Aplastic, Hemolytic   493
Sickle Cell Crisis   503
Adult Leukemias   516
Lymphomas   525

CHAPTER 10
Renal and Urinary Tract   **536**
Renal Failure: Acute   536
Renal Failure: Chronic   548
Renal Dialysis—General Considerations   560
Peritoneal Dialysis (PD)   570
Hemodialysis (HD)   575
Urinary Diversions/Urostomy (Postoperative
   Care)   578
Benign Prostatic Hyperplasia (BPH)   588
Prostatectomy   596
Urolithiasis (Renal Calculi)   603

CHAPTER 11
Women's Reproductive   **611**
Hysterectomy   611
Mastectomy   619

CHAPTER 12
Orthopedic   **632**
Fractures   632
Amputation   646
Total Joint Replacement   655

CHAPTER 13
Integumentary   **667**
Burns: Thermal, Chemical, and
   Electrical—Acute and Convalescent
   Phases   667

CHAPTER 14
Systemic Infections and
Immunological Disorders   **686**
Sepsis/Septicemia   686
The HIV-Positive Client   697
Acquired Immunodeficiency Syndrome
   (AIDS)   709
Rheumatoid Arthritis (RA)   729
Transplantation Considerations—
   Postoperative and Lifelong   739

CHAPTER 15
General   **749**
Psychosocial Aspects of Care   749
Dementia of the Alzheimer's
   Type/Vascular Dementia   764
Surgical Intervention   782
Extended Care   801
Alcohol: Acute Withdrawal   819
Substance Dependence/Abuse
   Rehabilitation   835
Cancer   846
End-of-Life Care/Hospice   866
Disaster Considerations   876
Pediatric Considerations   890
Fluid and Electrolyte Imbalances   903

BIBLIOGRAPHY 935

INDEX OF NURSING
DIAGNOSES 958

**A table of contents including nursing
diagnoses follows.**

DETAILED CONTENTS

INDEX OF NURSING DIAGNOSES
APPEARS ON PAGES   958–961

INTRODUCTION   xv

CHAPTER 1

**Issues and Trends in Nursing and
  Healthcare Delivery**   1
The Ever-Changing Healthcare
  Environment   1
Healthcare Costs and the Allocation of
  Resources   1
Restructuring Healthcare   2
Nursing Care Costs   3
Early Discharge   4
Aging Population   4
Technological Advances   5
Future of Nursing   5
Conclusion   6

CHAPTER 2

**The Nursing Process: Planning Care
  Using Nursing Diagnoses**   7
Planning Care   10
Components of the Plan of Care   10
  Client Database   10
  Interviewing   10
  Physical Assessment   10
  Diagnostic Studies   10
  Nursing Priorities   11
  Discharge Goals   11
  Nursing Diagnosis (Problem and Need
    Identification)   11
  Desired Client Outcomes   12
  Planning (Goals and Actions/Interventions) 12
Rationale   13
Conclusion   13

CHAPTER 3

**Critical Thinking: Adaptation of Theory
  to Practice**   14
Client Situation: Diabetes Mellitus   23
  Admitting Physician's Orders   23
  Client Assessment Database   23
  Mind Map   27
Evaluation   28
Documentation   28
  Sample Clinical Pathway   30
  Plan of Care: Mr. R. S.   32

CHAPTER 4

Cardiovascular   37
Hypertension: Severe   37
  Cardiac Output, risk for decreased   41
  Activity Intolerance   43
  Pain, acute   43
  Nutrition: More than Body Requirements,
    imbalanced   44
  Coping, ineffective   45
  Knowledge, deficient [Learning Need]   46
Heart Failure: Chronic   48
  Cardiac Output, decreased   53
  Activity Intolerance   56
  Fluid Volume, excess   57
  Gas Exchange, risk for impaired   58
  Pain, risk for chronic   59
  Skin Integrity, risk for impaired   60
  Knowledge, deficient [Learning Need]   60
  Sample Clinical Pathway   62
Angina (Coronary Artery Disease, Acute
  Coronary Syndrome)   64
  Pain, acute   68
  Cardiac Output, risk for decreased   70
  Anxiety [specify level]   72
  Knowledge, deficient [Learning Need]   73
Myocardial Infarction   74
  Pain, acute   79
  Activity Intolerance   81
  Anxiety [specify level]/Fear   82
  Cardiac Output, risk for decreased   83
  Perfusion, ineffective tissue (specify) 84
  Fluid Volume, risk for excess   86
  Knowledge, deficient [Learning Need]   87
Dysrhythmias   88
  Cardiac Output, risk for decreased   93
  Poisoning, risk for [Digoxin Toxicity] 97
  Knowledge, deficient [Learning Need]   98
Cardiac Surgery: Postoperative
  Care—Coronary Artery Bypass Graft
  (CABG), Minimally Invasive Direct
  Coronary Artery Bypass (MIDCAB),
  Cardiomyoplasty, Valve Replacement   100
  Cardiac Output, risk for decreased   104
  Pain, acute/Comfort, impaired   106
  Breathing Pattern, risk for ineffective 107
  Skin Integrity, impaired   108
  Knowledge, deficient [Learning Need]   109
Thrombophlebitis: Deep Vein
  Thrombosis (Including Pulmonary
  Emboli Considerations)   111
  Perfusion, ineffective peripheral tissue 114
  Pain, acute/Comfort, impaired   116

Gas Exchange, impaired (in presence of pulmonary embolus) 117
Knowledge, deficient [Learning Need] 118

CHAPTER 5

Respiratory 120

Chronic Obstructive Pulmonary Disease (COPD) and Asthma 120
Airway Clearance, ineffective 124
Gas Exchange, impaired 126
Nutrition: Less than Body Requirements, imbalanced 128
Knowledge, deficient [Learning Need] 129
Pneumonia 131
Airway Clearance, ineffective 135
Gas Exchange, impaired 136
Infection, risk for [spread] 137
Activity Intolerance 138
Pain, acute 138
Nutrition: Less than Body Requirements, risk for imbalanced 139
Fluid Volume, risk for deficient 140
Knowledge, deficient [Learning Need] 141
Sample Clinical Pathway 142
Lung Cancer: Postoperative Care 144
Gas Exchange, impaired 148
Airway Clearance, ineffective 149
Pain, acute 150
Fear/Anxiety [specify level] 151
Knowledge, deficient [Learning Need] 152
Pneumothorax/Hemothorax 154
Breathing Pattern, ineffective 156
Trauma/Suffocation, risk for 159
Knowledge, deficient [Learning Need] 160
Radical Neck Surgery: Laryngectomy (Postoperative Care) 160
Airway Clearance, ineffective 164
Communication, impaired verbal 165
Skin/Tissue Integrity, impaired 166
Oral Mucous Membrane, impaired 167
Pain, acute 168
Nutrition: Less than Body Requirements, imbalanced 169
Body Image, disturbed/Role Performance, ineffective 170
Knowledge, deficient [Learning Need] 171
Ventilatory Assistance (Mechanical) 173
Breathing Pattern, ineffective/Spontaneous Ventilation, impaired 175
Airway Clearance, ineffective 178
Communication, impaired verbal 179
Fear/Anxiety [specify level] 180
Oral Mucous Membrane, impaired 181
Nutrition: Less than Body Requirements, imbalanced 181
Infection, risk for 182
Ventilatory Weaning Response, risk for dysfunctional 183
Knowledge, deficient [Learning Need] 185
Pulmonary Tuberculosis (TB) 186
Infection, risk for [spread/reactivation] 190
Airway Clearance, ineffective 191
Gas Exchange, risk for impaired 192
Nutrition: Less than Body Requirements, imbalanced 193
Knowledge, deficient [Learning Need] 194

Respiratory Acid-Base Imbalances 195
Respiratory Acidosis (Primary Carbonic Acid Excess) 195
Gas Exchange, impaired 199
Respiratory Alkalosis (Primary Carbonic Acid Deficit) 200
Gas Exchange, impaired 202

CHAPTER 6

Neurological/Sensory Disorders 204

Glaucoma 204
Sensory Perception, disturbed visual 207
Anxiety [specify level] 208
Knowledge, deficient [Learning Need] 209
Seizure Disorders 210
Trauma/Suffocation, risk for 215
Airway Clearance/Breathing Pattern, risk for ineffective 217
Self-Esteem, [specify situational or chronic] low 218
Knowledge, deficient [Learning Need] 219
Craniocerebral Trauma—Acute Rehabilitative Phase 220
Perfusion, ineffective cerebral tissue 226
Breathing Pattern, risk for ineffective 229
Sensory Perception, disturbed (specify) 230
Thought Processes, disturbed 231
Mobility, impaired physical 233
Infection, risk for 234
Nutrition: Less than Body Requirements, risk for imbalanced 235
Family Processes, interrupted 236
Knowledge, deficient [Learning Need] 237
Cerebrovascular Accident (CVA)/Stroke 238
Perfusion, ineffective cerebral tissue 242
Mobility, impaired physical 244
Communication, impaired verbal [and/or written] 246
Sensory Perception, disturbed [specify] 247
Self-Care Deficit [specify] 248
Coping, ineffective 249
Swallowing, risk for impaired 250
Knowledge, deficient [Learning Need] 252
Neglect, unilateral 253
Herniated Nucleus Pulposus (Ruptured Intervertebral Disc) 254
Pain, acute/chronic 257
Mobility, impaired physical 259
Anxiety [specify level]/Coping, ineffective 259
Knowledge, deficient [Learning Need] 260
Disc Surgery 262
Perfusion, ineffective tissue [specify] 263
Trauma, risk for [spinal] 264
Breathing Pattern/Airway Clearance, risk for ineffective 265
Pain, acute 265
Mobility, impaired physical 266
Constipation 267
Urinary Retention, risk for 268
Knowledge, deficient [Learning Need] 268
Sample Clinical Pathway 270

Spinal Cord Injury (Acute Rehabilitative
  Phase) 271
  Breathing Pattern, risk for ineffective 275
  Trauma, risk for [additional spinal] 277
  Mobility, impaired physical 277
  Sensory Perception, disturbed 279
  Pain, acute 280
  Grieving 281
  Self-Esteem, situational low 282
  Bowel Incontinence/Constipation 283
  Urinary Elimination, impaired 284
  Autonomic Dysreflexia, risk for 286
  Skin/Tissue Integrity, risk for impaired 287
  Knowledge, deficient [Learning Need] 288
Multiple Sclerosis (MS) 290
  Fatigue 294
  Self-Care Deficit [specify] 296
  Self-Esteem, low (specify situational/
    chronic) 297
  Powerlessness [specify degree]/
    Hopelessness 298
  Coping, risk for ineffective 299
  Coping, compromised/disabled family 300
  Urinary Elimination, impaired 301
  Caregiver Role Strain, risk for 302
  Knowledge, deficient [Learning Need] 303

CHAPTER 7

Gastrointestinal Disorders 306
  Upper Gastrointestinal/Esophageal
    Bleeding 306
    Bleeding, risk for 310
    Shock, risk for 313
    Fear/Anxiety [specify level] 313
    Pain, acute/chronic 314
    Knowledge, deficient [Learning Need] 315
  Gastrectomy/Gastric Resection 317
    Nutrition: Less than Body Requirements,
      risk for imbalanced 318
    Knowledge, deficient [Learning Need] 319
  Inflammatory Bowel Disease (IBD):
    Ulcerative Colitis, Crohn's Disease 321
    Diarrhea 327
    Fluid Volume, risk for deficient 328
    Nutrition: Less than Body Requirements,
      imbalanced 328
    Anxiety [specify level] 330
    Pain, acute 331
    Coping, ineffective 332
    Knowledge, deficient [Learning Need] 333
  Fecal Diversions: Postoperative Care
    of Ileostomy and Colostomy 334
    Skin Integrity, risk for impaired 335
    Body Image, disturbed 336
    Pain, acute 337
    Skin/Tissue Integrity, impaired 338
    Fluid Volume, risk for deficient 338
    Nutrition: Less than Body Requirements,
      risk for imbalanced 339
    Sleep Deprivation 340
    Constipation/Diarrhea, risk for 341
    Sexual Dysfunction, risk for 341
    Knowledge, deficient [Learning Need] 342
  Appendectomy 344
    Infection, risk for 346

Fluid Volume, risk for deficient 347
Pain, acute 348
Knowledge, deficient [Learning Need] 348
Peritonitis 349
  Infection, risk for [septicemia] 352
  Fluid Volume, deficient [mixed] 353
  Pain, acute 354
  Nutrition: Less than Body Requirements,
    risk for imbalanced 355
  Anxiety [specify level]/Fear 356
  Knowledge, deficient [Learning Need] 356
Cholecystitis With Cholelithiasis 357
  Pain, acute 360
  Fluid Volume, risk for deficient 361
  Nutrition: Less than Body Requirements,
    risk for imbalanced 362
  Knowledge, deficient [Learning Need] 363
Cholecystectomy 364
  Breathing Pattern, ineffective 365
  Fluid Volume, risk for deficient 366
  Skin/Tissue Integrity, impaired 367
  Knowledge, deficient [Learning Need] 368

CHAPTER 8

Metabolic and Endocrine Disorders 369
  Eating Disorders: Anorexia Nervosa/
    Bulimia Nervosa 369
    Nutrition: Less than Body Requirements,
      imbalanced 374
    Fluid Volume, [actual/]risk for deficient 377
    Thought Processes, disturbed 377
    Body Image, disturbed/Self-Esteem,
      chronic low 378
    Parenting, impaired 380
    Skin Integrity, risk for impaired 381
    Knowledge, deficient [Learning Need] 381
    Sample Clinical Pathway 383
  Eating Disorders: Obesity 387
    Nutrition: More than Body Requirements,
      imbalanced 390
    Lifestyle, sedentary 392
    Body Image, disturbed/Self-Esteem,
      chronic low 393
    Social Interaction, impaired 394
    Knowledge, deficient [Learning Need] 395
  Obesity: Bariatric Surgery—Gastric
    Partitioning/Gastroplasty, Gastric
    Bypass 396
    Breathing Pattern, ineffective 399
    Perfusion, risk for ineffective tissue 400
    Fluid Volume, risk for deficient 400
    Nutrition: Less than Body Requirements,
      risk for imbalanced 401
    Skin Integrity, [actual/]risk for impaired 402
    Infection, risk for 403
    Diarrhea 403
    Knowledge, deficient [Learning Need] 404
  Diabetes Mellitus/Diabetic Ketoacidosis 405
    Fluid Volume, deficient [specify] 410
    Glucose Level, unstable blood 411
    Infection, risk for [sepsis] 413
    Sensory Perception, risk for disturbed
      (specify) 414
    Fatigue 415

Powerlessness	415
Knowledge, deficient [Learning Need]	416
Hyperthyroidism (Graves' Disease, Thyrotoxicosis)	419
Cardiac Output, risk for decreased	422
Fatigue	425
Nutrition: Less than Body Requirements, risk for imbalanced	425
Anxiety [specify level]	426
Thought Processes, risk for disturbed	427
Tissue Integrity, risk for impaired	427
Knowledge, deficient [Learning Need]	428
Thyroidectomy	429
Airway Clearance, risk for ineffective	430
Communication, impaired verbal	431
Injury, risk for [tetany, thyroid storm]	431
Pain, acute	432
Knowledge, deficient [Learning Need]	433
Hepatitis	434
Liver Function, impaired	437
Fatigue	439
Nutrition: Less than Body Requirements, imbalanced	440
Fluid Volume/Bleeding, risk for deficient	441
Self-Esteem, situational low	442
Infection, risk for [secondary/spread]	442
Skin/Tissue Integrity, risk for impaired	443
Knowledge, deficient [Learning Need]	444
Cirrhosis of the Liver	445
Nutrition: Less than Body Requirements, imbalanced	449
Fluid Volume, excess	451
Skin Integrity, risk for impaired	452
Breathing Pattern, risk for ineffective	453
Bleeding, risk for	454
Confusion, risk for acute	455
Self-Esteem [specify]/Body Image, disturbed	456
Knowledge, deficient [Learning Need]	457
Pancreatitis	458
Pain, acute	463
Fluid Volume, risk for deficient/Bleeding	464
Nutrition: Less than Body Requirements, imbalanced	465
Glucose Level, risk for unstable blood	466
Infection, risk for [sepsis]	467
Breathing Pattern, risk for ineffective/Gas Exchange, impaired	468
Knowledge, deficient [Learning Need]	468
Total Nutritional Support: Parenteral/ Enteral Feeding	469
Nutrition: Less than Body Requirements, imbalanced	474
Infection, risk for	477
Injury, risk for [multifactor]	478
Aspiration, risk for	479
Fluid Volume, risk for imbalanced	480
Fatigue	481
Knowledge, deficient [Learning Need]	482
Metabolic Acid-Base Imbalances	483
Metabolic Acidosis—Primary Base Bicarbonate (HCO_3^-) Deficiency	483
Metabolic Alkalosis—Primary Base Bicarbonate Excess	488

CHAPTER 9
Diseases of the Blood/Blood-Forming Organs — 493

Anemias—Iron Deficiency, Anemia of Chronic Disease, Pernicious, Aplastic, Hemolytic	493
Activity Intolerance	498
Nutrition: Less than Body Requirements, imbalanced	499
Constipation/Diarrhea	500
Infection, risk for	501
Knowledge, deficient [Learning Need]	501
Sickle Cell Crisis	503
Gas Exchange, impaired	507
Pain, acute/chronic	509
Perfusion, ineffective tissue (specify)	510
Fluid Volume, risk for deficient	511
Mobility, impaired physical	512
Skin Integrity, risk for impaired	513
Infection, risk for [sepsis]	513
Knowledge, deficient [Learning Need]	514
Adult Leukemias	516
Infection, risk for	520
Fluid Volume, risk for deficient	521
Pain, acute	523
Activity Intolerance	524
Knowledge, deficient [Learning Need]	524
Lymphomas	525
Gas Exchange, risk for impaired	530
Nausea	532
Sexual Dysfunction	533
Knowledge, deficient [Learning Need]	534

CHAPTER 10
Renal and Urinary Tract — 536

Renal Failure: Acute	536
Fluid Volume, excess	541
Cardiac Output, risk for decreased	543
Nutrition: Less than Body Requirements, risk for imbalanced	545
Infection, risk for	546
Fluid Volume, risk for deficient	546
Knowledge, deficient [Learning Need]	547
Renal Failure: Chronic	548
Cardiac Output, risk for decreased	553
Protection, risk for ineffective	555
Thought Processes, disturbed	556
Skin Integrity, risk for impaired	557
Oral Mucous Membrane, risk for impaired	557
Knowledge, deficient [Learning Need]	558
Renal Dialysis—General Considerations	560
Nutrition: Less than Body Requirements, imbalanced	562
Mobility, impaired physical	563
Self-Care Deficit (specify)	564
Constipation, risk for	565
Thought Processes, risk for disturbed	565
Anxiety [specify level]/Fear	566
Body Image, disturbed/Self-Esteem, situational low	567
Knowledge, deficient [Learning Need]	568
Peritoneal Dialysis (PD)	570
Fluid Volume, risk for excess	570
Fluid Volume, risk for deficient	571

Trauma, risk for 572
Pain, acute 572
Infection, risk for [peritonitis] 573
Breathing Pattern, risk for ineffective 574
Hemodialysis (HD) 575
Injury, risk for [loss of vascular access] 575
Fluid Volume, risk for deficient 577
Fluid Volume, risk for excess 578
Urinary Diversions/Urostomy (Postoperative Care) 578
Skin Integrity, risk for impaired 580
Body Image, disturbed 582
Pain, acute 583
Infection, risk for 584
Urinary Elimination, impaired 585
Sexual Dysfunction, risk for 586
Knowledge, deficient [Learning Need] 587
Benign Prostatic Hyperplasia (BPH) 588
Urinary Retention, [acute/chronic] 591
Pain, acute 593
Fluid Volume, risk for deficient 593
Fear/Anxiety [specify level] 594
Knowledge, deficient [Learning Need] 594
Prostatectomy 596
Urinary Elimination, impaired 597
Fluid Volume/Bleeding, risk for deficient 598
Infection, risk for 599
Pain, acute 600
Sexual Dysfunction, risk for 600
Knowledge, deficient [Learning Need] 601
Sample Clinical Pathway 602
Urolithiasis (Renal Calculi) 603
Pain, acute 606
Urinary Elimination, impaired 607
Fluid Volume, risk for deficient 609
Knowledge, deficient [Learning Need] 609

CHAPTER 11
Women's Reproductive 611
Hysterectomy 611
Self-Esteem, situational low 613
Urinary Elimination, impaired/Urinary Retention, [acute] 613
Constipation/Diarrhea, risk for 614
Perfusion, risk for ineffective tissue (specify) 615
Sexual Dysfunction, risk for 616
Grieving, risk for 616
Knowledge, deficient [Learning Need] 617
Mastectomy 619
Anxiety/Anxiety, death 623
Skin/Tissue Integrity, impaired 624
Pain, acute 624
Self-Esteem, situational low 625
Mobility, impaired physical 626
Knowledge, deficient [Learning Need] 627
Sample Clinical Pathway 629

CHAPTER 12
Orthopedic 632
Fractures 632
Trauma, risk for [additional] 635
Pain, acute 636
Peripheral Neurovascular Dysfunction, risk for 637

Gas Exchange, risk for impaired 639
Mobility, impaired physical 640
Skin/Tissue Integrity, [actual]/risk for impaired 641
Infection, risk for 643
Knowledge, deficient [Learning Need] 644
Amputation 646
Self-Esteem, situational low 648
Pain, acute 649
Perfusion, risk for ineffective peripheral tissue 650
Infection, risk for 651
Mobility, impaired physical 652
Knowledge, deficient [Learning Need] 653
Total Joint Replacement 655
Pain, acute 657
Infection, risk for 658
Peripheral Neurovascular Dysfunction, risk for 658
Mobility, impaired physical 660
Constipation, risk for 661
Knowledge, deficient [Learning Need] 662
Sample Clinical Pathway 663

CHAPTER 13
Integumentary 667
Burns: Thermal, Chemical, and Electrical—Acute and Convalescent Phases 667
Airway Clearance, risk for ineffective 672
Fluid Volume, risk for deficient 673
Pain, acute 675
Infection, risk for 676
Perfusion, ineffective tissue/Peripheral Neurovascular Dysfunction, risk for 678
Nutrition: Less than Body Requirements, imbalanced 679
Mobility, impaired physical 680
Skin Integrity, impaired [grafts] 681
Fear/Anxiety 682
Body Image, disturbed/Role Performance, ineffective 683
Knowledge, deficient [Learning Need] 684

CHAPTER 14
Systemic Infections and Immunological Disorders 686
Sepsis/Septicemia 686
Infection, risk for [progression of sepsis to septic shock, development of opportunistic infections] 690
Hyperthermia 691
Shock, risk for 692
Fluid Volume, risk for deficient 694
Gas Exchange, risk for impaired 695
Knowledge, deficient [Learning Need] 696
The HIV-Positive Client 697
Behavaior, risk-prone health 699
Fatigue 701
Nutrition: Less than Body Requirements, risk for imbalanced 702
Knowledge, deficient [Learning Need] 703
Social Isolation, risk for 706

Health Management, ineffective
  self/Therapeutic Regimen Management,
  family 707

Acquired Immunodeficiency Syndrome (AIDS) 709
Infection, risk for [progression to sepsis/
  onset of new opportunistic infection] 714
Fluid Volume, risk for deficient 715
Breathing Pattern, ineffective/Gas
  Exchange, risk for impaired 717
Bleeding, risk for 718
Nutrition: Less than Body Requirements,
  imbalanced 718
Pain, acute/chronic 720
Skin Integrity, [actual]/risk for impaired 721
Oral Mucous Membrane, impaired 722
Fatigue 723
Thought Processes, disturbed 723
Anxiety, death 725
Social Isolation 726
Powerlessness 727
Knowledge, deficient [Learning Need] 727

Rheumatoid Arthritis (RA) 729
Pain, acute/chronic 732
Mobility, impaired physical/Walking,
  impaired 734
Body Image, disturbed/Role Performance,
  ineffective 735
Self-Care Deficit (specify) 736
Home Maintenance, risk for impaired 737
Knowledge, deficient [Learning Need] 737

Transplantation Considerations—
Postoperative and Lifelong 739
Infection, risk for 742
Anxiety [specify level]/Fear 743
Coping, risk for ineffective/compromised
  [or] disabled family 744
Knowledge, deficient [Learning Need] 745

CHAPTER 15
General 749
Psychosocial Aspects of Care 749
Coping, ineffective/Conflict, decisional
  (specify) 751
Coping, risk for compromised family 752
Coping, readiness for enhanced family 753
Anxiety [specify level]/Fear 754
Self-Esteem, situational low 756
Grieving [specify] 757
Religiosity, risk for impaired 759
Health Management, risk for ineffective self 760
Violence, risk for self-directed/
  other-directed 761
Post-Trauma Syndrome, risk for 762

Dementia of the Alzheimer's
Type/Vascular Dementia 764
Injury/Trauma, risk for 768
Confusion, chronic 770
Sensory Perception, disturbed (specify) 772
Fear 773
Grieving 774
Sleep Deprivation 774
Self-Care Deficit (specify type/level) 775

Nutrition: Less/More than Body
  Requirements, risk for imbalanced 776
Constipation (specify)/Bowel
  Incontinence/Urinary Elimination,
  impaired 777
Sexual Dysfunction, risk for 778
Coping, compromised/disabled family 779
Home Maintenance, impaired/Health
  Maintenance, ineffective 780
Caregiver Role Strain, risk for 781
Relocation Stress Syndrome, risk for 782

Surgical Intervention 782
Knowledge, deficient [Learning Need] 786
Fear/Anxiety [specify level] 787
Injury, risk for perioperative positioning 788
Injury, risk for 789
Infection, risk for 791
Body Temperature, risk for imbalanced 792
Breathing Pattern, ineffective 793
Sensory Perception, disturbed (specify)/
  Thought Processes, disturbed 794
Fluid Volume, risk for deficient 795
Pain, acute 796
Skin/Tissue Integrity, impaired 798
Perfusion, risk for ineffective tissue 799
Knowledge, deficient [Learning Need] 800

Extended Care 801
Relocation Stress Syndrome, risk for 803
Grieving 804
Memory, impaired/Thought Processes,
  disturbed 805
Coping, compromised family 806
Poisoning, risk for [drug toxicity] 807
Communication, impaired verbal 808
Sleep Pattern, disturbed 809
Nutrition: Less [or] More than Body
  Requirements, imbalanced 810
Self-Care Deficit [specify] 812
Skin Integrity, risk for impaired 812
Urinary Elimination, risk for impaired 814
Constipation/Diarrhea, risk for 815
Mobility, impaired physical/Falls, risk for 816
Diversional Activity, deficient 817
Sexual Dysfunction, risk for 818
Health Maintenance, ineffective 818

Alcohol: Acute Withdrawal 819
Breathing Pattern, risk for ineffective 825
Cardiac Output, risk for decreased 826
Injury, risk for [specify] 827
Sensory Perception, disturbed [specify] 828
Anxiety [severe/panic]/Fear 829
Sample Clinical Pathway 831

Substance Dependence/Abuse
Rehabilitation 835
Denial 837
Coping, ineffective 838
Powerlessness 839
Nutrition: Less than Body Requirements,
  imbalanced 840
Self-Esteem, chronic low 841
Family Processes, dysfunctional 843
Sexual Dysfunction 844
Knowledge, deficient [Learning Need] 845

Cancer 846
Fear/Anxiety [specify level] 850
Grieving 852
Self-Esteem, situational low 853
Pain, acute/chronic 854
Nutrition: Less than Body Requirements, imbalanced 856
Fluid Volume, risk for deficient 857
Fatigue 858
Infection, risk for 859
Oral Mucous Membrane, risk for impaired 860
Skin/Tissue Integrity, risk for impaired 861
Constipation/Diarrhea, risk for 862
Sexual Dysfunction, risk for 863
Family Processes, risk for interrupted 864
Knowledge, deficient [Learning Need] 865

End-of-Life Care/Hospice 866
Pain, acute/chronic 869
Activity Intolerance/Fatigue 870
Grieving/Anxiety, death 871
Coping, compromised [or] disabled family/Caregiver Role Strain 873
Spiritual Distress, risk for 874

Disaster Considerations 876
Injury—Trauma, Suffocation, Poisoning, risk for[/or actual] 878
Infection, risk for 879
Anxiety [severe/panic]/Fear 881
Spiritual Distress 882
Post-Trauma Syndrome, risk for 883
Coping, ineffective community 884
Coping, readiness for enhanced community 885

Pediatric Considerations 890
Pain, acute/chronic 893
Anxiety/Fear; Coping, ineffective 894
Activity Intolerance, [specify level]/Fatigue 895
Growth and Development, risk for delayed 896
Nutrition: Less than Body Requirements, risk for imbalanced 897

Injury, risk for (specify: Trauma, Suffocation, Poisoning) 898
Fluid Volume, risk for imbalanced 899
Family Processes, interrupted/Parenting, impaired 900
Body Temperature, risk for imbalanced 901
Health Maintenance, risk for ineffective 902

Fluid and Electrolyte Imbalances 903
Fluid Balance 904
Hypervolemia (Extracellular Fluid Volume Excess) 905
Fluid Volume, excess 907
Hypovolemia (Extracellular Fluid Volume Deficit) 908
Fluid Volume, deficient 910
Sodium 911
Hyponatremia (Sodium Deficit) 911
Electrolyte Imbalance, risk for 914
Hypernatremia (Sodium Excess) 915
Electrolyte Imbalance, risk for 917
Potassium 918
Hypokalemia (Potassium Deficit) 918
Electrolyte Imbalance, risk for 920
Hyperkalemia (Potassium Excess) 921
Electrolyte Imbalance, risk for 923
Calcium 924
Hypocalcemia (Calcium Deficit) 924
Electrolyte Imbalance, risk for 926
Hypercalcemia (Calcium Excess) 927
Electrolyte Imbalance, risk for 928
Magnesium 930
Hypomagnesemia (Magnesium Deficit) 930
Electrolyte Imbalance, risk for 931
Hypermagnesemia (Magnesium Excess) 932
Electrolyte Imbalance, risk for 933

Bibliography 935
Index of Nursing Diagnoses 958

CONTENTS OF THE CD-ROM

Medical/Surgical Care Plans (includes all care plans from the book)
Cardiovascular
Respiratory
Neurological/Sensory Disorders
Gastrointestinal Disorders
Metabolic and Endocrine Disorders
Diseases of the Blood/Blood-Forming
   Organs
Renal and Urinary Tract
Women's Reproductive
Orthopedic
Integumenatry
Systemic Infections and Immunological
   Disorders
General

Psychiatric Care Plans
Childhood and Adolescent Disorders
Pervasive Developmental Disorders
Attention-Deficit/Hyperactivity Disorder
   (ADHD)
Conduct Disorder
Oppositional Defiant Disorder
Elimination Disorders: Enuresis/Encopresis
Parenting: Growth-Promoting Relationship

Dementia and Amnestic and Other
Cognitive Disorders
Dementia of Alzheimer's Type/Vascular
   Dementia
Dementia Due to HIV Disease

Substance-Related Disorders
Alcohol-Related Disorders
Stimulants (Amphetamines, Cocaine, Caffeine,
   and Nicotine) and Inhalant-Related
   Disorders
Depressants (Barbiturates, Nonbarbiturates,
   Hypnotics and Anxiolytics, Opioids)
Hallucinogen-, Phencyclidine-, and Cannabis-
   Related Disorders
Substance Dependence/Abuse Rehabilatation

Schizophrenia and Other Psychotic
Disorders
Schizophrenia
Schizoaffective Disorder
Delusional Disorder

Mood Disorders
Major Depressive/Dysthymic Disorder
Bipolar Disorders

Anxiety Disorders
Generalized Anxiety Disorder
Panic Disorders/Phobias
Obsessive-Compulsive Disorder
Posttraumatic Stress Disorder

Somatoform Disorders
Dissociative Disorders
Sexual and Gender Identity Disorders
Sexual Dysfunctions and Paraphilias
Gender Identity Disorder

Eating Disorders
Anorexia Nervosa/Bulimia Nervosa
Obesity

Adjustment Disorders
Personality Disorders
Antisocial Personality Disorder
Borderline Personality Disorder
Passive-Aggressive Personality Disorder

Other Conditions That May Be a Focus of
Attention
Psychological Factors Affecting Medical
   Condition
Problems Related to Abuse or Neglect
Premenstrual Dysphoric Disorder
   (Premenstrual Syndrome)

Maternal/Newborn Care Plans
Prenatal Concepts
Genetic Counseling
First Trimester
Second Trimester
Third Trimester
The High-Risk Pregnancy
Prenatal Substance Dependence/Abuse
The Pregnant Adolescent
Cardiac Conditions
Pregnancy-Induced Hypertension
Diabetes Mellitus: Prepregnancy/Gestational
Prenatal Hemorrhage
Prenatal Infection
Premature Dilation of the Cervix
   (Incompetent/Dysfunctional Cervix)
Spontaneous Termination
Elective Termination
Preterm Labor/Prevention of Delivery

Intrapartal Concepts
Labor Stage I—Latent Phase
Labor Stage I—Active Phase
Labor Stage I—Transition Phase (Deceleration)
Labor Stage II—Expulsion
Labor Stage III—Placental Expulsion
Dysfunctional Labor/Dystocia
Labor: Induced/Augmented
Cesarean Birth
Precipitous Labor/Delivery or Unplanned/
   Out-of-Hospital Delivery
Intrapartal Hypertension
Intrapartal Diabetes Mellitus

Maternal Postpartal Concepts
  Stage IV—First 4 Hours Following Delivery of
    the Placenta
  The Client at 4 Hours to 2 Days Postpartum
  Care Following Cesarean Birth (4 Hours to
    3 Days Postpartum)
  The Client at 24–48 Hours Following Early
    Discharge
  The Client at 1 Week Following Discharge
  The Client at 4–6 Weeks Following Discharge
  Postpartal Hemorrhage
  Postpartal Diabetes Mellitus
  Puerperal Infection
  Postpartal Thrombophlebitis
  The Parents of a Child With Special Needs
  Perinatal Loss
Newborn Concepts
  The First Hour of Life
  The Neonate at 2 Hours to 2 Days of Age

  The Neonate at 24–48 Hours Following Early
    Discharge
  The Neonate at 1 Week Following Discharge
  The Infant at 4 Weeks Following Birth
  The Preterm Infant
  Deviations in Growth Patterns
  Circumcision
  Hyperbilirubinemia
  The Infant of an Addicted Mother
  The Infant of an HIV-Positive Mother

Pediatric Considerations
500 Health Conditions and Client Concerns With Associated Nursing Diagnoses

CHAPTER 1

Issues and Trends in Nursing and Healthcare Delivery

In order for nurses to be actively involved in restructuring and maximizing healthcare delivery systems, they must possess current knowledge of trends in the healthcare environment and issues in nursing practice that relate to overall healthcare practice.

The Ever-Changing Healthcare Environment

The Center for American Nurses cites the American Nurses Association's (ANA) *Code of Ethics for Nurses* (2001) and *Nursing: Scope and Standards of Practice* (2004) as proof that nurses have a professional responsibility to be involved in the planning and delivery of nursing practice.

According to Rivera and Halvorson (2008), "the fundamental focus of healthcare reform must be on quality of care." This is not new to nurses. Quality of care has always been a major focus of the profession. And we agree that it is a critical issue in healthcare reform, but it is by no means the only issue.

Healthcare is impacted by many other factors, including poverty, the escalating cost of healthcare, the ever-increasing numbers of uninsured or underinsured healthcare consumers, and the need for allocation of limited healthcare dollars and resources. According to The World Health Organization, the United States is 37th in their ranking of health among nations worldwide, even though the United States spends a larger percentage of its wealth on healthcare than any other industrialized nation (Rivera & Halvorson, 2008). While left to ponder the possible reasons for that ranking, healthcare providers realize that issues about socioeconomic status, ethnicity, and culture impact the disparity in healthcare and will continue to have an effect on nursing practice and job satisfaction.

In addition, technological advances, as well as the ethical and liability issues associated with living in a technological age, will continue to affect nursing practice now and in the future.

Nurses must be aware of these varied influences and take an active role in the formulation of policies and legislation affecting their practice. The Center for American Nurses (2007) strongly supports nurses' active participation in the assessment, restructuring, and redesign of their work to ensure that nursing practice is evidence-based and positively impacts healthcare consumers' and providers' safety and satisfaction. Furthermore, as nurses define their practice, they must set the standards of practice to provide quality nursing care with a high degree of client satisfaction and within the constraints of available resources, such as shortages and changing roles for healthcare providers.

Healthcare Costs and the Allocation of Resources

Nurses have a responsibility to be aware of how the cost of healthcare impacts clients' choices and well-being. Healthcare-funding issues are constantly in the news, and cuts threaten the health of our nation. As healthcare expenditures continue to rise, both government and private payers of healthcare costs are pursuing various methods of cost containment.

Modern reforms began in the 1980s when the Medicare payment system for inpatient healthcare services changed from a cost-based retrospective payment system to a prospective payment system based on diagnosis-related groups (DRGs). This change meant that reimbursement for services followed specific guidelines and restrictions, including the requirement of prior approval for treatment. Since then, many changes and upgrades have been made in this payment system, such as all-patient refined DRGs (or APR-DRGs) and severity DRGs, to better reflect the complexity of a client's condition or care needs; however, reimbursement still remains below billed costs. Now, as a result of budgetary concerns, most states are considering or have already developed options to similarly curb Medicaid reimbursement. These changes have widely affected both access to healthcare and healthcare delivery systems.

One of the most far-reaching solutions for cost containment has been the implementation of managed care services and the building of health maintenance organizations

1

(HMOs) or physician provider organizations (PPOs). The high prevalence of unhealthy behaviors of healthcare consumers (such as smoking, lack of exercise, poor dietary habits, and obesity) causes concern for healthcare policymakers as well as healthcare providers. In some managed care systems, special financial incentives (such as paid health club memberships, substance abuse programs, smoking cessation programs, etc.) are provided to consumers to promote health or to manage their disease risk factors. The expectation is that health promotion will reduce future healthcare expenditures.

Healthcare financing will always be an issue. In the United States, healthcare has largely been based on employer-sponsored insurance coverage, which has seen a significant increase in the average premium levels for individual coverage accompanied by a decline in the percentage of eligible private-sector employees enrolled in health insurance programs (State Health, 2006b). The high cost of insurance has prompted many employers to pursue other methods of providing benefits, such as self-funded insurance plans in which the employer sets aside funds to pay for anticipated employee healthcare claims instead of paying premiums to a health insurance carrier. This method reduces overhead costs and permits employers to try innovative approaches, such as on-site walk-in clinics managed by nurse practitioners.

Most insurance plans require preauthorization for services and/or procedures based on established protocols. In addition, they encourage early discharge from hospital care, preferring to provide payment for outpatient healthcare providers with whom they have contracted services.

Service fees are also subject to capitation, which means providing services for a preset fee regardless of actual cost. This affects both the healthcare provider and the healthcare consumer. Healthcare providers must pick and choose between procedures and treatments they deem necessary and those that the client can pay for, whether by their insurance plan or out of pocket. Many healthcare providers have been unable to operate their businesses under the reduced payment for services resulting in the provider limiting services offered or leaving private practice altogether. Inversely, many healthcare consumers are unable to pay for services not included in their insurance plans or cannot afford the high premiums required to maintain health insurance.

Thus there are a rising number of underinsured and uninsured healthcare consumers impacting both access to healthcare and the cost of healthcare. Studies have shown that adults who lack health insurance coverage are more likely to rate their health status as poor or fair and are less likely to receive preventive services and cancer screenings than adults with insurance (State Health, 2006a). Uninsured individuals are more likely to seek healthcare from hospital emergency departments. The high cost of emergent care has required some hospitals to engage in cost-shifting to cash or self-pay clients, or in some cases, to even close emergency departments.

Major disparities exist in health and healthcare based on socioeconomic status, race, ethnicity, and insurance status. Disparities in risk factors and morbidity also exist and vary by race and ethnicity. Socioeconomic status, health practices, psychosocial stress, limited resources, environmental exposures, discrimination, and access to healthcare are all issues that the policymakers and the healthcare profession must address (Health, United States, 2007).

Nurses need to be familiar with the agencies that are involved in the trends and responses to healthcare reform. The Centers for Medicare and Medicaid Services (CMS) has a strategic action plan entitled "Achieving a Transformed and Modernized Healthcare System for the 21st Century." The CMS vision of modernizing healthcare will have a huge impact on the recipients of nursing care. Specific areas of concentration of the CMS strategic plan publicized by the U.S. Department of Health and Human Services (HHS) include

1. implementing the Medicare Modernization Act successfully by energizing broad participation, emphasizing preventive care, reaching out to those eligible for low-income subsidies, and stimulating a competitive market;
2. modernizing Medicaid to ensure program dollars are used appropriately, to make consumers more cost-conscious, to tailor benefits to need, to allow home and community care for the elderly and persons with disabilities, and to stop inappropriate intergovernmental transfers;
3. creating workable methods of rewarding healthcare providers for positive outcomes; and
4. positioning HHS at the forefront of the health information technology interoperability movement.

Legislation related to these initiatives will impact nursing and healthcare and requires that nurses be involved.

Restructuring Healthcare

In recent years, changes in reimbursement and the practice of managed healthcare delivery have required hospitals to change the way they operate. They adopted methods used in industry, such as reengineering and work redesign. Restructuring the workforce and the client care system was initially accomplished through mergers, consolidation of services, and downsizing of professional staff.

Healthcare professionals expressed great concern regarding the effect of downsizing on the quality of care provided, noting the decline in healthcare consumer satisfaction reported on discharge surveys and research studies (e.g., Blegen et al, 1998; Yang, 2003). Additionally, various research studies have shown that in-hospital client mortality increases by 7% for each additional client added to the average RN workload (Aiken et al, 2002), and there are higher fall rates associated with fewer nursing hours per patient day and a lower percentage of RNs in the staffing mix (Dunton et al, 2004). Responding to these concerns, many healthcare providers formed collaborative practice teams whose goal is to revise the healthcare delivery system by reducing redundancy of services, eliminating nonproductive activities, and relocating ancillary services. Employers also implemented cross-training of staff to enhance provider scope of services and qualifications; however, this was not sufficient to solve the problem. An increase of RNs in the staffing mix was supported by additional studies that reported decreased lengths of stay and decreased rates of complications with a higher proportion of RNs in the staffing mix and more RN hours per patient day (Needleman et al, 2002; Mark et al, 2007).

Shifting the focus to the work of providing healthcare, the federal government has directed facilities to expand computer capabilities to reduce errors and untoward outcomes by improving order entry, streamlining documentation, facilitating data retrieval, and developing structured care methodologies. This push to implement computers is supported by studies such as that of Leape and Berwick (2005), which found that computerizing physician order entry could reduce prescription errors by as much as 81%.

Access to computers, whether by central location, bedside terminal, or handheld units, allows the immediate entry and retrieval of client data by care providers. Pagers, cell phones, and voice-activated devices facilitate communication between healthcare team members and clients, reducing response time for meeting client needs. Documentation time can be reduced by using detailed flow sheets, charting by exception, standardized and computerized plans of care, and developing clinical pathways or care maps.

Clinical pathways support the coordination and evaluation of interdisciplinary care through the identification of specific outcomes, which are important in today's focus on "outcomes-based" client care, and the corresponding activities for a given condition or procedure based on the DRG or the facility's definition of expected length of stay (ELOS). Clinical pathways provide a mechanism for modifying care to reflect current clinical practice expectations based on clinical innovations and research findings. They may also be useful for timely identification of actual or potential outliers, thus allowing reallocation of resources to maximize client outcomes while controlling costs.

Other structured care methodologies promoting standardization of care processes include the use of algorithms, guidelines, or protocols (standing orders). In the field of medicine, criteria have been developed, such as the APACHE (Acute Physiology and Chronic Health Evaluation) computer programs, to assist providers in choosing appropriate treatment options and to help allocate resources. APACHE programs provide data on the likely outcomes of various treatments in specific client populations. Thus, reimbursement could conceivably be tied to a scoring system reflecting the likelihood of survival and corresponding treatment protocols.

The advancement of knowledge continues with the work of the U.S. Department of Health and Human Services' Agency for Healthcare Research and Quality (formerly the Agency for Health Care Policy and Research), whose purpose is to enhance the quality, appropriateness, and effectiveness of healthcare services. Multidisciplinary panels of clinicians, including nurses, created clinical practice and client teaching guidelines addressing specific client care situations. These guidelines not only assist in the prevention, diagnosis, and management of clinical conditions, but also provide a resource by which client care can be evaluated, the provider held accountable, and reimbursement justified. The agency now serves as a repository for research resources and documents that provide a comprehensive database for the development of evidence-based clinical practice guidelines.

Nurses and healthcare organizations are being encouraged to focus more attention on evidenced-based practice in all settings. These processes tend to stabilize care practices and system processes and are designed to improve outcomes.

The need to provide services at lower costs has forced providers to seek alternatives to inpatient care. Currently, the emphasis is on outpatient services and affiliations with other provider groups to provide a wider continuum of client care. Significant changes in client care management are taking place because of the implementation of case management, disease-state management, and evidence-based care. Case management services are now provided across all settings, from case managers employed by insurers to entrepreneurial individuals engaged in "continuum of care" specialty areas, as well as from alternate sites, including outpatient, subacute, and home care.

In addition, promoting client self-care and family support through their participation in the planning of care and mutual goal setting, as well as the self-administration of some therapies and medications, provides opportunities for the client and family to maximize their control of and contribution to their health status, demonstrate newly learned skills, and improve their acute care experience.

Even with these changes and advancements, the ANA believes these attempts at restructuring have not provided the desired improvement in the access to and overall quality of healthcare. The ANA's Health Care Agenda 2005, states that "The U.S. health care system remains in a state of crisis. Despite incremental efforts at reform, the number of uninsured continues to grow, the cost of care continues to rise, and the safety and quality of care is questioned."

The ANA Health Care Agenda 2005 supports a restructured healthcare system that assures universal access to a standard package of essential healthcare services for all citizens and residents. This package would focus more on primary care, thereby reducing the overuse of expensive, technology-driven, acute hospital-based services.

Nursing Care Costs

Nurses have always been the mainstay of care for people throughout their life span, especially at the end of their lives. Nurses continue to play a vital role in promoting responsible, appropriate, and ethical healthcare.

Today, the nurse's attention is focused on providing nursing care to more severely ill clients within the constraints of scarce dollars, limited inpatient stays, reduced staff, and restricted numbers of health-monitoring visits.

Quantifying the contribution of nursing to client care requires identification of the level of nursing care necessary for each client and translating that into direct billing of services rendered. In those facilities or agencies already billing for nursing services, the client plan of care is an integral part of the justification of nursing care costs.

A recent focus of growth in the profession has been the effort to standardize nursing language to better demonstrate what nursing is and what nurses do. Currently, 13 classification systems or standardized nursing languages have been recognized by the ANA and submitted to the National Library of Medicine for inclusion in the Unified Medical Language System Metathesaurus. These nursing languages (e.g., NANDA; NIC/NOC, or Nursing Interventions Classification/Nursing Outcomes Classification; Omaha System; Clinical Care Classification; Perioperative Nursing Data Set; and International Classification for Nursing Practice) can enhance the ability of nurses to communicate and document the care they provide and charge for these services. A standardized nursing language facilitates the recognition of nursing's contribution to client care and promotes the view that nursing is a revenue-generating center.

NANDA International is one organization helping to operationalize the work of nursing by categorizing and classifying labels describing human responses to health, illness, and life processes that are amenable to treatment by nurses. Also helpful in this area are two other groups. The Iowa Intervention Project: Nursing Interventions Classification (NIC) has focused attention on the content and process of nursing care by identifying and standardizing the direct and indirect care activities that nurses perform, and the Iowa Outcomes Project: Nursing Outcomes Classification (NOC) has addressed client outcomes responsive to and associated with nursing interventions. The linking of these three standardized languages, nursing diagnoses, interventions, and outcomes, has provided a comprehensive language included in the Systematized Nomenclature of Medicine (SNOMED), an international coding system in support of the electronic health record that is applicable in multiple healthcare settings.

Nursing research has studied ways to improve the delivery and coordination of healthcare. HANDS (Hands-on Automated Nursing Data System) is a method for the automated collection of a cross-setting clinical data set to support interdisciplinary care and evidence-based practice. Regardless of the client's entry point into healthcare, this plan of care history is readily available to assist providers with decisions regarding immediate and future care (Keenan et al, 2002). The HANDS Project Research Team concluded that the standardized terminologies of NANDA, NIC, and NOC can be successfully used to transform nursing practice and that the development of these standardized nursing terminologies has provided a consistent way to describe nursing practice, which is important because nurses coordinate and provide more than 80% of the healthcare in the United States (Keenan et al, 2008).

Early Discharge

Clients are discharged from acute care as soon as their condition is stabilized, but they may still require specialized care. Subacute or transitional units provide routine services such as monitoring, ongoing therapies, and complex care that may include intravenous therapy, pain management, wound care, airway management, and ventilator weaning, as well as rehabilitation services and postsurgical recovery care.

Shorter hospital stays have also shifted recovery care to the home setting. Families are expected to be more involved in postdischarge care. Although the rate of healthcare facility-acquired infections may decline, clients may feel abandoned or recovery may be delayed or prolonged if the family's personal resources cannot meet the new challenges associated with the recovery process.

In the acute care setting, early discharge allows for a greater volume of admissions while actually reducing the number of beds and staff required to provide care. As a result, in the future the majority of nursing care will likely be provided outside the confines of an acute care hospital setting.

Aging Population

Individuals are living longer and, often, more active lives. As a result, they expect access to procedures such as coronary artery bypass, total joint replacements, aggressive cancer care, and other interventions that in the past were not recommended in the presence of advanced age and comorbidities. The increased mean age of clients requiring hospitalization necessitates some changes in the way their healthcare is provided. Optimal client care requires general knowledge regarding special needs of the elderly, along with resources to meet these needs and to reduce the incidence of adverse events, including confusion, falls, and incontinence. At the least, these factors can cause prolonged facility stays and increase the number and complexity of treatments, readmissions, and adverse outcomes.

To this end, the nursing profession is working to develop models such as the Nurses Improving Care to the Hospitalized Elderly (NICHE) Project that will improve the care provided to this population. The provision of primary nurse case managers to follow chronically ill clients across the continuum of care attempts to ensure that elderly clients are not lost to follow-up and receive ongoing monitoring for timely, cost-effective intervention.

Healthcare decision making has changed dramatically in recent decades, with an explicit acknowledgment of the client's right to determine the course of care. In the nursing profession, there has been a long-standing allegiance to the client's role in decision making, but nurses, especially those in elder care, fear that the interpretation and use of advance directives can create ethical conflicts regarding the withdrawal or withholding of treatment or care, especially when the client is concerned about being a "burden to others." Living wills and advance directives cannot be expected to address all situations that clients may encounter; however, they can provide information to a proxy who is named the medical durable power of attorney to help in the decision-making process. Even with advance directives in place, nurses need to be sensitive to clients' rights to change their minds and redefine their wishes based on changes in their health status or availability of care options.

Technological Advances

The purpose of medical technology is to improve clinical decision making and symptom management, and technology continues to evolve at an astounding rate in both treatment and equipment. Robots are being used to dispense medications in pharmacies and to assist with surgical procedures such as coronary artery bypass, mitral valve repair, and prostate removal. And with the projection of large increases in the aging population, robots such as the Nursebot Project and DO-U-MI are also being developed to assist with activities of daily living (ADLs) and transfers and to provide mobility assistance, companionship, and entertainment for the elderly and disabled (Matthews, 2002; Park, 2001; Pineau, 2003; Pollack, 2002).

The use of in-room cameras and computers, combined with video conferencing (eICU), to monitor the vital signs and status of multiple clients in intensive care units promotes earlier recognition of changes and timely response by nurses and physicians, improving client outcomes and reducing mortality rates (Kohl, 2007). Clients undergoing minimally invasive surgery (e.g., laparoscopy) report lower pain levels, have less blood loss and scarring, have shorter lengths of stay, and report faster healing. Other equipment developments that allow clients to leave acute care settings more quickly include user-friendly ventilators, smaller implantable ventilator-assist devices, and artificial hearts. Biventricular pacing for cardiac resynchronization is available, although underused, for the treatment of clients with class III and IV heart failure. Brain stimulators are treating movement disorders such as Parkinson's disease, dystonia, and essential tremors. Implantable insulin pumps are reducing or delaying the complications associated with type 1 diabetes mellitus.

In the near future, the expanded use of monoclonal antibodies to carry chemotherapy agents or radionuclides to cancer cells will reduce adverse reactions and possibly the need for acute care. Endotoxin antibodies (immune system molecules that can mediate sepsis) and gene therapies are being developed that, it is hoped, can manage or even eliminate hereditary/degenerative diseases, thereby reducing high-cost therapy needs.

Work is also progressing toward the creation of a computerized patient record (CPR) or electronic health record (EHR) that will provide a composite "cradle to grave" record for each individual accessing healthcare in this country. And in support of nursing, point-of-care computer systems are being refined in an effort to cut documentation time and to track nursing time for the costing of care. Computers providing real-time updating of the client plan of care enable the nurse to process data from monitoring activities and facilitate evaluation of the effectiveness of nursing actions and other therapies.

In another arena, telehealth is being used to not only triage the needs of large populations, but also to provide direct client care to underserved areas via long-distance communication lines. Video conferencing, the Internet, and interactive voice-response systems are being used to monitor chronically ill clients in their own homes to promote timely intervention and reduce hospitalizations.

As technology advances and more people become knowledgeable partners in healthcare, clients are choosing to direct their own therapies, challenging therapeutic plans developed by healthcare providers or withdrawing from established medical care in favor of alternative therapies and modalities. Nurses need to be knowledgeable and open-minded regarding complementary/alternative therapies, supporting client choices and learning and evaluating new techniques to help educate clients.

And finally, although nurses and clients alike are turning to the Internet for medical information and therapeutic options, this resource can be a double-edged sword because data provided may or may not be accurate. Therefore, nurses need to be aware of and knowledgeable about various Web sites in order to direct their clients to reputable and valid resources.

Future of Nursing

Healthcare reform remains the focus of much writing, debate, and litigation in this new century. Questions still abound regarding what constitutes healthcare reform. Whether brought about by statute, insurance payers, or healthcare providers, the changes in healthcare delivery are continuing and far-reaching. These changes are, and should be, of great concern to nurses.

Nurses should be supportive of the American Nurses' Health Care Agenda, which documents the commitment to the principle that all persons are entitled to ready access to affordable quality healthcare services and that nurses are well positioned to advocate on behalf of and in concert with individuals, families, and communities.

We, the authors, are nurses who still believe that a nursing perspective is essential if nurses are to position themselves for a role in future healthcare-delivery systems. As Virginia Henderson said, "The beauty of nursing is the combination of the heart, head, and hands" (Buerhaus, 1998). We are opposed to any system that reduces or eliminates the role of nursing. And we believe that clients depend on nurses to advocate for their rights, as well as to provide them with quality nursing care when they are ill.

Although the public expects nurses to demonstrate technical competence and academic knowledge, it is also now demanding better consumer service, that is, friendliness, attention to the client's personal or special needs, concern for privacy, information about tests and therapies, and inclusion of the family in the information loop.

To ensure that clients are getting what they need without wasting healthcare dollars, nurses must be knowledgeable about costs and reimbursement plans, as well as the relative benefits of treatment options.

Healthcare systems can no longer employ RNs in roles that do not directly, critically, and clearly contribute to the outcomes of the organization. Today's nurse must be technically competent, skilled at critical thinking and problem-solving, able to work with a variety of people, and fiscally responsible.

This is not enough, however. The outcomes of nursing care are the true measurement of the ability to provide care. Nurses are entering (and even creating) new practice environments in which to use their skills. They are also working to further define nursing practice and the special contribution that nursing will continue to offer, because that is how services will be evaluated and reimbursed.

In the midst of this whirlwind of change, as we experiment with new ways to provide cost-effective care within a specified time frame, it is imperative that we build on the foundation of the profession: nursing is a science as well as an art, and nursing practice is rooted in the scientific process. Whether or not we choose to rename the steps we routinely engage in—assessing clients, determining their needs, choosing actions to meet those needs, and evaluating the effectiveness of those actions—our purpose remains the same: the diagnosis and treatment of human responses to health, illness, and life processes.

Conclusion

We are living in an age of escalating uncertainty and tension. Rapid and continuous changes in the healthcare environment have greatly increased the responsibilities facing today's nurse. The scientific and technological advances that we so covet are the same advances that can strip life of its simplicity. In the future, technologies can and will be created to support and, in some cases, replace dependent and interdependent activities of nursing.

As a result of the efficiencies afforded by advances in automation and information management, the focus of nursing practice could shift away from primarily task-oriented client interactions. However, inserting an intravenous line, assessing for respiratory sounds, and providing client teaching, although vital, do not entirely reflect what nurses believe and value as the most important elements of practice. Nurses have long placed emphasis on the psychosocial, spiritual, and physical needs of their clients within the medical regimen. Even in a technologically driven healthcare system, clients will always feel the need to be comforted, listened to, and treated with dignity and respect.

Both planning and documentation of care are essential to satisfy client needs and meet legal obligations. Documentation of the impact of nursing on desired client outcomes provides a basis for evaluating continuing care needs, dealing with legal concerns, and determining payment. The handoff of nursing care involves sharing information on each client, unit, and organization (workflow), and the plan of care has been identified as an ideal source of information that facilitates that transfer of care, providing the best continuity for the system and client (Solovy et al, 2007).

Therefore, as nurses work collaboratively with other disciplines to provide client care, we need to continue to identify and document the nursing care needs of clients through the use of the nursing process and nursing diagnosis. Although this journey into change is not optional, nurses have the opportunity and responsibility to take an active role in shaping that change.

What lies ahead for nursing and planning of client care? Definitely, it will be a tremendously exciting and exacting challenge!

CHAPTER 2

The Nursing Process: Planning Care Using Nursing Diagnoses

Nurses and healthcare consumers agree that nursing care is a key factor in achieving positive outcomes and enhancing client satisfaction. Nursing care is instrumental in all phases of acute care as well as in the maintenance of general well-being, in such areas as prevention of illness, rehabilitation, and maximization of health, or where a return to health is not possible, the relief of pain and discomfort and a peaceful death. To this end, the nursing profession has identified a problem-solving process that "combines the most desirable elements of the art of nursing with the most relevant elements of systems theory, using the scientific method" (Shore, 1988).

The original concept of the nursing process was introduced in the 1950s as a three-step process of assessment, planning, and evaluation based on the scientific method of observing, measuring, gathering data, and analyzing the findings. Over time, this process became part of the conceptual framework of all nursing curricula and is included in the legal definition of nursing in the nurse practice acts of most states. After years of study, use, and refinement, the three-step process was expanded. The five steps—(1) assessment (systematic collection of data relating to clients and their problems and needs), (2) diagnosis (analysis and interpretation of data), (3) planning (prioritizing needs, identifying goals, and choosing solutions), (4) implementation (putting the plan into action), and (5) evaluation (assessing the effectiveness of the plan and changing the plan as indicated by current needs)—are central to nursing actions and the delivery of high-quality, individualized client care in any setting.

When a client enters the healthcare system, the nurse uses the steps of the nursing process to work toward achieving the desired outcomes and goals identified for the client. The effectiveness of the plan of care is evaluated by ascertaining whether or not the desired outcomes and goals have been attained (client's problems and needs have been resolved) or whether problems remain at the time of discharge. If problems are unresolved, plans need to be made for further follow-up, including assessment, additional problem and need identification, alteration of desired outcomes and goals, and changes of interventions in the next care setting.

Although some nurses view the nursing process as separate, progressive steps, the elements are actually interrelated. Taken together, they form a continuous circle of thought and action throughout the client's contact with the healthcare system. The process combines all the skills of critical thinking and good nursing care because it creates a method of active problem-solving that is both dynamic and cyclic. Figure 2.1 demonstrates the way this cyclic process works. As we learn more about diagnostic reasoning and critical thinking, some scholars are proposing a new model to describe what nurses do. With the emphasis on healthcare outcomes, the American Nurses Association's (ANA) 1995 Social Policy Statement focused on outcomes and deemphasized problem-focused approaches to nursing care. Through ongoing research into the nature of thinking and reasoning, the nursing process continues to be redefined (Pesut & Herman, 1999).

The "what" and "how" of the work of nursing have been explained in part in a number of existing publications that help operationalize the work of nursing. The ANA Social Policy Statement (1980) defined nursing as the "diagnosis and treatment of human responses to actual and potential health problems." The statement represents a framework for understanding nursing's relationship with society and nursing's obligations to those who receive nursing care. In 1991, the ANA *Standards of Clinical Nursing Practice* described the client care process and standards for professional performance, providing impetus and support for the use of nursing diagnosis in the practice setting. The work of NANDA (formerly North American Nursing Diagnosis Association) has been ongoing for more than 25 years, beginning with efforts to identify client problems and needs for which nurses are accountable. NANDA-I (NANDA International) continues to support the development of nursing diagnosis labels (Table 2.1), which are now being complemented by the Iowa Intervention Project: Nursing Interventions Classification (NIC) and the Iowa Outcomes Project: Nursing Outcomes Classification (NOC). NIC directs our focus to the content and process of nursing care by identifying and standardizing the care activities nurses perform, and NIC describes

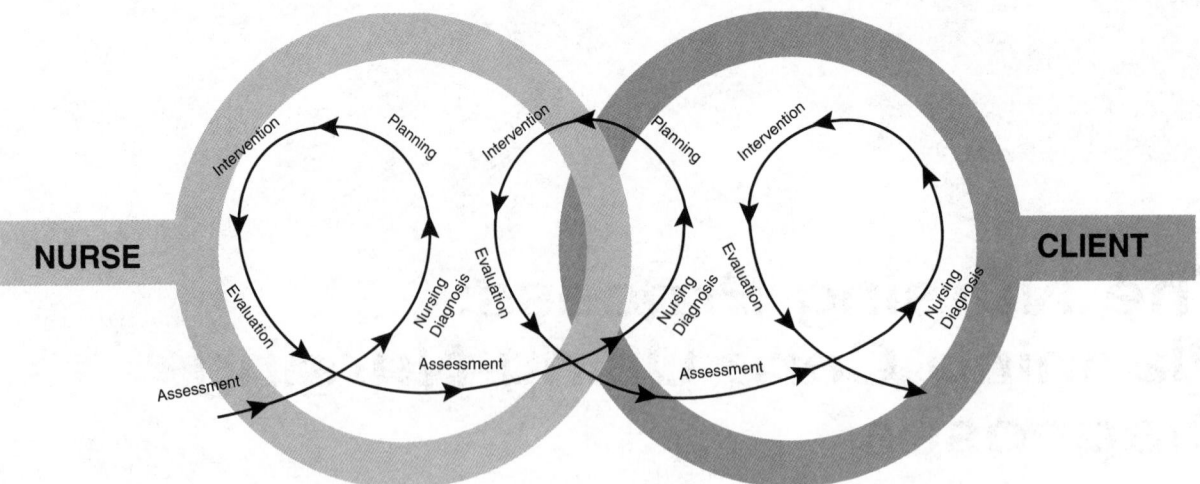

Figure 2.1 Diagram of the nursing process. The steps of the nursing process are interrelated, forming a continuous circle of thought and action that is both dynamic and cyclic.

TABLE 2.1 Nursing Diagnoses Accepted for Use and Research Through 2009

Activity Intolerance [specify level]
Activity Intolerance, risk for
Activity Planning, ineffective
Airway Clearance, ineffective
Allergy Response, latex
Allergy Response, risk for latex
Anxiety [specify level]
Anxiety, death
Aspiration, risk for
Attachment, risk for impaired
Autonomic Dysreflexia
Autonomic Dysreflexia, risk for

Behavior, risk-prone health
Bleeding, risk for
Body Image, disturbed
Body Temperature, risk for imbalanced
Bowel Incontinence
Breastfeeding, effective
Breastfeeding, ineffective
Breastfeeding, interrupted
Breathing Pattern, ineffective

Cardiac Output, decreased
Caregiver Role Strain
Caregiver Role Strain, risk for
Childbearing Process, readiness for enhanced
Comfort, impaired
Comfort, readiness for enhanced
Communication, impaired verbal
Communication, readiness for enhanced
Conflict, decisional (specify)
Conflict, parental role
Confusion, acute
Confusion, risk for acute
Confusion, chronic
Constipation
Constipation, perceived
Constipation, risk for
Contamination
Contamination, risk for
Coping, compromised family

Coping, defensive
Coping, disabled family
Coping, ineffective
Coping, ineffective community
Coping, readiness for enhanced
Coping, readiness for enhanced community
Coping, readiness for enhanced family

Death Syndrome, risk for sudden infant
Decision Making, readiness for enhanced
Denial, ineffective
Dentition, impaired
Development, risk for delayed
Diarrhea
Dignity, risk for compromised human
Distress, moral
Disuse Syndrome, risk for
Diversional Activity, deficient

Electrolyte Imbalance, risk for
Energy Field, disturbed
Environmental Interpretation Syndrome, impaired

Failure to Thrive, adult
Falls, risk for
Family Processes, dysfunctional
Family Processes, interrupted
Family Processes, readiness for enhanced
Fatigue
Fear [specify focus]
Feeding Pattern, ineffective infant
Fluid Balance, readiness for enhanced
[Fluid Volume, deficient hypertonic/hypotonic]
Fluid Volume, deficient [isotonic]
Fluid Volume, excess
Fluid Volume, risk for deficient
Fluid Volume, risk for imbalanced

Gas Exchange, impaired
Glucose Level, risk for unstable blood
Grieving
Grieving, complicated
Grieving, risk for complicated
Growth, risk for disproportionate
Growth and Development, delayed

Health Maintenance, ineffective
Health Management, ineffective self
Health Management, readiness for enhanced self
Home Maintenance, impaired
Hope, readiness for enhanced
Hopelessness
Hyperthermia
Hypothermia

Identity, disturbed personal
Immunization Status, readiness for enhanced
Infant Behavior, disorganized
Infant Behavior, risk for disorganized
Infant Behavior, readiness for enhanced organized
Infection, risk for
Injury, risk for
Injury, risk for perioperative positioning
Insomnia
Intracranial Adaptive Capacity, decreased

Jaundice, neonatal

Knowledge, deficient [Learning Need] [specify]
Knowledge [specify], readiness for enhanced

Lifestyle, sedentary
Liver Function, risk for impaired
Loneliness, risk for

TABLE 2.1 **Nursing Diagnoses Accepted for Use and Research Through 2009** (continued)

Maternal/Fetal Dyad, risk for disturbed
Memory, impaired
Mobility, impaired bed
Mobility, impaired physical
Mobility, impaired wheelchair
Motility, dysfunctional gastrointestinal
Motility, risk for dysfunctional
    gastrointestinal

Nausea
Neglect, self
Neglect, unilateral
Noncompliance, [ineffective Adherence]
    [specify]
Nutrition, readiness for enhanced
Nutrition: less than body requirements,
    imbalanced
Nutrition: more than body requirements,
    imbalanced
Nutrition: more than body requirements, risk
    for imbalanced

Oral Mucous Membrane, impaired

Pain, acute
Pain, chronic
Parenting, impaired
Parenting, readiness for enhanced
Parenting, risk for impaired
Perfusion, ineffective peripheral tissue
Perfusion, risk for ineffective cardiac
    tissue
Perfusion, ineffective cerebral tissue
Perfusion, risk for ineffective gastrointestinal
Perfusion, risk for ineffective renal
Peripheral Neurovascular Dysfunction,
    risk for
Poisoning, risk for
Post-Trauma Syndrome [specify stage]
Post-Trauma Syndrome, risk for
Power, readiness for enhanced
Powerlessness [specify level]
Powerlessness, risk for

Protection, ineffective

Rape-Trauma Syndrome
Relationship, readiness for
    enhanced
Religiosity, impaired
Religiosity, readiness for enhanced
Religiosity, risk for impaired
Relocation Stress Syndrome
Relocation Stress Syndrome,
    risk for
Resilience, impaired individual
Resilience, readiness for enhanced
Resilience, risk for compromised
Role Performance, ineffective

Self-Care, readiness for enhanced
Self-Care Deficit, bathing
Self-Care Deficit, dressing
Self-Care Deficit, feeding
Self-Care Deficit, toileting
Self-Concept, readiness for
    enhanced
Self-Esteem, chronic low
Self-Esteem, situational low
Self-Esteem, risk for situational low
Self-Mutilation
Self-Mutilation, risk for
Sensory Perception, disturbed
    [specify: visual, auditory,
    kinesthetic, gustatory, tactile,
    olfactory]
Sexual Dysfunction
Sexuality Pattern, ineffective
Shock, risk for
Skin Integrity, impaired
Skin Integrity, risk for impaired
Sleep, readiness for enhanced
Sleep Deprivation
Sleep Pattern, disturbed
Social Interaction, impaired
Social Isolation
Sorrow, chronic

Spiritual Distress
Spiritual Distress, risk for
Spiritual Well-Being, readiness for
    enhanced
Stress Overload
Suffocation, risk for
Suicide, risk for
Surgical Recovery, delayed
Swallowing, impaired

[Therapeutic Regimen Management,
    ineffective community]
Therapeutic Regimen Management,
    ineffective family
Thermoregulation, ineffective
[Thought Processes, disturbed]
Tissue Integrity, impaired
Transfer Ability, impaired
Trauma, risk for
Trauma, risk for vascular

Urinary Elimination, impaired
Urinary Elimination, readiness for
    enhanced
Urinary Incontinence, functional
Urinary Incontinence, overflow
Urinary Incontinence, reflex
Urinary Incontinence, stress
[Urinary Incontinence, total]
Urinary Incontinence, urge
Urinary Incontinence, risk for urge
Urinary Retention [acute/chronic]

Ventilation, impaired spontaneous
Ventilatory Weaning Response,
    dysfunctional
Violence, [actual/] risk for
    other-directed
Violence, [actual/] risk for
    self-directed

Walking, impaired
Wandering [specify sporadic or
    continual]

[ ] author recommendations
Used with permission from NANDA International: Definitions and Classification, 2009–2010. NANDA, Philadelphia, 2009.

client outcomes that are responsive to nursing intervention and developing corresponding measurement scales.

The implementation of prospective and capitated payment plans has moved a greater portion of healthcare delivery away from acute care hospitals into the community, with an emphasis on multifaceted free-standing care centers and home health services. Standards of care such as those published by the American Association of Critical-Care Nurses (AACN) and the Joint Commission on Accreditation of Healthcare Organizations (JCAHO) emphasize that even in these environments nursing must meet standards that further specify the parameters of client assessment and documentation of care.

Changes in the healthcare system continue to occur at an ever-increasing rate, requiring the profession of nursing

to define itself in a way that will complement and facilitate the provision of appropriate, cost-effective, evidenced-based care to all persons. Nurses need a common framework of communication and documentation so that their contribution to healthcare is recognized as being essential and they are remunerated appropriately. At the very least, nursing requires a commonality of terms describing practice so it can be captured and is visible in the healthcare databases (Aquilino, 2000; Delany, 2000).

The linkage of nursing diagnoses to specific nursing interventions and client outcomes has led to the development of a number of standardized nursing languages, for instance Omaha System, Clinical Care Classification (formerly Home Healthcare Classification), Ozbolt Patient Care Data

Set, and Perioperative Minimum Data Set. The purpose of these languages is to help ensure continuity of appropriate high-quality nursing care for the client regardless of setting. This is accomplished in part through enhanced communication, standardization of the process evaluating the care provided, and facilitation of documentation.

Planning Care

Medicine and nursing, as well as other healthcare disciplines, are interrelated, and therefore the actions for each discipline have implications for the others. This interrelationship allows for exchange of information and ideas and for development of plans of care that include all data pertinent to the individual client and family. In this book, the plan of care contains not only the actions initiated by medical and nursing orders, but also the coordination of care provided by all related healthcare disciplines. The nurse is often the person responsible for coordinating these various activities into a comprehensive functional plan, essential in providing holistic care for the client. Although independent nursing actions are an integral part of this process, collaborative actions are present based on the medical regimen or orders from other disciplines participating in the care of the client. We believe that nursing is an essential part of collaborative practice, and as such, nursing has a responsibility and accountability in every collaborative problem in which the nurse interacts with the client. The educational background and expertise of the nurse, standing protocols, delegation of tasks, the use of care partners, and the area of practice—for example rural or urban, acute care or community care settings—influence whether an intervention is actually an independent nursing function or requires collaboration.

The well-developed plan of care communicates the client's past and present health status and current needs to all members of the healthcare team involved in providing care. It identifies problems solved and those yet to be solved, can provide information about approaches that have been successful, and notes patterns of client responses to interventions. In legal terms, the plan of care documents client care in areas of liability, accountability, and quality improvement. It also provides a mechanism to help ensure continuity of care when the client leaves a care setting while still needing services.

Components of the Plan of Care

The critical element for providing effective planned nursing care is its relevance as identified in client assessments. ANA's 1991 *Standards of Clinical Nursing Practice* determined that client assessment is required in the following areas and abilities: physical, psychological, sociocultural, spiritual, cognitive, functional, developmental, economic, and lifestyle. These assessments, combined with the results of medical findings and diagnostic studies, are documented in the client database and form the foundation for development of the client's plan of care. For each plan of care presented in this book, a client assessment database is created from information that would likely be obtained from the history, physical examination, and related diagnostic studies. Nursing priorities are then determined and ranked. Priorities are simply stated and represent a general ranking system for the nursing diagnoses in the plan of care. They can be reworded and reorganized, along with their timelines, to create short- and long-term goals. Next, the nursing diagnosis statements, which include possible related factors (etiology) and corresponding signs and symptoms (cues) when appropriate, are presented. Desired client outcomes are then identified and followed by appropriate independent and collaborative interventions with accompanying rationales.

Client Database

In this book, each selected medical condition has an accompanying client database that includes subjective ("may report") and objective ("may exhibit") data that would likely be collected through the history-taking interview, physical assessment, diagnostic studies, and review of prior records. The client database is organized within the 13 categories of the Diagnostic Divisions. A sample medical/surgical assessment tool, definitions of the Divisions, and a client situation are included in Chapter 3. As the nurse develops the plan of care, it will also be individualized to the client's situation.

Interviewing

Interviewing the client and significant other(s) provides data that the nurse obtains through conversation and observation. This information includes the individual's perceptions, that is, what the client perceives to be a problem or need and typically what he or she wants to share. Data may be collected during one or more contact periods and should include all relevant information. All participants in the interview process need to know that collected data are used in planning the client's care. Organizing and updating the data assists in the ongoing identification of client care needs and nursing diagnoses.

Physical Assessment

During information gathering, the nurse exercises perceptual and observational skills, assessing the client through the senses of sight, hearing, touch, and smell. The duration and depth of any physical assessment depend on the current condition of the client and the urgency of the situation, but it usually includes inspection, palpation, percussion, and auscultation. In this book, the physical assessment data are presented within the client database as objective data.

Diagnostic Studies

Interpretation of diagnostic test results is integrated with the history and physical findings as part of objective findings. Some tests are used to diagnose disease, whereas others are useful in following the course of a disease or in adjusting therapies. The nurse needs to be aware of significant test results that require reporting to the physician and/or initiation of specific nursing interventions. In many cases, the relationship of the test to the pathological physiology is clear, but in other cases it is not. This is the result of the interrelationship between various organs and body systems.

Nursing Priorities

In this book, nursing priorities are listed in a certain order to facilitate the linking and ranking of selected associated nursing diagnoses that appear in the plan of care guidelines. In any given client situation, nursing priorities are based on the client's specific needs and can vary from minute to minute. A nursing diagnosis that is a priority today may be less of a priority tomorrow, depending on the fluctuating physical and psychosocial condition of the client or the client's changing responses to the existing condition.

An example of nursing priorities for a client diagnosed with severe hypertension would include the following:

1. Maintain and enhance cardiovascular functioning.
2. Prevent complications.
3. Provide information about disease process, prognosis, and treatment regimen.
4. Support active client control or management of the condition.

Discharge Goals

Once the nursing priorities are determined, the next step is to establish goals of treatment. In this book, each medical condition has established discharge goals, which are broadly stated and reflect the desired general status of the client on discharge or transfer to another care setting.

Discharge goals for a client with severe hypertension would include the following:

1. Blood pressure within acceptable limits for individual
2. Cardiovascular and systemic complications prevented or minimized
3. Disease process and prognosis and therapeutic regimen understood
4. Necessary lifestyle and behavioral changes initiated

Nursing Diagnosis (Problem and Need Identification)

Nursing diagnoses are a uniform way of identifying, focusing on, and dealing with specific client needs and responses to actual and high-risk problems. Nursing diagnosis labels (see Table 2.1) provide a format for expressing the problem-identification portion of the nursing process. In 1989, NANDA developed a taxonomy or classification scheme to categorize and classify nursing diagnostic labels. (This was replaced by a new taxonomy in 2000.) The NANDA definition of nursing diagnosis approved in 1990 further clarified the second step of the nursing process (i.e., diagnosis or problem and need identification). The definition of nursing diagnosis developed by NANDA is presented in Box 2.1.

> **Box 2.1   NANDA-I Definition of Nursing Diagnosis**
>
> A nursing diagnosis is a clinical judgment about individual, family, or community responses to actual or potential health problems/life processes. A nursing diagnosis provides the basis for selection of nursing interventions to achieve outcomes for which the nurse is accountable.

There are several steps involved in the process of problem and need identification. Integrating these steps provides a systematic approach to accurately identifying nursing diagnoses using the process of critical thinking.

1. Collect a client database (nursing interview, physical assessment, and diagnostic studies) combined with information collected by other healthcare providers.
2. Review and analyze the client data.
3. Synthesize the gathered client data as a whole and then label the clinical judgment about the client's responses to these actual or high-risk problems and life processes.
4. Compare and contrast the relationships of clinical judgments with related factors and define characteristics for the selected nursing diagnosis. This step is crucial to choosing and validating the appropriate nursing diagnosis label that will be used to create a specific client diagnostic statement.
5. Combine the nursing diagnosis with the related factors and define characteristics to create the client diagnostic statement. For example, the diagnostic statement for a paraplegic client with a decubitus ulcer could read as follows: impaired Skin Integrity related to pressure, circulatory impairment, and decreased sensation evidenced by draining wound, sacral area.

The nursing diagnosis is as correct as the present information allows because it is supported by the immediate data collected. It documents the client's situation at the present time and should reflect changes as they occur in the client's condition. Accurate need identification and diagnostic labeling provide the basis for selecting nursing interventions.

The nursing diagnosis may be a physical or a psychosocial response. Physical nursing diagnoses include those that pertain to physical processes, such as circulation (ineffective renal Tissue Perfusion), ventilation (impaired Gas Exchange), and elimination (Constipation). Psychosocial nursing diagnoses include those that pertain to the mind (acute Confusion), emotions (Fear), or lifestyle and relationships (ineffective Role Performance). Unlike medical diagnoses, nursing diagnoses change as the client progresses through various stages of illness and/or maladaptation to resolution of the problem or to the conclusion of the condition. Each decision the nurse makes is time dependent, and with additional information gathered at a later time, decisions may change. For example, the initial problems and needs for a client undergoing cardiac surgery may be acute Pain, decreased Cardiac Output, ineffective Airway Clearance, and risk for

Infection. As the client progresses, problems and needs are likely to shift to Activity Intolerance, deficient Knowledge, and ineffective Role Performance.

Diagnostic reasoning is used to ensure the accuracy of the client diagnostic statement. The defining characteristics and related factors associated with the chosen nursing diagnosis are reviewed and compared with the client data. If the diagnosis is not consistent with a majority of the cues or is not supported by relevant cues, additional data may be required or another nursing diagnosis considered.

Desired Client Outcomes

The nurse identifies outcomes for a plan of care individualized for a specific client (ANA, 2004). A desired client outcome is defined as the result of achievable nursing interventions and client responses that is desired by the client or caregiver and attainable within a defined time period, given the current situation and resources. These desired outcomes are the measurable steps toward achieving the previously established discharge goals and are used to evaluate the client's response to nursing interventions. (The fifth step of the nursing process, evaluation, is addressed in the sample client situation provided in Chapter 3.) Useful desired client outcomes must have the following characteristics:

1. Be specific
2. Be realistic or achievable
3. Be measurable
4. Indicate a definite time frame for achievement
5. Consider client's desires and resources

Desired client outcomes are created by listing items and behaviors that can be observed or heard. They are monitored to determine whether an acceptable outcome has been achieved within a specified time frame. Action verbs and time frames are used, for example, "client will ambulate, using cane, within 48 hours of surgery." The action verbs describe the client's behavior to be evaluated. Time frames are dependent on the client's projected or anticipated length of stay, often determined by diagnosis-related group (DRG) classification and considering the presence of complications or extenuating circumstances, such as age, debilitating disease process, and so on. The ongoing work of NOC in identifying 385 outcomes now also addresses client groups or aggregates. Although the NOC outcomes are listed in general terms such as Ambulation, 16 indicators are included for this outcome that can be measured by a five-point Likert-type scale, ranging from "severely compromised" to "not compromised." This facilitates tracking clients across care settings and can demonstrate client progress even when outcomes are not met.

When outcomes are properly written, they provide direction for planning and validating the selected nursing interventions. Consider the two following client outcomes: "Client will identify individual nutritional needs within 36 hours" and ". . . formulate a dietary plan based on identified nutritional needs within

72 hours." Based on the clarity of these outcomes, the nurse can select nursing interventions to ensure that the client's dietary knowledge is assessed, individual needs identified, and nutritional education presented. Often, the client outcomes identified are not unique to nursing because we provide care in a team approach with other disciplines. However, the NOC indicators for outcomes are generally more sensitive to nursing interventions. Other team members can use the majority of NOC labels and identify different indicators relative to their specialty focus to demonstrate their contribution to client improvement or to track deterioration. In this book, the identified outcomes in each plan of care are stated in more specific terms but are organized by using NOC labels (which are boxed to call attention to this language).

Planning (Goals and Actions/Interventions)

Once outcomes are identified, the nurse develops strategies or interventions and alternatives to achieve the outcomes (ANA, 2004). Nursing interventions are prescriptions for specific behaviors expected from the client and actions to be carried out or facilitated by nurses. These actions and interventions are selected to assist the client in achieving the stated desired client outcomes and discharge goals. The expectation is that the prescribed behavior will benefit the client and family in a predictable way related to the identified problem, need, and chosen outcomes. These interventions have the intent of individualizing care by meeting a specific client need and should incorporate identified client strengths when possible.

Nursing interventions should be specific and clearly stated, beginning with an action verb indicating what the nurse is expected to do. Qualifiers of how, when, where, time, frequency, and amount provide the content of the planned activity, for example, "Assist as needed with self-care activities each morning"; "Record respiratory and pulse rates before, during, and after activity"; and "Instruct family in postdischarge care."

The NIC project has identified 542 interventions (both direct and indirect) that are stated in general terms, such as Respiratory Monitoring. Each label has a varied number of activities that may be chosen to accomplish the intervention. The interventions encompass a broad range of nursing practice, with some requiring specialized training or advanced certification. Others may be appropriate for delegation to other care providers, for example, licensed practical nurses (LPNs) or vocational nurses (LVNs), nursing assistants, and unlicensed personnel, but still require planning and evaluation by registered nurses. In this text, these NIC labels are boxed to help the user identify how they can be used.

This book divides the nursing interventions and actions into independent (nurse initiated) and collaborative (initiated by and/or performed in conjunction with other care providers) under the appropriate NIC labels. Examples of these two different professionally initiated actions are as follows:

- Independent: Provide calm, restful surroundings, minimize environmental activity and noise, and limit numbers of visitors and length of stay.
- Collaborative: Administer antianxiety medication as indicated.

Rationale

Although rationales do not appear on regular plans of care, they are included in this book to assist the student and practicing nurse in associating the pathophysiological and psychological principles with the selected nursing intervention. This will help the nurse determine whether an intervention is appropriate for a specific client.

Conclusion

This book is intended to facilitate the application of the nursing process and the use of nursing diagnosis in medical and surgical clients. (The enclosed CD-ROM also contains plan of care guides for maternity, newborn, and psychiatric clients.) Each plan of care guideline was designed to provide generalized information on the associated medical condition. The guidelines can be modified either by using portions of the information provided or by adding more client care information to the existing guides. The plan of care guidelines were developed using the NANDA-I recommendations, except in a few examples where the authors believed more clarification and enhancement were required. The ongoing controversy on the validity of the NANDA-I-approved nursing diagnosis of deficient Knowledge is one example where further clarification was added. The term "Learning Need" has been added to the nursing diagnosis label. Also, some diagnoses, such as Anxiety/Fear, have been combined for convenience; the combination indicates that two or more factors may be involved, and the nurse can then choose the most appropriate diagnosis for a specific client. We recognize that not all of the NANDA-I-approved nursing diagnoses have been used in these plan of care guidelines, but we hope that these guidelines will assist you in determining your clients' needs, outcomes, and nursing interventions.

Next, Chapter 3 will assist you in applying and adapting theory to practice.

CHAPTER 3

Critical Thinking: Adaptation of Theory to Practice

Critical thinking is defined as the "intellectually disciplined process of actively and skillfully conceptualizing, applying, analyzing, synthesizing, and evaluating information gathered from or generated by observation, experience, reflection, reasoning, or communication, as a guide to belief and action" (Scriven, 1987). Critical thinking requires cognitive, psychomotor, and affective skills in order to use the tools of a comprehensive knowledge base, the nursing process, and established standards of care, as well as nursing research, to analyze data and plan a course of action based on new insights and conclusions. To this end, the nurse defines the problem, selects pertinent information for the solution, recognizes stated and unstated assumptions, formulates and selects relevant and promising hypotheses, draws conclusions, and judges the validity of the inferences (Hickman, 1993). Although critical thinking skills are used in all aspects of nursing practice, they are most evident when assessment data are analyzed to identify relevant information, make decisions about client needs, and develop an individualized plan of care. Therefore, client assessment is the foundation on which identification of individual needs, responses, and problems is based. Nurses of the future will still manage and interpret data and evaluate nursing activities and interventions. They will also need competencies in case and financial management, healthcare policy and economics, legislative outcomes, and research methods. Additionally, they will need skills of delegation and the ability to think and reason across diverse settings in which they will practice (Pesut & Herman, 1999).

To facilitate the steps of assessing and diagnosing in the nursing process and to aid in the critical thinking process, assessment databases have been developed (Fig. 3.1) that use a nursing focus instead of the traditional medical approach of a review of systems. To achieve this nursing focus, we have grouped NANDA-I (NANDA International, formerly the North American Nursing Diagnosis Association) nursing diagnoses into related categories titled Diagnostic Divisions (Box 3.1). These categories reflect a blending of theories, primarily Maslow's Hierarchy of Needs and a self-care philosophy. These divisions serve as the framework or outline for data collection and direct the nurse to the corresponding nursing diagnosis labels.

Because these divisions are based on human responses and needs and are not specific systems, data may be recorded in more than one area. For this reason, the nurse is encouraged to keep an open mind and to collect as much information as possible before choosing the nursing diagnosis label. The results (synthesis) of the collected data are written concisely (client diagnostic statements) to best reflect the client's situation.

From the specific data recorded in the database, the related or risk factors (etiology) and signs and symptoms can be identified, and an individualized client diagnostic statement can be formulated according to the problem, etiology, and signs and symptoms (PES) format to accurately represent the client's situation. For example, the diagnostic statement may read as follows: "ineffective peripheral tissue Perfusion related to decreased arterial flow, evidenced by decreased pulses, pale and cool feet, thick brittle nails, numbness and tingling of feet when walks 1/4 mile."

Outcomes are identified to facilitate choosing appropriate interventions and to serve as evaluators of both nursing care and client response. In addition to being measurable, outcomes must be achievable and desired by the client. These outcomes also form the framework for documentation.

Interventions are designed to specify the action of the nurse, the client, and significant other(s). They are not all-inclusive because such basic nursing actions as "bathe the client" or "notify the physician of changes" have been omitted. It is expected that these actions are included in routine client care. On occasion, controversial issues or treatments are presented for the sake of information and because different therapies may be used in different care settings or geographic locations.

Interventions need to promote the client's movement toward health and independence. This requires involvement of the client in his or her own care, including participation in decisions about the care activities and projected outcomes. This promotes client responsibility, negating the idea that healthcare providers control clients' lives.

(text continues on page 22)

ADULT MEDICAL/SURGICAL ASSESSMENT TOOL

General Information

Name: _____

Age: _____ DOB: _____ Gender: _____ Race: _____

Admission Date: _____ Time: _____ From: _____

Reason for this visit (primary concern): _____

Cultural concerns (relating to healthcare decisions, religious concerns, pain, childbirth, family involvement, communication, etc.):
_____

Source of information: _____ Reliability (1–4 with 4 = very reliable): _____

Activity/Rest

Subjective (Reports)

Occupation: _____

Able to participate in usual activities/hobbies: _____

Ambulatory: _____ Gait (describe): _____

Activity level (sedentary to very active): _____

Daily exercise/type: _____

Muscle mass/tone/strength (e.g., normal,
   increased, decreased): _____

History of problems/limitations imposed by condition
   (e.g., immobility, can't transfer, weakness,
   breathlessness): _____

Feelings (e.g., exhaustion, restlessness, can't concentrate,
   dissatisfaction): _____

Developmental factors (e.g., delayed/age): _____

Sleep: Hours: _____ Naps: _____

   Insomnia: _____ Related to: _____

   Difficulty falling asleep: _____

   Difficulty staying asleep: _____

   Rested on awakening: _____

   Excessive grogginess: _____

Bedtime rituals: _____

Relaxation techniques: _____

Sleeps on more than one pillow: _____

Oxygen use (type): _____When used: _____

Medications or herbals for/affecting sleep:_____

   _____

Objective (Exhibits)

Observed response to activity: Heart rate:_____

   Rhythm (reg/irreg): _____

   Blood pressure: _____

   Respiration rate: _____

   Pulse oximetry: _____

Mental status (i.e., cognitive impairment,
   withdrawn/lethargic): _____

Muscle mass/tone: _____

   Posture (e.g., normal, stooped, curved spine): _____

   Tremors: _____

      (location): _____

   ROM: _____

   Strength: _____

   Deformity: _____

Uses mobility aid (list): _____

Circulation

Subjective (Reports)

History of/treatment for (date): High blood pressure: _____

   Brain injury: _____ Stroke: _____

   Heart problems/surgery: _____ Palpitations: _____

   Syncope: _____ Cough/hemoptysis: _____ Blood clots: _____

   Bleeding tendencies/episodes: _____

   Pain in legs w/activity _____

Extremities: Numbness: _____ (location): _____

   Tingling: _____ (location): _____

Slow healing (describe): _____

Change in frequency/amount of urine:_____

History of spinal cord injury/dysreflexia episodes: _____

Medications/herbals:_____

Objective (Exhibits)

Color (e.g., pale, cyanotic, jaundiced, mottled, ruddy):

   Skin: _____ Mucous membranes: _____ Lips: _____

   Nail beds:_____ Conjunctiva: _____ Sclera: _____

Skin moisture (e.g., dry, diaphoretic): _____

BP: Lying: R_____ L_____ Sitting: R_____ L_____

   Standing: R_____ L_____

   Pulse pressure: _____ Auscultatory gap: _____

Pulses (palpated 1–4 strength): Carotid: _____ Temporal: _____

   Jugular: _____ Radial: _____ Femoral: _____ Popliteal: _____

   Post-tibial: _____ Dorsalis pedis: _____

Cardiac (palpation): Thrill: _____ Heaves: _____

Heart sounds (auscultation): Rate: _____ Rhythm: _____

   Quality: _____ Friction rub: _____

   Murmur (describe location/sounds): _____

Vascular bruit (location): _____ Jugular vein distention: _____

Breath sounds (location/describe): _____

Extremities: Temperature: _____ Color: _____

   Capillary refill (1–3 sec): _____ Homans' sign: _____

   Varicosities (location): _____

Edema (location/severity +1– +4): _____

   Distribution/quality of hair: _____

   Trophic skin changes: _____ Nail abnormalities: _____

Ego Integrity

Subjective (Reports)

Relationship status: _____

Expression of concerns (e.g., financial, lifestyle
   or role changes): _____

Stress factors: _____

Usual ways of handling stress: _____

Expression of feelings: Anger: _____ Anxiety: _____
   Fear: _____ Grief: _____ Helplessness: _____
   Hopelessness: _____ Powerlessness: _____

Cultural factors/ethnic ties: _____

Religious affiliation: _____ Active/practicing: _____
   Practices prayer/meditation: _____
   Religious/spiritual concerns: _____
   Desires clergy visit: _____

Expression of sense of connectedness/harmony
   with self and others: _____

Medications/herbals: _____

Objective (Exhibits)

Emotional status (check those that apply):
   Calm: _____ Anxious: _____
   Angry: _____ Withdrawn: _____
   Fearful: _____ Irritable: _____
   Restive: _____ Euphoric: _____

Observed body language: _____

Observed physiological responses (e.g., palpitations, crying,
   change in voice quality/volume): _____

Changes in energy field:
   Temperature: _____
   Color: _____
   Distribution: _____
   Movement: _____
   Sounds: _____

Elimination

Subjective (Reports)

Usual bowel elimination pattern: _____
   Character of stool (e.g., hard, soft, liquid): _____
   Stool color (e.g., brown, black, yellow,
   clay colored, tarry): _____

Date of last BM and character of stool: _____

History of bleeding: _____ Hemorrhoids/fistula: _____

Constipation: acute: _____ or chronic: _____
   Diarrhea: acute: _____ or chronic: _____
   Bowel incontinence: _____

Laxative: _____ (how often): _____
   Enema/suppository: _____ (how often): _____

Usual voiding pattern and character of urine: _____

Difficulty voiding: _____ Urgency: _____
   Frequency: _____ Retention: _____
   Bladder spasms: _____ Burning: _____

Urinary incontinence (type/time of day usually occurs): _____
_____

History of kidney/bladder disease: _____

Diuretic use: _____ Herbals: _____

Objective (Exhibits)

Abdomen (auscultation): Bowel sounds (location/type): _____

Abdomen (palpation): Soft/firm: _____
   Tenderness/pain (quadrant location): _____
   Distention: _____ Palpable mass/location: _____
   Size/girth: _____ CVA tenderness: _____

Bladder palpable: _____ Overflow voiding: _____

Rectal sphincter tone (describe): _____

Hemorrhoids/fistulas: _____ Stool in rectum: _____
   Impaction: _____ Occult blood (+ or −): _____

Presence/use of catheter or continence devices: _____

Ostomy appliances (describe appliance and location): _____
_____

Food/Fluid

Subjective (Reports)

Usual diet (type): _____
   Calorie, carbohydrate, protein, fat intake (g/day): _____

# of meals daily: ____ Snacks (number/time consumed): ____

Dietary pattern/content:
   B _____
   L: _____
   D: _____
   Snacks: _____

Last meal consumed/content: _____

Food preferences: _____

Food allergies/intolerances: _____

Cultural or religious food preparation
   concerns/prohibitions: _____

Usual appetite: _____ Change in appetite: _____

Usual weight: _____
   Unexpected/undesired weight loss or gain: _____

Nausea/vomiting: ____ (related to): _____
   Heartburn/indigestion: _____
   (related to): _____ (relieved by): _____

Chewing/swallowing problems: _____
   Gag/swallow reflex present: _____

Objective (Exhibits)

Current weight: _____ Height: _____
   Body build: _____ Body fat %: _____

Skin turgor (e.g., firm, supple, dehydrated): _____

Mucous membranes (moist/dry): _____

Edema: Generalized: _____
   Dependent: _____
   Feet/ankles: _____
   Periorbital: _____
   Abdominal/ascites: _____

Jugular vein distention: _____

Breath sounds (auscultate)/location: _____
   Faint/distant: _____ Crackles: _____ Wheezes: _____

Condition of teeth/gums: _____ Appearance of tongue: _____
   Mucous membranes: _____

Abdomen: Bowel sounds (quadrant location/type): _____

Hernia/masses: _____

Urine S/A or Chemstix: _____
   Blood glucose (Glucometer): _____

Food/Fluid (continued)

Subjective (Reports)

Facial injury/surgery: _____

  Stroke/other neurological deficit: _____

Teeth: Normal: ____ Dentures (full/partial):_____

  Loose/absent teeth/poor dental care: _____

  Sore mouth/gums:_____

Diabetes: _____ Controlled with diet/pills/insulin: _____

Vitamin/food supplements: _____

Medications/herbals: _____

Hygiene

Subjective (Reports)

Ability to carry out activities of daily living: _____

  Independent/dependent (level 1 = no assistance needed

  to level 4 = completely dependent): _____

Mobility: ___ Assistance needed (describe): _____

  Assistance provided by: _____

  Equipment/prosthetic devices required: _____

Feeding: ___ Help with food preparation: _____

  Help with eating utensils: _____

Hygiene: ____ Get supplies: ____ Wash body/body parts: ___

  Regulate bath water temperature: ___ Get in/out alone: ___

  Preferred time of personal care/bath: _____

Dressing: ___ Can select clothing: ____ Can dress self: _____

  Needs assistance with(describe): _____

Toileting: ___ Can get to toilet/commode alone: _____

  Needs assistance with (describe): _____

Objective (Exhibits)

General appearance: Manner of dress: _____

  Grooming/personal habits: _____

  Condition of hair/scalp: _____

  Body odor: _____

Presence of vermin (e.g., lice, scabies): _____

Neurosensory

Subjective (Reports)

History of brain injury, trauma, stroke (residual effects): ____

Fainting spells/dizziness: _____

Headaches (location/type/frequency): _____

Tingling/numbness/weakness (location): _____

Seizures: ____ History or new onset seizures: _____

  Type (e.g., grandmal, partial): _____ Frequency: _____

  Aura: _____ Postictal state: _____ How controlled: ___

Vision: Loss/changes in vision: _____ Date last exam: ___

  Glaucoma: ____ Cataract: ____ Eye surgery (type/date): ___

Hearing loss: ____ Sudden or gradual: _____

  Date last exam:_____

Sense of smell (changes): _____

Sense of taste (changes): _____ Epistaxis:_____

Other: _____

Objective (Exhibits)

Mental status (note duration of change):_____

  Oriented/disoriented: Time: _____ Place:_____

  Person: _____

  Situation: _____

Check all that apply: Alert: _____ Drowsy: _____ Lethargic: _____

  Stupor: __ Comatose: __ Cooperative: __ Agitated/Restless: __

  Combative: _____ Follows commands: _____

Delusions (describe): _____ Hallucinations (describe):_____

Affect (describe): _____ Speech Pattern: _____

Memory: Recent: _____ Remote: _____

Pupil shape: _____ Size/reaction: R/L: _____

Facial droop: _____ Swallowing: _____

Hand grasp/release: R: _____ L: _____

Coordination: _____ Balance: _____ Walking: _____

Deep tendon reflexes (present/absent/location): _____

Tremors: _____ Paralysis (R/L): _____ Posturing: _____

Wears glasses: _____ Contacts: _____ Hearing aids: _____

Pain/Discomfort

Subjective (Reports)

Primary focus: _____ Location: _____

Intensity (use pain scale or pictures): _____

  Quality (e.g., stabbing, aching, burning): _____

  Radiation: _____ Duration: _____ Frequency: _____

Precipitating factors: _____

Relieving factors (including nonpharmaceuticals/therapies):

_____

Associated symptoms (e.g., nausea, sleep problems, crying):

_____

  Effect on daily activities: _____

  Relationships: _____ Job:_____

  Enjoyment of life:_____

Additional pain focus (describe): _____

Medications: _____ Herbals: _____

Objective (Exhibits)

Facial grimacing: _____ Guarding affected area: _____

  Emotional response (e.g., crying, withdrawal, anger): _____

  Narrowed focus:_____

Vitals sign changes (acute pain):

  BP: _____

  Pulse:_____

  Respirations: _____

Respiration

Subjective (Reports)

Dyspnea/related to: _____
  Precipitating factors: _____ Relieving factors: _____
Airway clearance (e.g., spontaneous/device): _____
Cough (e.g., hard, persistent, croupy): _____
  Produces sputum (describe color/character): _____
  Requires suctioning: _____
History of (year): Bronchitis: _____ Asthma: _____
  Emphysema: _____ Tuberculosis: _____
  Recurrent pneumonia: _____
  Exposure to noxious fumes/allergens, infectious agents/
  diseases, poisons/pesticides: _____
Smoker: _____ packs/day: _____ # of years: _____
Use of respiratory aids: _____ Oxygen (type/frequency): _____
Medications/herbals: _____

Objective (Exhibits)

Respirations (spontaneous/assisted): _____ Rate: _____
  Depth: _____ Chest excursion (e.g., equal/unequal): _____
  Use of accessory muscles: _____
  Nasal flaring: _____ Fremitus: _____
Breath sounds (presence/absence; crackle, wheezes): _____
  Egophony: _____
Skin/mucous membrane color (e.g., pale, cyanotic): _____
Clubbing of fingers: _____
Sputum characteristics: _____
Mentation (e.g., calm, anxious, restless): _____
Pulse oximetry: _____

Safety

Subjective (Reports)

Allergies/sensitivity (medications, foods, environment, latex):
_____
  Type of reaction: _____
Blood transfusion/number: ____ Date: _____
  Reaction (describe): _____
Exposure to infectious diseases (e.g., measles, influenza,
  pink eye): _____
Exposure to pollution, toxins, poisons/pesticides, radiation:
_____
  (describe reactions): _____
Geographic areas lived in/visited: _____
Immunization history: Tetanus:____ MMR: ____ Polio: _____
  Influenza: ____ Pneumonia: ____ Hepatitis: _____ HPV: _____
Altered/suppressed immune system (list cause): _____
History of sexually transmitted disease (date/type): _____
  Testing: _____
High risk behaviors: _____
Uses seat belt regularly: _____ Bike helmets: _____
  Other safety devices: _____
Workplace safety/health issues (describe): _____
  Currently working: _____
  Rate working conditions (e.g., safety, noise, heating,
  water, ventilation): _____
History of accidental injuries: _____
Fractures/dislocations: _____
Arthritis/unstable joints: _____ Back problems: _____
Skin problems (e.g., rashes, lesions, moles, breast lumps,
  enlarged nodes) describe: _____
Delayed healing (describe): _____
Cognitive limitations (e.g., disoriented, confusion): _____
Sensory limitations (e.g., impaired vision/hearing, detecting
  heat/cold, taste, smell, touch): _____
Prostheses: _____ Ambulatory devices: _____
Violence (episodes or tendencies): _____

Objective (Exhibits)

Body temperature/method: (e.g., **o**ral, **r**ectal, **t**ympanic): _____
Skin integrity (mark location on diagram): Scars: _____
  Bruises: _____ Rashes: _____ Abrasions: _____
  Lacerations: _____ Ulcerations: _____ Blisters: _____
  Drainage: _____ Burns [degree/%]: _____

Musculoskeletal: General strength: _____ Muscle tone: _____
Gait: _____ ROM: _____ Paresthesia/paralysis: _____
Results of testing (e.g., cultures, immune function, TB, hepatitis):
_____

Sexuality [Component of Social Interaction]

Subjective (Reports)

Sexually active: _____ Birth control method: _____
  Use of condoms: _____
Sexual concerns/difficulties (e.g., pain, relationship, role):
_____
Recent change in frequency/interest: _____

Male: Subjective (Reports)

Circumcised: ____ Vasectomy (date): _____
Prostate disorder: _____
Practice self-exam: Breast: _____ Testicles: _____
Last proctoscopic/prostate exam: _____ Last PSA/date: _____
Medications/herbals: _____

Objective (Exhibits)

Genitalia: Penis: Circumcised: _____ Warts/lesions: _____
  Bleeding/discharge: _____ Testicles (e.g., lumps): _____
  Vasectomy: _____
Breasts examination: _____
Test results: PSA: _____ STD: _____

Sexuality [Component of Social Interaction] (continued)

Female: Subjective (Reports)

Menstruation: Age at menarche: ____ Length of cycle: _____
  Duration: _____ Number of pads/tampons used/day: _____
  Last menstrual period: _____
  Bleeding between periods: _____
Reproductive: Infertility concerns: _____
  Type of therapy: _____ Pregnant now: _____
  Para: _____ Gravida: _____ Due date: _____
Menopause: ____ Last period: _____
  Hysterectomy (type/date): _____
  Problem with: Hot flashes: _____ Night sweats: _____
  Vaginal lubrication: ____ Vaginal discharge: _____
Hormonal therapies: _____
  Osteoporosis medications: _____
Breasts: Practices breast self-exam: _____
  Last mammogram: _____
Last PAP smear: _____

Objective (Exhibits)

Breasts examination: _____
Genitalia: Warts/lesions: _____
  Vaginal bleeding/discharge: _____
Test results: PAP: _____
  Mammogram: _____
  STD: _____

Social Interactions

Subjective (Reports)

Relationship status (check): Single: _____ Married: _____
  Living with partner: ____ Divorced: _____ Widowed: _____
  Years in relationship: ____ Perception of relationship: ____
  Concerns/stresses: _____
Role within family structure: _____
Number/age of children: _____
Perception of relationship with family members: _____
Extended family: _____
  Other support person(s): _____
Ethnic/cultural affiliations: _____
  Strength of ethnic identity: _____
  Lives in ethnic community: _____
Feelings of (describe): Mistrust: _____ Rejection: _____
  Unhappiness: _____ Loneliness/isolation: _____
Problems related to illness/condition: _____
Problems with communication (e.g., speech, another
  language, brain injury): _____
  Use of speech/communication aids (list): _____
  Interpreter needed: ____ Primary language: _____
Genogram: Diagram on separate page

Objective (Exhibits)

Communication/speech: Clear: _____
  Slurred: _____
  Unintelligible: _____
  Aphasic: _____
  Unusual speech pattern/impairment: _____
  Laryngectomy present: _____
Verbal/nonverbal communication with family/SO(s): _____
  _____
  Family interaction (behavioral) pattern: _____

Teaching/Learning

Subjective (Reports)

Communication: Dominant language (specify): _____
  Second language: _____ Literate (reading/writing): _____
  Education level: _____
  Learning disabilities (specify): _____
  Cognitive limitations: _____
Culture/ethnicity: Where born: _____
  If immigrant, how long in this country: _____
Health and illness beliefs/practices/customs: _____
Which family member makes healthcare decisions/is
  spokesperson for client: _____
Presence of Advance Directives: _____ Code status: _____
  Durable Medical Power of Attorney: _____
  Designee: _____
Health goals: _____
Current health problem: _____
Client understanding of problem: _____
Special healthcare concerns (e.g., impact of
  religious/cultural practices): _____

Prescribed medications: Drug: _____ Dose: _____
  Times (circle last dose): _____ Take regularly: _____
  Purpose: _____ Side effects/problems: _____
Nonprescription drugs/frequency: OTC drugs: _____
  Vitamins: _____ Herbals: _____
Street drugs: _____ Alcohol (amount/frequency): _____
  Tobacco: _____ Smokeless tobacco: _____
Admitting diagnosis per provider: _____
Reason for hospitalization/visit per client: _____
History of current problem: _____
Expectations of this hospitalization/visit: _____
Will admission cause any lifestyle changes (describe): _____
  _____
Previous illnesses and/or hospitalizations/surgeries: _____
  _____
Evidence of failure to improve: _____
Last complete physical exam: _____

Teaching/Learning (continued)

Subjective (Reports)

Familial risk factors (indicate relationship):
Diabetes: _____ Thyroid (specify): _____
Tuberculosis: _____Heart disease: _____ Stroke: _____
Hypertension: _____Epilepsy/seizures:_____
Kidney disease: _____ Cancer: _____
Mental illness/depression: _____ Other: _____

Discharge Plan Considerations

Projected length of stay (days or hours):_____
Anticipated date of discharge: _____
Date information obtained: _____
Resources available: Persons: _____
  Financial: _____
Community supports: _____
  Groups: _____
Areas that may require alteration/assistance
  Food preparation: ____ Shopping:_____Transportation: __
  Ambulation: ____Medication/IV therapy: _____
  Treatments: _____ Wound care: _____
  Supplies: _____Self-care (specify): _____
  Homemaker/maintenance (specify): ____Socialization:____
  Physical layout of home (specify): _____

Anticipated changes in living situation after discharge: _____
  Living facility other than home (specify): _____
Referrals (date/source/services): Social Services: _____
  Rehab services: _____ Dietary: _____ Home care: _____
  Resp/O_2: _____ Equipment: _____
  Supplies: _____ Other: _____

Figure 3.1 Adult medical-surgical assessment tool. This is a suggested guide and tool for creating a database reflecting a nursing focus. Although the diagnostic divisions are alphabetized here for ease of presentation, they can be prioritized or rearranged in any manner to meet individual needs. In addition, this assessment tool can be adapted to meet the needs of specific client populations.

Box 3.1 Nursing Diagnoses Organized According to Diagnostic Divisions

After data are collected and areas of concern or need identified, the nurse is directed to the Diagnostic Divisions to review the list of nursing diagnoses that fall within the individual categories. This will assist the nurse in choosing the specific diagnostic label to accurately describe the data. Then, with the addition of etiology or related/risk factors (when known), and signs and symptoms, or cues (defining characteristics), the client diagnostic statement emerges.

Activity/Rest—ability to engage in necessary or desired activities of life (work and leisure) and to obtain adequate sleep and rest

- Activity Intolerance
- Activity Intolerance, risk for
- Activity Planning, ineffective
- Disuse Syndrome, risk for
- Diversional Activity, deficient
- Fatigue
- Insomnia
- Lifestyle, sedentary
- Mobility, impaired bed
- Mobility, impaired wheelchair
- Sleep, readiness for enhanced
- Sleep Deprivation
- Sleep Pattern, disturbed
- Transfer Ability, impaired
- Walking, impaired

Circulation—ability to transport oxygen and nutrients necessary to meet cellular needs

- Autonomic Dysreflexia
- Autonomic Dysreflexia, risk for
- Bleeding, risk for
- Cardiac Output, decreased
- Intracranial Adaptive Capacity, decreased
- Perfusion, ineffective peripheral tissue
- Perfusion, risk for decreased cardiac tissue
- Perfusion, risk for ineffective cerebral tissue
- Perfusion, risk for ineffective gastrointestinal
- Perfusion, risk for ineffective renal
- Shock, risk for

Ego Integrity—ability to develop and use skills and behaviors to integrate and manage life experiences

- Anxiety [specify level]
- Anxiety, death
- Behavior, risk-prone health
- Body Image, disturbed
- Conflict, decisional (specify)
- Coping, defensive
- Coping, ineffective
- Coping, readiness for enhanced
- Decision Making, readiness for enhanced
- Denial, ineffective

- Dignity, risk for compromised human
- Distress, moral
- Energy Field, disturbed
- Fear
- Grieving
- Grieving, complicated
- Grieving, risk for complicated
- Hope, readiness for enhanced
- Hopelessness
- Identity, disturbed personal
- Post-Trauma Syndrome
- Post-Trauma Syndrome, risk for
- Power, readiness for enhanced
- Powerlessness
- Powerlessness, risk for
- Rape-Trauma Syndrome
- Relationships, readiness for enhanced
- Religiosity, impaired
- Religiosity, risk for impaired
- Religiosity, readiness for enhanced
- Relocation Stress Syndrome
- Relocation Stress Syndrome, risk for
- Resilience, impaired individual
- Resilience, readiness for enhanced
- Resilience, risk for compromised
- Self-Concept, readiness for enhanced
- Self-Esteem, chronic low
- Self-Esteem, situational low
- Self-Esteem, risk for situational low
- Sorrow, chronic
- Spiritual Distress
- Spiritual Distress, risk for
- Spiritual Well-Being, readiness for enhanced

Elimination—ability to excrete waste products

- Bowel Incontinence
- Constipation
- Constipation, perceived
- Constipation, risk for
- Diarrhea
- Motility, dysfunctional gastrointestinal
- Motility, risk for dysfunctional gastrointestinal
- Urinary Elimination, impaired
- Urinary Elimination, readiness for enhanced
- Urinary Incontinence, functional
- Urinary Incontinence, overflow
- Urinary Incontinence, reflex
- Urinary Incontinence, stress
- Urinary Incontinence, urge
- Urinary Incontinence, risk for urge
- Urinary Retention [acute/chronic]

Food/Fluid—ability to maintain intake of and utilize nutrients and liquids to meet physiological needs

- Breastfeeding, effective
- Breastfeeding, ineffective
- Breastfeeding, interrupted
- Dentition, impaired
- Electrolyte Imbalance, risk for
- Failure to Thrive, adult

- Feeding Pattern, ineffective infant
- Fluid Balance, readiness for enhanced
- [Fluid Volume, deficient hypertonic or hypotonic]
- Fluid Volume, deficient [isotonic]
- Fluid Volume excess
- Fluid Volume, risk for deficient
- Fluid Volume, risk for imbalanced
- Glucose Level, risk for unstable blood
- Liver Function, risk for impaired
- Nausea
- Nutrition: less than body requirements, imbalanced
- Nutrition: more than body requirements, imbalanced
- Nutrition: more than body requirements, risk for imbalanced
- Nutrition, readiness for enhanced
- Oral Mucous Membrane, impaired
- Swallowing, impaired

Hygiene—ability to perform activities of daily living

- Neglect, self
- Self-Care, readiness for enhanced
- Self-Care Deficit: bathing
- Self-Care Deficit: dressing
- Self-Care Deficit: feeding
- Self-Care Deficit: toileting

Neurosensory—ability to perceive, integrate, and respond to internal and external cues

- Confusion, acute
- Confusion, risk for acute
- Confusion, chronic
- Infant Behavior, disorganized
- Infant Behavior, risk for disorganized
- Infant Behavior, readiness for enhanced organized
- Memory, impaired
- Neglect, unilateral
- Peripheral Neurovascular Dysfunction, risk for
- Sensory Perception, disturbed (specify: visual, auditory, kinesthetic, gustatory, tactile, olfactory)
- Stress Overload
- [Thought Processes, disturbed]

Pain/Discomfort—ability to control internal/external environment to maintain comfort

- Comfort, impaired
- Comfort, readiness for enhanced
- Pain, acute
- Pain, chronic

Respiration—ability to provide and use oxygen to meet physiological needs

- Airway Clearance, ineffective
- Aspiration, risk for
- Breathing Pattern, ineffective
- Gas Exchange, impaired
- Ventilation, impaired spontaneous
- Ventilatory Weaning Response, dysfunctional

Safety—ability to provide safe, growth-promoting environment

- Allergy Response, latex
- Allergy Response, risk for latex

(continues on page 22)

- Body Temperature, risk for imbalanced
- Contamination
- Contamination, risk for
- Death Syndrome, risk for sudden infant
- Environmental Interpretation Syndrome, impaired
- Falls, risk for
- Health Maintenance, ineffective
- Home Maintenance, impaired
- Hyperthermia
- Hypothermia
- Immunization Status, readiness for enhanced
- Infection, risk for
- Injury, risk for
- Injury, risk for perioperative positioning
- Jaundice, neonatal
- Maternal/Fetal Dyad, risk for disturbed
- Mobility, impaired physical
- Poisoning, risk for
- Protection, ineffective
- Self-Mutilation
- Self-Mutilation, risk for
- Skin Integrity, impaired
- Skin Integrity, risk for impaired
- Suffocation, risk for
- Suicide, risk for
- Surgical Recovery, delayed
- Thermoregulation, ineffective
- Tissue Integrity, impaired
- Trauma, risk for
- Trauma, risk for vascular
- Violence, [actual/] risk for other-directed
- Violence, [actual/] risk for self-directed
- Wandering [specify sporadic or continual]

Sexuality [Component of Ego Integrity and Social Interaction]—ability to meet requirements/characteristics of male/female role

- Childbearing Process, readiness for enhanced

- Sexual Dysfunction
- Sexuality Pattern, ineffective

Social Interaction—ability to establish and maintain relationships

- Attachment, risk for impaired
- Caregiver Role Strain
- Caregiver Role Strain, risk for
- Communication, impaired verbal
- Communication, readiness for enhanced
- Conflict, parental role
- Coping, ineffective community
- Coping, readiness for enhanced community
- Coping, compromised family
- Coping, disabled family
- Coping, readiness for enhanced family
- Family Processes, dysfunctional
- Family Processes, interrupted
- Family Processes, readiness for enhanced
- Loneliness, risk for
- Parenting, impaired
- Parenting, risk for impaired
- Parenting, readiness for enhanced
- Role Performance, ineffective
- Social Interaction, impaired
- Social Isolation

Teaching/Learning—ability to incorporate and use information to achieve healthy lifestyle and optimal wellness

- Development, risk for delayed
- Growth, risk for disproportionate
- Growth and Development, delayed
- Health Management, ineffective self
- Health Management, readiness for enhanced self
- Knowledge, deficient (specify)
- Knowledge (specify), readiness for enhanced
- Noncompliance [Adherence, ineffective] [specify]
- [Therapeutic Regimen Management, ineffective community]
- Therapeutic Regimen Management, ineffective family

To assist in visualizing this critical thinking process, a prototype client situation (Fig. 3.2) is provided as an example of data collection and construction of a plan of care. As the client assessment database is reviewed, the nurse can identify the related or risk factors, and defining characteristics (signs and symptoms) if present, that were used to formulate the client diagnostic statements. The addition of timelines to specific client outcomes and goals reflects the anticipated length of stay and individual client-nurse expectations. Interventions are based on concerns and needs identified by the client and nurse during data collection. In addition, physician and other discipline orders are also considered when identifying interventions. Although not normally included in a plan of care, rationales are included in this sample for the purpose of explaining or clarifying the choice of interventions.

Another way to conceptualize the client's care needs is to create a Mind Map (Fig. 3.3). This new technique and learning tool has been developed to help visualize the linkages or interconnections between various client symptoms, interventions, or problems as they impact each other. The best parts of the traditional care plans (problem-solving and categorizing) are retained, but the linear and columnar nature of the plan is changed to a design that uses the whole brain—a design that brings left-brained, linear problem-solving thinking together with the free-wheeling, interconnected, creative right brain. Joining mind mapping and care planning enables the nurse to create a holistic view of a client, strengthening critical thinking skills and facilitating the creative process of planning client care.

(text continues on page 28)

Client Situation: Diabetes Mellitus

Mr. R.S., a client with type 2 diabetes (non–insulin-dependent) for 8 years, presented to his physician's office with a nonhealing ulcer of 3 weeks' duration on his left foot. Screening studies done in the doctor's office revealed blood glucose (BG) of 356/fingerstick and urine Chemstix of 2%. Because of distance from medical provider and lack of local community services, he is admitted to the hospital.

Admitting Physician's Orders

Culture/sensitivity and Gram's stain of foot ulcer
Random blood glucose on admission and fingerstick BG qid
CBC, electrolytes, serum lipid profile, glycosylated Hb in AM
Chest x-ray and ECG in AM
DiaBeta 10 mg, PO BID
Glucophage 500 mg, PO daily to start—will increase gradually
Humulin N 10 U SC q AM and HS. Begin insulin instruction for post-discharge self-care if necessary
Dicloxacillin 500 mg PO q6h, start after culture obtained
Darvocet-N 100 mg PO q4h prn pain
Diet—2400 calories, 3 meals with 2 snacks
Up in chair ad lib with feet elevated
Foot cradle for bed
Irrigate lesion L foot with NS tid, then cover with wet to dry sterile dressing
Vital signs qid

Client Assessment Database

Name: R.S.   Informant: Client Reliability (Scale 1–4): 3   Age: 72   DOB: 5/3/36   Race: Caucasion
Gender: M   Adm. date: 6/28/2007   Time: 7 PM   From: Home

ACTIVITY/REST

Subjective (Reports): Occupation: Farmer
Usual activities/hobbies: reading, playing cards. "Don't have time to do much. Anyway, I'm too tired most of the time to do anything after the chores."
Limitations imposed by illness: "Have to watch what I order if I eat out."
Sleep: Hours: 6 to 8 hr/night Naps: No Aids: No
    Insomnia: "Not unless I drink coffee after supper."
    Usually feels rested when awakens at 4:30 AM

Objective (Exhibits): Observed response to activity: Limps, favors L foot when walking
Mental status: Alert/active
Neuro/muscular assessment: Muscle mass/tone:
    Bilaterally equal/firm   Posture: Erect
    ROM: Full Strength: Equal 4 extremities/(favors L foot currently)

CIRCULATION

Subjective (Reports): History of slow healing: Lesion L foot, 3 weeks' duration
Extremities: Numbness/tingling: "My feet feel cold and tingly like sharp pins poking the bottom of my feet when I walk the quarter mile to the mailbox."
Cough/character of sputum: Occ./white
Change in frequency/amount of urine: Yes/voiding more lately

Objective (Exhibits): Peripheral pulses: Radials 3+; popliteal, dorsalis, post-tibial/pedal, all 1+
BP: R: Lying: 146/90 Sitting: 140/86 Standing: 138/90
    L: Lying: 142/88 Sitting: 138/88 Standing: 138/84
Pulse: Apical: 86 Radial: 86   Quality: Strong Rhythm: Regular
Chest auscultation: Few wheezes clear with cough, no murmurs/rubs
Jugular vein distention: 0
Extremities: Temperature: Feet cool bilaterally/legs warm
    Color: Skin: Legs pale Capillary refill: Slow both feet (approx. 4 seconds)
    Homans' sign: 0 Varicosities: Few enlarged superficial veins both calves
    Nails: Toenails thickened, yellow, brittle
    Distribution and quality of hair: Coarse hair to midcalf, none on ankles/toes
Color: General: Ruddy face/arms Mucous membranes/lips: Pink
    Nailbeds: Blanch well   Conjunctiva and sclera: White

EGO INTEGRITY

Subjective (Reports):
Report of stress factors: "Normal farmer's problems: weather, pests, bankers, etc."
Ways of handling stress: "I get busy with the chores and talk things over with my livestock. They listen pretty good."
Financial concerns: No insurance; needs to hire someone to do chores while here
Relationship status: Married
Cultural factors: Rural/agrarian, eastern European descent, "American," no ethnic ties
Religion: Protestant/practicing
Lifestyle: Middle class/self-sufficient farmer
Recent changes: No
Feelings: "I'm in control of most things, except the weather and this diabetes now."
Concerned re possible therapy change "from pills to shots."

Objective (Exhibits):
Emotional status: Generally calm, appears frustrated at times
Observed physiological response(s): Occasionally sighs deeply/frowns, fidgeting with coin, shoulders tense/shrugs shoulders, throws up hands

ELIMINATION

Subjective (Reports):
Usual bowel pattern: almost every PM
Last BM: Last night   Character of stool: Firm/brown
Bleeding: 0   Hemorrhoids: 0   Constipation: occ.
Laxative used: Hot prune juice on occ.
Urinary: No problems   Character of urine: Pale yellow

Objective (Exhibits):
Abdomen tender: No   Soft/firm: Soft   Palpable mass: 0
Bowel sounds: Active all 4 quads

FOOD/FLUID

Subjective (Reports):
Usual diet (type): 2400 calorie (occ. "cheats" with dessert; "My wife watches it pretty closely.")
No. of meals daily: 3/1 snack
Dietary pattern: B: Fruit juice/toast/ham/decaf coffee
  L: Meat/potatoes/veg/fruit/milk D: ½ meat sandwich/soup/fruit/decaf coffee
  Snack: Milk/crackers at HS. Usual beverage: Skim milk, 2 to 3 cups decaf coffee, drinks "lots of water"— several quarts
Last meal/intake: Dinner: Roast beef sandwich, vegetable soup, pear with cheese, decaf coffee
Loss of appetite: "Never, but lately I don't feel as hungry as usual."
Nausea/vomiting: 0   Food allergies: None
Heartburn/food intolerance: Cabbage causes gas, coffee after supper causes heartburn
Mastication/swallowing problems: 0
  Dentures: Partial upper plate—fits well
Usual weight: 175 lb   Recent changes: Has lost about 6 lb this month
Diuretic therapy: No

Objective (Exhibits):
Wt: 171 lb   Ht: 5 ft 10 in   Build: Stocky
Skin turgor: Good/leathery   Mucous membranes: Moist
Condition of teeth/gums: Good, no irritation/bleeding noted
  Appearance of tongue: Midline, pink
  Mucous membranes: Pink, intact
Breath sounds: Few wheezes cleared with cough
Bowel sounds: Active all 4 quads
Urine Chemstix: 2%   Fingerstick: 356 (Dr. office) 450 random BG on adm

HYGIENE

Subjective (Reports):
Activities of daily living: Independent in all areas
Preferred time of bath: PM

Objective (Exhibits):
General appearance: Clean, shaven, short-cut hair; hands rough and dry; skin on feet dry, cracked, and scaly
Scalp and eyebrows: Scaly white patches
No body odor

NEUROSENSORY

Subjective (Reports):
Headache: "Occasionally behind my eyes when I worry too much."
Tingling/numbness: Feet, 4 or 5 times/week (as noted)
Eyes: Vision loss, farsighted, "Seems a little blurry now." Examination: 2 yr ago
Ears: Hearing loss R: "Some"   L: No (has not been tested)
Nose: Epistaxis: 0   Sense of smell: "No problem."

Objective (Exhibits):
Mental status: Alert, oriented to time, place, person, situation
Affect: Concerned   Memory: Remote/recent: Clear and intact
Speech: Clear/coherent, appropriate
Pupil reaction: PERRLA/small
Glasses: Reading   Hearing aid: No
Handgrip/release: Strong/equal

PAIN/DISCOMFORT

Subjective (Reports):
Primary focus: L foot   Location: Medial aspect, L heel
Intensity (0–10): 4 to 5   Quality: Dull ache with occ. sharp stabbing sensation
Frequency/duration: "Seems like all the time."   Radiation: No
Precipitating factors: Shoes, walking   How relieved: ASA, not helping
Other complaints: Sometimes has back pain following chores/heavy lifting, relieved
    by ASA/liniment rubdown

Objective (Exhibits):
Facial grimacing: When lesion border palpated
Guarding affected area: Pulls foot away
Narrowed focus: No
Emotional response: Tense, irritated

RESPIRATION

Subjective (Reports):
Dyspnea: 0   Cough: Occ. morning cough, white sputum
Emphysema: 0   Bronchitis: 0   Asthma: 0   Tuberculosis: 0
Smoker: Filters pk/day: 1/2   No. yrs: 25+
Use of respiratory aids: 0

Objective (Exhibits):
Respiratory rate: 22   Depth: Good   Symmetry: Equal, bilateral
Auscultation: Few wheezes, clear with cough
Cyanosis: 0   Clubbing of fingers: 0
Sputum characteristics: None to observe
Mentation/restlessness: Alert/oriented/relaxed

SAFETY

Subjective (Reports):
Allergies: 0   Blood transfusions: 0
Sexually transmitted disease: 0
Wears seat belt
Fractures/dislocations: L clavicle, 1960s, fell getting off tractor
Arthritis/unstable joints: "Some in my knees."
Back problems: Occ. lower back pain
Vision impaired: Requires glasses for reading
Hearing impaired: Slightly (R), compensates by turning "good ear" toward speaker
Immunizations: Current flu/pneumonia 3 yrs ago/tetanus maybe 8 yrs ago

Objective (Exhibits):
Temperature: 99.4°F (37.4°C) tympanic
Skin integrity: Impaired L foot   Scars: R inguinal, surgical
Rashes: 0   Bruises: 0   Lacerations: 0   Blisters: 0
Ulcerations: Medial aspect L heel, 2.5-cm diameter, approx. 3 mm deep, wound
    edges inflamed, draining small amount cream-color/pink-tinged matter, slight
    musty odor noted
Strength (general): Equal all extremities   Muscle tone: firm
ROM: Good   Gait: Favors L foot   Paresthesia/paralysis: Tingling, prickly sensation
    in feet after walking ¼ mile

SEXUALITY: MALE

Subjective (Reports):
Sexually active: Yes   Use of condoms: No (monogamous)
Recent changes in frequency/interest: "I've been too tired lately."
Penile discharge: 0   Prostate disorder: 0   Vasectomy: 0

SEXUALITY: MALE (continued)

Subjective (Reports): Last proctoscopic examination: 2 yr ago   Prostate examination: 1 yr ago
Practice self-examination: Breast/testicles: No
Problems/complaints: "I don't have any problems, but you'd have to ask my wife if there are any complaints."

Objective (Exhibits): Examination: Breast: No masses   Testicles: Deferred   Prostate: Deferred

SOCIAL INTERACTIONS

Subjective (Reports): Marital status: Married 45 yr   Living with: Wife
Report of problems: None
Extended family: 1 daughter lives in town (30 miles away);
    1 daughter married/grandson, living out of state
Other: Several couples, he and wife play cards/socialize with 2 to 3 times/mo
Role: Works farm alone; husband/father/grandfather
Report of problems related to illness/condition: None until now
Coping behaviors: "My wife and I have always talked things out. You know the 11th
    commandment is 'Thou shalt not go to bed angry.'"

Objective (Exhibits): Speech: Clear, intelligible
Verbal/nonverbal communication with family/SO(s): Speaks quietly with wife,
    looking her in the eye; relaxed posture
Family interaction patterns: Wife sitting at bedside, relaxed, both reading paper,
    making occasional comments to each other

TEACHING/LEARNING

Subjective (Reports): Dominant language: English   Second language: 0   Literate: Yes
Education level: 2-yr college
Health and illness/beliefs/practices/customs: "I take care of the minor problems and
    see the doctor only when something's broken."
Presence of Advance Directives: Yes—wife to bring in
Durable Medical Power of Attorney: Wife
Familial risk factors/relationship:
    Diabetes: Maternal uncle
    Tuberculosis: Brother died, age 27
    Heart disease: Father died, age 78, heart attack
    Strokes: Mother died, age 81
    High BP: Mother
Prescribed medications:
    Drug: Diabeta Dose: 10 mg bid
    Schedule: 8 AM/6 PM, last dose 6 PM today
    Purpose: Control diabetes
    Takes medications regularly? Yes
Home urine/glucose monitoring: "Only using TesTape, stopped some months ago
    when I ran out. It was always negative, anyway."
Nonprescription (OTC) drugs: Occ. ASA
Use of alcohol (amount/frequency): Socially, occ. beer
Tobacco: 1/2 pk/day
Admitting diagnosis (physician): Hyperglycemia with nonhealing lesion L foot
Reason for hospitalization (client): "Sore on foot and the doctor is concerned about
    my blood sugar, and says I'm supposed to learn this fingerstick test now."
History of current complaint: "Three weeks ago I got a blister on my foot from
    breaking in my new boots. It got sore so I lanced it but it isn't getting any better."
Client's expectations of this hospitalization: "Clear up this infection and
    control my diabetes."
Other relevant illness and/or previous hospitalizations/surgeries: 1960s, R inguinal
    hernia repair
Evidence of failure to improve: Lesion L foot, 3 wk
Last physical examination: Complete 1 yr ago, office follow-up 5 mo ago

DISCHARGE CONSIDERATIONS (AS OF 6/28)

Anticipated discharge: 7/1/07 (3 days)
Resources: Self, wife

DISCHARGE CONSIDERATIONS (AS OF 6/28) (continued)

Financial: "If this doesn't take too long to heal, we got some savings to cover things."

Community supports: Diabetic support group (has not participated)

Anticipated lifestyle changes: Become more involved in management of condition

Assistance needed: May require farm help for several days

Teaching: Learn new medication regimen and wound care; review diet; encourage smoking cessation

Referral: Supplies: Downtown Pharmacy or AARP

Equipment: Glucometer-AARP

Follow-up: Primary care provider 1 wk after discharge to evaluate wound healing and potential need for additional changes in diabetic regimen

Figure 3.2 Client situation: Diabetes Mellitus.

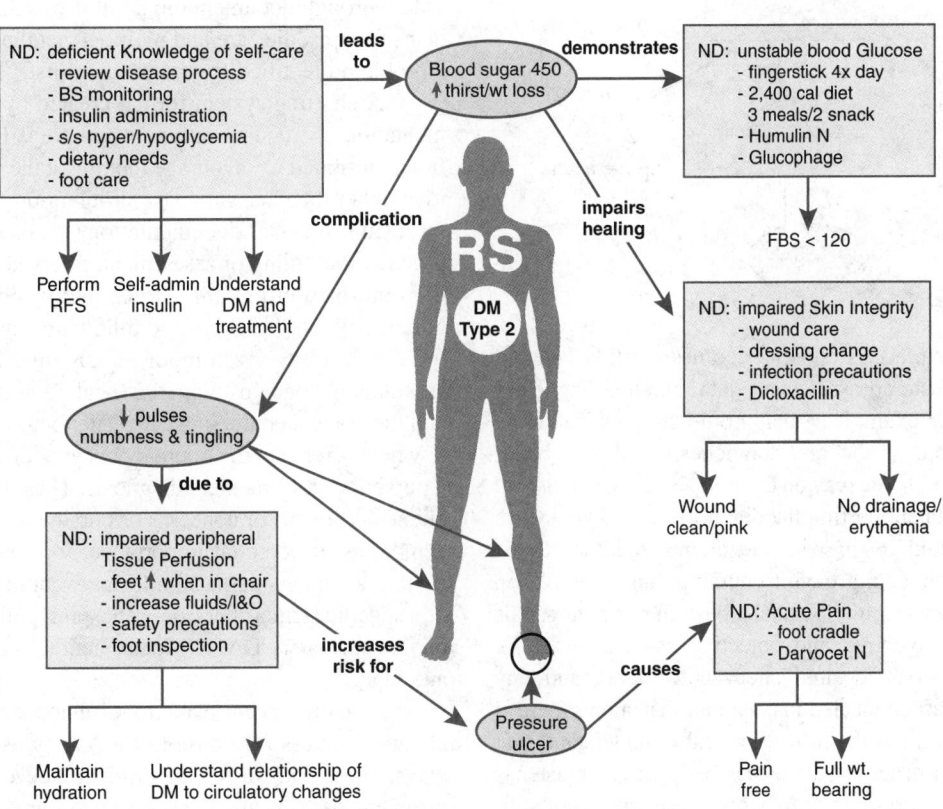

Figure 3.3 Mind map for Mr. R.S.

Mind mapping starts in the center of the page with a representation of the main concept—the client. (This helps keep in mind that the client is the focus of the plan, not the medical diagnosis or condition.) From that central thought, other main ideas that relate to the client radiate out from the center similar to spokes of a wheel (however, they do not have to be added in a balanced manner; it does not have to be a round "wheel"). Different concepts can be grouped together by geometric shapes, color coding, or by placement on the page. Connections and interconnections between groups of ideas are represented by the use of arrows or lines, with defining phrases added that explain how the interconnected thoughts relate to one another. In this manner, many different pieces of information *about* the client can be connected directly *to* the client.

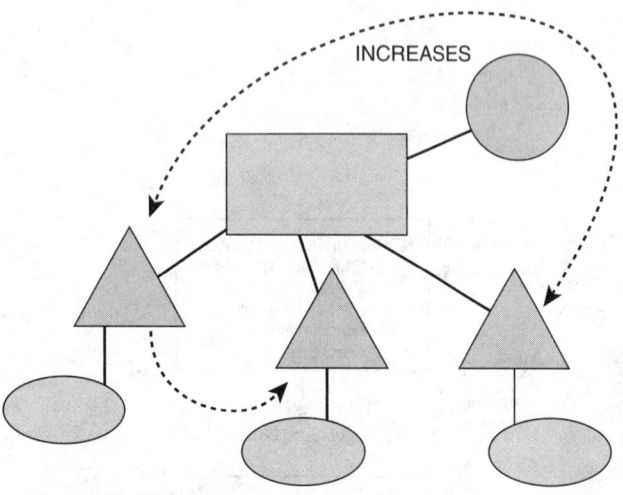

Whichever piece is chosen becomes the first layer of connections—clustered assessment data, nursing diagnoses, or outcomes. For example, a map could start with nursing diagnoses featured as the first "branches," each one being listed separately in some way on the map. Next, the signs and symptoms or data supporting the diagnoses could be added. Or, the plan could begin with the client outcomes to be achieved then connecting them to nursing diagnoses. When the plan is completed, there should be a nursing diagnosis (supported by subjective and objective assessment data), nursing interventions, desired client outcome(s), and any evaluation data, all connected in a manner that shows there is a relationship between them. It is critical to understand that there is no preset order for the pieces because one cluster is not more or less important than another (or one is not subsumed under another). It is important, however, that those pieces within a branch be in the same order in each branch.

Finally, to complete the learning experience, samples of the evaluation step based on the client situation are presented.

Evaluation

As nursing care is provided, ongoing assessment evaluates the client's response to therapy and progress toward accomplishing the desired outcomes. This activity serves as the

feedback and control part of the nursing process through which the status of the individual client diagnostic statement is judged to be resolved, continuing, or requiring revision.

This process is visualized in Figure 3.4. Observation of Mr. R.S.'s wound reveals that edges are clean and pink and drainage is scant. Therefore, he is progressing toward achieving wound healing; this problem will continue to be addressed, although no revision in the treatment plan is required at this time.

Documentation

To date, a number of charting formats have been used for documentation. These include block notes, with a single entry covering an entire shift (e.g., 7 to 3 p.m.); narrative timed notes (e.g., 8:30 a.m., ate 100% of breakfast); the problem-oriented medical record system (POMR or PORS) to record the subjective and objective data, analysis of the data, and the resulting plan (SOAP); and flow sheets with charting by exception, to name a few. The POMR can provide thorough documentation, but it was designed by physicians for episodic care and requires that the entries be tied to a problem identified from a problem list.

A charting system format created by nurses for documentation of frequent or repetitive care is Focus Charting®. It was designed to encourage looking at the client from a positive rather than a negative (or problem-oriented) perspective by using precise documentation to record the nursing process. Recording of assessment, interventions, and evaluation information in *data, action,* and *response* (DAR) categories facilitates tracking and following what is happening to the client at any given moment. Charting focuses on client and nursing concerns, with the focal point being client status and the associated nursing care. The focus is always stated in a way that reflects the client's concerns or needs rather than a nursing task or medical diagnosis. Thus, the focus can be a client's problems or concerns or nursing diagnosis; signs and symptoms of potential importance, for instance, fever, dysrhythmia, and edema; a significant event or change in status; or a specific standard of care or hospital policy. An expansion of this format is DATRP: data, action, teaching, response, and plan.

A more recent way to evaluate and document the client's progress (response to care) is by using clinical pathways. These pathways were originally developed as tools for providing care in case management systems and are now used in many settings. A clinical pathway is a type of abbreviated plan of care that is event oriented (task oriented) and provides outcome-based guidelines for goal achievement within a designated length of stay. The pathway incorporates agency and professional standards of care and may be interdisciplinary, depending on the care setting. As a rule, however, the standardized clinical pathways address a specific diagnosis, condition, or procedure, such as myocardial infarction, total hip replacement, or chemotherapy, and do not provide for inclusion of secondary diagnoses or complications, such as an asthmatic client in alcohol withdrawal. In short, if the client

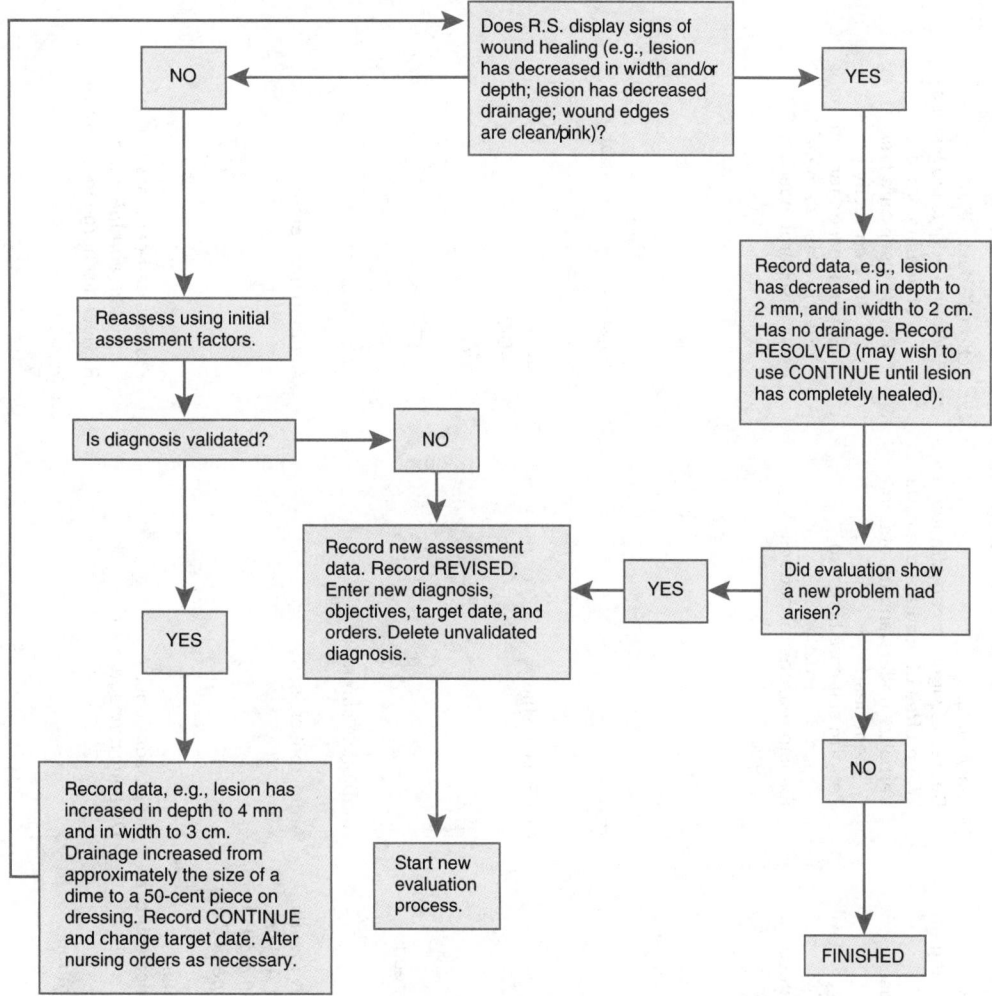

●Figure 3.4 Outcome-based evaluation of the client's response to therapy. (Adapted from Cox, HC, et al: Clinical Applications of Nursing Diagnosis, ed 3. FA Davis, Philadelphia, 1996.)

does not achieve the daily outcomes or goals of care, the variance is identified and a separate plan of care must be developed to meet the client's individual needs. Therefore, although clinical pathways are becoming more common in the clinical setting, they have limited value (in place of more individualized plans of care) as learning tools for students who are working to practice the nursing process, critical thinking, and a holistic approach to meeting client needs. A sample clinical pathway (Fig. 3.5) reflects Mr. R.S.'s primary diagnostic problem: nonhealing Lesion, diabetic.

CP: Non-healing Lesion—Diabetic. ELOS: 3 Days—Variations from Designated Pathway Should Be Documented in Progress Notes

ND and Categories of Care	Adm Day 6/28 7pm	Day 1 6/29	Day 2 6/30	Day 3 7/1 Discharge
Impaired skin/ tissue integrity	Actions/Goals:	Actions/Goals: Verbalize understanding of condition Display blood glucose WNL (ongoing)	Actions/Goals: Be free of signs of dehydration Wound free of purulent drainage Verbalize understanding of treatment need Perform self-care tasks No. 1 and 3 correctly Explain reasons for actions	Actions/Goals: Wound edges show signs of healing process Perform self-care task No. 2 correctly Explain reason for actions Plan in place to meet discharge needs
Referrals		Dietician & determine need for: Home care Physical therapy Visiting nurse		
Diagnostic studies	Wound culture/sensitivity Gram's stain Random blood glucose Fingerstick BG hs	CBC, electrolytes Glycosylated Hb Serum lipid profile →Fingerstick BG qid Chest x-ray (if indicated) ECG (if indicated)	↑	Fingerstick BG bid if stable
Additional assessments	VS qid I&O/level of hydration qd Character of wound tid Level of knowledge and priorities of learning needs Observe for signs of antibiotic hypersensitivity reaction	↑ ↑ ↑	→VS each shift ↑ ↑ ↑	↑ →D/C ↑
Medications	Antibiotic: *Dicloxacillin 500 mg PO q6h* Antidiabetic: *Humulin N insulin 0 units SC hs*	Antibiotic: same Antidiabetic: *Humulin N insulin 10 U SC q AM/hs DiaBeta 10 mg PO bid Glucophage 500 mg PO qd*	Antibiotic: same Antidiabetic: same	Antibiotic: same Antidiabetic: same
Client education	Provide: *Understanding Your Diabetes*	Film *Living With Diabetes* Demonstrate and practice self-care activities: 1. Fingerstick BG 2. Insulin administration 3. Wound care 4. Routine foot care	Group sessions: *Diabetic management*	Practice self-care task No. 2: *insulin administration* Review discharge instructions
Additional nursing actions	Up ad lib NS soaks/dressing change tid Goals:	↑ ↑	↑ ↑	↑ ↑

CP: Non-healing Lesion—Diabetic. ELOS: 3 Days—Variations from Designated Pathway Should Be Documented in Progress Notes (Continued)

ND and Categories of Care	Adm Day 6/28 7pm	Day 1 6/29	Day 2 6/30	Day 3 7/1 Discharge
Acute Pain	Actions/Goals: State pain relieved or minimized with 1 hr of analgesic administration (ongoing) Verbalize understanding of when to report pain and rating scale used Verbalize understanding of self-care measures No. 1 and 2 Explain reason for actions	Actions/Goals: Verbalize understanding of self-care measure No. 3 Explain reason for actions	Actions/Goals: Able to participate in usual level: *ambulate full weight bearing*	Actions/Goals: State pain-free/controlled with medication Verbalize understanding of correct medication use
Additional assessments	Characteristics of pain Level of participation activities Individual analgesic needs	↑ ↑ ↑ ↑ ↑ ↑	↑ ↑ ↑ ↑ ↑ ↑	↑ ↑ ↑ ↑ ↑ ↑
Medications Allergies: -0- Client education	Analgesic: Darvocet-N 100 mg PO q4h PRN Orient to unit/room Guidelines for self-report of pain and rating scale 0–10	Analgesic: same	Analgesic: same	Analgesic: same Review discharge medication instructions: dosage, route, frequency, side effects
Additional nursing actions	Safety/comfort measures: *1 elevation of feet 2 proper footwear* Bed cradle as indicated	Safety/comfort measures: *3 prevention of injury*		

Figure 3.5 Sample clinical pathway.

PLAN OF CARE: Mr R.S.

Client Diagnostic Statement

impaired Skin Integrity related to pressure, altered metabolic state, circulatory impairment, and decreased sensation, as evidenced by draining wound L foot.

Outcome

Wound Healing: Secondary Intention (NOC) Indicators:

Client Will

Be free of purulent drainage within 48 hours (6/30, 7 p.m.). Display signs of healing with wound edges clean and pink within 60 hours (7/1, 7 a.m.).

ACTIONS/INTERVENTIONS	RATIONALE
Wound Care (NIC)	
Irrigate wound with room-temperature sterile normal saline (NS) tid.	Cleans wound without harming delicate tissues.
Assess wound with each dressing change. Obtain wound tracing on admission and at discharge.	Provides information about effectiveness of therapy and identifies additional needs.
Apply wet to dry sterile dressing. Use paper tape.	Keeps wound clean, minimizes cross-contamination. Adhesive tape may be abrasive to fragile tissues.
Infection Control (NIC)	
Follow wound precautions.	Use of gloves and proper handling of contaminated dressings reduces likelihood of spread of infection.
Obtain sterile specimen of wound drainage on admission.	Culture/sensitivity identifies pathogens and therapy of choice.
Administer dicloxacillin 500 mg PO q6h, starting at 10 p.m.	Treatment of infection and prevention of complications. Food interferes with drug absorption, requiring scheduling around meals.
Observe for signs of hypersensitivity: pruritus, urticaria, rash.	Although no prior history of penicillin reaction, it may occur at any time.

PLAN OF CARE:

Client Diagnostic Statement

unstable blood Glucose related to lack of adherence to diabetes management and inadequate blood glucose monitoring as evidenced by fingerstick 450/adm.

Outcome

Blood Glucose Control (NOC) Indicators:

Client Will

Demonstrate correction of metabolic state as evidenced by fasting blood sugar (FBS) less than 120 mg/dL within 36 hours (6/30, 7 a.m.).

ACTIONS/INTERVENTIONS	RATIONALE
Hyperglycemia Management (NIC)	
Perform fingerstick BG qid.	Bedside analysis of blood glucose levels is a more timely method for monitoring effectiveness of therapy and provides direction for alteration of medications.
Administer antidiabetic medications.	Treats underlying metabolic dysfunction, reducing hyperglycemia and promoting healing.
10 units Humulin N insulin SC q AM/hs after fingerstick BG.	Intermediate-acting preparation with onset of 2 to 4 hr, peak 4 to 10 hr, and duration 10 to 16 hr. Increases transport of glucose into cells and promotes the conversion of glucose to glycogen.
DiaBeta 10 mg PO bid.	Lowers blood glucose by stimulating the release of insulin from the pancreas and increasing the sensitivity to insulin at the receptor sites.

ACTIONS/INTERVENTIONS (continued)	RATIONALE (continued)
Glucophage 500 mg PO daily. Note onset of side effects.	Glucophage lowers serum glucose levels by decreasing hepatic glucose production and intestinal glucose absorption and increasing sensitivity to insulin. By using in conjunction with DiaBeta, client may be able to discontinue insulin once target dosage is achieved (e.g., 2,000 mg/day). Increase of 1 tablet per week is necessary to limit side effects of diarrhea, abdominal cramping, and vomiting, possibly leading to dehydration and prerenal azotemia.
Provide diet 2,400 cal—three meals/two snacks.	Proper diet decreases glucose levels and insulin needs, prevents hyperglycemic episodes, reduces serum cholesterol levels, and promotes satiation.
Schedule consultation with dietitian to restructure meal plan and evaluate food choices.	Calories are unchanged on new orders but have been redistributed to two meals and two snacks. Dietary choices (e.g., increased vitamin C) may enhance healing.

PLAN OF CARE:

Client Diagnostic Statement

acute Pain related to physical agent (open wound L foot) as evidenced by verbal report of pain and guarding behavior.

Outcome

Pain Self-Control (NOC) Indicators:

Client Will

Report pain is minimized/relieved within 1 hr of analgesic administration (ongoing).
Report absence or control of pain by discharge (7/1).

Outcome

Pain Disruptive Effects (NOC) Indicators:

Client Will

Ambulate normally, full weight-bearing by discharge (7/1).

ACTIONS/INTERVENTIONS	RATIONALE
Pain Management (NIC)	
Determine pain characteristics through client's description.	Establishes baseline for assessing improvement and changes.
Place foot cradle on bed; encourage use of loose-fitting slipper when up.	Avoids direct pressure to area of injury, which could result in vasoconstriction and increased pain.
Administer Darvocet-N 100 mg PO every 4 hr as needed. Document effectiveness.	Provides relief of discomfort when unrelieved by other measures.

PLAN OF CARE:

Client Diagnostic Statement

ineffective peripheral tissue Perfusion related to decreased arterial flow as evidenced by decreased pulses, pale and cool feet, thick brittle nails, numbness and tingling of feet "when walks 1/4 mile."

Outcomes

Knowledge: Diabetes Management (NOC) Indicators:

Client Will

Verbalize understanding of relationship between chronic disease (diabetes mellitus) and circulatory changes within 48 hr (6/30, 7 p.m.).

Demonstrate awareness of safety factors and proper foot care within 48 hr (6/30, 7 p.m.).

Maintain adequate level of hydration to maximize perfusion (ongoing), as evidenced by balanced intake/output, moist skin and mucous membranes, and capillary refill less than 3 sec (ongoing).

ACTIONS/INTERVENTIONS	RATIONALE
CIRCULATORY CARE: Arterial Insufficiency (NIC)	
Elevate feet when up in chair. Avoid long periods with feet in dependent position.	Minimizes interruption of blood flow and reduces venous pooling.
Assess for signs of dehydration. Monitor intake/output. Encourage oral fluids.	Glycosuria may result in dehydration with consequent reduction of circulating volume and further impairment of peripheral circulation.
Instruct client to avoid constricting clothing and socks and ill-fitting shoes.	Compromised circulation and decreased pain sensation may precipitate or aggravate tissue breakdown.
Reinforce safety precautions regarding use of heating pads, hot water bottles, or soaks.	Heat increases metabolic demands on compromised tissues. Vascular insufficiency alters pain sensation, increasing risk of injury.
Recommend cessation of smoking.	Vascular constriction associated with smoking and diabetes impairs peripheral circulation.
Discuss complications of disease that result from vascular changes: ulceration, gangrene, and muscle or bony structure changes.	Although proper control of diabetes mellitus may not prevent complications, severity of effects may be minimized. Diabetic foot complications are the leading cause of non-traumatic lower extremity amputations. *Note:* Skin dry, cracked, scaly; feet cool; and pain when walking a distance suggest mild to moderate vascular disease (autonomic neuropathy) that can limit response to infection, impair wound healing, and increase risk of bony deformities.
Review proper foot care as outlined in teaching plan.	Altered perfusion of lower extremities may lead to serious or persistent complications at the cellular level.

PLAN OF CARE:

Client Diagnostic Statement

Learning Need regarding diabetic condition, related to misinterpretation of information and/or lack of recall as evidenced by inaccurate follow-through of instructions regarding home glucose monitoring and foot care and failure to recognize signs and symptoms of hyperglycemia.

Outcomes

Knowledge: Diabetes Management (NOC) Indicators:

Client Will

Perform procedure of home glucose monitoring correctly within 36 hr (6/30, 7 a.m.).
Verbalize basic understanding of disease process and treatment within 38 hr (6/30, 9 a.m.).
Explain reasons for actions within 38 hr (6/30, 9 a.m.).
Perform insulin administration correctly within 60 hr (7/1, 7 a.m.).

ACTIONS/INTERVENTIONS	RATIONALE

TEACHING: Disease Process (NIC)

Determine client's level of knowledge, priorities of learning needs, and desire and need for including wife in instruction.

Establishes baseline and direction for teaching and planning. Involvement of wife, if desired, will provide additional resource for recall and understanding and may enhance client's follow-through.

Provide teaching guide, "Understanding Your Diabetes," 6/28 p.m. Show film *Living With Diabetes,* 6/29, 4 p.m., when wife is visiting. Include in group teaching session, 6/30 a.m. Review information and obtain feedback from client and wife.

Provides different methods for accessing and reinforcing information and enhances opportunity for learning and understanding.

Discuss factors related to and altering diabetic control, such as stress, illness, and exercise.

Drug therapy and diet may need to be altered in response to both short- and long-term stressors and changes in activity level.

Review signs and symptoms of hyperglycemia (e.g., fatigue, nausea, vomiting, polyuria, polydipsia). Discuss how to prevent and evaluate this situation and when to seek medical care. Have client identify appropriate interventions.

Recognition and understanding of these signs and symptoms and timely intervention will aid client in avoiding recurrences and preventing complications.

Review and provide information about necessity for routine examination of feet and proper foot care (e.g., daily inspection for injuries, pressure areas, corns, calluses; proper nail cutting; daily washing; application of good moisturizing lotion such as Eucerin, Keri, or Nivea bid). Recommend loose-fitting socks and shoes that fit (break new shoes in gradually), and avoid going barefoot. If foot injury or skin break occurs, wash with soap or dermal cleanser and water, cover with sterile dressing, inspect wound, and change dressing daily; report redness, swelling, or presence of drainage.

Reduces risk of tissue injury and promotes understanding and prevention of stasis ulcer formation and wound healing difficulties.

TEACHING: Prescribed Medication (NIC)

Instruct regarding prescribed insulin therapy:

May be a temporary treatment of hyperglycemia with infection or may be permanent replacement of oral hypoglycemic agent.

Humulin N insulin, SC.

Intermediate-acting insulin generally lasts 18 to 28 hr, with peak effect 6 to 12 hr.

Keep vial in current use at room temperature (if used within 30 days).

Cold insulin is poorly absorbed.

Store extra vials in refrigerator.

Refrigeration prolongs the drug shelf-life by preventing wide fluctuations in temperature.

Roll bottle and invert to mix, or shake gently, avoiding bubbles.

Vigorous shaking may create foam, which can interfere with accurate dose withdrawal and damage the insulin molecule. *Note:* New research suggests that gently shaking the vial may be more effective in mixing suspension.

Choice of injection sites (e.g., across lower abdomen in Z pattern).

Provides for steady absorption of medication. Site is easily visualized and accessible by client, and Z pattern minimizes tissue damage.

Demonstrate, then observe client in drawing insulin into syringe, reading syringe markings, and administering dose. Assess for accuracy.

May require several instruction sessions and practice before client and wife feel comfortable drawing up and injecting medication.

Instruct in signs and symptoms of insulin reaction and hypoglycemia: fatigue, nausea, headache, hunger, sweating, irritability, shakiness, anxiety, and difficulty concentrating.

Knowing what to watch for and appropriate treatment such as $\frac{1}{2}$ cup grape juice for immediate response and snack within 30 min (e.g., one slice bread with peanut butter or cheese, fruit and slice of cheese for sustained effect) may prevent or minimize complications.

Review "sick day rules," for example, call doctor if too sick to eat normally or stay active; take insulin as ordered. Keep record as noted in Sick Day Guide.

Understanding of necessary actions in the event of mild to severe illness promotes competent self-care and reduces risk of hyperglycemia or hypoglycemia.

Instruct client and wife in fingerstick glucose monitoring to be done four times per day until stable, then B.I.D. at rotating times, such as FBS and before dinner, before lunch, and at bedtime. Observe return demonstrations of the procedure.

Fingerstick monitoring provides accurate and timely information regarding diabetic control. Return demonstration verifies correct learning.

(continues on page 36)

Recommend client maintain record or log of fingerstick testing, antidiabetic medication and insulin dosage/site, unusual physiological response, and dietary intake. Outline desired goals, for example, FBS 80 to 110, premeal 80 to 120.

Provides accurate record for review by caregivers for assessment of therapy effectiveness and needs.

Discuss other healthcare issues, such as smoking habits, self-monitoring for cancer (breasts and testicles), and reporting changes in general well-being.

Encourages client involvement, awareness, and responsibility for own health; promotes wellness. *Note:* Smoking tends to increase client's resistance to insulin.

CHAPTER 4

Cardiovascular

HYPERTENSION: SEVERE

I. Pathophysiology
  a. Multifactoral
    i. Complex interactions between the vasculature, kidneys, sympathetic nervous system, baroreceptors, renin-angiotensin-aldosterone system, and insulin resistance
  b. Mosaic theory
    i. Genetic disposition
    ii. Environmental: dietary Na^+/fat intake, trace metals, stress, smoking
    iii. Anatomical: abnormalities of vascular system
    iv. Adaptive: e.g., regulation of intracellular Na^+ and Ca^{++} by cell membrane ion pumps
    v. Neural: variety of complex nerve mechanisms
    vi. Endocrine: pheochromocytoma, primary aldosteronism
    vii. Humoral: varied agents that constrict and dilate blood vessels
    viii. Hemodynamic: blood volume or viscosity, intrarenal hemodynamics

II. Classification—2003 Guidelines National Heart, Lung, and Blood Institute (NHLBI)
  a. Normal blood pressure (BP)—less than 120/80 mm Hg
  b. Prehypertension—120/80 to 139/89 mm Hg
  c. Hypertension—greater than 140/90 mm Hg

III. Degree of Severity
  a. Stage I (mild)—140/90 to 159/99 mm Hg
  b. Stage II (moderate)—160/100 mm Hg or greater
  c. Stage III (severe)—systolic pressure greater than 180 and diastolic pressure greater than 110
  d. Stage IV (very severe)—systolic pressure 210 or greater with diastolic pressure greater than 120

IV. Etiology
  a. Primary (essential), which accounts for approximately 85% to 95% of all cases, has no identifiable cause
  b. Secondary, which occurs as a result of an identifiable, sometimes correctable, pathological condition, such as kidney disorders, adrenal gland tumors, or primary aldosteronism, medications, drugs, or other chemicals

V. Statistics (NHLBI, 2006; Centers for Disease Control and Prevention [CDC], CDC, 2006b; 2007a)
  a. Morbidity: 72 million Americans are hypertensive (nearly 1 in 3).
    i. 23% of adults aged 20 to 75 are hypertensive.
    ii. 70% of adults over age 75 are hypertensive.
    iii. Approximately 20% are undiagnosed.
    iv. Prevalence: African Americans 32%, whites 23%, Hispanics 23%
  b. Mortality: There are more than 19,000 deaths per year.
  c. Cost: $47.2 billion is spent per year.

GLOSSARY

Atrial hypertrophy: Increased atrial volume and pressure.
Hyperglycemia: Increased serum glucose.
Hypertension: Blood pressure (BP) greater than 140/90 mm Hg.
Hypokalemia: Low serum potassium.
Prehypertension: BP in range of 120/80 to 139/89 mm Hg.
Stroke: Cellular death of cerebral tissue caused by obstruction of blood flow to sections of the brain, which results in neurological deficits.

Systemic vascular resistance (SVR): An index of arterial compliance or constriction throughout the body; equal to BP divided by cardiac output.
Target organ disease or damage (TOD): Organ or system of organs that are primarily affected by hypertension, such as the heart, kidneys, and brain.
Transient ischemic attack (TIA): Brief periods of confusion or difficulty with speech caused by an intermittent reduction in blood flow to the brain.

Care Setting

Although hypertension is usually treated in a community setting, management of stages III and IV with symptoms of complications or compromise may require inpatient care, especially when target organ disease (TOD) is present. The majority of interventions included here can be used in either setting.

Related Concerns

Cerebrovascular accident (CVA)/stroke, page 238
Myocardial infarction, page 74
Psychosocial aspects of care, page 749
Renal failure: acute, page 536
Renal failure: chronic, page 548

Client Assessment Database

DIAGNOSTIC DIVISION MAY REPORT	MAY EXHIBIT
ACTIVITY/REST • Sedentary lifestyle, which is a major risk factor for hypertension • Weakness, fatigue • Shortness of breath	• Elevated heart rate • Change in heart rhythm • Tachypnea • Dyspnea with exertion
CIRCULATION • History of elevated BP over time • Presence of TOD, such as atherosclerotic, valvular, or coronary artery heart disease, including myocardial infarction (MI), angina, heart failure (HF), and cerebrovascular disease • Episodes of palpitations, diaphoresis	• *Pulses:* Bounding carotid, jugular, radial pulsations • Pulse disparities, particularly femoral delay as compared with radial or brachial pulsation and absence of or diminished popliteal, posterior tibial, pedal pulses • *Apical pulse:* Point of maximal impulse (PMI) possibly displaced or forceful • *Heart rate and rhythm:* Tachycardia, various dysrhythmias • *Heart sounds:* Accentuated S_2 at base; S_3 in early HF; S_4, which reflects rigid left ventricle and left ventricular hypertrophy; murmurs of valvular stenosis; vascular bruits audible over carotid, femoral, or epigastrium • Jugular vein distension (JVD) • *Extremities:* Discoloration of skin, cool temperature indicating peripheral vasoconstriction and slow or delayed capillary refill indicating vasoconstriction • *Skin:* Pallor, cyanosis, and diaphoresis, suggesting pulmonary congestion and hypoxemia, or flushing, suggesting pheochromocytoma
EGO INTEGRITY • History of personality changes, anxiety, depression, euphoria, or chronic anger that may indicate cerebral impairment • Multiple stress factors, such as relationship, financial, or job-related concerns	• Mood swings, restlessness, irritability • Narrowed focus
ELIMINATION • Past or present renal insult, such as kidney infection, renovascular obstruction, or past history of kidney disease	• May have decreased urinary output, if kidney failure is present, or increased output, if taking diuretics
FOOD/FLUID • Food preferences that are high-calorie, high-salt, high-fat, and high-cholesterol, such as fried foods, cheese, eggs, or licorice • Low dietary intake of potassium, calcium, and magnesium • Nausea, vomiting • Recent weight changes • Current or history of diuretic use	• Normal weight or obesity • Presence of edema • Venous congestion, JVD • Glycosuria—almost 10% of hypertensive clients are diabetic, reflecting renal TOD
NEUROSENSORY • History of numbness or weakness on one side of the body; TIA or stroke • Fainting spells or dizziness	• *Mental status:* Changes in alertness, orientation, speech pattern and content, affect, thought process, or memory

Client Assessment Database (continued)

<table>
<tr><th>DIAGNOSTIC DIVISION
MAY REPORT (continued)</th><th>MAY EXHIBIT (continued)</th></tr>
<tr><td>

• Throbbing, suboccipital headaches, usually present on awakening and disappearing spontaneously after several hours
• Visual disturbances, such as diplopia and blurred vision
• Episodes of epistaxis

</td><td>

• *Motor responses:* Decreased strength, hand grip, and deep tendon reflexes
• *Optic retinal changes:* From mild sclerosis and arterial narrowing to marked retinal and sclerotic changes with edema or papilledema, exudates, hemorrhages, and arterial nicking, although dependent on severity and duration of hypertension and resulting TOD

</td></tr>
<tr><td>

PAIN/DISCOMFORT
• Severe, throbbing occipital headaches located in suboccipital region, present on awakening, and disappearing spontaneously after several hours
• Stiffness of neck, dizziness, and blurred vision
• Abdominal pain or masses, suggesting pheochromocytoma

</td><td>

• Relu-ctance to move head, rubbing head, avoidance of bright lights and noise, wrinkled brow, clenched fists; grimacing and guarding behaviors

</td></tr>
<tr><td>

RESPIRATION
• Dyspnea associated with activity or exertion
• Tachypnea, orthopnea, paroxysmal nocturnal dyspnea
• Cough with or without sputum production
• Smoking history, which is a major risk factor

</td><td>

• Respiratory distress or use of accessory muscles
• Adventitious breath sounds, such as crackles or wheezes
• Pallor or cyanosis generally associated with advanced cardiopulmonary effects of sustained or severe hypertension

</td></tr>
<tr><td>

SAFETY
• Transient episodes of numbness, unilateral paresthesias
• Light-headedness with position changes

</td><td>

• Impaired coordination or gait

</td></tr>
<tr><td>

SEXUALITY
• Postmenopausal, which is a major risk factor
• Erectile dysfunction (ED), which may be associated with hypertension or antihypertensive medications

TEACHING/LEARNING
• Familial risk factors, including hypertension, atherosclerosis, heart disease, diabetes mellitus, and cerebrovascular or kidney disease
• Ethnic or racial risk factors, such as increased prevalence in African American and Southeast Asian populations
• Use of birth control pills or other hormone replacement therapy
• Drug and alcohol use
• Use of herbal supplements to manage BP, such as garlic, hawthorn, black cohash, celery seed, coleus, and evening primrose

DISCHARGE PLAN CONSIDERATIONS
• May require assistance with self-monitoring of BP as well as periodic evaluation of and alterations in medication therapy

▶ Refer to section at end of plan for postdischarge considerations.

</td><td>

</td></tr>
</table>

TEST WHY IT IS DONE	WHAT IT TELLS ME
BLOOD TESTS	
• *Hemoglobin/hematocrit:* Assesses relationship of red blood cells (RBCs) to fluid volume or viscosity and may indicate risk factors, such as anemia or hypercoagulability.	Hematocrit rises when the number of RBCs increases or when the plasma volume is reduced, as in dehydration.
• *Platelets:* Platelets have an essential function in coagulation, hemostasis, and thrombus formation. An elevated platelet count can cause increased clotting.	May show abnormalities leading to clotting and increased risk for heart attack or stroke, particularly in persons with diabetes.
• *Blood urea nitrogen (BUN) and creatinine (Cr):* BUN measures the amount of urea nitrogen in the blood. Cr measures the amount of creatinine in blood or urine.	Provides information about renal perfusion and function and can reveal cause if hypertension is related to kidney dysfunction.
• *Glucose:* Measures the amount of glucose in the blood right at the time of sample collection.	Hyperglycemia may result from elevated catecholamine levels, which increases BP, and use of thiazide diuretics. Also, diabetes mellitus can be associated with hypertension.
• *Serum potassium:* Potassium is an electrolyte that helps regulate the amount of fluid in the body, stimulate muscle contraction, and maintain a stable acid-base balance.	Hypokalemia may indicate the presence of primary aldosteronism as a possible cause of hypertension or it may be a side effect of diuretic therapy.
• *Lipid panel, including total lipids, high-density lipoprotein (HDL) cholesterol, low-density lipoprotein (LDL) cholesterol, total cholesterol, triglycerides:* The group of tests that make up a lipid profile have been shown to be good indicators of risk for heart attack or stroke.	A predisposition for or presence of atheromatous plaque is indicated by the following: HDL levels that are less than 40 mg/dL in men and less than 50 mg/dL in women, triglycerides that are more than 150 mg/dL, and an increase in small-particle LDL.
• *Thyroid studies:* Blood test and scan to evaluate thyroid function; most commonly used laboratory test is the measurement of thyroid-stimulating hormone (TSH).	Hypertension is present in approximately 3% of clients with hypothyroidism and 20% to 30% in those with thyrotoxicosis (Hix & Vidt, 2004).
• *Serum/urine aldosterone level:* May be done to assess for primary aldosteronism as cause of hypertension.	Elevated in primary aldosteronism.
• *Renin:* An enzyme that activates the renin-angiotensin system and screens for essential, renal, or renovascular hypertension.	Elevated in renovascular and malignant hypertension and salt-wasting disorders.
• *C-reactive protein (CRP):* A member of the class of acute phase reactants. Serum levels rise dramatically during inflammatory processes occurring in the body. Monitoring serial CRP values can help determine disease progress or the effectiveness of treatment.	Research suggests that patients with elevated basal levels of CRP are at increased risk for hypertension (Sesso et al, 2003).
URINE TESTS	
• *Urinalysis:* Screening tool to determine effectiveness of kidney function and to monitor fluid imbalances and treatment.	Presence of blood, protein, or white blood cells (WBCs) suggests renal dysfunction; glucose suggests presence of diabetes.
• *Creatinine clearance:* Determines extent of nephron damage in known kidney disease.	Reduced in hypertensive patient with renal damage.
• *Urine vanillylmandelic acid (VMA) (catecholamine metabolite):* 24-hour urine VMA may be done for assessment of intermittent hypertension.	Elevation may indicate presence of pheochromocytoma.
• *Uric acid:* Measures end product of purine metabolism, providing one index of renal function.	Hyperuricemia has been implicated as a risk factor for the development of hypertension.
OTHER DIAGNOSTIC STUDIES	
• *Intravenous pyelogram (IVP):* Visualizes kidneys, ureters, bladder, and renal pelvis to determine urinary tract dysfunction or kidney disease.	May identify cause of secondary hypertension, such as renal parenchymal disease and renal or urethral obstruction.
• *Kidney and renography nuclear scan (also called renogram):* Assists in diagnosing renal disorders.	Determines if hypertension is due to kidney disease.
• *Chest x-ray:* Evaluates organs and structures within the chest.	May demonstrate calcification in valve areas or aorta causing blood flow obstruction or cardiac enlargement, indicating heart failure.

TEST WHY IT IS DONE (continued)	WHAT IT TELLS ME (continued)
• *Computed tomography (CT) scan:* Noninvasive procedure, done with or without contrast media, to enhance certain anatomic views of cerebral structures and locate abnormalities.	Assesses for cerebral tumor or stroke; also rules out pheochromocytoma or encephalopathy as contributing factors for hypertension.
• *Electrocardiogram (ECG):* Record of the electrical activity of the heart that can demonstrate conduction disturbances, enlarged heart, and chamber strain patterns.	Broad, notched P wave is one of the earliest signs of hypertensive heart disease.

Nursing Priorities

1. Maintain or enhance cardiovascular functioning.
2. Prevent complications.
3. Provide information about disease process, prognosis, and treatment regimen.
4. Support active client control of condition.

Discharge Goals

1. BP within acceptable limits for individual.
2. Cardiovascular and systemic complications prevented or minimized.
3. Disease process, prognosis, and therapeutic regimen understood.
4. Necessary lifestyle or behavioral changes initiated.
5. Plan in place to meet needs after discharge.

NURSING DIAGNOSIS: risk for decreased Cardiac Output

Risk factors may include
Increased vascular resistance, vasoconstriction
Myocardial ischemia
Ventricular hypertrophy or rigidity

Possibly evidenced by
(Not applicable; presence of signs and symptoms establishes an *actual* diagnosis)

Desired Outcomes/Evaluation Criteria—Client Will

Circulation Status (NOC)
Participate in activities that reduce BP and cardiac workload.
Maintain BP within individually acceptable range.
Demonstrate stable cardiac rhythm and rate within normal range.

ACTIONS/INTERVENTIONS	RATIONALE
Hemodynamic Regulation (NIC) *Independent* Measure BP in both arms or thighs. Take three readings, 3 to 5 minutes apart while client is at rest, then sitting, and then standing for initial evaluation. Use correct cuff size and accurate technique. Take note of elevations in systolic as well as diastolic readings.	Serial measurements using correct equipment provide a more complete picture of vascular involvement and scope of problem. Progressive diastolic readings above 120 mm Hg are considered first accelerated, then malignant (very severe). Systolic hypertension also is an established risk factor for cerebrovascular disease and ischemic heart disease even when diastolic pressure is not elevated. In younger client with normal systolic readings, elevated diastolic numbers may indicate prehypertension.
Note presence and quality of central and peripheral pulses.	Bounding carotid, jugular, radial, and femoral pulses may be observed and palpated. Pulses in the legs and feet may be diminished, reflecting effects of vasoconstriction and venous congestion.

(continues on page 42)

ACTIONS/INTERVENTIONS (continued)

Auscultate heart tones and breath sounds.

Observe skin color, moisture, temperature, and capillary refill time.

Note dependent and generalized edema.

Provide calm, restful surroundings, minimize environmental activity and noise. Consider limiting the number of visitors or length of visitation.

Maintain activity restrictions during crisis situation such as bedrest or chair rest and schedule periods of uninterrupted rest; assist client with self-care activities as needed.

Provide comfort measures, such as back and neck massage or elevation of head.

Instruct in relaxation techniques, guided imagery, and distractions.

Monitor response to medications that control BP.

Collaborative

Administer medications, as indicated:

Diuretics, for example, thiazide, such as chlorothiazide (Diuril), hydrochlorothiazide (Esidrix, HydroDIURIL), hydrochlorothiazide with triamterene (Diazide, Maxide) or amiloride (Modiuretic), bendroflumethiazide (Naturetin), indapamide (Lozol), metolazone (Mykrox, Zaroxolyn); and loop diuretics, such as furosemide (Lasix), bumetanide (Bumex), and torsemide (Demadex)

Potassium-sparing diuretics, such as spironolactone (Aldactone), triamterene (Dyrenium), and amiloride (Midamor)

Beta blockers, such as doxazosin (Cardura), acebutolol (Sectral), metoprolol (Lopressor), labetalol (Normodyne), atenolol (Tenormin), nadolol (Corgard), carvedilol (Coreg), propranolol (Inderal), methyldopa (Aldomet), clonidine (Catapres), prazosin (Minipress), terazosin (Hytrin), pindolol (Visken), and timolol (Blocarden)

Calcium channel blockers, such nifedipine (Adalat, Procardia), verapamil (Calan, Isoptin, Verelan), diltiazem (Cardizem), amlodipine (Norvasc), isradipine (DynaCirc), nicardipine (Cardene), and felodipine (Plendil)

Direct-acting oral vasodilators, such as hydralazine (Apresoline) and minoxidil (Loniten)

Direct-acting parenteral vasodilators, such as diazoxide (Hyperstat), nitroprusside (Nitropress), and labetalol (Normodyne)

Angiotensin-converting enzyme (ACE) inhibitors, such as captopril (Capoten), enalapril (Vasotec), benazepril (Lotensin), lisinopril (Zestril), fosinopril (Monopril), ramipril (Altace), moexipril (Univasc), and trandolapril (Mavik)

Angiotensin II receptor blockers (ARBs), such as candesartan (Atacand), olmesartan (Benicar), valsartan (Diovan), losartan (Cozaar), and irbesartan (Avapro)

RATIONALE (continued)

S_4 is commonly heard in severely hypertensive clients because of the presence of atrial hypertrophy. Development of S_3 indicates ventricular hypertrophy and impaired cardiac functioning. Presence of crackles or wheezes may indicate pulmonary congestion secondary to developing or chronic heart failure.

Presence of pallor; cool, moist skin; and delayed capillary refill time may be due to peripheral vasoconstriction or reflect cardiac decompensation and decreased output.

Indicates heart or kidney failure or vascular impairment.

Helps reduce sympathetic stimulation and promotes relaxation.

Reduces physical stress and tension that affect BP and the course of hypertension.

Decreases discomfort and may reduce sympathetic stimulation.

Can reduce stressful stimuli and produce calming effect, thereby reducing BP.

Response to drug therapy is dependent on both the individual drugs and their synergistic effects. Because of potential side effects and drug interactions, it is important to use the smallest number and lowest dosage of medications possible.

Diuretics are considered first-line medications for uncomplicated hypertension and may be used alone or in association with other drugs, such as beta blockers, to reduce BP in clients with relatively normal renal function. These diuretics also potentiate the effects of other antihypertensive agents by limiting fluid retention and may reduce the incidence of stroke and heart failure.

These drugs produce marked diuresis by inhibiting resorption of sodium and chloride and are effective antihypertensives, especially in clients who are resistant to thiazides or have renal impairment. May be given in combination with a thiazide diuretic to minimize potassium loss.

Beta blockers are recommended for BP control in clients with heart failure and cardiovascular disease. Cardioselective beta blockers, such as acebutolol, atenolol, and metroprolol, primarily affect β-1 receptors in the heart, slowing heart rate and decreasing the heart's workload. Nonselective beta blockers, such as propranolol and timolol, also decrease the heart's workload and promote vasodilation, but they exert effects on the β-2 receptors on the bronchioles as well, potentially increasing symptoms of reactive airway disease and chronic obstructive pulmonary disease. Cardioselective beta blockers are safer choices for patients with pulmonary disorders (Woods & Moshang, 2006).

Calcium channel blockers are categorized into two types. One group, such as amlodipine, diltiazem, and isradipine, primarily affects blood vessels and can be used to treat severe hypertension when a combination of a diuretic and a sympathetic inhibitor does not sufficiently control BP.

Action is to relax vascular smooth muscle, thereby reducing vascular resistance.

These are given intravenously (IV) for management of hypertensive emergencies.

ACE inhibitors are generally considered first-line drugs for clients with documented congestive heart failure (CHF), diabetes, and those at risk for renal failure.

ARBs block the action of angiotensin II. As a result, blood vessels dilate and BP is reduced.

ACTIONS/INTERVENTIONS (continued)

Aldosterone blockers, such as eplerenone (Inspra) and spironolactone

Implement dietary restrictions, as indicated, such as reducing calories and avoiding refined carbohydrates, sodium, fat, and cholesterol. (Refer to ND, imbalanced Nutrition.)

Prepare for surgery when indicated.

RATIONALE (continued)

Aldosterone antagonists block the effects of aldosterone on the kidneys, allowing the kidneys to excrete extra sodium and water, thereby reducing BP.

Limiting sodium and sodium-rich processed foods can help manage fluid retention and, with associated hypertensive response, decrease myocardial workload. A diet rich in calcium, potassium, and magnesium may help lower BP.

When hypertension is due to pheochromocytoma, removing the tumor corrects the condition.

NURSING DIAGNOSIS: Activity Intolerance

May be related to
Generalized weakness
Imbalance between oxygen supply and demand

Possibly evidenced by
Verbal report of fatigue or weakness
Abnormal heart rate or BP response to activity
Exertional discomfort or dyspnea
ECG changes reflecting ischemia, dysrhythmias

Desired Outcomes/Evaluation Criteria—Client Will

Endurance (NOC)
Participate in necessary and desired activities.
Report a measurable increase in activity tolerance.
Demonstrate a decrease in physiological signs of intolerance.

ACTIONS/INTERVENTIONS

Energy Management (NIC)
Independent
Assess the client's response to activity, noting pulse rate more than 20 beats per minute faster than resting rate; marked increase in BP (systolic increases more than 40 mm Hg or diastolic increases more than 20 mm Hg) during and after activity, dyspnea or chest pain, excessive fatigue and weakness, and diaphoresis, dizziness, and syncope.

Instruct client in energy-conserving techniques, such as using chair when showering, sitting to brush teeth or comb hair, and carrying out activities at a slower pace.

Encourage progressive activity and self-care when tolerated. Provide assistance as needed.

RATIONALE

Changes in baseline are helpful in assessing physiological responses to the stress of activity and, if present, are indicators of overexertion.

Energy-saving techniques reduce the energy expenditure, thereby assisting in equalization of oxygen supply and demand.

Gradual activity progression prevents a sudden increase in cardiac workload. Provide assistance only as needed, which encourages independence in performing activities.

NURSING DIAGNOSIS: acute Pain

May be related to
Increased cerebral vascular pressure

Possibly evidenced by
Reports of throbbing pain located in suboccipital region, present on awakening, and disappearing spontaneously after being up and about
Reluctance to move head, rubbing head, avoidance of bright lights and noise, wrinkled brow, clenched fists
Reports of stiffness of neck, dizziness, blurred vision, nausea, and vomiting

Desired Outcomes/Evaluation Criteria—Client Will

Pain Control (NOC)
Report pain or discomfort is relieved or controlled.
Verbalize methods that provide relief.
Follow prescribed pharmacological regimen.

ACTIONS/INTERVENTIONS

Pain Management (NIC)
Independent

Determine specifics of pain, such as location, characteristics, intensity (on a 0 to 10 scale), onset, and duration. Note nonverbal cues.

Encourage and maintain bedrest during acute phase, if indicated.

Provide or recommend nonpharmacological measures for relief of headache, such as placing a cool cloth to forehead; back and neck rubs; quiet, dimly lit room; relaxation techniques, such as guided imagery and distraction; and diversional activities.

Eliminate or minimize vasoconstricting activities that may aggravate headache, such as straining at stool, prolonged coughing, and bending over.

Assist client with ambulation, as needed.

Provide liquids, soft foods, and frequent mouth care if nosebleeds occur or nasal packing has been done to stop bleeding.

Collaborative

Administer analgesics, as indicated.

Administer anti-anxiety agents, such as lorazepam (Ativan), alprazolam (Xanax), and diazepam (Valium).

RATIONALE

Facilitates diagnosis of problem and initiation of appropriate therapy. Helpful in evaluating effectiveness of therapy.

Minimizes stimulation and promotes relaxation.

Measures that reduce cerebral vascular pressure and that slow or block sympathetic response are effective in relieving headache and associated complications.

Activities that increase vasoconstriction accentuate the headache in the presence of increased cerebral vascular pressure.

Dizziness and blurred vision frequently are associated with vascular headache. Client may also experience episodes of postural hypotension, causing weakness when ambulating.

Promotes general comfort. Nasal packing may interfere with swallowing or require mouth breathing, leading to stagnation of oral secretions and drying of mucous membranes.

Reduce or control pain and decrease stimulation of the sympathetic nervous system.

May aid in the reduction of tension and discomfort that is intensified by stress.

NURSING DIAGNOSIS: **imbalanced Nutrition: More than Body Requirements**

May be related to
Excessive intake in relation to metabolic need
Sedentary activity level and lifestyle
Cultural preferences

Possibly evidenced by
Weight that is 10% to 20% more than ideal for height and frame
Triceps skinfold that is more than 15 mm in men and 25 mm in women, the maximum for age and sex
Reported or observed dysfunctional eating patterns

Desired Outcomes/Evaluation Criteria—Client Will

Knowledge: Treatment Regimen (NOC)
Identify correlation between hypertension and obesity.

Weight Control (NOC)
Demonstrate change in eating patterns, such as food choices and quantity, to attain desirable body weight with optimal maintenance of health.
Initiate and maintain individually appropriate exercise program.

ACTIONS/INTERVENTIONS

Weight Reduction Assistance (NIC)
Independent

Assess client's understanding of direct relationship between hypertension and obesity.

RATIONALE

Obesity is an added risk with hypertension because of the disproportion between fixed aortic capacity and increased cardiac output associated with increased body mass. Reduction in weight may reduce or eliminate the need for drug therapy needed to control BP. *Note:* Recent research suggests that bringing weight within 15% of ideal weight can result in a drop of 10 mm Hg in both systolic and diastolic BP (Khan et al, 2004).

ACTIONS/INTERVENTIONS (continued)

Discuss necessity for decreased caloric intake and limited intake of fats, salt, and sugar, as indicated.

Determine client's desire to lose weight.

Review usual daily caloric intake and dietary choices.

Establish a realistic weight reduction plan with the client, such as weight loss of 1 pound per week.

Encourage client to maintain a diary of food intake, including when and where eating takes place and the circumstances and feelings around which the food was eaten.

Instruct and assist client in appropriate food selections, such as implementing a diet rich in fruits, vegetables, and low-fat dairy foods referred to as the Dietary Approaches to Stop Hypertension (DASH) diet. Help the client identify—and thus avoid—foods high in saturated fat, such as butter, cheese, eggs, ice cream, and meat, and those that are high in cholesterol, such as whole dairy products, shrimp, and organ meats.

Collaborative

Refer to dietitian or weight management programs, as indicated.

RATIONALE (continued)

Faulty eating habits contribute to atherosclerosis and obesity that can predispose to hypertension and subsequent complications, such as stroke, kidney disease, and heart failure. Excessive salt intake expands the intravascular fluid volume and may damage kidneys, which can further aggravate hypertension.

Motivation for weight reduction is internal. The individual must want to lose weight or the program most likely will not succeed.

Identifies current strengths and weaknesses in dietary program. Aids in determining individual need for adjustment and teaching.

Slow reduction in weight is associated with fat loss with muscle sparing and generally reflects a change in eating habits.

Provides a database for both the adequacy of nutrients eaten and the relationship of emotion to eating. Helps focus attention on factors that client can control or change.

Moderation and use of low-fat products in place of total abstinence from certain food items may prevent client's sense of deprivation and enhance commitment to achieving health goals. Avoiding foods high in saturated fat and cholesterol is important in preventing progressing atherogenesis. The DASH diet, in conjunction with exercise, weight loss, and limits on salt intake, may reduce or even eliminate the need for drug therapy in early stages of hypertension (Elmer et al, 2006).

Can provide additional counseling and assistance with meeting individual dietary needs.

NURSING DIAGNOSIS: ineffective Coping

May be related to
Situational or maturational crisis, multiple life changes
Inadequate relaxation, little or no exercise; work overload
Inadequate support systems
Poor nutrition
Unmet expectations, unrealistic perceptions
Inadequate coping methods

Possibly evidenced by
Verbalization of inability to cope or ask for help
Inability to meet role expectations, basic needs, or problem-solve
Destructive behavior toward self, overeating or lack of appetite, excessive smoking and drinking, and proneness to alcohol abuse
Chronic fatigue, insomnia, muscular tension, frequent headaches and neck aches, chronic worry, irritability, anxiety, emotional tension, and depression

Desired Outcomes/Evaluation Criteria—Client Will

Coping (NOC)
Identify ineffective coping behaviors and consequences.
Verbalize awareness of own coping abilities and strengths.
Identify potential stressful situations and steps to avoid or modify them.
Demonstrate the use of effective coping skills.

ACTIONS/INTERVENTIONS

RATIONALE

Coping Enhancement (NIC)
Independent

Assess effectiveness of coping strategies by observing behaviors, such as ability to verbalize feelings and concerns, and willingness to participate in the treatment plan.

Adaptive mechanisms are necessary to appropriately alter one's lifestyle, deal with the chronicity of hypertension, and integrate prescribed therapies into daily living.

(continues on page 46)

ACTIONS/INTERVENTIONS (continued)

Note reports of sleep disturbances, increasing fatigue, impaired concentration, irritability, decreased tolerance of headache, and inability to cope or problem-solve.

Assist client to identify specific stressors and possible strategies for coping with them.

Include client in planning of care and encourage maximum participation in treatment plan and with the interdisciplinary team.

Encourage client to evaluate life priorities and personal goals. Ask questions such as, "Is what you are doing getting you what you want?"

Assist client to identify and begin planning for necessary lifestyle changes. Assist to adjust, rather than abandon, personal and family goals.

RATIONALE (continued)

Manifestations of maladaptive coping mechanisms may be indicators of repressed anger and have been found to be major determinants of diastolic BP (Shapiro et al, 1995).

Recognition of stressors is often the first step in altering one's response to the stressor.

Involvement provides client with an ongoing sense of control, improves coping skills, and enhances commitment to achieving health goals. Ongoing intensive assessment and management by an interdisciplinary team promotes timely adjustments to therapeutic regimen.

Focuses client's attention on reality of present situation relative to client's goals. Strong work ethic, need for "control," and outward focus may have led to lack of attention to personal needs.

Necessary changes should be realistically prioritized so client can avoid being overwhelmed and feeling powerless.

NURSING DIAGNOSIS: **deficient Knowledge [Learning Need] regarding condition, treatment plan, self-care, and discharge needs**

May be related to
Lack of knowledge and recall
Information misinterpretation
Cognitive limitation
Denial of diagnosis

Possibly evidenced by
Verbalization of the problem
Request for information
Statement of misconception
Inaccurate follow-through of instructions, inadequate performance of procedures
Inappropriate or exaggerated behaviors, such as hostility, agitation, or apathy

Desired Outcomes/Evaluation Criteria—Client Will

Knowledge: Hypertension Management (NOC)
Verbalize understanding of disease process and treatment regimen.
Identify drug side effects and possible complications that necessitate medical attention.
Maintain BP within individually acceptable parameters.
Describe reasons for therapeutic actions and treatment regimen.

ACTIONS/INTERVENTIONS

Teaching: Disease Process (NIC)
Independent
Assist client in identifying modifiable risk factors, such as obesity; diet high in sodium, saturated fats, and cholesterol; sedentary lifestyle; smoking; alcohol intake of more than 2 ounces per day on a regular basis; and a stressful lifestyle.

Problem-solve with client to identify ways in which appropriate lifestyle changes can be made to reduce modifiable risk factors.

Discuss importance of eliminating smoking, and assist client in formulating a plan to quit smoking. Refer to smoking cessation program or healthcare provider for helpful medications.

Reinforce the importance of adhering to treatment regimen and keeping follow-up appointments.

RATIONALE

These risk factors contribute to hypertension and cardiovascular and renal disease.

Changing "comfortable or usual" behavior patterns can be very difficult and stressful. Support, guidance, and empathy can enhance client's success in accomplishing his or her health goals.

Nicotine increases catecholamine discharge, resulting in increased heart rate, BP, vasoconstriction, and myocardial workload, and reduces tissue oxygenation.

Lack of engagement in the treatment plan is a common reason for failure of antihypertensive therapy. Therefore, ongoing evaluation for client participation is critical to successful treatment. When client understands causative factors and consequences of inadequate intervention and is motivated to achieve health, the client typically participates in treatment interventions.

ACTIONS/INTERVENTIONS (continued)

Instruct and demonstrate BP self-monitoring technique. Evaluate client's hearing, visual acuity, manual dexterity, and coordination.

Help client develop a simple, convenient schedule for taking medications.

Explain prescribed medications along with their rationale, dosage, expected and adverse side effects, and particular traits, such as the following:

Diuretics:
Take daily or larger dose in the early morning.
Weigh self on a regular schedule and record.
Avoid or limit alcohol intake.

Notify physician if unable to tolerate food or fluid.

Antihypertensives:
Take prescribed dose on a regular schedule; avoid skipping, altering, or making up doses; and do not discontinue without notifying the healthcare provider. Review potential side effects and drug interactions, and discuss need for informing healthcare provider about onset of adverse effects such as ED.

Rise slowly from a lying to standing position, sitting for a few minutes before standing. Sleep with the head slightly elevated. Suggest frequent position changes and leg exercises when lying down.

Recommend avoiding hot baths, steam rooms, and saunas, especially with concomitant use of alcoholic beverages.

Instruct client to consult healthcare provider before taking other prescription or over-the-counter (OTC) medications.

As indicated, instruct client about increasing intake of foods and fluids high in potassium, such as oranges, bananas, figs, dates, tomatoes, potatoes, raisins, apricots, Gatorade, and fruit juices, and foods and fluids high in calcium, such as low-fat milk, yogurt, or calcium supplements.

Review the signs and symptoms that require the client to notify the healthcare provider, such as headache present on awakening that does not abate; sudden and continued increase of BP; chest pain; shortness of breath; irregular or increased pulse rate; significant weight gain (2 lb/day or 5 lb/wk); peripheral or abdominal swelling; visual disturbances; frequent, uncontrollable nosebleeds; depression or emotional lability; severe dizziness or episodes of fainting; muscle weakness or cramping; nausea or vomiting; or excessive thirst.

Explain rationale for prescribed dietary regimen—usually a diet low in sodium, saturated fat, and cholesterol.

Help client identify sources of sodium intake, such as table salt, salty snacks, processed meats and cheeses, sauerkraut, sauces, canned soups and vegetables, baking soda, baking powder, and monosodium glutamate. Stress the importance of reading ingredient labels of foods and OTC drugs.

Encourage foods rich in essential fatty acids, such as salmon, cod, mackerel, and tuna.

RATIONALE (continued)

Monitoring BP at home is reassuring to client because it provides visual feedback to determine treatment outcomes and helps promote early detection of deleterious changes.

Individualizing schedule to fit client's personal habits may make it easier to get in the habit of including antihypertensives in healthcare management activities.

Adequate information and understanding about side effects can enhance client's commitment to the treatment plan. For instance, mood changes, initial weight gain, and dry mouth are common and often subside with time.

Scheduling doses early in the day minimizes nighttime urination.
Primary indicator of effectiveness of diuretic therapy.
The combined vasodilating effect of alcohol and the volume-depleting effect of a diuretic greatly increase the risk of orthostatic hypotension.

Dehydration can develop rapidly if intake is poor and client continues to take a diuretic.

Because clients often cannot feel the difference the medication is making in BP, it is critical that there be understanding about the medication's actions and side effects. For example, abruptly discontinuing a drug may cause rebound hypertension leading to severe complications, or medication may need to be altered to reduce adverse effects. *Note:* Many drugs used to treat hypertension have been linked to ED. Drugs may need to be changed or dose adjusted.

Measures reduce potential for orthostatic hypotension associated with the use of vasodilators and diuretics.

Prevents vasodilation with potential for dangerous side effects of syncope and hypotension.

Any drug that contains a sympathetic nervous stimulant may increase BP or counteract effects of antihypertensive medications.

Some diuretics can deplete potassium levels. Dietary potassium is desirable means of correcting deficits and may be more palatable to the client than drug supplements. Correcting mineral deficiencies can also affect BP.

Early detection and reporting of developing complications, decreased effectiveness of drug regimen, or adverse reactions allows for timely intervention.

Excess saturated fats, cholesterol, sodium, alcohol, and calories have been defined as nutritional risks in hypertension. A diet low in fat and high in polyunsaturated fat reduces BP, possibly through prostaglandin balance in both normotensive and hypertensive people.

A moderately low-salt diet may be sufficient to control mild hypertension or reduce or eliminate the need for drug therapy needed to control BP.

Omega-3 fatty acids in fish tend to relax artery walls, reducing blood pressure. They also make blood thinner and less likely to clot.

(continues on page 48)

Encourage client to establish a regular exercise program, incorporating aerobic exercise within client's capabilities. Stress the importance of avoiding isometric activity.

Demonstrate application of ice pack to the back of the neck and pressure over the distal third of nose, and recommend that client lean head forward if nosebleed occurs.

Provide information regarding community resources, and support client in making lifestyle changes. Initiate referrals, as indicated.

Besides helping to lower BP, aerobic activity aids in toning the cardiovascular system. Isometric exercise can increase serum catecholamine levels, further elevating BP.

Nasal capillaries may rupture as a result of excessive vascular pressure. Cold temperature and pressure constrict capillaries to slow or halt bleeding. Leaning forward reduces the amount of blood that is swallowed.

Community resources, such as the American Heart Association, "coronary clubs," stop smoking clinics, alcohol or drug rehabilitation, weight loss programs, stress management classes, and counseling services may be helpful in client's efforts to initiate and maintain lifestyle changes.

POTENTIAL CONSIDERATIONS following acute hospitalization (dependent on client's age, physical condition and presence of complications, personal resources, and life responsibilities)

- *Activity Intolerance*—frequently occurs as a result of alterations in cardiac output and side effects of medication
- *imbalanced Nutrition: More than Body Requirements*—obesity is often present and a factor in BP control
- *ineffective self Health Management*—result of the complexity of the therapeutic regimen, required lifestyle changes, side effects of medication, and frequent feelings of general well-being, such as reports of "I'm not really sick."
- *Sexual Dysfunction*—interference in sexual functioning may occur because of activity intolerance and side effects of medication
- *readiness for enhanced family Coping*—opportunity exists for family members to support client while reducing risk factors for themselves and improving quality of life for family as a whole

---

HEART FAILURE: CHRONIC

I. Pathophysiology

a. Remodeling of the myocardium (as a structural response to injury) changes the heart from an efficient football shape to an inefficient basketball shape, making coordinated contractility difficult.
   i. Ventricular dilation (systolic dysfunction) results in poor contractility and inadequate emptying of chamber.
   ii. Ventricular stiffening (diastolic dysfunction) impairs ability of chamber to relax and receive and eject blood.

b. Failure of the left and/or right chambers of the heart results in insufficient output to meet metabolic needs of organ and tissues.

c. Cardiac-related elevation of pulmonary or systemic venous pressures leads to organ congestion.

d. Backward heart failure (HF): passive engorgement of the veins caused by elevated systemic venous pressure or a "backward" rise in pressure proximal to the failing cardiac chambers (right ventricular failure)

e. Forward HF: decreased cardiac output with reduced forward flow into the aorta, systemic circulation (inadequate renal blood flow leads to sodium and water retention), and increasing pulmonary venous pressure results in fluid accumulation in alveoli (left ventricular failure)

f. Myocardial muscle dysfunction associated with left ventricular hypertrophy (LVH) causes decreased cardiac output, activating neurohormones.

g. Elevated circulating or tissue levels of neurohormones, norepinephrine, angiotensin II, aldosterone, endothelin, vasopressin, and cytokines, causes sodium retention and peripheral vasoconstriction, increasing hemodynamic stresses on the ventricle.

II. Classification

a. New York Heart Association Functional Classification System for HF (9th ed, 1994)
   i. Class I—normal physical activity is not limited by symptoms.
   ii. Class II—ordinary physical activity results in fatigue, dyspnea, or other symptoms.
   iii. Class III—marked limitation in normal physical activity
   iv. Class IV—symptoms at rest or with any physical activity

b. American College of Cardiology/American Heart Association (ACC/AHA) 2005 Guidelines include specific recommendations for each stage (Hunt et al, 2005).
   i. Stage A—high risk for HF associated with such conditions as hypertension, diabetes, and obesity. Treatment is focused on comorbidity.
   ii. Stage B—presence of structural heart disease, such as left ventricular remodeling, LVH, or previous myocardial infarction (MI), but is asymptomatic. Treatment is focused on retarding the progression of ventricular remodeling and delaying the onset of HF symptoms.
   iii. Stage C—clients with past or current HF symptoms associated with structural heart disease, such as advanced ventricular remodeling. Treatment is focused on modifying fluid and dietary intake and drug therapies as well as nonpharmacological measures, such as biventricular pacing and valvular or revascularization surgery.

iv. Stage D—refractory advanced HF symptoms at rest or with minimal exertion and frequently requiring intervention in the acute setting. Treatment is focused on promoting clinical stability including supportive therapy to sustain life, such as left ventricular assist device, continuous intravenous (IV) inotropic therapy, experimental surgery or drugs, a heart transplant, or end-of-life or hospice care.

III. Etiology
a. Multifactoral
  i. Complex clinical syndrome resulting from any structural or functional cardiac disorder that impairs the ability of the ventricle to fill with or eject blood (ACC/AHA 2005 Guidelines; see Hunt et al, 2005).
  ii. Risk factors and comorbidities—hypertension; obesity; diabetes; coronary artery disease (CAD); peripheral and cerebrovascular disease; valvular heart disease with onset of atrial fibrillation (AF); sleep disorders such as sleep apnea; history of exposure to cardiotoxins, for example, chemotherapy, alcohol, and cocaine; family history of cardiomyopathy

IV. Statistics
  a. High morbidity and mortality, particularly in clients with New York Heart Association Class IV symptoms (Hunt et al, 2005)
  b. Morbidity: 5.2 million Americans have HF. (National Heart, Lung and Blood Institute [NHLBI], 2007)
    i. Approximately 550,000 new cases reported annually (Centers for Disease Control and Prevention [CDC], 2006b).
    ii. 1.1 million hospitalizations reported annually (CDC, 2006b).
  c. Mortality: 287,000 deaths reported annually (CDC, 2006b).
  d. Cost: $29.6 billion spent in 2006, making HF the most common reason for hospitalization of Medicare clients (CDC, 2006b).

GLOSSARY

Angiotensin converting enzyme inhibitor (ACEI) (also called ACE inhibitors): Medication that blocks the action of the angiotensin-converting enzyme in the lungs so that angiotensin I is not converted into angiotensin II. The production of this powerful blood vessel constrictor is thereby prevented and blood vessels remain dilated, which results in lower blood pressure.

Angiotensin receptor blocker (ARB): Medication that blocks the chemical receptors for angiotensin II on the small arteries. Therefore, the angiotensin cannot cause these arteries to constrict, which lowers blood pressure.

Ascites: Accumulation of fluid in the abdominal cavity can be associated with increased blood pressure in the veins draining the liver, with impaired drainage in the lymph system, and with low levels of albumin and other proteins in the blood.

Cardiac remodeling: The left ventricular chamber dilates and becomes more spherical. This condition increases the stress on the myocardial walls and depresses cardiac performance. Remodeling often precedes symptoms and may contribute to worsening of symptoms despite treatment (Hunt et al, 2005).

Heart failure (HF): A clinical syndrome characterized by inadequate systemic perfusion to meet the body's metabolic demands as a result of impaired cardiac pump function (Hobbs & Boye, 2004).

Heart sounds: S_1 corresponds to the closure of mitral and tricuspid valves. S_2 corresponds to closure of the aortic and pulmonary valves. S_3, heard mid-diastolic at the apex, is a low-pitched gallop or blowing sound sometimes called a ventricular gallop and is a common sign of left ventricular failure or distension in adults (Karmath & Thornton, 2002).

Positive hepatojugular reflex: An elevation of venous pressure, visible in the jugular veins and measurable in the veins of the arm, which is produced by firm pressure with the flat hand over the abdomen in active or impending congestive heart failure.

Pulsas alternans: Alternating weak and strong beats of the pulse associated with weak left ventricular function.

Pulse pressure: Difference between systolic and diastolic blood pressures.

Care Setting

Although generally managed at the community level, an in-client stay may be required for periodic exacerbation of failure or development of complications.

Related Concerns

Myocardial infarction, page 74
Hypertension: severe, page 37
Cardiac surgery, page 100
Dysrhythmias, page 88
Psychosocial aspects of care, page 749

DIAGNOSTIC DIVISION MAY REPORT	MAY EXHIBIT
ACTIVITY/REST • Fatigue, exhaustion progressing throughout the day • Inability to perform normal daily activities, such as making bed, climbing stairs, and so on • Exercise intolerance • Dyspnea at rest or with exertion • Insomnia, inability to sleep flat	• Limited exercise tolerance • Fatigue • Restlessness, mental status changes, such as anxiety and lethargy • Vital sign changes with activity
CIRCULATION • History of hypertension, recent or past MIs, multiple MIs, previous episodes of HF, valvular heart disease, cardiac surgery, endocarditis, systemic lupus erythematosus, anemia, septic shock • Swelling of feet, legs, abdomen, or "belt too tight"	• Blood pressure (BP) may be low with cardiac pump failure; in normal range with mild or chronic HF; or high with fluid overload, left-sided HF, and increased systemic vascular resistance (SVR) • Pulse pressure narrow, reflecting reduced ventricular stroke volume • *Heart rate and rhythm:* Tachycardia; dysrhythmias such as atrial fibrillation, premature ventricular contractions, heart blocks • *Apical pulse:* Point of maximal intensity (PMI) diffuse and displaced to the left • *Heart sounds:* S_1 and S_2 possibly softened; S_3 gallop rhythm diagnostic of congestive HF; S_4 occurring with hypertension; systolic and diastolic murmurs indicating the presence of valvular stenosis or insufficiency, causing or exacerbating heart failure • *Pulses:* Peripheral pulses diminished; central pulses may be bounding, for example, visible jugular, carotid, abdominal pulsations • Pulsus alternans may be noted • Skin tissue color pale, ashen, dusky, or cyanotic • Nail beds pale or cyanotic, with slow capillary refill • Liver enlarged and palpable; positive hepatojugular reflex may be present in right-sided HF • Edema dependent, generalized, or pitting, especially in extremities • Bulging neck veins (jugular vein distention [JVD])
EGO INTEGRITY • Anxiety, apprehension, fear • Stress related to illness or financial concerns (job, cost of medical care)	• Various behavioral manifestations, for example, anxiety, anger, fear, irritability
ELIMINATION • Decreased voiding, dark urine • Night voiding	• Decreased daytime urination and increased nighttime urination (nocturia)
FOOD/FLUID • History of diet high in salt and processed foods, fat, sugar, and caffeine • Loss of appetite, anorexia • Nausea, vomiting • Significant weight gain (may not respond to diuretic use) • Tight clothing or shoes • Use of diuretics	• Rapid or continuous weight gain • Generalized edema, including whole body or lower extremity swelling—edema generalized, dependent, pitting, brawny • Abdominal distention, suggesting ascites or liver engorgement
HYGIENE • Fatigue, weakness, exhaustion during self-care activities	• Appearance indicative of neglect of personal care

DIAGNOSTIC DIVISION MAY REPORT (continued)	MAY EXHIBIT (continued)
NEUROSENSORY • Weakness • Dizziness • Fainting episodes	• Lethargy, confusion, disorientation • Behavior changes, irritability
PAIN/DISCOMFORT • Chest pain • Chronic or acute angina • Right upper abdominal pain (right-sided HF) • Generalized muscle aches and pains	• Restlessness • Narrowed focus and withdrawal • Guarding behavior
RESPIRATION • Dyspnea with exertion or rest • Nocturnal dyspnea that interrupts sleep • Sleeping sitting up or with several pillows • Cough with or without sputum production, especially when recumbent • Use of respiratory aids, for example, oxygen or medications	• Tachypnea • Shallow, labored breathing • Use of accessory muscles, nasal flaring • Moist cough with left-sided HF • Sputum may be blood-tinged, pink and frothy (pulmonary edema) • Breath sounds may be diminished, with bibasilar crackles and wheezes • Mentation may be diminished; lethargy, restlessness present • Pallor or cyanosis
SAFETY	• Changes in mentation and confusion • Loss of strength or muscle tone • Increasing risk for falls • Skin excoriations, rashes
SOCIAL INTERACTION • Decreased participation in usual social activities	
TEACHING/LEARNING • Family history of developing HF at young age (genetic form) • Family risk factors, such as heart disease, hypertension, diabetes • Use or misuse of cardiac medications • Use of vitamins, herbal supplements, for example, niacin, coenzyme Q10, garlic, ginkgo, black hellebore, dandelion, or aspirin • Recent or recurrent hospitalizations • Evidence of failure to improve	
DISCHARGE PLAN CONSIDERATIONS • Assistance with shopping, transportation, self-care needs, homemaker and maintenance tasks • Alteration in medication use or therapy • Changes in physical layout of home • May need oxygen at home ⬦ Refer to section at end of plan for postdischarge considerations.	

TEST WHY IT IS DONE	WHAT IT TELLS ME
BLOOD TESTS	
• *Atrial natriuretic peptide (ANP):* Hormone secreted from right atrial cells when pressure increases.	Increased in congestive HF.
• *Beta-type natriuretic peptide (BNP):* Neurohormone secreted from the cardiac ventricles as a response to ventricular volume and fluid overload.	The level of BNP in the blood increases when symptoms of HF worsen and decreases when symptoms of HF improve to stable condition. Elevation of BNP correlates with both the severity of symptoms and the prognosis in congestive HF. A level of BNP that is greater than 100 pg/mL is predictive of HF and increased risk of sudden death (Berger et al, 2002).
• *Complete blood count (CBC):* Battery of screening tests that includes hemoglobin (Hgb); hematocrit (Hct); red blood cell (RBC) count; morphology, indices, and distribution width index; platelet count and size; white blood cell (WBC) count and differential tests.	May reveal anemia (major contributor and exacerbating factor in HF), polycythemia, or dilutional changes indicating water retention. WBCs may be elevated, reflecting recent or acute MI, pericarditis, or other inflammatory or infectious states. *Note:* Anemia may be a sign of disease progression and is associated with impaired survival.
• *Liver enzyme tests, alanine aminotransferase (ALT) and aspartate aminotransferase (AST) (formally referred to as SPGT and SGOT):* To determine degree of end-organ involvement.	Elevated in liver congestion, which may be present in right-sided HF.
• *Digoxin and other cardiac drug levels:* Monitored to determine therapeutic range of medications.	Correlation of expected response with client response permits adjustment of medication regimen.
• *Erythrocyte sedimentation rate (ESR):* Shows the alteration of blood proteins caused by inflammatory and necrotic processes.	May be elevated, indicating acute systemic inflammatory reaction, especially if viral infection is cause of HF.
• *Bleeding and clotting times:* Clotting factors, prothrombin time (PT), partial thromboplastin time (PTT), platelets.	Identifies those at risk for excessive clot formation and identifies therapeutic range for anticoagulant therapy.
• *Electrolytes (sodium, potassium, chloride, magnesium, calcium):* Elements or chemicals needed for the body and heart to work properly.	Electrolytes may be altered because of fluid shifts and decreased renal function associated with HF and medications (e.g., diuretics, ACE inhibitors) used in HF treatment.
• *Blood urea nitrogen (BUN) and creatinine:* BUN levels reflect the balance between production and excretion of urea. Creatine is end-product of creatinine metabolism and must be cleared from blood via the kidneys.	Elevated BUN suggests decreased renal perfusion as may occur with HF or as a side effect of prescribed medications (e.g., diuretics and ACE inhibitors). Elevation of both BUN and creatinine is typical in HF.
• *Albumin and transferrin, total protein:* Plasma proteins exert oncotic pressure needed to keep fluid in the capillaries.	May be decreased as a result of reduced protein intake (nutritional) or reduced protein synthesis (congested liver associated with HF).
• *Thyroid studies:* Blood test and scan to evaluate thyroid function. The most commonly used laboratory screening test is the measurement of thyroid-stimulating hormone (TSH).	Increased thyroid activity suggests thyroid hyperactivity as precipitator of HF. Hypothyroidism can also cause or exacerbate HF.
• *Arterial blood gas (ABG) value:* Measures arterial pH, PCO_2, and PO_2. Evaluates respiratory function and provides a measure for determining acid-base balance.	Left ventricular failure is characterized by mild respiratory alkalosis (early); respiratory acidosis, with hypoxemia; and increased PCO_2, with decompensated HF.
OTHER DIAGNOSTIC STUDIES	
• *Chest x-ray:* Evaluates organs and structures within the chest.	May demonstrate calcification in valve areas or aorta, causing blood flow obstruction, or cardiac enlargement, indicating HF. Infiltrates in the lungs indicate presence of congestion.
• *Electrocardiogram (ECG):* Record of the electrical activity of the heart.	An abnormal ECG can point out the underlying cause of HF, such as ventricular hypertrophy, valvular dysfunction, ischemia, and myocardial damage patterns. Dysrhythmias, such as tachycardia, atrial fibrillation, and conduction delays, especially left bundle branch block and frequent premature ventricular contractions (PVCs), may be present. Persistent ST-T segment abnormalities and decreased QRS amplitude may be present.

Diagnostic Studies (continued)

TEST WHY IT IS DONE (continued)	WHAT IT TELLS ME (continued)
• *Echocardiography (also called two-dimensional echocardiogram or Doppler ultrasound):* Evaluates the left ventricle, including size, valvular function, wall thickness, and pumping action as measured by the ejection fraction (EF).	May reveal enlarged chamber dimensions, alterations in valvular and ventricular function and structure. EF is reduced (less than 50%) indicating systolic dysfunction or "preserved" (normal is 50% to 65%) indicating diastolic dysfunction (Cunningham, 2006).
• *Stress test (also called exercise treadmill or exercise ECG):* Raises heart rate and BP by means of exercise; heart rate can also be raised pharmacologically through the use of such drugs as dobutamine or dipyridamol.	Helps detect valvular heart disease, ventricular remodeling and structural anomalies, and problems with coronary circulation affecting heart function.
• *Cardiac angiography (also called cardiac catheterization):* Assesses patency of coronary arteries, reveals abnormal heart and valve size or shape, and evaluates ventricular contractility. Pressures can be measured within each chamber of the heart and across the valves.	Abnormal pressures indicate problems with ventricular function, helping to identify valvular stenosis or insufficiency and differentiating right-sided versus left-sided HF.
• *Pulse oximetry:* Noninvasive study that provides continuous readings of arterial blood oxygen saturation.	Oxygen saturation (SPO_2) may be low, especially when acute HF is imposed on chronic obstructive pulmonary disease (COPD) or chronic HF.

Nursing Priorities

1. Improve myocardial contractility and systemic perfusion.
2. Reduce fluid volume overload.
3. Prevent complications.
4. Provide information about disease and prognosis, therapy needs, and prevention of recurrences.

Discharge Goals

1. Cardiac output adequate for individual needs.
2. Complications prevented or resolved.
3. Optimum level of activity and functioning attained.
4. Disease process, prognosis, and therapeutic regimen understood.
5. Plan in place to meet needs after discharge.

NURSING DIAGNOSIS: decreased Cardiac Output

May be related to
Altered myocardial contractility, inotropic changes
Alterations in rate, rhythm, electrical conduction
Structural changes, such as valvular defects and ventricular aneurysm

Possibly evidenced by
Increased heart rate (tachycardia), dysrhythmias, ECG changes
Changes in BP (hypotension, hypertension)
Extra heart sounds (S_3, S_4)
Decreased urine output
Diminished peripheral pulses
Cool, ashen skin and diaphoresis
Orthopnea, crackles, JVD, liver engorgement, edema
Chest pain

Desired Outcomes/Evaluation Criteria—Client Will

Cardiac Pump Effectiveness (NOC)
Display vital signs within acceptable limits, dysrhythmias absent or controlled, and no symptoms of failure, for example, hemodynamic parameters within acceptable limits and urinary output adequate.
Report decreased episodes of dyspnea and angina.

Cardiac Disease Self-Management (NOC)
Participate in activities that reduce cardiac workload.

ACTIONS/INTERVENTIONS	RATIONALE

Hemodynamic Regulation (NIC)

Independent

Auscultate apical pulse; assess heart rate, rhythm, and document dysrhythmia if telemetry available.	Tachycardia is usually present, even at rest, to compensate for decreased ventricular contractility. Premature atrial contractions (PACs), paroxysmal atrial tachycardia (PAT), PVCs, multifocal atrial tachycardia (MAT), and AF are common dysrhythmias associated with HF, although others may also occur. *Note:* Intractable ventricular dysrhythmias unresponsive to medication suggest ventricular aneurysm.
Note heart sounds.	S_1 and S_2 may be weak because of diminished pumping action. Gallop rhythms are common (S_3 and S_4), produced as blood flows into noncompliant, distended chambers. Murmurs may reflect valvular incompetence and stenosis.
Palpate peripheral pulses.	Decreased cardiac output may be reflected in diminished radial, popliteal, dorsalis pedis, and post-tibial pulses. Pulses may be fleeting or irregular to palpation, and pulsus alternans may be present.
Monitor BP.	In early, moderate, or chronic HF, BP may be elevated because of increased SVR. In advanced HF, the body may no longer be able to compensate, and profound or irreversible hypotension may occur. *Note:* Many clients with HF have consistently low systolic BP (80 to 100 mm Hg) due to their disease process and the medications they take, and most tolerate these BPs without incident (Wingate, 2007).
Inspect skin for pallor and cyanosis.	Pallor is indicative of diminished peripheral perfusion secondary to inadequate cardiac output, vasoconstriction, and anemia. Cyanosis may develop in refractory HF. Dependent areas are often blue or mottled as venous congestion increases.
Monitor urine output, noting decreasing output and dark or concentrated urine.	Kidneys respond to reduced cardiac output by retaining water and sodium. Urine output is usually decreased during the day because of fluid shifts into tissues, but may be increased at night because fluid returns to circulation when client is recumbent.
Note changes in sensorium, for example, lethargy, confusion, disorientation, anxiety, and depression.	May indicate inadequate cerebral perfusion secondary to decreased cardiac output.
Encourage rest, semirecumbent in bed or chair. Assist with physical care, as indicated.	Physical rest should be maintained during acute or refractory HF to improve efficiency of cardiac contraction and to decrease myocardial oxygen consumption and workload.
Provide quiet environment, explain medical and nursing management, help client avoid stressful situations, listen and respond to expressions of feelings or fears.	Physical and psychological rest helps reduce stress, which can produce vasoconstriction, elevating BP and increasing heart rate and work.
Provide bedside commode. Have client avoid activities eliciting a vasovagal response, for instance, straining during defecation and holding breath during position changes.	Commode use decreases work of getting to bathroom or struggling to use bedpan. Vasovagal maneuver causes vagal stimulation followed by rebound tachycardia, which further compromises cardiac function and output.
Elevate legs, avoiding pressure under knee. Encourage active and passive exercises. Increase ambulation and activity as tolerated.	Decreases venous stasis and may reduce incidence of thrombus and embolus formation.
Check for calf tenderness; diminished pedal pulse; and swelling, local redness, or pallor of extremity.	Reduced cardiac output, venous pooling and stasis, and enforced bedrest increases risk of thrombophlebitis.
Withhold digoxin, as indicated, and notify physician if marked changes occur in cardiac rate or rhythm or signs of digoxin toxicity occur.	Incidence of toxicity is high (20%) because of narrow margin between therapeutic and toxic ranges. Digoxin may have to be discontinued in the presence of toxic drug levels, a slow heart rate, or low potassium level. (Refer to CP: Dysrhythmias; ND: risk for Poisoning: digoxin toxicity.)

Collaborative

Administer supplemental oxygen, as indicated.	Increases available oxygen for myocardial uptake to combat effects of hypoxia and ischemia.
Administer medications, as indicated, for example:	A variety of medications (usually a combination of a diuretic, an ACEI, or ARB and beta blocker) may be used to increase stroke volume, improve contractility, and reduce congestion.

ACTIONS/INTERVENTIONS (continued)	RATIONALE (continued)
Loop diuretics, such as furosemide (Lasix), ethacrynic acid (Edecrin), and bumetanide (Bumex); thiazide and thiazide-like diuretics, such as hydrocholorothiazide (HydroDiuril) and metolazone (Zaroxolyn)	Diuretics, in conjunction with restriction of dietary sodium and fluids, often lead to clinical improvement in clients with stages I and II HF. In general, type and dosage of diuretic depend on cause and degree of HF and state of renal function. Preload reduction is most useful in treating clients with a relatively normal cardiac output accompanied by congestive symptoms. Loop diuretics block chloride reabsorption, thus interfering with the reabsorption of sodium and water.
ACE inhibitors, such as benazepril (Lotensin), captopril (Capoten), lisinopril (Prinivil), enalapril (Vasotec), quinapril (Accupril), ramipril (Altace), and moexipril (Univasc)	ACE inhibitors represent first-line therapy to control HF by decreasing ventricular filling pressures and SVR, while increasing cardiac output with little or no change in BP and heart rate.
ARBs (also known as angiotensin II receptor antagonists), such as candesartan (Atacand), losartan (Cozaar), eprosartan (Teveten), ibesartan (Avapro), and valsartan (Diovan)	Antihypertensive and cardioprotective effects are attributable to selective blockade of AT_1 (angiotensin II) receptors and angiotensin II synthesis. *Note:* ARBs used in combination with ACE inhibitors and beta blockers are thought to have decreased hospitalizations for HF clients.
Vasodilators, such as nitrates (Nitro-Dur, Isordil); arteriodilators such as hydralazine (Apresoline); combination drugs, such as prazosin (Minipress) and nesiritide (Natrecor)	Vasodilators are used to increase cardiac and renal output, reducing circulating volume (preload and afterload), and decreasing SVR, thereby reducing ventricular workload. *Note:* Nesiritide is used in acutely decompensated congestive HF and has been used with digoxin, diuretics, and ACE inhibitors. Parenteral vasodilators are reserved for clients with severe HF or those unable to take oral medications.
β-adrenergic receptor antagonists (also called beta blockers), such as carvedilol (Coreg), bisoprolol (Zebeta), and metoprolol (Lopressor)	Useful in the treatment of HF by blocking the cardiac effects of chronic adrenergic stimulation. Many clients experience improved activity tolerance and EF.
Digoxin (Lanoxin)	Increases force of myocardial contraction when diminished contractility is the cause of HF and slows heart rate by decreasing conduction velocity and prolonging refractory period of the atrioventricular (AV) junction to increase cardiac efficiency and output.
Inotropic agents, such as amrinone (Inocor), milrinone (Primacor), and vesnarinone (Arkin-Z)	These medications are useful for short-term treatment of HF unresponsive to cardiac glycosides, vasodilators, and diuretics in order to increase myocardial contractility and produce vasodilation. Positive inotropic properties have reduced mortality rates (by 50%) and improved quality of life.
Aldosterone antagonist, such as eplerenone (Inspra)	Approved by the Food and Drug Administration (FDA) in 2003, eplerenone has been shown to improve survival in HF, especially following MI.
Morphine sulfate	Decreases vascular resistance and venous return, reducing myocardial workload, especially when pulmonary congestion is present.
Anti-anxiety agents and sedatives	Allays anxiety and breaks the feedback cycle of anxiety to catecholamine release to anxiety. Promotes rest and relaxation, reducing oxygen demand and myocardial workload.
Anticoagulants, such as low-dose heparin and warfarin (Coumadin)	May be used prophylactically to prevent thrombus and embolus formation in the presence of risk factors, such as venous stasis, enforced bedrest, cardiac dysrhythmias, and history of previous thrombolic episodes.
Administer IV solutions, restricting total amount, as indicated. Avoid saline solutions.	Because of existing elevated left ventricular pressure, client may not tolerate increased fluid volume (preload). Clients with HF also excrete less sodium, which causes fluid retention and increases myocardial workload.
Monitor and replace electrolytes, as indicated.	Fluid shifts and use of diuretics can alter electrolytes (especially potassium and chloride), which affect cardiac rhythm and contractility.
Monitor serial ECG and chest x-ray changes.	ST-segment depression and T-wave flattening can develop because of increased myocardial oxygen demand, even if no CAD is present. Chest x-ray may show enlarged heart and changes of pulmonary congestion.
Measure cardiac output and other functional parameters, as indicated.	Cardiac index, preload and afterload, contractility, and cardiac work can be measured noninvasively by using thoracic electrical bioimpedance (TEB) technique. TEB is useful in determining effectiveness of therapeutic interventions and response to activity.

(continues on page 56)

Prepare for insertion and maintain pacemaker or pacemaker/defibrillator, if indicated.	May be necessary to correct bradydysrhythmias unresponsive to drug intervention, which can aggravate congestive failure and produce pulmonary edema. *Note:* Biventricular pacemaker and cardiac defibrillators are designed to provide resynchronization for the heart by simultaneous electrical activation of both the right and left sides of the heart, thereby creating a more effective and efficient pump.
Prepare for surgery, such as valve replacement, angioplasty, coronary artery bypass grafting (CABG), as indicated:	HF due to ventricular aneurysm or valvular dysfunction may require aneurysmectomy or valve replacement to improve myocardial contractility and function. Revascularization of cardiac muscle by CABG may be done to improve cardiac function.
Cardiomyoplasty	Cardiomyoplasty, an experimental procedure in which the latissimus dorsi muscle is wrapped around the heart and electrically stimulated to contract with each heartbeat, may be done to augment ventricular function while the client is awaiting cardiac transplantation or when transplantation is not an option.
Transmyocardial revascularization	Other new surgical techniques include transmyocardial revascularization, such as percutaneous transmyocardial revascularization (PTMR), using CO_2 laser technology, in which a laser is used to create multiple 1-mm-diameter channels in viable but underperfused cardiac muscle.
Assist with and maintain mechanical circulatory support system, such as intra-aortic balloon pump (IABP) or left-ventricular assist device (LVAD), when indicated.	An IABP may be inserted as a temporary support to the failing heart in the critically ill client with potentially reversible HF. A battery-powered LVAD may also be used positioned between the cardiac apex and the descending thoracic or abdominal aorta. This device receives blood from the left ventricle and ejects it into the systemic circulation, often allowing client to resume a nearly normal lifestyle while awaiting heart transplantation, or in some instances, allowing the heart to recover and regain its function. With end-stage HF, cardiac transplantation may be indicated.

NURSING DIAGNOSIS: Activity Intolerance

May be related to
Imbalance between oxygen supply and demand
Generalized weakness
Prolonged bedrest, immobility

Possibly evidenced by
Weakness, fatigue
Changes in vital signs, presence of dysrhythmias
Dyspnea
Pallor, diaphoresis

Desired Outcomes/Evaluation Criteria—Client Will

Endurance (NOC)
Participate in desired activities; meet own self-care needs.
Achieve measurable increase in activity tolerance, evidenced by reduced fatigue and weakness and by vital signs within acceptable limits during activity.

ACTIONS/INTERVENTIONS | RATIONALE

Energy Management (NIC)
Independent

Check vital signs before and immediately after activity during acute episode or exacerbation of HF, especially if client is receiving vasodilators, diuretics, or beta blockers.	Orthostatic hypotension can occur with activity because of medication effect (vasodilation), fluid shifts (diuresis), or compromised cardiac pumping function.
Document cardiopulmonary response to activity. Note tachycardia, dysrhythmias, dyspnea, diaphoresis, and pallor.	Compromised myocardium and inability to increase stroke volume during activity may cause an immediate increase in heart rate and oxygen demands, thereby aggravating weakness and fatigue.

ACTIONS/INTERVENTIONS (continued)

Assess level of fatigue, and evaluate for other precipitators and causes of fatigue, for example, HF treatments, pain, cachexia, anemia, and depression.

Evaluate accelerating activity intolerance.

Provide assistance with self-care activities, as indicated. Intersperse activity with rest periods.

Collaborative
Implement graded cardiac rehabilitation and activity program.

RATIONALE (continued)

Fatigue because of advanced HF can be profound and is related to hemodynamic, respiratory, and peripheral muscle abnormalities. Fatigue is also a side effect of some medications (e.g., beta blockers). Other key causes of fatigue should be evaluated and treated as appropriate and desired.

May denote increasing cardiac decompensation rather than overactivity.

Meets client's personal care needs without undue myocardial stress or excessive oxygen demand.

Strengthens and improves cardiac function under stress if cardiac dysfunction is not irreversible. Gradual increase in activity avoids excessive myocardial workload and oxygen consumption.

NURSING DIAGNOSIS: excess Fluid Volume

May be related to
Reduced glomerular filtration rate (decreased cardiac output), increased antidiuretic hormone (ADH) production, and sodium and water retention

Possibly evidenced by
Orthopnea, S_3 heart sound
Oliguria, edema, JVD, positive hepatojugular reflex
Weight gain
Hypertension
Respiratory distress, abnormal breath sounds

Desired Outcomes/Evaluation Criteria—Client Will

Fluid Overload Severity (NOC)
Demonstrate stabilized fluid volume with balanced intake and output, breath sounds clear or clearing, vital signs within acceptable range, stable weight, and absence of edema.
Verbalize understanding of individual dietary and fluid restrictions.

ACTIONS/INTERVENTIONS

Fluid Management (NIC)
Independent
Monitor urine output, noting amount and color, as well as time of day when diuresis occurs.

Monitor 24-hour intake and output (I&O) balance.

Maintain chair rest or bedrest in semi-Fowler's position during acute phase.
Establish fluid intake schedule if fluids are medically restricted, incorporating beverage preferences when possible.
Give frequent mouth care and ice chips as part of fluid allotment.
Weigh daily.

Assess for distended neck and peripheral vessels. Inspect dependent body areas for edema with and without pitting; note presence of generalized body edema (anasarca).

RATIONALE

Urine output may be scanty and concentrated (especially during the day) because of reduced renal perfusion. Recumbency favors diuresis; therefore, urine output may be increased at night or during bedrest.

Diuretic therapy may result in sudden or excessive fluid loss, creating a circulating hypovolemia, even though edema and ascites remains in the client with advanced HF or CHF.

Recumbency increases glomerular filtration and decreases production of ADH, thereby enhancing diuresis.

Involving client in therapy regimen may enhance sense of control and cooperation with restrictions.

Documents changes in or resolution of edema in response to therapy. A gain of 5 lb represents approximately 2 L of fluid. Conversely, diuretics can result in rapid and excessive fluid shifts and weight loss.

Excessive fluid retention may be manifested by venous engorgement and edema formation. Peripheral edema begins in feet and ankles, or dependent areas, and ascends as failure worsens. Pitting edema is generally obvious only after retention of at least 10 lb of fluid. Increased vascular congestion—associated with right-sided HF—eventually results in systemic tissue edema.

(continues on page 58)

ACTIONS/INTERVENTIONS (continued)	RATIONALE (continued)
Change position frequently. Elevate feet when sitting. Inspect skin surface, keep dry, and provide padding, as indicated. (Refer to ND: risk for impaired Skin Integrity.)	Edema formation, slowed circulation, altered nutritional intake, and prolonged immobility or bedrest are cumulative stressors that affect skin integrity and require close supervision and preventive interventions.
Auscultate breath sounds, noting decreased and adventitious sounds, for example, crackles and wheezes. Note presence of increased dyspnea, tachypnea, orthopnea, paroxysmal nocturnal dyspnea, and persistent cough.	Excess fluid volume often leads to pulmonary congestion. Symptoms of pulmonary edema may reflect acute left-sided HF. With right-sided HF, respiratory symptoms of dyspnea, cough, and orthopnea may have slower onset, but are more difficult to reverse. *Note:* Among clients with advanced HF, 60% experience significant dyspnea (Pantilat & Steimle, 2004), usually related to volume overload.
Investigate reports of sudden extreme dyspnea and air hunger, need to sit straight up, sensation of suffocation, feelings of panic or impending doom.	May indicate development of complications, such as pulmonary edema or embolus, which differs from orthopnea or paroxysmal nocturnal dyspnea in that it develops much more rapidly and requires immediate intervention.
Monitor BP and central venous pressure (CVP) (if available).	Hypertension and elevated CVP suggest fluid volume excess and may reflect developing or increasing pulmonary congestion, HF.
Assess bowel sounds. Note complaints of anorexia, nausea, abdominal distention, and constipation.	Visceral congestion, occurring in progressive HF, can alter gastrointestinal function.
Provide small, frequent, easily digestible meals.	Reduced gastric motility can adversely affect digestion and absorption. Small, frequent meals may enhance digestion and prevent abdominal discomfort.
Measure abdominal girth, as indicated.	In progressive right-sided HF, fluid may shift into the peritoneal space, causing increasing abdominal girth (ascites).
Encourage verbalization of feelings regarding limitations.	Expression of feelings or concerns may decrease stress and anxiety, which is an energy drain that can contribute to feelings of fatigue.
Palpate abdomen. Note reports of right upper-quadrant pain or tenderness.	Advancing HF leads to venous congestion, resulting in abdominal distention, liver engorgement (hepatomegaly), and pain. This can alter liver function and impair or prolong drug metabolism.
Note increased lethargy, hypotension, and muscle cramping.	These are signs of potassium and sodium deficits that may occur because of fluid shifts and diuretic therapy.
Fluid [or] Electrolyte Management (NIC) *Collaborative* Administer medications, as indicated, for example:	
Diuretics, such as furosemide (Lasix) and bumetanide (Bumex)	Increases rate of urine flow and may inhibit reabsorption of sodium and chloride in the renal tubules.
Thiazides with potassium-sparing agents, such as spironolactone (Aldactone)	Promotes diuresis without excessive potassium losses.
Potassium supplements, such as K-Dur	Replaces potassium that is lost as a common side effect of diuretic therapy, which can adversely affect cardiac function.
Maintain fluid and sodium restrictions, as indicated.	Reduces total body water and prevents fluid reaccumulation.
Consult with dietitian.	May be necessary to provide diet acceptable to client that meets caloric needs within sodium restriction.
Monitor chest x-ray.	Reveals changes indicative of increase or resolution of pulmonary congestion.
Assist with rotating tourniquets and phlebotomy, dialysis, or ultrafiltration, as indicated.	Although not frequently used, mechanical fluid removal rapidly reduces circulating volume, especially in pulmonary edema refractory to other therapies.

NURSING DIAGNOSIS: risk for impaired Gas Exchange

Risk factors may include
Alveolar-capillary membrane changes such as fluid collection and shifts into interstitial space or alveoli

Possibly evidenced by
(Not applicable; presence of signs and symptoms establishes an *actual* diagnosis)

Desired Outcomes/Evaluation Criteria—Client Will

Respiratory Status: Gas Exchange (NOC)
Demonstrate adequate ventilation and oxygenation of tissues by ABG values and oximetry within client's normal ranges and be free of symptoms of respiratory distress.
Participate in treatment regimen within level of ability and situation.

ACTIONS/INTERVENTIONS

RATIONALE

Airway Management (NIC)
Independent

Auscultate breath sounds, noting crackles and wheezes.

Instruct client in effective coughing and deep breathing.
Encourage frequent position changes.
Maintain chair rest and bedrest in a semi-Fowler's position, with head of bed elevated 20 to 30 degrees. Support arms with pillows.

Collaborative

Monitor and graph serial ABG values and pulse oximetry.

Administer supplemental oxygen, as indicated.

Administer medications, as indicated, such as the following:
Diuretics, for example, furosemide (Lasix)
Bronchodilators, for example, aminophylline

Reveals presence of pulmonary congestion or collection of secretions, indicating need for further intervention.
Clears airways and facilitates oxygen delivery.
Helps prevent atelectasis and pneumonia.
Reduces oxygen consumption and demands and promotes maximal lung inflation.

Hypoxemia can be severe during pulmonary edema. Compensatory changes are usually present in chronic HF.
Increases alveolar oxygen concentration, which may correct or reduce tissue hypoxemia.

Reduce alveolar congestion, enhancing gas exchange.
Increase oxygen delivery by dilating small airways and exert mild diuretic effect to aid in reducing pulmonary congestion.

NURSING DIAGNOSIS: risk for chronic Pain

Risk factors may include
Chronic physical disease or condition
Altered ability to continue previous activities

Possibly evidenced by
(Not applicable; presence of signs and symptoms establishes an *actual* diagnosis)

Desired Outcomes/Evaluation Criteria—Client Will

Pain Control (NOC)
Verbalize and demonstrate relief or control of pain or discomfort.
Demonstrate and initiate behavioral modifications of lifestyle and appropriate use of therapeutic interventions.

ACTIONS/INTERVENTIONS

RATIONALE

Pain Management (NIC)
Independent

Assess for presence of pain.

Note coexisting condition(s).

Assess for lifestyle effects of pain, such as deconditioning, severe fatigue, weight loss or gain, sleep difficulties, and depression.

Provide anticipatory guidance.

Collaborative

Assist with treatment of underlying or coexisting conditions.
Administer analgesics, as indicated.

Pain, physical discomfort, or both are reported by 30% to 80% of clients with advanced HF (Walke et al, 2004). It is unknown whether pain occurs because of the HF itself, due to edema, chest fullness, and underperfused organs (Wingate, 2007).
Many HF clients are elderly and have multiple chronic conditions, such as angina, arthritis, gout, back pain, claudication, and neuropathies.
Pain issues should be addressed and managed, when present, even though it may not be possible to determine if pain is a result of the HF itself (associated with underperfused organs) or be related to other conditions.
In client with HF in which pain is common (Wingate, 2007), educating client and significant other (SO) about when, where, and how to seek interventions or treatment may reduce limitations imposed by pain. If pain is present, pain management should be initiated.

Promotes comfort and general well-being.
Promotes rest and relaxation and enhances ability to engage in activity.

NURSING DIAGNOSIS: risk for impaired Skin Integrity

Risk factors may include
Prolonged bedrest
Edema, decreased tissue perfusion

Possibly evidenced by
(Not applicable; presence of signs and symptoms establishes an *actual* diagnosis)

Desired Outcomes/Evaluation Criteria—Client Will

Tissue Perfusion: Peripheral (NOC)
Maintain skin integrity.
Demonstrate behaviors or techniques to prevent skin breakdown.

ACTIONS/INTERVENTIONS	RATIONALE
Pressure Management (NIC)	
Independent	
Inspect skin, noting skeletal prominences, presence of edema, and areas of altered circulation and pigmentation.	Skin is at risk because of impaired peripheral circulation, obesity or emaciation, edema, physical immobility, and alterations in nutritional status.
Provide gentle massage around reddened or blanched areas.	Improves blood flow, minimizing tissue hypoxia. *Note:* Direct massage of compromised area may cause tissue injury.
Encourage frequent position changes in bed and chair. Assist with active or passive range of motion (ROM) exercises.	Reduces pressure on tissues, improving circulation and reducing time any one area is deprived of full blood flow.
Provide frequent skin care; minimize contact with moisture or excretions.	Excessive dryness or moisture damages skin and hastens breakdown.
Check fit of shoes or slippers and change as needed.	Dependent edema may cause shoes to fit poorly, thereby increasing risk of pressure and skin breakdown on feet.
Avoid intramuscular route for medication administration.	Interstitial edema and impaired circulation impede drug absorption and predispose to tissue breakdown and development of infection.
Collaborative	
Provide alternating pressure or egg-crate mattress and sheepskin elbow and heel protectors.	Reduces pressure to skin and may improve circulation.

NURSING DIAGNOSIS: deficient Knowledge [Learning Need] regarding condition, treatment regimen, self-care, and discharge needs

May be related to
Lack of understanding, misconceptions about interrelatedness of cardiac function, disease, and failure

Possibly evidenced by
Questions
Statements of concern, misconceptions
Recurrent, preventable episodes of HF

Desired Outcomes/Evaluation Criteria—Client Will

Knowledge: Cardiac Disease Management (NOC)
Identify relationship of ongoing therapies (treatment program) to reduction of recurrent episodes and prevention of complications.
List signs and symptoms that require immediate intervention.
Identify own stress and risk factors and some techniques for handling them.
Initiate necessary lifestyle and behavioral changes.

ACTIONS/INTERVENTIONS	RATIONALE
Teaching: Disease Process (NIC)	
Independent	
Discuss normal heart function. Include information regarding client's variance from normal function. Explain difference between heart attack and HF.	Knowledge of disease process and expectations can facilitate client's participation in management of HF, including prescribed treatment regimen (Tenenbaum, 2003).

ACTIONS/INTERVENTIONS (continued)	**RATIONALE** (continued)
Reinforce treatment rationale. Include SO and family members in teaching as appropriate, especially for complicated regimens such as management of technology, for example, implantable cardioverter-defibrillator (ICD) or LVAD, dobutamine infusion home therapy when client does not respond to customary combination therapy or cannot be weaned from dobutamine, or in those awaiting heart transplant.	Client may believe it is acceptable to alter postdischarge regimen when feeling well and symptom-free or when feeling below par, which can increase the risk of exacerbation of symptoms. Understanding of regimen, medications, technology, and restrictions may augment cooperation with control of symptoms. Home IV therapy requires a significant commitment by caregivers to operate and troubleshoot infusion pump, change dressing for peripherally inserted central catheter (PICC) line, and monitor I&O and signs and symptoms of HF.
Encourage developing a regular home exercise program and provide guidelines for sexual activity.	Promotes maintenance of muscle tone and organ function for overall sense of well-being. Changing sexual habits, for example, sex in morning when well rested, client on top, inclusion of other physical expressions of affection, may be difficult, but provides opportunity for continuing satisfying sexual relationship.
Discuss importance of being as active as possible without becoming exhausted and need for rest between activities.	Excessive physical activity or overexertion can further weaken the heart, exacerbating failure, and necessitates adjustment of exercise program.
Discuss importance of sodium limitation. Provide list of sodium content of common foods that are to be avoided or limited. Encourage reading of labels on food and drug packages.	Dietary intake of sodium of more than 3 g/day can offset effect of diuretic. Most common source of sodium is table salt and obviously salty foods, although canned soups and vegetables, luncheon meats, and dairy products also may contain high levels of sodium.
Refer to dietitian for counseling specific to individual needs and dietary customs.	Identifies dietary needs, especially in presence of obesity (major risk factor for developing HF), diabetes, or presence of nausea and vomiting and resulting wasting syndrome (cardiac cachexia). Eating six small meals and using liquid dietary supplements and vitamin supplements can limit inappropriate weight loss.
Review medications, purpose, and side effects. Provide both oral and written instructions.	Understanding therapeutic needs and importance of prompt reporting of side effects can prevent occurrence of drug-related complications. Anxiety may block comprehension of input or details, and client and SO may refer to written material at later date to refresh memory.
Recommend taking diuretic early in morning.	Provides adequate time for drug effect before bedtime to prevent or limit interruption of sleep.
Instruct and receive return demonstration of ability to take and record daily pulse and BP and when to notify healthcare provider, for example, parameters above or below preset rate and changes in rhythm or regularity.	Promotes self-monitoring of condition and drug effect. Early detection of changes allows for timely intervention and may prevent complications, such as digoxin toxicity.
Explain and discuss client's role in control of risk factors, such as smoking and alcohol abuse, and precipitating or aggravating factors, such as high-salt diet, inactivity or overexertion, and exposure to extremes in temperature.	Adds to body of knowledge and permits client to make informed decisions regarding control of condition and prevention of recurrence or complications. Smoking potentiates vasoconstriction; sodium intake promotes water retention and edema formation. Improper balance between activity and rest and exposure to temperature extremes may result in exhaustion, increased myocardial workload, and increased risk of respiratory infections. Alcohol can depress cardiac contractility. Limitation of alcohol use to social occasions or maximum of one drink per day may be tolerated unless cardiomyopathy is alcohol induced, which requires complete abstinence.
Review signs and symptoms that require immediate medical attention, such as rapid and significant weight gain, edema, shortness of breath, increased fatigue, cough, hemoptysis, and fever.	Self-monitoring increases client responsibility in health maintenance and aids in prevention of complications such as pulmonary edema, pneumonia. Weight gain of more than 3 lb in 1 week requires medical evaluation or adjustment of diuretic therapy. *Note:* Client should weigh self daily in morning without clothing, after voiding, and before eating.
Provide opportunities for client and SO to ask questions, discuss concerns, and make necessary lifestyle changes.	Chronicity and recurrent, debilitating nature of HF often exhausts coping abilities and supportive capacity of both client and SO, leading to depression.
Address caregiver's concerns and needs. Refer for support, assistance, and resources, as indicated.	Caregiver burden can exhaust SO's coping capabilities and health, especially when client has advanced HF, has a ventricular assist device, or is awaiting heart transplantation. (Refer to CP: Multiple Sclerosis, ND: risk for Caregiver Role Strain.)

(continues on page 62)

ACTIONS/INTERVENTIONS (continued)

Discuss general health risks, such as infection, and recommend avoidance of crowds and individuals with respiratory infections and obtaining yearly influenza immunization and one-time pneumonia immunization.

Stress importance of reporting signs and symptoms of digoxin toxicity: development of gastrointestinal and visual disturbances, changes in pulse rate and rhythm, and worsening of HF.

Identify community resources or support groups and visiting home health nurse, as indicated.

Discuss importance of advance directives and of communicating plan and wishes to family and primary care providers.

RATIONALE (continued)

This population is at increased risk for infection because of circulatory compromise.

Early recognition of developing complications and involvement of healthcare provider may prevent toxicity and hospitalization.

May need additional assistance with self-monitoring and home management, especially when HF is progressive.

Up to 50% of all deaths from HF are sudden, with many occurring at home, possibly without significant worsening of symptoms. If client chooses to refuse life-support measures, an alternative contact person (rather than 911) needs to be designated, should cardiac arrest occur.

POTENTIAL CONSIDERATIONS following discharge from care setting (dependent on client's age, physical condition and presence of complications, personal resources, and life responsibilities)
- *Activity Intolerance*—poor cardiac reserve, side effects of medication, generalized weakness
- *excess or deficient Fluid Volume*—changes in glomerular filtration rate, diuretic use, individual fluid and salt intake
- *impaired Skin Integrity*—decreased activity level, prolonged sitting, presence of edema, altered circulation
- *ineffective self Health Management*—complexity of regimen, economic limitations
- *impaired Home Maintenance*—chronic and debilitating condition, insufficient finances, inadequate support systems
- *Self-Care Deficit*—decreased strength and endurance, depression

---

Sample clinical pathway follows in Table 4.1.

TABLE 4.1 **Sample CP: Heart Failure, Hospital. ELOS 4 Days Cardiology or Medical Unit**

ND and Categories of Care	Day 1 _____	Day 2 _____	Day 3 _____	Day 4 _____
Decreased cardiac output R/T decreased myocardial contractility, altered electrical conduction, structural changes	Goals Participate in actions to reduce cardiac workload	Display VS within acceptable limits; dysrhythmias controlled; pulse oximetry within acceptable range Meets own self-care needs with assistance as necessary	→ Dysrhythmias controlled or absent Free of signs of respiratory distress Demonstrate measureable increase in activity tolerance	→ → →
Fluid volume excess R/T compromised regulatory mechanisms—hypertension, sodium/water retention	Verbalize understanding of fluid/food restrictions	Verbalize understanding of general condition and healthcare needs Breath sounds clearing Urinary output adequate Weight loss (reflecting fluid loss)	Plan for lifestyle/behavior changes Breath sounds clear Balanced I&O Edema resolving	Plan in place to meet postdischarge needs Weight stable or continued loss if edema present
Referrals	Cardiology Dietitian	Cardiac rehabilitation Occupational therapist (for ADLs) Social services Home care	Community resources	
Diagnostic studies	ECG, echo-Doppler ultrasound, stress test, cardiac scan CXR ABGs/pulse oximetry Cardiac enzymes; ANP, BNP	Echo-Doppler (if not done day 1) or other cardiac scans Cardiac enzymes (if ↑)	CXR	

TABLE 4.1 **Sample CP: Heart Failure, Hospital. ELOS 4 Days Cardiology or Medical Unit** (continued)

ND and Categories of Care	Day 1 _____	Day 2 _____	Day 3 _____	Day 4 _____
	BUN/Cr			
	CBC/electrolytes, MG++	BUN/Cr	BUN/Cr	
		Electrolytes	Electrolytes	
	PT/aPTT	PT/aPTT (if taking anticoagulants)	PT/aPTT (as indicated)	
	Liver function studies			
	Serum glucose			
	Albumin/total protein			
	Thyroid studies			
	Digoxin level (as indicated)		Repeat digoxin level (if indicated)	
	UA			
Additional assessments	Apical pulse, heart/breath sounds q8h	→	→ bid	→
	Cardiac rhythm (telemetry) q4h	→	→ D/C	
	BP, P, R q2h until stable, q4h	→ q8h	→	→
	Temp q8h	→	→	→
	I&O q8h	→	→	→ D/C
	Weight qAM	→	→	→
	Peripheral edema 8h	→	→ bid	→ qd
	Peripheral pulses 8h	→	→ bid	→ D/C
	Sensorium q8h	→	→ bid	→ D/C
	DVT check qd	→	→	→
	Response to activity	→	→	→
	Response to therapeutic interventions	→	→	→
Medications	IV diuretic	→ PO	→	→
Allergies:	ACEI, ARB, vasodilators, beta blocker	→	→	→
	IV/PO potassium	→	→ D/C	
_____	Digoxin	→	→	→
_____	PO/cutaneous nitrates	→	→	→
	Morphine sulfate	→	→ D/C	
	Daytime hours sedation	→	→	→ D/C
	PO/low-dose anticoagulant	→	→ PO or D/C	→
	Stool softener/laxative	→	→	→
Client education	Orient to unit/room	Cardiac education per protocol	Signs/symptoms to report to healthcare provider	Provide written instructions for homecare
	Review advance directives	Review medications: Dose, times, route, purpose, side effects	Plan for homecare needs	Schedule for follow-up appointments
	Discuss expected outcomes, diagnostic tests/results	Progressive activity program		
	Fluid/nutritional restrictions/needs	Skin care		
Additional nursing actions	Bedrest/chair rest	→ BPR/Ambulate as tolerated, cardiac program	→ Up ad lib/graded program	→
	Assist with physical care	→	→	→
	Pressure-relieving mattress	→	→	→ (send home)

(continues on page 64)

ND and Categories of Care	Day 1 _____	Day 2 _____	Day 3 _____	Day 4 _____
Dysrythmia/angina care per protocol	→		→	→
Supplemental	→			
O₂	→		→ D/C if able	→
Cardiac diet	→		→	

Key: ABG, arterial blood gas; ACEI, angiotensin converting enzyme inhibitor; ad lib, as needed; ADLs, activities of daily living; ANP, atrial natriuretic peptide; aPTT, activated prothrombin time; ARB, angiotensin II receptor blockers; bid, twice a day; BNP, beta-type natriuretic peptide; BP, blood pressure; BRP, bathroom privileges; BUN, blood urea nitrogen; CBC, complete blood count; Cr, creatinine; CXR, chest x-ray; D/C, discontinue; ECG, electrocardiogram; ELOS, estimated length of stay; I&O, intake and output; MG++, magnesium; P, pulse; PO, by mouth; PT, prothrombin time; q2h, every 2 hours; q4h, every 4 hours; q8h, every 8 hours; qAM, every morning; qd, every day; R, respirations; R/T, related to; UA, urinalysis; VS, vital signs.

ANGINA (CORONARY ARTERY DISEASE, ACUTE CORONARY SYNDROME)

I. Pathophysiology
a. The disorder is characterized by a narrowing of coronary arteries due to atherosclerosis, spasm or, rarely, embolism.
b. Atherosclerotic changes in coronary arteries results in damage to the inner layers of the coronary arteries with stiffening of vessels and diminished dilatory response.
c. Accumulation of fatty deposits and lipids, along with development of fibrous plaques over the damaged areas in the vessels, causes narrowing of the arteries, thus reducing the size of the vessel's lumen and impeding blood flow to the myocardial tissues.
d. Decreased delivery of oxygen and nutrients to the tissues causes transient myocardial ischemia and pain.
e. Hard plaque causes hardened arteries, whereas soft plaque can cause formation of blood clots.

II. Types
a. Stable
  i. Most common type, precipitated by physical exertion, emotional stress, exposure to hot or cold temperatures, heavy meals, and smoking
  ii. Occurs in a regular pattern, usually lasts 5 minutes or less, and is easily relieved by medications
b. Unstable
  i. May be new onset of pain with exertion or at rest, or recent acceleration in severity of pain
  ii. Occurs in no regular pattern, usually lasts longer (30 minutes), not generally relieved with rest or medications
  iii. Sometimes grouped with myocardial infarction (MI) under the diagnosis of acute coronary syndrome (ACS)
c. Variant (Prinzmetal's)
  i. Rare, usually occurs at rest—midnight to early morning hours
  ii. Pain possibly severe
  iii. Electrocardiogram (ECG) changes due to coronary artery spasm

III. Classification
a. New York Heart Association Classification (9th edition update, 1994) quantifies the functional limitation imposed by patients' symptoms:
  i. Class I—no limitation of ordinary physical activity
  ii. Class II—slight limitation of ordinary physical activity
  iii. Class III—moderate limitation of activity; comfortable at rest, but less than ordinary activities cause symptoms
  iv. Class IV—unable to perform any physical activity without discomfort, therefore severe limitation and may be symptomatic even at rest
b. Canadian Cardiovascular Society Functional Classification (CCSC) System of unstable angina aids in determining the risk of adverse outcomes and level of treatment needs:
  i. Class 1—no angina with usual physical activities such as walking, climbing stairs; occurs with strenuous, rapid, or prolonged exertion at work or recreation
  ii. Class 2—slight limitation of ordinary activity with angina occurring with moderate exertion such as walking or climbing stairs rapidly, walking uphill, activity after meals, activity in cold or wind, during emotional stress, or during the few hours after awakening
  iii. Class 3—marked limitations of ordinary physical activity with angina occurring during mild exertion, such as walking one to two level blocks or climbing one flight of stairs at a normal pace
  iv. Class 4—angina at any level of physical exertion; may be present even at rest

IV. Etiology
a. Increased cardiac workload: exertion, hypertension, aortic stenosis or regurgitation, hypertrophic cardiomyopathy
b. Decreased O₂ supply: severe anemia, hypoxia
c. Risk factors: being overweight and obese, smoking, sedentary lifestyle, diabetes, family history of early heart disease, metabolic syndrome (fasting hyperglycemia and insulin resistance, hypertension, central obesity, decreased high-density lipoprotein [HDL] and elevated low-density lipoprotein [LDL] cholesterol, elevated triglycerides)

V. Statistics (National Heart, Lung and Blood Institute [NHLBI], 2007; Centers for Disease Control and Prevention [CDC], 2007b)
a. Morbidity: There are an estimated 79.4 million Americans with some form of cardiovascular disease.
  i. Coronary artery disease (CAD) accounting for 15.8 million; angina, approximately 9 million
  ii. 400,000 new cases annually, most are over age 65

b. Prevalence: leading cause of death in Caucasians, African Americans, Hispanics, and American Indians for both males and females

c. Mortality: There were 872,000 deaths from cardio-vascular disease in 2004; accounts for approximately 36% of total deaths.

d. Cost: An estimated $432 billion was spent in 2007.

GLOSSARY

Angioplasty (also called percutaneous transluminal coronary angioplasty, or PTCA): Procedure that increases coronary blood flow by compression of atheromatous lesions and dilation of the vessel lumen in an occluded coronary artery.

Cardiovascular disease (CVD): Diseases of the heart and blood vessels.

Coronary artery disease (CAD): A disease in which there is a narrowing or blockage of the coronary arteries that carry blood and oxygen to the heart muscle.

Ejection fraction (EF): Percentage of blood ejected from the left ventricle; normal is 50% or higher.

Hypertension (HTN): High blood pressure.

Myocardial infarction (MI): An occlusion or blockage of arteries supplying the muscles of the heart, resulting in injury or necrosis of the heart muscle (heart attack).

Thoracic electrical bioimpedance (TEB): Continuous noninvasive real-time monitoring of stroke volume and cardiac output.

Care Setting

Clients judged to be at intermediate or high risk for MI are often hospitalized for further evaluation and therapeutic intervention.

Related Concerns

Cardiac surgery: postoperative care, page 100
Dysrhythmias, page 88
Heart failure: chronic, page 48
Myocardial infarction, page 74
Psychosocial aspects of care, page 749

Client Assessment Database

DIAGNOSTIC DIVISION MAY REPORT	MAY EXHIBIT
ACTIVITY/REST • Sedentary lifestyle • Weakness, feeling incapacitated after exercise • Fatigue • Activities and sleep disrupted by pain	• Exertional dyspnea
CIRCULATION • History of heart disease, hypertension in self or family	• Tachycardia, dysrhythmias • Blood pressure (BP) normal, elevated, or decreased • *Heart sounds:* May be normal, late S_4 or transient late systolic murmur—suggesting papillary muscle dysfunction—that may be evident during pain • Moist, cool, pale skin, mucous membranes in presence of vasoconstriction • Orthostatic blood pressure changes
EGO INTEGRITY • Stressors of work, family, others, and financial concerns	• Apprehension, uneasiness
FOOD/FLUID • Nausea, "heartburn," or epigastric distress with eating, bloating, gas • Diet high in cholesterol and fats, salt, caffeine, liquor	• Belching, gastric distention

(continues on page 66)

NEUROSENSORY
- History of dizziness, fainting spells, transient numbness, tingling in extremities (ischemia anywhere in the body can produce transient neurological symptoms)

PAIN
Note: Reports of pain location and severity differ between men and women.
- Substernal or anterior chest pain that may radiate to jaw, neck, shoulders, and upper extremities, often to left side more than right. Women may report pain between shoulder blades, back pain.
- *Quality:* Varies from transient and mild to moderate, heavy pressure, tightness, squeezing, burning. Women may report dull aching pain.
- *Duration:* Usually less than 15 minutes, rarely more than 30 minutes (average of 3 minutes).
- *Precipitating factors:* Physical exertion or great emotion, such as anger or sexual arousal; exercise in weather extremes; or may be unpredictable or occur during rest or sleep in unstable angina
- *Relieving factors:* Pain may be responsive to particular relief mechanisms, such as rest and anti-anginal medications. Women may not respond to these.
- New or ongoing chest pain that has changed in frequency, duration, character, or predictability, especially unstable, variant, or Prinzmetal's type.

- Facial grimacing, restlessness
- Placing fist over midsternum
- Rubbing left arm, muscle tension
- Autonomic responses, for example tachycardia, blood pressure changes

RESPIRATION
- Dyspnea associated with activity or rest
- Cough with or without sputum
- Smoking history

- Increased rate and rhythm, alteration in depth

SAFETY
- History of falls, fainting spells, or light-headedness with change of positions

SEXUALITY
- History of erectile dysfunction (ED), decreased libido
- Chest pain during sex

TEACHING/LEARNING
- Family history or risk factors of CAD; obesity, sedentary lifestyle, HTN, stroke, diabetes, smoking, hyperlipidemia
- Use or misuse of cardiac, antihypertensive, and over-the-counter (OTC) drugs
- History of hormone replacement therapy (HRT) in postmenopausal women
- Use of vitamins or herbal supplements, such as niacin, coenzyme Q10, ginger, bilberry, comfrey, garlic, or L-carnitine
- Use or misuse of alcohol or illicit drug use, such as cocaine or amphetamines

DISCHARGE PLAN CONSIDERATIONS
- Assistance with homemaker or maintenance tasks
- Changes in physical layout of home

♦ Refer to section at end of plan for postdischarge considerations.

Diagnostic Studies

TEST / WHY IT IS DONE	WHAT IT TELLS ME

BLOOD TESTS

- *Cardiac enzymes, including troponin I and cardiac troponin T, CPK, CK and CK-MB, LDH and isoenzymes LD_1, LD_2:* Substances released from heart muscle when it is damaged.

Usually within normal limits. Any elevation indicates myocardial damage.

- *Serum lipids, including total lipids, lipoprotein electrophoresis, isoenzymes, cholesterols (HDL, LDL, very low density lipoprotein [VLDL]), triglycerides, phospholipids:* A group of tests that make up a lipid profile.

The presence of lipid abnormalities can increase the risk of CAD.

- *Homocysteine:* Amino acid that plays an important role in blood clotting.

An elevated level results in increased platelet aggregation. A positive test indicates a potentially increased risk for cardiovascular disease (CVD).

- *C-reactive protein (CRP):* A marker for inflammation.

CRP levels have been shown to predict risk of both recurrent ischemia and death among those with stable and unstable angina (Ridker, 2003).

- *Hemoglobin (Hgb) and hematocrit (Hct):* Hgb measures the amount of oxygen-carrying capacity of the red blood cells (RBCs), and the Hct level looks at the relative proportion of RBCs and plasma.

Low Hgb and Hct levels can aggravate angina because of potential for ischemia.

- *Coagulation studies, including partial thromboplastin time (PTT), activated partial thromboplastin time (aPPT), and platelets:* Injury to a vessel wall or the tissue initiates the coagulation cascade and formation of a thrombus.

Thrombus formation can potentiate ischemic damage to the myocardium as blood flow is blocked.

- *PCO_2, potassium, and myocardial lactate:* Markers for metabolic acidity.

May be elevated during anginal attack (all play a role in myocardial ischemia and may perpetuate it).

OTHER DIAGNOSTIC STUDIES

- *Electrocardiogram (ECG):* Record of the electrical activity of the heart to detect dysrhythmias, to identify electrolyte imbalance, to identify any myocardial ischemia present or any damage to myocardial tissue from the past.

Often normal when client at rest or when pain-free; depression of the ST segment or T-wave inversion signifies ischemia. Dysrhythmias and heart block may also be present. Significant Q waves are consistent with a prior MI. ST depression without pain is highly indicative of ischemia.

- *Exercise or pharmacological stress electrocardiography (also called stress test, exercise treadmill, or exercise ECG):* Raises heart rate and blood pressure by means of exercise. Heart can also be stressed with drugs such as dobutamine or persantine.

Useful in screening for CAD, evaluating myocardial perfusion, differentiating between ischemia and scar area of the myocardium, developing a cardiac rehabilitation program, evaluating cardiac status for work capability, and evaluating drug efficacy. Provides other diagnostic information, such as duration and level of activity attained before onset of angina. A markedly positive test is indicative of severe CAD.

- *24-hour ECG monitoring (Holter):* Ambulatory ECG recording.

Can determine whether pain episodes correlate with or change during exercise or activity.

- *Echocardiography (also called two-dimensional echocardiogram and Doppler ultrasound):* Evaluates the left ventricle, including size, valvular function, wall thickness, and pumping action as measured by the EF. May be done at rest or during exercise.

Detects changes in heart wall motion that occur during myocardial ischemia. Normal myocardium becomes hyperdynamic during exercise; ischemic segments become hypokinetic or akinetic. Helps diagnose cardiomyopathy, heart failure (HF), pericarditis, and abnormal valvular action that might be cause of chest pain.

- *Coronary magnetic resonance (CMR) scan:* Test that uses magnetic fields to produce two- or three-dimensional images of the heart.

Assesses cardiac chamber volumes and function, as well as muscle mass and is particularly valuable for distinguishing ischemic from nonischemic cardiomyopathy.

- *Myocardial perfusion imaging (MPI) scans, which may include stress MPI and single-photon emission computed tomography (SPECT):* Scans the heart using radioactive dyes to show areas of increased metabolic activity and decreased blood flow.

MPI is the most widely used imaging test for the evaluation of suspected myocardial ischemia. SPECT is capable of assessing cardiovascular risk with a high degree of accuracy, measuring both ventricular function and relative regional perfusion at rest and with stress.

(continues on page 68)

TEST WHY IT IS DONE (continued)	WHAT IT TELLS ME (continued)
• *Calcium scoring (also called coronary artery calcium scoring computed tomography, or CT, scan):* Ultrafast CT scan that measures the amount of calcium in the coronary arteries.	Elevated calcium scoring in client with other risk factors, such as family history, hypertension, diabetes, or hypercholesterolemia, is an indication of some level of CAD.
• *Coronary computed tomography angiography (CTA):* High-resolution, three-dimensional pictures of the moving heart and great vessels.	Defines the presence and extent of coronary artery luminal narrowing.
• *Cardiac catheterization with angiography:* Assesses patency of coronary arteries, reveals abnormal heart and valve size or shape, and evaluates ventricular contractility. Pressures can be measured within each chamber of the heart and across the valves.	Definitive test for CAD in clients with known ischemic disease with angina or incapacitating chest pain, in clients with cholesterolemia and familial heart disease who are experiencing chest pain, and in clients with abnormal resting ECGs. Abnormal results are present in valvular disease, altered contractility, ventricular failure, and circulatory abnormalities. *Note:* Ten percent of clients with unstable angina have normal-appearing coronary arteries.
• *Chest x-ray:* Visualize any infiltrates that may be present in the lung.	Any changes from normal may indicate pulmonary complications or decompensation of cardiac status such as congestive heart failure (CHF).

Nursing Priorities

1. Relieve or control pain.
2. Prevent or minimize development of myocardial complications.
3. Provide information about disease process, prognosis, and treatment.
4. Support client or significant other (SO) in initiating necessary lifestyle or behavioral changes.

Discharge Goals

1. Desired activity level achieved, with return to activity baseline, and self-care needs met with minimal or no pain.
2. Remains free of complications.
3. Disease process, prognosis, and therapeutic regimen understood.
4. Participates in treatment program and behavioral changes.
5. Plan in place to meet needs after discharge.

NURSING DIAGNOSIS: acute Pain

May be related to
Increased cardiac workload and oxygen consumption
Decreased myocardial blood flow, tissue ischemia

Possibly evidenced by
Reports of pain varying in frequency, duration, and intensity, especially as condition worsens
Narrowed focus
Distraction behaviors, such as moaning, crying, pacing, or restlessness
Autonomic responses, such as diaphoresis, BP and pulse rate changes, pupillary dilation, increased or decreased respiratory rate

Desired Outcomes/Evaluation Criteria—Client Will

Pain Level (NOC)
Report anginal episodes decreased in frequency, duration, and severity.
Demonstrate relief of pain as evidenced by stable vital signs and absence of muscle tension and restlessness.

ACTIONS/INTERVENTIONS	RATIONALE

Pain Management (NIC)

Independent

Instruct client to notify nurse immediately when chest pain occurs.

Pain and decreased cardiac output may stimulate the sympathetic nervous system to release excessive amounts of norepinephrine, which increases platelet aggregation, and release of thromboxane A2. This potent vasoconstrictor causes coronary artery spasm, which can precipitate, complicate, and prolong an anginal attack. Unbearable pain may cause vasovagal response, thus decreasing BP and heart rate.

Assess and document client response and effects of medication.

Provides information about disease progression. Aids in evaluating effectiveness of interventions and may indicate need for change in therapeutic regimen.

Identify precipitating event, if any; identify frequency, duration, intensity, and location of pain.

Helps differentiate chest pain and aids in evaluating possible progression to unstable angina. Stable angina usually lasts 3 to 15 minutes and is often relieved by rest and sublingual nitroglycerin (NTG); unstable angina is more intense, occurs unpredictably, may last longer, and is not usually relieved by NTG or rest.

Observe for associated symptoms, such as dyspnea, nausea, vomiting, dizziness, palpitations, and desire to urinate.

Decreased cardiac output, which may occur during ischemic myocardial episode, stimulates sympathetic or parasympathetic nervous system, causing a variety of vague sensations that client may not identify as related to anginal episode.

Evaluate reports of pain in jaw, neck, shoulder, arm, or hand (typically on left side).

Cardiac pain may radiate; for example, pain is often referred to more superficial sites served by the same spinal cord nerve level.

Place client at complete rest during anginal episodes.

Reduces myocardial oxygen demand to minimize risk of tissue injury and necrosis.

Elevate head of bed if client is short of breath.

Facilitates gas exchange to decrease hypoxia and resultant shortness of breath.

Monitor heart rate and rhythm.

Clients with unstable angina have an increased risk of acute life-threatening dysrhythmias, which occur in response to ischemic changes and stress.

Monitor vital signs every 5 minutes during initial anginal attack.

BP may initially rise because of sympathetic stimulation and then fall if cardiac output is compromised. Tachycardia also develops in response to sympathetic stimulation and may be sustained as a compensatory response if cardiac output falls.

Stay with client who is experiencing pain or appears anxious.

Anxiety releases catecholamines, which increase myocardial workload and can escalate or prolong ischemic pain. Presence of nurse can reduce feelings of fear and helplessness.

Maintain quiet, comfortable environment; restrict visitors as necessary.

Mental or emotional stress increases myocardial workload.

Provide light meals. Have client rest for 1 hour after meals.

Decreases myocardial workload associated with work of digestion, reducing risk of anginal attack.

Collaborative

Provide supplemental oxygen, as indicated.

Increases oxygen available for myocardial uptake and reversal of ischemia.

Administer anti-anginal medication(s) promptly, as indicated, for example:
Nitrates: NTG sublingual (Nitrostat, NitroQuick); extended release tablets and capsules, such as Nitrong and Nitrogard SR; metered-dose spray (Nitrolingual); transdermal patch (Minitran, Nitrodisc); transdermal ointment (Nitrol, Nitro-Bid); isosorbide (Isordil, Imdur)

NTG has been the standard for treating and preventing anginal pain for more than 100 years. Today, it is available in many forms and is still the cornerstone of anti-anginal therapy. Rapid vasodilator effect lasts 10 to 30 minutes and can be used prophylactically to prevent, as well as abort, anginal attacks. Long-acting preparations are used to prevent recurrences by reducing coronary vasospasms and reducing cardiac workload. May cause headache, dizziness, and light-headedness—symptoms that usually pass quickly. If headache is intolerable, alteration of dose or discontinuation of drug may be necessary. *Note:* Isordil may be more effective for clients with variant form of angina.

(continues on page 70)

Beta blockers, such as atenolol (Tenormin), carteolol (Cartrol), labetalol (Normodyne), nadolol (Corgard), metroprolol (Tropol XL), and propranolol (Inderal)

Reduce angina by reducing the heart's workload. (Refer to ND: risk for decreased Cardiac Output following.) *Note:* Often, these drugs alone are sufficient to relieve angina in less severe conditions.

Calcium channel blockers, such as bepridil (Vascor), amlodipine (Norvasc), nicardipine (Cardene), nifedipine (Procardia), felodipine (Plendil), isradipine (DynaCirc), and diltiazem (Cardizem)

Produce relaxation of coronary vascular smooth muscle, dilate coronary arteries, and decrease peripheral vascular resistance.

Analgesics, such as acetaminophen (Tylenol)

Usually sufficient analgesia for relief of headache caused by dilation of cerebral vessels in response to nitrates.

Morphine sulfate (MS)

Potent opioid analgesic may be used in acute onset because of its beneficial effects. Such effects include peripheral vasodilatation and reduced myocardial workload; sedation, which produces relaxation; and interrupted flow of vaso-constricting catecholamines, thereby effectively relieving severe chest pain. MS is given intravenously (IV) for rapid action and because decreased cardiac output compromises peripheral tissue absorption.

Monitor serial ECG changes.

Ischemia during anginal attack may cause transient ST-segment depression or elevation and T-wave inversion. Serial tracings verify ischemic changes, which may disappear when client is pain free. They also provide a baseline against which to compare later pattern changes.

NURSING DIAGNOSIS: risk for decreased Cardiac Output

Risk factors may include
Inotropic changes, such as transient or prolonged myocardial ischemia and effects of medications
Alterations in rate, rhythm, and electrical conduction

Possibly evidenced by
(Not applicable; presence of signs and symptoms establishes an *actual* diagnosis)

Desired Outcomes/Evaluation Criteria—Client Will

Cardiac Pump Effectiveness (NOC)
Demonstrate increased activity tolerance.
Report or display decreased episodes of dyspnea, angina, and dysrhythmias.
Participate in behaviors and activities that reduce the workload of the heart.

ACTIONS/INTERVENTIONS　　　　**RATIONALE**

Hemodynamic Regulation (NIC)
Independent

Maintain bedrest or chair rest in position of comfort during acute episodes.

Decreases oxygen consumption and demand, reducing myocardial workload and risk of decompensation.

Monitor vital signs and cardiac rhythm.

Tachycardia and changes in blood pressure (hypotension or hypertension) may be present because of pain, anxiety, hypoxemia, and reduced cardiac output. ECG changes reflecting ischemia and dysrhythmias indicate need for additional evaluation and therapeutic intervention.

Auscultate breath sounds and heart sounds. Listen for murmurs.

S_3, S_4, or crackles may occur with cardiac decompensation or some medications, especially beta blockers. Development of murmurs may reveal a valvular cause for chest pain, such as aortic or mitral stenosis or papillary muscle rupture.

Provide for adequate rest periods. Assist with or perform self-care activities, as indicated.

Conserves energy and reduces cardiac workload.

Stress importance of avoiding straining and bearing down, especially during defecation.

Valsalva's maneuver causes bradycardia, which may be followed by rebound tachycardia, both of which may impair cardiac output.

Encourage immediate reporting of pain for prompt administration of medications, as indicated.

Timely interventions can reduce oxygen consumption and myocardial workload and may prevent or minimize cardiac complications.

ACTIONS/INTERVENTIONS (continued)

Monitor for and document effects of and adverse response to medications, noting BP, heart rate, and rhythm (especially when giving combination of calcium antagonists, beta blockers, and nitrates).

Assess for signs and symptoms of heart failure.

Evaluate mental status, noting development of confusion and disorientation.
Note skin color and presence and quality of pulses.

Assess lung for adventitious sounds, such as crackles.

Collaborative
Administer supplemental oxygen as needed.

Monitor pulse oximetry or arterial blood gases (ABGs), as indicated.

Measure cardiac output and other functional parameters, as indicated.

Administer medications, as indicated, for example:
  Calcium channel blockers, such as diltiazem (Cardizem), nifedipine (Procardia), verapamil (Calan), bepridil (Vascor), amlodipine (Norvasc), felodipine (Plendil), and isradipine (DynaCirc)
  Beta blockers, such as atenolol (Tenormin), nadolol (Corgard), propranolol (Inderal), and esmolol (Brevibloc)

  Antiplatelets, such as aspirin (ASA), clopidogrel (Plavix), ticlopidine (Ticlid), tirofiban (Aggrastat), and eptifibatide (Integrilin)

  IV heparin

Monitor laboratory studies, such as PTT and aPTT.
Discuss purpose and prepare for stress testing and cardiac catheterization when indicated.
Prepare for surgical interventions such as angioplasty with or without intracoronary stent placement, valve replacement, and coronary artery bypass grafting (CABG), if indicated.

RATIONALE (continued)

Desired effect is to decrease myocardial oxygen demand by decreasing ventricular stress. Drugs with negative inotropic properties can decrease perfusion to an already ischemic myocardium. Combination of nitrates and beta blockers may have cumulative effect on cardiac output.
Angina is only a symptom of underlying pathology causing myocardial ischemia. Disease may compromise cardiac function to point of decompensation.
Reduced perfusion of the brain can produce observable changes in sensorium.
Peripheral circulation is reduced when cardiac output falls, giving the skin a pale or gray color depending on level of hypoxia and diminishing the strength of peripheral pulses.
Respiratory system may become decompensated with anginal attack.

Increases oxygen available for myocardial uptake to improve contractility, reduce ischemia, and reduce lactic acid levels.
Oxygen saturation may decrease as oxygen demands increase for heart muscle and systemic circulation. Monitoring determines adequacy of respiratory function and O$_2$ therapy.
Cardiac index, preload and afterload, contractility, and cardiac work may be measured noninvasively through various means, including TEB technique, and is useful in evaluating response to therapeutic interventions and identifying need for more aggressive emergency care. *Note:* Evaluation of changes in heart rate, BP, and cardiac output requires consideration of client's circadian hemodynamic variability. These measurements are normally expected to be lower at night in clients who are active during the day.

Although differing in mode of action, calcium channel blockers play a major role in preventing and terminating ischemia induced by coronary artery spasm and in reducing vascular resistance, thereby decreasing BP and cardiac workload.
These medications decrease cardiac workload by reducing heart rate and systolic BP. *Note:* Overdose produces cardiac decompensation.
Aspirin is proven beneficial in primary and secondary prevention of coronary artery disease. For clients with major gastrointestinal intolerance, alternative drugs may be indicated. Newer antiplatelets, especially Plavix, are frequently used in conjunction with angioplasty and stent placement for relief of angina.
Bolus followed by continuous infusion is recommended to help reduce risk of subsequent MI by reducing the thrombotic complications of plaque rupture for clients diagnosed with intermediate or high-risk unstable angina. *Note:* Use of low-molecular-weight heparin is increasing because it is more efficacious and predictable and has fewer adverse effects, such as less risk of bleeding and longer half-life. It also does not require anticoagulation monitoring.
Evaluates anticoagulation therapy needs and effectiveness.
Stress testing provides information about the health or strength of the ventricles.
Angioplasty, also called percutaneous transluminal coronary angioplasty (PTCA), increases coronary blood flow by compression of atheromatous lesions and dilation of the vessel lumen in an occluded coronary artery. Intracoronary stints may be placed at the time of PTCA to provide structural support within the coronary artery and improve the odds of long-term patency. This procedure is preferred over the more invasive CABG surgery. Drug-coated stents may be considered for clients at high risk for thrombosis, acute

(continues on page 72)

closure, and for diabetics. Several different drugs are available to help decrease restenosis after insertion of stents or angioplasty. Stent placement may also be effective for the variant form of angina where periodic vasospasms impair arterial flow. *Note:* A recent innovation in thrombolytic therapy associated with angioplasty and use of stents is the Anjiojet (a device approved for removing blood clots from coronary arteries), which can reduce risk of heart attack or death. CABG is the recommended treatment when testing confirms myocardial ischemia due to left main coronary artery disease or symptomatic three-vessel disease, especially in those with left ventricular dysfunction.

Prepare for transfer to critical care unit if condition warrants.

Profound or prolonged chest pain with decreased cardiac output reflects development of complications requiring more intense or emergency interventions.

NURSING DIAGNOSIS: Anxiety [specify level]

May be related to
Situational crises
Threat to self-concept, such as altered image or abilities
Underlying pathophysiological response
Threat to or change in health status, such as a disease course that can lead to further compromise, debility, and even death
Negative self-talk

Possibly evidenced by
Expressed concern regarding changes in life events
Increased tension and helplessness
Apprehension, uncertainty, restlessness
Association of diagnosis with loss of healthy body image, loss of place or influence
View of self as noncontributing member of family or society
Fear of death as an imminent reality

Desired Outcomes/Evaluation Criteria—Client Will

Anxiety Self-Control (NOC)
Verbalize awareness of feelings of anxiety and healthy ways to deal with them.
Report that anxiety is reduced to a manageable level.
Express concerns about effect of disease on lifestyle and position within family and society.
Demonstrate effective coping strategies and problem-solving skills.

ACTIONS/INTERVENTIONS	RATIONALE
Anxiety Reduction (NIC)	
Independent	
Explain purpose of tests and procedures.	Reduces anxiety attributable to fear of unknown diagnosis and prognosis.
Promote expression of feelings and fears such as denial, depression, and anger. Let client or SO know these are normal reactions. Note statements of concern, such as, "heart attack is inevitable."	Unexpressed feelings may create internal turmoil and affect self-image. Verbalization of concerns reduces tension, verifies level of coping, and facilitates dealing with feelings. Presence of negative self-talk can increase level of anxiety and may contribute to exacerbation of anginal attacks.
Encourage family and friends to treat client as before.	Reassures client that role in the family and business has not been altered.
Tell client the medical regimen has been designed to reduce or limit future attacks and increase cardiac stability.	Encourages client to test symptom control such as no angina with certain levels of activity, to increase confidence in medical program, and to integrate abilities into perceptions of self. (Refer to CP: Psychosocial Aspects of Care, ND: Anxiety [specify level]/Fear for additional considerations.)
Collaborative	
Administer sedatives and tranquilizers, as indicated.	May be desired to help client relax until physically able to reestablish adequate coping strategies.

NURSING DIAGNOSIS: deficient Knowledge [Learning Need] regarding condition, treatment needs, self-care, and discharge needs

May be related to
Lack of exposure
Inaccurate information or misinterpretation of information
Unfamiliarity with information resources

Possibly evidenced by
Questions, statement of concerns
Request for information
Inaccurate follow-through of instructions

Desired Outcomes/Evaluation Criteria—Client Will

Participate in learning process.
Assume responsibility for own learning, looking for information and asking questions.

Knowledge: Cardiac Disease Management (NOC)
Verbalize understanding of condition, disease process, and potential complications.
Verbalize understanding of and participate in therapeutic regimen.
Initiate necessary lifestyle changes.

ACTIONS/INTERVENTIONS	RATIONALE
Teaching: Disease Process (NIC) *Independent* Discuss pathophysiology of condition. Stress need for preventing and managing anginal attacks.	Clients with angina need to learn why it occurs and what they can do to control it. This is the focus of therapeutic management to reduce likelihood of MI and promote heart-healthy lifestyle.
Review significance of cholesterol levels and differentiate between LDL and HDL factors. Emphasize importance of periodic laboratory measurements and use of cholesterol-lowering drugs.	Although the American Heart Association recommended LDL is ±130 mg/dL, clients with two or more risk factors, including smoking, hypertension, diabetes mellitus, and positive family history, should keep LDL ±100 mg/dL, and those with diagnosis of CAD need to keep LDL below 100 mg/dL. HDL below 35 to 45 is considered a risk factor; a level above 60 mg/dL is considered an advantage. *Note:* The National Cholesterol Education Program Guidelines now state that all adult high-risk clients with LDL of 100 mg/dL should be treated with drug therapy.
Encourage avoidance of factors or situations that may precipitate anginal episode, such as emotional stress, extensive or intense physical exertion, ingestion of large or heavy meal (especially close to bedtime), and exposure to extremes in environmental temperature.	May reduce incidence or severity of ischemic episodes. Helps client manage symptoms.
Assist client or SO to identify sources of physical and emotional stress and discuss ways that they can be avoided.	This is a crucial step in limiting or preventing anginal attacks.
Review importance of cessation of smoking, weight control, dietary changes, and exercise.	Knowledge of the significance of risk factors provides client with opportunity to make needed changes. Clients with high cholesterol who do not respond to a 6-month program of low-fat diet and regular exercise will require medication.
Encourage client to follow prescribed reconditioning program; caution client to avoid exhaustion.	Fear of triggering attacks may cause client to avoid participation in activity that has been prescribed to enhance recovery by increasing myocardial strength and forming collateral circulation. Cardiac rehabilitation programs provide a phased approach to increasing client's activity and exercise tolerance.
Discuss impact of condition on desired lifestyle and activities, including work, driving, sexual activity, and hobbies. Provide information, privacy, or consultation, as indicated.	Client may be reluctant to resume or continue usual activities because of fear of anginal attack or death. Client should take nitroglycerin prophylactically before any activity that is known to precipitate angina. *Note:* ED can be sign of CAD or diabetes in men. Use of Viagra, or similar drugs, is contraindicated with nitrates, which are usually used with angina.

(continues on page 74)

ACTIONS/INTERVENTIONS (continued)	RATIONALE (continued)
Demonstrate how and encourage client to monitor own pulse and BP during and after activities, when appropriate, and to schedule and simplify activities, avoid strain, and take rest periods.	Allows client to identify those activities that can be modified to avoid cardiac stress and stay below the anginal threshold.
Discuss steps to take when anginal attacks occur, such as cessation of activity, keeping "rescue" NTG on hand, administration of PRN medication, and use of relaxation techniques.	Being prepared for an event takes away the fear that client will not know what to do if attack occurs.
Review prescribed medications for control and prevention of anginal attacks as previously presented:	Angina is a complicated condition that often requires the use of many drugs to decrease myocardial workload, improve coronary circulation, and control the occurrence of attacks.
ASA and other antiplatelet agents	May be given prophylactically on a daily basis to decrease platelet aggregation and improve coronary circulation. May prolong survival rate of clients with unstable angina.
Lipid-lowering agents: bile acid sequestrants, such as cholestyramine (Questran), colestipol (Colestid), and nicotinic acid (Niacin); fibrates, such as fenofibrate (Tricor) and gemfibrozil (Lopid); and HMG-CoA reductase inhibitors, such as lovastatin (Lipitor), fluvastatin (Lescol), pravastatin (Pravachol), and simvastatin (Zocor)	These drugs are considered first-line agents for lowering serum cholesterol levels. *Note:* Questran and Colestid may inhibit absorption of fat-soluble vitamins and some drugs, such as Coumadin, Lanoxin, and Inderal. The HMG-CoA reductase inhibitors may cause photosensitivity. Most lipid-lowering agents are inhibited by grapefruit juice.
Stress importance of checking with physician before taking OTC drugs.	OTC drugs may potentiate or negate effects of prescribed medications.
Discuss use of herbals such as ginseng, garlic, ginkgo, hawthorn, and bromelain, as indicated.	Some herbals, such as ginkgo, ginseng, and bromelain can affect bleeding and clotting, especially when added to medications such as Plavix or Coumadin, which increase bleeding. Others, such as hawthorn, can increase the effects of certain heart medications.
Review symptoms to be reported to physician, particularly an increase in frequency and duration of attacks and changes in response to medications.	Knowledge of expectations can avoid undue concern for insignificant reasons or delay in treatment of important symptoms.
Discuss importance of follow-up appointments.	Angina is a symptom of progressive CAD that should be monitored and may require occasional adjustment of treatment regimen.

POTENTIAL CONSIDERATIONS following discharge from care setting (dependent on client's age, physical condition and presence of complications, personal resources, and life responsibilities)
- *acute Pain*—episodes of decreased myocardial blood flow and ischemia
- *Activity Intolerance*—imbalance between oxygen supply and demand, sedentary or stressful lifestyle
- *ineffective Denial*—learned response patterns, such as avoidance, cultural factors, and personal and family value systems
- *interrupted Family Processes*—situational transition and crisis
- *impaired Home Maintenance*—altered ability to perform tasks, inadequate support systems, reluctance to request assistance

---

MYOCARDIAL INFARCTION

I. Pathophysiology
a. Marked reduction or loss of blood flow through one or more of the coronary arteries, resulting in cardiac muscle ischemia, and over a finite period, resulting in necrosis
b. Occurs most often due to coronary artery disease (CAD)
c. Cellular ischemia and necrosis can affect the heart's rhythm, pumping action, and blood circulation.
d. Other problems may also ensue, such as heart failure, life-threatening arrhythmias, and death.
e. Delay in seeking treatment is the largest barrier to receiving therapy quickly.

II. Classification
a. Type of myocardial infarction (MI) can be identified on the electrocardiogram (ECG).
  i. ST-segment elevation (also called STEMI)
  ii. Non-ST elevation
b. Location of MI can be identified on the ECG.
  i. Anterior wall of the ventricle
  ii. Inferior wall of the ventricle
  iii. Posterior wall of the ventricle
  iv. Lateral wall of the ventricle

c. Infarcts are usually classified by size.
   i. Microscopic (focal necrosis)
   ii. Small (<10% of the left ventricle)
   iii. Medium (10% to 30% of the left ventricle)
   iv. Large (>30% of the left ventricle)
d. Point of time can be identified on the ECG by the Q wave and the client's history.
   i. Acute or evolving infarction is characterized by the presence of polymorphonuclear leukocytes unless the interval between the onset of infarction and death is brief (e.g., 6 hours), minimal, or no polymorphonuclear leukocytes may be seen.
   ii. Old or healed infarction is manifested as scar tissue without cellular infiltration, a process usually requiring 5 to 6 weeks or more.

III. Etiology
a. CAD common cause with plaque formation narrowing vessels and pieces of plaque breaking off, creating emboli
b. Severe spasm of a coronary artery is less common cause
c. Risk factors—age, being overweight or obese, smoking, hyperlipidemia, family history
d. Greater risk in presence of kidney problems, peripheral arterial disease, or prior MI

IV. Statistics (Centers for Disease Control and Prevention [CDC],2007b; National Heart, Lung and Blood Institute [NHLBI], 2007)
a. Morbidity: Approximately 1.1 million people in the United States suffer from MI annually.
b. Mortality: almost 50% die, approximately 460,000 annually.
   i. CAD is leading killer of both men and women in the United States.
   ii. Leading cause of death for American Indians, Alaskan Natives, African Americans, Hispanics, and whites, and second leading cause of death for Asians and Pacific Islanders
c. Cost: Projected $258 billion spent for heart disease in 2006.

GLOSSARY

Acute coronary syndrome (ACS): Signs and symptoms that indicate unstable angina or acute myocardial infarction.

Atherosclerosis: Abnormal accumulation of lipid deposits and fibrous tissue within the arterial walls and lumen.

Coronary artery bypass graft (CABG): Surgical procedure in which a blood vessel from another part of the body is grafted onto the occluded coronary artery above and below the occlusion in such a way that blood flow bypasses the blockage.

Creatine kinase (CK): Enzyme found in human tissues. One of the three types of CK is specific to the heart muscle and may be used as an indicator of heart muscle injury.

Myocardial infarction (MI, also called acute MI orAMI): Reduced myocardial perfusion and death of heart tissue caused by lack of oxygenated blood flow.

Percutaneous transluminal coronary angioplasty (PTCA): Type of percutaneous coronary intervention in which a balloon is inflated within a coronary artery to break an atheroma and open the vessel lumen, improving coronary artery blood flow.

Stent: Woven mesh that provides structural support to a coronary vessel, preventing its closure.

Thrombolytic: Agent or process that breaks down blood clots.

Troponin: Myocardial protein; measurement is used to assess heart muscle injury.

Care Setting

Myocardial infarctions are treated in the emergency room, inpatient acute hospital, critical care unit (CCU), intensive care unit (ICU), step-down unit, or medical unit.

Related Concerns

Angina, page 64
Dysrhythmias, page 88
Heart failure: chronic, page 48
Psychosocial aspects of care, page 749
Thrombophlebitis: deep vein thrombosis, page 111

DIAGNOSTIC DIVISION MAY REPORT	MAY EXHIBIT
ACTIVITY/REST • History of sedentary lifestyle, sporadic exercise schedule • Weakness, fatigue, intolerance to usual activities	• Chest pain with activity or rest • Tachycardia, dyspnea with rest or activity • Fatigue with normal daily activities
CIRCULATION • History of previous MI, CAD, heart failure, hypertension, diabetes mellitus, hypercholesterolemia	• *Color:* Pallor or cyanosis; mottling of the skin, nail beds, mucous membranes, and lips • Blood pressure (BP) normal, increased, or decreased; orthostatic changes may occur • Pulse normal, full, bounding, or have a weak or thready quality with delayed capillary refill • Dysrhythmias, tachycardia, or bradycardia • *Heart sounds:* S_3 and S_4, reflecting a pathological condition such as cardiac failure, decreased ventricular contractility, or compliance • Murmurs reflecting valvular insufficiency or papillary muscle dysfunction • Friction rub suggests pericarditis • *Edema:* Signs of jugular vein distention (JVD), peripheral edema, dependent edema, generalized edema
EGO INTEGRITY • Denial of significance of symptoms and presence of condition • Fear of dying, feelings of impending doom • Anger at inconvenience of illness and the "unnecessary" attention and hospitalization • Worry about family, employment, finances, childcare, elders at home, and pets at home	• Withdrawal, anxiety, lack of eye movements • Irritability, anger, combative behavior; may refuse emergent care • Focus on self and pain
ELIMINATION • History of straining with bowel movements • Syncopal events with bowel movements	• Normal or decreased bowel sounds
FOOD/FLUID • History of reflux disease, obesity • Nausea, vomiting, belching, heartburn • Recent history of eating large fatty meals, alcohol consumption, antacid use	• Vomiting • Poor skin turgor, dry or diaphoretic skin • Decreased urine output
HYGIENE • Recent history of not being able to care for self due to fatigue, chest pains, or shortness of breath	• Signs of not being able to perform self-care tasks, evidenced by body odor, dirty clothes, soiled undergarments
NEUROSENSORY • History of dizziness, fainting spells, falling	• Mentation changes such as disorientation, poor memory, changes in personality or thought processes • Motor weakness • Unsteady gait
PAIN/DISCOMFORT • Sudden onset of chest pain unrelieved by rest or nitroglycerin • *Location:* Typically, anterior chest including substernal and precordium pain that may radiate to arms, jaw, face • May have atypical location, such as pain in epigastric or abdominal area, elbow, jaw, back, neck, between shoulder blades, or throat	• Facial grimacing, changes in body posture; may place clenched fist on midsternum when describing pain • Crying, groaning, squirming, stretching • Withdrawal, lack of eye contact • *Autonomic responses:* Changes in heart rate and rhythm, blood pressure, respirations, skin color and moisture, and level of consciousness

Client Assessment Database (continued)

DIAGNOSTIC DIVISION MAY REPORT (continued)	MAY EXHIBIT (continued)
• Women may report pain between shoulder blades, back pain, tiredness, and throat fullness. • *Quality:* Crushing, constricting, squeezing, heavy, steady pain. Women may report dull aching pain. • *Intensity:* Usually a 10 on a scale of 0 to 10 or the "worst pain ever experienced" • Pain sometimes absent in women, postoperative clients, those with prior stroke or heart failure, diabetes, hypertension, or the elderly • *Precipitating factors:* May or may not be associated with activity or increased stress	

RESPIRATION
- Recent history of dyspnea with or without exertion, nocturnal dyspnea, unable to sleep flat
- Recent history of cough with or without sputum production
- History of smoking, chronic respiratory disease

- Increased respiratory rate, shallow and labored breathing
- *Color:* Pallor or cyanosis
- Decreased oxygen saturation on pulse oximetry
- *Breath sounds:* May be clear, or crackles and wheezes present
- *Sputum:* Clear, possible pink-tinged

SOCIAL INTERACTION
- Recent history of stressors such as work, family, financial, caretaking
- Difficulty coping with recent or current stressors
- May be worried about current hospitalization's effect on self and family and question coping abilities

- Difficulty resting quietly
- Overemotional responses such as intense anger or fear
- Withdrawal from family
- Not willing to cooperate with treatment recommendations; not responsive to teaching

SEXUALITY
- Postmenopausal; past history of hormone replacement therapy
- *Erectile dysfunction (ED):* May be associated with hypertension or antihypertensive medications

TEACHING/LEARNING
- Family history of heart disease, MI, diabetes, stroke, hypertension, peripheral vascular disease, hypercholesterolemia
- Use of tobacco; may express desire or attempts at smoking cessation
- Use of alcohol or other drugs
- Use or misuse of cardiac medications, over-the-counter (OTC) preparations
- Use of vitamins and herbal supplements such as vitamin E, ginseng, garlic, ginkgo, hawthorn, bromelain

DISCHARGE PLAN CONSIDERATIONS
- May require assistance with activities of daily living (ADLs), food preparation, shopping, transportation, homemaking or maintenance tasks, modifications of physical layout of home

▶ Refer to section at end of plan for postdischarge considerations.

TEST WHY IT IS DONE	WHAT IT TELLS ME
BLOOD TESTS • **Cardiac Enzymes and Isoenzymes** • *Troponin 1 (cTnl) and Troponin (cTn):* Contractile proteins found in the myocardium with nearly absolute myocardial tissue specificity, as well as high sensitivity, thereby reflecting even microscopic zones of myocardial necrosis. Troponins increase within 3 to 4 hours, peak in 4 to 24 hours, and return to normal in 1 to 3 weeks.	Troponins are a critical and reliable marker of myocardial injury.
• *Creatine kinase (CK) and its isoenzyme CK-MB:* Released after tissue necrosis. Serum CK levels initially rise within 4 to 6 hours of tissue injury, peak at 12 to 24 hours, and return to normal in 72 to 96 hours. Serum CK-MB levels increase within 2 to 6 hours, peak at 18 hours, and return to normal within 24 hours.	Helps determine extent and timing of muscle damage.
• *Myoglobin:* A heme protein of small molecular weight that is more rapidly released from damaged muscle tissue, with elevation in 1 to 3 hours, peaking in 4 to 12 hours, and lasting 12 hours.	If increased, it is not specific for cardiac muscle tissue; but, if negative, it can help rule out MI.
• *Lipid profile:* Includes total cholesterol, high-density lipoprotein (HDL), low-density lipoprotein (LDL), and triglycerides.	The lipid profile may be low during an acute MI; therefore, it is important to follow up. It may show that the client has hyperlipidemia that was not identified or was uncontrolled in the past, which would be a risk factor for CAD and MI.
• *Electrolytes:* A substance that, in solution, conducts an electric current and is decomposed by its passage. Sodium, potassium, and calcium are examples of common electrolytes.	Imbalances of sodium and potassium can alter conduction and compromise contractility.
• **Complete blood count:** Battery of screening tests that typically includes hemoglobin (Hgb); hematocrit (Hct); red blood cell (RBC) count, morphology, indices, and distribution width index; platelet count and size; white blood cell (WBC) count; and differential.	Leukocytosis (WBC count of 10,000 to 20,000) usually appears on the second day after acute MI due to inflammatory process.
OTHER DIAGNOSTIC STUDIES • *ECG:* Record of the electrical activity of the heart showing rhythm and rate, electrical conduction, signs of ischemia, and muscle damage to heart.	The 12-lead ECG is central to diagnosing acute MI. ST-segment elevation greater than 0.1 mV in two or more precordial contiguous leads or at least two adjacent limb leads is considered significant for myocardial injury. If the client has a new left bundle branch block (LBBB) and other signs and symptoms of acute MI, he or she should be evaluated immediately for reperfusion therapy (Lackey, 2006).
• **Echocardiography, also called two-dimensional echocardiogram and Doppler ultrasound:** Evaluates the left ventricle, including size, valvular function, wall thickness, and pumping action as measured by the ejection fraction (EF).	Reveals abnormalities in chambers, septal and ventricular wall motion, blood flow, and valve functions.
NUCLEAR IMAGING STUDIES • **Persantine or thallium scan:** Evaluates myocardial blood flow and status of myocardial cells.	Abnormalities in the blood flow, location, and extent of MI (acute or previous).
• **Cardiac blood imaging, also called multiple-gated acquisition (MUGA):** Evaluates specific and general ventricular performance.	Abnormalities of ventricular performance, wall motion, and ejection fraction.
• **Technetium:** Accumulates in ischemic cells, outlining necrotic areas.	Shows necrotic areas.
• **Digital subtraction angiography (DSA):** A form of digital radiography that delineates blood vessels by subtracting a digitized tissue background image from an image of tissue injected with an intravascular contrast.	Technique used to visualize status of arterial bypass grafts and to detect peripheral artery disease.

Diagnostic Studies (continued)

TEST WHY IT IS DONE (continued)	WHAT IT TELLS ME (continued)
• *Magnetic resonance imaging (MRI):* Allows visualization of blood flow, cardiac chambers, intraventricular septum, valves, vascular lesions, plaque formation, areas of necrosis and infarction, and blood clots.	Abnormalities of heart.
• *Cardiac angiography (also called cardiac catheterization):* Gold standard for the assessment of coronary blood flow and ventricular function. Blood flow of coronary arteries may be restored by means of angioplasty with or without stent placement, although procedure is not usually done in acute phase of MI unless angioplasty or emergency heart surgery is imminent.	Demonstrates patency of coronary arteries, reveals abnormal heart and valve size or shape, measures pressures within each chamber of the heart, calculates ventricular contractility, and identifies location of MI.
• *Magnetic resonance angiography (MRA):* Allows visualization of blood flow and differentiates diseased from normal blood vessels.	May be used in place of angiography in client who is allergic to contrast medium to identify areas of occluded blood flow.
• *Chest x-ray:* Evaluates organs and structures within the chest	May be normal or show an enlarged cardiac shadow, suggestive of heart failure, or show ventricular aneurysm, affecting ventricular wall motion.

Nursing Priorities

1. Relieve pain and anxiety.
2. Reduce myocardial workload.
3. Prevent, detect, and assist in treatment of life-threatening dysrhythmias or complications.
4. Promote cardiac health and self-care.

Discharge Goals

1. Chest pain absent or controlled.
2. Heart rate and rhythm sufficient to sustain adequate cardiac output and tissue perfusion.
3. Achievement of activity level sufficient for basic self-care.
4. Anxiety reduced and managed.
5. Disease process, treatment plan, and prognosis understood.
6. Plan in place to meet needs after discharge, including follow-up appointments.

NURSING DIAGNOSIS: acute Pain

May be related to
Tissue ischemia (coronary artery occlusion)

Possibly evidenced by
Reports of chest pain with or without radiation
Facial grimacing
Restlessness, changes in level of consciousness
Changes in pulse, BP

Desired Outcomes/Evaluation Criteria—Client Will

Pain Level (NOC)
Verbalize relief or control of chest pain within appropriate period for administered medications.
Display reduced tension, relaxed manner, and ease of movement.

Pain Control (NOC)
Demonstrate use of relaxation techniques.

ACTIONS/INTERVENTIONS

Pain Management (NIC)

Independent

Monitor and document characteristics of pain, noting verbal reports, nonverbal cues, for example, moaning, crying, restlessness, diaphoresis, clutching chest, rapid breathing, and hemodynamic response (BP and heart rate changes).

Obtain full description of pain from client including location, intensity (0 to 10), duration, characteristics (dull or crushing), and radiation. Assist client to quantify pain by comparing it to other experiences.

Review history of previous angina, anginal equivalent, or MI pain. Discuss family history if pertinent.

Instruct client to report pain immediately.

Provide quiet environment, calm activities, and comfort measures, for instance, dry or wrinkle-free linens and backrub. Approach client calmly and confidently.

Assist or instruct in relaxation techniques, such as deep, slow breathing and distraction.

Check vital signs before and after administration of opioid medication.

Collaborative

Administer supplemental oxygen by means of nasal cannula or face mask, as indicated.

Administer medications, as indicated, for example:
Aspirin (ASA)

Anti-anginals, such as nitroglycerin (Nitro-Bid, Nitrostat, Nitro-Dur), isosorbide dinitrate (Isordil), and mononitrate (Imdur)

Angiotensin-converting enzyme (ACE) inhibitors, such as lisinopril (Zestril), captopril (Capoten), and benazepril (Lotensin)

Angiotensin receptor blockers (ARBs), such as candesartan (Atacand), olmesartan (Benicar), and valsartan (Diovan)

Aldosterone blockers, such as eplerenone (Inspra) and spironolactone

RATIONALE

Variation of appearance and behavior of clients in pain may present a challenge in assessment. For example, men and women consistently present differently, or an individual may present differently from one episode to another. However, most clients with an acute MI appear ill, distracted, and focused on pain. Verbal history and deeper investigation of precipitating factors should be postponed until pain is relieved. Respirations may be increased as a result of pain and associated anxiety; release of stress-induced catecholamines increases heart rate and BP.

Pain is a subjective experience and must be described by client. Provides baseline for comparison to aid in determining effectiveness of therapy, resolution or progression of problem.

May differentiate current pain from preexisting patterns as well as identify complications, such as extension of infarction, pulmonary embolus, or pericarditis.

Delays in reporting pain hinders pain relief and may necessitate increased dosage of medication to achieve relief. In addition, severe pain may induce shock by stimulating the sympathetic nervous system, thereby creating further damage and interfering with diagnostics and relief of pain.

Decreases external stimuli, which may aggravate anxiety and cardiac strain and limit coping abilities and adjustment to current situation.

Helpful in decreasing perception of or response to pain. Provides a sense of having some control over the situation, increase in positive attitude.

Hypotension and respiratory depression can occur as a result of opioid administration. These problems may increase myocardial damage in presence of ventricular insufficiency.

Increases amount of oxygen available for myocardial uptake and thereby may relieve discomfort associated with tissue ischemia.

Giving aspirin as soon as possible (unless contraindicated) inhibits platelet activity, interrupting platelet aggregation at the site of plaque rupture—a key mechanism in the unfolding acute MI. Patients who receive aspirin in the acute phase have a 15% lower mortality rate than those who don't (Lackey, 2006).

Nitrates are useful for pain control by coronary vasodilating effects, which increase coronary blood flow and myocardial perfusion. Peripheral vasodilation effects reduce the volume of blood returning to the heart (preload), thereby decreasing myocardial workload and oxygen demand.

May be given to reduce hypertension and reduce risk of developing heart failure following MI in client with diminished ventricular EF and in those with hypertension, diabetes, or chronic kidney disease, unless contraindicated (Smith et al, 2006).

May be used in patients who are intolerant to ACE inhibitors and have heart failure (HF) or have had an MI with left ventricular EF less than or equal to 40%. They block the action of angiotensin II that causes the blood vessels to dilate and reduce BP.

May be used in post-MI patients who have had an MI, ACS, or left ventricular dysfunction with or without HF symptoms, unless contraindicated. They block the effects of aldosterone on the kidneys, allowing the kidneys to excrete extra sodium and water, thereby reducing BP.

ACTIONS/INTERVENTIONS (continued)	RATIONALE (continued)
Analgesics, such as morphine sulfate	Although intravenous (IV) morphine is the usual drug of choice, other injectable opioids may be used in acute-phase or recurrent chest pain unrelieved by nitroglycerin to reduce severe pain, provide sedation, and decrease myocardial workload. IM injections should be avoided, if possible, because they can alter the CPK diagnostic indicator and are not well absorbed in underperfused tissue.

NURSING DIAGNOSIS: Activity Intolerance

May be related to
Imbalance between myocardial oxygen supply and demand
Presence of ischemia and necrotic myocardial tissues
Cardiac depressant effects of certain drugs, such as beta blockers, antidysrhythmics

Possibly evidenced by
Alterations in heart rate and BP with activity
Development of dysrhythmias
Changes in skin color and moisture
Exertional angina
Generalized weakness

Desired Outcomes/Evaluation Criteria—Client Will

Activity Tolerance (NOC)
Demonstrate measurable, progressive increase in tolerance for activity with heart rate and rhythm, BP within client's normal limits, and skin warm, pink, and dry.
Report absence of angina with activity.

ACTIONS/INTERVENTIONS	RATIONALE
Energy Management (NIC)	
Independent	
Record and document heart rate and rhythm and BP changes before, during, and after activity, as indicated. Correlate with reports of chest pain or shortness of breath. (Refer to ND: risk for decreased Cardiac Output.)	Trends determine client's response to activity and may indicate myocardial oxygen deprivation that may require decrease in activity level, return to bedrest, changes in medication regimen, or use of supplemental oxygen.
Encourage bedrest to chair rest initially. Thereafter, limit activity on basis of pain or adverse cardiac response. Provide nonstress diversional activities.	Reduces myocardial workload and oxygen consumption, reducing risk of complications, such as extension of MI. Clients with uncomplicated MI are encouraged to engage in mild activity out of bed, including short walks 12 hours after incident.
Instruct client to avoid increasing abdominal pressure, such as straining during defecation.	Activities that require holding the breath and bearing down, such as Valsalva's maneuver, can result in bradycardia with temporarily reduced cardiac output and rebound tachycardia with elevated BP.
Explain pattern of graded increase of activity level, such as getting up to commode or sitting in chair, progressive ambulation, and resting after meals.	Progressive activity provides a controlled demand on the heart, increasing strength and preventing overexertion.
Review signs and symptoms reflecting intolerance of present activity level or requiring notification of nurse or physician.	Palpitations, pulse irregularities, development of chest pain, or dyspnea may indicate need for changes in exercise regimen or medication.
Collaborative	
Refer to cardiac rehabilitation program.	Provides continued support and additional supervision and promotes participation in recovery and wellness process.

Anxiety [specify level]/Fear

May be related to
Threat to or change in health and socioeconomic status
Threat of loss or death
Unconscious conflict about essential values, beliefs, and goals of life
Interpersonal transmission or contagion

Possibly evidenced by
Fearful attitude
Apprehension, increased tension, restlessness, facial tension
Uncertainty, feelings of inadequacy
Somatic complaints and sympathetic stimulation
Focus on self, expressions of concern about current and future events
Fight- (e.g., belligerent attitude) or-flight behavior

Desired Outcomes/Evaluation Criteria—Client Will

Anxiety Self-Control [or] Fear Self-Control (NOC)
Recognize and verbalize feelings.
Identify causes and contributing factors.
Verbalize reduction of anxiety or fear.
Demonstrate positive problem-solving skills.
Identify and use resources appropriately.

ACTIONS/INTERVENTIONS	RATIONALE
Anxiety Reduction (NIC)	
Independent	
Identify and acknowledge client's perception of threat or situation. Encourage expressions of, and avoid denying feelings of anger grief, sadness, and fear.	Coping with the pain and emotional trauma of an MI is difficult. Client may fear death or be anxious about immediate environment. Ongoing anxiety related to concerns about impact of heart attack on future lifestyle, matters left unattended or unresolved, and effects of illness on family may be present in varying degrees for some time and may be manifested by symptoms of depression.
Note presence of hostility, withdrawal, and denial—inappropriate affect or refusal to comply with medical regimen.	Research into survival rates between type A and type B individuals and the impact of denial has been ambiguous; however, studies show some correlation between degree and expression of anger or hostility and an increased risk for MI.
Maintain confident manner, without false reassurance.	Client and SO may be affected by the anxiety or uneasiness displayed by health team members. Honest explanations can alleviate anxiety.
Observe for verbal and nonverbal signs of anxiety, and stay with client. Intervene if client displays destructive behavior.	Client may not express concern directly, but words or actions may convey sense of agitation, aggression, and hostility. Intervention can help client regain control of own behavior.
Accept but do not reinforce use of denial. Avoid confrontations.	Denial can be beneficial in decreasing anxiety but can postpone dealing with the reality of the current situation. Confrontation can promote anger and increase use of denial, reducing cooperation and possibly impeding recovery.
Orient client and SO to routine procedures and expected activities. Promote participation when possible.	Predictability and information can decrease anxiety for client.
Answer all questions factually. Provide consistent information; repeat as indicated.	Accurate information about the situation reduces fear, strengthens nurse-client relationship, and assists client and SO to deal realistically with situation. Attention span may be short, and repetition of information helps with retention.
Encourage client and SO to communicate with one another, sharing questions and concerns.	Sharing information elicits support and comfort and can relieve tension of unexpressed worries.
Provide privacy for client and SO.	Allows needed time for personal expression of feelings; may enhance mutual support and promote more adaptive behaviors.
Provide rest periods and uninterrupted sleep time and quiet surroundings, with client controlling type and amount of external stimuli.	Conserves energy and enhances coping abilities.
Support normality of grieving process, including time necessary for resolution.	Can provide reassurance that feelings are normal response to situation and perceived changes.

ACTIONS/INTERVENTIONS (continued)	RATIONALE (continued)
Encourage independence, self-care, and decision making within accepted treatment plan.	Increased independence from staff promotes self-confidence and reduces feelings of abandonment that can accompany transfer from coronary unit and discharge from hospital.
Encourage discussion about postdischarge expectations.	Helps client and SO identify realistic goals, thereby reducing risk of discouragement in face of the reality of limitations of condition and pace of recuperation.
Collaborative
Administer anti-anxiety or hypnotics, as indicated, such as alprazolam (Xanax) and lorazepam (Ativan).	Promotes relaxation and rest and reduces feelings of anxiety.

NURSING DIAGNOSIS: risk for decreased Cardiac Output

Risk factors may include
Changes in rate, rhythm, electrical conduction
Reduced preload and increased systemic vascular resistance (SVR)
Infarcted or dyskinetic muscle, structural defects—ventricular aneurysm, septal defects

Possibly evidenced by
(Not applicable; presence of signs and symptoms establishes *actual* diagnosis)

Desired Outcomes/Evaluation Criteria—Client Will

Cardiac Pump Effectiveness (NOC)
Maintain hemodynamic stability, such as BP, cardiac output within normal range, adequate urinary output, decreased frequency or absence of dysrhythmias.
Report decreased episodes of dyspnea and angina.
Demonstrate an increase in activity tolerance.

ACTIONS/INTERVENTIONS	RATIONALE
Cardiac Care: Acute (NIC)
Independent
Obtain BP readings. Compare both arms and obtain lying, sitting, and standing pressures when able.	Hypotension may occur related to ventricular dysfunction, hypoperfusion of the myocardium, and vagal stimulation. However, hypertension is also a common phenomenon, possibly related to pain, anxiety, catecholamine release, and preexisting vascular problems. Orthostatic (postural) hypotension may be associated with complications of infarct, such as heart failure.
Evaluate quality and equality of pulses, as indicated.	Decreased cardiac output results in diminished, weak, or thready pulses. Irregularities suggest dysrhythmias, which may require further evaluation and monitoring.
Auscultate heart sounds:
Note development of S_3 and S.	S_3 is usually associated with heart failure, but it may also be noted with the mitral insufficiency (regurgitation) and left ventricular overload that can accompany severe infarction. S_4 may be associated with myocardial ischemia, ventricular stiffening, and pulmonary or systemic hypertension.
Note presence of murmurs and rubs.	Indicates disturbances of normal blood flow within the heart, such as incompetent valve, septal defect, or vibration of papillary muscle and chordae tendineae (complication of MI). Presence of rub with an infarction is also associated with inflammation, such as pericardial effusion and pericarditis.
Auscultate breath sounds.	Crackles reflect pulmonary congestion; may develop because of depressed myocardial function.
Monitor heart rate and rhythm. Document dysrhythmias via telemetry.	Heart rate and rhythm respond to medication, activity, and developing complications. Dysrhythmias, especially premature ventricular contractions or progressive heart blocks, can compromise cardiac function or increase ischemic damage. Acute or chronic atrial flutter or fibrillation may be seen with coronary artery or valvular involvement and may or may not be pathological.

(continues on page 84)

ACTIONS/INTERVENTIONS (continued)

Note response to activity and promote rest appropriately. (Refer to ND: Activity Intolerance.)

Provide small, easily digested meals. Limit caffeine intake, such as coffee, chocolate, and cola, as indicated.

Have emergency equipment and medications available.

Collaborative

Administer supplemental oxygen, as indicated.

Measure cardiac output and other functional parameters as appropriate.

Maintain IV and saline-lock access, as indicated.

Review serial ECGs.

Review chest x-ray.

Monitor laboratory data, such as cardiac enzymes, arterial blood gases (ABGs), and electrolytes.

Administer medications, as indicated:
  Antidysrhythmic drugs (refer to CP: Dysrhythmias)

  Antiemetics and stool softener

Assist with insertion and maintain pacemaker or automatic internal cardiac defibrillator (AICD) when used.

RATIONALE (continued)

Overexertion increases oxygen consumption and demand and can compromise myocardial function.

Large meals may increase myocardial workload and cause vagal stimulation, resulting in bradycardia or ectopic beats. Caffeine is a direct cardiac stimulant that can increase heart rate, but may not be a problem for everyone, such as for some clients with regular daily caffeine intake.

Sudden coronary occlusion, lethal dysrhythmias, extension of infarct, and unrelenting pain are situations that may precipitate cardiac arrest, requiring immediate life-saving therapies or transfer to CCU.

Increases amount of oxygen available for myocardial uptake, reducing ischemia and resultant cellular irritation and dysrhythmias.

Cardiac index, preload and afterload, contractility, and cardiac work can be measured noninvasively with thoracic electrical bioimpedance (TEB) technique. Useful in evaluating response to therapeutic interventions and identifying need for more aggressive or emergency care.

Patent line is important for administration of emergency drugs in presence of persistent lethal dysrhythmias or chest pain.

Provides information regarding progression or resolution of infarction, status of ventricular function, electrolyte balance, and effect of drug therapies.

May reflect pulmonary edema related to ventricular dysfunction.

Enzymes monitor resolution or extension of infarction. Presence of hypoxia indicates need for supplemental oxygen. Electrolyte imbalances, such as hypo- or hyperkalemia, adversely affect cardiac rhythm and contractility.

Dysrhythmias are usually treated symptomatically. Early inclusion of ACE inhibitor therapy, especially in presence of large anterior MI, ventricular aneurysm, or heart failure, enhances ventricular output, increases survival, and may slow progression of heart failure.

Vomiting (vasovagal reflex) or bearing down to pass stool (Valsalva's maneuver) can result in bradycardia, temporarily reducing cardiac output followed by rebound tachycardia.

Pacing may be a temporary support measure during acute phase or may be needed permanently if infarction severely damages conduction system, impairing systolic function. Use of AICD is currently advocated in client who has had ventricular fibrillation or tachycardia resulting in arrest. Strong supporting data document the benefits of ICDs for the primary prevention of sudden cardiac death.

NURSING DIAGNOSIS: ineffective tissue Perfusion (specify)

May be related to

Reduction or interruption of blood flow—vasoconstriction, hypovolemia, shunting, thromboembolic, atherosclerotic plaque formation

Possibly evidenced by

(Not applicable; presence of signs and symptoms establishes an *actual* diagnosis)

Desired Outcomes/Evaluation Criteria—Client Will

Cardiac Pump Effectiveness (NOC)

Demonstrate adequate perfusion as individually appropriate, such as skin warm and dry, peripheral pulses present and strong, vital signs within client's normal range, client alert or oriented, balanced intake and output (I&O), absence of edema, free of pain or discomfort, stable, improving ECG, vitals, and mentation.

ACTIONS/INTERVENTIONS	RATIONALE
Hemodynamic Regulation (NIC)	
Independent	
Investigate sudden changes or continued alterations in mentation, such as anxiety, confusion, lethargy, and stupor.	Cerebral perfusion is directly related to cardiac output and is influenced by electrolyte and acid-base variations, hypoxia, and systemic emboli.
Inspect for pallor, cyanosis, mottling, and cool or clammy skin. Note strength of peripheral pulses.	Systemic vasoconstriction resulting from diminished cardiac output may be evidenced by decreased skin perfusion and diminished pulses. (Refer to ND: risk for decreased Cardiac Output.)
Monitor respirations, noting work of breathing.	Cardiac pump failure and ischemic pain may precipitate respiratory distress; however, sudden or continued dyspnea may indicate thromboembolic pulmonary complications.
Monitor intake, noting changes in urine output. Record urine specific gravity, as indicated.	Decreased intake or persistent nausea may result in reduced circulating volume, which negatively affects perfusion and organ function. Specific gravity measurements reflect hydration status and renal function.
Assess gastrointestinal function, noting anorexia, decreased or absent bowel sounds, nausea and vomiting, abdominal distention, and constipation.	Reduced blood flow to mesentery can produce gastrointestinal dysfunction, such as loss of peristalsis. Problems may be potentiated or aggravated by use of analgesics, decreased activity, and dietary changes.
Circulatory Care: Venous Insufficiency (NIC)	
Encourage active or assist with passive leg exercises, with avoidance of isometric exercises.	Enhances venous return, reduces venous stasis, and decreases risk of thrombophlebitis; however, isometric exercises can adversely affect cardiac output by increasing myocardial work and oxygen consumption.
Assess for pain in lower extremity and Homans' sign, erythema, and edema.	Indicators of deep vein thrombosis (DVT), although calf pain is not always present.
Instruct client in application and periodic removal of antiembolic hose when used.	Limits venous stasis, improves venous return, and reduces risk of thrombophlebitis in client who is limited in activity.
Collaborative	
Apply elastic compression stockings or intermittent pneumatic compression devices, as indicated.	May be desired to prevent DVT, especially in client who is unable to be out of bed or cannot ambulate freely.
Cardiac Care: Acute (NIC)	
Obtain a 12-lead ECG recording.	Determines extension of infarction.
Monitor laboratory data, such as ABGs, blood urea nitrogen (BUN), creatinine, electrolytes, and coagulation studies (prothrombin time [PT], activated prothrombin time [aPTT], clotting times).	Indicators of organ perfusion and function. Abnormalities in coagulation may occur as a result of therapeutic measures, such as heparin or Coumadin use and some cardiac drugs.
Provide supplemental oxygen as prescribed.	Increases oxygen supply to the myocardium.
Administer medications, as indicated, for example:	
Antiplatelet agents, such as aspirin, abciximab (ReoPro), clopidogrel (Plavix), and eptifibatide (Integrilin)	Reduces mortality in MI clients and is taken daily. Aspirin also reduces coronary reocclusion after percutaneous transluminal coronary angioplasty (PTCA). IV antiplatelet drugs such as ReoPro and Integrilin are used as adjuncts to PTCA to decrease complication of platelet clumping within stent when placed.
Anticoagulants, such as heparin/enoxaparin (Lovenox)	Low-dose heparin is given during PTCA and may be given prophylactically in high-risk clients, such as those with atrial fibrillation, obesity, ventricular aneurysm, or history of thrombophlebitis, to reduce risk of thrombophlebitis or mural thrombus formation.
Cimetidine (Tagamet), ranitidine (Zantac), and antacids	May occasionally be used to reduce or neutralize gastric acid, preventing discomfort and gastric irritation, especially in presence of reduced mucosal circulation.
Assist with reperfusion therapy:	
Administer thrombolytic agents: alteplase (Activase, rt-PA), reteplase (Retavase), streptokinase (Streptase), anistreplase (Eminase), and urokinase (Abbokinase).	Thrombolytic therapy is the treatment of choice if angioplasty is not immediately available within 90 minutes. The goal is to restore perfusion to the myocardium.

(continues on page 86)

ACTIONS/INTERVENTIONS (continued)	RATIONALE (continued)
Prepare for procedures such as balloon PTCA, with or without intracoronary stents.	Angioplasty is used to open blocked coronary arteries and immediately restore myocardial perfusion. The mechanism includes a combination of vessel stretching and plaque compression and removal of thrombotic material. Intracoronary stents may be placed at the time of PTCA to provide structural support within the coronary artery. Drug-eluting (drug-coated) stents may be used to decrease risk of restenosis and improve long-term patency.
Transfer to CCU or step-down unit.	Depending on client's condition—degree of heart damage or other chronic health conditions—telemetry or more intensive monitoring and aggressive interventions may be necessary to promote optimum outcome.

NURSING DIAGNOSIS: risk for excess Fluid Volume

Risk factors may include
Decreased organ perfusion (renal)
Increased sodium and water retention
Increased hydrostatic pressure or decreased plasma proteins—sequestering of fluid in interstitial space and tissues

Possibly evidenced by
(Not applicable; presence of signs and symptoms establishes an *actual* diagnosis)

Desired Outcomes/Evaluation Criteria—Client Will

Fluid Balance (NOC)
Maintain fluid balance as evidenced by BP within client's normal limits.
Have no signs of fluid overload such as edema, weight gain, shortness of breath, and lung sounds with crackles.

ACTIONS/INTERVENTIONS	RATIONALE
Fluid Management (NIC)	
Independent	
Auscultate breath sounds for presence of crackles.	May indicate pulmonary edema secondary to cardiac decompensation.
Note JVD and development of dependent edema.	Suggests developing congestive failure or fluid volume excess.
Measure I&O, noting decrease in output and concentrated urine. Calculate fluid balance.	Decreased cardiac output results in impaired kidney perfusion, sodium and water retention, and reduced urine output.
Weigh daily at the same time on the same scale.	Sudden changes in weight reflect alterations in fluid balance.
Maintain total fluid intake at 2,000 mL every 24 hours within cardiovascular tolerance.	Meets normal adult body fluid requirements, but may require alteration or restriction in presence of cardiac decompensation.
Collaborative	
Provide low-sodium, low-caffeine diet, including beverages.	Sodium enhances fluid retention and should therefore be restricted during active MI phase or if heart failure is present. Caffeine may cause vasospasm.
Administer diuretics, such as furosemide (Lasix), spironolactone with hydrochlorothiazide (Aldactazide), hydralazine (Apresoline).	May be necessary to correct fluid overload. Drug choice is usually dependent on acute or chronic nature of symptoms.
Monitor potassium, as indicated.	Hypokalemia can limit effectiveness of therapy and can occur with use of potassium-depleting diuretics.

NURSING DIAGNOSIS: **deficient Knowledge [Learning Need] regarding cause and treatment of condition, self-care, and discharge needs**

May be related to
Lack of information, misunderstanding of medical condition or therapy needs
Unfamiliarity with information resources
Lack of recall

Possibly evidenced by
Questions, statement of misconception
Failure to improve on previous regimen
Development of preventable complications

Desired Outcomes/Evaluation Criteria—Client Will

Knowledge: Cardiac Disease Management (NOC)
Verbalize understanding of condition, potential complications, individual risk factors, and function of pacemaker (if used).
Relate signs of pacemaker failure.
Verbalize understanding of therapeutic regimen.
List desired action and possible adverse side effects of medications.

Cardiac Disease Self-Management (NOC)
Correctly perform necessary procedures and explain reasons for actions.
Keep follow-up appointments.

ACTIONS/INTERVENTIONS	RATIONALE
Teaching: Individual (NIC)	
Independent	
Assess client and SO level of knowledge and ability or desire to learn.	Necessary for creation of individual instruction plan. Reinforces expectation that this will be a "learning experience." Verbalization identifies misunderstandings and allows for clarification.
Be alert to signs of avoidance, such as changing subject away from information being presented or extremes of behavior, such as withdrawal or euphoria.	Natural defense mechanisms, such as anger or denial of significance of situation, can block learning, affecting client's response and ability to assimilate information. Changing to a less formal or structured style may be more effective until client and SO is ready to accept or deal with current situation.
Present information in varied learning formats, such as programmed books, audiovisual tapes, question-and-answer sessions, and group activities.	Using multiple learning methods enhances retention of material.
Cardiac Care: Rehabilitation (NIC)	
Reinforce explanations of risk factors, dietary and activity restrictions, medications, and symptoms requiring immediate medical attention.	Provides opportunity for client to retain information and to assume control and participate in rehabilitation program.
Review activity limitations, such as refraining from strenuous activities until first checking with provider. Avoid exertion in extreme heat or cold. Stop any activity if chest pain, unusual shortness of breath, dizziness, lightheadedness, or nausea occurs.	During healing phase, restrictions may be needed to limit amount of myocardial workload and oxygen consumption.
Explain rationale of dietary regimen, diet low in sodium, saturated fats, and cholesterol.	Excess saturated fats, cholesterol, calories, and sodium increases BP and risk for heart disease. Excess of cholesterol builds plaque in arteries.
Instruct client to consult healthcare provider before taking other prescription or OTC medications.	Many drugs may contain sympathetic nervous stimulants and may increase BP or counteract other medications.
Discuss use of herbals, such as ginseng, garlic, ginkgo, hawthorn, and bromelain, as indicated.	Use of supplements or herbal remedies can result in alterations in blood clotting, especially when anticoagulant therapy, such as Plavix or ASA, is prescribed. Hawthorn can increase the effect of certain cardiac medications.
Encourage identification and reduction of individual risk factors, such as smoking and alcohol consumption and obesity.	These behaviors and chemicals have direct adverse effects on cardiovascular function and may impede recovery and increase risk for complications.
Warn against isometric activity, Valsalva's maneuver, and activities requiring arms positioned above head.	These activities greatly increase cardiac workload and myocardial oxygen consumption and may adversely affect myocardial contractility and output.

(continues on page 88)

Review programmed increases in levels of activity. Educate client regarding gradual resumption of activities, such as walking, work, and recreational and sexual activity. Provide guidelines for gradually increasing activity and instruction regarding target heart rate and pulse taking, as appropriate.

Identify alternative activities for "bad weather" days, such as measured walking in house or shopping mall.

Review signs and symptoms requiring reduction in activity and notification of healthcare provider. Differentiate between increased heart rate that normally occurs during various activities and worsening signs of cardiac stress: chest pain, dyspnea, palpitations, increased heart rate lasting more than 15 minutes after cessation of activity, and excessive fatigue the following day.

Stress importance of follow-up care, and identify community resources and support groups, such as cardiac rehabilitation programs, "coronary clubs," and smoking cessation clinics.

Recommend client receive annual influenza and periodic pneumonia vaccination unless otherwise contraindicated.

Emphasize importance of contacting physician if chest pain, change in anginal pattern, or other symptoms recur.

Stress importance of reporting development of fever in association with diffuse or atypical chest pain (pleural, pericardial) and joint pain.

Encourage client and SO to share concerns and feelings. Discuss signs of pathological depression versus transient feelings frequently associated with major life events. Recommend seeking professional help if feelings of depression persist.

Gradual increase in activity increases strength and prevents overexertion, may enhance collateral circulation, and promotes return to normal lifestyle. *Note:* Sexual activity can be safely resumed once client can accomplish activity equivalent to climbing two flights of stairs without adverse cardiac effects.

Provides for continuing daily activity program.

Pulse elevations beyond established limits, development of chest pain, or dyspnea may require changes in exercise and medication regimen.

Reinforces that this is an ongoing or continuing health problem for which support and assistance is available after discharge. *Note:* After discharge, client may encounter limitations in physical functioning and often incur difficulty with emotional, social, and role functioning requiring ongoing support.

Helps protect against viral and bacterial cardiorespiratory illnesses that can negatively impact client's heart health.

Timely evaluation and intervention may prevent complications.

Post-MI complication of pericardial inflammation (Dressler's syndrome) requires further medical evaluation and intervention.

Depressed clients have a greater risk of dying 6 to 18 months following a heart attack. Timely intervention may be beneficial. *Note:* Selective serotonin reuptake inhibitors (SSRIs), such as paroxetine (Paxil), have been found to be as effective as tricyclic antidepressants but with significantly fewer adverse cardiac complications.

POTENTIAL CONSIDERATIONS following discharge from care setting (dependent on client's age, physical condition and presence of complications, personal resources, and life responsibilities)

- *Activity Intolerance*—imbalance between myocardial oxygen supply and demand
- *Grieving*—perceived loss of general well-being, required changes in lifestyle, confronting mortality
- *decisional Conflict regarding treatment*—multiple or divergent sources of information, perceived threat to value system, support system deficit
- *interrupted Family Processes*—situational transition and crisis
- *impaired Home Management*—altered ability to perform tasks, inadequate support systems, reluctance to request assistance

---

DYSRHYTHMIAS

I. Pathophysiology
  a. Abnormal formation or conduction of the electrical impulses within the heart
    i. Bradyarrhythmias: decreased intrinsic pacemaker function or block in conduction, often at atrioventricular (AV) junction or His-Purkinje system
    ii. Tachyarrhythmias: caused by reentry, often due to enhanced or abnormal automaticity
  b. Causes abnormalities of the heart rate, rhythm, or both
  c. Change in conduction may alter pumping action of heart, affecting blood pressure and perfusion of body organs.

II. Classification: Types of Dysrhythmias (Wedro, 2007)
  a. Named according to the site of origination and the mechanism of conduction involved:
    i. Sinus or sinoatrial (SA) node
    ii. AV node
    iii. Involved heart chamber—atrial or ventricular
    iv. Between the atria and ventricles—supraventricular or junctional dysrhythmias
  b. Differentiated by rate
    i. Slow: bradycardia, pulse below 60 in adult
    ii. Fast: tachycardia, pulse above 100 in adult
  c. Rhythm disturbances can be regular (e.g., sinus tachycardia) or irregular (e.g., atrial fibrillation).

III. Etiology

a. Primary cardiac disorder: coronary artery disease (CAD), myocardial infarction (MI), heart valve dysfunction, coronary artery bypass (CABG) surgery, or valve replacement surgery

b. Systemic conditions: hypothyroidism and hyperthyroidism; fever and dehydration; sepsis; shock states (hypovolemic, cardiogenic); anemia; pulmonary diseases; brain injury; catecholamine release, such as occurs in intense emotional stress or vigorous exercise; anxiety disorders and panic attacks

c. Electrolyte imbalances, such as with potassium

d. Effects of drugs and drug toxicity, such as with digoxin, aminophylline, atropine, and caffeine

e. Illicit drug use, such as cocaine, methamphetamines

IV. Statistics

a. Atrial fibrillation is a frequent complication of cardiac surgery, occurring in 30% of patients after CABG surgery and up to 50% of patients following valve surgery (Yee, 2006).

b. Mortality: 350,000 to 400,000 Americans die annually from sudden cardiac death (Coughlin, 2007).

COMMON DYSRHYTHMIAS

Tachycardias

I. Sinus Tachycardia

a. Sinus node creates rate that is faster than normal (greater than 100)

b. Associated with physiological or psychological stress; medications, such as catecholamines, aminophylline, atropine, stimulants, and illicit drugs; enhanced automaticity; and autonomic dysfunction

II. Atrial Flutter

a. Occurs in the atrium and creates regular atrial rates between 250 and 400. Because AV node cannot keep up with conduction of all these impulses, not all atrial impulses are conducted into the ventricle, causing a therapeutic block at the AV node.

III. Atrial Fibrillation (AF)

a. Rapid, irregular twitching of the atrial musculature with an atrial rate of 300 to 600 and a ventricular rate of 120 to 200 if untreated

b. Associated with advanced age, valvular heart disease, hyperthyroidism, pulmonary disorder, pulmonary disease, alcohol ingestion ("holiday heart syndrome"), hypertension, diabetes, CAD, or after open-heart surgery

IV. Paroxysmal Supraventricular Tachycardia (PSVT, also called SVT)

a. Pathways in the AV node or atrium allow an altered conduction of electricity, causing a regular and fast rate of sometimes more than 150 to 200.

b. Ventricle, sensing the electrical activity coming through the AV node, beats along with each stimulation.

c. Rarely a life-threatening event, but most people feel uncomfortable when PSVT occurs.

V. Ventricular Tachycardia (VT)

a. Rapid heartbeat initiated within the ventricles, characterized by three or more consecutive premature ventricular beats with elevated and regular heart rate (such as 160 to 240 beats per minute)

b. Heart rate sustained at a high rate causes symptoms such as weakness, fatigue, dizziness, fainting, or palpitations

c. Potentially lethal disruption of normal heartbeat that can degenerate to ventricular fibrillation

VI. Ventricular Fibrillation (VF)

a. Aside from myocardial ischemia, other causes of ventricular fibrillation may include severe weakness of the heart muscle, electrolyte disturbances, drug overdose, and poisoning.

b. Electrical signal is sent from the ventricles at a very fast and erratic rate, impairing the ability of ventricles to fill with blood and pump it out, markedly decreasing cardiac output, and resulting in very low blood pressure and loss of consciousness.

c. Sudden death will occur if VF not corrected.

Bradycardias

I. Sinus Bradycardia

a. Rarely symptomatic until heart rate drops below 50, then fainting or syncope may be reported

b. Causes include hypothyroidism, athletic training, sleep, vagal stimulation, increased intracranial pressure, MI, hypovolemia, hypoxia, acidosis, hypokalemia and hyperkalemia, hyperglycemia, hypothermia, toxins, tamponade, tension pneumothorax, thrombosis (cardiac or pulmonary), and trauma.

c. Medications, such as beta blockers, calcium channel blockers, and amiodarone, also slow the heart rate (AHA, 2005).

II. Sick Sinus Syndrome (SSS)

a. Varity of conditions affecting SA node function, including bradycardia, sinus arrest, sinoatrial block, episodes of tachycardia, and carotid hypersensitivity

b. Signs and symptoms related to cerebral hypoperfusion

c. May be associated with rapid rate (tachycardia) or alternate between too fast and too slow (bradycardia-tachycardia syndrome). A long pause (asystole) may occur between heartbeats, especially after an episode of tachycardia.

III. Heart Blocks

a. First-degree AV block

i. Asymptomatic; usually an incidental finding on electrocardiogram (ECG)

b. Second-degree AV (type I and type II)

i. Usually asymptomatic, although some clients can feel irregularities (palpitations) of the heartbeat, or syncope may occur, which usually is observed in more advanced conduction disturbances such as Mobitz II AV block

ii. Medications affecting AV node function, such as digoxin, beta blockers, calcium channel blockers, may contribute

(text continues on page 90)

c. Third-degree AV block (also called complete heart block)
   i. May be associated with acute MI either causing the block or related to reduced cardiac output from bradycardia in the setting of advanced atherosclerotic CAD

   ii. Symptomatic with fatigue, dizziness, and syncope and possible loss of consciousness
   iii. Can be life-threatening, especially if associated with heart failure

Other Dysrhythmias

I. Premature Atrial Complex (PAC)
a. Electrical impulse starts in the atrium before the next normal impulse of the sinus node.
b. Causes include caffeine, alcohol, and nicotine use, stretched atrial myocardium; anxiety; hypokalemia; and hypermetabolic states (pregnancy), or may be related to atrial ischemia, injury, or infarction.

II. Premature Ventricular Contraction (PVC)
a. Electrical signal originates in the ventricles, causing them to contract before receiving the electrical signal from the atria.
b. PVCs not uncommon and are often asymptomatic.
c. Increase to several per minute may cause symptoms such as weakness, fatigue, dizziness, fainting, or palpitations.
d. Irritability of the heart demonstrated by frequent and or multiple back-to-back PVCs can lead to VF.

GLOSSARY

Arrhythmias (also called dysrhythmias): Heart rhythm disturbances classified by rate (normal, tachycardia, bradycardia); mechanism (automaticity, reentry, fibrillation); and by site of origin (atrial, ventricular, junctional).

AV node: The electrical relay station between the atria (the upper) and the ventricles (the lower chambers of the heart).

Bigeminal pulse: Irregular strong beat alternating with weak beat.

Bradycardias: Abnormally slow rhythms may be ascribed to two general mechanisms—failure of the sinoatrial (SA) node to generate impulses, such as in sinus bradycardia, or failure of the impulses to conduct normally to the ventricles, such as in heart blocks.

Pacemaker: A system that sends electrical impulses to the heart in order to set the heart rhythm. The pacemaker can be the natural pacemaker of the heart or it can be an artificial electronic device.

Palpitations: An increased awareness of the heartbeat and palpitations can result from many dysrhythmias, including any bradycardia and tachycardia, premature

ventricular and atrial contractions, sick sinus syndrome (SSS), advanced arteriovenous block, or ventricular tachycardia (VT). Palpitations associated with dizziness, near-syncope, or syncope suggest tachyarrhythmia and are potentially more serious.

Pulse deficit: Difference between apical pulse and radial pulse.

Pulsus alternans: Regular strong beat, alternating with weak beat.

Sinoatrial (SA) node: One of the major elements in the cardiac conduction system that controls the heart rate. The SA node generates electrical impulses and conducts them throughout the muscle of the heart, stimulating the heart to contract and pump blood.

Sudden cardiac death (also known as cardiac arrest): A sudden, unexpected death caused by loss of heart function. Most sudden cardiac deaths are caused by dysrhythmias, such as ventricular fibrillation (VF). The only treatment is defibrillation with an electrical shock.

Tachycardias: Rapid heart rates originating from either the atrium or the ventricle.

Care Settings

Generally, minor dysrhythmias are monitored and treated in the community setting; however, potential life-threatening situations (including heart rates above 150 beats per minute) may require a short inpatient stay.

Related Concerns

Angina, page 64
Heart failure: chronic, page 48
Myocardial infarction, page 74
Psychosocial aspects of care, page 749

Client Assessment Database

DIAGNOSTIC DIVISION MAY REPORT	MAY EXHIBIT
ACTIVITY/REST • Generalized weakness • Exertional fatigue	• Changes in heart rate/blood pressure (BP) with activity or exercise
CIRCULATION • History of previous or acute MI (90% to 95% experience dysrhythmias), cardiac surgery, cardiomyopathy, rheumatic heart disease and heart failure (HF), valvular heart disease, long-standing hypertension, use of pacemaker • *Pulse:* Fast, slow, or irregular; palpitations, skipped beats	• BP changes (hypertension or hypotension) during episodes of dysrhythmia • Pulses may be irregular, for example, skipped beats; pulsus alternans, bigeminal pulse • Pulse deficit • *Heart sounds:* irregular rhythm, extra sounds, dropped beats • Skin color and moisture changes, such as pallor, cyanosis, diaphoresis (HF, shock) • Edema dependent, generalized, jugular vein distention (JVD) (in presence of HF) • Urine output decreased if cardiac output is severely diminished
EGO INTEGRITY • Feeling nervous (certain tachydysrhythmias), sense of impending doom • Stressors related to current medical problems	• Anxiety, fear, withdrawal, anger, irritability, crying • Denial of health problems
FOOD/FLUID • Loss of appetite, anorexia • Food intolerance (with certain medications) • Nausea or vomiting • Changes in weight	• Weight gain or loss • Edema • Changes in skin moisture or turgor • Lung sounds have crackles
NEUROSENSORY • Dizzy spells, fainting, headaches • Numbness or tingling of fingers or toes	• Mental status or sensorium changes, such as disorientation, confusion, loss of memory; changes in usual speech pattern and consciousness, stupor, coma • Behavioral changes, such as combativeness, lethargy, hallucinations • Pupil changes (equality and reaction to light) • Loss of deep tendon reflexes with life-threatening dysrhythmias (VT, severe bradycardia)
PAIN/DISCOMFORT • Chest pain (mild to severe) that may or may not be relieved by anti-anginal medication	• Distraction behaviors, such as restlessness
RESPIRATION • Chronic lung disease • History of or current tobacco use • Shortness of breath • Coughing with or without sputum production	• Changes in respiratory rate and depth during dysrhythmia episode • *Breath sounds:* Adventitious sounds such as crackles, rhonchi, or wheezing, indicating respiratory complications, such as left-sided heart failure (pulmonary edema) or pulmonary thromboembolic phenomena • Hemoptysis • Abnormal pulse oximetry or blood gases
SAFETY	• Fever • *Skin:* Rashes (medication reaction) • Loss of muscle tone and strength

(continues on page 92)

TEACHING/LEARNING
- Familial risk factors, such as heart disease, stroke
- Use or misuse of prescribed medications, such as heart medications, anticoagulants, or over-the-counter (OTC) medications, for example, cough syrup, analgesics containing aspirin (ASA), and decongestants
- Use of vitamins and herbal supplements for heart rhythm, such as belladonna, camphor, dong quai, ginseng, goldenseal
- Stimulant abuse, including caffeine and nicotine; street drugs, including cocaine derivitives, methamphetamines, ecstasy, inhalants
- Lack of understanding about disease process and therapeutic regimen
- Evidence of failure to improve, such as recurrent or intractable dysrhythmias that are life-threatening

DISCHARGE PLAN CONSIDERATIONS
- Alteration of medication use and therapy
- Coumadin precautions
- Teaching regarding pacemaker or other device

▶ Refer to section at end of plan for postdischarge considerations.

Diagnostic Studies

TEST WHY IT IS DONE	WHAT IT TELLS ME
BLOOD TESTS	
Electrolytes: Substances that, in solution, conduct an electric current and are decomposed by its passage. Sodium, potassium, calcium, and magnesium are common electrolytes.	Imbalance of electrolytes, such as potassium, magnesium, and calcium, adversely affects cardiac rhythm and contractility.
Drug screen: Laboratory procedure that checks blood or urine sample for presence of certain medications or drugs of abuse.	May reveal therapeutic or toxic levels of prescription medications; suggest interaction of drugs, such as digoxin and quinidine; or detect presence of street drugs that can affect or contribute to dysrhythmias.
Thyroid studies: Blood test and/or scan to evaluate thyroid function. The most commonly used laboratory test is the measurement of thyroid-stimulating hormone (TSH).	Hyperthyroidism or hypothyroidism can cause or aggravate dysrhythmias.
C-reactive protein (CRP): Blood test shows presence of affected cardiac tissue.	Elevation may indicate acute or active inflammatory process, such as endocarditis, as a precipitating factor for dysrhythmias.
Arterial blood gas (ABG) and pulse oximetry: Blood test or peripheral scan to measure oxygen content and saturation of the blood.	Hypoxemia can cause or exacerbate dysrhythmias.
OTHER DIAGNOSTIC STUDIES	
Electrocardiogram (ECG): Record of the electrical activity of the heart.	Reveals type and source of dysrhythmia and effects of electrolyte imbalances and cardiac medications. Demonstrates patterns of ischemic injury and conduction aberrance. *Note:* Exercise ECG reveals dysrhythmias occurring only when client is not at rest (can be diagnostic for cardiac cause of syncope).

TEST WHY IT IS DONE (continued)	WHAT IT TELLS ME (continued)
• *Extended or event monitoring (Holter monitor):* Extended ECG tracing (24 hours to weeks).	May be used to determine which dysrhythmias may be causing specific symptoms when client is active at home or work or at rest. May also be used to evaluate pacemaker function, antidysrhythmic drug effect, or effectiveness of cardiac rehabilitation.
• *Signal-averaged ECG (SAE):* May be used to screen high-risk clients especially, with post-MI or unexplained syncope.	May reveal ventricular dysrhythmias, presence of delayed conduction, and late potentials—as occurs with sustained ventricular tachycardia.
• *Electrophysiological (EP) studies:* Test that records the electrical activity and the electrical pathways of the heart. During the EP study, the tester safely reproduces the abnormal heart rhythm.	Used to diagnose dysrhythmias and evaluate effectiveness of medication or pacemaker therapies.
• *Myocardial imaging scans, such as myocardial perfusion imaging (MPI) or cardiac computed tomography (CT):* Uses radioactive isotopes to gauge the blood supply and viability of regions or walls of the heart, often in conjunction with exercise tolerance tests.	May demonstrate ischemic or damaged myocardial areas that could impede normal conduction or impair wall motion and pumping capabilities.
• *Chest x-ray:* Procedure used to evaluate organs and structures within the chest.	May show enlarged cardiac shadow due to ventricular or valvular dysfunction.

Nursing Priorities

1. Prevent or treat life-threatening dysrhythmias.
2. Support client and significant other (SO) in dealing with anxiety and fear of potentially life-threatening situation.
3. Assist in identification of cause or precipitating factors.
4. Review information regarding condition, prognosis, and treatment regimen.

Discharge Goals

1. Free of life-threatening dysrhythmias and complications of impaired cardiac output and tissue perfusion.
2. Anxiety reduced and managed.
3. Disease process, therapy needs, and prevention of complications understood.
4. Plan in place to meet needs after discharge.

NURSING DIAGNOSIS: **risk for decreased Cardiac Output**

Risk factors may include
Altered electrical conduction
Reduced myocardial contractility

Possibly evidenced by
(Not applicable; presence of signs and symptoms establishes an *actual* diagnosis)

Desired Outcomes/Evaluation Criteria—Client Will

Cardiac Pump Effectiveness (NOC)
Maintain or achieve adequate cardiac output as evidenced by BP and pulse within normal range, adequate urinary output, palpable pulses of equal quality, and usual level of mentation.
Display reduced frequency or absence of dysrhythmia(s).
Participate in activities that reduce myocardial workload.

ACTIONS/INTERVENTIONS	RATIONALE
Dysrhythmia Management (NIC) *Independent* Palpate radial, carotid, femoral, and dorsalis pedis pulses, noting rate, regularity, amplitude (full or thready), and symmetry. Document presence of pulsus alternans, bigeminal pulse, or pulse deficit.	Differences in equality, rate, and regularity of pulses are indicative of the effect of altered cardiac output on systemic and peripheral circulation.

(continues on page 94)

ACTIONS/INTERVENTIONS (continued)

Auscultate heart sounds, noting rate, rhythm, presence of extra heartbeats, and dropped beats.

Monitor vital signs. Assess adequacy of cardiac output and tissue perfusion, noting significant variations in BP, pulse rate equality, respirations, changes in skin color and temperature, level of consciousness and sensorium, and urine output during episodes of dysrhythmias.

Determine type of dysrhythmia and document with rhythm strip if cardiac or telemetry monitoring is available:

Sinus tachycardia

Sinus bradycardia

Atrial dysrhythmias, such as PACs, atrial flutter, AF, and atrial supraventricular tachycardias (i.e., paroxysmal atrial tachycardia [PAT], multifocal atrial tachycardia [MAT], SVT)

Ventricular dysrhythmias, such as PVCs and ventricular premature beats (VPBs), VT, and ventricular flutter and VF

Heart blocks

Provide calm and quiet environment. Review reasons for limitation of activities during acute phase.

Demonstrate and encourage use of stress management behaviors such as relaxation techniques; guided imagery; and slow, deep breathing.

Investigate reports of chest pain, documenting location, duration, intensity (0 to 10 scale), and relieving or aggravating factors. Note nonverbal pain cues, such as facial grimacing, crying, changes in BP and heart rate.

RATIONALE (continued)

Specific dysrhythmias are more clearly detected audibly than by palpation. Hearing extra heartbeats or dropped beats helps identify dysrhythmias in the unmonitored client.

Although not all dysrhythmias are life-threatening, immediate treatment may be required to terminate dysrhythmia in the presence of alterations in cardiac output and tissue perfusion.

Useful in determining need and type of intervention required.

Tachycardia can occur in response to stress, pain, fever, infection, coronary artery blockage, valvular dysfunction, hypovolemia, hypoxia, or as a result of decreased vagal tone or of increased sympathetic nervous system activity associated with the release of catecholamines. Although it generally does not require treatment, persistent tachycardia may worsen underlying pathology in clients with ischemic heart disease because of shortened diastolic filling time and increased oxygen demands. These clients may require medications.

Bradycardia is common in clients with acute MI (especially anterior and inferior) and is the result of excessive parasympathetic activity, blocks in conduction to the SA or AV nodes, or loss of automaticity of the heart muscle. Clients with severe heart disease may not be able to compensate for a slow rate by increasing stroke volume; therefore, decreased cardiac output, HF, and potentially lethal ventricular dysrhythmias may occur.

PACs can occur as a response to ischemia and are normally harmless, but can precede or precipitate AF. Acute and chronic atrial flutter or fibrillation (the most common dysrhythmia) can occur with coronary artery or valvular disease and may or may not be pathological. Rapid atrial flutter or fibrillation reduces cardiac output as a result of incomplete ventricular filling (shortened cardiac cycle) and increased oxygen demand.

PVCs or VPBs reflect cardiac irritability and are commonly associated with MI, digoxin toxicity, coronary vasospasm, and misplaced temporary pacemaker leads. Frequent, multiple, or multifocal PVCs result in diminished cardiac output and may lead to potentially lethal dysrhythmias, such as VT or sudden death or cardiac arrest from ventricular flutter or VF. *Note:* Intractable ventricular dysrhythmias unresponsive to medication may reflect ventricular aneurysm. Polymorphic VT (torsades de pointes) is recognized by inconsistent shape of QRS complexes and is often related to use of drugs such as procainamide (Pronestyl), quinidine (Quinaglute), disopyramide (Norpace), and sotalol (Betapace).

Reflect altered transmission of impulses through normal conduction channels (slowed, altered) and may be the result of MI, CAD with reduced blood supply to SA or AV nodes, drug toxicity, and sometimes cardiac surgery. Progressing heart block is associated with slowed ventricular rates, decreased cardiac output, and potentially lethal ventricular dysrhythmias or cardiac standstill.

Reduces stimulation and release of stress-related catecholamines, which can cause or aggravate dysrhythmias and vasoconstriction, increasing myocardial workload.

Promotes client participation in exerting some sense of control in a stressful situation.

Reasons for chest pain are variable and depend on underlying cause. However, chest pain may indicate ischemia due to altered electrical conduction, decreased myocardial perfusion, or increased oxygen need, such as impending or evolving MI.

ACTIONS/INTERVENTIONS (continued)

Be prepared to initiate cardiopulmonary resuscitation (CPR), as indicated.

Collaborative

Monitor laboratory studies, such as the following:
Electrolytes

Medication and drug levels

Administer supplemental oxygen, as indicated.

Prepare for and assist with diagnostic and treatment procedures such as EP studies, radiofrequency ablation (RFA), and cryoablation (CA).

Administer medications, as indicated, for example:
Potassium

Antidysrhythmics, such as the following:
Class I drugs:

Class Ia, such as disopyramide (Norpace), procainamide (Procan SR), quinidine (Cardioquin), and moricizine (Ethmozine)

Class Ib, such as lidocaine (Xylocaine), phenytoin (Dilantin), tocainide (Tonocard), and mexiletine (Mexitil)

Class Ic, such as flecainide (Tambocor) and propafenone (Rhythmol)

Class II drugs, such as atenolol (Tenormin), propranolol (Inderal), nadolol (Corgard), acebutolol (Sectral), esmolol (Brevibloc), sotalol (Betapace), and bisoprolol (Zebeta)

RATIONALE (continued)

Development of life-threatening dysrhythmias requires prompt intervention to prevent ischemic damage or death.

Imbalance of electrolytes, such as potassium, magnesium, and calcium, adversely affects cardiac rhythm and contractility.
Reveal therapeutic and toxic level of prescription medications or street drugs that may affect or contribute to presence of dysrhythmias.
Increases amount of oxygen available for myocardial uptake, reducing irritability caused by hypoxia.
Treatment for several tachycardia dysrhythmias, including SVT, atrial flutter, Wolf-Parkinson-White (WPW) syndrome, AF, and VT, is often carried out as first-line treatment via heart catheterization or angiographic procedures. After rhythm is confirmed with EP study, the client will then often have either an RFA or CA to terminate or disrupt the dysfunctional pattern. Medications may be tried first or added after ablation for increased treatment success.

Correction of hypokalemia may be sufficient to terminate some ventricular dysrhythmias. *Note:* Potassium imbalance is the number one cause of AF.

Class I drugs depress depolarization and alter repolarization, stabilizing the cell. These drugs are divided into groups a, b, and c, based on their unique effects.
These drugs increase action potential, duration, and effective refractory period and decrease membrane responsiveness, prolonging both QRS complex and QT interval. This also results in decreasing myocardial conduction velocity and excitability in the atria, ventricles, and accessory pathways. They suppress ectopic focal activity. Useful for treatment of atrial and ventricular premature beats and repetitive dysrhythmias, such as atrial tachycardias and atrial flutter and AF. *Note:* Myocardial depressant effects may be potentiated when class Ia drugs are used in conjunction with any drugs possessing similar properties.
These drugs shorten the duration of the refractory period (QT interval), and their action depends on the tissue affected and the level of extracellular potassium. These drugs have little effect on myocardial contractility, AV and intraventricular conduction, and cardiac output. They also suppress automaticity in the His-Purkinje system. Drugs of choice for ventricular dysrhythmias, they are also effective for automatic and re-entrant dysrhythmias and digoxin-induced dysrhythmias. *Note:* These drugs may aggravate myocardial depression.
These drugs slow conduction by depressing SA node automaticity and decreasing conduction velocity through the atria, ventricles, and Purkinje's fibers. The result is prolongation of the PR interval and lengthening of the QRS complex. They suppress and prevent all types of ventricular dysrhythmias. *Note:* Flecainide increases risk of drug-induced dysrhythmias post-MI. Propafenone can worsen or cause new dysrhythmias, a tendency called the "pro-arrhythmic effect."
Beta-adrenergic blockers have antiadrenergic properties and decrease automaticity. They reduce the rate and force of cardiac contractions, which in turn decrease cardiac output, blood pressure, and peripheral vascular resistance. Therefore, they are useful in the treatment of dysrhythmias caused by SA and AV node dysfunction, including SVTs, atrial flutter and AF. *Note:* These drugs may exacerbate bradycardia and cause myocardial depression, especially when combined with drugs that have similar properties.

(continues on page 96)

Class III drugs, such as bretylium tosylate (Bretylol), amio-darone (Cordarone), sotalol (Betapace), ibutilide (Corvert), and dofetilide (Tikosyn)

These drugs prolong the refractory period and action potential duration, consequently prolonging the QT interval. They decrease peripheral resistance and increase coronary blood flow. They have anti-anginal and anti-adrenergic properties. They are used to terminate VF and other life-threatening ventricular dysrhythmias and sustained ventricular tachy-arrhythmias, especially when lidocaine and procainamide are not effective. *Note:* Sotalol is a nonselective beta blocker with characteristics of both class II and class III.

Class IV drugs, such as verapamil (Calan), nifedipine (Procardia), and diltiazem (Cardizem)

Calcium antagonists, or calcium channel blockers, slow conduction time through the AV node, prolonging PR inter-val to decrease ventricular response in SVTs, atrial flutter and AF. Calan and Cardizem may be used for bedside conversion of acute AF.

Class V drugs, such as atropine sulfate, isoproterenol (Isuprel), and cardiac glycosides (digoxin [Lanoxin])

Miscellaneous drugs useful in treating bradycardia by increas-ing SA and AV conduction and enhancing automaticity. Cardiac glycosides may be used alone or in combination with other antidysrhythmic drugs to reduce ventricular rate in presence of uncontrolled or poorly tolerated atrial tachycardias or atrial flutter and AF.

Adenosine (Adenocard)

First-line treatment for PSVT. Slows conduction and interrupts reentry pathways in AV node. *Note:* Contraindicated in clients with second- or third-degree heart block or those with SSS who do not have a functioning pacemaker.

Prepare for and assist with elective cardioversion.

May be used in AF after trials of first-line drugs, such as atenolol, metoprolol, diltiazem, and verapamil, have failed to control heart rate or in certain unstable dysrhythmias to restore normal heart rate or relieve symptoms of heart failure.

Assist with insertion and maintain pacemaker (external or tem-porary, internal or permanent) function.

Temporary pacing may be necessary to accelerate impulse formation in bradydysrhythmias, synchronize electrical impulsivity, or override tachydysrhythmias and ectopic activity to maintain cardiovascular function until sponta-neous pacing is restored or permanent pacing is initiated. These devices may include atrial and ventricular pacemak-ers and may provide single chamber or dual chamber pacing. The placement of implantable cardioverter defibril-lators (ICDs) is on the rise.

Insert and maintain intravenous (IV) access.

Patent access line may be required for administration of emer-gency drugs.

Prepare for surgery, such as aneurysmectomy, CABG, and Maze, as indicated.

Differential diagnosis of underlying cause may be required to formulate appropriate treatment plan. Resection of ventricular aneurysm may be required to correct intractable ventricular dysrhythmias unresponsive to medical therapy. Surgery such as CABG may be indicated to enhance circulation to myocardium and conduction system. *Note:* A Maze procedure is an open heart surgical procedure sometimes used to treat refractory AF by surgically redirect-ing electrical conduction pathways.

Prepare for placement of ICD when indicated.

This device may be surgically implanted in those clients with recurrent, life-threatening ventricular dysrhythmias unre-sponsive to tailored drug therapy. The latest generation of devices can provide multilevel or "tiered" therapy, that is, antitachycardia and antibradycardia pacing, cardiover-sion, or defibrillation depending on how each device is programmed.

NURSING DIAGNOSIS: risk for Poisoning [Digoxin Toxicity]

Risk factors may include
Limited range of therapeutic effectiveness, lack of education or proper precautions, reduced vision, cognitive limitations

Possibly evidenced by
(Not applicable; presence of signs and symptoms establishes an *actual* diagnosis)

Desired Outcomes/Evaluation Criteria—Client Will

Knowledge: Medication (NOC)
Verbalize understanding of individual prescription, how it interacts with other drugs or substances, and importance of maintaining prescribed regimen.
Recognize signs of digoxin overdose and developing heart failure and identify what to report to physician.

Cardiac Pump Effectiveness (NOC)
Be free of signs of toxicity; display serum drug level within individually acceptable range.

ACTIONS/INTERVENTIONS	RATIONALE
Medication Management (NIC)	
Independent	
Explain client's specific type of digoxin preparation and its specific therapeutic use.	Reduces confusion due to digoxin preparations varying in name (although they may be similar), dosage strength, and onset and duration of action. Up to 15% of all clients receiving digoxin develop toxicity at some time during the course of therapy because of its narrow therapeutic range.
Instruct client not to change dose for any reason, not to omit dose—unless instructed to, based on pulse rate—not to increase dose or take extra doses, and to contact physician if more than one dose is omitted.	Alterations in drug regimen can reduce therapeutic effects, result in toxicity, and cause complications.
Advise client that digoxin may interact with many other drugs, such as barbiturates, neomycin, cholestyramine, quinidine, and antacids, and that physician should be informed that digoxin is taken whenever new medications are prescribed. Advise client not to use OTC drugs, such as laxatives, antidiarrheals, antacids, cold remedies, diuretics, and herbals, without first checking with the pharmacist or healthcare provider.	Knowledge may help prevent dangerous drug interactions.
Review importance of dietary and supplemental intake of potassium, calcium, and magnesium.	Maintaining electrolytes at normal ranges may prevent or limit development of toxicity and correct many associated dysrhythmias.
Provide information and have the client and SO verbalize understanding of toxic signs and symptoms to report to the healthcare provider.	Nausea, vomiting, diarrhea, unusual drowsiness, confusion, very slow or very fast irregular pulse, thumping in chest, double or blurred vision, yellow or green tint or halos around objects, flickering color forms or dots, altered color perception, and worsening HF, such as dependent or generalized edema, dyspnea, decreased amount or frequency of voiding, indicate need for prompt evaluation and intervention. Mild symptoms of toxicity may be managed with a brief drug holiday. *Note:* In severe or refractory heart failure, altered cardiac binding of digoxin may result in toxicity even with previously appropriate drug doses.
Discuss necessity of periodic laboratory evaluations, as indicated:	
Serum digoxin (Lanoxin) or digitoxin (Crystodigin) level	Digoxin has a narrow therapeutic serum range, with toxicity occurring at levels that are dependent on individual response. Laboratory levels are evaluated in conjunction with clinical manifestations and ECG to determine individual therapeutic levels and resolution of toxicity.
Electrolytes, blood urea nitrogen (BUN), creatinine, and liver function studies	Abnormal levels of potassium, calcium, or magnesium increase the heart's sensitivity to digoxin. Impaired kidney function can cause digoxin (mainly excreted by the kidney) to accumulate to toxic levels. Digitoxin levels (mainly excreted by the bowel) are affected by impaired liver function.

(continues on page 98)

Collaborative

Administer medications, as appropriate, for example:
   Other antidysrhythmia medications, such as lidocaine
   (Xylocaine), propranolol (Inderal), and procainamide
   (Pronestyl)

   Digoxin immune Fab (Digibind)

Prepare client for transfer to critical care unit (CCU), as
   indicated, such as for dangerous dysrhythmias, exacerbation of heart failure.

May be necessary to maintain and improve cardiac output in
   presence of excess effect of digoxin.

A digoxin/digitoxin antagonist that increases drug excretion by
   the kidneys in acute or severe toxicity when standard therapies are unsuccessful.
In the presence of digoxin toxicity, clients frequently require
   intensive monitoring until therapeutic levels have been
   restored. Because all digoxin preparations have long serum
   half-lives, stabilization can take several days.

NURSING DIAGNOSIS: deficient Knowledge [Learning Need] regarding cause, treatment, self-care, and discharge needs

May be related to
Lack of information, misunderstanding of medical condition or therapy needs
Unfamiliarity with information resources
Lack of recall

Possibly evidenced by
Questions, statement of misconception
Failure to improve on previous regimen
Development of preventable complications

Desired Outcomes/Evaluation Criteria—Client Will

Knowledge: Disease Process (NOC)
Verbalize understanding of condition, prognosis, and function of pacemaker (if used).
Relate signs of pacemaker failure.

Knowledge: Treatment Regimen (NOC)
Verbalize understanding of therapeutic regimen.
List desired action and possible adverse side effects of medications.
Correctly perform necessary procedures and explain reasons for actions.

ACTIONS/INTERVENTIONS

RATIONALE

Teaching: Individual (NIC)
Independent
Assess client and SO level of knowledge and ability and desire
   to learn.

Be alert to signs of avoidance, such as changing subject away
   from information being presented or extremes of behavior
   (withdrawal or euphoria).

Present information in varied learning formats, for example,
   programmed books, audiovisual tapes, question-and-
   answer sessions, and group activities.
Provide information in written form for client and SO to take
   home.

Teaching: Disease Process (NIC)
Reinforce explanations of risk factors, dietary and activity restrictions, medications, and symptoms requiring immediate medical attention.
Encourage identification and reduction of individual risk
   factors, such as smoking and alcohol consumption and
   obesity.

Necessary for creation of individual instruction plan.
   Reinforces expectation that this will be a "learning
   experience." Verbalization identifies misunderstandings and
   allows for clarification.
Natural defense mechanisms, such as anger or denial of significance of situation, can block learning, affecting client's
   response and ability to assimilate information. Changing to
   a less formal or structured style may be more effective until
   client and SO are ready to accept and deal with current
   situation.
Multiple learning methods may enhance retention of material.

Follow-up reminders may enhance client's understanding and
   cooperation with the desired regimen. Written instructions
   are a helpful resource when client is not in direct contact
   with healthcare team.

Provides opportunity for client to retain information and to
   assume control and participate in rehabilitation program.

These behaviors and chemicals have direct adverse effect on
   cardiovascular function and may impede recovery and
   increase risk for complications.

ACTIONS/INTERVENTIONS (continued)

Review normal cardiac function and electrical conduction.

Explain and reinforce specific dysrhythmia problem and therapeutic measures to client and SO.

Identify adverse effects and complications of specific dysrhythmias, such as fatigue, dependent edema, progressive changes in mentation, vertigo, and psychological manifestations.

Instruct and document teaching regarding medications. Include the desired action, how and when to take the drug, what to do if a dose is forgotten (dosage and usage information), and expected side effects or possible adverse reactions or interactions with other prescribed and OTC drugs or substances (alcohol, tobacco, herbal remedies), as well as what and when to report to the healthcare provider.

Encourage development of regular exercise routine, avoiding overexertion. Identify signs and symptoms requiring immediate cessation of activities, such as dizziness, lightheadedness, dyspnea, and chest pain.

Review individual dietary needs and restrictions, such as potassium and caffeine.

Demonstrate proper pulse-taking technique. Recommend weekly checking of pulse for 1 full minute or daily recording of pulse before medication and during exercise as appropriate. Identify situations requiring immediate medical intervention, for example, dizziness or irregular heartbeat, fainting, and chest pain.

Review safety precautions, techniques to evaluate and maintain pacemaker or ICD function, and symptoms requiring medical intervention; for example, report pulse rate below set limit for demand pacing or less than low-limit rate for rate-adaptive pacers and prolonged hiccups.

Recommend wearing medical alert bracelet or necklace and carrying pacemaker ID card.

Discuss monitoring and environmental safety concerns in presence of pacemaker or ICD, for example, microwave ovens and other electrical appliances (including electrical blankets, razors, radio/TV) can be safely operated if they are properly grounded and in good repair; there is no problem with metal detectors, although pacemaker may trigger sensitive detectors. Cordless phones are safe, although cellular phones held directly over pacemaker may cause interference; it is recommended that client not carry phone in shirt pocket when phone is on. High-voltage areas, magnetic fields, and radiation can interfere with optimal pacemaker function, so client should avoid high-tension electric wires, arc welding, and large industrial magnets, such as demolition sites and magnetic resonance imaging (MRI).

RATIONALE (continued)

Provides a knowledge base to understand individual variations and reasons for therapeutic interventions.

Ongoing and updated information, such as whether the problem is resolving or may require long-term control measures, can decrease anxiety associated with the unknown and prepare client and SO to make necessary lifestyle adaptations. Educating the SO may be especially important if client is elderly, visually or hearing impaired, or unable or even unwilling to learn or follow instructions. Repeated explanations may be needed because anxiety and bulk of new information can block or limit learning.

Dysrhythmias may decrease cardiac output, manifested by symptoms of developing cardiac failure and altered cerebral perfusion. Tachydysrhythmias may also be accompanied by debilitating anxiety and feelings of impending doom.

Information necessary for client to make informed choices and to manage medication regimen. *Note:* Use of herbal remedies in conjunction with drug regimen may result in adverse effects, for example, cardiac stimulation and impaired clotting, necessitating evaluation of product for safe use.

When dysrhythmias are properly managed, normal activity should not be affected. Exercise program is useful in improving overall cardiovascular well-being.

Depending on specific problem, client may need to increase dietary potassium, such as when potassium-depleting diuretics are used. Caffeine may be limited to prevent cardiac excitation.

Continued self-observation or monitoring provides for timely intervention to avoid complications. Medication regimen may be altered or further evaluation may be required when heart rate varies from desired rate or pacemaker's preset rate.

Promotes self-care, provides for timely interventions to prevent serious complications. Instructions or concerns depend on function and type of device as well as client's condition and presence or absence of family or caregivers.

Allows for appropriate evaluation and timely intervention, especially if client is unable to respond in an emergency situation.

Aids in clarifying misconceptions and fears and encourages client to be proactive in avoiding potentially harmful situations.

CARDIAC SURGERY: POSTOPERATIVE CARE— CORONARY ARTERY BYPASS GRAFT (CABG), MINIMALLY INVASIVE DIRECT CORONARY ARTERY BYPASS (MIDCAB), CARDIOMYOPLASTY, VALVE REPLACEMENT

I. **Purpose:** to maximize cardiac output by improving blood flow and myocardial muscle function

II. **Types**
   a. Reparative: closure of atrial or ventricular septal defect or repair of stenotic mitral valve; reparative surgeries more likely to produce cure or prolonged improvement
   b. Reconstructive: coronary artery bypass grafting (CABG), restructure of incompetent valve leaflets
   c. Substitutional: valve replacement, cardiac transplant

III. **Procedures**
   a. Procedures requiring use of cardiopulmonary bypass (CPB)
      i. CABG has an average patency rate of 20 years and decreased overall mortality from coronary heart disease, relief from angina, improved functional status, and may improve quality of life due to decreased need for pharmacological therapy and a reduction in frequency of interventional procedures (Kark, 2008).
      ii. Open heart valve repair or replacement using natural (biological) or artificial (mechanical) valves are the most common minimally invasive heart surgery procedures (Cleveland Clinic, 2007).
      iii. Port-access coronary artery bypass (PACAB) is a minimally invasive option in certain conditions, such as single bypass from left mammary artery to left anterior descending coronary artery.
   b. Procedures not requiring use of CPB (heart-lung) machine
      i. Off-pump coronary artery bypass (OPCAB) or beating heart bypass surgery may be an option for client with single-vessel disease, such as the left anterior descending artery or right coronary artery.
      ii. Minimally invasive direct coronary bypass (MIDCAB)
      iii. Robotic-assisted coronary artery bypass (RACAB), also called closed-chest heart surgery
      iv. Totally endoscopic coronary artery bypass (TECAB) using a port access, which may be video and robotic assisted—primarily carried out in large heart centers where specialized equipment and training are available
      v. Percutaneous mitral, aortic, and pulmonic valvotomy for stenosis; transapical aortic valve implant
      vi. Transmyocardial laser revascularization (TMR) uses lasers to create channels in heart muscle to improve direct blood flow.
      vii. Endoscopic pulmonary vein isolation for the treatment of atrial fibrillation, thoracic endografting for the treatment of aortic aneurysmal disease

IV. **Statistics**
   a. 46,900 CAB procedures and 106,000 valve replacements were performed in the United States in 2005 (American Heart Association [AHA], 2007).
   b. Cost: The mean charge per CABG procedure in 2001 was $60,853 (AHA, 2004).

GLOSSARY

Anastomosis: Surgical connection created between tubular structures, such as blood vessels, that are grafted into the coronary arteries to create a bypass channel for circulation around a blocked artery.

Cardiopulmonary bypass (CBP) (also called heart-lung machine): Mechanical means of circulating and oxygenating the blood through the body when it's diverted from the heart and lungs. The heart's beating is stopped so the surgeon can perform the bypass procedure on a still heart.

Coronary artery bypass grafting (CABG): Procedure in which one or more blocked coronary arteries are bypassed by a blood vessel graft to restore normal blood flow to the heart. These grafts usually come from the client's own arteries and veins located in the leg (saphenous vein), internal mammary artery (IMA), or arm (radial artery). The graft goes around the blocked artery (or arteries) to create new pathways for oxygen-rich blood to flow to the heart.

Minimally invasive direct coronary bypass (MIDCAB): Requires a smaller incision and may be done for CABG and some valve remodeling and replacement procedures.

Off-pump coronary artery bypass (OPCAB) (also called off-pump coronary revascularization): Similar to the conventional CABG procedure. OPCAB still uses a medial sternotomy; however, CPB pump is no longer employed. Off-pump procedures can offer certain advantages in low-risk populations, such as decreased cost, reduced length of stay, reduced postoperative complications, and avoidance of blood transfusions.

They also reduce surgical trauma to the client as well as risk of stroke and kidney failure.

Percutaneous transmyocardial revascularization (PTMR) (also called transmyocardial laser revascularization, or TMR): Laser surgery that opens tiny new pathways within the heart muscle to treat the symptoms of angina in a client who cannot withstand more conventional treatments such as bypass surgery or balloon angioplasty.

Robotic-assisted coronary artery bypass (RACAB): Surgeon views the procedure on a video screen, uses a robot to perform the bypass, and has no direct contact with the client.

Sternotomy: Surgical incision made in the breastbone (mediastinum).

Totally endoscopic coronary artery bypass (TECAB): Robotic-assisted procedure in which small-port incisions are made in intercostal spaces. TECAB is performed on the beating heart using a stabilization device that holds the anastomosis site steady and removes the need for CPB.

Care Setting

Client is cared for at inpatient acute hospital on a surgical or post-intensive care unit (ICU) step-down unit.

Related Concerns

Angina, page 64

Heart failure: chronic, page 48

Dysrhythmias, page 88

Myocardial infarction, page 74

Pneumothorax/hemothorax, page 154

Psychosocial aspects of care, page 749

Surgical intervention, page 782

Transplantation considerations—postoperative and lifelong, page 739

Client Assessment Database

The preoperative data presented here depend on the specific disease process and underlying cardiac condition and reserve.

DIAGNOSTIC DIVISION MAY REPORT	MAY EXHIBIT
ACTIVITY/REST	
• Exercise intolerance	• Abnormal heart rate, blood pressure (BP) changes with activity
• Generalized weakness, fatigue	• Exertional dyspnea
• Inability to perform expected or usual life activities	• Electrocardiogram (ECG) changes and dysrhythmias with activity
• Insomnia and sleep disturbances	
CIRCULATION	
• History of recent or acute MI (three or more), vessel coronary artery disease, valvular heart disease, hypertension	• Variations in BP, heart rate and rhythm
• History of inherited clotting disorders, such as hemophilia, and acquired clotting disorders, such as acute lymphocytic leukemia or lupus (which can affect postoperative bleeding)	• Abnormal heart sounds: S_3/S_4, murmurs
• History of abnormal bleeding with previous surgeries, dental procedures, or childbirth	• Pallor and cyanosis of skin or mucous membranes
• Current use of antithrombotic drugs, including those that inhibit the production of clotting factors in the liver, such as warfarin (Coumadin); those that interfere with blood clotting by blocking thrombin activity, such as heparin and lepirudin (Refludan); and antiplatelet drugs, such as aspirin, clopidogrel (Plavix), tirofiban (Aggrastat), and eptifibatide (Integrilin), which keep platelets from aggregating into clots. *Note:* Cardiac patients taking these drugs preoperatively require various interventions to ensure their safety for CPB and to reduce postoperative bleeding complications	• Cool and clammy skin
	• Edema, jugular vein distention (JVD)
	• Diminished peripheral pulses
	• Abnormal breath sounds, such as crackles
	• Restlessness and other changes in mentation or sensorium (severe cardiac decompensation)
• Recent use of over-the-counter (OTC) drugs, such as ibuprofen, and dietary supplements, such as vitamin E, garlic, ginseng, and ginkgo (can inhibit clotting)	

(continues on page 102)

DIAGNOSTIC DIVISION MAY REPORT (continued)	MAY EXHIBIT (continued)

EGO INTEGRITY
- Feeling frightened, apprehensive, or helpless
- Distress over current events
- Fear of death or eventual outcome of surgery or possible complications
- Fear about changes in lifestyle and role functioning

- Apprehension, restlessness
- Facial or general tension
- Withdrawal and lack of eye contact
- Focus on self, hostility, anger, crying

FOOD/FLUID
- Change in weight
- Loss of appetite
- Nausea or vomiting
- Change in urine frequency or amount

- Weight gain or loss
- Dry skin, poor skin turgor
- Postural hypotension
- Edema—generalized, dependent, pitting

NEUROSENSORY
- Fainting spells, vertigo

- Changes in orientation or usual response to stimuli
- Restlessness, irritability, apathy

PAIN/DISCOMFORT
- Chest pain, angina

RESPIRATION
- Shortness of breath

- Dyspnea
- Abnormal breath sounds, such as crackles
- Productive cough

SAFETY
- Infectious episode with valvular involvement or myopathy

TEACHING/LEARNING
- Familial risk factors of diabetes, heart disease, hypertension, strokes
- Use of various cardiovascular drugs
- Failure to improve

POSTOPERATIVE ASSESSMENT
Pain/Discomfort
- Incisional discomfort
- Pain or paresthesia of shoulders, arms, hands, legs

- Guarding of incisional areas
- Facial mask of pain, grimacing
- Distraction behaviors, moaning, restlessness
- Changes in BP, pulse, respiratory rate

Respiration
- Inability to cough or take a deep breath

- Decreased chest expansion
- Splinting or muscle guarding
- Dyspnea—normal response to thoracotomy
- Areas of diminished or absent breath sounds (atelectasis)
- Changes in arterial blood gas (ABG) levels or pulse oximetry

Safety
- Oozing or bleeding from chest or donor site incisions

TEACHING/LEARNING
- Modifiable risk factors for sternal wound infection, such as obesity, diabetes, and smoking
- Postoperative incision care to minimize or prevent infection

DISCHARGE PLAN CONSIDERATIONS
- Short-term assistance with food preparation, shopping, transportation, self-care needs, and homemaker and home maintenance tasks

▶ Refer to section at end of plan for postdischarge considerations.

Diagnostic Studies (Postoperative)

TEST WHY IT IS DONE	WHAT IT TELLS ME
BLOOD TEST	
• *Hemoglobin (Hgb) and hematocrit (Hct):* To identify red blood cell (RBC) and fluid replacement needs.	Whether heart surgery is performed on or off CPB equipment, clients develop moderate hemodilution from the fluids given perioperatively, thus lowering the Hct and platelet count. A low Hgb reduces oxygen-carrying capacity and indicates need for RBC replacement. Elevation of Hct suggests dehydration and need for fluid replacement.
• *Coagulation studies:* Various studies may be done, such as platelet count and bleeding and clotting time	Platelet function and coagulation factors are altered as a result of CPB and don't normalize for up to 12 hours after surgery. Body temperature is also lowered for open heart surgery, which can depress normal platelet function for a time, even after the client is rewarmed, raising the risk of abnormal bleeding (Sorensen et al, 2006).
• *Electrolytes:* A substance that, in solution, conducts an electric current and is decomposed by its passage. Sodium (Na), potassium (K⁺), and calcium (Ca) are common electrolytes.	Imbalances—hyperkalemia or hypokalemia, hypernatremia or hyponatremia, and hypocalcemia—can affect cardiac function and fluid balance.
• *Arterial blood gas (ABG) analysis:* Assessment of levels of oxygen (PaO_2) and carbon dioxide ($PaCO_2$)	Verifies oxygenation status, effectiveness of respiratory function, and acid-base balance.
• *Blood urea nitrogen (BUN) and creatinine (Cr):* Elevated BUN can occur with dehydration, shock due to too much blood being lost, or any condition that decreases blood flow to the kidneys. Often, an additional test is done to measure Cr.	Considered together, the BUN-Cr ratio gives very good evidence of the filtering function of the kidneys and a measure of the degree of bodily hydration.
• *Glucose:* Blood glucose levels should be controlled in all patients with diabetes to avoid hyperglycemia perioperatively.	Fluctuations may occur because of preoperative nutritional status, presence of diabetes or organ dysfunction, and rate of dextrose infusions.
• *Cardiac enzyme and isoenzymes Troponin 1 (cTnl) and Troponin T (cTnT):* Contractile proteins found in the myocardium with nearly absolute myocardial tissue specificity, as well as high sensitivity, thereby reflecting even microscopic zones of myocardial necrosis. Troponins increase within 3 to 4 hours of myocardial injury.	Elevated in the presence of acute, recent, or perioperative myocardial infarction (MI). Troponins are a critical and reliable marker of myocardial injury.
OTHER DIAGNOSTIC STUDIES	
• *Chest x-ray:* Evaluates organs and structures within the chest.	Reveals heart size and position, pulmonary vasculature, and changes indicative of pulmonary complications, such as atelectasis. Verifies condition of valve prosthesis and sternal wires, position of pacing leads, intravascular or cardiac lines.
• *Electrocardiogram (ECG):* Record of the electrical activity of the heart; provides important information concerning the spread of electricity to the different parts of the heart.	Identifies changes in electrical and mechanical function such as might occur in immediate postoperative phase, acute or perioperative MI, valve dysfunction, and pericarditis.
• *Transesophageal echocardiography:* Invasive procedure in which a transducer is placed inside the esophagus to provide clear images of the heart's movement.	Useful in diagnosing cardiac valve and chamber abnormalities, such as regurgitation, shunting, or stenosis in client in whom transthoracic approach is not feasible.
• *Nuclear studies (thallium-201, DPY-thallium and Persantine):* Evaluates myocardial blood flow and status of myocardial contractility.	Heart scans that reveal status of coronary artery bypass grafts, heart chamber dimensions, and pre- or postsurgical functional capabilities.

Nursing Priorities

1. Support hemodynamic stability and ventilatory function.
2. Promote relief of pain and discomfort.
3. Promote healing.
4. Provide information about postoperative expectations and treatment regimen.

Discharge Goals

1. Activity tolerance adequate to meet self-care needs.
2. Pain alleviated or managed.
3. Complications prevented or minimized.
4. Incisions healing.
5. Postdischarge medications, exercise, diet, and therapy understood.
6. Plan in place to meet needs after discharge.

NURSING DIAGNOSIS: **risk for decreased Cardiac Output**

Risk factors may include
Altered myocardial contractility secondary to temporary factors, such as ventricular wall surgery, recent MI, response to certain medications and drug interactions
Altered preload (hypovolemia) and afterload (systemic vascular resistance)
Altered heart rate or rhythm (dysrhythmias)

Possibly evidenced by
(Not applicable; presence of signs and symptoms establishes an *actual* diagnosis)

Desired Outcomes/Evaluation Criteria—Client Will

Tissue Perfusion: Cardiac (NOC)
Display hemodynamic stability, such as stable blood pressure, cardiac output.
Report and display decreased episodes of angina and dysrhythmias.
Demonstrate an increase in activity tolerance.
Participate in activities that maximize and enhance cardiac function.

ACTIONS/INTERVENTIONS	RATIONALE
Hemodynamic Regulation (NIC) *Independent* Monitor and document trends in heart rate and BP, especially noting hypertension. Be aware of specific systolic and diastolic limits defined for client.	Tachycardia is a common response to discomfort, inadequate blood or fluid replacement, and the stress of surgery. However, sustained tachycardia increases cardiac workload and can decrease effective cardiac output. Hypotension may result from fluid deficit, dysrhythmias, heart failure, and shock. Hypertension can occur (fluid excess or preexisting condition), placing stress on suture lines of new grafts and changing blood flow or pressure within heart chambers and across valves, with increased risk for various complications.
Monitor and document cardiac dysrhythmias. Observe client response to dysrhythmias, such as drop in BP, chest pain, and dyspnea.	Life-threatening dysrhythmias can occur because of electrolyte imbalance, myocardial ischemia, or alterations in the heart's electrical conduction. Atrial fibrillation and atrial flutter are the most common dysrhythmias occurring around the second or third day after CABG (older clients or presence of right coronary artery disease increases risk). Decreased cardiac output and hemodynamic compromise that occur with dysrhythmias require prompt intervention. *Note:* This is the most frequently occurring postoperative complication, often prolonging hospital stay.
Observe for bleeding from incisions and chest tube (if in place).	Helps identify bleeding complications that can reduce circulating volume, organ perfusion, and cardiac function.
Observe for changes in usual mental status, orientation, and body movement or reflexes, such as onset of confusion, disorientation, restlessness, reduced response to stimuli, and stupor.	May indicate decreased cerebral blood flow or oxygenation as a result of diminished cardiac output—sustained or severe dysrhythmias, low BP, heart failure, or thromboembolic phenomena.
Record skin temperature and color and quality and equality of peripheral pulses.	Warm, pink skin and strong, equal pulses are general indicators of adequate cardiac output.
Measure and document intake and output (I&O) and calculate fluid balance.	Useful in determining fluid needs or identifying fluid excesses, which can compromise cardiac output and oxygen consumption.

ACTIONS/INTERVENTIONS (continued)

Schedule uninterrupted rest and sleep periods. Assist with self-care activities as needed.

Monitor graded activity program. Note client response; vital signs before, during, and after activity; and development of dysrhythmias.

Evaluate presence and degree of anxiety or emotional duress. Encourage the use of relaxation techniques such as deep breathing and diversional activities.

Inspect for JVD, peripheral or dependent edema, congestion in lungs, shortness of breath, and change in mental status.

Investigate reports of angina or severe chest pain accompanied by restlessness, diaphoresis, and ECG changes.

Investigate and report profound hypotension and unresponsiveness to fluid challenge, tachycardia, distant heart sounds, and stupor or coma.

Collaborative

Review serial ECGs.

Measure cardiac output and other functional parameters, as indicated.

Monitor Hgb, Hct, and coagulation studies, such as activated prothrombin time (aPTT), international normalized ratio (INR), activated clotting time (ACT), and platelet count.

Monitor results of thromboelastography (TEG), as indicated.

Administer intravenous (IV) fluids or blood products as needed.

Administer supplemental oxygen as appropriate.

Administer electrolytes and medications, as indicated, such as potassium, antidysrhythmics, digoxin preparations, diuretics, and anticoagulants.

Maintain surgically placed pacing wires (atrial or ventricular) and initiate pacing if indicated.

RATIONALE (continued)

Prevents fatigue or exhaustion and excessive cardiovascular stress.

Regular exercise stimulates circulation and promotes feeling of well-being. Progression of activity depends on cardiac tolerance.

Excessive or escalating emotional reactions can negatively affect vital signs and systemic vascular resistance, eventually affecting cardiac function.

May be indicative of acute or chronic heart failure.

Although not a common complication of CABG, perioperative or postoperative MI can occur.

Development of cardiac tamponade can rapidly progress to cardiac arrest because of the heart's inability to fill adequately for effective cardiac output. *Note:* This is a relatively rare, life-threatening complication that usually occurs in the immediate postoperative period but can occur later in the recovery phase.

Most frequently done to follow the progress in normalization of electrical conduction patterns and ventricular function after surgery or to identify complications such as perioperative MI.

Useful in evaluating response to therapeutic interventions and identifying need for more aggressive or emergency care.

Help to identify bleeding or clotting problems associated with the surgery. *Note:* Diverting the client's blood through the CPB machine activates the clotting cascade and decreases the number (as well as the function) of platelets. Hemodilution occurs when the client's blood mixes with the crystalloid solution used to prime the CPB machine. Because blood is being diluted, the Hct drops, as does the concentration of coagulation factors, fibrinogen, and platelets. In addition, the use of hypothermia during surgery to decrease tissue oxygen requirements slows down the process of clotting and decreases platelet function.

TEG is a point-of-care test that can rapidly identify whether the client has a normal hemostasis or is bleeding and whether it is due to surgery, coagulopathy, or residual anticoagulation therapy. Results will identify the specific therapy to treat it, whether client needs fresh frozen plasma (FFP), platelets, antifibrinolytic drugs, or thrombolytic drugs (Sorensen et al, 2006).

Clients who have surgery on CPB equipment are more likely to bleed excessively than those who have off-bypass cardiac surgery. RBC replacement is often indicated to restore and maintain adequate circulating volume and enhance oxygen-carrying capacity. IV fluids may be discontinued before discharge from the ICU or may remain in place for fluid replacement and emergency cardiac medications.

Promotes maximal oxygenation to reduce cardiac workload and aid in resolving myocardial irritability and dysrhythmias.

Client needs are variable, depending on type of surgery, client's response to surgical intervention, and preexisting conditions, such as general health, age, and type of heart disease. Electrolytes, antidysrhythmics, and other heart medications may be required on a short-term or long-term basis to maximize cardiac contractility and output.

May be required to support cardiac output in presence of conduction disturbances (severe dysrhythmias) that compromise cardiac function.

NURSING DIAGNOSIS: acute Pain/impaired Comfort

May be related to
Sternotomy (mediastinal incision) or donor site (leg or arm incision)
Myocardial ischemia (acute MI, angina)
Tissue inflammation, edema formation
Intraoperative nerve trauma

Possibly evidenced by
Reports of incisional discomfort or pain; paresthesia; pain in hand, arm, shoulder
Anxiety, restlessness, irritability
Distraction behaviors
Increased heart rate

Desired Outcomes/Evaluation Criteria—Client Will

Pain Level (NOC)
Verbalize relief or absence of pain.
Demonstrate relaxed body posture and ability to rest and sleep appropriately.

Pain Control (NOC)
Differentiate surgical discomfort from angina or preoperative heart pain.

ACTIONS/INTERVENTIONS	RATIONALE
Pain Management (NIC) *Independent* Note type and location of incision(s).	Newer procedures, such as MIDCAB, require smaller chest and leg incisions, with less significant pain. Many CABG clients do not experience severe discomfort in chest incision and may complain more often of donor site incision discomfort. Severe pain in either area should be investigated further for possible complications.
Encourage client to report type, location, and intensity of pain, rating it on a scale. Note associated symptoms. Ascertain how this compares with preoperative chest pain.	Pain is perceived, manifested, and tolerated individually. It is important for client to differentiate incisional pain from other types of chest pain, such as angina or discomfort from chest tubes.
Observe for anxiety, irritability, crying, restlessness, and sleep disturbances.	These nonverbal cues may indicate the presence or degree of pain being experienced.
Monitor vital signs.	Heart rate usually increases with acute pain, although a bradycardiac response can occur in a severely diseased heart. BP may be elevated slightly with incisional discomfort, but may be decreased or unstable if chest pain is severe or myocardial damage is occurring.
Identify and promote position of comfort, using adjuncts as necessary.	Pillows or blanket rolls are useful in supporting extremities, maintaining body alignment, and splinting incisions to reduce muscle tension and promote comfort.
Provide comfort measures, such as back rubs and position changes, assist with self-care activities, and encourage diversional activities, as indicated.	May promote relaxation, redirect attention, and reduce analgesic dosage needs or frequency.
Schedule care activities to balance with adequate periods of sleep and rest.	Rest and sleep are vital for cardiac healing (balance between oxygen demand and consumption) and can enhance coping with stress and discomfort.
Identify and encourage use of behaviors such as guided imagery, distractions, visualizations, and deep breathing.	Relaxation techniques aid in management of stress, promote sense of well-being, may reduce analgesic needs, and promote healing.
Tell client that it is acceptable, even preferable, to request analgesics as soon as discomfort becomes noticeable.	Presence of pain causes muscle tension, which can impair circulation, slow healing process, and intensify pain.
Medicate before procedures and activities, as indicated.	Client participation in respiratory treatments, ambulation, and procedures, such as removal of chest tubes, pacemaker wires, and sutures, are facilitated by maximum analgesic blood level.
Investigate reports of pain in unusual areas, for instance, calf of leg or abdomen, or vague complaints of discomfort, especially when accompanied by changes in mentation, vital signs, and respiratory rate.	May be an early manifestation of developing complication, such as thrombophlebitis, infection, and gastrointestinal dysfunction.

ACTIONS/INTERVENTIONS (continued)

Note reports of pain or numbness in ulnar area (fourth and fifth digits) of the hand, often accompanied by pain and discomfort of the arms and shoulders. Tell client that the problem usually resolves with time.

Collaborative

Administer medications, as indicated: propoxyphene and acetaminophen (Darvocet-N), acetaminophen and oxycodone (Tylox), and ketorolac (Toradol).

RATIONALE (continued)

Indicative of a stretch injury of the brachial plexus as a result of the position of the arms during surgery. No specific treatment is currently useful.

Usually provides for adequate control of pain and inflammation and reduces muscle tension, which improves client comfort and promotes healing.

NURSING DIAGNOSIS: risk for ineffective Breathing Pattern

Risk factors may include
Inadequate ventilation (pain, muscular weakness)
Diminished oxygen-carrying capacity (blood loss)
Decreased lung expansion (atelectasis or pneumothorax and hemothorax)

Possibly evidenced by
(Not applicable; presence of signs and symptoms establishes an *actual* diagnosis.)

Desired Outcomes/Evaluation Criteria—Client Will

Respiratory Status: Ventilation (NOC)
Maintain an effective respiratory pattern free of cyanosis and other signs and symptoms of hypoxia, with breath sounds equal bilaterally, lung fields clearing.
Display complete reexpansion of lungs with absence of pneumothorax and hemothorax.

ACTIONS/INTERVENTIONS

Respiratory Monitoring (NIC)
Independent
Evaluate respiratory rate and depth. Note respiratory effort, for example, presence of dyspnea, use of accessory muscles, and nasal flaring.

Auscultate breath sounds. Note areas of diminished or absent breath sounds and presence of adventitious sounds, such as crackles or rhonchi.

Observe chest excursion. Investigate decreased expansion or lack of symmetry in chest movement.

Observe character of cough and sputum production.

Inspect skin and mucous membranes for cyanosis.

Elevate head of bed, place in upright or semi-Fowler's position. Assist with early ambulation and increased time out of bed.
Encourage client participation in and responsibility for deep-breathing exercises, use of adjuncts, and coughing, as indicated.

RATIONALE

Client responses are variable. Rate and effort may be increased by pain, fear, fever, diminished circulating volume due to blood or fluid loss, accumulation of secretions, hypoxia, or gastric distention. Respiratory suppression can occur from long time period under anesthesia, or heavy use of opioid analgesics. Early recognition and treatment of abnormal ventilation may prevent complications.
Breath sounds are often diminished in lung bases for a period of time after surgery because of normally occurring atelectasis. Loss of active breath sounds in an area of previous ventilation may reflect collapse of the lung segment, especially if chest tubes have recently been removed. Crackles or rhonchi may be indicative of fluid accumulation due to interstitial edema, pulmonary edema, or infection, or partial airway obstruction with pooling of secretions.
Air or fluid in the pleural space prevents complete expansion (usually on one side) and requires further assessment of ventilation status.
Frequent coughing may simply be throat irritation from operative endotracheal tube (ET) placement or can reflect pulmonary congestion. Purulent sputum suggests onset of pulmonary infection.
Cyanosis of lips, nail beds, or earlobes, or general duskiness may indicate a hypoxic condition due to heart failure or pulmonary complications. General pallor, commonly present in immediate postoperative period, may indicate anemia from blood loss or insufficient blood replacement or RBC destruction from CPB pump.
Stimulates respiratory function and lung expansion. Effective in preventing and resolving pulmonary congestion.
Aids in lung reexpansion and maintaining patency of small airways, especially after removal of chest tubes. Coughing is not necessary unless wheezes and rhonchi are present, indicating retention of secretions.

(continues on page 108)

ACTIONS/INTERVENTIONS (continued)

Reinforce splinting of chest with pillows during deep breathing or coughing.

Explain that coughing and respiratory treatments will not loosen or damage grafts or reopen chest incision.

Encourage maximal fluid intake within cardiac reserves.

Medicate with analgesic before respiratory treatments, as indicated.

Record response to deep-breathing exercises or other respiratory treatment, noting breath sounds before and after treatment, as well as cough and sputum production.

Investigate and report respiratory distress, diminished or absent breath sounds, tachycardia, severe agitation, and drop in BP.

Collaborative

Review chest x-ray reports and laboratory studies (such as ABGs, Hgb), as indicated.

Instruct in and assist with use of incentive spirometer.

Administer supplemental oxygen by cannula or mask, as indicated.

Assist with reinsertion of chest tubes or thoracentesis if indicated.

RATIONALE (continued)

Reduces incisional tension, promotes maximal lung expansion, and may enhance effectiveness of cough effort.

Provides reassurance that injury will not occur and may enhance cooperation with therapeutic regimen.

Adequate hydration helps liquefy secretions, facilitating expectoration.

Allows for easier chest movement and reduces discomfort related to incisional pain, facilitating client cooperation with and effectiveness of respiratory treatments.

Documents effectiveness of therapy or need for more aggressive interventions.

Although not a common complication, hemothorax or pneumothorax may occur following removal of the chest tubes and requires prompt intervention to maintain respiratory function.

Monitors effectiveness of respiratory therapy and documents developing complications. A blood transfusion may be needed if blood loss is the reason for respiratory hypoxemia.

Maximizes lung inflation, reduces atelectasis, and prevents pulmonary complications.

Enhances oxygen delivery to the lungs for circulatory uptake, especially in presence of reduced and altered ventilation.

Reexpands lung by removal of accumulated blood and air and restoration of negative pleural pressure.

NURSING DIAGNOSIS: **impaired Skin Integrity**

May be related to
Surgical incisions, puncture wounds

Possibly evidenced by
Disruption of skin surface

Desired Outcomes/Evaluation Criteria—Client Will

Wound Healing: Primary Intention (NOC)
Demonstrate behaviors and techniques to promote healing and prevent complications.
Display timely wound healing.

ACTIONS/INTERVENTIONS

Incision Site Care (NIC)
Independent

Inspect all incisions. Evaluate healing progress. Review expectations for healing with client.

Suggest wearing soft cotton shirts and loose-fitting clothing, leaving incisions open to air as much as possible, covering and padding portion of incisions as necessary.

Have client shower in warm water, washing incisions gently. Instruct client to avoid tub baths until approved by physician.

Encourage ankle exercises and elevation of legs when sitting in chair.

Review normal signs of healing, such as itching along wound line, bruising, slight redness, and scabbing.

RATIONALE

Healing begins immediately, but complete healing takes time. Chest incision heals first (minimal muscle tissue), but donor site incision requires more time (more muscle tissue, longer incision, slower circulation). As healing progresses, the incision lines may appear dry, with crusty scabs. Underlying tissue may look bruised and feel tense, warm, and lumpy, suggesting resolving hematoma.

Reduces suture line irritation and pressure from clothing. Leaving incisions open to air promotes healing process and may reduce risk of infection.

Keeps incision clean and promotes circulation and healing. *Note:* Climbing out of tub requires use of arms and pectoral muscles, which can put undue stress on sternotomy.

Promotes circulation and reduces edema to improve tissue healing.

Helps client understand expected progression of healing and recognize signs of complications or nonhealing requiring further evaluation and intervention.

ACTIONS/INTERVENTIONS (continued)

Instruct to watch for and report to physician places in incision that do not heal; reopening of healed incision; bloody or purulent drainage; localized area that is swollen with redness, feels increasingly painful, and is hot to touch; and temperature greater than 101.5°F (38.6°C) for longer than 24 hours.

Promote adequate nutritional and fluid intake.

Collaborative
Obtain specimen of wound drainage, as indicated. Administer antimicrobials and local treatments, as indicated.

RATIONALE (continued)

Incisional problems rank second behind chest pain as cause of readmission after CABG. The incidence of sternal infection (mediastinitis) following coronary artery bypass graft surgery is less than 5% (Keib, 2006); however, this devastating complication results in significant mortality and morbidity and financial and care burden.

Helps maintain good circulating volume for tissue perfusion and meets cellular energy requirements to facilitate tissue regeneration and healing process.

If infection occurs, local and systemic treatments may be required.

NURSING DIAGNOSIS: **deficient Knowledge [Learning Need] regarding condition, postoperative care, self-care, and discharge needs**

May be related to
Lack of exposure or recall
Information misinterpretation

Possibly evidenced by
Questions and requests for information
Verbalization of problem, statement of misconception
Inaccurate follow-through of instructions

Desired Outcomes/Evaluation Criteria—Client Will

Cardiac Disease Self-Management (NOC)
Participate in learning process.
Assume responsibility for own learning.
Begin to ask questions and look for information.

Knowledge: Treatment Regimen (NOC)
Verbalize understanding of condition, prognosis, and potential complications.
Describe reasons for therapeutic actions.

ACTIONS/INTERVENTIONS

Teaching: Disease Process (NIC)
Independent
Reinforce surgeon's explanation of particular surgical procedure, providing diagram as appropriate.

Discuss importance of reporting changes in memory or mentation.

Cardiac Care: Rehabilitation (NIC)
Reinforce continuation of breathing exercises, incentive spirometry, and coughing with splinting incision.
Discuss routine and prophylactic medications and OTC drug use. Stress importance of checking with physician before taking any drugs. Reinforce need for routine laboratory tests, outpatient education, and community resources when client with valve replacement will be taking warfarin (Coumadin).
Review prescribed cardiac rehabilitation or exercise program and progress to date. Assist client and significant other (SO) to set realistic goals.

RATIONALE

Provides individually specific information, creating knowledge base for subsequent learning regarding home management. Length of rehabilitation and prognosis are dependent on type of surgical procedure, preoperative physical condition, and duration and severity of any complications.
Cerebral dysfunction ranging from focal ischemic injury to encephalopathy has been associated with CPB and may present from 1 to several days after the procedure, thus affecting length of stay and mortality rates (McKhann et al, 2002, 2006).

Promotes alveolar ventilation, reducing risk of lung congestion.
Depending on type of valve replacement (i.e., synthetic), life-long anticoagulant therapy may be indicated. Potential for drug interactions must be considered before adding therapeutic agents to regimen. *Note:* Using herbal products, such as ginkgo, garlic, and vitamins, can alter coagulation and have an adverse effect when taken with anticoagulants.
Individual capabilities and expectations depend on type of surgery, underlying cardiac function, and prior physical conditioning. *Note:* Obesity is a predictor of hospital readmission and may require additional interventions.

(continues on page 110)

ACTIONS/INTERVENTIONS (continued)

Encourage participation in home routines, such as self-care and cooking. Suggest alternating rest periods with activity, and light tasks with heavy tasks. Avoid heavy lifting and isometric and strenuous upper-body exercise.

Problem-solve with client and SO ways to continue progressive activity program during temperature extremes and high wind or pollution days, such as walking predetermined distance within own house, in local indoor shopping mall, or on exercise track.

Reinforce physician's time limitations about lifting, driving, returning to work, resuming sexual activity, and exercising that involves upper extremities.

Assist client and SO to develop strategies for dealing with changes during recovery period, such as shifting responsibilities to other family members, friends, or neighbors; acquiring temporary assistance for housekeeping; and investigating avenues for financial assistance.

Discuss issues concerning resumption of sexual activity, such as comparison of stress of sexual intercourse with other activities:

Position recommendations

Expectations of sexual performance

Appropriate timing, for example, avoid sexual intercourse following heavy meal, during periods of emotional distress, when client is fatigued or exhausted

Pharmacological considerations

Identify services and resources available after discharge. Provide telephone contact number or schedule follow-up calls as appropriate. Include referral names for home care services, as indicated.

RATIONALE (continued)

Prevents excessive fatigue and exhaustion. Scheduling rest periods and short naps several times a day enhances coping abilities, reduces nervousness (common in this phase), and promotes healing. *Note:* Strenuous use of arms can place undue stress on sternotomy.

Having a plan forestalls giving up exercise because of interferences such as weather.

These restrictions are present until after the first postoperative office visit for assessment of sternum healing.

Planning for changes that may occur or be required promotes sense of control and accomplishment without loss of self-esteem.

Concerns about sexual activity often go unexpressed, but clients usually desire information about what to expect. In general, client can safely engage in sex when activity level has advanced to point at which client can climb two flights of stairs, which is about the same amount of energy expenditure.

Client should avoid positions that restrict breathing (sexual activity increases oxygen demand and consumption). Client with sternotomy should not support self or partner with arms (breast bone healing, support muscles stretched).

Impotence appears to occur with some regularity in postoperative cardiac surgery clients. Although etiology is unknown, condition usually resolves in time without specific intervention. If situation persists, it may require further evaluation.

Timing of activity may reduce occurrence of complications or angina.

Some clients may benefit from prophylactic use of anti-anginal medications for sexual activity.

Facilitates transition to home and provides for ongoing monitoring, continuation of prescribed therapies, and opportunity to discuss concerns and alleviate anxiety.

POTENTIAL CONSIDERATIONS following discharge from care setting (dependent on client's age, physical condition and presence of complications, personal resources, and life responsibilities)
- *Activity Intolerance*—generalized weakness, sedentary lifestyle
- *impaired Skin/Tissue Integrity*—surgical incisions, puncture wounds
- *impaired Home Maintenance*—altered ability to perform tasks, inadequate support systems, reluctance to request assistance
- *risk for Infection*—broken skin, traumatized tissue, invasive procedures, decreased hemoglobin
- *Self-Care Deficit*—decreased strength and endurance, discomfort
- *risk for ineffective Role Performance*—situational crisis and recuperative process, uncertainty about future

THROMBOPHLEBITIS: DEEP VEIN THROMBOSIS (INCLUDING PULMONARY EMBOLI CONSIDERATIONS)

I. Pathophysiology: Related to three factors known as the Virchow triad—stasis of blood flow, vessel wall injury, and alterations in the clotting mechanism.

  a. Mechanical (e.g., trauma, surgery) or physiological (e.g., hypertension, phlebitis) damage to the vessel wall leads to platelet activation, with platelets adhering to one another and clumping together forming a thrombus.

  b. The thrombus either dissolves over time or grows and becomes large enough to occlude a vessel, which causes blood flow to slow, expands the veins to accommodate the increased volume, and causes more clots to form.

  c. Proximal deep vein thrombosis (DVT) (extending to the popliteal, femoral, or iliofemoral vessels)—more likely to break away from the vessel and cause pulmonary embolism (PE).

  d. Approximately 50% of clients with DVT are asymptomatic.

II. Etiology

  a. Thromboembolism can affect superficial or deep veins although DVT is more serious in terms of potential complications, including PE, postphlebotic syndrome, chronic venous insufficiency, and vein valve destruction.

  b. Predisposing and risk factors

    i. Major surgery, especially orthopedic; trauma; prolonged immobilization for any cause; spinal cord injury; extended travel

    ii. Cardiovascular conditions such as valvular heart disease with dysrhythmias, myocardial infarction (MI), heart failure, stroke

    iii. Cancer; central venous catheter use

    iv. Obesity; age greater than 40

    v. Pregnancy-related complications

    vi. Intravenous (IV) drug users, hormone replacement therapy, oral estrogen birth control pills

III. Statistics

  a. Morbidity: Approximately 2.5 million people experience DVT/PE (Day, 2003) with 600,000 hospitalizations annually (Schreiber, 2007); risk for hospitalized medical and surgical clients at 10% to 40% and orthopedic surgery clients at 40% to 60% (Geerts et al, 2004).

  b. Mortality: Initial and recurrent thromboembolic events are estimated to cause 300,000 deaths annually (Bussey, 2007).

  c. Cost: Estimates vary; de Lissovoy (2001) suggests $3 to $4 billion annually for DVT/PE.

GLOSSARY

Coagulation: Complex process or cascade of events involving more than 30 types of cells and substances by which blood cells clump together to form a clot via one of two pathways: extrinsic (blood is exposed to a subendothelial tissue factor) or intrinsic (triggered when the blood is exposed to a foreign substance). Disorders of coagulation can lead to an increased risk of bleeding and clotting or thrombus formation.

Deep vein thrombosis (DVT): A blood clot (thrombus) in a deep vein in the thigh or leg. The clot can break off as an embolus and make its way to the lung, where it can cause respiratory distress and respiratory failure.

Embolus: Something that travels through the bloodstream, lodges in a blood vessel, and blocks it. Examples of emboli are a detached blood clot, a clump of bacteria, and foreign material such as air.

Homans' sign: Deep calf pain in affected leg upon dorsiflexion of foot, which is present in approximately 50% of cases of DVT.

Post-thrombotic syndrome: Occurs when blood can no longer circulate properly because venous circulation is impaired from veins and valves that have been damaged by thrombosis. It can mimic recurrent DVT.

Pulmonary embolism (PE): A thrombus that dislodges from a vessel wall and travels through the right side of the heart into the pulmonary artery, thereby obstructing blood flow.

Recurrent DVT: Occurs within a year after the initial event. Because of persistent abnormalities in effected vasculature after the initial DVT, it can be difficult to clinically differentiate acute DVT from ipsilateral limb DVT recurrence. Diagnosis requires evidence of new clot formation.

Thrombophlebitis: Inflammation of a vein that occurs when a blood clot develops in the vein.

Venous thromboembolism (VTE): Broader term referring to DVT, PE, or to a combination of both.

Care Settings

Primarily treated at the community level, with short inpatient stay generally indicated in the presence of embolization.

Related Concerns

Cancer, page 846

Fractures, page 632

Spinal cord injury, page 271

Surgical intervention, page 782

Ventilatory assistance (mechanical), page 173

DIAGNOSTIC DIVISION MAY REPORT	MAY EXHIBIT
ACTIVITY/REST • Occupation that requires sitting or standing for long periods of time • Prolonged immobility • Leg pain with activity • Fatigue, general malaise • Weakness of affected extremity	• Generalized or extremity weakness
CIRCULATION • History of previous peripheral vascular disease, venous thrombosis, varicose veins • Presence of other predisposing factors, such as pregnancy-induced hypertension, diabetes mellitus, MI or valvular heart disease, thrombotic stroke, or blood dyscrasias	• Tachycardia • Peripheral pulse may be diminished in the affected extremity • Varicosities • Hardened, bumpy or knotty vein • Skin color and temperature in affected extremity pale, cool, edematous (deep vein), pinkish red, warm along the superficial vein • Positive Homans' sign (absence does not rule out DVT because less than 50% of clients have a positive sign) • Edema of affected extremity, ankle engorgement • Differences in leg circumferences bilaterally from thigh to ankle
FOOD/FLUID	• Poor skin turgor, dry mucous membranes (dehydration predisposes to hypercoagulability) • Obesity (predisposes to stasis and pelvic vein pressure)
PAIN/DISCOMFORT • Throbbing, tenderness, aching pain aggravated by standing or movement of affected extremity • Groin tenderness	• Guarding of affected extremity
SAFETY • History of direct or indirect injury to extremity or vein, such as major trauma or fractures, orthopedic or pelvic surgery, surgical procedures longer than 2 hours, urologic surgery, pregnancy, prolonged labor with fetal head pressure on pelvic veins, heart failure, venous cannulation or catheterization or IV therapy • Presence of malignancy, particularly neoplasms of the pancreas, lung, gastrointestinal system, prostate • Sepsis	• Fever, chills
TEACHING/LEARNING • Use of oral contraceptives and estrogens; recent anticoagulant therapy predisposes to hypercoagulability • Use of vitamins and herbal supplements, such as vitamin B_6, vitamin E, niacin, magnesium, L-carnitine, and bromelain, for heart or blood pressure health • Recurrence and lack of resolution of previous thrombophlebotic episode	
DISCHARGE PLAN CONSIDERATIONS • Temporary assistance with shopping, transportation, and homemaker and maintenance tasks • Properly fitted antiembolic hose	

◗ Refer to section at end of plan for postdischarge considerations.

Diagnostic Studies

TEST WHY IT IS DONE	WHAT IT TELLS ME
BLOOD TESTS • *Complete blood count (CBC):* Battery of screening tests, which typically includes hemoglobin (Hgb), hematocrit (Hct), red blood cell (RBC) count, morphology, indices, and distribution width index; platelet count and size; and white blood cell (WBC) count and differential.	Hemoconcentration (elevated Hct) potentiates risk of thrombus formation.
• *Coagulation profile:* Tests that measure the speed of blood coagulation at different steps of the coagulation pathway. There are many types of coagulation tests. Some are general and tell only whether a person's blood is clotting normally. Other tests can identify which element within the blood is causing abnormal clotting.	Identifies clotting problems that may increase one's risk of DVT. For example, antithrombin is useful in determining cause of hypercoagulation; inherited biochemical conditions; and deficits in certain other coagulation modulators, such as antithrombin III, protein S, or protein C, that can predispose client to thrombus formation.
• *D-Dimer Assay:* Measures fibrin degradation fragments generated by fibrinolysis.	An elevated D-dimer level indicates a thrombotic process but is not specific to DVT. This test is useful as an adjunct to noninvasive testing (Stockman, 2008).
OTHER DIAGNOSTIC STUDIES • *Noninvasive flow studies (Doppler ultrasound, duplex venous ultrasound):* Detects and measures blood flow.	Ultrasound imagery can reveal a thrombus in a deep vein, especially above the knee. The Doppler ultrasound measures the blood flow velocity in veins and can detect flow abnormalities (Stockman, 2008). Duplex venous ultrasonography appears to be the most accurate noninvasive method for diagnosing multiple proximal DVT in iliac, femoral, popliteal veins, but is less reliable in detecting isolated calf vein thrombi.
• *Impedance plethysmography (IPG):* Noninvasive test that uses a blood pressure cuff and electrodes to assess blood flow and volume of body fluid based on the idea that changes in volume cause electrical resistance.	Abnormal readings coupled with a high clinical suspicion of DVT are sufficient for diagnosis of DVT. *Note:* Abnormal findings include a fully occluded vessel, although IPG does not detect most calf vein thrombi and may not detect partially occlusive thrombi (Crowther & McCourt, 2005).
• *Venography:* A special x-ray of the veins that is performed by first injecting a radiopaque contrast into the vein in question and then taking a conventional x-ray.	Used to demonstrate a vein blockage. Radiographically confirms diagnosis through changes in blood flow and size of channels. *Note:* Although considered the diagnostic gold standard, this study carries a risk of inducing DVT and therefore is reserved for the client with negative or difficult to interpret noninvasive studies.
• *Magnetic resonance imaging (MRI):* Technique that uses the properties of magnetic fields to provide images of the body.	May be done for diagnosis of both proximal and distal DVT and is believed to be superior to other diagnostic tests for detection of pelvic DVT or suspected DVT of the inferior vena cava or pelvic veins (Stockman, 2008).

Nursing Priorities

1. Maintain or enhance tissue perfusion and facilitate resolution of thrombus.
2. Promote optimal comfort.
3. Prevent complications.
4. Provide information about disease process, prognosis, and treatment regimen.

Discharge Goals

1. Tissue perfusion improved in affected limb.
2. Pain or discomfort relieved.
3. Complications prevented or resolved.
4. Disease process, prognosis, and therapeutic needs understood.
5. Plan in place to meet needs after discharge.

NURSING DIAGNOSIS: ineffective peripheral tissue Perfusion

May be related to
Decreased blood flow and venous stasis (partial or complete venous obstruction)

Possibly evidenced by
Tissue edema, pain
Diminished peripheral pulses, slow or diminished capillary refill
Skin color changes—pallor, erythema

Desired Outcomes/Evaluation Criteria—Client Will

Tissue Perfusion: Peripheral (NOC)
Demonstrate improved perfusion as evidenced by peripheral pulses present, equal skin color, and temperature normal and absence of edema.
Engage in behaviors or actions to enhance tissue perfusion.
Display increasing tolerance to activity.

ACTIONS/INTERVENTIONS	RATIONALE
Embolus Care: Peripheral (NIC) *Independent*	
Evaluate circulatory and neurological studies of involved extremity, both sensory and motor. Inspect legs from groin to foot for skin color and temperature changes as well as edema. Note symmetry of calves; measure and record calf circumference. Report proximal progression of inflammatory process and traveling pain.	Symptoms help distinguish between thrombophlebitis and DVT. Redness, heat, tenderness, and localized edema are characteristic of superficial involvement. *Note:* Unilateral edema is one of the most reliable physical findings in DVT. Calf vein involvement is associated with absence of edema; femoral vein involvement is associated with mild to moderate edema; and iliofemoral vein thrombosis is characterized by severe edema.
Examine extremity for obviously prominent veins. Palpate gently for local tissue tension, stretched skin, and knots or bumps along course of vein.	Distention of superficial veins can occur in DVT because of backflow through communicating veins. Thrombophlebitis in superficial veins may be visible or palpable.
Assess capillary refill and check for Homans' sign.	Diminished capillary refill usually present in DVT. *Note:* Homans' sign is unreliable because it is not present in many clients with DVT.
Promote early ambulation.	Short, frequent walks are better for extremities and prevention of pulmonary complications than one long walk. If client is confined to bed, ensure range-of-motion exercises.
Elevate legs when in bed or chair, as indicated.	Reduces tissue swelling and rapidly empties superficial and tibial veins, preventing overdistention and thereby increasing venous return. *Note:* Some physicians believe that elevation may potentiate release of thrombus, thus increasing risk of embolization and decreasing circulation to the most distal portion of the extremity.
Initiate active or passive exercises while in bed, for example, flex, extend, and rotate feet periodically. Assist with gradual resumption of ambulation as soon as client is permitted out of bed.	These measures are designed to increase venous return from lower extremities and reduce venous stasis as well as improve general muscle tone and strength. They also promote normal organ function and enhance general well-being.
Caution client to avoid crossing legs or hyperflex at knee, such as seated position with legs dangling or lying in jackknife position.	Physical restriction of circulation impairs blood flow and increases venous stasis in pelvic, popliteal, and leg vessels, thus increasing swelling and discomfort.
Instruct client to avoid rubbing or massaging the affected extremity.	This activity potentiates risk of fragmenting and dislodging thrombus, causing embolization, and increasing risk of complications.
Encourage deep-breathing exercises.	Increases negative pressure in thorax, which assists in emptying large veins.
Increase fluid intake to at least 1,500 to 2,000 mL/day, within cardiac tolerance.	Dehydration increases blood viscosity and venous stasis, predisposing to thrombus formation.

ACTIONS/INTERVENTIONS (continued)

RATIONALE (continued)

Collaborative

Apply warm, moist compresses or heat cradle to affected extremity if indicated.

May be prescribed to promote vasodilation and venous return for resolution of local edema and to enhance comfort (Breen, 2000; Earhart & Tomlinson, 2007). *Note:* May be contraindicated in presence of arterial insufficiency, in which heat can increase cellular oxygen consumption and nutritional needs, furthering imbalance between supply and demand.

Administer pharmacological measures, as indicated:

Pharmacological measures involve various types of anticoagulation in order to reduce blood coagulability.

Heparin sodium via continuous or intermittent IV and intermittent subcutaneous (SC) injections

Heparin may be used initially because of its prompt, predictable, antagonistic action on thrombin as it is formed and also because it removes activated coagulation factors XII, XI, IX, and X (intrinsic pathway), preventing further clot formation.

Low-molecular-weight heparin (LMWH) preparations, such as enorxaparin (Lovenox) and dalteparin (Fragmin) via SC injections

Anticoagulant of choice after major orthopedic surgery and major trauma due to a lower risk of bleeding, more predictable dose response, and longer half-life than heparin sodium.

Oral coumarin derivatives, such as warfarin (Coumadin) or dicumarol (Sintrom)

Coumadin has a potent depressant effect on liver formation of prothrombin from vitamin K and impairs formation of factors VII, IX, and X (extrinsic pathway). Coumadin is generally used for long-term postdischarge therapy to keep international normalized ratio (INR) at 2 to 3. However, it does have a narrow therapeutic window and requires frequent monitoring. A large number of foods, drugs, and disease processes alter Coumadin's effectiveness, making it difficult to regulate. The elderly client should be started on lower doses and monitored more frequently (Kehl-Pruett, 2006).

Thrombolytic agents, such as activase (Alteplase) and reteplase (Retavase)

Thrombolytic therapy dissolves thrombi in 50% of patients (Stockman, 2008) if given within first 3 days after acute thrombosis. May be used in hemodynamically unstable client with PE or massive DVT to reduce risk of developing PE, or in the presence of valvular damage or chronic venous insufficiency. *Note:* Catheter-directed fibrinolysis may be used to infuse a fibrinolytic agent directly into a thrombus in order to reduce the risks associated with systemic fibrinolytic therapy.

Monitor laboratory studies, as indicated:
Prothrombin time (PT), partial thromboplastin time (PTT), and activated prothrombin time (aPTT)

Monitors anticoagulant therapy and presence of risk factors, such as hemoconcentration and dehydration, which potentiate clot formation. *Note:* Lovenox does not require serial monitoring because PT and aPTT are not affected.

Platelet count, platelet function or aggregation test, and anti-heparin antibody assay

On occasion, platelet count may decrease as a result of an immune reaction leading to platelet aggregation or the formation of "white clots." If bacteremia and disseminated intravascular coagulation (DIC) have been ruled out, condition may be the result of heparin-induced thrombocytopenia and thrombosis (HITT), requiring a change to Coumadin or other agents.

Apply and regulate graduated compression stockings and intermittent pneumatic compression if indicated.

Sequential compression devices may be used to improve blood flow velocity and empty vessels by providing artificial muscle-pumping action.

Apply elastic support hose following acute phase. Take care to avoid tourniquet effect.

Properly fitted support hose are useful, once ambulation has begun, to minimize or delay development of postphlebotic syndrome. They must exert a sustained, evenly distributed pressure over entire surface of calves and thighs to reduce the caliber of superficial veins and increase blood flow to deep veins.

(continues on page 116)

ACTIONS/INTERVENTIONS (continued)

Prepare for and assist with procedures, such as the following:
Percutaneous mechanical thrombectomy (PMT)

Surgical intervention, such as thrombectomy and vena cava screen, when indicated

RATIONALE (continued)

PMT has generally replaced the open surgical approach. This technology was designed primarily to eliminate the bleeding risks associated with catheter-directed thrombolysis. As an endovascular technique, PMT employs rotational or hydrodynamic mechanisms to fragment and aspirate thrombi, thus reducing thrombus burden (Marchigiano et al, 2006).

Thrombectomy (excision of thrombus) is occasionally necessary if inflammation extends proximally or circulation is severely restricted. Multiple or recurrent thrombotic episodes unresponsive to medical treatment (or when anticoagulant therapy is contraindicated) may require insertion of a vena cava screen or umbrella.

NURSING DIAGNOSIS: acute **Pain/impaired Comfort**

May be related to
Diminished arterial circulation and oxygenation of tissues with production and accumulation of lactic acid in tissues
Inflammatory process

Possibly evidenced by
Reports of pain, tenderness, aching or burning
Guarding of affected limb
Restlessness, distraction behaviors

Desired Outcomes/Evaluation Criteria—Client Will

Pain Control (NOC)
Report that pain or discomfort is alleviated or controlled.
Verbalize methods that provide relief.
Display relaxed manner; be able to sleep or rest and engage in desired activity.

ACTIONS/INTERVENTIONS

Pain Management (NIC)
Independent

Assess degree and characteristics of discomfort and pain. Note guarding of extremity. Palpate leg with caution.

Maintain bedrest during acute phase.

Elevate affected extremity.

Provide foot cradle.

Encourage client to change position frequently.

Monitor vital signs, noting elevated temperature.

Investigate reports of sudden or sharp chest pain, accompanied by dyspnea, tachycardia, and apprehension, or development of a new pain with signs of another site of vascular involvement.

Collaborative

Administer medications, as indicated, for example, analgesics (opioid and nonopioid) and antipyretics, such as acetaminophen (Tylenol).

Apply moist heat to extremity if indicated.

RATIONALE

Degree of pain is directly related to extent of circulatory deficit, inflammatory process, degree of tissue ischemia, and extent of edema associated with thrombus development. Changes in characteristics of pain may indicate development of complications.

Reduces discomfort associated with muscle contraction and movement.

Encourages venous return to facilitate circulation, reducing stasis and edema formation.

Cradle keeps pressure of bedclothes off the affected leg, thereby reducing pressure discomfort.

Reduces muscle fatigue, helps minimize muscle spasm, and maximizes circulation to tissues.

Elevations in heart rate may indicate increased discomfort or may occur in response to fever and inflammatory process. Fever can also increase client's discomfort.

These signs and symptoms suggest the presence of PE as a complication of DVT or peripheral arterial occlusion associated with HITT. Both conditions require prompt medical evaluation and treatment.

Relieves pain and decreases muscle tension. Reduces fever and inflammation. *Note:* Risk of bleeding may be increased by concurrent use of drugs that affect platelet function, such as aspirin and NSAIDs.

Causes vasodilation, which increases circulation, relaxes muscles, and may stimulate release of natural endorphins.

NURSING DIAGNOSIS: **impaired Gas Exchange (in presence of pulmonary embolus)**

May be related to
Altered blood flow to alveoli or to major portions of the lung
Alveolar-capillary membrane changes—atelectasis, airway or alveolar collapse, pulmonary edema or effusion, excessive secretions or active bleeding

Possibly evidenced by
Profound dyspnea, restlessness, apprehension, somnolence, cyanosis
Changes in arterial blood gases (ABGs) or pulse oximetry, such as hypoxemia and hypercapnia

Desired Outcomes/Evaluation Criteria—Client Will

Respiratory Status: Gas Exchange (NOC)
Demonstrate adequate ventilation and oxygenation by ABGs within client's normal range.
Report or display resolution or absence of symptoms of respiratory distress.

ACTIONS/INTERVENTIONS	RATIONALE
Embolus Care: Pulmonary (NIC)	
Independent	
Note respiratory rate and depth and work of breathing, such as use of accessory muscles or nasal flaring and pursed-lip breathing.	Tachypnea and dyspnea accompany pulmonary obstruction. Dyspnea and increased work of breathing may be first or only sign of subacute PE. Severe respiratory distress and failure accompanies moderate to severe loss of functional lung units.
Auscultate lungs for areas of decreased and absent breath sounds and the presence of adventitious sounds, such as crackles.	Nonventilated areas may be identified by absence of breath sounds. Crackles occur in fluid-filled tissues and airways or may reflect cardiac decompensation.
Observe for generalized duskiness and cyanosis in "warm tissues," such as earlobes, lips, tongue, and buccal membranes.	Indicative of systemic hypoxemia.
Monitor vital signs. Note changes in cardiac rhythm.	Tachycardia, tachypnea, and changes in BP are associated with advancing hypoxemia and acidosis. Rhythm alterations and extra heart sounds may reflect increased cardiac workload related to worsening ventilation imbalance.
Assess level of consciousness and evaluate mentation changes.	Systemic hypoxemia may be demonstrated initially by restlessness and irritability, then by progressively decreased mentation.
Assess activity tolerance, such as reports of weakness and fatigue, vital sign changes, or increased dyspnea during exertion. Encourage rest periods, and limit activities to client tolerance.	These parameters assist in determining client response to resumed activities and ability to participate in self-care.
Airway Management (NIC)	
Institute measures to restore or maintain patent airways, such as deep-breathing exercises, coughing, and suctioning.	Plugged or collapsed airways reduce number of functional alveoli, negatively affecting gas exchange.
Elevate head of bed as client tolerates.	Promotes maximal chest expansion, making it easier to breathe and enhancing physiological and psychological comfort.
Assist with frequent changes of position, and get client out of bed to ambulate as tolerated.	Turning and ambulation enhance aeration of different lung segments, thereby improving oxygen diffusion.
Assist client to deal with fear and anxiety that may be present:	Feelings of fear and severe anxiety are associated with inability to breathe and may actually increase oxygen consumption and demand.
Encourage expression of feelings and inform client and SOs of normalcy of anxious feelings and sense of impending doom.	Understanding basis of feelings may help client regain some sense of control over emotions.
Provide brief explanations of what is happening and expected effects of interventions.	Allays anxiety related to unknown and may help reduce fears concerning personal safety.
Monitor frequently, and arrange for someone to stay with client, as indicated.	Provides assurance that changes in condition will be noted and that assistance is readily available.

(continues on page 118)

Embolus Care: Pulmonary (NIC)
Collaborative

Prepare for lung scan.

May reveal pattern of abnormal perfusion in areas of ventilation, reflecting ventilation and perfusion mismatch, confirming diagnosis of PE and degree of obstruction. Absence of both ventilation and perfusion reflects alveolar congestion or airway obstruction.

Monitor serial ABGs or pulse oximetry.

Hypoxemia is present in varying degrees, depending on the amount of airway obstruction, usual cardiopulmonary function, and presence and degree of shock. Respiratory alkalosis and metabolic acidosis may also be present.

Airway Management (NIC)

Administer supplemental oxygen by appropriate method.

Maximizes available oxygen for gas exchange, reducing work of breathing. *Note:* If obstruction is large or hypoxemia does not respond to supplemental oxygenation, it may be necessary to move client to critical care area for intubation and mechanical ventilation.

Administer fluids, IV or by mouth (PO), as indicated.

Increased fluids may be given to reduce hyperviscosity of blood, which can potentiate thrombus formation, or to support circulating volume and tissue perfusion.

Administer medications, as indicated, for example:
  Thrombolytic agents, such as alteplase (Activase, t-PA), anistreplase (APSAC, Eminase), reteplase (Retavase), streptokinase (Kabbikinase, streptase), tenecteplase (TNKase), and urokinase (Abbokinase)

Indicated in massive pulmonary obstruction when client is seriously hemodynamically threatened. *Note:* These clients will probably be initially cared for in, or transferred to, the critical care setting.

  Morphine sulfate and anti-anxiety agents

May be necessary initially to control pain or anxiety and improve work of breathing, maximizing gas exchange.

Provide supplemental humidification, such as ultrasonic nebulizers.

Delivers moisture to mucous membranes and helps liquefy secretions to facilitate airway clearance.

Assist with chest physiotherapy, such as postural drainage and percussion of nonaffected area, blow bottles, and incentive spirometer.

Facilitates deeper respiratory effort and promotes drainage of secretions from lung segments into bronchi, where they may more readily be removed by coughing or suctioning.

Prepare for and assist with bronchoscopy.

May be done to remove blood clots and clear airways.

Prepare for surgical intervention, if indicated.

Vena caval ligation or insertion of an intracaval umbrella may be useful for clients who experience recurrent emboli despite adequate anticoagulation, when anticoagulation is contraindicated, or when septic emboli arising from below the renal veins do not respond to treatment. Additionally, pulmonary embolectomy may be considered in life-threatening situations.

NURSING DIAGNOSIS: **deficient Knowledge [Learning Need] regarding condition, treatment program, self-care, and discharge needs**

May be related to
Lack of exposure or recall
Misinterpretation of information
Unfamiliarity with information resources

Possibly evidenced by
Request for information, statement of misconception
Inaccurate follow-through of instructions
Development of preventable complications

Desired Outcomes/Evaluation Criteria—Client Will

Knowledge: Disease Process (NOC)
Verbalize understanding of disease process, treatment regimen, and limitations.
Participate in learning process.
Identify signs and symptoms requiring medical evaluation.

Knowledge: Treatment Regimen (NOC)
Correctly perform therapeutic actions and explain reasons for actions.

ACTIONS/INTERVENTIONS	RATIONALE

Teaching: Disease Process (NIC)
Independent

Review pathophysiology of condition and signs and symptoms of possible complications, such as PE, chronic venous insufficiency, and venous stasis ulcers (postphlebitic syndrome).

Provides a knowledge base from which client can make informed choices and understand and identify healthcare needs. A significant number of clients experience a recurrence of DVT. *Note:* Genetic blood testing may help identify inherited thrombotic disorders. Screening tests should be done when venous thrombosis occurs in those aged 45 years or younger; when a thrombus occurs at an unusual location such as in gastrointestinal tract, brain, or arm; and when there is an immediate family history of DVT.

Explain purpose of activity restrictions and need for balance between activity and rest.

Rest reduces oxygen and nutrient needs of compromised tissues and decreases risk of fragmentation of thrombosis. Balancing rest with activity prevents exhaustion and further impairment of cellular perfusion.

Establish appropriate exercise and activity program.

Aids in developing collateral circulation, enhances venous return, and prevents recurrence.

Problem-solve solutions to predisposing factors that may be present, such as employment that requires prolonged standing or sitting, wearing restrictive clothing, use of oral contraceptives, obesity, prolonged immobility, and dehydration.

Actively involves client in identifying and initiating lifestyle and behavior changes to promote health and prevent recurrence of condition or development of complications.

Recommend sitting with feet touching the floor, avoiding crossing of legs.

Prevents excess pressure on the popliteal space.

Review purpose and demonstrate correct application and removal of antiembolic hose.

Understanding may enhance cooperation with prescribed therapy and prevent improper or ineffective use.

Instruct in meticulous skin care of lower extremities, such as prevent or promptly treat breaks in skin and report development of ulcers or changes in skin color.

Chronic venous congestion and postphlebitic syndrome may develop, especially in presence of severe vascular involvement and recurrent DVT, potentiating risk of stasis ulcers.

Teaching: Prescribed Medication (NIC)

Discuss purpose and dosage of anticoagulant. Emphasize importance of taking drug as prescribed.

Promotes client safety by reducing risk of inadequate therapeutic response and deleterious side effects.

Identify safety precautions, such as use of soft toothbrush, electric razor for shaving, gloves for gardening, avoiding sharp objects (including toothpicks), walking barefoot, engaging in rough sports and activities, or forceful blowing of nose.

Reduces the risk of traumatic injury, which potentiates bleeding or clot formation.

Review client's usual medications and foods when on oral anticoagulants, stress need to read ingredient labels of over-the-counter (OTC) drugs and herbal supplements, and discuss use with healthcare provider prior to starting new medications.

Warfarin (Coumadin) interacts with many foods and drugs, either increasing or decreasing the anticoagulant effect. Salicylates and excess alcohol decrease prothrombin activity, whereas vitamin K (multivitamins, bananas, leafy green vegetables) increases prothrombin activity and can cause a higher or lower INR, possibly outside the therapeutic range. Barbiturates increase metabolism of coumarin drugs; antibiotics alter intestinal flora and may interfere with vitamin K synthesis.

Identify untoward anticoagulant effects requiring medical attention, such as bleeding from mucous membranes (nose, gums), continued oozing from cuts and punctures, severe bruising after minimal trauma, and development of petechiae.

Early detection of deleterious effects of therapy, such as prolongation of clotting time, allows for timely intervention and may prevent serious complications. *Note:* Even regular use of acetaminophen may prolong clotting times. In addition, use of herbal products, such as ginkgo, garlic, and vitamin E, also impairs clotting and should be avoided during anticoagulant therapy.

Stress importance of medical follow-up and laboratory testing.

Understanding that close supervision of anticoagulant therapy is necessary (therapeutic dosage range is narrow and complications may prove fatal) promotes client participation.

Encourage wearing of medical ID bracelet or tag, as indicated.

Alerts emergency healthcare providers to history of thrombotic problems or current use of or need for anticoagulants, such as prophylactic before and after any procedure or event with an increased risk of venous thromboembolism.

POTENTIAL CONSIDERATIONS following discharge from care setting (dependent on client's age, physical condition and presence of complications, personal resources, and life responsibilities)
• **ineffective self Health Management**—perceived seriousness of condition, susceptibility to recurrence, benefit of therapy

CHAPTER 5

Respiratory

CHRONIC OBSTRUCTIVE PULMONARY DISEASE (COPD) AND ASTHMA

I. Pathophysiology
a. Chronic obstructive pulmonary disease (COPD): chronic obstructive bronchitis and emphysema
   - i. Chronic airflow limitations (CAL): caused by a mixture of small airway disease (obstructive bonchiolitis) and parenchymal destruction (emphysema)
   - ii. Airway inflammation: causes structural changes, narrowing of lumina, and loss of elastic recoil in parenchyma
b. Asthma (also called chronic reactive airway disease)
   - i. Chronic inflammatory disorder—episodic exacerbations of reversible inflammation and hyperreactivity and variable constriction of bronchial smooth muscle, hypersecretion of mucus, and edema

II. Spirometric Classification of Severity of COPD—2007 Global Initiative for Chronic Obstructive Lung Disease
a. Stage I (mild COPD)—mild airflow limitation (FEV_1/FVC < 0.70; $FEV_1 \geq$ to 80% predicted)
b. Stage II (moderate COPD)—worsening airflow limitation (FEV_1/FVC < 0.70; 50% $\leq$ to $FEV_1 < 80\%$ predicted); shortness of breath on exertion, and cough and sputum production may be present
c. Stage III (severe COPD)—continued worsening of airflow limitation (FEV_1/FVC < 0.70; 30% $\leq$ to $FEV_1 < 50\%$ predicted); increasing shortness of breath, reduced exercise capacity, fatigue, and repeated exacerbations
d. Stage IV (very severe COPD)—severe airflow limitation (FEV_1/FVC < 0.70; $FEV_1 < 30\%$ predicted or $FEV_1 < 50\%$ predicted plus presence of chronic respiratory failure)

III. Etiology
a. COPD
   - i. Risk factors: smoking (primary irritant), air pollution, secondhand smoke, history of childhood respiratory infections, heredity—α_1-antitrypsin deficiency
   - ii. Acute exacerbations usually due to pulmonary infections
b. Asthma
   - i. Tends to be acute and intermittent or episodic
   - ii. Genetic and environmental: household substances (such as dust mites, pets, cockroaches, mold), pollen, foods, latex, emotional upheaval, air pollution, cold weather, exercise, chemicals, medications, viral infections

IV. Statistics (American Lung Association, 2006, 2007a; National Heart, Lung and Blood Institute [NHLBI], 2008b)
a. COPD
   - i. Morbidity: COPD affects more than 12 million people.
   - ii. Mortality: It is the fourth leading cause of death in the United States with 122,000 deaths in 2003; women's deaths exceed that of men (63,000 females to 59,000 males).
   - iii. Cost: $37.2 billion is spent each year.
b. Asthma
   - i. Morbidity: Asthma is most common chronic disorder in children, affecting 6.8 million under age 18; affects 15.4 million adults.
   - ii. Cost: $14.7 billion is spent each year.

GLOSSARY

Asthma: Chronic, reversible inflammation of the airways caused by a reaction of the airways to various stimuli.

Chronic bronchitis: Inflammation and scarring of the lining of the bronchi.

Chronic obstructive pulmonary disease (COPD): Disease state characterized by an airflow limitation that is not fully reversible. It is usually progressive and associated with an abnormal inflammatory response to noxious particles or gases (Global Initiative for Chronic Obstructive Lung Disease [GOLD], 2007).

Emphysema: Destruction of the alveoli, which leads to overdistention of the air spaces. Damage is irreversible.

FEV_1: Forced expired volume in 1 second.

FVC: Forced vital capacity.

Care Setting

Primarily community level; however, severe exacerbations may necessitate emergency or inpatient hospital stay.

Related Concerns

Heart failure: chronic, page 48
Pneumonia, page 131
Psychosocial aspects of care, page 749
Ventilatory assistance (mechanical), page 173
Surgical intervention, page 782

Client Assessment Database

DIAGNOSTIC DIVISION MAY REPORT	MAY EXHIBIT
ACTIVITY/REST • Fatigue, exhaustion, malaise • Inability to perform basic activities of daily living (ADLs) because of breathlessness • Inability to sleep, need to sleep sitting up • Dyspnea at rest or in response to activity or exercise	• Fatigue • Restlessness, insomnia • General debilitation or loss of muscle mass
CIRCULATION • Swelling of lower extremities	• Elevated blood pressure (BP) • Elevated heart rate or severe tachycardia, dysrhythmias • Distended neck veins, with advanced disease • Dependent edema, which may not be related to heart disease • Faint heart sounds due to increased anteroposterior (AP) chest diameter • Skin color and mucous membranes may be pale or bluish and cyanotic, clubbing of nails and peripheral cyanosis, pallor (can indicate anemia)
EGO INTEGRITY • Increased stress factors • Changes in lifestyle • Feelings of hopelessness, loss of interest in life	• Anxious, fearful, irritable behavior, emotional distress • Apathy, change in alertness, dull affect, withdrawal
FOOD/FLUID • Nausea—side effect of medication or mucus production • Poor appetite, anorexia (emphysema) • Inability to eat because of respiratory distress • Persistent weight loss, decreased muscle mass or subcutaneous fat (emphysema) • Weight gain reflecting edema (bronchitis, prednisone use)	• Poor skin turgor • Dependent edema • Diaphoresis • Abdominal palpation may reveal hepatomegaly
HYGIENE • Decreased ability and increased need for assistance with ADLs	• Poor hygiene
RESPIRATION • Variable levels of dyspnea, with insidious and progressive onset (predominant symptom in emphysema), especially on exertion • Seasonal or episodic occurrence of breathlessness (asthma); sensation of chest tightness, inability to breathe (asthma); chronic "air hunger"	• Respirations are usually rapid and may be shallow: • Prolonged expiratory phase with grunting, pursed-lip breathing (emphysema) • Assumption of three-point ("tripod") position for breathing—especially with acute exacerbation of chronic bronchitis

(continues on page 122)

DIAGNOSTIC DIVISION **MAY REPORT** (continued)	**MAY EXHIBIT** (continued)

MAY REPORT (continued)

- Persistent cough with sputum production (gray, white, or yellow), which may be copious (chronic bronchitis)
- Intermittent cough episodes, usually nonproductive in early stages, although they may become productive (emphysema)
- Paroxysms of cough (asthma)
- History of recurrent pneumonia, long-term exposure to chemical pollution or respiratory irritants, such as with cigarette smoke; or, occupational dust and fumes, such as with cotton, hemp, asbestos, coal dust, sawdust
- Familial and hereditary factors, that is, deficiency of α_1-antitrypsin (emphysema)
- Use of oxygen at night or continuously

SAFETY
- History of allergic reactions or sensitivity to substances or environmental factors
- Recent or recurrent infections

SEXUALITY
- Decreased libido

SOCIAL INTERACTION
- Dependent relationship(s)
- Insufficient support from or to partner or significant other (SO), lack of support systems
- Prolonged disease or disability progression

TEACHING/LEARNING
- Use or misuse of respiratory drugs
- Use of herbal supplements, such as astragalus, coleus, echinacea, elderberry, elecampe, ephedra, garlic, ginkgo, horehound, licorice, marshmallow, mullein, onion, turmeric, goldenseal, Oregon grape root, wild cherry bark, peppermint, hyssop
- Smoking or difficulty stopping smoking, chronic exposure to secondhand smoke, smoking substances other than tobacco
- Regular use of alcohol
- Failure to improve over long period of time

DISCHARGE PLAN CONSIDERATIONS
- Episodic or long-term assistance with shopping, transportation, self-care needs, homemaker or home maintenance tasks
- Changes in medication and therapeutic treatments, use of supplemental oxygen, ventilator support; end-of-life issues

▶ Refer to section at end of plan for postdischarge considerations.

MAY EXHIBIT (continued)

- Use of accessory muscles for respiration, such as elevated shoulder girdle, retraction of supraclavicular fossae, flaring of nares
- Chest may appear hyperinflated with increased AP diameter (barrel-shaped), minimal diaphragmatic movement
- Breath sounds may be faint with expiratory wheezes (emphysema):
  - Scattered, fine, or coarse moist crackles (bronchitis)
  - Rhonchi, wheezing throughout lung fields on expiration, and possibly during inspiration, progressing to diminished or absent breath sounds (asthma)
- Percussion may reveal hyperresonance over lung fields (air-trapping with emphysema) or dullness over lung fields (consolidation, fluid, mucus)
- Difficulty speaking sentences of more than four or five words at one time, loss of voice
- *Color:* Pallor, with cyanosis of lips, nailbeds; overall duskiness; ruddy color (chronic bronchitis, "blue bloaters"):
  - Normal skin color despite abnormal gas exchange and rapid respiratory rate (moderate emphysema, known as "pink puffers")
- Clubbing of fingernails (not characteristic of emphysema, and if present, should alert clinician to another condition such as pulmonary fibrosis, cystic fibrosis, lung cancer, or asbestosis)

- Flushing, perspiration (asthma)

- Inability to converse or maintain voice because of respiratory distress
- Limited physical mobility
- Neglectful relationships with other family members
- Inability to perform or inattention to employment responsibilities, absenteeism, confirmed disability

TEST WHY IT IS DONE	WHAT IT TELLS ME
BLOOD TESTS • *Arterial blood gases (ABGs):* Measures oxygen and carbon dioxide levels to rule out hypoxemia or hypercapnia.	Most often PaO_2 is decreased, and $PaCO_2$ is normal or increased in chronic bronchitis and emphysema, but is often decreased in asthma; pH normal or acidotic, mild respiratory alkalosis secondary to hyperventilation (moderate emphysema or asthma).
• *Complete blood count (CBC) and differential:* Provides baseline data about the hematologic system and yields information related to oygenation and infection.	Increased hemoglobin (advanced emphysema) and increased eosinophils (asthma); white blood cells (WBCs) can be elevated in severe respiratory infection.
• *α-₁ antitrypsin (A1AT):* Verify deficiency of this enzyme and diagnosis of primary emphysema.	Decreased levels are seen in early onset emphysema in adults; increased levels are present in acute and chronic inflammatory disorders.
PULMONARY STUDIES • *Spirometry testing, including FVC and FEV₁:* Measures lung function; recommended for diagnosis and management of persons with COPD, those at risk for COPD, and follow-up of persons with documented COPD. Used to stage COPD (GOLD, 2007).	Provides information on the degree of obstruction or restriction and evaluates effects of therapy, for example, bronchodilators.
• *Total lung capacity (TLC), functional residual capacity (FRC), and residual volume (RV):* Provides information on the extent of the pulmonary abnormality and if there is air-trapping in the lungs.	May be increased, indicating air-trapping. In obstructive lung disease, the RV will make up the greater portion of the TLC.
• *Tidal volume (V_T) and minute volume (MV):* Measures respiratory function and extent of pulmonary abnormality.	Decreased V_T may indicate restrictive disease. Decreased MV may indicate pulmonary edema; increased MV can occur with acidosis, increased CO_2, decreased PaO_2, and low compliance states.
• *Thoracic gas volume (TCV):* Measures lung volumes and diffusing capacity of the lung.	Increased TCV indicates air-trapping, such as might occur with COPD.
• *Body plethysmography:* May be used to measure pressure and flow or volume changes, such as TCV, airway resistance, and conductance.	Measures changes in lung volumes, airway resistance, and compliance.
• *Diminished carbon monoxide diffusion in the lung (DLCO):* Assesses diffusion in lungs. Carbon monoxide is used to measure gas diffusion across the alveocapillary membrane. Because carbon monoxide combines with hemoglobin 200 times more easily than oxygen, it easily affects the alveoli and small airways where gas exchange occurs.	DLCO is seen in patients with emphysema. This helps distinguish COPD from asthma, as DLCO is normal in patients with asthma.
OTHER DIAGNOSTIC STUDIES • *Pulse oximetry:* Noninvasive measure of arterial blood oxygen diffusion and saturation.	The percentage expressed is the ratio of oxygen to hemoglobin. Abnormally low levels (<88%) indicate impaired gas exchange and impending respiratory failure.
• *Chest x-ray:* Evaluates organs or structures within the chest.	May reveal hyperinflation of lungs with increased AP diameter, flattened diaphragm, increased retrosternal air space, decreased vascular markings/bullae (emphysema), increased bronchovascular markings (bronchitis), and normal findings during periods of remission (asthma).
• *Sputum culture and cytological examination:* Rule out other causes of increased sputum production.	Determines presence of infection and identifies pathogen, if present. Cytological examination may reveal a malignancy or allergic disorder.
• *Electrocardiogram (ECG):* Record of the electrical activity of the heart, which can demonstrate conduction disturbances, enlarged heart, and chamber strain patterns.	Right axis deviation and peaked P waves are seen in severe asthma. Atrial dysrhythmias may be present in bronchitis. Tall, peaked P waves in leads II, III, AVF may be present in bronchitis or emphysema. Vertical QRS axis may be present in emphysema.

(continues on page 124)

TEST WHY IT IS DONE (continued)	WHAT IT TELLS ME (continued)
• *Exercise ECG, stress test (also called exercise treadmill or exercise ECG):* Raises heart rate and BP by means of exercise; or heart can also be stressed with drugs, such as dobutamine or dipyridamol.	May be done for evaluation of hypoxemia or desaturation in the presence of dyspnea, known pulmonary disease, and abnormal diagnostic tests such as diffusing capacity. Helps in assessing degree of pulmonary dysfunction, evaluating effectiveness of bronchodilator therapy, and planning and evaluating exercise program.

Nursing Priorities

1. Maintain airway patency.
2. Assist with measures to facilitate gas exchange.
3. Enhance nutritional intake.
4. Prevent complications and slow progression of condition.
5. Provide information about disease process, prognosis, and treatment regimen.

Discharge Goals

1. Ventilation/oxygenation adequate to meet self-care needs.
2. Nutritional intake meeting caloric needs.
3. Infection treated or prevented.
4. Disease process, prognosis, and therapeutic regimen understood.
5. Plan in place to meet needs after discharge.

NURSING DIAGNOSIS: **ineffective Airway Clearance**

May be related to
Bronchospasm
Increased production of secretions, retained secretions, thick, viscous secretions
Decreased energy or fatigue

Possibly evidenced by
Statement of difficulty breathing
Changes in depth and rate of respirations, use of accessory muscles
Abnormal breath sounds such as wheezes, rhonchi, crackles
Cough (persistent), with or without sputum production

Desired Outcomes/Evaluation Criteria—Client Will

Respiratory Status: Airway Patency (NOC)
Maintain patent airway with breath sounds clear or clearing.
Demonstrate behaviors to improve airway clearance.

ACTIONS/INTERVENTIONS	RATIONALE
Airway Management (NIC) *Independent* Auscultate breath sounds. Note adventitious breath sounds such as wheezes, crackles, or rhonchi.	Some degree of bronchospasm is present with obstructions in airway and may or may not be manifested in adventitious breath sounds, such as scattered, moist crackles (bronchitis); faint sounds, with expiratory wheezes (emphysema); or absent breath sounds (severe asthma).
Assess and monitor respiratory rate. Note inspiratory-to-expiratory ratio.	Tachypnea is usually present to some degree and may be pronounced on admission, during stress, or during concurrent acute infectious process. Respirations may be shallow and rapid, with prolonged expiration in comparison to inspiration.
Note presence and degree of dyspnea, for example, reports of "air hunger," restlessness, anxiety, respiratory distress, and use of accessory muscles. Use a 0 to 10 scale or American Thoracic Society's Grade of Breathlessness Scale to rate breathing difficulty. Ascertain precipitating factors when possible. Differentiate acute episode from exacerbation of chronic dyspnea.	Respiratory dysfunction is variable depending on the underlying process; for example, infection, allergic reaction, and the stage of chronicity in a client with established COPD. *Note:* Using a scale to rate dyspnea aids in quantifying and tracking changes in respiratory distress. Rapid onset of acute dyspnea may reflect pulmonary embolus.

ACTIONS/INTERVENTIONS (continued)

Assist client to maintain a comfortable position to facilitate breathing by elevating the head of bed, leaning on or over bed table, or sitting on edge of bed.

Keep environmental pollution from sources such as dust, smoke, and feather pillows to a minimum according to individual situation.

Encourage and assist with abdominal or pursed-lip breathing exercises.

Observe for persistent, hacking, or moist cough. Assist with measures to improve effectiveness of cough effort.

Increase fluid intake to 3,000 mL/day within cardiac tolerance. Provide warm or tepid liquids. Recommend intake of fluids between, instead of during, meals.

Collaborative

Administer medications, as indicated, for example:

Beta-agonists, such as epinephrine (Adrenalin, AsthmaNefrin, Primatene, Sus-Phrine), albuterol (Proventil, Velmax, Ventolin, AccuNeb, Airet), formoterol (Foradil), lev-albuterol (Xopenex); metaproterenol (Alupent), pirbuterol (Maxair), terbutaline (Brethine), and salmeterol (Serevent)

Bronchodilators, such as anticholinergic agents: ipratropium (Atrovent)

Leukotriene antagonists, such as montelukast (Singulair), zafirlukast (Accolate), and zileuton (Zyflo)

Anti-inflammatory drugs: oral, intravenous (IV), and inhaled steroids, such as prednisone (Cordrol, Deltasone, Pred-Pak, Liquid Pred), methylprednisolone (Medrol), dexamethasone (Decadron), beclomethasone (Beclovent, Vanceril), budesonide (Pulmacort), fluticasone (Flovent), and triamcinolone (Azmacort)

Antimicrobials

Methylxanthine derivatives, such as aminophylline, oxtriphylline (Choledyl), and theophylline (Bronkodyl, Theo-Dur, Elixophyllin, Slo-Bid, Slo-Phyllin)

RATIONALE (continued)

Elevation of the head of the bed facilitates respiratory function using gravity; however, client in severe distress will seek the position that most eases breathing. Supporting arms and legs with table, pillows, and so on helps reduce muscle fatigue and can aid chest expansion.

Precipitators of allergic type of respiratory reactions that can trigger or exacerbate onset of acute episode.

Provides client with some means to cope with and control dyspnea and reduce air-trapping.

Cough can be persistent but ineffective, especially if client is elderly, acutely ill, or debilitated. Coughing is most effective in an upright or in a head-down position after chest percussion.

Hydration helps decrease the viscosity of secretions, facilitating expectoration. Using warm liquids may decrease bronchospasm. Fluids during meals can increase gastric distention and pressure on the diaphragm.

Inhaled β_2-adrenergic agonists are first-line therapies for rapid symptomatic improvement of bronchoconstriction. These medications relax smooth muscles and reduce local congestion, reducing airway spasm, wheezing, and mucus production. Medications may be oral, injected, or inhaled. Inhalation by metered-dose inhaler (MDI) with a spacer is recommended, but medications may be nebulized in the event client has severe coughing or is too dyspneic to puff effectively.

Inhaled anticholinergic agents are now considered the first-line drugs for clients with stable COPD because studies indicate they have a longer duration of action with less toxicity potential, whereas still providing the effective relief of the beta-agonists. Some of these medications are available in combinations; for example, albuterol and Atrovent are available as Combivent.

Reduce leukotriene activity to limit inflammatory response. In mild to moderate asthma, reduces need for inhaled β_2-agonists and systemic corticosteroids. Not effective in acute exacerbations because there is no bronchodilator effect. *Note:* This drug class is not recommended for clients with COPD because of insufficient testing.

Decrease local airway inflammation and edema by inhibiting effects of histamine and other mediators to reduce severity and frequency of airway spasm, respiratory inflammation, and dyspnea. Studies have shown benefits of systemic steroids in the management of COPD exacerbations. Inhaled steroids may serve as a systemic steroid-sparing agent. *Note:* The aim of inhaled corticosteroids is to reduce exacerbation rates and slow decline in health status. Maintenance use of oral corticosteroids is not recommended unless absolutely necessary. Clients must be monitored for osteoporosis as a side effect. Clients over age 65 should be treated prophylactically to prevent osteoporosis.

Various antimicrobials may be indicated for control of bacterial exacerbations of COPD, such as pneumonia. (Refer to CP, Pneumonia.)

Decrease mucosal edema and smooth muscle spasm (bronchospasm) by indirectly increasing cyclic adenosine monophosphate (AMP). May also reduce muscle fatigue and respiratory failure by increasing diaphragmatic contractility. Use of theophylline may be of little or no benefit in the presence of adequate beta-agonist regimen; however, it may sustain bronchodilation because effect of beta-agonist diminishes between doses. *Note:* Theophylline products are used with less frequency now and are not recommended in older clients because of their potentially adverse cardiovascular effects.

(continues on page 126)

ACTIONS/INTERVENTIONS (continued)

Analgesics, cough suppressants, or antitussives, such as codeine and dextromethorphan products (Benylin DM, Comtrex, Novahistine)

Artificial surfactant such as colfosceril palmitate (Exosurf)

Provide supplemental humidification, such as ultrasonic nebulizer and aerosol room humidifier.

Assist with respiratory treatments, such as spirometry and chest physiotherapy.

Monitor and graph serial ABGs, pulse oximetry, and chest x-ray.

RATIONALE (continued)

Persistent, exhausting cough may need to be suppressed to conserve energy and permit client to rest. *Note:* Regular use of antitussives is not recommended for COPD clients as cough can have a significant protective effect.

Research suggests aerosol administration may enhance expectoration of sputum, improve pulmonary function, and reduce lung volumes (air-trapping).

Humidity helps reduce viscosity of secretions, facilitating expectoration, and may reduce or prevent formation of thick mucous plugs in bronchioles.

Breathing exercises help enhance diffusion; aerosol or nebulizer medications can reduce bronchospasm and stimulate expectoration. Postural drainage and percussion enhance removal of excessive and sticky secretions and improve ventilation of bottom lung segments. *Note:* Chest physiotherapy may aggravate bronchospasm in asthmatics.

Establishes baseline for monitoring progression or regression of disease process and complications. *Note:* Pulse oximetry readings detect changes in saturation as they are happening, helping to identify trends possibly before client is symptomatic. However, studies have shown that the accuracy of pulse oximetry may be questioned if client has severe peripheral vasoconstriction.

NURSING DIAGNOSIS: impaired Gas Exchange

May be related to
Altered oxygen supply—obstruction of airways by secretions, bronchospasm, air-trapping
Alveoli destruction

Possibly evidenced by
Dyspnea
Confusion, restlessness
Inability to move secretions
Abnormal ABGs—hypoxia and hypercapnia
Changes in vital signs
Reduced tolerance for activity

Desired Outcomes/Evaluation Criteria—Client Will

Respiratory Status: Gas Exchange (NOC)
Demonstrate improved ventilation and adequate oxygenation of tissues by ABGs within client's normal range and be free of symptoms of respiratory distress.
Participate in treatment regimen within level of ability and situation.

ACTIONS/INTERVENTIONS

Acid-Base Management (NIC)
Independent
Assess respiratory rate and depth. Note use of accessory muscles, pursed-lip breathing, and inability to speak or converse.

Elevate head of bed and assist client to assume position to ease work of breathing. Include periods of time in prone position as tolerated. Encourage deep, slow or pursed-lip breathing as individually needed and tolerated.

Assess and routinely monitor skin and mucous membrane color.

Encourage expectoration of sputum; suction when indicated.

RATIONALE

Useful in evaluating the degree of respiratory distress and chronicity of the disease process.

Oxygen delivery may be improved by upright position and breathing exercises to decrease airway collapse, dyspnea, and work of breathing. *Note:* Recent research supports use of prone position to increase PaO_2.

Cyanosis may be peripheral (noted in nailbeds) or central (noted around lips or earlobes). Duskiness and central cyanosis indicate advanced hypoxemia.

Thick, tenacious, copious secretions are a major source of impaired gas exchange in small airways. Deep suctioning may be required when cough is ineffective for expectoration of secretions.

ACTIONS/INTERVENTIONS (continued)

ACTIONS/INTERVENTIONS (continued)	RATIONALE (continued)
Auscultate breath sounds, noting areas of decreased airflow and adventitious sounds.	Breath sounds may be faint because of decreased airflow or areas of consolidation. Presence of wheezes may indicate bronchospasm or retained secretions. Scattered, moist crackles may indicate interstitial fluid or cardiac decompensation.
Palpate chest for fremitus.	Decrease of vibratory tremors suggests fluid collection or air-trapping.
Monitor level of consciousness and mental status. Investigate changes.	Restlessness and anxiety are common manifestations of hypoxia. Worsening ABGs accompanied by confusion and somnolence are indicative of cerebral dysfunction due to hypoxemia.
Evaluate level of activity tolerance. Provide calm, quiet environment. Limit client's activity or encourage bedrest or chair rest during acute phase. Have client resume activity gradually and increase as individually tolerated.	During severe, acute, or refractory respiratory distress, client may be totally unable to perform basic self-care activities because of hypoxemia and dyspnea. Rest interspersed with care activities remains an important part of treatment regimen. An exercise program is aimed at improving aerobic capacity and functional performance, increasing endurance and strength without causing severe dyspnea, and can enhance sense of well-being.
Evaluate sleep patterns, note reports of difficulties and whether client feels well rested. Provide quiet environment and group care and monitoring activities to allow periods of uninterrupted sleep. Limit stimulants such as caffeine. Encourage position of comfort.	Multiple external stimuli and presence of dyspnea and hypoxemia may prevent relaxation and inhibit sleep.
Monitor vital signs and cardiac rhythm.	Tachycardia, dysrhythmias, and changes in BP can reflect effect of systemic hypoxemia on cardiac function.

Collaborative

ACTIONS/INTERVENTIONS	RATIONALE
Monitor and graph serial ABGs and pulse oximetry.	$PaCO_2$ is usually elevated in bronchitis and emphysema, and PaO_2 is generally decreased, so that hypoxia is present in a greater or lesser degree. *Note:* A "normal" or increased $PaCO_2$ signals impending respiratory failure for asthmatics.
Administer supplemental oxygen judiciously via nasal cannula, mask, or mechanical ventilator, and titrate as indicated by ABG results and client tolerance.	Used to correct and prevent worsening of hypoxemia, improve survival, and quality of life. Supplemental oxygen can be provided during exacerbations only, or as a long-term therapy.
Administer antianxiety, sedative, or opioid agents, such as morphine, with caution.	May be used to reduce dyspnea by controlling anxiety and restlessness, which increases oxygen consumption and demand, exacerbating dyspnea. Must be monitored closely because depressive effect may lead to respiratory failure.
Assist with noninvasive (nasal or oronasal intermittent) positive-pressure ventilation (NIPPV) or intubation and institution and maintenance of mechanical ventilation; transfer to critical care unit depending on client directives.	Development of or impending respiratory failure requires prompt life-saving measures. *Note:* NIPPV provides ventilatory support by means of positive pressure, typically through a nasal mask. It may be useful in the home setting as well to treat chronic respiratory failure or limit acute exacerbations in clients who are able to maintain spontaneous respiratory effort.
Prepare for additional referrals and interventions, such as to a pulmonary specialist, to a pulmonary rehabilitation program, or for surgical intervention, as appropriate.	May be indicated to confirm diagnosis and optimize appropriate treatment. A multidisciplinary approach including education and exercise training may be helpful in improving client function and quality of life. Screened candidates—those with severe dyspnea or end-stage emphysema with FEV_1 less than 35% of the predicted value despite maximal medical therapy and with the ability to complete preoperative pulmonary rehabilitation programs—may benefit from lung volume reduction surgery (LVRS) in which hyperinflated giant bullae and cysts are removed. These bullae or cysts may occupy at least one-third of the involved lobe or areas of lung tissue with small cystic disease. In the absence of fibrosis, this procedure removes ineffective lung tissue, allowing for better lung expansion and elastic recoil, enhanced blood flow to healthy tissues (correction of ventilation-perfusion mismatch), improved respiratory muscle efficiency, and increased venous return.

ACTIONS/INTERVENTIONS	RATIONALE
Nutrition Therapy (NIC)	
Independent	
Assess dietary habits, recent food intake. Note degree of difficulty with eating. Evaluate weight and body size or mass.	Client in acute respiratory distress is often anorectic because of dyspnea, sputum production, and medication effects. In addition, many COPD clients habitually eat poorly even though respiratory insufficiency creates a hypermetabolic state with increased caloric needs. As a result, client often is admitted with some degree of malnutrition. People who have emphysema are often thin, with wasted musculature.
Auscultate bowel sounds.	Diminished or hypoactive bowel sounds may reflect decreased gastric motility and constipation (common complication) related to limited fluid intake, poor food choices, decreased activity, and hypoxemia.
Give frequent oral care, remove expectorated secretions promptly, and provide specific container for disposal of secretions and tissues.	Noxious tastes, smells, and sights are prime deterrents to appetite and can produce nausea and vomiting with increased respiratory difficulty.
Encourage a rest period of 1 hour before and after meals. Provide frequent small feedings.	Helps reduce fatigue during mealtime, and provides opportunity to increase total caloric intake.
Avoid gas-producing foods and carbonated beverages.	Can produce abdominal distention, which hampers abdominal breathing and diaphragmatic movement and can increase dyspnea.
Avoid very hot or very cold foods.	Extremes in temperature can precipitate or aggravate coughing spasms.
Weigh, as indicated.	Useful in determining caloric needs, setting weight goal, and evaluating adequacy of nutritional plan. *Note:* Weight loss may continue initially despite adequate intake, as edema is resolving.
Collaborative	
Consult dietitian or nutritional support team to provide easily digested, nutritionally balanced meals by mouth, supplemental or tube feedings, and parenteral nutrition. (Refer to CP: Total Nutritional Support: Parenteral/Enteral Feeding.)	Method of feeding and caloric requirements are based on individual situation and specific needs to provide maximal nutrients with minimal client effort and energy expenditure.
Review serum albumin or prealbumin, transferrin, amino acid profile, iron, nitrogen balance studies, glucose, liver function studies, and electrolyte laboratory values as ordered.	Determines deficits and monitors effectiveness of nutritional therapy.
Administer supplemental oxygen during meals, as indicated.	Decreases dyspnea and increases energy for eating, enhancing intake.

NURSING DIAGNOSIS: **deficient Knowledge [Learning Need] regarding condition, treatment, self-care, and discharge needs**

May be related to
Lack of information or unfamiliarity with information resources
Information misinterpretation
Lack of recall or cognitive limitation

Possibly evidenced by
Request for information
Statement of concerns and misconceptions
Inaccurate follow-through of instructions
Development of preventable complications

Desired Outcomes/Evaluation Criteria—Client Will

Knowledge: Illness Care (NOC)
Verbalize understanding of condition and disease process and treatment.
Identify relationship of current signs and symptoms to the disease process and correlate these with causative factors.
Initiate necessary lifestyle changes and participate in treatment regimen.

ACTIONS/INTERVENTIONS	RATIONALE
Teaching: Disease Process (NIC)	
Independent	
Explain and reinforce explanations of individual disease process, including factors that lead to exacerbation episodes. Encourage client and SO to ask questions.	Understanding decreases anxiety and can lead to improved participation in treatment plan.
Discuss self-management plan:	
Avoidance of triggers and education regarding zones, as appropriate	Avoiding triggers, such as known allergens, environmental temperature extremes, chemical products and fumes, is important in the self-management of asthma and in the prevention of acute exacerbations. Zones may be divided into green (peak expiratory flow rate [PEFR] 80% to 100% and no breathing difficulty), yellow (PEFR 50% to 80% of baseline and some difficulty breathing, with wheezing and coughing), and red (PEFR less than 50% baseline and does not respond to inhaled bronchodilators).
Review of breathing exercises, coughing effectively, and general conditioning exercises	Pursed-lip and abdominal or diaphragmatic breathing exercises strengthen muscles of respiration, help minimize collapse of small airways, and provide the individual with means to control dyspnea. General paced conditioning exercises, carried out regularly and perhaps timed with activity soon after taking medication or breathing treatments, can increase activity tolerance, muscle strength, and sense of well-being and quality of life.
Importance of regular oral care and dental hygiene	Decreases bacterial growth in the mouth, which can lead to pulmonary infections.
Importance of avoiding people with active respiratory infections; stress need for routine influenza and pneumococcal vaccinations	Decreases exposure to and incidence of acquired acute upper respiratory infections (URIs).
Identify individual environmental factors such as excessively dry air, wind, temperature extremes, pollen, tobacco smoke, aerosol sprays, and air pollution that may trigger or aggravate condition. Encourage client and SO to explore ways to control these factors in and around the home and work setting.	These can induce or aggravate bronchial irritation, leading to increased secretion production and airway blockage.
Review the harmful effects of smoking, and strongly advise cessation of smoking by client and SO. Provide information on QUITLINES, support groups, nicotine substitutes, and other resources that aid in smoking cessation.	Cessation of smoking may slow or halt progression of COPD. Even when client wants to stop smoking, support groups and medical monitoring may be needed. *Note:* Research studies suggest that sidestream or secondhand smoke can be as detrimental as actually smoking.

(continues on page 130)

Provide information about benefits of regular exercise while addressing individual activity limitations.

Having this knowledge can enable client and SO to make informed choices and decisions to reduce client's dyspnea, maximize functional level, perform most desired activities, and prevent complications. This may include alternating activities with rest periods to prevent fatigue, conserving energy during activities by pulling instead of pushing articles, sitting instead of standing while performing tasks; using pursed-lip breathing, side-lying position, and possible need for supplemental oxygen during sexual activity.

Discuss importance of regular medical follow-up care, when to notify healthcare professional of changes in condition, and periodic spirometry testing, chest x-rays, and sputum cultures.

Monitoring disease process allows for alterations in therapeutic regimen to meet changing needs and may help prevent complications.

Review oxygen requirements and dosage for client who is discharged on supplemental oxygen. Discuss safe use of oxygen and refer to supplier as indicated.

Reduces risk of misuse—too little or too much—and resultant complications. Promotes environmental and physical safety.

Instruct client and SO in use of NIPPV as appropriate. Problem-solve possible side effects, and identify adverse signs and symptoms such as increased dyspnea, fatigue, daytime drowsiness, or headaches on awakening.

NIPPV may be used at night and periodically during day to decrease CO_2 level, improve quality of sleep, and enhance functional level during the day. Signs of increasing CO_2 level indicate need for more aggressive therapy.

Instruct asthmatic client in use of peak flow meter as appropriate.

Peak flow level can drop before client exhibits any signs and symptoms of asthma after the "first time" the client is exposed to a trigger. Regular use of the peak flow meter may reduce the severity of the attack because of earlier intervention.

Provide information and encourage participation in support groups sponsored by the American Lung Association and public health department.

These clients and their SOs may experience anxiety, depression, and other reactions as they deal with a chronic disease that has an impact on their desired lifestyle. Support groups may be desired or needed to provide assistance, emotional support, and respite care.

Refer for evaluation of home care if indicated. Provide a detailed plan of care and baseline physical assessment to home care nurse as needed on discharge from acute care.

Provides for continuity of care. May help reduce frequency of hospitalization.

Assist client and SO in making arrangements for access to emergency assistance, such as a buddy system for getting help quickly, special phone numbers, and "panic button."

Client with chronic respiratory condition should have access to prompt assistance when needed. This is both necessary and psychologically comforting for self-management.

Facilitate discussion about healthcare directives and end-of-life wishes as indicated.

Although many clients have an interest in discussing living wills, their wishes may be unspoken. In client with severe pulmonary disease, it is helpful to discuss preferences regarding aggressive treatment, home care only, hospitalization for comfort care, and full life support. It is useful also to discuss the goals of care, such as functional independence or continuation of life support in an extended care nursing facility.

Discuss respiratory medications, side effects, drug interactions, and adverse reactions.

Frequently, these clients are simultaneously on several respiratory drugs that have similar side effects and potential drug interactions. It is important that the client understands the difference between nuisance side effects (medication continued) and untoward or adverse side effects (medication possibly discontinued or dosage changed).

Demonstrate correct technique for using an MDI, such as how to hold it, pausing 2 to 5 minutes between puffs, and cleaning the inhaler.

Proper administration of drug enhances delivery and effectiveness.

Devise system for recording prescribed intermittent drug and inhaler usage.

Reduces risk of improper use or overdosage of prn (as necessary) medications, especially during acute exacerbations, when cognition may be impaired.

Discuss use of herbals, especially when client is on multiple respiratory medications.

Many interactions can occur between herbals and medications used to treat respiratory disorders. Although most herbals do not have dangerous side effects, effects can be dangerous or lethal if combined with other substances or when taken in larger doses. Herbs, such as ephedra, should be used only in very small doses and for a short time. Echinacea can alter the actions of a variety of drugs and is not recommended for persons with HIV infection, multiple sclerosis (MS), and other autoimmune disorders.

ACTIONS/INTERVENTIONS (continued)

Recommend avoidance of sedative antianxiety agents unless specifically prescribed and approved by physician treating respiratory condition.

RATIONALE (continued)

Although client may be nervous and feel the need for sedatives, these can depress respiratory drive and protective cough mechanisms. *Note:* These drugs may be used prophylactically when client is unable to avoid situations known to increase stress and trigger respiratory response.

> **POTENTIAL CONSIDERATIONS** following acute hospitalization (dependent on client's age, physical condition and presence of complications, personal resources, and life responsibilities)
> - *Self-Care Deficit, specify*—intolerance to activity, decreased strength and endurance, depression, severe anxiety
> - *ineffective Home Maintenance*—intolerance to activity, inadequate support system, insufficient finances, unfamiliarity with neighborhood resources
> - *risk for Infection*—decreased ciliary action, stasis of secretions, tissue destruction, increased environmental exposure, chronic disease process, malnutrition

PNEUMONIA

I. Pathophysiology
a. Inflammation of the lung parenchyma associated with alveolar edema and congestion that impairs gas exchange
b. Common pathogens
   i. Viruses
      1. Common causative organisms include respiratory syncytial virus (RSV) and influenza
      2. Accounts for approximately half of all cases of community-acquired pneumonia (CAP)
   ii. Bacteria
      1. Divided into typical and atypical types
      2. Gram-positive *Streptococcus pneumoniae, Haemophilus,* and *Staphylococcus* most common bacterial causes
   iii. Fungus
      1. Most common causes *Histoplasma capsulatum* and *Coccidioides immitis*
      2. *Pneumocystis carinii* and cytomegalovirus (CMV) often occur in immunocompromised persons
   iv. Other
      1. Agents include *Mycoplasma, Mycobacterium tuberculosis, Coxiella burnetii, Chlamydia,* and *Legionella*

II. Classification
a. Site and causative agent
   i. Lobar, single lobe; broncho, smaller lung areas in several lobes; interstitial, tissues surrounding the alveoli and bronchi
   ii. Bacteria, viruses, and fungi
b. Distribution
   i. CAP commonly caused by *S. pneumoniae, Chlamydia pneumoniae, Haemophilus influenzae,* RSV, occasionally atypical pathogens
   ii. Nosocomial develops at least 48 hours after admission to an institution or care center; hospital-acquired pneumonia (HAP) and/or ventilator-associated pneumonia (VAP) is often caused by *Pseudomonas aeruginosa, Klebsiella pneumoniae, Staphylococcus aureus,* and both methicillin-sensitive and methicillin-resistant *S. aureus* (MRSA)

III. Etiology
a. Primary pneumonia is caused by the client's inhalation or aspiration of a pathogen (microaspiration).
b. Secondary pneumonia ensues from lung damage caused by the spread of an infectious agent—bacterial, viral, or fungal—from another site in the body or from various chemical irritants (including gastric reflux and aspiration, smoke inhalation) or radiation therapy.
c. Risk factors: comorbidities, such as heart or lung disease, compromised immune system, diabetes mellitus, liver or renal failure, malnutrition, smoking, over age 70, previous antibiotic therapy, abdominal or thoracic surgical procedures, endotracheal intubation with mechanical ventilation

IV. Statistics (American Lung Association, 2007c; National Center for Health Statistics [NCHS], 2007; National Heart, Lung and Blood Institute [NHLBI], 2008a)
a. Morbidity: An estimated 6 million cases are reported annually; hospital discharges attributed to pneumonia in 2005 were 651,000 males (44.9 per 10,000) and 717,000 females (47.7 per 10,000).
b. Mortality: Approximately 58,000 deaths per year; eighth leading cause of death in the United States (pneumonia and influenza combined, with pneumonia the leading cause); accounts for approximately 10% of all inpatient deaths.
c. Cost: Estimated annual cost is $8.4 billion for CAP (Lutfiyya, 2006); in excess of $1 billion per year for HAPs; up to $20,000 to $29,000 per episode of VAP, with length of stay increased by as much as 14 days (Niederman, 2001; Schleder, 2004).

Adventitious breath sounds: Abnormal breath sounds heard when listening to the chest. Adventitious sounds may include crackles or rales, rhonchi or wheezes, or pleural friction rubs.

Bronchial breath sounds: A harsh or blowing quality, made by air moving in the large bronchi and barely, if at all, modified by the intervening lung; may be heard over a consolidated lung.

Community-acquired pneumonia (CAP): Acquired outside healthcare organizations, including hospitals, nursing homes, and other long-term care facilities; includes the first 2 days of hospitalization.

Crackles: An adventitious breath sound produced by air passing over airway secretions; a discontinuous sound, as opposed to a wheeze, which is continuous. Crackles are classified as "fine" or "coarse"; also known as rales.

Empyema: A condition in which pus and fluid from infected tissue collects in a body cavity; most often used to refer to collections of pus in the space around the lungs (pleural cavity).

Fremitus: A palpable vibration, as felt by the hand placed on the chest during coughing or speaking.

Nosocomial pneumonia: Hospital-acquired form, which occurs 48 hours or longer after admission.

Percussion: An assessment method in which the surface of the body is struck with the fingertips to obtain sounds that can be heard or vibrations that can be felt. It can determine the position, size, and consistency of an internal organ. It is done over the chest to determine the presence of normal air content in the lungs.

Pleural effusion: Accumulation of fluid in the space between the membrane encasing the lung and lining the thoracic cavity.

Pleural friction rub: An abrasive sound that is synchronous with the respiratory movements, made by the rubbing together of two acutely inflamed serous surfaces, as in acute pleurisy.

Care Setting

Most clients are treated as outpatients in community settings; however, persons at higher risk, such as those older than 65 and persons with other chronic conditions such as chronic obstructive pulmonary disease (COPD), diabetes, cancer, and congestive heart failure, are treated in the hospital, as are those already hospitalized for other reasons and who have developed nosocomial pneumonia.

Related Concerns

Acquired immunodeficiency syndrome (AIDS), page 709

Chronic obstructive pulmonary disease (COPD) and asthma, page 120

Psychosocial aspects of care, page 749

Sepsis/septicemia, page 686

Surgical intervention, page 782

Client Assessment Database

DIAGNOSTIC DIVISION MAY REPORT	MAY EXHIBIT
ACTIVITY/REST • Fatigue, weakness • Insomnia • Prolonged immobility and bedrest	• Lethargy • Decreased tolerance to activity
CIRCULATION • History of recent or chronic heart failure (HF)	• Tachycardia • Flushed appearance, pallor, central cyanosis
FOOD/FLUID • Loss of appetite • Nausea, vomiting • May be receiving intestinal, gastric feedings	• Distended abdomen • Hyperactive bowel sounds • Dry skin with poor turgor • Cachectic appearance (malnutrition)
NEUROSENSORY • Frontal headache (influenza)	• Changes in mentation, such as confusion, somnolence • Changes in behavior such as irritability, restlessness, lethargy

DIAGNOSTIC DIVISION
MAY REPORT (continued)

MAY EXHIBIT (continued)

PAIN/DISCOMFORT
- Headache
- Chest pain (pleuritic) aggravated by cough
- Substernal chest pain (influenza)
- Myalgia, arthralgia
- Abdominal pain

- Splinting, guarding over affected area
- Position—commonly lies on affected side to restrict movement

RESPIRATION
- History of recurrent or chronic upper respiratory infections (URIs), tuberculosis, COPD, cigarette smoking
- Progressive shortness of breath
- Presence of tracheostomy, endotracheal tube
- Current treatment with mechanical ventilator
- Cough is dry and hacking (initially), progressing to productive cough

- *Respirations:* Tachypnea, shallow grunting respirations
- Use of accessory muscles, nasal flaring
- Breath sounds are diminished or absent over involved area
- Bronchial breath sounds over area(s) of consolidation
- Coarse inspiratory crackles
- *Color:* Pallor or cyanosis of lips or nailbeds
- *Sputum:* Scanty or copious; pink, rusty, or purulent (green, yellow, or white)
- *Percussion:* Dull over consolidated areas
- *Fremitus:* Tactile and vocal, gradually increases with consolidation
- Pleural friction rub

SAFETY
- Recurrent chills
- History of altered immune system, such as systemic lupus erythematosis (SLE), AIDS, active malignancies, neurological disease, HF, diabetes, steroid or chemotherapy use; institutionalization, general debilitation

- Diaphoresis
- Shaking
- Rash, in cases of rubeola or varicella
- Fever of 102°F to 104°F (39°C to 40°C)

TEACHING/LEARNING
- Recent surgery, chronic alcohol use or long history of alcoholism, intravenous (IV) drug therapy or abuse, chemotherapy or other immunosuppressive therapy
- Use of herbal supplements, such as garlic, ginkgo, licorice, onion, turmeric, horehound, marshmallow, mullein, wild cherry bark, astragalus, echinacea, elderberry, goldenseal, Oregon grape root

DISCHARGE PLAN CONSIDERATIONS
- Assistance with self-care, homemaker tasks
- Supplemental oxygen, especially if recovery is prolonged or other predisposing condition exists

▶ Refer to section at end of plan for postdischarge considerations.

TEST WHY IT IS DONE	WHAT IT TELLS ME
BLOOD TESTS	
• *Complete blood count (CBC):* Battery of screening tests that typically includes hemoglobin (Hgb); hematocrit (Hct); red blood cell (RBC) count, morphology, indices, and distribution width index; platelet count and size; white blood cell (WBC) count and differential. Provides baseline data about the hematologic system and yields information related to oxygenation and infection.	Leukocytosis with a left shift is usually present in bacterial pneumonia, although a low WBC count may be present in viral infection, immunosuppressed conditions such as AIDS, and overwhelming bacterial pneumonia.
• *Electrolytes:* An electrolyte is a substance that will dissociate into ions in solution and acquire the capacity to conduct electricity. Common electrolytes include sodium, potassium, chloride, calcium, and phosphate. Provides baseline data and can be used to evaluate and monitor fluid and electrolyte balance.	Sodium and chloride levels may be low.
• *Erythrocyte sedimentation rate (ESR):* Nonspecific test done to detect illnesses associated with acute infection and inflammation.	Elevated levels may be present in bacterial infections.
• *Serologic studies (viral or Legionella titers, cold agglutinins):* Assist in differential diagnosis of specific organism.	Provide information on the specific organism causing the pneumonia or can rule out other diseases.
• *Arterial blood gases (ABGs):* Measure oxygen and carbon dioxide levels to rule out hypoxemia or hypercapnia.	Abnormalities may be present, depending on extent of lung involvement and underlying lung disease.
OTHER DIAGNOSTIC STUDIES	
• *Chest x-ray:* Evaluates organs and structures within the chest.	Identifies structural distribution of pneumonia, such as lobar or bronchial. May show scattered or localized infiltration (bacterial) or diffuse and extensive nodular infiltrates (more often viral). In *Mycoplasma* pneumonia, chest x-ray may be clear.
• *Fiberoptic bronchoscopy:* Allows direct visualization of tracheobronchial tree for abnormalities and to obtain sputum for cytological examination.	May be both diagnostic (qualitative cultures) and therapeutic (reexpansion of lung segment).
• *Pulmonary function studies:* Various tests measure lung function, provide information on the extent of the pulmonary abnormality, and determine if there is airway obstruction or trapping in the lungs.	Lung volumes may be decreased (congestion and alveolar collapse). Airway pressure may be increased and compliance decreased. Shunting is present (hypoxemia).
• *Pulse oximetry:* Noninvasive measure of arterial blood oxygen diffusion and saturation.	The percentage expressed is the ratio of oxygen to Hgb. Pulse oximetry less than 90% indicates significant hypoxia. Abnormally low levels (<88%) indicate impaired gas exchange and impending respiratory failure.
• *Gram stain and cultures:* Sputum collection; needle aspiration of empyema, pleural, and transtracheal or transthoracic fluids; and lung biopsies and blood cultures may be done to recover causative organism.	More than one type of organism may be present; common bacteria include *Diplococcus pneumoniae, S. aureus,* α-hemolytic streptococcus, *H. influenzae,* and CMV. *Note:* Sputum cultures may not identify all offending organisms. Blood cultures may show transient bacteremia.

Nursing Priorities

1. Maintain or improve respiratory function.
2. Prevent complications.
3. Support recuperative process.
4. Provide information about disease process, prognosis, and treatment.

Discharge Goals

1. Ventilation and oxygenation adequate for individual needs.
2. Complications prevented or minimized.
3. Disease process, prognosis, and therapeutic regimen understood.
4. Lifestyle changes identified and initiated to prevent recurrence.
5. Plan in place to meet needs after discharge.

NURSING DIAGNOSIS: ineffective Airway Clearance

May be related to
Tracheal bronchial inflammation, edema formation, increased sputum production
Pleuritic pain
Decreased energy, fatigue

Possibly evidenced by
Changes in rate, depth of respirations
Abnormal breath sounds, use of accessory muscles
Dyspnea, cyanosis
Cough, effective or ineffective; with or without sputum production

Desired Outcomes/Evaluation Criteria—Client Will

Respiratory Status: Airway Patency (NOC)
Identify and demonstrate behaviors to achieve airway clearance.
Display patent airway with breath sounds clearing and absence of dyspnea and cyanosis.

ACTIONS/INTERVENTIONS	RATIONALE
Airway Management (NIC)	
Independent	
Assess rate and depth of respirations and chest movement. Monitor for signs of respiratory failure; for example, cyanosis and severe tachypnea.	Tachypnea, shallow respirations, and asymmetric chest movement are frequently present because of discomfort of moving chest wall or fluid in lung. When pneumonia is severe, the client may require endotracheal intubation and mechanical ventilation to keep airways clear.
Auscultate lung fields, noting areas of decreased or absent airflow and adventitious breath sounds, such as crackles and wheezes.	Decreased airflow occurs in areas consolidated with fluid. Bronchial breath sounds (normal over bronchus) can also occur in consolidated areas. Crackles, rhonchi, and wheezes are heard on inspiration and expiration in response to fluid accumulation, thick secretions, and airway spasm or obstruction.
Elevate head of bed; change position frequently.	Keeping the head elevated lowers diaphragm, promoting chest expansion, aeration of lung segments, and mobilization and expectoration of secretions to keep the airway clear.
Assist client with frequent deep-breathing exercises. Demonstrate and help client, as needed; learn to perform activity, such as splinting chest and effective coughing while in upright position.	Deep breathing facilitates maximum expansion of the lungs and smaller airways. Coughing is a natural self-cleaning mechanism, assisting the cilia to maintain patent airways. Splinting reduces chest discomfort, and an upright position favors deeper, more forceful cough effort. *Note:* Cough associated with pneumonias may last days, weeks, or even months.
Suction, as indicated; for example, oxygen desaturation related to airway secretions.	Stimulates cough or mechanically clears airway in client who is unable to do so because of ineffective cough or decreased level of consciousness.
Force fluids to at least 2,500 mL per day, unless contraindicated, as in HF. Offer warm, rather than cold, fluids.	Fluids, especially warm liquids, aid in mobilization and expectoration of secretions.
Collaborative	
Assist with and monitor effects of nebulizer treatments and other respiratory physiotherapy, such as incentive spirometer, intermittent positive-pressure breathing (IPPB), percussion, and postural drainage. Perform treatments between meals and limit fluids when appropriate.	Facilitates liquefaction and removal of secretions. Postural drainage may not be effective in interstitial pneumonias or those causing alveolar exudates or destruction. Coordination of treatments, schedules, and oral intake reduces likelihood of vomiting with coughing and expectorations.
Administer medications, as indicated, for example mucolytics, expectorants, bronchodilators, and analgesics.	Aids in reduction of bronchospasm and mobilization of secretions. Analgesics are given to improve cough effort by reducing discomfort, but should be used cautiously because they can decrease cough effort and depress respirations.
Provide supplemental fluids such as IV, humidified oxygen, and room humidification.	Fluids are required to replace losses, including insensible, and aid in mobilization of secretions. *Note:* Some studies indicate that room humidification has been found to provide minimal benefit and is thought to increase the risk of transmitting infection.
Monitor serial chest x-rays, ABGs, and pulse oximetry readings. (Refer to ND: impaired Gas Exchange, following.)	Follows progress and effects of disease process and therapeutic regimen, and facilitates necessary alterations in therapy.

NURSING DIAGNOSIS: impaired Gas Exchange

May be related to
Alveolar-capillary membrane changes—inflammatory effects
Altered oxygen-carrying capacity of blood or release at cellular level—fever, shifting oxyhemoglobin curve
Altered delivery of oxygen—hypoventilation

Possibly evidenced by
Dyspnea, cyanosis
Tachycardia
Restlessness and changes in mentation
Hypoxia

Desired Outcomes/Evaluation Criteria—Client Will

Respiratory Status: Gas Exchange (NOC)
Demonstrate improved ventilation and oxygenation of tissues by ABGs within client's acceptable range and absence of symptoms of respiratory distress.
Participate in actions to maximize oxygenation.

ACTIONS/INTERVENTIONS	RATIONALE
Respiratory Monitoring (NIC) *Independent* Assess respiratory rate, depth, and ease.	Manifestations of respiratory distress are dependent on, and indicative of, the degree of lung involvement and underlying general health status.
Observe color of skin, mucous membranes, and nailbeds, noting presence of peripheral cyanosis (nailbeds) or central cyanosis (circumoral).	Cyanosis of nailbeds may represent vasoconstriction or the body's response to fever or chills; however, cyanosis of earlobes, mucous membranes, and skin around the mouth ("warm membranes") is indicative of systemic hypoxemia.
Assess mental status.	Restlessness, irritation, confusion, and somnolence may reflect hypoxemia or decreased cerebral oxygenation.
Monitor heart rate and rhythm.	Tachycardia is usually present as a result of fever and dehydration, but may represent a response to hypoxemia.
Monitor body temperature, as indicated. Assist with comfort measures to reduce fever and chills, such as addition or removal of bedcovers, comfortable room temperature, and tepid or cool water sponge bath.	High fever, common in bacterial pneumonia and influenza, greatly increases metabolic demands and oxygen consumption and alters cellular oxygenation.
Maintain bedrest. Encourage use of relaxation techniques and diversional activities.	Prevents exhaustion and reduces oxygen consumption and demands to facilitate resolution of infection.
Elevate head and encourage frequent position changes, deep breathing, and effective coughing.	These measures promote maximal inspiration and enhance expectoration of secretions to improve ventilation. (Refer to ND: ineffective Airway Clearance.)
Assess level of anxiety. Encourage verbalization of concerns and feelings. Answer questions honestly. Visit frequently and arrange for significant other (SO) and visitors to stay with client as indicated.	Anxiety is a manifestation of psychological concerns and physiological responses to hypoxia. Providing reassurance and enhancing sense of security can reduce the psychological component, thereby decreasing oxygen demand and adverse physiological responses.
Observe for deterioration in condition, noting hypotension, copious amounts of pink or bloody sputum, pallor, cyanosis, change in level of consciousness, severe dyspnea, and restlessness.	Shock and pulmonary edema are the most common causes of death in pneumonia and require immediate medical intervention.
Collaborative Monitor ABGs and pulse oximetry.	Identifies problems, such as ventilatory failure; follows progress of disease process or improvement; and facilitates alterations in pulmonary therapy.
Oxygen Therapy (NIC) Administer oxygen therapy by appropriate means, for example, nasal prongs, mask, Venturi mask.	The purpose of oxygen therapy is to maintain PaO_2 above 60 mm Hg, or greater than 90% O_2 saturation. Oxygen is administered by the method that provides appropriate delivery within the client's tolerance.
Prepare for and transfer to critical care unit if indicated.	Intubation and mechanical ventilation may be required in the event of severe respiratory insufficiency. (Refer to CP: Ventilatory Assistance [Mechanical].)

NURSING DIAGNOSIS: risk for Infection [spread]

Risk factors may include
Inadequate primary defenses—decreased ciliary action, stasis of respiratory secretions
Inadequate secondary defenses—presence of existing infection, immunosuppression; chronic disease, malnutrition

Possibly evidenced by
(Not applicable; presence of signs and symptoms establishes an *actual* diagnosis)

Desired Outcomes/Evaluation Criteria—Client Will

Infection Status (NOC)
Achieve timely resolution of current infection without complications.

Knowledge: Infection Control (NOC)
Identify interventions to prevent and reduce risk and spread of a secondary infection.

ACTIONS/INTERVENTIONS

RATIONALE

Infection Control (NIC)
Independent

Monitor vital signs closely, especially during initiation of therapy.

During this period, potentially fatal complications, such as hypotension or shock, may develop.

Instruct client concerning the disposition of secretions (e.g., raising and expectorating versus swallowing) and reporting changes in color, amount, and odor of secretions.

Although client may find expectoration offensive and attempt to limit or avoid it, it is essential that sputum be disposed of in a safe manner. Changes in characteristics of sputum reflect resolution of pneumonia or development of secondary infection.

Demonstrate and encourage good hand-washing technique.

Effective means of reducing spread or acquisition of infection.

Change position frequently and provide good pulmonary toilet.

Promotes expectoration, clearing of infection.

Perform proper suctioning technique for ventilated clients as appropriate.

Secretions that accumulate below and above the endotracheal (ET) tube cuff are an ideal growth medium for pathogens. The ET tube also prevents normal closure of the epiglottis, resulting in an incomplete seal of the laryngeal structures that normally protect the lungs. This can contribute to aspiration and VAP (Pruitt & Jacobs, 2006).

Limit visitors as indicated.

Reduces likelihood of exposure to other infectious pathogens.

Institute isolation precautions as individually appropriate.

Depending on type of infection, response to antibiotics, client's general health, and development of complications, isolation techniques may be instituted to prevent spread and protect client from other infectious processes.

Encourage adequate rest balanced with moderate activity. Promote adequate nutritional intake.

Facilitates healing process and enhances natural resistance.

Monitor effectiveness of antimicrobial therapy.

Signs of improvement in condition should occur within 24 to 48 hours.

Investigate sudden changes or deterioration in condition, such as increasing chest pain, extra heart sounds, altered sensorium, recurring fever, and changes in sputum characteristics.

Delayed recovery or increase in severity of symptoms suggests resistance to antibiotics or secondary infection. Complications affecting any organ system include lung abscess, empyema, bacteremia, pericarditis, endocarditis, meningitis, encephalitis, and superinfections.

Collaborative

Administer antimicrobials, as indicated, by results of sputum and blood cultures: for example, macrolides such as azithromycin (Zithromax), clarithromycin (Biaxin), erythromycin (E-Mycin); penicillin combinations, for example, amoxicillin and clavulanate (Augmentin); tetracyclines, for example, doxycycline (Doryx, Bio-Tab); fluoroquinolones, for example, moxifloxacin (Avelox), levofloxacin (Levaquin), ciprofloxin (Cipro), gemifloxin (Factive); cephalosporins, for example, cefuroxime (Kefurox, Zinacef), cefaclor (Ceclor), ceftazidime (Ceptax, Fortaz); ketolides, for example, telithromycin (KETEK).

These drugs are used to combat most of the microbial pneumonias. Combinations of drugs can be used when the pneumonia is a result of mixed organisms.

Prepare for and assist with additional diagnostic studies, as indicated.

Fiberoptic bronchoscopy may be done for clients who do not respond in a reasonable amount of time to antimicrobial therapy to clarify diagnosis and therapeutic needs.

NURSING DIAGNOSIS: Activity Intolerance

May be related to
Imbalance between oxygen supply and demand
General weakness
Exhaustion associated with interruption in usual sleep pattern because of discomfort, excessive coughing, and dyspnea

Possibly evidenced by
Verbal reports of weakness, fatigue, exhaustion
Exertional dyspnea, tachypnea
Tachycardia in response to activity
Development of, or worsening of, pallor or cyanosis

Desired Outcomes/Evaluation Criteria—Client Will

Activity Tolerance (NOC)
Report and demonstrate a measurable increase in tolerance to activity with absence of dyspnea and excessive fatigue, with vital signs within client's acceptable range.

ACTIONS/INTERVENTIONS	RATIONALE
Energy Management (NIC)	
Independent	
Evaluate client's response to activity. Note reports of dyspnea, increased weakness and fatigue, and changes in vital signs during and after activities.	Establishes client's capabilities and needs and facilitates choice of interventions.
Provide a quiet environment and limit visitors during acute phase as indicated. Encourage use of stress management and diversional activities as appropriate.	Reduces stress and excess stimulation, promoting rest.
Explain importance of rest in treatment plan and necessity for balancing activities with rest.	Bedrest is maintained during acute phase to decrease metabolic demands, thus conserving energy for healing. Activity restrictions thereafter are determined by individual client response to activity and resolution of respiratory insufficiency.
Assist client to assume comfortable position for rest and sleep.	Client may be comfortable with head of bed elevated, sleeping in a chair, or leaning forward on over-bed table with pillow support.
Assist with self-care activities as necessary. Provide for progressive increase in activities during recovery phase.	Minimizes exhaustion and helps balance oxygen supply and demand.

NURSING DIAGNOSIS: acute Pain

May be related to
Inflammation of lung parenchyma
Cellular reactions to circulating toxins
Persistent coughing

Possibly evidenced by
Reports of pleuritic chest pain, headache, muscle or joint pain
Guarding of affected area
Distraction behaviors, restlessness

Desired Outcomes/Evaluation Criteria—Client Will

Pain Level (NOC)
Verbalize relief or control of pain.
Demonstrate relaxed manner, resting, sleeping, and engaging in activity appropriately.

ACTIONS/INTERVENTIONS

RATIONALE

Pain Management (NIC)
Independent

Determine pain characteristics, such as sharp, constant, and stabbing. Investigate changes in character, location, and intensity of pain.

Monitor vital signs.

Provide comfort measures, such as back rubs, change of position, and quiet music or conversation. Encourage use of relaxation and breathing exercises.

Offer frequent oral hygiene.

Instruct and assist client in chest-splinting techniques during coughing episodes. (Refer to ND: ineffective Airway Clearance.)

Collaborative

Administer analgesics and antitussives, as indicated.

Chest pain, usually present to some degree with pneumonia, may also herald the onset of complications of pneumonia, such as pericarditis and endocarditis.

Changes in heart rate or blood pressure (BP) may indicate that client is experiencing pain, especially when other reasons for changes in vital signs have been ruled out.

Nonanalgesic measures administered with a gentle touch can lessen discomfort and augment therapeutic effects of analgesics. Client involvement in pain control measures promotes independence and enhances sense of well-being.

Mouth breathing and oxygen therapy can irritate and dry out mucous membranes, potentiating general discomfort.

Aids in control of chest discomfort while enhancing effectiveness of cough effort.

These medications may be used to suppress nonproductive or paroxysmal cough or reduce excess mucus, thereby enhancing general comfort and rest.

NURSING DIAGNOSIS: **risk for imbalanced Nutrition: Less than Body Requirements**

Risk factors may include

Increased metabolic needs secondary to fever and infectious process

Anorexia associated with bacterial toxins, the odor and taste of sputum, and certain aerosol treatments

Abdominal distention and gas associated with swallowing air during dyspneic episodes

Possibly evidenced by

(Not applicable; presence of signs and symptoms establishes an *actual* diagnosis)

Desired Outcomes/Evaluation Criteria—Client Will

Nutritional Status (NOC)

Demonstrate increased appetite.

Maintain or regain desired body weight.

ACTIONS/INTERVENTIONS

RATIONALE

Nutrition Therapy (NIC)
Independent

Identify factors that are contributing to inability to eat, such as severe dyspnea, pain, nausea and vomiting, copious sputum, or respiratory treatments.

Provide covered container for sputum and replace at frequent intervals. Assist with and encourage oral hygiene after emesis, after aerosol and postural drainage treatments, and before meals.

Schedule respiratory treatments at least 1 hour before meals.

Auscultate for bowel sounds. Observe and palpate for abdominal distention.

Provide small, frequent meals, including dry foods, such as toast or crackers, and foods that are appealing to client.

Evaluate general nutritional state. Obtain baseline weight.

Choice of interventions depends on the underlying cause of the problem.

Eliminates noxious sights, tastes, and smells from the client's environment and can reduce nausea.

Reduces effects of nausea associated with these treatments.

Bowel sounds may be diminished or absent if the infectious process is severe or prolonged. Abdominal distention may occur because of air swallowing or reflect the influence of bacterial toxins on the gastrointestinal (GI) tract.

These measures may enhance intake even though appetite may be slow to return.

Lifestyle, financial, and socioeconomic conditions prior to present illness condition can contribute to malnutrition. Client may present with hypermetabolic state and lowered resistance to infection, which can exacerbate malnutrition and delay response to therapy.

(continues on page 140)

ACTIONS/INTERVENTIONS (continued)	RATIONALE (continued)
Weigh regularly and graph results.	Monitors effectiveness of nutritional therapy.
Collaborative	
Assist in treatment of underlying condition(s).	May promote healing and strengthen immune system, improve appetite, and enhance general well-being.
Consult dietitian and nutritional team.	To develop dietary plan individualized to client's specific needs and challenges.

NURSING DIAGNOSIS: **risk for deficient Fluid Volume**

Risk factors may include
Excessive fluid loss—fever, profuse diaphoresis, mouth breathing and hyperventilation, vomiting
Decreased oral intake

Possibly evidenced by
(Not applicable; presence of signs and symptoms establishes an *actual* diagnosis)

Desired Outcomes/Evaluation Criteria—Client Will

Fluid Balance NIC
Demonstrate fluid balance evidenced by individually appropriate parameters, such as moist mucous membranes, good skin turgor, prompt capillary refill, and stable vital signs.

ACTIONS/INTERVENTIONS	RATIONALE
Fluid Management NIC	
Independent	
Assess vital sign changes, such as increased temperature, prolonged fever, tachycardia, and orthostatic hypotension.	Elevated temperature or prolonged fever increases metabolic rate and fluid loss through evaporation. Orthostatic BP changes and increasing tachycardia may indicate systemic fluid deficit.
Assess skin turgor, moisture of mucous membranes—lips and tongue.	Indirect indicators of adequacy of fluid volume, although oral mucous membranes may be dry because of mouth breathing and supplemental oxygen.
Note reports of nausea and vomiting.	Presence of these symptoms reduces oral intake.
Monitor intake and output (I&O), noting color and character of urine. Calculate fluid balance. Be aware of insensible losses. Weigh as indicated.	Provides information about adequacy of fluid volume and replacement needs.
Force fluids to at least 3,000 mL per day or as individually appropriate.	Meets basic fluid needs, reducing risk of dehydration.
Collaborative	
Administer medications, as indicated, such as antipyretics, antiemetics.	Useful in reducing fluid losses.
Provide supplemental IV fluids as necessary.	In the presence of reduced intake or excessive loss, use of parenteral route may correct or prevent deficiency.

NURSING DIAGNOSIS: **deficient Knowledge [Learning Need] regarding condition, treatment, self-care, and discharge needs**

May be related to
Lack of exposure
Misinterpretation of information
Altered recall

Possibly evidenced by
Requests for information; statement of misconception
Failure to improve or a recurrence of the condition

Desired Outcomes/Evaluation Criteria—Client Will

Knowledge: Illness Care (NOC)
Verbalize understanding of condition, disease process, and prognosis.
Verbalize understanding of therapeutic regimen.
Initiate necessary lifestyle changes.
Participate in treatment program.

ACTIONS/INTERVENTIONS	RATIONALE
Teaching: Disease Process (NIC)	
Independent	
Review normal lung function and pathology of condition.	Promotes understanding of current situation and importance of cooperating with treatment regimen.
Discuss debilitating aspects of disease, length of convalescence, and recovery expectations. Identify self-care and homemaker needs and resources.	Information can enhance coping and help reduce anxiety and excessive concern. Respiratory symptoms may be slow to resolve, and fatigue and weakness can persist for an extended period. These factors may be associated with depression and the need for various forms of support and assistance.
Provide information in written and verbal form.	Fatigue and depression can affect ability to assimilate information and follow medical regimen.
Stress importance of continuing effective coughing and deep-breathing exercises.	During initial 6 to 8 weeks after discharge, client is at greatest risk for recurrence of pneumonia.
Emphasize necessity for continuing antibiotic therapy for prescribed period.	Early discontinuation of antibiotics may result in failure to completely resolve infectious process.
Review importance of cessation of smoking.	Smoking destroys tracheobronchial ciliary action, irritates bronchial mucosa, and inhibits alveolar macrophages, compromising body's natural defense against infection.
Outline steps to enhance general health and well-being, such as balanced rest and activity, well-rounded diet, program of aerobic exercise or strength training (particularly elderly individuals), and avoidance of crowds during cold and flu season and of persons with upper respiratory infections.	Increases natural defenses and immunity and limits exposure to pathogens. Recent research suggests elderly people with moderate physical limitations can significantly improve immunological defenses through exercise that increases levels of salivary IgA—immunoglobulin that aids in blocking infectious agents entering through mucous membranes.
Stress importance of continuing medical follow-up and obtaining vaccinations and immunizations as appropriate.	May prevent recurrence of pneumonia and related complications.
Identify signs and symptoms requiring notification of healthcare provider, such as increasing dyspnea, chest pain, prolonged fatigue, weight loss, fever or chills, persistence of productive cough, and changes in mentation.	Prompt evaluation and timely intervention may prevent or minimize complications.

POTENTIAL CONSIDERATIONS following acute hospitalization (dependent on client's age, physical condition and presence of complications, personal resources, and life responsibilities)
• *Fatigue*—increased energy requirements to perform activities of daily living (ADLs), discomfort, effects of antimicrobial therapy
• *risk for Infection*—inadequate secondary response (e.g., leukopenia, suppressed inflammatory response), chronic disease, malnutrition, current use of antibiotics
• *ineffective self Health Management*—complexity of therapeutic regimen, economic difficulties, perceived seriousness and susceptibility

Sample clinical pathway follows in Table 5.1.

TABLE 5.1 Sample CP: Bacterial Pneumonia, Hospital. ELOS: 5 Days Medical Unit

ND and Categories of Care	Day 1	Day 2	Day 3	Day 4	Day 5
Impaired gas exchange R/T alveolar congestion, inflammation, hypoventilation	Goals: Participate in activities to maximize oxygenation and airway clearance	Demonstrate improving ventilation and oxygenation by lessening symptoms of respiratory distress, ABGs approaching acceptable levels	Verbalize understanding of general healthcare needs	Initiate activities accepting responsibility for therapeutic regimen within level of ability; Plan in place to meet postdischarge needs	Demonstrate ABGs within client's acceptable range and absence of respiratory distress
Referrals	Pulmonary specialist		Home care; Home O₂/Resp. Therapist		
Diagnostic studies	CXR				
	ABGs CBC, electrolytes	→ Repeat if pulse oximetry < 87%	Repeat if WBC count elevated, febrile, or ABGs not WNL; Hb/Hct		
	Sputum C&S/Gram stain				
	Blood culture				
	Pulse oximetry q4h	→ D/C if 92%			
Additional assessments	Respiratory rate, rhythm, depth; use of accessory muscles; color of skin and mucous membranes q4h	→	→ q8h	→	→
	Breath sounds q4h	→	→ q8h	→ →	→ →
	Cough and sputum characteristics	→	→ q8h	→ → →	→ → →
	Vital signs q4h	→	→	→ → →	→ → →
	I&O q8h	→	→		
	Weight qd	→	→		
Medications	IV antibiotics	→	→ PO	→ →	→ →
	Bronchodilator via MDI or nebulizer	→ MDI	→		
	Mucolytic	→	→	→ →	→ →
	Antitussives—prn	→	→		
	Acetaminophen if temperature above 101°F	→	→ D/C		
	Analgesics—prn	→ D/C			
Allergies: ____ ____					

Client education				
Orient to unit and room	Adaptive breathing techniques as indicated	Individual risk factors, prevention of recurrence, vaccinations and immunizations	Medications postdischarge: dose, time, route, purpose, side effects	Provide written instructions
Review advance directives	Pacing of activities	Signs and symptoms to report to healthcare provider	Proper use and care of home care equipment (e.g., O$_2$ concentrator, nebulizer)	Schedule for follow-up appointments
Diagnostic tests and results	Smoking cessation fluid and nutritional needs, balancing activity and rest			
Pulmonary hygiene: T, C, DB, splinting techniques				
Position for maximal respiratory effort	→ per self	→	→ per self	↑
Additional nursing actions				
Assist with physical care	→	→ as necessary	→ per self	↑
Incentive spirometry q4h	→	→ per self WA	→ D/C	↑
Supplemental O$_2$	→ per self	→	→	
Oral care prn	→	→	→	
Suction as indicated	→	→	→ D/C	
Screen visitors and staff for URI	→	→	→ D/C	
Encourage fluid to 2,500 mL/day as tolerated	→	→	→ per self	↑

Key: ABG, arterial blood gas; C, cough; CBC, complete blood count; C&S, culture and sensitivity; CXR, chest x-ray; DB, deep breath; D/C, discontinue; ELOS, expected length of stay; Hb/Hct, hemoglobin/hemocrit; I&O, intake and output; qd, every day; MDI, metered-dose inhaler; prn, as necessary; q4h, every 4 hours; q8h, every 8 hours; R/T, related to; T, turn; URI, upper respiratory infection; WA, while awake; WBC, white blood cell; WNL, within normal limits.

LUNG CANCER: POSTOPERATIVE CARE

I. Pathophysiology
a. Usually develops within the wall or epithelium of the bronchial tree
b. Prolonged exposure to cancer-promoting agents causes damage to ciliated cells and mucus-producing cells, leading to genetic mutations and development of dysplastic cells.

II. Classification (Memorial Sloan-Kettering Cancer Center, 2008; National Cancer Institute, 2008)
a. Small cell lung cancers (SCLCs), or oat cell lung cancer
   i. Represent about 15% to 25% of lung cancer cases (Elias & Baldini, 2008)
   ii. Occur almost exclusively in smokers
   iii. Aggressive and fast growing with surgery seldom a treatment option
b. Non–small cell lung cancers (NSCLCs)
   i. Most common type of lung cancer (75% to 85%, Elias & Baldini, 2008)
   ii. Include adenocarcinoma, squamous cell, and large cell carcinomas
   iii. Frequently associated with metastases, but are generally slow growing

III. Staging (National Cancer Institute, 2008)
a. Stage 0—cancer cells only found in the innermost lining of the lung
b. Stage IA—tumor has grown through the innermost lining of the lung into deeper lung tissue, but does not invade the bronchus; no cancer cells found in nearby lymph nodes
c. Stage IB—tumor is larger, may be more than 3 cm across; may have grown into the main bronchus; may have grown into the pleura, but no cancer cells found in nearby lymph nodes
d. Stage IIB—tumor has invaded the chest wall, diaphragm, pleura, main bronchus, or tissue that surrounds the heart; cancer cells found in nearby lymph nodes
e. Stage IIIA—tumor may be any size; cancer cells found in the lymph nodes near the lungs and bronchi and between the lungs on the same side of the chest as the tumor
f. Stage IIIB—tumor may be any size; cancer cells found on the opposite side of the chest from the tumor, with possible invasion into nearby organs
g. Stage IV—malignant growths may be found in more than one lobe or may have metastasized to other organs

IV. Etiology (American Cancer Society, 2008)
a. Risk factors include cigarette smoking or being exposed to secondhand smoke; radon, asbestos, other occupational exposures, including radioactive ores such as uranium, inhaled chemicals or minerals, such as nickel compounds, silica, coal dust, and cromates, or diesel exhaust; high levels of arsenic in drinking water; and family history of lung cancer.
b. Chronic obstructive pulmonary disease (COPD) and pulmonary fibrosis may increase susceptibility.

V. Statistics
a. Morbidity: Second most commonly diagnosed cancer accounting for 13% of all cases (American Association for Cancer Research, 2005) with new cases of lung and bronchus cancer estimated at 172,570 for 2005 (Jemal et al, 2005).
b. Mortality: Number one cause of death in cancer patients; in 2004, death rates for men and women were 89,575 and 68,431, respectively; results in more deaths than breast cancer, prostate cancer, and colon cancer combined (U.S. Cancer Statistics Worling Group, 2007).
c. Cost: $9.6 billion was spent for treatment in 2004.

VI. Treatment Options
a. Depends upon staging—generally the lower the stage, the more favorable the prognosis
   i. Surgery is primary treatment for NSCLC stage I and stage II tumors.
   ii. Selected stage III carcinomas may be operable if the tumor is resectable.
b. Surgical procedures for operable tumors of the lung include:
   i. Pneumonectomy—performed for lesions originating in the main stem bronchus or lobar bronchus
   ii. Lobectomy—preferred for peripheral carcinoma localized in a lobe
   iii. Wedge or segmental resection—performed for lesions that are small and well contained within one segment
   iv. Endoscopic laser resection—may be done on peripheral tumors to reduce the necessity of cutting through ribs
   v. Photodynamic therapy—reduces symptoms such as bleeding or may be used to treat very small tumors

---

GLOSSARY

Clubbing: Broadening or thickening of the tips of the fingers (and toes) with increased lengthwise curvature of the nail and a decrease in the angle normally seen between the cuticle and the fingernail. Clubbing may be seen in a wide variety of conditions, most of which result in decreased blood oxygen.

Fremitus: Vibration in the chest over areas of consolidation, detectable by palpation.

Hemoptysis: Expectoration of blood or of blood-stained sputum.

Lobectomy: Removal of one lobe.

Photodynamic therapy (PTD): A two-step outpatient procedure where a photosensitizing agent, porfimer sodium (Photofrin), is injected into the bloodstream, specifically targeting cancer cells. The second part of the procedure—24 to 72 hours later—involves inserting a laser light through a scope to the cancerous cells. The light activates the drug, resulting in a chemical reaction that destroys cancerous cells and blood vessels supplying the tumor.

Pneumonectomy: Removal of an entire lung.

Staging: Classification as to the extent of disease, based on pathology report from tissue obtained during bronchoscopy, needle (or other) biopsy, blood work, and imaging studies to rule out distant metastases.

Wedge or segmental resection: Removal of the tumor and a small part of the lung.

Care Setting

Client is treated in inpatient surgical and possibly subacute units.

Related Concerns

Cancer, page 846
Pneumothorax/hemothorax, page 154
Psychosocial aspects of care, page 749
Radical neck surgery: laryngectomy (postoperative care), page 160
Surgical intervention, page 782

Client Assessment Database (Preoperative)

Findings depend on type, duration of cancer, and extent of metastasis.

DIAGNOSTIC DIVISION MAY REPORT	MAY EXHIBIT
ACTIVITY/REST • Fatigue, inability to maintain usual routine • Dyspnea with activity	• Lassitude—usually in advanced stage
CIRCULATION	• Jugular vein distention (JVD), with vena caval obstruction • *Heart sounds:* Pericardial rub, indicating effusion • Tachycardia and dysrhythmias • Clubbing of fingers
EGO INTEGRITY • Frightened feelings, fear of outcome of surgery • Denial of severity of condition and potential for malignancy	• Restlessness • Repetitive questioning
ELIMINATION • Intermittent diarrhea, due to hormonal imbalance, small cell lung cancer (SCLC) • Increased frequency and amount of urine, due to hormonal imbalance (epidermoid tumor)	
FOOD/FLUID • Weight loss • Poor appetite, decreased food intake • Difficulty swallowing • Thirst, increased fluid intake	• Thin, emaciated, or wasted appearance in late stages • Edema of face or neck, chest, back, due to vena caval obstruction; facial or periorbital edema, due to hormonal imbalance (SCLC) • Glucose in urine, due to hormonal imbalance (epidermoid tumor)
PAIN/DISCOMFORT • Chest pain—not usually present in early stages and not always present in advanced stages • Pain may or may not be affected by position • Shoulder or arm pain, particularly with large cell carcinoma or adenocarcinoma • Bone and joint pain—cartilage erosion secondary to increased growth hormones (large cell carcinoma or adenocarcinoma) • Intermittent abdominal pain	• Distraction behaviors, such as restlessness, withdrawal • Guarding and protective actions
RESPIRATION • History of smoking; occupational exposure to pollutants, industrial dusts, such as asbestos, iron oxides, coal dust, or to radioactive materials	• Dyspnea, aggravated by exertion • Increased tactile fremitus, indicating consolidation • Brief crackles or wheezes on inspiration or expiration

(continues on page 146)

DIAGNOSTIC DIVISION MAY REPORT (continued)	MAY EXHIBIT (continued)
• Mild cough or change in usual cough pattern, sputum production • Shortness of breath • Hoarseness or change in voice, such as with vocal cord paralysis	• Persistent crackles or wheezes; tracheal shift (space-occupying lesion) • Hemoptysis
SAFETY	• Fever may be present, with large cell carcinoma or adenocarcinoma • Bruising, discoloration of skin, due to hormonal imbalance (SCLC)
SEXUALITY	• Gynecomastia, due to neoplastic hormonal changes (large cell carcinoma) • Amenorrhea, impotence, due to hormonal imbalance (SCLC)
TEACHING/LEARNING • Familial risk factors—cancer, especially lung, tuberculosis • Failure to improve • Use of vitamins or herbal supplements, such as vitamins A, C, E; riboflavin; folic acid; ashwagandha; birch; yellow doc; milk thistle; turmeric; ginger; red clover; echinacea; astragalus; reishi and shiitake mushrooms; zedoary	
DISCHARGE PLAN CONSIDERATIONS • Assistance with transportation, medications, treatments, self-care, homemaker and maintenance tasks ▶ Refer to section at end of plan for postdischarge considerations.	

Diagnostic Studies

TEST WHY IT IS DONE	WHAT IT TELLS ME
BLOOD TESTS • *Carcinoembryonic antigen (CEA, also called carcinogenic antigen):* A cancer-specific immune system protein that is present in many adenocarcinomas, including lung adenocarcinoma. • *Parathyroid hormone protein-related (PTHrP):* Measures the release of a protein—similar to parathyroid hormone—produced by some cancers, including all lung cancers.	Increased preoperative levels of CEA usually suggest a poor prognosis. A CEA level greater than 50 may indicate advanced-stage lung cancer. Blood levels of PTHrP may help to distinguish lung cancer from cancer of the pleura or other diseases, is responsible for the clinical syndrome of hypercalcemia of malignancy, may stimulate proliferation of cancer cells, and is a factor in development of bone metastasis.
• *Lymphocyte count:* Determines number of white blood cells present.	Lymphocytopenia or decreased level of cells can occur with surgical procedures and is associated with shorter survival times for clients with advanced lung cancer. Preoperative treatment with recombinant human interleukin-2 (rhIL-2) may help prevent the lymphocyte decrease.
OTHER DIAGNOSTIC STUDIES • *Chest x-ray, posteroanterior (PA) and lateral:* Evaluates organs or structures within the chest.	Lung cancer is often discovered on chest x-ray. Size and location of mass can be determined. Peripheral nodules and hilar and mediastinal changes may suggest lymphadenopathy. Pleural effusions and endobronchial obstruction may be seen.
• *Thoracic computed tomography (CT):* Noninvasive procedure, done with or without contrast media, to enhance certain anatomic views of chest structures and locate abnormalities.	Used to confirm abnormalities seen on chest x-ray, to detect early (<1 cm) lesions not visible on chest x-ray, and to assess spread to the mediastinum. Outlines shape, size, and location of lesion. May reveal erosion of ribs or vertebrae.

Diagnostic Studies (continued)

TEST WHY IT IS DONE (continued)	WHAT IT TELLS ME (continued)
• *Positron emission tomography (PET) scan:* Based on the uptake of radioactive glucose in metabolically active cells, it is used to determine differences in the metabolism of normal and neoplastic cells.	Identifies occult metastatic disease in the mediastinum and distant sites. More sensitive and specific than CT scans.
• *Magnetic resonance imaging (MRI) scan:* Noninvasive procedure that uses magnetic fields to produce two- or three-dimensional images of organs inside the body. Provides valuable information on anatomic structures and provides better contrast between normal and pathological tissue than does a CT scan.	May be used in combination with, or instead of, CT scans to determine tumor size and location and for staging.
• *Fiberoptic bronchoscopy:* Allows for direct visualization of the larynx, trachea, and bronchial tree. The flexible bronchoscopy allows for tissue biopsy and bronchial washings and for obtaining specimens for cytological examination.	A large percentage of bronchogenic carcinomas may be visualized.
• *Cytological examinations (sputum, pleural, or lymph node):* Studies the origin, structure, function, and pathology of cells. Detects neoplastic cells in secretions	Performed to detect cell changes resulting from neoplastic conditions. Cytological sputum analysis is considered about 80% reliable (Springhouse, 2006). Assesses presence and stage of carcinoma and may identify tumors of the bronchial wall.
• *Biopsy:* A biopsy may be performed using forceps or needle or may be open surgical incision. Allows for direct and microscopic examination of tissue for presence of malignant cells.	Needle biopsy may be performed on scalene nodes, hilar lymph nodes, or pleura to establish diagnosis. Tissue biopsy of metastatic sites is used to stage disease and determine prognosis and treatment.
• *Mediastinoscopy:* Allows for direct visualization of structures behind the sternum and between lungs, including trachea, esophagus, heart, and major blood vessels and lymph nodes that receive drainage from the lungs. Evaluates mediastinal and hilar lymph nodes (especially for nodes larger than 1 cm).	May be performed to confirm radiological or cytological evidence of carcinoma, to detect metastasis, to determine stage of known bronchogenic carcinoma, and to aid in determining if client is good candidate for surgical intervention.
• *Video-assisted thoracoscopy (VATS):* Common thoracic surgical procedure that allows more complete staging for lung cancer, while reducing surgical trauma and postoperative pain associated with thoracotomy.	Allows assessment of suspicious adenopathy in areas inaccessible to conventional mediastinoscopy.
• *Pulmonary function studies:* These studies include total lung capacity (TLC), functional residual capacity (FRC), and residual volume (RV). They provide information on the extent of the pulmonary abnormality and if there is air-trapping in the lungs.	Volumes may be increased, indicating air-trapping, especially advanced disease. If airways are blocked by tumor, an obstructive pattern of pulmonary disease may lead to increased or decreased FRC (Schumann, 2005).
• *Bone scan:* Evaluates presence of bone metastases in client with bone pain, chest pain, or an elevated calcium or alkaline phosphatase level.	Determines if cancer has spread to the bones.
• *CT or MRI scan of brain:* Performed when central nervous system (CNS) signs or symptoms suggest brain metastases.	Determines if cancer has metastasized to the brain.

Nursing Priorities

1. Maintain or improve respiratory function.
2. Control or alleviate pain.
3. Support efforts to cope with diagnosis and situation.
4. Provide information about disease process, prognosis, and therapeutic regimen.

Discharge Goals

1. Oxygenation and ventilation adequate to meet individual activity needs.
2. Pain controlled.
3. Anxiety and fear decreased to manageable level.
4. Free of preventable complications.
5. Disease process, prognosis, and planned therapies understood.
6. Plan in place to meet needs after discharge.

NURSING DIAGNOSIS: impaired Gas Exchange

May be related to
Removal of lung tissue
Altered oxygen supply—hypoventilation
Decreased oxygen-carrying capacity of blood—blood loss

Possibly evidenced by
Dyspnea
Restlessness
Changes in mentation
Hypoxemia and hypercapnia
Cyanosis

Desired Outcomes/Evaluation Criteria—Client Will

Respiratory Status: Gas Exchange (NOC)
Demonstrate improved ventilation and adequate oxygenation of tissues by arterial blood gases (ABGs) within client's normal range.
Be free of symptoms of respiratory distress.

ACTIONS/INTERVENTIONS	RATIONALE
Respiratory Management (NIC)	
Independent	
Note respiratory rate, depth, and ease of respirations. Observe for use of accessory muscles, pursed-lip breathing, or changes in skin or mucous membrane color, such as pallor and cyanosis.	Respirations may be increased as a result of pain or as an initial compensatory mechanism to accommodate for loss of lung tissue. However, increased work of breathing and cyanosis may indicate increasing oxygen consumption and energy expenditures or reduced respiratory reserve, for example, in an elderly client or extensive COPD.
Auscultate lungs for air movement and abnormal breath sounds.	Consolidation and lack of air movement on operative side are normal in the client who has had a pneumonectomy; however, a client who has had a lobectomy should demonstrate normal airflow in remaining lobes.
Investigate restlessness and changes in mentation and level of consciousness.	May indicate increased hypoxia or complications such as mediastinal shift in a client who has had a pneumonectomy when accompanied by tachypnea, tachycardia, and tracheal deviation.
Assess client response to activity. Encourage rest periods, limiting activities to client tolerance.	Increased oxygen consumption and demand and stress of surgery may result in increased dyspnea and changes in vital signs with activity; however, early mobilization is desired to help prevent pulmonary complications and to obtain and maintain respiratory and circulatory efficiency. Adequate rest balanced with activity can prevent respiratory compromise.
Note development of fever.	Fever within the first 24 hours after surgery is frequently due to atelectasis. Temperature elevation within postoperative day 5 to 10 usually indicates an infection, such as wound or systemic.
Airway Management (NIC)	
Maintain patent airway by positioning, suctioning, and use of airway adjuncts.	Airway obstruction impedes ventilation, impairing gas exchange. (Refer to ND: ineffective Airway Clearance.)
Reposition frequently, placing client in sitting and supine to side positions.	Maximizes lung expansion and drainage of secretions.
Avoid positioning client with a pneumonectomy on the operative side; instead, favor the "good lung down" position.	Research shows that positioning clients following lung surgery with their "good lung down" maximizes oxygenation by using gravity to enhance blood flow to the healthy lung, thus creating the best possible match between ventilation and perfusion.
Encourage and assist with deep-breathing exercises and pursed-lip breathing, as appropriate.	Promotes maximal ventilation and oxygenation and reduces or prevents atelectasis.
Tube Care: Chest (NIC)	
Maintain patency of chest drainage system following lobectomy and segmental wedge resection procedures.	Drains fluid from pleural cavity to promote reexpansion of remaining lung segments.

ACTIONS/INTERVENTIONS (continued)

Note changes in amount or type of chest tube drainage.

Observe for presence of bubbling in water-seal chamber.

Airway Management (NIC)
Collaborative

Administer supplemental oxygen via nasal cannula, partial rebreathing mask, or high-humidity face mask, as indicated.

Assist with and encourage use of incentive spirometer.

Monitor and graph ABGs and pulse oximetry readings. Note hemoglobin (Hgb) levels.

RATIONALE (continued)

Bloody drainage should decrease in amount and change to a more serous composition as recovery progresses. A sudden increase in amount of bloody drainage or return to frank bleeding suggests thoracic bleeding or a hemothorax; sudden cessation suggests blockage of tube, requiring further evaluation and intervention.

Air leaks appearing immediately postoperatively are not uncommon, especially following lobectomy or segmental resection; however, this should diminish as healing progresses. Prolonged or new leaks require evaluation to identify problems in client versus a problem in the drainage system.

Maximizes available oxygen, especially while ventilation is reduced because of anesthetic, depression, or pain, and during period of compensatory physiological shift of circulation to remaining functional alveolar units.

Prevents or reduces atelectasis and promotes reexpansion of small airways.

Decreasing PaO_2 or increasing $PaCO_2$ may indicate need for ventilatory support. Significant blood loss results in decreased oxygen-carrying capacity, reducing PaO_2.

NURSING DIAGNOSIS: ineffective Airway Clearance

May be related to
Increased amount or viscosity of secretions
Restricted chest movement, pain
Fatigue, weakness

Possibly evidenced by
Changes in rate and depth of respiration
Abnormal breath sounds
Ineffective cough
Dyspnea

Desired Outcomes/Evaluation Criteria—Client Will

Respiratory Status: Airway Patency (NOC)
Demonstrate patent airway, with fluid secretions easily expectorated, clear breath sounds, and noiseless respirations.

ACTIONS/INTERVENTIONS

Airway Management (NIC)
Independent

Auscultate chest for character of breath sounds and presence of secretions.
Assist client with and provide instruction in effective deep breathing, coughing in upright position (sitting), and splinting of incision.

Observe amount and character of sputum and aspirated secretions. Investigate changes, as indicated.

Suction if cough is weak or breath sounds not cleared by cough effort. Avoid deep endotracheal and nasotracheal suctioning in client who has had pneumonectomy if possible.

RATIONALE

Noisy respirations, rhonchi, and wheezes are indicative of retained secretions or airway obstruction.
Upright position favors maximal lung expansion, and splinting improves force of cough effort to mobilize and remove secretions. Splinting may be done by nurse placing hands anteriorly and posteriorly over chest wall and by client, with pillows, as strength improves.

Increased amounts of colorless (or blood-streaked) or watery secretions are normal initially and should decrease as recovery progresses. Presence of thick, tenacious, bloody, or purulent sputum suggests development of secondary problems—for example, dehydration, pulmonary edema, local hemorrhage, or infection—that require correction or treatment.

"Routine" suctioning increases risk of hypoxemia and mucosal damage. Deep tracheal suctioning is generally contraindicated following pneumonectomy to reduce the risk of rupture of the bronchial stump suture line. If suctioning is unavoidable, it should be done gently and only to induce effective coughing.

(continues on page 150)

ACTIONS/INTERVENTIONS (continued)	RATIONALE (continued)
Encourage oral fluid intake, at least 2,500 mL/day, within cardiac tolerance.	Adequate hydration aids in keeping secretions loose and enhances expectoration.
Assess for pain and discomfort and medicate on a routine basis and before breathing exercises.	Encourages client to move, cough more effectively, and breathe more deeply to prevent respiratory insufficiency.
Collaborative	
Provide and assist client with incentive spirometer and postural drainage and percussion, as indicated.	Improves lung expansion and ventilation and facilitates removal of secretions. *Note:* Postural drainage may be contraindicated in some clients, and, in any event, must be performed cautiously to prevent respiratory embarrassment and incisional discomfort.
Use humidified oxygen and ultrasonic nebulizer. Provide additional fluids intravenously (IV), as indicated.	Providing maximal hydration helps loosen and liquefy secretions to promote expectoration. Impaired oral intake necessitates IV supplementation to maintain hydration.
Administer bronchodilators, expectorants, and analgesics, as indicated.	Relieves bronchospasm to improve airflow. Expectorants increase mucus production and liquefy and reduce viscosity of secretions, facilitating removal. Alleviation of chest discomfort promotes cooperation with breathing exercises and enhances effectiveness of respiratory therapies.

NURSING DIAGNOSIS: acute Pain

May be related to
Surgical incision, tissue trauma, and disruption of intercostal nerves
Presence of chest tube(s)
Cancer invasion of pleura, chest wall

Possibly evidenced by
Verbal reports of discomfort
Guarding of affected area
Distraction behaviors such as restlessness
Narrowed focus, withdrawal
Changes in blood pressure (BP), heart, or respiratory rate

Desired Outcomes/Evaluation Criteria—Client Will

Pain Level (NOC)
Report pain relieved or controlled.
Appear relaxed and sleep or rest appropriately.
Participate in desired as well as needed activities.

ACTIONS/INTERVENTIONS	RATIONALE
Pain Management (NIC)	
Independent	
Ask client about pain. Determine pain location and characteristics; for example, continuous, aching, stabbing, or burning. Have client rate intensity on a scale of 0 to 10.	Helpful in evaluating cancer-related pain symptoms, which may involve viscera, nerve, or bone tissue. Use of rating scale aids client in assessing level of pain and provides tool for evaluating effectiveness of analgesics, enhancing client control of pain.
Assess client's verbal and nonverbal pain cues.	Discrepancy between verbal and nonverbal cues may provide clues to degree of pain and need for and effectiveness of interventions.
Note possible pathophysiological and psychological causes of pain.	Fear, distress, anxiety, and grief over confirmed diagnosis of cancer can impair ability to cope. In addition, a posterolateral incision is more uncomfortable for client than an anterolateral incision. The presence of chest tubes can greatly increase discomfort.
Evaluate effectiveness of pain control. Encourage sufficient medication to manage pain; change medication or time span as appropriate.	Pain perception and pain relief are subjective, thus pain management is best left to client's discretion. If client is unable to provide input, the nurse should observe physiological and nonverbal signs of pain and administer medications on a regular basis.
Encourage verbalization of feelings about the pain.	Fears and concerns can increase muscle tension and lower threshold of pain perception. (Refer to ND: Fear/Anxiety [specify level], following.)

ACTIONS/INTERVENTIONS (continued) | RATIONALE (continued)

ACTIONS/INTERVENTIONS (continued) — RATIONALE (continued)

Provide comfort measures such as frequent changes of position, back rubs, and support with pillows. Encourage use of relaxation techniques including visualization, guided imagery, and appropriate diversional activities.

Promotes relaxation and redirects attention. Relieves discomfort and augments therapeutic effects of analgesia.

Schedule rest periods; provide quiet environment.

Decreases fatigue and conserves energy, enhancing coping abilities.

Assist with self-care activities, breathing, arm exercises, and ambulation.

Prevents undue fatigue and incisional strain. Encouragement and physical assistance and support may be needed for some time before client is able or confident enough to perform these activities because of pain or fear of pain.

Collaborative

Assist with patient-controlled analgesia (PCA) or analgesia through epidural catheter. Administer intermittent analgesics routinely, as indicated, especially 45 to 60 minutes before respiratory treatments, and deep-breathing and coughing exercises.

Maintaining a constant drug level avoids cyclic periods of pain, aids in muscle healing, and improves respiratory function and emotional comfort and coping.

NURSING DIAGNOSIS: Fear/Anxiety [specify level]

May be related to
Situational crises
Threat to or change in health status
Perceived threat of death

Possibly evidenced by
Withdrawal
Apprehension
Anger
Increased pain, sympathetic stimulation
Expressions of denial, shock, guilt, insomnia

Desired Outcomes/Evaluation Criteria—Client Will

Fear Self-Control [or] Anxiety Self-Control (NOC)
Acknowledge and discuss fears and concerns.
Demonstrate appropriate range of feelings and appear relaxed and resting appropriately.
Verbalize accurate knowledge of situation.
Report beginning use of individually appropriate coping strategies.

ACTIONS/INTERVENTIONS — RATIONALE

Anxiety Reduction (NIC)
Independent

Evaluate client and significant other (SO) level of understanding of diagnosis.

Client and SO are hearing and assimilating new information that includes changes in self-image and lifestyle. Understanding perceptions of those involved sets the tone for individualizing care and provides information necessary for choosing appropriate interventions.

Acknowledge reality of client's fears and concerns and encourage expression of feelings.

Support may enable client to begin exploring and dealing with the reality of cancer and its treatment. Client may need time to identify feelings and even more time to begin to express them.

Provide opportunity for questions and answer them honestly. Be sure that client and care providers have the same understanding of terms used.

Establishes trust and reduces misperceptions or misinterpretation of information.

Accept, but do not reinforce, client's denial of the situation.

When extreme denial or anxiety is interfering with progress of recovery, the issues facing client need to be explained and resolutions explored.

Note comments and behaviors indicative of beginning acceptance or use of effective strategies to deal with situation.

Fear and anxiety will diminish as client begins to accept and deal positively with reality. Indicator of client's readiness to accept responsibility for participation in recovery and to "resume life."

(continues on page 152)

Involve client and SO in care planning. Provide time to prepare for events and treatments.

May help restore some feeling of control and independence to client who feels powerless in dealing with diagnosis and treatment.

Provide for client's physical comfort.

It is difficult to deal with emotional issues when experiencing extreme or persistent physical discomfort.

NURSING DIAGNOSIS: **deficient Knowledge [Learning Need] regarding condition, treatment, prognosis, self-care, and discharge needs**

May be related to
Lack of exposure, unfamiliarity with information or resources
Information misinterpretation
Lack of recall

Possibly evidenced by
Statements of concern; request for information
Inadequate follow-through of instruction
Inappropriate or exaggerated behaviors—hysterical, hostile, agitated, apathetic

Desired Outcomes/Evaluation Criteria—Client Will

Knowledge: Disease Process (NOC)
Verbalize understanding of ramifications of diagnosis, prognosis, and possible complications.
Participate in learning process.

Knowledge: Treatment Regimen (NOC)
Verbalize understanding of therapeutic regimen.
Correctly perform necessary procedures and explain reasons for the actions.
Initiate necessary lifestyle changes.

ACTIONS/INTERVENTIONS

RATIONALE

Teaching: Disease Process (NIC)
Independent

Discuss diagnosis, current and planned therapies, and expected outcomes.

Provides individually specific information, creating knowledge base for subsequent learning regarding home management. Radiation or chemotherapy may follow surgical intervention, and information is essential to enable the client and SO to make informed decisions.

Reinforce surgeon's explanation of particular surgical procedure, providing diagram as appropriate. Incorporate this information into discussion about short- and long-term recovery expectations.

Length of rehabilitation and prognosis depend on type of surgical procedure, preoperative physical condition, and duration and degree of complications.

Discuss necessity of planning for follow-up care before discharge.

Follow-up assessment of respiratory status and general health is imperative to assure optimal recovery. Also provides opportunity to readdress concerns or questions at a less stressful time.

Identify signs and symptoms requiring medical evaluations, such as changes in appearance of incision, development of respiratory difficulty, fever, increased chest pain, and changes in appearance of sputum.

Early detection and timely intervention may prevent or minimize complications.

Stress importance of avoiding exposure to smoke, air pollution, and contact with individuals with upper respiratory infections (URIs).

Protects lung(s) from irritation and reduces risk of infection.

Review nutritional and fluid needs. Suggest increasing protein and use of high-calorie snacks as appropriate.

Meeting cellular energy requirements and maintaining good circulating volume for tissue perfusion facilitate tissue regeneration and healing process.

Identify individually appropriate community resources, such as American Cancer Society, visiting nurse, social services, and home care.

Agencies such as these offer a broad range of services that can be tailored to provide support and meet individual needs.

ACTIONS/INTERVENTIONS (continued) | **RATIONALE** (continued)

Prescribed Activity/Exercise (NIC)

Help client determine activity tolerance and set goals.

Weakness and fatigue should decrease as lung heals and respiratory function improves during recovery period, especially if cancer was completely removed. If cancer is advanced, it is emotionally helpful for client to be able to set realistic activity goals to achieve optimal independence.

Evaluate availability and adequacy of support system(s) and necessity for assistance in self-care and home management.

General weakness and activity limitations may reduce individual's ability to meet own needs.

Encourage alternating rest periods with activity and light tasks with heavy tasks. Stress avoidance of heavy lifting and isometric or strenuous upper body exercise. Reinforce physician's time limitations about lifting.

Generalized weakness and fatigue are usual in the early recovery period but should diminish as respiratory function improves and healing progresses. Rest and sleep enhance coping abilities, reduce nervousness (common in this phase), and promote healing. *Note:* Strenuous use of arms can place undue stress on incision because chest muscles may be weaker than normal for 3 to 6 months following surgery.

Recommend stopping any activity that causes undue fatigue or increased shortness of breath.

Exhaustion aggravates respiratory insufficiency.

Instruct and provide rationale for arm and shoulder exercises. Have client or SO demonstrate exercises. Encourage following graded increase in number and intensity of routine repetitions.

Simple arm circles and lifting arms over the head or out to the affected side are initiated on the first or second postoperative day to restore normal range of motion (ROM) of shoulder and to prevent ankylosis of the affected shoulder.

Incision Site Care (NIC)

Encourage inspection of incisions. Review expectations for healing with client.

Healing begins immediately, but complete healing takes time. As healing progresses, incision lines may appear dry with crusty scabs. Underlying tissue may look bruised and feel tense, warm, and lumpy (resolving hematoma).

Instruct client and SO to watch for and report places in incision that do not heal or reopening of healed incision, any drainage (bloody or purulent), and localized area of swelling with redness or increased pain that is hot to touch.

Signs and symptoms indicating failure to heal, development of complications requiring further medical evaluation and intervention.

Suggest wearing soft cotton shirts and loose-fitting clothing; cover portion of incision with pad, as indicated, and leave incision open to air as much as possible.

Reduces suture line irritation and pressure from clothing. Leaving incisions open to air promotes healing process and may reduce risk of infection.

Shower in warm water, washing incision gently. Avoid tub baths until approved by physician.

Keeps incision clean and promotes circulation and healing. *Note:* "Climbing" out of tub requires use of arms and pectoral muscles, which can put undue stress on incision.

Support incision with butterfly bandages as needed when sutures and staples are removed.

Aids in maintaining approximation of wound edges to promote healing.

POTENTIAL CONSIDERATIONS following hospitalization (dependent on client's age, physical condition and presence of complications, personal resources, and life responsibilities)

• *ineffective Airway Clearance*—increased amount or viscosity of secretions, restricted chest movement and pain, fatigue, weakness

• *acute Pain*—surgical incision, tissue trauma, disruption of intercostal nerves, presence of distress or anxiety

• *Self-Care Deficit*—decreased strength and endurance, presence of pain, intolerance to activity, depression, presence of therapeutic devices, such as IV lines.

Refer to CP, Cancer for other considerations.

PNEUMOTHORAX/HEMOTHORAX

I. Pathophysiology
  a. Partial or complete collapse of lung due to accumulation of air (pneumothorax), blood (hemothorax), or other fluid (pleural effusion) in the pleural space
  b. Intrathoracic pressure changes induced by increased pleural space volumes and reduced lung capacity, causing respiratory distress and gas exchange problems and producing tension on mediastinal structures that can impede cardiac and systemic circulation
  c. Complications include hypoxemia, respiratory failure, and cardiac arrest.

II. Classification
  a. Primary spontaneous pneumothorax
  b. Secondary spontaneous pneumothorax
  c. Iatrogenic pneumothorax
  d. Traumatic pneumothorax

III. Etiology
  a. Primary spontaneous: rupture of pleural blebs typically occurs in young people without parenchymal lung disease or occurs in the absence of traumatic injury to the chest or lungs
  b. Secondary spontaneous: occurs in the presence of lung disease, primarily emphysema, but can also occur with tuberculosis (TB), sarcoidosis, cystic fibrosis, malignancy, and pulmonary fibrosis
  c. Iatrogenic: complication of medical or surgical procedures, such as therapeutic thoracentesis, tracheostomy, pleural biopsy, central venous catheter insertion, positive pressure mechanical ventilation, inadvertent intubation of right mainstem bronchus
  d. Traumatic: most common form of pneumothorax and hemothorax, caused by open or closed chest trauma related to blunt or penetrating injuries

IV. Statistics (American Lung Association, June 2005)
  a. Morbidity: Primary spontaneous pneumothorax affects 9,000 persons per year and is more common in tall, thin men between 20 and 40 years of age.
  b. Recurrence rate: Is about 40% for both primary and secondary spontaneous pneumothorax, occurring in intervals of 1.5 to 2 years.
  c. Mortality: Rate is 15% for those with secondary pneumothorax.

GLOSSARY

Blunt force chest trauma: Closed trauma to the chest may result in laceration of lung tissue or an artery by a rib, causing blood to collect in the pleural space.

Chest tube drainage unit (CDU): Drainage system that is connected to a chest tube to remove air or fluids from the chest cavity or pleural space. The device consists of a water seal and collection chambers and a suction control chamber, or a one-way mechanical valve, depending on the amount of drainage anticipated and the client's level of mobility.

Crepitation: A dry, crackling sound or sensation on auscultation or palpation of the skin, indicating the presence of subcutaneous emphysema, or air trapped in the tissues, associated with a pneumothorax.

Empyema: Pus from an infection, such as pneumonia, in the pleural space.

Fremitus: Vibratory sensation or tremors felt through the chest wall during coughing or speaking.

Hemopneumothorax: Both air and blood in the pleural space.

Hemothorax: Collection of blood in the pleural space, which can exert pressure on the lung, causing it to collapse.

Hypercapnia: Increased level of carbon dioxide in the blood.

Hypoxemia: Decreased level of oxygen in the blood.

Penetrating chest trauma: Chest trauma in which a weapon, such as a knife, bullet, or needle, lacerates the lung.

Pleural effusion: Excessive fluid in the pleural space.

Pleural space: Area between the parietal pleura (membrane lining the chest cavity) and the visceral pleura, which surrounds the lungs. Normally, this potential space holds about 50 mL of lubricating fluid that prevents friction between the pleurae as they move during inhalation and exhalation.

Pneumothorax: Buildup of air in the pleural space, exerting pressure against the lung and causing it to collapse.

Tachypnea: Abnormally rapid respirations.

Tension pneumothorax: Unrelieved accumulation of air in the intrapleural space shifts mediastinum to unaffected side, thus impairing ventilation and compromising cardiac function and venous return.

Thoracentesis: Use of a needle to rapidly remove fluid from the pleural space.

Care Setting

Client is treated in inpatient medical or surgical unit.

Related Concerns

Cardiac surgery: postoperative care, page 100

Chronic obstructive pulmonary disease (COPD) and asthma, page 120

Psychosocial aspects of care, page 749

Pulmonary tuberculosis (TB), page 186

Ventilatory assistance (mechanical), page 173

Findings vary depending on the amount of air and/or fluid accumulation, rate of accumulation, and underlying lung function.

DIAGNOSTIC DIVISION MAY REPORT	MAY EXHIBIT
ACTIVITY/REST • Shortness of breath • Tiredness	• Dyspnea with activity or even at rest
CIRCULATION	• Tachycardia; irregular rate, dysrhythmias • S_3 or S_4 or gallop heart rhythm—heart failure (HF) secondary to effusion • Apical pulse reveals point of maximal impulse (PMI) displaced in presence of mediastinal shift with tension pneumothorax • Hamman's sign—crunching sound correlating with heartbeat, reflecting air in mediastinum • *Blood pressure (BP):* Hypertension or hypotension • Jugular vein distention (JVD), especially with tension pneumothorax
EGO INTEGRITY • Anxiety, apprehension	• Restlessness, irritability
PAIN/DISCOMFORT • Unilateral chest pain, aggravated by breathing, coughing, and movement • Sudden onset of symptoms while coughing or straining—spontaneous pneumothorax • Sharp, stabbing pain aggravated by deep breathing, possibly radiating to neck, shoulders, abdomen—pleural effusion	• Guarding affected area • Distraction behaviors • Facial grimacing
RESPIRATION • History of recent chest surgery or trauma; chronic lung disease, lung inflammation or infection (empyema or effusion); diffuse interstitial disease (sarcoidosis); malignancies (e.g., obstructive tumor) • Previous spontaneous pneumothorax; spontaneous rupture of emphysematous bulla, subpleural bleb in COPD • Difficulty breathing, "air hunger" • Coughing, which may be presenting symptom	• *Respirations:* Tachypnea • Increased work of breathing, use of accessory muscles in chest, neck; intercostal retractions; forced abdominal expiration • Breath sounds decreased or absent on involved side • Fremitus decreased on involved site • *Chest percussion:* Hyperresonance over air-filled area—pneumothorax; dullness over fluid-filled area—hemothorax • *Chest observation and palpation:* Unequal or paradoxical chest movement (if trauma, flail), reduced thoracic excursion on affected side • *Skin:* Pallor, cyanosis, diaphoresis, subcutaneous crepitation • *Mentation:* Anxiety, restlessness, confusion, stupor • Use of positive pressure mechanical ventilation or positive end-expiratory pressure (PEEP) therapy
SAFETY • Recent chest trauma, such as fractured ribs, penetrating wound • Radiation and chemotherapy for malignancy • Presence of central intravenous (IV) line	
TEACHING/LEARNING • History of familial risk factors, such as TB, cancer • Recent intrathoracic surgery or lung biopsy	
DISCHARGE PLAN CONSIDERATIONS • Temporary assistance with self-care, homemaker and maintenance tasks ▶ Refer to section at end of plan for postdischarge considerations.	

TEST WHY IT IS DONE	WHAT IT TELLS ME
BLOOD TESTS • *Arterial blood gases (ABGs):* Measures oxygen and carbon dioxide levels to rule out hypoxemia or hypercapnia.	Variable depending on degree of compromised lung function, altered breathing mechanics, and ability to compensate. $PaCO_2$ occasionally elevated. PaO_2 may be normal or decreased; oxygen saturation usually decreased.
• *Hemoglobin/hematocrit (Hgb/Hct):* Assesses relationship of red blood cells (RBCs) to fluid volume or viscosity.	May be decreased, indicating blood loss.
OTHER DIAGNOSTIC STUDIES • *Chest x-ray:* Evaluates organs or structures within the chest and is the initial study of choice in blunt force chest trauma.	May show chest wall fractures, injuries to the heart or great vessels, and reveal air and fluid accumulation in the pleural space; may show shift of mediastinal structures (heart).
• *Thoracic computed tomography (CT):* Enhance anatomic views of the chest and locates abnormalities. Early CT may influence therapeutic management.	CT is more sensitive than x-ray in detecting thoracic injuries, lung contusion, hemothorax, and pneumothorax.
• *Thoracic ultrasound:* Assists in determining abnormalities in the chest.	Can be used in emergency department to quickly and reliably diagnose a hemothorax associated with chest trauma.
• *Thoracentesis:* Performed to relieve the intrathoracic pressure due to accumulation of fluid in the pleural space.	Presence of blood or serosanguinous fluid indicates hemothorax.

Nursing Priorities

1. Promote or maintain lung reexpansion for adequate oxygenation and ventilation.
2. Minimize or prevent complications.
3. Reduce discomfort and pain.
4. Provide information about disease process, treatment regimen, and prognosis.

Discharge Goals

1. Adequate ventilation and oxygenation maintained.
2. Complications prevented or resolved.
3. Pain absent or controlled.
4. Disease process, prognosis, and therapy needs understood.
5. Plan in place to meet needs after discharge.

NURSING DIAGNOSIS: **ineffective Breathing Pattern**

May be related to
Decreased lung expansion due to air or fluid accumulation
Musculoskeletal impairment
Pain and anxiety
Inflammatory process

Possibly evidenced by
Dyspnea, tachypnea
Changes in depth or equality of respirations; altered chest excursion
Use of accessory muscles, nasal flaring
Cyanosis, abnormal ABGs

Desired Outcomes/Evaluation Criteria—Client Will

Respiratory Status: Ventilation (NOC)
Establish a normal and effective respiratory pattern with ABGs within client's normal range.
Be free of cyanosis and other signs or symptoms of hypoxia.

ACTIONS/INTERVENTIONS	RATIONALE

Respiratory Monitoring (NIC)
Independent

Identify etiology or precipitating factors, such as spontaneous collapse, trauma, malignancy, infection, and complication of mechanical ventilation.

Understanding the cause of lung collapse is necessary for proper chest tube placement and choice of other therapeutic measures.

Evaluate respiratory function, noting rapid or shallow respirations, dyspnea, reports of "air hunger," development of cyanosis, and changes in vital signs.

Respiratory distress and changes in vital signs occur because of physiological stress and pain or may indicate development of shock due to hypoxia or hemorrhage.

Monitor for synchronous respiratory pattern when using mechanical ventilator. Note changes in airway pressures.

Difficulty breathing with ventilator or increasing airway pressures suggests worsening of condition and development of complications, such as spontaneous rupture of a bleb creating a new pneumothorax.

Auscultate breath sounds.

Breath sounds may be diminished or absent in a lobe, lung segment, or entire lung field (unilateral). Atelectatic area will have no breath sounds, and partially collapsed areas have decreased sounds. Regularly scheduled evaluation also helps determine areas of good air exchange and provides a baseline to evaluate resolution of pneumothorax.

Note chest excursion and position of trachea.

Chest excursion is unequal until lung reexpands. Trachea deviates from affected side with tension pneumothorax.

Assess fremitus.

Voice and tactile fremitus (vibration) is reduced in fluid-filled or consolidated tissue.

Ventilation Assistance (NIC)

Assist client with splinting painful area when coughing, or during deep breathing.

Supporting chest and abdominal muscles makes coughing more effective and less traumatic.

Maintain position of comfort, usually with head of bed elevated. Turn to affected side. Encourage client to sit up as much as possible.

Promotes maximal inspiration; enhances lung expansion and ventilation in unaffected side.

Maintain a calm attitude, assisting client to "take control" by using slower, deeper respirations.

Assists client to deal with the physiological effects of hypoxia, which may be manifested as anxiety or fear.

Tube Care: Chest (NIC)

Once chest tube is inserted:
  Determine if dry seal chest drain or water seal system is used.

Some chest drains use a mechanical one-way valve in place of a conventional water seal. The one-way valve allows air to escape from the chest and prevents air from entering the chest. Dry suction control systems regulate suction pressure mechanically rather than with a column of water. Some dry suction systems use a screw-type valve that varies the size of the opening to the vacuum source, thereby limiting the amount of negative pressure that can be transmitted to the chest. These valves narrow the opening of the chest drain in order to adjust the level of negative pressure; therefore, the total amount of air that can flow out of the chest drain is also limited. Thus, this type of dry suction control mechanism is impractical for clients with significant pleural air leaks (Atrium, 2007b).

If water seal system is used:
  Check suction control chamber for correct amount of suction, as determined by water level, wall or table regulator, at correct setting.

Maintains prescribed intrapleural negativity, which promotes optimum lung expansion and fluid drainage. *Note:* Dry-seal setups are also used with an automatic control valve (AVC), which provides a one-way valve seal similar to that achieved with the water-seal system.

  Check fluid level in water-seal chamber; maintain at prescribed level.

Water in a sealed chamber serves as a barrier that prevents atmospheric air from entering the pleural space should the suction source be disconnected and aids in evaluating whether the chest drainage system is functioning appropriately. *Note:* Underfilling the water-seal chamber leaves it exposed to air, putting client at risk for pneumothorax or tension pneumothorax. Overfilling, a more common mistake, prevents air from easily exiting the pleural space, thus preventing resolution of pneumothorax and possibly creating a tension pneumothorax.

(continues on page 158)

Observe for bubbling in water-seal chamber.

Evaluate for abnormal or continuous water-seal chamber bubbling.

Determine location of air leak (client or system centered) by clamping thoracic catheter just distal to exit from chest.

Place petrolatum gauze or other appropriate material around the insertion as indicated.

Clamp tubing in stepwise fashion downward toward drainage unit if air leak continues.

Seal drainage tubing connection sites securely with lengthwise tape or bands according to established policy.

Monitor water-seal chamber "tidaling." Note whether change is transient or permanent.

Position drainage system tubing for optimal function; for example, shorten tubing or coil extra tubing on bed, making sure tubing is not kinked or hanging below entrance to drainage container. Drain accumulated fluid as necessary.

Note character and amount of chest tube drainage, whether tube is warm and full of blood and whether bloody fluid level in water-seal bottle is rising.

Evaluate need for gentle "milking" of chest tube per protocol.

If thoracic catheter is disconnected or dislodged:
Observe for signs of respiratory distress. If possible, reconnect thoracic catheter to tubing and suction, using clean technique. If the catheter is dislodged from the chest, cover insertion site immediately with petrolatum dressing and apply firm pressure. Notify physician at once.

After thoracic catheter is removed:
Cover insertion site with sterile occlusive dressing. Observe for signs or symptoms that may indicate recurrence of pneumothorax, such as shortness of breath and reports of pain. Inspect insertion site, noting character of drainage.

Collaborative

Assist with and prepare for reinflation procedures; for example, simple aspiration, Heimlich valve, and chest tube placement with chest tube drainage unit (CDU).

Bubbling during expiration reflects venting of pneumothorax (desired action). Bubbling usually decreases as the lung expands or may occur only during expiration or coughing as the pleural space diminishes. Absence of bubbling may indicate complete lung reexpansion (normal) or represent complications, such as obstruction, in the tube.

With suction applied, this indicates a persistent air leak that may be from a large pneumothorax at the chest insertion site (client centered) or chest drainage unit (system centered).

If bubbling stops when catheter is clamped at insertion site, leak is client centered at insertion site or within the client.

Usually corrects insertion site air leak.

Isolates location of a system-centered air leak. *Note:* As a rule, clamping for a suspected leak is the only time that chest tube should be clamped.

Prevents or corrects air leaks at connector sites.

The water-seal chamber serves as an intrapleural manometer (gauges intrapleural pressure); therefore, fluctuation, or tidaling, reflects pressure differences between inspiration and expiration. Tidaling of 2 to 6 cm during inspiration is normal and may increase briefly during coughing episodes. Continuation of excessive tidal fluctuations may indicate existence of airway obstruction or presence of a large pneumothorax.

Improper position, kinking, or accumulation of clots and fluid in the tubing changes the desired negative pressure and impedes air or fluid evacuation. *Note:* If a dependent loop in the drainage tube cannot be avoided, lifting and draining it every 15 minutes will maintain adequate drainage in the presence of a hemothorax.

Useful in evaluating resolution of pneumothorax or development of hemorrhage requiring prompt intervention. *Note:* Some drainage systems are equipped with an autotransfusion device, which allows for salvage of shed blood.

May be indicated to maintain drainage in the presence of fresh bleeding, large blood clots, or purulent exudates (empyema). Caution is necessary to prevent undue discomfort or injury, such as invagination of tissue into catheter eyelets and rupture of small blood vessels.

Pneumothorax may recur, requiring prompt intervention to prevent fatal pulmonary and circulatory impairment.

Early detection of a developing complication, such as recurrence of pneumothorax or presence of infection, is essential.

Treatment goals include air evacuation, lung reinflation, and prevention of recurrence. Although simple aspiration or Heimlich one-way valve procedures may be useful for small uncomplicated pneumothorax with little or no drainage, chest tube placement is the treatment of choice for traumatic hemopneumothoraces. CDUs include a collection chamber, a water-seal chamber, and a suction-control regulator. A dry suction system can also be used. *Note:* Tension pneumothorax requires immediate needle depression, followed by chest tube placement.

ACTIONS/INTERVENTIONS (continued)

Obtain postplacement x-rays and review serial chest x-rays.

Ventilation Assistance (NIC)
Monitor and graph serial ABGs and pulse oximetry. Review vital capacity and tidal volume measurements.
Administer supplemental oxygen via cannula, mask, or mechanical ventilation, as indicated.
Administer analgesics and sedatives, as indicated.

RATIONALE (continued)

Placement of tube(s) is determined by the cause of the problem; for example, anterior chest near apex of lung, or one tube at the apex and one at posterior fifth to sixth intercostal space. X-rays confirm proper placement and monitor progress of reexpansion of lung.

Assesses status of gas exchange and ventilation and need for continuation or alterations in therapy.
Aids in reducing work of breathing; promotes relief of respiratory distress and cyanosis associated with hypoxemia.
Given to manage pleuritic pain and reduce anxiety and tachycardia associated with impaired respiratory function, especially when client is on a ventilator.

NURSING DIAGNOSIS: risk for Trauma/Suffocation

Risk factors may include
Concurrent disease or injury process
Dependence on external device—chest drainage system
Lack of safety education and precautions

Possibly evidenced by
(Not applicable; presence of signs and symptoms establishes an *actual* diagnosis)

Desired Outcomes/Evaluation Criteria—Client Will

Risk Control (NOC)
Recognize need for and seek assistance to prevent complications.

Caregiver Will

Correct and avoid environmental and physical hazards.

ACTIONS/INTERVENTIONS

Teaching: Procedure/Treatment (NIC)
Independent
Review with client purpose and function of CDU, taking note of safety features.
Instruct client to refrain from lying or pulling on tubing.

Identify changes and situations that should be reported to caregivers, such as change in sound of bubbling, sudden "air hunger" and chest pain, and disconnection of equipment.

Tube Care: Chest (NIC)
Anchor thoracic catheter to chest wall and provide extra length of tubing before turning or moving client.

Secure tubing connection sites.
Pad banding sites with gauze or tape.
Secure drainage unit to client's bed or on stand or cart placed in low-traffic area.
Provide safe transportation if client is sent off unit for diagnostic purposes. Before transporting, check water-seal chamber for correct fluid level; presence or absence of bubbling; and presence, degree, and timing of tidaling. Ascertain whether chest tube can be clamped or disconnected from suction source.

Monitor thoracic insertion site, noting condition of skin and presence and characteristics of drainage from around the catheter. Change and reapply sterile occlusive dressing as needed.
Observe for signs of respiratory distress if thoracic catheter is disconnected or dislodged. (Refer to ND: ineffective Breathing Pattern.)

RATIONALE

Information on how system works provides reassurance, reducing client anxiety.
Reduces risk of obstructing drainage or inadvertently disconnecting tubing.
Timely intervention may prevent serious complications.

Prevents thoracic catheter dislodgment or tubing disconnection and reduces pain and discomfort associated with pulling or jarring of tubing.
Prevents tubing disconnection.
Protects skin from irritation and pressure.
Maintains upright position and reduces risk of accidental tipping and breaking of unit.
Promotes continuation of optimal evacuation of fluid or air during transport. If client is draining large amounts of chest fluid or air, tube should not be clamped or suction interrupted because of risk of accumulating fluid or air, compromising respiratory status.

Provides for early recognition and treatment of developing skin or tissue erosion or infection.

Pneumothorax may recur or worsen, compromising respiratory function and requiring emergency intervention.

deficient Knowledge [Learning Need] regarding condition, treatment regimen, self-care, and discharge needs

May be related to
Lack of exposure to information

Possibly evidenced by
Expressions of concern, request for information
Recurrence of problem

Desired Outcomes/Evaluation Criteria—Client Will

Knowledge: Disease Process (NOC)
Verbalize understanding of cause of problem (when known).
Identify signs or symptoms requiring medical follow-up.

Knowledge: Treatment Regimen (NOC)
Follow therapeutic regimen and demonstrate lifestyle changes, if necessary, to prevent recurrence.

ACTIONS/INTERVENTIONS	RATIONALE
Teaching: Disease Process (NIC)	
Independent	
Review pathology of individual problem.	Information reduces fear of unknown. Provides knowledge base for understanding underlying dynamics of condition and significance of therapeutic interventions.
Identify likelihood for recurrence or long-term complications.	Certain underlying lung diseases, such as severe COPD and malignancies, may increase incidence of recurrence. In otherwise healthy clients who suffered a spontaneous pneumothorax, incidence of recurrence is 10% to 50%. Those who have a second spontaneous episode are at high risk for a third incident (60%).
Review signs and symptoms requiring immediate medical evaluation, for example, sudden chest pain, dyspnea, air hunger, and progressive respiratory distress.	Recurrence of pneumothorax and hemothorax requires medical intervention to prevent and reduce potential complications.
Review significance of good health practices, such as adequate nutrition, rest, and exercise.	Maintenance of general well-being promotes healing and may prevent or limit recurrences.
Emphasize need for smoking cessation when indicated.	Prevents recurrence of pneumothorax or respiratory complications, such as fibrotic changes.

POTENTIAL CONSIDERATIONS following acute hospitalization (dependent on client's age, physical condition and presence of complications, personal resources, and life responsibilities)
- *risk for Infection*—may occur as a result of invasive procedure, traumatized tissue or broken skin, decreased ciliary action
- *ineffective Breathing Pattern*—may indicate recurrence of condition, inflammatory process

RADICAL NECK SURGERY: LARYNGECTOMY (POSTOPERATIVE CARE)

I. Pathophysiology

a. Malignancy lies above the clavicle, for instance lip, mouth, nasal cavity, paranasal sinuses, pharynx, larynx, but excludes the brain, spinal cord, axial skeleton, and vertebrae.

b. Cancers limited to the vocal cords (intrinsic) tend to spread slowly, whereas cancers involving the epiglottis (extrinsic) are more likely to metastasize to lymph nodes of neck.

c. 90% to 95% of laryngeal neoplasms are squamous cell carcinomas that arise from the oral cavity (Campbell & de le Torre, 2008; Oral Cancer Foundation, 2008).

d. Rate of disability is high because of the potential loss of voice, disfigurement, and social consequences.

II. Treatment

a. Radiation alone is the most common treatment for early stages of some head and neck cancers, such as those affecting the nasopharynx, larynx, and oropharynx.

b. Combination of radiation and chemotherapy is increasing in use to preserve structures.

c. Surgery remains mainstay of treatment for advanced-stage laryngeal cancer, often in combination with radiation.

   i. Total laryngectomy (TL), resulting in a permanent tracheostomy, with normal speech and swallowing no longer possible

   ii. Near total laryngectomy (NTL) or conservation laryngeal surgery, with swallowing function and some speech retained

III. Etiology

a. Between 85% to 90% of all head and neck cancers can be traced to the use of tobacco products or excessive consumption of alcohol (American Association for Cancer Research, 2008).

b. Additional risk factors include chronic candidiasis, poor oral hygiene, ill-fitting dentures, human papillomavirus (HPV), Epstein-Barr virus (EBV), and acid reflux disease (Campbell & de la Torre, 2008).

IV. Statistics (National Cancer Institute [NCI], 2007b)

a. Morbidity: Head and neck cancers compose approximately 4% of all cancer cases in the United States, with an estimated 40,000 men and women diagnosed in 2004.
  i. Peak incidence between ages 50 and 60
  ii. Male-to-female rates greater than 2:1 (Campbell & de la Torre, 2008)

b. Mortality: 5-year survival rate is at 50% (Mouth Cancer Foundation, 2008).

c. Cost: In 2001, lifetime economic burden in the United States was estimated at $976 billion (Lee et al, n.d.) and the annual cost for treatment in the United States was approximately $3.2 billion.

GLOSSARY

Diplopia: Double vision.
Dysphagia: Difficulty in swallowing.
Near total laryngectomy (NTL): Partial or hemilaryngectomy—one vocal cord is retained, also called subtotal laryngectomy; other conservation laryngeal surgical procedures include supracricoid partial laryngectomy (SCPL) and supraglottic laryngectomy (SGL).

Total laryngectomy (TL): Removal of the entire larynx, hyoid bone, cricoid cartilage, two or three tracheal rings, and the strap muscles connected to the larynx.

Care Settings

Client is treated in inpatient surgical and possibly subacute units.

Related Concerns

Cancer, page 846
Psychosocial aspects of care, page 749
Surgical intervention, page 782
Total nutritional support: parenteral/enteral feeding, page 469

Client Assessment Database (Preoperative and Postoperative)

Preoperative data presented here depend on the specific type and location of cancer process and underlying complications.

DIAGNOSTIC DIVISION MAY REPORT	MAY EXHIBIT
ACTIVITY/REST • Weakness, fatigue	• Weakness, fatigue, lethargy
EGO INTEGRITY • Feelings of fear about loss of voice, dying, occurrence or recurrence of cancer • Concern about how surgery will affect family relationships, ability to work, and finances	• Anxiety • Depression • Anger • Withdrawal • Denial
FOOD/FLUID • Difficulty swallowing, chokes easily, taste changes	• Swelling, ulcerations, masses may be noted depending on location of cancer • Oral inflammation and drainage, poor dental hygiene • Leukoplakia, erythroplasia of oral cavity • Halitosis • Swelling of tongue • Altered gag reflex and facial paralysis • Difficulty handling oral secretions, or dry mouth (postoperative)
HYGIENE • Neglect of dental hygiene	• Need for assistance in basic care

(continues on page 162)

DIAGNOSTIC DIVISION MAY REPORT (continued)	MAY EXHIBIT (continued)

NEUROSENSORY
- Double vision
- Deafness, involved side
- Tingling, paresthesia of facial muscles

- Hemiparalysis of face with parotid and submandibular involvement
- Persistent hoarseness or loss of voice—dominant and earliest symptom of intrinsic laryngeal cancer
- Difficulty swallowing
- Conduction deafness
- Disruption of mucous membranes

PAIN/DISCOMFORT
Preoperative:
- Chronic sore throat, "lump in throat"
- Referred pain to ear, facial pain (late stage, probably metastatic)
- Pain or burning sensation with swallowing, especially with hot liquids or citrus juices
- Sore throat or mouth

Postoperative:
- Surgical site pain
- Shoulder pain on affected side

- Guarding behaviors
- Restlessness
- Facial mask of pain
- Alteration in facial muscle tone

RESPIRATION
- History of tobacco use including cigars and chewing tobacco
- Occupation working with hardwood sawdust, toxic chemicals and fumes, heavy metals
- History of voice overuse, for example, professional singer or auctioneer
- History of chronic lung disease
- Cough with or without sputum
- Blood-tinged sputum or nasal drainage

- Hemoptysis
- Dyspnea (late)

SAFETY
- Excessive sun exposure over a period of years
- Radiation therapy
- Visual or hearing changes

- Masses or enlarged nodes

SOCIAL INTERACTION
- Lack of family or support system—may be result of age group or behaviors such as alcoholism
- Concerns about ability to communicate, engage in social interactions

- Persistent hoarseness, change in voice pitch
- Muffled or garbled speech, reluctance to speak
- Hesitancy or reluctance of significant others (SOs) to provide care or be involved in rehabilitation

TEACHING/LEARNING
- Nonhealing of oral lesions
- Concurrent use of alcohol or history of alcohol abuse

DISCHARGE PLAN CONSIDERATIONS
- May require assistance with wound care, treatments, supplies, transportation, shopping, food preparation, self-care, homemaker and maintenance tasks

▶ Refer to section at end of plan for postdischarge considerations.

TEST WHY IT IS DONE	WHAT IT TELLS ME
BLOOD TESTS	
• *Complete blood count (CBC):* Battery of screening tests that typically includes hemoglobin (Hgb), hematocrit (Hct), red blood cell (RBC) count and morphology, indices, and distribution width index; platelet count and size; white blood cell (WBC) count and differential.	May reveal anemia, which is a common problem. Folate deficiency is very common in clients with history of alcoholism and malnutrition.
• *Immunological surveys:* Measure levels of T cells, natural killer (NK) cells, macrophages, and so on.	May be done for clients receiving chemotherapy or immunotherapy to determine status of immune system and to assist with use of vaccines for manipulation of cancer-directed immune response therapy.
• *Human papillomavirus (HPV; particularly for type 16) test:* To screen for presence of HPV.	HPV-related cancers tend to occur on the tonsillar area and the base of the tongue and the oropharynx, whereas non–HPV-related tumors tend to involve the anterior tongue, floor of the mouth, and the mucosa that covers the inside of the cheeks and alveolar ridges where the teeth are located.
• *Biochemical profile:* Battery of tests including electrolytes, glucose, total protein, amylase, blood urea nitrogen (BUN)/creatinine (Cr), bilirubin, total CO_2, cholesterol, lipids, and aspartate aminotransferase (AST)/alinine aminotransferase (ALT) to evaluate general status of organ function.	Changes may occur in organ function as a result of cancer, metastasis, and therapies.
OTHER DIAGNOSTIC STUDIES	
• *Direct/indirect laryngoscopy:* Provides direct visualization of structures of the mouth and throat by means of either a rigid or flexible endoscope. Allows for biopsy and aspiration of secretions for cytology.	Visualizes local or regional cancers of the oropharynx and upper airways and allows staging.
• *Laryngeal computed tomography (CT) scan:* X-ray procedure that uses a computer to produce a detailed picture of a cross-section of the body.	Defines tumor extension deep in the laryngeal mucosal surface, cartilaginous invasion, and metastatic disease to the lymph nodes of the neck. Has largely replaced contrast laryngography as the primary method for staging laryngeal carcinoma (Silverman et al, 1984).
• *Magnetic resonance imaging (MRI) scan:* Evaluates tumor status and treatment options.	MRI is most often used as the primary imaging modality when evaluating tumor spread in nasopharynx, oropharynx, palate, base of tongue, and floor of mouth.
• *Positron emission tomography (PET) scan:* Measures the activity or functional level of the brain by measuring its use of glucose.	Because cancer cells are dividing rapidly, they break down glucose much faster than do normal cells. The increased activity will show up on a PET scan and can indicate both primary and metastatic tumors. PET scan allows identification of tumor, especially in difficult cases where no obvious mass was seen clinically or on either CT or MRI (American Head and Neck Society, n.d.).
• *Single photon-emission tomography (SPECT) scan:* Nuclear medicine procedure in which a gamma camera rotates around the client and takes pictures.	SPECT is particularly useful for detection of occult head and neck tumors and for assessing possibility of recurrence. It may also help stage primary tumors, differentiate metastatic from reactive lymph nodes in the neck, and screen for distant metastases (Olmos et al, 1997).
• *Laryngography:* X-ray examination of the larynx after the insertion of a contrast medium.	May be performed to study blood vessels and lymph nodes.
• *Chest x-ray:* Evaluates organs and structures within the chest.	Done to establish baseline lung status and to identify metastases.
• *Pulmonary function studies, including spirometry, lung volumes, and perfusion:* Measure how well the lungs take in and release air and how well they move oxygen into the blood.	Chronic obstructve pulmonary disease (COPD) is common in this group of clients. Abnormal findings may indicate need for additional interventions to improve pulmonary reserve prior to surgery.
• *Arterial blood gases (ABGs)/pulse oximetry:* Blood test or peripheral scan to measure oxygen content and saturation of the blood	May be done to establish baseline and monitor status of lungs.

Nursing Priorities ─────────

1. Maintain patent airway and adequate ventilation.
2. Assist client in developing alternative communication methods.
3. Restore or maintain skin integrity.
4. Reestablish or maintain adequate nutrition.
5. Provide emotional support for acceptance of altered body image.
6. Provide information about disease process, prognosis, and treatment.

Discharge Goals ─────────

1. Ventilation and oxygenation adequate for individual needs.
2. Communicate effectively.
3. Complications prevented or minimized.
4. Begin to cope with change in body image.
5. Disease process, prognosis, and therapeutic regimen understood.
6. Plan in place to meet needs after discharge.

NURSING DIAGNOSIS: **ineffective Airway Clearance**

May be related to
Partial or total removal of the glottis, altering ability to breathe, cough, and swallow
Temporary or permanent change to neck breathing—dependent on patent stoma
Edema formation—surgical manipulation and lymphatic accumulation
Copious and thick secretions

Possibly evidenced by
Dyspnea and difficulty breathing
Changes in rate and depth of respiration; use of accessory respiratory muscles
Abnormal breath sounds
Cyanosis

Desired Outcomes/Evaluation Criteria—Client Will

Respiratory Status: Airway Patency (NOC)
Maintain patent airway with breath sounds clear or clearing.
Clear secretions and be free of aspiration.

ACTIONS/INTERVENTIONS	RATIONALE
Airway Management (NIC)	
Independent	
Monitor respiratory rate and depth; note ease of breathing. Auscultate breath sounds. Investigate restlessness, dyspnea, and development of cyanosis.	Changes in respirations, use of accessory muscles, and presence of crackles or wheezes suggest retention of secretions. Airway obstruction (even partial) can lead to ineffective breathing patterns and impaired gas exchange, resulting in complications, such as pneumonia and respiratory arrest.
Elevate head of bed 30 to 45 degrees.	Facilitates drainage of secretions, work of breathing, and lung expansion. *Note:* Increase elevation when oral intake is provided.
Encourage swallowing, if client is able.	Prevents pooling of oral secretions, reducing risk of aspiration. *Note:* Swallowing is impaired when the epiglottis is removed and/or significant postoperative edema and pain are present.
Encourage effective coughing and deep breathing.	Mobilizes secretions to clear airway and helps prevent respiratory complications.
Suction laryngectomy and tracheostomy tube and oral and nasal cavities. Note amount, color, and consistency of secretions.	Prevents secretions from obstructing airway, especially when swallowing ability is impaired and client cannot blow nose. Changes in character of secretions may indicate developing problems, such as dehydration and infection, and need for further evaluation and treatment.
Demonstrate and encourage client to begin self-suction procedures as soon as possible. Educate client in "clean" techniques.	Assists client to exercise some control in postoperative care and prevention of complications. Reduces anxiety associated with difficulty in breathing or inability to handle secretions when alone.
Maintain proper position of laryngectomy or tracheostomy tube. Check and adjust ties as indicated.	As edema develops or subsides, tube can be displaced, compromising airway. Ties should be snug but not constrictive to surrounding tissue or major blood vessels.
Observe tissues surrounding tube for bleeding. Change client's position to check for pooling of blood behind neck or on posterior dressings.	Small amount of oozing may be present; however, continued bleeding or sudden eruption of uncontrolled hemorrhage presents a sudden and real possibility of airway obstruction and suffocation.

ACTIONS/INTERVENTIONS (continued)

Change tube and inner cannula, as indicated. Instruct client in cleaning procedures.

Collaborative

Provide supplemental humidification, such as compressed air or oxygen mist collar and increased fluid intake.

Resume oral intake with caution. (Refer to ND: imbalanced Nutrition: Less than Body Requirements.)
Monitor serial ABGs or pulse oximetry and chest x-ray.

RATIONALE (continued)

Prevents accumulation of secretions and thick mucous plugs from obstructing airway. *Note:* This is a common cause of respiratory distress and arrest in later postoperative period.

Normal physiological (nasal passages) means of filtering and humidifying air are bypassed. Supplemental humidity decreases mucous crusting and facilitates coughing or suctioning of secretions through stoma.
Changes in muscle mass and strength and nerve innervation increase likelihood of aspiration.
Pooling of secretions or presence of atelectasis may lead to pneumonia, requiring more aggressive therapeutic measures.

NURSING DIAGNOSIS: **impaired Verbal Communication**

May be related to
Anatomical deficit—removal of vocal cords
Physical barrier—tracheostomy tube
Required voice rest

Possibly evidenced by
Inability to speak
Change in vocal characteristics

Desired Outcomes/Evaluation Criteria—Client Will

Communication (NOC)
Communicate needs in an effective manner.
Identify and plan for appropriate alternative speech methods after healing.

ACTIONS/INTERVENTIONS

Communication Enhancement: Speech Deficit (NIC)
Independent
Review preoperative instructions and discussion of why speech and breathing are altered, using anatomic drawings or models to assist in explanations.

Determine whether client has other communication impairments, such as hearing, vision, and literacy.
Provide immediate and continual means to summon nurse, for example, a call bell. Let client know the summons will be answered immediately. Stop by to check on client periodically without being summoned. Post notice at central answering system or nursing station that client is unable to speak.
Prearrange signals for obtaining immediate help.
Provide alternative means of communication appropriate to client need, such as pad and pencil, magic slate, alphabet or picture board, and sign language. Consider placement of intravenous (IV) line.
Allow sufficient time for communication.

Provide nonverbal communication, such as touching and physical presence. Anticipate needs.

Encourage ongoing communication with "outside world," such as newspapers, television, radio, calendar, and clock.

RATIONALE

Reinforces teaching at a time when fear of surviving surgery is past. *Note:* Following NTL procedure and the passage of time, the client may experience voice and ease of swallowing, although this depends entirely on multiple factors, including type and invasiveness of cancer, type and success of reconstructive surgery, and response to radiation and chemotherapy.
Presence of other problems influences plan for alternative communication.
Client needs assurance that nurse is vigilant and will respond to summons. Trust and self-esteem are fostered when the nurse cares enough to come at times other than when called by client.

May decrease client's anxiety about inability to speak.
Permits client to express needs and concerns. *Note:* IV positioned in hand or wrist may limit ability to write or sign.

Loss of speech and stress of alternative communication can cause frustration and block expression, especially when caregivers seem "too busy" or preoccupied.
Communicates concern and meets need for contact with others. Touch is believed to generate complex biochemical events, with possible release of endorphins contributing to reduction of anxiety.
Maintains contact with "normal lifestyle" and continued communication through other avenues.

(continues on page 166)

ACTIONS/INTERVENTIONS (continued)

Refer to loss of speech as temporary after a partial laryngectomy, as appropriate, for instance if client may have return of voice, or be candidate for voice prosthetics or vocal cord transplant.

Caution client not to use voice until physician gives permission.

Arrange for meeting with other persons who have experienced this procedure, as appropriate.

Collaborative

Consult with appropriate healthcare team members, therapists, speech pathologist, and social services. Refer to hospital-based rehabilitation, and community resources, such as Lost Chord or New Voice Club, International Association of Laryngectomees, and American Cancer Society.

RATIONALE (continued)

Provides encouragement and hope for future with the thought that alternative means of communication and speech are available and possible. *Note:* Some procedures allow for return of voice function, either by means of an artificial larynx (neck or intraoral); a tracheoesophageal puncture (TEP) and prosthesis, which allows lung-powered speech; or a form not requiring a prosthesis—esophageal speech through air forced into the top of the esophagus.

Promotes healing of vocal cord and limits potential for permanent cord dysfunction.

Provides role model, enhancing motivation for problem-solving and learning new ways to communicate.

Ability to use alternative voice and speech methods, such as electrolarynx, TEP, voice prosthesis, and esophageal speech, varies greatly, depending on extent of surgical procedures, client's age and emotional state, and motivation to return to an active life. Rehabilitation time may be lengthy and require a number of agencies and resources to facilitate or support learning process. *Note:* Some clients may be candidates for vocal cord transplant at a future date.

NURSING DIAGNOSIS: impaired Skin/Tissue Integrity

May be related to
Surgical removal of tissues and grafting
Radiation or chemotherapeutic agents
Altered circulation or reduced blood supply
Compromised nutritional status
Edema formation
Pooling or continuous drainage of secretions—oral, lymph, or chyle

Possibly evidenced by
Disruption of skin and tissue surface
Destruction of skin and tissue layers

Desired Outcomes/Evaluation Criteria—Client Will

Wound Healing: Primary Intention (NOC)
Display timely wound healing without complications.
Demonstrate techniques to promote healing and prevent complications.

ACTIONS/INTERVENTIONS

Skin Surveillance (NIC)
Independent

Assess skin color, temperature, and capillary refill in operative and skin graft areas.

Keep head of bed elevated 30 to 45 degrees. Monitor facial edema—usually peaks by third to fifth postoperative day.

Protect skin flaps and suture lines from tension or pressure. Provide pillow or rolls and instruct client to support head and neck during activity.

Monitor bloody drainage from surgical sites, suture lines, and drains. Measure drainage from collection device, such as Hemovac, if used.

Note and report any milky-appearing drainage.

RATIONALE

Skin should be pink or similar to color of surrounding skin. Skin graft flaps should be pink and warm and should blanch when gentle finger pressure is applied, with return to color within seconds. Cyanosis and slow refill may indicate venous congestion, which can lead to tissue ischemia and necrosis.

Minimizes postoperative tissue congestion and edema related to excision of lymph channels.

Pressure from tubing and tracheostomy tapes or tension on suture lines can alter circulation and cause tissue injury.

Bloody drainage usually declines steadily after first 24 hours. Steady oozing or frank bleeding indicates problem requiring medical attention.

Milky drainage may indicate thoracic lymph duct leakage, which can result in depletion of body fluids and electrolytes. Such a leak may heal spontaneously or require surgical closure.

ACTIONS/INTERVENTIONS (continued)

Wound Care (NIC)
Change dressings, as indicated.

Cleanse incisions with sterile saline and peroxide (mixed 1:1), or per protocal, after dressings have been removed.

Monitor donor site if graft performed; check dressings as indicated.

Cleanse thoroughly around stoma and neck tubes (if in place), avoiding soap or alcohol. Show client how to do self-care of stoma and tube with clean water and peroxide, using soft, lint-free cloth, not tissue or cotton.

Monitor all sites for signs of wound infection, such as unusual redness; increasing edema, pain, exudates; and temperature elevation.

Collaborative
Cover donor sites with petroleum gauze or moisture-impermeable dressing.
Administer oral, IV, and topical antibiotics, as indicated.

RATIONALE (continued)

Damp dressings increase risk of tissue damage and infection. *Note:* Pressure dressings are not used over skin flaps because blood supply is easily compromised.
Prevents crust formation, which can trap purulent drainage, destroy skin edges, and increase size of wound. Peroxide is not used full strength because it may cauterize wound edges and impair healing.
Donor site may be adjacent to operative site or a distant site, such as the thigh. Pressure dressings are usually removed within 24 to 48 hours, and the wound is left open to air to promote healing.
Keeping area clean promotes healing and comfort. Soap and other drying agents can lead to stomal irritation and possible inflammation. Materials other than cloth may leave fibers in stoma that can irritate or be inhaled into lungs.
Impedes healing, which may already be slow because of changes induced by cancer, cancer therapies, or malnutrition.

Nonadherent dressing covers exposed sensory nerve endings and protects site from contamination.
Prevents or controls infection.

NURSING DIAGNOSIS: impaired Oral Mucous Membrane

May be related to
Dehydration or absence of oral intake, decreased saliva production secondary to radiation (common) or surgical procedure (rare)
Poor or inadequate oral hygiene
Pathological condition (oral cancer), mechanical trauma (oral surgery)
Difficulty swallowing and pooling of secretions and drooling
Nutritional deficits

Possibly evidenced by
Xerostomia (dry mouth), oral discomfort
Thick, mucoid saliva; decreased saliva production
Dry, crusted, coated tongue; inflamed lips
Absent teeth and gums, poor dental health, halitosis

Desired Outcomes/Evaluation Criteria—Client Will

Tissue Integrity: Skin and Mucous Membranes (NOC)
Report or demonstrate a decrease in symptoms.
Identify specific interventions to promote healthy oral mucosa.
Demonstrate techniques to restore and maintain mucosal integrity.

ACTIONS/INTERVENTIONS

Oral Health Restoration (NIC)
Independent
Inspect oral cavity and note changes in:
  Saliva

  Tongue

  Lips

RATIONALE

Damage to salivary glands may decrease production of saliva, resulting in dry mouth. Pooling and drooling of saliva may occur because of compromised swallowing capability or pain in throat and mouth.
Surgery may have included partial resection of tongue, soft palate, and pharynx. This client has decreased sensation and movement of tongue, with difficulty swallowing and increased risk of aspiration of secretions, as well as potential for hemorrhage.
Surgical removal of part of lip may result in uncontrollable drooling.

(continues on page 168)

ACTIONS/INTERVENTIONS (continued)

Teeth and gums

Mucous membranes

Suction oral cavity gently and frequently. Have client perform self-suctioning when possible or use gauze wick to drain secretions.

Show client how to brush inside of mouth, palate, tongue, and teeth.

Apply lubrication to lips; provide oral irrigations as indicated.

Avoid alcohol-based mouthwashes. Use normal saline or mixture of salt water and baking soda for rinsing. Suggest use of artificial saliva preparations, such as pilocarpine hydrochloride (Salagen), if mucous membranes are dry.

RATIONALE (continued)

Teeth may not be intact (surgical) or may be in poor condition because of malnutrition, chemical therapies, and neglect. Gums may also be surgically altered or inflamed because of poor hygiene, long history of smoking or chewing tobacco, or chemical therapies.

May be excessively dry, ulcerated, erythematous, and edematous.

Saliva contains digestive enzymes that may be erosive to exposed tissues. Because drooling may be constant, client can promote own comfort and enhance oral hygiene by performing self-suctioning.

Frequent oral care reduces bacteria and risk of infection and promotes tissue healing and comfort.

Counteracts drying effects of therapeutic measures and negates erosive nature of secretions.

Alcohol can be drying and irritating. Salt and soda rinses return mouth to neutral rather than acidic environment. Although drooling is often present and abundant immediately postoperatively, surgical or radiation damage to the parotid glands can drastically reduce saliva production on a permanent basis. Cholinergic effect of medication can increase saliva production.

NURSING DIAGNOSIS: acute Pain

May be related to
Surgical incisions
Tissue swelling
Presence of nasogastric or orogastric feeding tube

Possibly evidenced by
Discomfort in surgical areas
Pain with swallowing
Facial mask of pain
Distraction behaviors, restlessness; guarding behavior

Desired Outcomes/Evaluation Criteria—Client Will

Pain Level (NOC)
Report pain is relieved or controlled.
Demonstrate relief of pain and discomfort by reduced tension and relaxed manner and sleeping or resting appropriately.

ACTIONS/INTERVENTIONS

Pain Management (NIC)
Independent
Support head and neck with pillows. Show client how to support neck during activity.

Provide comfort measures, such as back rub and position change, and diversional activities, such as television, visiting, and reading.

Encourage client to expectorate saliva or to suction mouth gently if unable to swallow.

Evaluate pain level frequently.

Investigate changes in characteristics of pain. Check mouth and throat suture lines for fresh trauma.

Note nonverbal indicators and autonomic responses to pain. Evaluate effects of analgesics.

RATIONALE

Muscle weakness results from muscle and nerve resection in the structures of the neck and shoulders. Lack of support aggravates discomfort and may result in injury to suture areas.

Promotes relaxation and helps client refocus attention on something beside self and discomfort. May reduce analgesic dosage frequency.

Swallowing causes muscle activity that may be painful because of edema or strain on suture lines.

Pain is a major concern for clients undergoing laryngectomy and it is believed as many as 32% still suffer severe distress, with the administered dosing less than needed to obtain optimal pain relief (Orgill et al, 2002).

May reflect developing complications requiring further evaluation or intervention. Tissues are inflamed and congested and may be easily traumatized by suction catheter or feeding tube.

Aids in determining presence of pain, effectiveness of medication, or the need for pain relief.

ACTIONS/INTERVENTIONS (continued)

Medicate before activity and treatments, as indicated.

Schedule care activities to balance with adequate periods of sleep or rest.
Recommend use of stress management behaviors, such as relaxation techniques and guided imagery.

Collaborative
Provide oral irrigations, anesthetic sprays, and gargles. Instruct client in self-irrigations.

Administer analgesics such as on a scheduled basis and prn (as necessary) or via patient-controlled analgesia; adjust dosages according to pain level per protocols.

Avoid medications containing aspirin.

RATIONALE (continued)

May enhance cooperation and participation in therapeutic regimen.
Prevents fatigue or exhaustion and may enhance coping with stress or discomfort.
Promotes sense of well-being and may reduce analgesic needs and enhance healing.

Improves comfort, promotes healing, and reduces halitosis. *Note:* Commercial mouthwashes containing alcohol or phenol are to be avoided because of their drying effect.
Degree of pain is related to extent and psychological impact of surgery as well as general body condition. Allowing client to control medication or giving medications on schedule rather than just prn and using report of pain level to adjust dosage minimizes chance that pain escalates "out of control."
Products containing aspirin are contraindicated because they potentiate bleeding.

NURSING DIAGNOSIS: **imbalanced Nutrition: Less than Body Requirements**

May be related to
Temporary or permanent alteration in mode of food intake
Altered feedback mechanisms of desire to eat, taste, and smell because of surgical or structural changes, radiation, or chemotherapy

Possibly evidenced by
Inadequate food intake, perceived inability to ingest food
Aversion to eating, lack of interest in food, reported altered taste sensation
Weight loss
Weakness of muscles required for swallowing or mastication

Desired Outcomes/Evaluation Criteria—Client Will

Nutritional Status (NOC)
Indicate understanding of importance of nutrition to healing process and general well-being.
Make dietary choices to meet nutrient needs within individual situation.
Demonstrate progressive weight gain toward goal, with normalization of laboratory values and timely healing of tissues and incisions.

ACTIONS/INTERVENTIONS

Nutrition Therapy (NIC)
Independent
Auscultate bowel sounds.

Maintain feeding tube: check for tube placement and flush with warm water, as indicated.

Monitor intake and weigh as indicated. Show client how to monitor and record weight on a scheduled basis.
Instruct client or SO/caregiver in self-feeding techniques—bulb syringe, bag and funnel method—and processing soft foods if client is to go home with a feeding tube. Make sure client and caregiver are able to perform this procedure before discharge and that appropriate food and equipment are available at home.
Begin with small feedings and advance as tolerated. Note signs of gastric fullness, regurgitation, and diarrhea.

RATIONALE

Feedings are usually begun after bowel sounds are restored postoperatively. *Note:* In more aggressive therapy, tube feeding may be started earlier if gastric residuals are closely monitored.
Tube is inserted during surgery and usually sutured in place. Initially, the tube may be attached to suction to reduce nausea or vomiting. Flushing aids in maintaining patency of tube.
Provides information regarding nutritional needs and effectiveness of therapy.
Helps promote nutritional success and preserves dignity in the adult who is now forced to depend on others for very basic needs in the social setting of meals.

Content of feeding may result in gastrointestinal (GI) intolerance, requiring change in rate or type of formula.

(continues on page 170)

ACTIONS/INTERVENTIONS (continued)	RATIONALE (continued)
Provide supplemental water by feeding tube or orally if client can swallow.	Keeps client hydrated to offset insensible losses and drainage from surgical areas. Meets free water needs associated with enteral feeding.
Encourage client when relearning swallowing—maintain quiet environment, have suction equipment on standby, and demonstrate appropriate breathing techniques.	Helps client deal with the frustration and safety concerns involved with swallowing. Provides reassurance that measures are available to prevent or limit aspiration.
Resume oral feedings when feasible. Stay with client during meals the first few days.	Oral feedings can usually resume after suture lines are healed (8 to 10 days) unless further reconstruction is required or client is going home with feeding tube. Client may experience pain or difficulty with chewing and swallowing initially and may require suctioning during meals in addition to support and encouragement.
Develop and encourage a pleasant environment for meals.	Promotes socialization and maximizes client comfort when eating difficulties cause embarrassment.
Help client and caregiver to develop nutritionally balanced home meal plans.	Promotes understanding of individual needs and significance of nutrition in healing and recovery process.
Collaborative	
Consult with dietitian or nutritional support team, as indicated. Incorporate and reinforce dietitian's teaching.	Useful in identifying individual nutritional needs to promote healing and tissue regeneration. Discharge teaching and follow-up by the dietitian may be needed to evaluate client needs for diet, equipment modifications, and meal planning in the home setting.
Provide nutritionally balanced diet with semisolid or soft foods or tube feedings and blended soft food or commercial preparations, as indicated.	Variations can be made to add or limit certain factors, such as fat and sugar, or to provide a food that client prefers.
Monitor laboratory studies, such as BUN, glucose, liver function, prealbumin, protein, and electrolytes.	Indicators of utilization of nutrients and organ function.

NURSING DIAGNOSIS: **disturbed Body Image/ineffective Role Performance**

May be related to
Loss of voice
Changes in anatomical contour of face and neck—disfigurement or severe functional impairment
Presence of chronic illness

Possibly evidenced by
Report of fear of rejection or reaction of others, change in social involvement, discomfort in social situations
Negative feelings about body change
Refusal to verify actual change or preoccupation with change or loss, not looking at self in mirror
Change in self or others' perception of role
Anxiety, depression, lack of eye contact
Failure of family members to adapt to change or deal with experience constructively

Desired Outcomes/Evaluation Criteria—Client Will

Body Image (NOC)
Identify feelings and methods for coping with negative perception of self.
Demonstrate initial adaptation to body changes as evidenced by participating in self-care activities and positive interactions with others.

Role Performance (NOC)
Communicate with SO about changes in role that have occurred.
Begin to develop plans for altered lifestyle.
Participate in team efforts toward rehabilitation.

ACTIONS/INTERVENTIONS	RATIONALE

Body Image [or] Role Enhancement (NIC)
Independent

Discuss meaning of loss or change with client, identifying perceptions of current situation and future expectations.

Note nonverbal body language, negative attitudes, and self-talk. Assess for self-destructive or suicidal behavior.

Note emotional reactions, such as grieving, depression, and anger. Allow client to progress at own rate.

Maintain calm, reassuring manner. Acknowledge and accept expression of feelings of grief and hostility.

Allow, but do not participate in, client's use of denial; for example, when client is reluctant to participate in self-care such as suctioning stoma. Provide care in a nonjudgmental manner.

Set limits on maladaptive behaviors, assisting client to identify positive behaviors that will aid recovery.

Encourage caregiver to treat client normally and not as an invalid.

Alert staff that facial expressions and other nonverbal behaviors need to convey acceptance and not revulsion.

Encourage identification of anticipated personal and work conflicts that may arise.

Recognize behavior indicative of overconcern with future lifestyle and relationship functioning.

Encourage client to deal with situation in small steps.

Provide positive reinforcement for efforts and any progress made.

Encourage client and SO to communicate feelings to each other.

Collaborative

Refer client and SO to supportive resources, such as psychotherapy, social worker, family counseling, and pastoral care.

Aids in identifying or defining the problem(s) to focus attention and interventions constructively.

May indicate depression and despair and need for further assessment or more intense intervention.

Client may experience immediate depression after surgery or react with shock and denial. Acceptance of changes cannot be forced, and the grieving process needs time for resolution.

May help allay client's fears of dying, suffocation, inability to communicate, or mutilation. Client and SO need to feel supported and know that all feelings are appropriate for the type of experience they are going through.

Denial may be the most helpful defense for client in the beginning, permitting the individual to begin to deal slowly with difficult adjustment.

Acting out can result in lowered self-esteem and impede adjustment to new self-image.

Distortions of body image may be unconsciously reinforced.

Client is very sensitive to nonverbal communication and may make negative assumptions about others' body language.

Expressions of concern bring problems into the open where they can be examined or dealt with.

Ruminating about anticipated losses and reactions of others is nonproductive and is a block to problem-solving.

May feel overwhelmed and have difficulty coping with larger picture, but can manage one piece at a time.

Encourages client to feel a sense of movement toward recovery.

All those involved may have difficulty in this area because of client's loss of voice function or disfigurement, but need to understand that they may gain courage and help from one another.

A multifaceted approach is required to assist client toward rehabilitation and wellness. Families need assistance in understanding the processes that client is going through and to help them with their own emotions. The goal is to enable them to guard against the tendency to withdraw or isolate client from social contact.

NURSING DIAGNOSIS: **deficient Knowledge [Learning Need] regarding prognosis, treatment, self-care, and discharge needs**

May be related to
Lack of information or recall
Misinterpretation of information
Poor assimilation of material presented; lack of interest in learning

Possibly evidenced by
Indications of concern, request for information
Inaccurate follow-through of instructions
Inappropriate or exaggerated behavior, such as hostile, agitated, apathetic

Desired Outcomes/Evaluation Criteria—Client Will

Knowledge: Disease Process (NOC)
Indicate basic understanding of disease process, surgical intervention, and prognosis.
Identify symptoms requiring medical evaluation and intervention.
Verbalize understanding of treatment regimen and rationale for actions.
Demonstrate ability to provide safe care.
Use resources, such as rehabilitation team members, appropriately.
Develop plan for and schedule follow-up appointments.

ACTIONS/INTERVENTIONS	RATIONALE

Learning Facilitation (NIC)

Independent

Ascertain amount of preoperative preparation and retention of information. Assess level of anxiety related to diagnosis and surgery.

Provide and repeat explanations at client's level of acceptance.

Provide written directions for client and caregiver to read and have available for future reference.

Information provides clues to client's postoperative reactions. Anxiety may have interfered with understanding of information given before surgery.

Limited knowledge is often present and presence of overwhelming stressors may impede understanding.

Reinforces proper information and may be used as a home reference.

Teaching: Disease Process (NIC)

Discuss inaccuracies in perception of disease process and therapies with client and SO.

Reinforce necessity of not smoking.

Discuss inability to smell and taste as before surgery.

Stress importance of reporting to physician immediately such symptoms as stoma narrowing, presence of "lump" in throat, dysphagia, or bleeding as well as changes in characteristics of pain.

Give careful attention to the provision of needed rehabilitative measures, such as temporary or permanent prosthesis, dental care, speech therapy, surgical reconstruction; vocational, sexual or marital counseling; and financial assistance.

Recommend wearing medical alert ID bracelet, identifying client as a neck breather. Encourage family members to become certified in cardiopulmonary resuscitation (CPR) if they are interested and able to do so.

Educate client and SO and caregiver about basic care and safety regarding stoma:

Shower with stoma collar; shampoo by leaning forward; no swimming or water sports

Cover stoma with foam or fiber filter, such as cotton or silk
Cover stoma when coughing or sneezing

Clean and maintain valve and prosthesis as indicated

Develop a means of emergency communication at home.
Identify homecare needs and available resources, such as supplies, support, and assistance.

Misconceptions are inevitable, but failure to explore and correct them can result in client's failing to progress toward health.

Necessary to preserve lung function. *Note:* Client may need extra support and encouragement to understand that respiratory function and quality of life can be improved by cessation of smoking.

Safety issues surround the inability to smell, including smoke from fire or odor from infection in stoma. Also, the loss of taste affects the desire to resume eating when client is otherwise able to do so.

May be signs of tracheal stenosis, recurrent cancer, or carotid erosion. *Note:* Postoperative myofascial pain dysfunction syndrome (MPDS), characterized by trigger points in muscle or at the junction of muscle and fascia that refer pain to other areas of the body, is often associated with head and neck surgery in cancer survivors (Polomano & Farrar, 2006).

These services can contribute to client's well-being and have a positive effect on client's quality of life.

Provides for appropriate care if client becomes unconscious or suffers a cardiopulmonary arrest.

Although the extra humidity provided by a shower can be beneficial by loosening secretions and enhancing expectoration, excessive water entering airway via stoma is detrimental.

Prevents dust and particles from being inhaled.
Normal airways are bypassed, and mucus will exit from stoma.

Stoma may be fitted with a valve or other type of prosthesis for maintaining the stoma opening, and in preparation of future speech.

Permits client to summon assistance when needed.
Provides support for transition from hospital setting.

POTENTIAL CONSIDERATIONS following acute hospitalization (dependent on client's age, physical condition and presence of complications, personal resources, and life responsibilities)

- *risk for Aspiration*—presence of tracheostomy, tube feedings, impaired swallowing, decreased muscle mass and strength (status after neck surgery)
- *impaired Verbal Communication*—anatomic presence of tracheostomy
- *risk for Infection*—broken skin and traumatized tissue, stasis of secretions, suppressed inflammatory response, chronic disease, malnutrition
- *imbalanced Nutrition: Less than Body Requirements*—temporary alteration in mode of food intake, altered feedback mechanisms relative to senses of taste and smell
- *Self-Care Deficit*—decreased strength and endurance, presence of pain, depression

VENTILATORY ASSISTANCE (MECHANICAL)

I. Pathophysiology—impairment of respiratory function affecting O_2 uptake and CO_2 elimination, requiring mechanical assist to support or replace spontaneous breathing

a. Inability to maintain adequate oxygenation (hypoxemia)

b. Inability to maintain adequate ventilation due to apnea or alveolar hypoventilation causing a rise in $PaCO_2$ and a fall in serum pH (respiratory acidosis)

c. Inability to continue the work of breathing (respiratory muscle weakness or failure)

II. Mechanical Ventilators

a. Classified by method of *cycling* from the inspiratory phase to the expiratory phase with signal to terminate the inspiratory activity of the machine:

  i. Preset volume (volume-cycled ventilator)

  ii. Preset pressure limit (pressure-cycled ventilator)

  iii. Preset time factor (time-cycled ventilator)

b. Mode of ventilation

  i. Assist control: provides a breath with either a preset volume for ventilator-initiated breaths or peak pressure every time client takes a breath

  ii. Pressure support ventilation: delivers preset level of positive airway pressure, rather than volume, to decrease work of breathing between ventilator-initiated breaths

  iii. Continuous positive airway pressure (CPAP): continuous level of elevated pressure during client-initiated breaths to maintain adequate oxygenation and decrease the work of breathing and the work of the heart

  iv. Positive end-expiratory pressure (PEEP): adjunct to mechanical ventilation using elevated pressure during the expiratory phase of the ventilatory cycle to increase functional residual capacity and surface area for gas exchange

c. Complications

  i. Associated with endotracheal (ET) tube: tissue damage to lips, tongue, throat; mucous plugs impairing ventilation and obstruction caused by client biting tube; auto PEEP; sinusitis or otitis; cuff herniation (rare)

  ii. Associated with the ventilator: infection, hemodynamic instability from positive-pressure ventilation, barotrauma, gastrointestinal (GI) bleeding due to stress ulcer

III. Etiology

a. Acute respiratory hypoxemia: pulmonary edema, severe pneumonia, sepsis, shock, acute respiratory distress syndrome (ARDS), embolism, drug reaction of overdose, lung trauma, high altitude

b. Acute respiratory acidosis: acute exacerbation of chronic emphysema or asthma

c. Respiratory muscle weakness or failure: paralysis of the diaphragm due to Guillain-Barré syndrome, myasthenia gravis, spinal cord injury, or the affects of anesthetic and muscle relaxant drugs; central nervous system (CNS) conditions, such as stroke, brain tumor, infections, sleep apnea; chest trauma, including fractures, pneumothorax

IV. Statistics

a. Morbidity: Acute respiratory failure requiring mechanical ventilation accounts for approximately 30% of admissions to intensive care units (ICUs) (Esteban et al, 2002).

b. Mortality: Hospital rate is 36%; 6-month mortality rate is approximately 67% for ages 65 and older (Seneff et al, 2000).

c. Cost: Mean ICU cost in United States is $31,574 to $42,570 per year (Dasta et al, 2005); average total hospital stay, $78,474; daily costs, $2,655; estimated cost for long-term acute-care facility admissions, $56,825 (Seneff, 2000).

GLOSSARY

Assist-control (AC) ventilation: Ventilator provides full mechanical support, delivering a preset rate or (if the client initiates a breath) a preset tidal volume or peak pressure. If the client fails to initiate a breath, the ventilator delivers the preset ventilator breath.

Assisted breath: Initiated by the client, but controlled and ended by the ventilator.

Auto-positive end-expiratory pressure (PEEP): Complication of mechanical ventilation where gas is trapped in alveoli at end expiration due to inadequate time for expiration, bronchoconstriction, or mucus plugging. It increases the work of breathing.

Barotrauma: Injury to the lungs due to local overinflation caused by high distending pressure in the intrapulmonary airways.

Cycling: Ventilator switches from inspiration to expiration; the flow has been delivered to the volume or pressure target.

Endotracheal (ET) tube: Tube inserted through the mouth into the trachea to facilitate passage of air into and out of the lungs.

Flow: Ventilator delivers a constant flow around the circuit throughout the respiratory cycle (flow-by). A deflection in this flow-by inspiration is monitored by the ventilator and it delivers a breath. This mechanism requires less work by the client than pressure triggering.

Hypercarbia: High level of carbon dioxide in the circulating blood.

Hyperventilation: Fast rate of respiration, which results in loss of carbon dioxide from the blood.

Hypoventilation: High partial pressure of alveolar CO_2 ($PaCO_2$).

Hypoxemia: Low oxygen levels in the blood.

Mandatory breath: Started, controlled, and ended by the ventilator.

Peak inspiratory pressure: Pressure in the lungs at the end of inspiration.

PEEP: Adjuvant to mode of ventilation used to help maintain functional residual capacity (FRC). At the end of expiration, PEEP exerts pressure to oppose passive emptying of lung, opening up collapsed alveoli and increasing surface area for gas exchange.

Positive-pressure ventilation: Increases pressure in airway, thus forcing air into lungs.

(text continues on page 174)

Care Setting

The focus of this plan of care is the client with invasive mechanical ventilation who remains on a ventilator, whether in an acute or postacute care setting. The expectation is that the majority of clients will be weaned before discharge. However, some clients are either unsuccessful at weaning or are not candidates for weaning. For these clients, portions of this plan of care would need to be modified for the discharge care setting, whether it be an extended care facility or home.

Related Concerns

Cardiac surgery: postoperative care, page 100
Chronic obstructive pulmonary disease (COPD) and asthma, page 120
Craniocerebral trauma (acute rehabilitative phase), page 220
Pneumothorax/hemothorax, page 154
Spinal cord injury (acute rehabilitative phase), page 271
Total nutritional support: parenteral/enteral feeding, page 469
Psychosocial aspects of care, page 749

Client Assessment Database

Gathered data depend on the underlying pathophysiology and reason for ventilatory support. Refer to the appropriate plan of care.

Discharge Plan Considerations

If ventilator-dependent, the plan may require changes in physical layout of home, acquisition of equipment and supplies, provision of a back-up power source, instruction of significant other (SO) and caregivers, provision for continuation of plan of care, assistance with transportation, and coordination of resources and support systems.

Refer to section at end of plan for postdischarge considerations.

Diagnostic Studies

TEST WHY IT IS DONE	WHAT IT TELLS ME
PULMONARY FUNCTION STUDIES Determine the ability of the lungs to exchange oxygen and carbon dioxide and include, but are not limited to, the following:	
• *Vital capacity (VC):* The total amount of air that can be exhaled after a maximum inspiration; the sum of the inspiratory reserve volume, the tidal volume, and the expiratory reserve volume.	Reduced in restrictive chest or lung conditions; normal or increased in COPD; normal to decreased in neuromuscular diseases, such as Guillain-Barré syndrome; and decreased in conditions limiting thoracic movement, such as kyphoscoliosis.
• *Forced vital capacity (FVC):* Total amount of air that can forcibly be blown out after full inspiration.	Reduced in restrictive conditions and in asthma and is normal to reduced in COPD.
• *Tidal volume (V_t):* Specific volume of air that is drawn into and then expired out of the lungs.	May be decreased in both restrictive and obstructive processes. *Note:* Negative inspiratory force (NIF) can be substituted for VC to help determine whether client can initiate a breath.
• *Minute ventilation (V_E):* Measures volume of air inhaled and exhaled in 1 minute of normal breathing.	This reflects muscle endurance and is a major determinant of work of breathing.
• *Inspiratory pressure (Pi_{max}); also called maximum inspiratory force (MIF):* Measures respiratory muscle strength upon inspiration.	Normal values should roughly equal the residual volume. Pi_{max} of less than 20 cm H_2O is considered insufficient for weaning.
• *Forced expiratory volume (FEV_1):* Measures amount of air in liters that a person can forcibly blow out in 1 second. Along with FVC, it is considered one of the primary indicators of lung function.	Usually decreased in obstructive and restrictive lung disorders.

Diagnostic Studies (continued)

TEST WHY IT IS DONE (continued)	WHAT IT TELLS ME (continued)
• *Flow-volume (F-V) loops:* Graphic record of lung function in which the amount of gas inhaled and exhaled is recorded on the horizontal axis and the rate at which the gas moves on the vertical axis.	Abnormal loops are indicative of large and small airway obstructive disease and restrictive diseases when far advanced.
OTHER DIAGNOSTIC STUDIES • *Arterial blood gases (ABGs):* Assesses status of oxygenation, ventilation, and acid-base balance via arterial blood.	ABG results help determine the settings for the ventilator, such as partial pressure of arterial oxygen (PaO_2), arterial oxygen saturation (SaO_2), and partial pressure of arterial carbon dioxide ($PaCO_2$).
• *Chest x-ray:* Procedure used to evaluate organs and structures within the chest.	Monitors resolution and progression of underlying condition, such as ARDS, atelectasis, and pneumonia.
• *Nutritional assessment:* Assesses albumin, prealbumin, serum transferrin, complete blood count (CBC), electrolytes, lipid profile, iron tests, blood urea nitrogen (BUN)/creatinine (Cr), glucose, and so on.	Done to identify nutritional imbalances that might prolong time on ventilator or interfere with successful weaning.

Nursing Priorities

1. Promote adequate ventilation and oxygenation.
2. Prevent complications.
3. Provide emotional support for client and SO.
4. Provide information about disease process, prognosis, and treatment needs.

Discharge Goals

1. Respiratory function maximized and adequate to meet individual needs
2. Complications prevented or minimized.
3. Effective means of communication established.
4. Disease process, prognosis, and therapeutic regimen understood, including home ventilatory support if indicated.
5. Plan in place to meet needs after discharge.

NURSING DIAGNOSIS: **ineffective Breathing Pattern/impaired Spontaneous Ventilation**

May be related to
Respiratory center depression
Respiratory muscle weakness or paralysis
Noncompliant lung tissue (decreased lung expansion)
Alteration of client's usual O_2/CO_2 ratio

Possibly evidenced by
Changes in rate and depth of respirations
Dyspnea and increased work of breathing, use of accessory muscles
Reduced VC and total lung volume
Tachypnea and bradypnea or cessation of respirations when off the ventilator
Cyanosis
Decreased PO_2 and SaO_2, increased PCO_2
Increased restlessness, apprehension, and metabolic rate

Desired Outcomes/Evaluation Criteria—Client Will

Respiratory Status: Ventilation (NOC)
Reestablish and maintain effective respiratory pattern via ventilator with absence of retractions and use of accessory muscles, cyanosis, or other signs of hypoxia; ABGs and oxygen saturation within acceptable range.
Participate in efforts to wean (as appropriate) within individual ability.

Caregiver Will

Demonstrate behaviors necessary to maintain client's respiratory function.

ACTIONS/INTERVENTIONS	RATIONALE

Mechanical Ventilation Management: Invasive (NIC)

Independent

Investigate etiology of respiratory failure.	Understanding the underlying cause of client's particular ventilatory problem is essential to the care of client, for example, decisions about future capabilities and ventilation needs and most appropriate type of ventilatory support.
Observe overall breathing pattern. Note respiratory rate, distinguishing between spontaneous respirations and ventilator breaths.	Client on a ventilator can experience hyperventilation, hypoventilation, or dyspnea and "air hunger" and attempt to correct deficiency by overbreathing.
Auscultate chest periodically, noting presence or absence and equality of breath sounds, adventitious breath sounds, and symmetry of chest movement.	Provides information regarding airflow through the tracheo-bronchial tree and the presence or absence of fluid, mucous obstruction. *Note:* Frequent crackles or rhonchi that do not clear with coughing or suctioning may indicate developing complications, such as atelectasis, pneumonia, acute bronchospasm, and pulmonary edema. Changes in chest symmetry may indicate improper placement of the ET tube or development of barotrauma.
Count client's respirations for 1 full minute and compare with desired respirations and ventilator set rate.	Respirations vary depending on problem requiring ventilatory assistance; for example, client may be totally ventilator dependent or be able to take breath(s) on own between ventilator-delivered breaths. Rapid client respirations can produce respiratory alkalosis and prevent desired volume from being delivered by ventilator. Slow client respirations and hypoventilation increases $PaCO_2$ levels and may cause acidosis.
Verify that client's respirations are in phase with the ventilator.	Adjustments may be required in flow, tidal volume, respiratory rate, and dead space of the ventilator, or client may need sedation to synchronize respirations and reduce work of breathing and energy expenditure.
Position client by elevating head of bed or chair if possible; place in prone position, as indicated.	Elevating the client's head and helping client get out of bed while still on the ventilator is both physically—helps decrease risk of aspiration—and psychologically beneficial. *Note:* Use of prone position is thought to improve oxygenation in client with severe hypoxic respiratory failure. However, it is not widely used due to the difficulties associated with placing and providing care to the intubated client in prone position as well as lack of studies showing its benefit in reducing mortality or duration of ventilation (Sud et al, 2008).
Inflate tracheal or ET tube cuff properly, using minimal leak and occlusive technique. Check cuff inflation every 4 to 8 hours and whenever cuff is deflated and reinflated.	The cuff must be properly inflated to ensure adequate ventilation and delivery of desired tidal volume and to decrease risk of aspiration. *Note:* In long-term clients, the cuff may be deflated most of the time or a noncuffed tracheostomy tube used if the client's airway is protected.
Check tubing for obstruction, such as kinking or accumulation of water. Drain tubing as indicated, avoiding draining toward client or back into the reservoir.	Kinks in tubing prevent adequate volume delivery and increase airway pressure. Condensation in tubing prevents proper gas distribution and predisposes to bacterial growth.
Check ventilator alarms for proper functioning. Do not turn off alarms, even for suctioning. Remove from ventilator and ventilate manually if source of ventilator alarm cannot be quickly identified and rectified. Ascertain that alarms can be heard in the nurses' station.	Ventilators have a series of visual and audible alarms, such as oxygen, low volume or apnea, high pressure, and inspiratory/expiratory (I:E) ratio. Turning off or failure to reset alarms places client at risk for unobserved ventilator failure or respiratory distress or arrest.
Keep resuscitation bag at bedside and ventilate manually whenever indicated.	Provides or restores adequate ventilation when client or equipment problems require client to be temporarily removed from the ventilator.
Assist client in "taking control" of breathing if weaning is attempted or ventilatory support is interrupted during procedure or activity.	Coaching client to take slower, deeper breaths; practice abdominal or pursed-lip breathing; assume position of comfort; and use relaxation techniques can be helpful in maximizing respiratory function.

Collaborative

Assess ventilator settings routinely and readjust, as indicated:	Controls or settings are adjusted according to client's primary disease and results of diagnostic testing to maintain parameters within appropriate limits.
Note operating mode of ventilation, that is, AC, pressure support (PS), and so on.	Client's respiratory requirements, presence or absence of an underlying disease process, and the extent to which client can participate in ventilatory effort determine parameters of each setting. PS has advantages for client on long-term ventilation because it allows client to strengthen pulmonary musculature without compromising oxygenation and ventilation during the weaning process.

ACTIONS/INTERVENTIONS (continued)	RATIONALE (continued)
Observe oxygen concentration percentage (FiO_2); verify that oxygen line is in proper outlet or tank; and monitor in-line oxygen analyzer or perform periodic oxygen analysis.	FiO_2 is adjusted (21% to 100%) to maintain an acceptable oxygen percentage and saturation, for example, 90%, for client's condition.
Observe end-tidal CO_2 ($ETCO_2$) values.	Measures the amount of exhaled CO_2 with each breath and is displayed graphically to spot CO_2 exchange problems early before they show up on ABGs. In some cases, a slightly higher level of CO_2 can be beneficial, such as for the client with long-standing emphysema. In this instance, elevated PCO_2 is accepted without correction, leading to the term "permissive hypercapnia" (Byrd et al, 2006).
Assess set respiratory frequency (f).	Respiratory rate of 10 to 15 per minute may be appropriate except for client with COPD and CO_2 retention. In these individuals, rate and volume should be adjusted to achieve personal baseline $PaCO_2$, not necessarily a "normal" $PaCO_2$.
Assess V_T. Verify proper function of spirometer, bellows, or computer readout of delivered volume; note alterations from desired volume delivery.	Monitors amount of air inspired and expired. Changes may indicate alteration in lung compliance or leakage through machine or around tube cuff. *Note:* For the client without preexisting lung disease, the V_T and rate are traditionally selected by using V_T of 12 mL/kg delivered 12 times per minute in the AC mode. For clients with COPD, the V_T and rate are slightly reduced to 10 mL/kg at 10 breaths per minute to prevent overinflation and hyperventilation (Girard & Bernard, 2007). Many clinicians now use a smaller V_T (6 to 8 mL/kg), especially in clients with ARDS and sometimes in obstructive and restrictive lung disease, in order to reduce air-trapping and mechanical stress on the lung.
Flow rate	Speed with which the V_T is delivered is usually about 50 L/min, but is variable in order to maintain I:E ratio appropriate for specific situation.
Pressure limit	Regulates the amount of pressure the volume-cycled ventilator can generate to deliver the preset V_T with usual setting at 10 to 20 cm H_2O above the client's peak inspiratory pressure. Airway pressure should remain relatively constant. Increased pressure alarm reading reflects (1) increased airway resistance as may occur with bronchospasm; (2) retained secretions; and (3) decreased lung compliance as may occur with obstruction of the ET tube, development of atelectasis, ARDS, pulmonary edema, worsening COPD, or pneumothorax. Low airway-pressure alarms may be triggered by pathophysiological conditions causing hypoventilation, such as disconnection from ventilator, low ET cuff pressure, ET tube displaced above the vocal cords, client "overbreathing," or out of phase with the ventilator.
Monitor I:E ratio	Expiratory phase is usually twice the length of the inspiratory rate, but may be longer to compensate for air-trapping to improve gas exchange in the client with COPD.
Set sigh rate, when used	Clinicians once recommended that periodic machine breaths that were 1.5 to 2 times the preset V_T be given 6 to 8 times per hour. At present, accounting for sighs is not recommended if the client is receiving V_T of 10 to 12 mL/kg or if PEEP is required. When a low V_T is used, sighs are preset at 1.5 to 2 times the V_T and delivered 6 to 8 times per hour if the peak and plateau pressures are within acceptable limits (Byrd et al, 2006).
Note inspired humidity and temperature; use heat moisture exchanger (HME), as indicated.	Usual warming and humidifying function of nasopharynx is bypassed with intubation. Dehydration can dry up normal pulmonary fluids, cause secretions to thicken, and increase risk of infection. Temperature should be maintained at about body temperature to reduce risk of damage to cilia and hyperthermia reactions. The introduction of a heated wire circuit to the traditional system significantly reduces the problem of "rainout" or condensation in the tubing.
Monitor serial ABGs and pulse oximetry.	Adjustments to ventilator settings may be required, depending on client's response and trends in gas exchange parameters.

NURSING DIAGNOSIS: ineffective Airway Clearance

May be related to
Foreign body (artificial airway) in the trachea
Inability to cough or ineffective cough

Possibly evidenced by
Changes in rate or depth of respiration
Cyanosis
Abnormal breath sounds
Anxiety and restlessness

Desired Outcomes/Evaluation Criteria—Client Will

Respiratory Status: Airway Patency (NOC)
Maintain patent airway with breath sounds clear.
Be free of aspiration.

Caregiver Will

Identify potential complications and initiate appropriate actions.

ACTIONS/INTERVENTIONS	RATIONALE
Artificial Airway Management (NIC) *Independent* Assess airway patency.	Obstruction may be caused by accumulation of secretions, mucous plugs, hemorrhage, bronchospasm, and problems with the position of tracheostomy or ET tube.
Evaluate chest movement and auscultate for bilateral breath sounds.	Symmetrical chest movement with breath sounds throughout lung fields indicates proper tube placement and unobstructed airflow. Lower airway obstruction, such as pneumonia or atelectasis, produces changes in breath sounds, such as rhonchi and wheezing.
Monitor ET tube placement. Note lip line marking and compare with desired placement. Secure tube carefully with tape or tube holder. Obtain assistance when retaping or repositioning tube.	The ET tube may slip into the right main-stem bronchus, thereby obstructing airflow to the left lung and putting client at risk for a tension pneumothorax.
Note excessive coughing, increased dyspnea (using a 0 to 10 scale), high-pressure alarm sounding on ventilator, visible secretions in endotracheal or tracheostomy tube, and increased rhonchi.	The intubated client often has an ineffective cough reflex, or client may have neuromuscular or neurosensory impairment, altering ability to cough. Client is usually dependent on suctioning to remove secretions. *Note:* Research supports use of a dyspnea rating scale (like those used to measure pain) to more accurately quantify and measure changes in dyspnea as experienced by client.
Suction as needed when client is coughing or experiencing respiratory distress, limiting duration of suction to 15 seconds or less. Choose appropriate suction catheter. Hyperventilate before and after each catheter pass, using 100% oxygen if appropriate, using vent rather than Ambu bag, which has an increased risk of barotrauma. Suction continuously or intermittently during withdrawal.	Suctioning should not be routine, and duration should be limited to reduce hazard of hypoxia. Suction catheter diameter should be less than 50% of the internal diameter of the ET or tracheostomy tube for prevention of hypoxia. Hyperoxygenation with ventilator sigh on 100% oxygen may be desired to reduce atelectasis and to reduce accidental hypoxia. *Note:* Instilling normal saline (NS) is no longer recommended (although it persists in practice) because research reveals that the fluid pools at the distal end of the ET or tracheal tube, impairing oxygenation and increasing bronchospasm and the risk of infection.
Use inline catheter suction when available.	Reduces risk of infection for healthcare workers and helps maintain oxygen saturation and PEEP when used.
Instruct client in coughing techniques during suctioning, such as splinting, timing of breathing, and "quad cough," as indicated.	Enhances effectiveness of cough effort and secretion clearing.
Reposition or turn periodically.	Promotes drainage of secretions and ventilation to all lung segments, reducing risk of atelectasis.
Encourage the client to drink fluids and provide fluids within individual capability.	Helps liquefy secretions, enhancing expectoration.

ACTIONS/INTERVENTIONS (continued)

Collaborative

Provide chest physiotherapy as indicated, such as postural drainage and percussion.

Administer intravenous (IV) and aerosol bronchodilators as indicated: aminophylline, albuterol sulfate (Proventil); albuterol/atrovent combination (such as Duoneb); inhaled steroids (such as Pulmicort, Flovent, etc.).

Assist with fiber-optic bronchoscopy, if indicated.

RATIONALE (continued)

Promotes ventilation of all lung segments and aids drainage of secretions.

Promotes ventilation and removal of secretions by relaxation of smooth muscle or bronchospasm.

May be performed to remove secretions and mucous plugs.

NURSING DIAGNOSIS: impaired verbal Communication

May be related to

Physical barrier, such as ET or tracheostomy tube

Neuromuscular weakness or paralysis

Possibly evidenced by

Inability to speak

Desired Outcomes/Evaluation Criteria—Client Will

Communication: Expressive Ability (NOC)

Establish method of communication in which needs can be understood.

ACTIONS/INTERVENTIONS

RATIONALE

Communication Enhancement: Speech Deficit (NIC)

Independent

Assess client's ability to communicate by alternative means.

Reasons for long-term ventilatory support are various; client may be alert and be adept at writing (such as chronic COPD with inability to be weaned) or may be lethargic, comatose, or paralyzed. Method of communicating with client is therefore highly individualized. *Note:* The inability to talk while intubated is a primary cause of feelings of fear.

Establish means of communication, for example, maintain eye contact; ask yes/no questions; provide magic slate, paper and pencil, or picture or alphabet board; use sign language as appropriate; and validate meaning of attempted communications.

Eye contact assures client of interest in communicating; if client is able to move head, blink eyes, or is comfortable with simple gestures, a great deal can be done with yes/no questions. Pointing to letter boards or writing is often tiring to client, who can then become frustrated with the effort needed to attempt conversations. Use of picture boards that express a concept or routine needs may simplify communication. Family members and other caregivers may be able to assist and interpret needs.

Consider form of communication when placing IV.

Place call light or bell within reach, making certain client is alert and physically capable of using it. Answer call light or bell immediately. Anticipate needs. Tell client that nurse is immediately available should assistance be required.

IV positioned in hand or wrist may limit ability to write or sign.

Ventilator-dependent client may be better able to relax, feel safe (not abandoned), and breathe with the ventilator knowing that nurse is vigilant and needs will be met.

Place note at central call station informing staff that client is unable to speak.

Alerts all staff members to respond to client at the bedside instead of over the intercom.

Encourage family and SO to talk with client, providing information about family and daily happenings.

SO may feel self-conscious in one-sided conversation, but knowledge that he or she is assisting client to regain or maintain contact with reality and enabling client to feel part of family unit can reduce feelings of awkwardness.

Collaborative

Evaluate need for or appropriateness of talking tracheostomy tube.

Client with adequate cognitive and muscular skills may have the ability to manipulate talking tracheostomy tube.

NURSING DIAGNOSIS: Fear/Anxiety [specify level]

May be related to
Situational crises; threat to self-concept
Threat of death, dependency on mechanical support
Change in health, socioeconomic status, or role functioning
Interpersonal transmission or contagion

Possibly evidenced by
Increased muscle and facial tension
Insomnia and restlessness
Hypervigilance
Feelings of inadequacy
Fearfulness, uncertainty, apprehension
Focus on self and negative self-talk
Expressed concern regarding changes in life events

Desired Outcomes/Evaluation Criteria—Client Will

Fear Self-Control [or] Anxiety Self-Control (NOC)
Verbalize or communicate awareness of feelings and healthy ways to deal with them.
Demonstrate problem-solving skills or behaviors to cope with current situation.
Report that anxiety or fear is reduced to manageable level.
Appear relaxed and sleeping or resting appropriately.

ACTIONS/INTERVENTIONS	RATIONALE
Anxiety Reduction (NIC)	
Independent	
Identify client's perception of threat represented by situation. Determine current respiratory status and adequacy of ventilation.	Defines scope of individual problem separate from physiological causes, and influences choice of interventions.
Observe and monitor physical responses, such as restlessness, changes in vital signs, and repetitive movements. Note congruency of verbal/nonverbal communication.	Useful in evaluating extent or degree of concerns, especially when compared with "verbal" comments.
Encourage client and SO to acknowledge and express fears.	Provides opportunity for dealing with concerns, clarifies reality of fears, and reduces anxiety to a more manageable level.
Acknowledge the anxiety and fear of the situation. Avoid meaningless reassurance that everything will be all right.	Validates the reality of the situation without minimizing the emotional impact. Provides opportunity for client and SO to accept and begin to deal with what has happened, reducing anxiety.
Identify and review with client and SO the safety precautions being taken, such as backup power and oxygen supplies and emergency equipment at hand for suctioning. Discuss or review the meanings of alarm system.	Provides reassurance to help allay unnecessary anxiety, reduce concerns of the unknown, and preplan for response in emergency situation.
Note reactions of SO. Provide opportunity for discussion of personal feelings, concerns, and future expectations.	Family members have individual responses to what is happening, and their anxiety may be communicated to client, intensifying these emotions.
Identify previous coping strengths of client and SO and current areas of control and ability.	Focuses attention on own capabilities, increasing sense of control.
Demonstrate and encourage use of relaxation techniques, such as focused breathing, guided imagery, and progressive relaxation. Provide music therapy and biofeedback as appropriate.	Provides active management of situation to reduce feelings of helplessness.
Provide and encourage sedentary diversional activities within individual capabilities, such as handicrafts, writing, and television.	Although handicapped by dependence on ventilator, activities that are normal or desired by the individual should be encouraged to enhance quality of life.
Collaborative	
Refer to support individuals, groups, and therapy, as needed.	May be necessary to provide additional assistance if client and SO are not managing anxiety or when client is "identified with the machine."

NURSING DIAGNOSIS: impaired Oral Mucous Membrane

Risk factors may include
Inability to swallow oral fluids
Presence of tube in mouth
Lack of or decreased salivation
Ineffective oral hygiene

Possibly evidenced by
(Not applicable; presence of signs and symptoms establishes an *actual* diagnosis)

Desired Outcomes/Evaluation Criteria—Client Will

Tissue Integrity: Skin and Mucous Membrane (NOC)
Report or demonstrate a decrease in symptoms.

Caregiver Will

Identify specific interventions to promote healthy oral mucosa as appropriate.

ACTIONS/INTERVENTIONS	RATIONALE
Oral Health Maintenance (NIC)	
Independent	
Routinely inspect oral cavity, teeth, gums for sores, lesions, and bleeding.	Early identification of problems provides opportunity for appropriate intervention and preventive measures.
Administer mouth care routinely per protocol and as needed, especially in client with an oral intubation tube; for example, cleanse mouth with water, saline, or preferred alcohol-free mouthwash. Brush teeth with soft toothbrush, WaterPik, or moistened swab.	Prevents drying and ulceration of mucous membrane and reduces medium for bacterial growth. Promotes comfort.
Change position of ET tube and airway on a regular and prn (as necessary) schedule as appropriate.	Reduces risk of lip and oral mucous membrane ulceration.
Apply lip balm; administer oral lubricant solution.	Maintains moisture and prevents drying.

NURSING DIAGNOSIS: imbalanced Nutrition: Less than Body Requirements

May be related to
Altered ability to ingest and properly digest food
Increased metabolic demands

Possibly evidenced by
Weight loss and poor muscle tone
Aversion to eating; reported altered taste sensation
Sore, inflamed buccal cavity
Absence of or hyperactive bowel sounds

Desired Outcomes/Evaluation Criteria—Client Will

Nutritional Status (NOC)
Indicate understanding of individual dietary needs.
Demonstrate progressive weight gain toward goal with normalization of laboratory values.

ACTIONS/INTERVENTIONS	RATIONALE
Nutrition Therapy (NIC)	
Independent	
Evaluate ability to eat.	Client with a tracheostomy tube may be able to eat, but client with ET tube must be tube fed or parenterally nourished.
Observe and monitor for generalized muscle wasting and loss of subcutaneous fat.	These symptoms are indicative of depletion of muscle energy and can reduce respiratory muscle function.
Weigh, as indicated.	Significant and recent weight loss (7% to 10% body weight) and poor nutritional intake provide clues regarding catabolism, muscle glycogen stores, and ventilatory drive sensitivity.
Document oral intake if and when resumed. Offer foods that client enjoys.	Appetite is usually poor and intake of essential nutrients may be reduced. Offering favorite foods can enhance oral intake.

(continues on page 182)

Provide small frequent feedings of soft and easily digested foods if able to swallow.

Prevents excessive fatigue, enhances intake, and reduces risk of gastric distress.

Encourage or administer fluid intake of at least 2,500 mL/day within cardiac tolerance.

Prevents dehydration that can be exacerbated by increased insensible losses (ventilator or intubation) and reduces risk of constipation.

Assess GI function: presence and quality of bowel sounds and changes in abdominal girth, nausea, and vomiting. Observe and document changes in bowel movements, such as diarrhea and constipation. Test all stools for occult blood.

A functioning GI system is essential for the proper utilization of enteral feedings. Mechanically ventilated clients are at risk of developing abdominal distention (trapped air or ileus) and gastric bleeding (stress ulcers).

Collaborative

Adjust diet to meet respiratory needs, as indicated.

High intake of carbohydrates, protein, and calories may be desired or needed during ventilation to improve respiratory muscle function. Carbohydrates may be reduced and fat somewhat increased just before weaning attempts to prevent excessive CO_2 production and reduced respiratory drive.

Administer tube feeding or hyperalimentation, as needed. (Refer to CP: Total Nutritional Support: Parenteral/Enteral Feeding.)

Provides adequate nutrients to meet individual needs when oral intake is insufficient or not appropriate.

Monitor laboratory studies as indicated, such as prealbumin, serum transferrin, BUN/Cr, and glucose.

Provides information about adequacy of nutritional support or need for change.

NURSING DIAGNOSIS: **risk for Infection**

Risk factors may include

Inadequate primary defenses—traumatized lung tissue, decreased ciliary action, stasis of body fluids

Inadequate secondary defenses—immunosuppression

Chronic disease, malnutrition

Invasive procedure—intubation

Possibly evidenced by

(Not applicable; presence of signs and symptoms establishes an *actual* diagnosis)

Desired Outcomes/Evaluation Criteria—Client Will

Knowledge: Infection Control (NOC)

Indicate understanding of individual risk factors.

Identify interventions to prevent or reduce risk of infection.

Demonstrate techniques to promote safe environment.

ACTIONS/INTERVENTIONS

RATIONALE

Infection Protection (NIC)

Independent

Note risk factors for occurrence of infection.

Intubation interferes with the normal defense mechanisms that keep microorganisms out of the lungs. ET tubes, especially cuffed ones, interfere with the mucociliary transport system that helps clear airway secretions. Secretions that accumulate below and above the ET tube cuff are ideal growth medium for pathogens. The ET tube also prevents normal closure of the epiglottis, resulting in an incomplete seal of the laryngeal structures that normally protect the lungs. This can contribute to aspiration, which often leads to ventilator-associated pneumonia (VAP) (Pruitt & Jacobs, 2006). VAP is the primary cause of hospital-acquired pneumonia (HAP) reportedly occurring in 10% to 25% of individuals receiving mechanical ventilation (Byrd et al, 2006). Other factors include prolonged mechanical ventilation, trauma, general debilitation, malnutrition, age, and invasive procedures. Awareness of individual risk factors provides opportunity to limit effects and helps prevent VAP.

Observe color, odor, and characteristics of sputum. Note drainage around tracheostomy tube.

Yellow or green, purulent odorous sputum is indicative of infection; thick, tenacious sputum suggests dehydration.

ACTIONS/INTERVENTIONS (continued)

Engage in proper hand washing or alcohol-based hand rubs, wear gloves when handling respiratory secretions and equipment contaminated with respiratory secretions, maintain sterile suction techniques in open system, use closed-system ET tube allowing for continuous removal of secretions, reduce the number of times the ventilator tubes are open, and provide clean nebulizer and tubing changes.

Encourage deep breathing, coughing, and frequent position changes.

Auscultate breath sounds.

Provide or instruct client and SO in proper oral care and secretion disposal, such as disposing of tissues and soiled tracheostomy dressings.

Monitor and screen visitors. Avoid contact with persons with respiratory infections.

Provide respiratory isolation when indicated.

Maintain adequate hydration and nutrition. Encourage fluids to 2,500 mL/day within cardiac tolerance.

Measure pH of gastric secretions, and monitor use of antacid medications, as indicated.

Encourage self-care and activities to limit of tolerance. Assist with graded exercise program.

Collaborative

Obtain sputum cultures as indicated.

Administer antimicrobials, as indicated.

RATIONALE (continued)

These factors may be the simplest but are the most important keys to prevention of hospital-acquired infection. *Note:* The Centers for Disease Control and Prevention's (CDC) (2005) guidelines recommend changing tubing no more often than every 48 hours. Research indicates that less frequent tubing changes (every 5 to 7 days) may be acceptable.

Maximizes lung expansion and mobilization of secretions to prevent or reduce atelectasis and accumulation of sticky, thick secretions.

Presence of rhonchi and wheezes suggests retained secretions requiring expectoration or suctioning.

Reduces risk of pneumonia associated with aspiration of oral bacteria, as well as transmission of fluidborne organisms. *Note:* Chlorhexidine mouth rinse has been found to reduce plaque and gingival inflammation as a means of preventing VAP.

Individual is already compromised and is at increased risk with exposure to infections.

Depending on specific diagnosis, client may require protection from others or must prevent transmission of infection, for example, tuberculosis (TB) to others.

Helps improve general resistance to disease and reduces risk of infection from static secretions.

Maintaining acid level of stomach about pH of 7.2 may help reduce risk of nosocomial infection and stress ulcers and contamination of respiratory tract by means of reflux and aspiration.

Improves general well-being and muscle strength and may stimulate immune system recovery.

May be needed to identify pathogens and appropriate antimicrobials. *Note:* Bacteria are the most frequently isolated pathogens for VAP.

If infection does occur, one or more agents may be used, depending on identified pathogen(s).

NURSING DIAGNOSIS: **risk for dysfunctional Ventilatory Weaning Response**

Risk factors may include

Sleep disturbance

Limited or insufficient energy stores

Pain or discomfort

Adverse environment, such as inadequate monitoring or support

Client-perceived inability to wean; decreased motivation

History of extended weaning

Possibly evidenced by

(Not applicable; presence of signs and symptoms establishes an *actual* diagnosis)

Desired Outcomes/Evaluation Criteria—Client Will

Respiratory Status: Ventilation (NOC)

Actively participate in the weaning process.

Reestablish independent respiration with ABGs within acceptable range and free of signs of respiratory failure.

Demonstrate increased tolerance for activity and participate in self-care within level of ability.

ACTIONS/INTERVENTIONS	RATIONALE

Mechanical Ventilatory Weaning (NIC)

Independent

Assess physical factors involved in weaning as follows:

Stable heart rate/rhythm, blood pressure (BP), and clear breath sounds

The heart has to work harder to meet increased energy needs associated with weaning. Physician may defer weaning if tachycardia, pulmonary crackles, or hypertension are present.

Fever

Increase of 1°F (0.6°C) in body temperature raises metabolic rate and oxygen demands by 7%.

Nutritional status and muscle strength

Weaning is hard work. Client not only must be able to withstand the stress of weaning but also must have the stamina to breathe spontaneously for extended periods.

Determine psychological readiness

Weaning provokes anxiety for client regarding concerns about ability to breathe on own and long-term need of ventilator.

Explain weaning techniques, for example, spontaneous breathing trial (SBT), T-piece, pressure support ventilation (PSV), and spontaneous intermittent maximal ventilation (SIMV). Discuss individual plan and expectations.

Assists client to prepare for weaning process, helps limit fear of unknown, promotes cooperation, and enhances likelihood of a successful outcome. *Note:* Current guidelines recommend SBT as the preferred method of weaning as it withdraws ventilatory support while oxygenation is continued. The simplest form of SBT is the T-piece trial. In PSV weaning, all breaths are spontaneous and combined with enough pressure support to ensure that each breath is a reasonable tidal volume. Findings from randomized trials suggest that SIMV weaning delays extubation compared with PSV and SBT and that it should not be the primary mode of weaning in most clients (Byrd et al, 2006).

Provide undisturbed rest and sleep periods. Avoid stressful procedures or situations and nonessential activities.

Maximizes energy for weaning process; limits fatigue and oxygen consumption. *Note:* It takes approximately 12 to 14 hours of respiratory rest to rejuvenate tired respiratory muscles. For clients on AC, raising the rate to 20 breaths per minute can also provide respiratory rest.

Evaluate and document client's progress. Note restlessness; changes in BP, heart rate, and respiratory rate; use of accessory muscles; discoordinated breathing with ventilator; increased concentration on breathing (mild dysfunction); client's concerns about possible machine malfunction; inability to cooperate or respond to coaching; and color changes.

Indicators that client may require slower weaning and an opportunity to stabilize, or may need to stop program. *Note:* Moving from pressure/volume (such as assist/control) ventilator to T-piece may precipitate a "flash" form of heart failure requiring prompt intervention.

Recognize and provide encouragement for client's efforts.

Positive feedback provides reassurance and support for continuation of weaning process.

Monitor cardiopulmonary response to activity.

Excessive oxygen consumption and demand increases the possibility of failure.

Collaborative

Consult with dietitian and nutritional support team for adjustments in composition of diet.

Reduction of carbohydrates and fats may be required to prevent excessive production of CO_2, which could alter respiratory drive.

Monitor CBC, serum albumin and prealbumin, transferrin, total iron-binding capacity, and electrolytes, especially potassium, calcium, and phosphorus.

Verifies that nutrition is adequate to meet energy requirements for weaning.

Review chest x-ray and ABGs.

Chest x-rays should show clear lungs or marked improvement in pulmonary congestion or infiltrates. ABGs should document satisfactory oxygenation on an Fio_2 of 40% or less.

NURSING DIAGNOSIS: **deficient Knowledge [Learning Need] regarding condition, prognosis and therapy, self-care, and discharge needs**

May be related to
Lack of exposure or recall
Misinterpretation of information; unfamiliarity with information resources
Stress of situational crisis

Possibly evidenced by
Questions about care, request for information
Reluctance to learn new skills
Inaccurate follow-through of instructions
Development of preventable complications

Desired Outcomes/Evaluation Criteria—Client/SO/Caregiver Will

Health-Seeking Behavior (NOC)
Participate in learning process.
Exhibit increased interest, shown by verbal or nonverbal cues.
Assume responsibility for own learning and begin to look for information and to ask questions.

Knowledge: Treatment Regimen (NOC)
Indicate understanding of mechanical ventilation therapy.
Demonstrate behaviors or new skills to meet individual needs and prevent complications.

ACTIONS/INTERVENTIONS	RATIONALE
Learning Facilitation (NIC)	
Independent	
Determine ability and willingness to learn.	Physical condition may preclude client involvement in care before and after discharge. SO/caregiver may feel inadequate, afraid of machinery, and have reservations about ability to learn or deal with overall situation.
Schedule teaching sessions for quiet, nonstressful times when all participants are well rested.	Enhances learners' ability to focus on and absorb content provided.
Arrange information in logical sequence, progressing from simple to more complex material at learners' pace.	Allows learner to build on information learned in previous sessions; is less threatening and overwhelming.
Knowledge: Disease Process (NIC)	
Provide material in multiple formats, such as books and pamphlets, audiovisuals, hands-on demonstrations, and take-home instruction sheets, as appropriate.	Uses multiple senses to stimulate learning and retention of information. Provides resources for review following discharge.
Discuss specific condition requiring ventilatory support, what measures are being tried for weaning, and short- and long-term goals of treatment.	Provides knowledge base to aid client and SO in making informed decisions. Weaning efforts may continue for several weeks (extended period of time). Dependence is evidenced by repeatedly increased PCO_2 and decline in PaO_2 during weaning attempts, presence of dyspnea, anxiety, tachycardia, perspiration, and cyanosis.
Encourage client and SO to evaluate impact of ventilatory dependence on their lifestyle and what changes they are willing or unwilling to make. Problem-solve solutions to issues raised.	Quality of life must be resolved by the ventilator-dependent client and caregivers who need to understand that home ventilatory support is a 24-hour job that affects everyone.
Promote participation in self-care and diversional activities and socialization, as appropriate.	Refocuses attention toward more normal life activities, increases endurance, and helps prevent depersonalization.
Review issues of general well-being: role of nutrition, assistance with feeding and meal preparation, graded exercise and specific restrictions, and rest periods alternated with activity.	Enhances recuperation and ensures that individual needs will be met.
Recommend that SO and caregivers learn cardiopulmonary resuscitation (CPR).	Provides sense of security about ability to handle emergency situations that might arise until help can be obtained.
Schedule team conference. Establish in-hospital training for caregivers if client is to be discharged home on ventilator.	Team approach is needed to coordinate client's care and teaching program to meet individual needs.
Instruct caregiver and client in hand-washing techniques, use of sterile technique for suctioning, tracheostomy or stoma care, and chest physiotherapy.	Reduces risk of infection and promotes optimal respiratory function.
Provide demonstration and "hands-on" sessions, as well as written material, about specific type of ventilator to be used, including function and care of equipment.	Enhances familiarity, reducing anxiety and promoting confidence in implementation of new tasks and skills.

(continues on page 186)

Discuss what and when to report to the healthcare provider, for example, signs of respiratory distress and infection.

Helps reduce general anxiety while promoting timely and appropriate evaluation and intervention to prevent complications.

Ascertain that all needed equipment is in place and that safety concerns have been addressed, such as alternative power source (generator, batteries), back-up equipment, and client call and alarm system.

Predischarge preparations can ease the transfer process. Planning for potential problems increases sense of security for client and SO.

Contact community or hospital-based services.

Suppliers of home equipment, physical therapy, care providers, emergency power provider, and social services, such as financial assistance, aid in procuring equipment and personnel and facilitate transition to home.

Refer to vocational or occupational therapist.

Some ventilator-dependent clients are able to resume vocations either while on the ventilator or during the day (while ventilator-dependent at night).

POTENTIAL CONSIDERATIONS following acute hospitalization (dependent on client's age, physical condition and presence of complications, personal resources, and life responsibilities)

If client is discharged on ventilator, the client's needs and concerns remain the same as noted in this plan of care, in addition to the following:

- *Self-Care Deficit*—decreased strength and endurance, inability to perform activities of daily living (ADLs), depression, restrictions imposed by therapeutic intervention
- *interrupted Family Processes*—situational crisis
- *risk for Relocation Stress Syndrome*—feelings of powerlessness, concern about adequacy of support, unpredictability of experiences
- *risk for Caregiver Role Strain*—severity of illness of care receiver, discharge of family member with significant home care needs, presence of situational stressors (economic vulnerability, changes in roles and responsibilities), duration of caregiving required, inexperience in caregiving

---

PULMONARY TUBERCULOSIS (TB)

I. Pathophysiology
  a. Bacterial infection by *Mycobacterium tuberculosis* bacilli (TB)
    i. Primarily affects the lungs (70% per Centers for Disease Control and Prevention [CDC], 2004) although it can invade other body systems
    ii. Airborne droplets are inhaled, with the droplet nuclei deposited within the alveoli of the lung.
  b. Primary infection followed by a latent or dormant phase, or by active disease in some individuals
  c. When the immune system weakens, dormant TB organisms can reactivate and multiply (reactivation TB).

II. Classifications
  a. Latent: Body's immune system has encapsulated the bacteria into tiny capsules called tubercles, infection not transmissible to others.
  b. Active: Infection is spreading in the body and can be transmitted to others.

III. Etiology
  a. Following exposure, the bacilli may (1) be killed by the immune system, (2) multiply and cause primary TB, (3) become dormant and remain asymptomatic, or (4) proliferate after a latency period (reactivation disease) (Herchline & Amorosa, 2007).
  b. Multidrug-resistant tuberculosis (MDR-TB)
    i. Primary: caused by person-to-person transmission of a drug-resistant organism

    ii. Secondary: usually the result of nonadherence to therapy or inappropriate treatment
    iii. On the rise especially in large cities, in those previously treated with antitubercular drugs, or in those who failed to follow or complete a drug regimen
    iv. Can progress from diagnosis to death in as little as 4 to 6 weeks
  c. Risk factors: individuals with weakened immune systems due to chronic conditions, advanced age, and malnutrition; higher among persons with HIV infection, the homeless, drug-addicted, and impoverished populations, as well as among immigrants from or visitors to countries in which TB is endemic

IV. Statistics (Centers for Disease Control and Prevention [CDC], 2005, 2007)
  a. Morbidity: In 2005, 14,903 cases of TB were reported in the United States (down from a peak of 25,287 cases in 1993), with foreign-born individuals accounting for a steadily increasing proportion (54%) of all reported TB cases (Herschline, 2007); globally, 9.2 million new cases reported annually.
  b. Morbidity: Globally, 1.7 million deaths from TB occurred in 2006, of which 0.2 million deaths were in HIV-positive individuals (World Health Organization [WHO], 2008).

Acid-fast bacilli (AFB): Rod-shaped bacteria that can be seen and counted under the microscope on a specially stained sputum sample on a glass slide, called an AFB smear. The most common AFB are members of the genus *Mycobacterium*.

Cavitation: The formation of cavities in a body tissue or an organ, especially those formed in the lung as a result of TB. In cavitary disease, breath sounds are high pitched and hollow (like blowing over the end of an empty bottle).

Directly observed treatment (DOT): Healthcare worker observes client taking antitubercular medications. DOT provides a mechanism for early detection of adverse medication reactions or nonadherence with medication regimen in high-risk clients or environments, such as jails, homeless shelters, crowded worksites, among others.

Fremitus: Sensation felt by a hand placed on the chest that vibrates during speech.

Tubular breath sounds: Low pitched and sticky and occurs over areas of consolidation.

Whispered pectoriloquies: Transmission of the voice sound through the pulmonary structures so that it is unusually audible on auscultation of the chest, indicating either consolidation of the lung parenchyma or the presence of a large cavity.

Care Setting

Most clients are treated in community clinics, but may be hospitalized for diagnostic evaluation or initiation of therapy, adverse drug reactions, or severe illness or debilitation. This plan of care is intended to reflect care of the person with active (rather than latent) TB, although if latent, when TB is diagnosed, treatment will be initiated.

Related Concerns

Extended care, page 801
Pneumonia, page 131
Psychosocial aspects of care, page 749

Client Assessment Database

Data depend on stage of disease and degree of involvement.

DIAGNOSTIC DIVISION MAY REPORT	MAY EXHIBIT
ACTIVITY/REST • Generalized weakness and fatigue • Shortness of breath with exertion • Difficulty sleeping, with evening or night fever, chills, and sweats • Nightmares	• Tachycardia, tachypnea/dyspnea on exertion • Muscle wasting, pain, and stiffness (advanced stages)
EGO INTEGRITY • Recent or long-standing stress factors • Financial concerns, poverty • Feelings of helplessness and hopelessness	• Denial (especially during early stages) • Anxiety, apprehension, irritability • Inattention, marked irritability, change in mentation (advanced stages)
FOOD/FLUID • Loss of appetite • Indigestion • Weight loss • Night sweats	• Poor skin turgor, dry and flaky skin • Muscle wasting and loss of subcutaneous fat
PAIN/DISCOMFORT • Chest pain aggravated by recurrent cough	• Guarding of affected area • Distraction behaviors, restlessness

(continues on page 188)

DIAGNOSTIC DIVISION MAY REPORT (continued)	MAY EXHIBIT (continued)
RESPIRATION • History of TB or exposure to infected individual • Persistent cough, productive or nonproductive • Shortness of breath	*Breath sounds:* • Diminished bilaterally or unilaterally (pleural effusion or pneumothorax); tubular breath sounds and/or whispered pectoriloquies over large lesions; crackles may be noted over apex of lungs during quick inspiration after a short cough (post-tussive crackles) • Increased respiratory rate is associated with extensive disease or fibrosis of the lung parenchyma and pleura • Asymmetry in respiratory excursion (pleural effusion) • Dullness to percussion and decreased fremitus (pleural fluid or pleural thickening) • *Sputum characteristics:* may be green, or purulent, mucoid, or blood tinged
SAFETY • Presence of immunosuppressed conditions, such as AIDS, cancer • Positive HIV test; HIV infection • Visit to, immigration from, or close contact with persons in countries with high prevalence of TB, such as Central America, Southeast Asia, subcontinental India, Russia	• Low-grade fever or acute febrile illness • Enlarged lymph nodes in neck
SOCIAL INTERACTION • Feelings of isolation and rejection because of communicable disease • Change in usual patterns of responsibility or change in physical capacity to resume role	
TEACHING/LEARNING • Familial history of TB • General debilitation and poor health status • Use or abuse of substances such as intravenous (IV) drugs, cocaine, and crack • Failure to improve or reactivation of TB • Nonparticipation in therapy	
DISCHARGE PLAN CONSIDERATIONS • Assistance with or alteration in drug therapy • Temporary assistance in self-care and homemaker and maintenance tasks ◗ Refer to section at end of plan for postdischarge considerations.	

Diagnostic Studies

TEST WHY IT IS DONE	WHAT IT TELLS ME
BLOOD TESTS • *Enzyme-linked immunosorbent assay (ELISA) and Western blot:* Detects antibodies to a foreign substance, such as a bacterium.	May reveal presence of HIV, which is a strong risk factor in development of TB.
• *Arterial blood gases (ABGs):* Assess levels of oxygen (PaO_2) and carbon dioxide ($PaCO_2$) in arterial blood.	May be abnormal, depending on location, severity, and residual damage to the lungs.

Diagnostic Studies (continued)

TEST WHY IT IS DONE (continued)	WHAT IT TELLS ME (continued)
• *Electrolytes:* Substances that, in solution, conduct an electric current and are decomposed by its passage. Sodium, potassium, and magnesium are common electrolytes.	May be abnormal, depending on the location and severity of infection; for example, low sodium (hyponatremia) caused by abnormal water retention may be found in extensive chronic pulmonary TB.
• *QuantiFERON TB Gold Test (QFT-G):* Measures immune reactivity to *M. tuberculosis.*	Helps confirm or rule out a latent or active TB infection. Results are usually available within 24 hours. Does not boost responses measured by subsequent tests, which can happen with other tuberculin skin tests (CDC, 2005).
OTHER DIAGNOSTIC STUDIES • *TB skin tests (TST), such as purified protein derivative (PPD) administered by single-needle intradermal injection (Mantoux test), multiple-puncture tests (tine, Aplitest):* Determines past or present exposure to TB.	A positive reaction—area of induration 10 mm or greater, occurring 48 to 72 hours after intradermal injection of the antigen—indicates past infection and the presence of antibodies, but is not necessarily indicative of active disease. Factors associated with a suppressed response to tuberculin skin tests include underlying viral or bacterial infections, malnutrition, lymphadenopathy, current use of corticosteroids or other immunosuppressants or exposure to live vaccine viruses, such as measles, mumps, and rubella, within last 4 to 6 weeks. A significant reaction in a client who is clinically ill means that active TB cannot be dismissed as a diagnostic possibility. A significant reaction in healthy persons usually signifies dormant TB or an infection caused by a different mycobacterium.
• *Chest x-ray:* Evaluates organs and structures within the chest for evidence of disease.	May show small, patchy infiltrations of early lesions in the upper-lung field, calcium deposits of healed primary lesions, or fluid of an effusion. Changes indicating more advanced TB may include cavitation, scar tissue, and fibrotic areas.
• *Sputum TB culture:* AFB are rod-shaped bacteria that can be identified through sputum culture and smear. *M. tuberculosis* is the most prevalent species of mycobacteria and the most infectious.	Positive for *M. tuberculosis* in the active stage of the disease. Sputum cultures will be repeated 3 months into therapy to evaluate for possible nonadherence to treatment or to identify drug-resistant bacilli.
• *Computed tomography (CT) scan:* Procedure that uses a computer to produce a detailed picture of a cross-section of the lungs.	Determines degree of lung damage and may confirm a difficult diagnosis.
• *Bronchoscopy:* Procedure used to view lungs, airways, voice box, vocal cord, trachea, and many branches of bronchi. There are two types of bronchoscopes: flexible fiber-optic and rigid.	Shows inflammation and altered lung tissue. May also be performed to obtain sputum if client is unable to produce an adequate specimen.
• *Needle biopsy of lung tissue:* Aspirates cells from a suspicious lesion in the lung to identify pathology.	Positive for granulomas of TB; presence of giant cells indicating necrosis.
• *Histologic or tissue cultures (including gastric washings, urine and cerebrospinal fluid [CSF], skin biopsy):* Identify presence of organism.	Positive for *M. tuberculosis* and may indicate extrapulmonary involvement.
• *Pulmonary function studies:* Group of tests that measure lung capacity and volumes as well as gas distribution, diffusion, and expiration.	Decreased vital capacity, increased dead space, increased ratio of residual air to total lung capacity, and decreased oxygen saturation are secondary to parenchymal infiltration and fibrosis, loss of lung tissue, and pleural disease (extensive chronic pulmonary TB).

Nursing Priorities

1. Achieve and maintain adequate ventilation and oxygenation.
2. Prevent spread of infection.
3. Support behaviors and tasks to maintain health.
4. Promote effective coping strategies.
5. Provide information about disease process, prognosis, and treatment needs.

Discharge Goals

1. Respiratory function adequate to meet individual need.
2. Complications prevented.
3. Lifestyle and behavior changes adopted to prevent spread of infection.
4. Disease process, prognosis, and therapeutic regimen understood.
5. Plan in place to meet needs after discharge.

NURSING DIAGNOSIS: risk for Infection [spread/reactivation]

Risk factors may include
Inadequate primary defenses, decreased ciliary action and stasis of secretions
Tissue destruction, extension of infection
Lowered resistance, suppressed inflammatory process
Malnutrition
Environmental exposure
Insufficient knowledge to avoid exposure to pathogens

Possibly evidenced by
(Not applicable; presence of signs and symptoms establishes an *actual* diagnosis)

Desired Outcomes/Evaluation Criteria—Client Will

Risk Control (NOC)
Identify interventions to prevent or reduce risk of spread of infection.
Demonstrate techniques and initiate lifestyle changes to promote safe environment.

ACTIONS/INTERVENTIONS	RATIONALE
Infection Control (NIC)	
Independent	
Review pathology of disease—active or inactive phases, dissemination of infection through bronchi to adjacent tissues or via bloodstream and lymphatic system—and potential spread of infection via airborne droplet during coughing, sneezing, spitting, talking, laughing, and singing.	Helps client realize and accept necessity of adhering to medication regimen to prevent reactivation and complications. Understanding of how the disease is passed and awareness of transmission possibilities help client and significant other (SO) take steps to prevent infection of others.
Identify others at risk, such as household members, close associates, and friends.	Those exposed may require a course of drug therapy to prevent development of infection.
Instruct client to cough, sneeze, and expectorate into tissue and to refrain from spitting. Review proper disposal of tissue and good hand-washing techniques. Request return demonstration.	Behaviors necessary to prevent spread of infection.
Review necessity of infection control measures, such as temporary respiratory isolation.	May help client understand need for protecting others while acknowledging client's sense of isolation and social stigma associated with communicable diseases. *Note:* AFB can pass through standard masks; therefore, particulate respirators are required.
Monitor temperature, as indicated.	Febrile reactions are indicators of continuing presence of infection.
Identify individual risk factors for reactivation of tuberculosis, such as lowered resistance associated with alcoholism, malnutrition, intestinal bypass surgery, use of immunosuppressant drugs, presence of diabetes mellitus or cancer, or postpartum.	Knowledge about these factors helps client alter lifestyle and avoid or reduce incidence of exacerbation.
Stress importance of uninterrupted drug therapy. Evaluate client's potential for cooperation.	Contagious period may last only 2 to 3 days after initiation of drug regimen, but in the presence of cavitation or moderately advanced disease, risk of spread of infection may continue up to 3 months. Compliance with multidrug regimens for prolonged periods is difficult; therefore, DOT should be considered.
Review importance of follow-up and periodic reculturing of sputum for the duration of therapy.	Aids in monitoring the effects of medications and client's response to therapy.
Encourage selection and ingestion of well-balanced meals. Provide frequent small "snacks" in place of large meals as appropriate.	Presence of anorexia or preexisting malnutrition lowers resistance to infectious process and impairs healing. Small snacks may enhance overall intake.
Collaborative	
Administer anti-infective agents, as indicated, for example:	The goals for treatment of TB are to cure the individual and to minimize transmission to other persons. It is essential that treatment be tailored and supervision be based on each client's clinical and social circumstances. DOT may be the most effective way to maximize the completion of therapy.

ACTIONS/INTERVENTIONS (continued)

Primary drugs: isoniazid (INH, Liniazid), rifampin (RIF, Rifadin, Rimactane), pyrazinamide (PZA, Tebrazid), and ethambutol (Etbi, Myambutol)

Rufabutin (Mucobutin)

Second-line drugs, such as ethionamide (Trecator-SC), para-aminosalicylate (PAS), cycloserine (Seromycin), amikacin (Amikin), and levofloxacin (Levoquin)

Investigational agents such as diarylquinoline (R207910)

Monitor laboratory studies, such as the following:
Sputum smear results

Liver function studies, such as aspartate aminotransferase (AST), alinine aminotransferase (ALT)

Notify local health department.

RATIONALE (continued)

These four drugs should not be given in divided doses; all four drugs should be given together. Evidence shows this promotes the therapy's effectiveness (CDC, 2005). INH is usually drug of choice for those exposed and who are at risk for developing TB. Extended therapy for up to 24 months is indicated for reactivation cases, extrapulmonary reactivated TB, or in the presence of other medical problems, such as diabetes mellitus or silicosis. Prophylaxis with INH for 12 months should be considered in HIV-positive clients with positive PPD test.

Therapeutic agent for atypical mycobacterium. May be used in client with advanced HIV disease with TB.

These second-line drugs may be required when infection is resistant to or intolerant of primary drugs or may be used concurrently with primary antitubercular drugs. *Note:* MDR-TB requires minimum of 18 to 24 months' therapy with at least three drugs in the regimen known to be effective against the specific infective organism and that client has not previously taken. Treatment is often extended to 24 months in clients with severe symptoms or HIV infection.

Innovative compounds are being developed based on new drug targets and structure to provide shorter and more effective treatment options. This agent, currently starting human trials, cuts off the energy supply of the mycobacterium and may be effective against drug-resistant forms of TB.

Client who has three consecutive negative sputum smears over a 3- to 5-month period is adhering to drug regimen and who is asymptomatic will be classified as a nontransmitter.

The most common serious adverse effect of drug therapy—particularly RIF, but possibly others as well—is drug-induced hepatitis.

Required by law, and should be reported within 1 week of diagnosis. Helpful in identifying contacts to reduce spread of infection. Treatment course is long and usually handled in the community, with public health nurse monitoring.

NURSING DIAGNOSIS: ineffective Airway Clearance

May be related to
Thick, viscous, or bloody secretions
Fatigue, poor cough effort
Tracheal or pharyngeal edema

Possibly evidenced by
Abnormal respiratory rate, rhythm, depth
Abnormal breath sounds—rhonchi, wheezes, stridor
Dyspnea

Desired Outcomes/Evaluation Criteria—Client Will

Respiratory Status: Airway Patency (NOC)
Maintain patent airway.
Expectorate secretions without assistance.
Demonstrate behaviors to improve or maintain airway clearance.
Participate in treatment regimen, within the level of ability and situation.
Identify potential complications and initiate appropriate actions.

ACTIONS/INTERVENTIONS	RATIONALE

Airway Management (NIC)
Independent

Assess respiratory function, such as breath sounds, rate, rhythm, and depth, and use of accessory muscles.	Diminished breath sounds may reflect atelectasis. Rhonchi and wheezes indicate accumulation of secretions and inability to clear airways, which may lead to use of accessory muscles and increased work of breathing.
Note ability to expectorate mucus and cough effectively; document character and amount of sputum and presence of hemoptysis.	Expectoration may be difficult when secretions are very thick as a result of infection or inadequate hydration. Blood-tinged or frankly bloody sputum results from tissue breakdown in the lungs and may require further evaluation and intervention.
Place client in semi- or high-Fowler's position. Assist client with coughing and deep-breathing exercises.	Positioning helps maximize lung expansion and decreases respiratory effort. Maximal ventilation may open atelectatic areas and promote movement of secretions into larger airways for expectoration.
Clear secretions from mouth and trachea; suction as necessary.	Prevents obstruction and aspiration. Suctioning may be necessary if client is unable to expectorate secretions.
Maintain fluid intake of at least 2,500 mL/day unless contraindicated.	High fluid intake helps thin secretions, making them easier to expectorate.

Collaborative

Humidify inspired oxygen.	Prevents drying of mucous membranes and helps thin secretions.
Administer medications, as indicated, for example: Mucolytic agents, such as acetylcysteine (Mucomyst)	Reduces the thickness and stickiness of pulmonary secretions to facilitate clearance.
Bronchodilators, such as oxtriphylline (Choledyl) and theophylline (Theo-Dur)	Increases lumen size of the tracheobronchial tree, thus decreasing resistance to airflow and improving oxygen delivery.
Corticosteroids (prednisone)	May be useful in the presence of extensive involvement with profound hypoxemia and when inflammatory response is life-threatening.
Be prepared for and assist with emergency intubation.	Intubation may be necessary in rare cases of bronchogenic TB accompanied by laryngeal edema or acute pulmonary bleeding.

NURSING DIAGNOSIS: risk for impaired Gas Exchange

Risk factors may include
Decrease in effective lung surface, atelectasis
Destruction of alveolar-capillary membrane
Thick, viscous secretions
Bronchial edema

Possibly evidenced by
(Not applicable; presence of signs and symptoms establishes an *actual* diagnosis)

Desired Outcomes/Evaluation Criteria—Client Will

Respiratory Status: Gas Exchange (NOC)
Report absence of or decreased dyspnea.
Demonstrate improved ventilation and adequate oxygenation of tissues by ABGs within acceptable ranges.
Be free of symptoms of respiratory distress.

ACTIONS/INTERVENTIONS	RATIONALE

Respiratory Monitoring (NIC)
Independent

Assess for dyspnea (using 0 to 10 scale), tachypnea, abnormal breath sounds, increased respiratory effort, limited chest wall expansion, and fatigue.	Pulmonary TB can cause a wide range of effects in the lungs, ranging from a small patch of bronchopneumonia to diffuse intense inflammation, caseous necrosis, pleural effusion, and extensive fibrosis. Respiratory effects can range from mild dyspnea to profound respiratory distress. *Note:* Using a scale to evaluate dyspnea helps clarify degree of difficulty and changes in condition.
Evaluate change in level of mentation. Note cyanosis or change in skin color, including mucous membranes and nailbeds.	Accumulation of secretions and airway compromise can impair oxygenation of vital organs and tissues. (Refer to ND: ineffective Airway Clearance.)

ACTIONS/INTERVENTIONS (continued)

Demonstrate and encourage pursed-lip breathing during exhalation, especially for clients with fibrosis or parenchymal destruction.

Promote bedrest, or limit activity and assist with self-care activities as necessary.

Collaborative

Monitor serial ABGs and pulse oximetry.

Provide supplemental oxygen as appropriate.

RATIONALE (continued)

Creates resistance against outflowing air to prevent collapse of the airways, thereby helping to distribute air throughout the lungs and relieve or reduce shortness of breath.

Reducing oxygen consumption and demand during periods of respiratory compromise may reduce severity of symptoms.

Decreased oxygen content (PaO_2) and saturation or increased $PaCO_2$ indicate need for change in therapeutic regimen.

Aids in correcting the hypoxemia that may occur secondary to decreased ventilation and diminished alveolar lung surface.

NURSING DIAGNOSIS: **imbalanced Nutrition: Less than Body Requirements**

May be related to
Fatigue
Frequent cough and sputum production; dyspnea
Anorexia
Insufficient financial resources

Possibly evidenced by
Weight 10% to 20% below ideal for frame and height
Reported lack of interest in food, altered taste sensation
Poor muscle tone

Desired Outcomes/Evaluation Criteria—Client Will

Nutritional Status (NOC)

Demonstrate progressive weight gain toward goal with normalization of laboratory values and be free of signs of malnutrition.
Initiate behaviors or lifestyle changes to regain and to maintain appropriate weight.

ACTIONS/INTERVENTIONS

Nutrition Management (NIC)
Independent

Document client's nutritional status on admission, noting skin turgor, current weight and degree of weight loss, integrity of oral mucosa, ability to swallow, presence of bowel tones, and history of nausea, vomiting, or diarrhea.

Ascertain client's usual dietary pattern and likes and dislikes.

Monitor intake and ouput (I&O) and weight periodically.

Investigate anorexia, nausea, and vomiting. Note possible correlation to medications. Monitor frequency, volume, and consistency of stools.

Encourage and provide for frequent rest periods.

Provide oral care before and after respiratory treatments.

Encourage small, frequent meals with foods high in protein and carbohydrates.

Encourage SO to bring foods from home and to share meals with client unless contraindicated.

Collaborative

Refer to dietitian for adjustments in dietary composition.

Consult with respiratory therapy to schedule treatments 1 to 2 hours before or after meals.

Monitor laboratory studies, such as blood urea nitrogen (BUN), serum protein, and prealbumin and albumin.

Administer antipyretics, as appropriate.

RATIONALE

Useful in defining extent of problem and appropriate choice of interventions.

Helps to identify specific needs or strengths. Consideration of individual preferences may improve dietary intake.

Useful in measuring effectiveness of nutritional and fluid support.

Affects dietary choices and can identify areas for problem-solving to enhance intake of nutrients.

Helps conserve energy, especially when metabolic requirements are increased by fever.

Reduces bad taste left from sputum or medications used for respiratory treatments that can stimulate the vomiting center.

Maximizes nutrient intake without undue energy expenditure from eating large meals.

Creates a more normal social environment during mealtime and helps meet personal and cultural preferences.

Provides assistance in planning a diet with nutrients adequate to meet client's metabolic requirements, dietary preferences, and financial resources postdischarge.

May help reduce the incidence of nausea and vomiting associated with medications or the effects of respiratory treatments on a full stomach.

Low values reflect malnutrition and indicate need for change in therapeutic regimen.

Fever increases metabolic needs and therefore calorie consumption.

deficient Knowledge [Learning Need] regarding condition, treatment, prevention, self-care, and discharge needs

May be related to
Lack of exposure to or misinterpretation of information
Cognitive limitations
Inaccurate or incomplete information presented

Possibly evidenced by
Request for information
Expressed misconceptions about health status
Lack of or inaccurate follow-through of instructions or behaviors
Expressing or exhibiting feelings of being overwhelmed

Desired Outcomes/Evaluation Criteria—Client Will

Knowledge: Illness Care (NOC)
Verbalize understanding of disease process, prognosis, and prevention.
Initiate behaviors or lifestyle changes to improve general well-being and reduce risk of reactivation of TB.
Identify symptoms requiring evaluation and intervention.
Describe a plan for receiving adequate follow-up care.
Verbalize understanding of therapeutic regimen and rationale for actions.

ACTIONS/INTERVENTIONS	RATIONALE
Learning Facilitation (NIC)	
Independent	
Assess client's ability to learn, such as level of fear, concern, fatigue, participation level; best environment in which client can learn; how much content the client can learn; best media and language to teach the client; and determine who should be included.	Learning depends on emotional and physical readiness and is achieved at an individual pace.
Provide instruction and specific written information for client to refer to, such as schedule for medications and follow-up sputum testing for documenting response to therapy.	Written information relieves client of the burden of having to remember large amounts of information. Repetition strengthens learning.
Encourage client and SO to verbalize fears and concerns. Answer questions factually. Note prolonged use of denial.	Provides opportunity to correct misconceptions that may alleviate anxiety. Prolonged denial may affect coping with and managing the tasks necessary to regain health.
Teaching: Disease Process (NIC)	
Identify symptoms that should be reported to healthcare provider, such as hemoptysis, chest pain, fever, difficulty breathing, hearing loss, and vertigo.	May indicate progression or reactivation of disease or side effects of medications, requiring further evaluation.
Emphasize the importance of maintaining high-protein and carbohydrate diet and adequate fluid intake. (Refer to ND: imbalanced Nutrition: Less than Body Requirements.)	Meeting metabolic needs helps minimize fatigue and promotes recovery. Fluids aid in liquefying and expectorating secretions.
Explain medication dosage, frequency of administration, expected action, and the reason for long treatment period. Review potential interactions with other drugs and substances. Emphasize reportable side effects.	Enhances cooperation with therapeutic regimen and may prevent client from discontinuing medication before cure is truly effected. DOT is the treatment of choice when client is unable or unwilling to take medications as prescribed. *Note:* Clients with HIV infection and TB are particularly susceptible to drug interactions because they are typically taking numerous medications, some of which react with antituberculosis medications.
Review potential side effects of treatment, such as dry mouth, gastrointestinal (GI) upset, constipation, visual disturbances, headache, and orthostatic hypertension, and problem-solve solutions.	It is important that antituberculosis drugs not be discontinued because of "nuisance" side effects. Problem-solving, such as taking medication with food and changing the hour of dosing, may reduce discomfort associated with therapy and enhance cooperation with regimen. Severe reactions must be reported to physician.
Stress need to abstain from alcohol while on INH.	Combination of INH and alcohol has been linked to increased incidence of hepatitis.
Refer for eye examination after starting and then monthly during the course of ethambutol (EMB).	Major side effect is reduced visual acuity; initial sign may be decreased ability to perceive the color green.
Encourage abstaining from smoking.	Although smoking does not stimulate recurrence of TB, it does increase the likelihood of respiratory dysfunction.

ACTIONS/INTERVENTIONS (continued)

Review that TB is transmitted primarily by inhalation of airborne organisms, but may also spread through stools or urine if infection is present in these systems; also review hazards of reactivation.

Discuss and reinforce concerns, such as treatment failure, drug-resistant TB, and relapse.

Refer to public health agency as appropriate.

RATIONALE (continued)

Knowledge may reduce risk of transmission or reactivation. Complications associated with reactivation include cavitation, abscess formation, destructive emphysema, spontaneous pneumothorax, diffuse interstitial fibrosis, serous effusion, empyema, bronchiectasis, hemoptysis, GI ulceration, bronchopleural fistula, tuberculosis laryngitis, and miliary spread.

Treatment failure most often occurs because client is not adhering to treatment regimen, but can also be due to drug resistance, malabsorption of drugs, laboratory error, and extreme biological variation in response. Most relapses or recurrence of positive cultures or radiographic deterioration occur 6 to 12 months after completion of therapy. Continuous monitoring by healthcare providers can identify these concerns early and alter the plan accordingly.

DOT by community nurses is often the most effective way to ensure client adherence to therapy. Monitoring may include pill counts and urine dipstick testing for presence of antitubercular drug. Clients with MDR-TB may be monitored with monthly sputum specimens for AFB smear and culture. *Note:* In some states, there are legal means for involuntary confinement for care if efforts to ensure client adherence are ineffective.

POTENTIAL CONSIDERATIONS following acute hospitalization (dependent on client's age, physical condition and presence of complications, personal resources, and life responsibilities)
- *ineffective self Health Management*—complexity of therapeutic regimen, economic difficulties, family patterns of healthcare, perceived seriousness and benefits
- *risk for Infection (secondary)*—decrease in ciliary action, stasis of body fluids, suppressed inflammatory response, tissue destruction, chronic disease, malnutrition, increased environmental exposure
- *Fatigue*—increased energy requirements to perform activities of daily living (ADLs), discomfort
- *ineffective family Therapeutic Regimen Management*—complexity of therapeutic regimen, decisional conflicts, economic difficulties, family conflict

---

RESPIRATORY ACID-BASE IMBALANCES

I. Pathophysiology—the body has the remarkable ability to maintain plasma pH within a narrow range of 7.35 to 7.45.
  a. Accomplished by chemical buffering mechanisms involving the lungs and kidneys
   i. Lungs compensate for acid-base imbalances resulting from altered levels of metabolic acids.
   ii. Kidneys compensate for acid-base imbalances resulting from altered levels of carbonic acid.
  b. Although simple acid-base imbalances (e.g., respiratory acidosis) do occur, mixed acid-base imbalances are more common (e.g., the respiratory acidosis and metabolic acidosis that occur with cardiac arrest).

RESPIRATORY ACIDOSIS (PRIMARY CARBONIC ACID EXCESS)

I. Types
  a. Acute respiratory acidosis: develops when an abrupt failure of ventilation occurs
   i. Due to rapid development of problem, metabolic compensation is ineffective.
   ii. $PaCO_2$ greater than 47 mm Hg with accompanying acidemia (pH 7.25)
  b. Chronic respiratory acidosis: progressive failure of ventilation over time
   i. Allows for some degree of compensation through increased renal reabsorption of HCO_3
   ii. $PaCO_2$ greater than 47 mm Hg, normal or near normal pH, and elevated serum bicarbonate (HCO_3 greater than 30 mm Hg)

(text continues on page 196)

II. Compensatory Mechanisms—occurs over 3 to 5 days
  a. Increased respiratory rate
  b. Hemoglobin (Hgb) buffering
  c. Forming bicarbonate ions and deoxygenated Hgb
  d. Increased renal ammonia acid excretions with reabsorption of bicarbonate

III. Etiology
  a. Alveolar hypoventilation, reduced CO_2 elimination, excess of carbonic acid (H_2CO_3)
  b. Conditions causing a decrease in respiratory rate and volume:
    i. Central nervous system (CNS) disorders, such as with depression of the central respiratory center; for example, brainstem disease or trauma, tumors, encephalitis, stroke, or drugs such as use of "downers" or overdose of sedatives or barbiturate poisoning
    ii. Pulmonary disorders of the airways or those causing airway obstruction, such as asthma or chronic obstructive pulmonary disease (COPD) exacerbation, bronchiectasis, aspiration of foreign body, acute pulmonary edema, acute laryngospasm, smoke inhalation, excessive CO_2 intake (for example, use of rebreathing mask, CO_2 therapy)
    iii. Neuromuscular disorders restricting chest movement and inability to ventilate adequately, such as myasthenia gravis, amyotrophic lateral sclerosis (ALS), Guillain-Barré syndrome, muscular dystrophy, botulism
    iv. Severe restrictive ventilatory defects, such as interstitial fibrosis, thoracic deformities, hemothorax and pneumothorax, atelectasis, acute respiratory distress syndrome (ARDS), spinal cord injuries, anesthesia and surgery, severe obesity (Pickwickian syndrome)

GLOSSARY

Acid: A substance that, when dissolved in water, dissociates and can donate a hydrogen (proton) to another molecule.

Acidosis: Increased acidity (i.e., an increased hydrogen [H^+] ion concentration). If not further qualified, it refers to acidity of the blood plasma. Acidosis is said to occur when arterial pH falls below 7.35.

Alkalosis: A dangerous decrease in the normal acidity of the blood, where there is too much base in the blood.

Base excess/deficit: A calculated number that represents a sum total of the metabolic buffering agents (anions) in the blood; these anions include hemoglobin, proteins, phosphates, and bicarbonate (HCO_3^-, dominant anion); these anions try to compensate for imbalances in the pH caused by diseases or conditions that affect the lungs (respiratory acidosis or alkalosis) or kidneys (metabolic acidosis or alkalosis).

Base: Chemical opposite of acid.

Buffers: Chemicals that help control the pH of body fluids. Each buffer system consists of a weak acid, which releases H^+ when the fluid is too alkaline and a base when the fluid is too acidic. H^+ ions are buffered by extracellular (such as bicarbonate, ammonia) and intracellular buffering agents (including proteins and phosphate).

Carbonic acid (H_2CO_3): If too much acid is present, the bicarbonate ions take up the hydrogen ions and become H_2CO_3, which is then excreted through the lungs in the form of carbon dioxide (CO_2) and water (H_2O^+). Conversely, if too little acid is present in extracellular fluid, the carbonic acid portion of the bicarbonate buffer system releases hydrogen ions. For the pH to remain within normal range (7.35 to 7.45), the ratio of bicarbonate ions to H_2CO_3 must be 20:1 (Felver, 2005).

Circumoral paresthesias: Numbness, stinging, or burning sensation around the mouth.

CO_2: Respiratory acid, which is the only acid that can be exhaled via the lungs.

H^+: The ion that is left when the hydrogen atom loses its electron, forming a proton.

HCO_3^-: Measurement of the metabolic component of the acid-base balance. HCO_3^- is excreted and reabsorbed (conserved) by the kidneys in response to pH imbalances and is directly related to the pH level; as the amount of HCO_3^- rises, so does the pH.

Hypercapnia: Increased amount of CO_2 in the blood.

Hyperventilation: Increased rate and depth of breathing that causes a decrease in CO_2.

Hypoventilation: Reduced rate and depth of breathing that causes an increase in CO_2.

Hypoxemia: Low level of oxygen (O_2) in the blood.

O_2 saturation: Percentage of hemoglobin saturation or how much O_2 is bound to hemoglobin in the red blood cells and available to be carried through the arteries to cells.

Partial pressure of carbon dioxide ($PaCO_2$): Reflects the balance between the production of CO_2 and its elimination. Unless the metabolic rate changes, the amount of CO_2 produced is roughly constant and determines the amount of ventilation required and the level of $PaCO_2$. The normal value in arterial blood is 40 mm Hg. In the healthy, awake individual, the end-exhaled value is usually similar.

Partial pressure of O_2 (PaO_2): Amount of oxygen gas dissolved in blood.

pH: A measure of the level of H^+, which indicates the acid-base status of blood; the pH decreases (becomes more acidic) with increased amounts of $PaCO_2$ and other acids, and the pH increases (blood becomes more alkaline) with decreased $PaCO_2$ or increased amounts of HCO_3^-.

Respiratory acidosis: Acute or chronic condition that occurs when the lungs cannot remove all the CO_2 the body produces.

Respiratory alkalosis: Condition marked by low levels of CO_2 in the blood.

Tachypnea: Rapid, shallow respirations.

Care Setting

This condition does not occur in isolation; rather, it is a complication of a broader health problem, disease, or condition for which the severely compromised client requires admission to a medical-surgical or subacute unit.

Related Concerns

Plans of care specific to predisposing factors and disease or medical condition, such as the following:

Cerebrovascular accident (CVA)/stroke, page 238
Chronic obstructive pulmonary disease (COPD) and
asthma, page 120

Craniocerebral trauma (acute rehabilitative phase),
page 220
Eating disorders: obesity, page 387
Alcohol: acute withdrawal, page 819
Spinal cord injury (acute rehabilitative phase), page 271
Surgical intervention, page 782
Ventilatory assistance (mechanical), page 173

Other Concerns

Fluid and electrolyte imbalances, page 903
Metabolic acidosis—primary base bicarbonate deficiency,
page 483
Metabolic alkalosis—primary base bicarbonate excess,
page 488

Client Assessment Database

DIAGNOSTIC DIVISION MAY REPORT	MAY EXHIBIT
ACTIVITY/REST • Fatigue, mild to profound • Sleep disturbances	• Generalized weakness • Ataxia or staggering • Loss of coordination • Stupor
CIRCULATION	• Blood pressure (BP) may be low, with bounding pulses, pinkish color, warm skin • Dilation of conjunctival and superficial facial blood vessels, reflecting vasodilation of severe acidosis • Tachycardia, irregular pulse, various dysrhythmias • Diaphoresis, pallor, and cyanosis—late stage of respiratory failure
FOOD/FLUID • Nausea, vomiting	
NEUROSENSORY • Feeling of fullness in head (acute—associated with vasodilation) • Headache (acute) • Dizziness • Visual disturbances	• Anxiety, confusion, apprehension, agitation, restlessness, delirium, depressed mental status, somnolence (CO_2 narcosis), coma (acute) • Tremors, decreased reflexes, or asterixis, myoclonus, and seizures (severe)
RESPIRATION • Shortness of breath with exertion	• Respirations dependent on underlying cause: • Tachypnea can occur often with prolonged expiration • Hypoventilation can be associated with depression of respiratory center (as in head trauma and respiratory failure), or with muscle paralysis, oversedation, general anesthesia, metabolic alkalosis • Increased respiratory effort with nasal flaring or yawning, use of neck and upper body muscles • Decreased breath sounds • Hyperresonance on percussion • Adventitious breath sounds—wheezes; stridor, crowing

(continues on page 198)

DIAGNOSTIC DIVISION MAY REPORT (continued)

TEACHING/LEARNING
Refer to specific plans of care reflecting individual predisposing or contributing factors.

DISCHARGE PLAN CONSIDERATIONS
May require assistance with changes in therapies for underlying disease process/condition.

▶ Refer to section at end of plan for postdischarge considerations.

MAY EXHIBIT (continued)

Diagnostic Studies

TEST WHY IT IS DONE	WHAT IT TELLS ME
BLOOD TESTS	
• Arterial blood gases (ABGs): Measure how much O_2 and CO_2 is in arterial blood. They also look at the acidity (pH) of the blood. *Normal ABGs at sea level:*	*PaO2:* Normal or may be low. Oxygen saturation (SaO_2) decreased. *PaCO2:* Increased, greater than 45 mm Hg (primary acidosis). *HCO3:* Normal or increased, greater than 26 mEq/L (compensated/ chronic stage).
• PaO_2: 75 to 100 mm Hg	*Arterial pH:* Decreased, less than 7.35.
• $PaCO_2$: 35 to 45 mm Hg	
• pH: 7.35 to7.45	
• SaO_2: 94 to 100%	
• HCO_3: 22 to 26 mEq/L	
Note: At altitudes of 3,000 feet and above, the oxygen values are lower.	
• *Capnography:* Monitors the concentration or PCO_2 in the respiratory gases.	Provides information about CO_2 production, lung perfusion, alveolar ventilation, respiratory patterns, and elimination of CO_2.
• *Electrolyte tests:* The electrolyte panel is composed of the individual tests for sodium, potassium, chloride, and total carbon dioxide. A related "test" is the anion gap, which is actually a value calculated using the results of an electrolyte panel.	*Serum potassium:* Typically increased. *Serum chloride:* Decreased. *Serum calcium:* Increased.
OTHER DIAGNOSTIC STUDIES	
• *Urinalysis:* Measures level of pH in the urine.	*pH:* Typically decreased.
• *Other screening tests:* As indicated by underlying illness or condition, including chest x-ray, chest computed tomography (CT), brain magnetic resonance imaging (MRI), pulmonary function studies, drug and toxicology screens, and tests to measure diaphragmatic function.	To determine underlying cause and treatment needs.

Nursing Priorities

1. Achieve homeostasis.
2. Prevent or minimize complications.
3. Provide information about condition, prognosis, and treatment needs as appropriate.

Discharge Goals

1. Physiological balance restored.
2. Free of complications.
3. Condition, prognosis, and treatment needs understood.
4. Plan in place to meet needs after discharge.

NURSING DIAGNOSIS: impaired Gas Exchange

May be related to
Ventilation perfusion imbalance—altered oxygen-carrying capacity of blood, altered oxygen supply, alveolar-capillary membrane changes, or altered blood flow

Possibly evidenced by
Dyspnea with exertion, tachypnea
Changes in mentation, irritability
Tachycardia
Hypoxia, hypercapnia

Desired Outcomes/Evaluation Criteria—Client Will

Electrolyte and Acid-Base Balance (NOC)
Demonstrate improved ventilation and adequate oxygenation of tissues as evidenced by ABGs within client's acceptable limits and absence of symptoms of respiratory distress.

Knowledge: Disease Process (NOC)
Verbalize understanding of causative factors and appropriate interventions.
Participate in treatment regimen within level of ability or situation.

ACTIONS/INTERVENTIONS	RATIONALE
Acid-Base Management: Respiratory Acidosis (NIC)	
Independent	
Monitor respiratory rate, depth, and effort.	Alveolar hypoventilation and associated hypoxemia lead to respiratory failure.
Auscultate breath sounds.	Identifies area(s) of decreased ventilation, such as atelectasis, or airway obstruction and changes as client deteriorates or improves, reflecting effectiveness of treatment and dictating therapy needs.
Note declining level of awareness or consciousness.	Signals severe acidotic state, which requires immediate attention. *Note:* In recovery, sensorium clears slowly because hydrogen ions are slow to cross the blood-brain barrier and clear from cerebrospinal fluid (CSF) and brain cells.
Monitor heart rate and rhythm.	Tachycardia develops early because the sympathetic nervous system is stimulated, resulting in the release of catecholamines, epinephrine, and norepinephrine in an attempt to increase oxygen delivery to the tissues. Dysrhythmias that may occur are due to hypoxia (myocardial ischemia) and electrolyte imbalances.
Note skin color, temperature, and moisture.	Diaphoresis, pallor, and cool, clammy skin are late changes associated with severe or advancing hypoxemia.
Encourage and assist with deep-breathing exercises, turning, and coughing. Suction as necessary. Provide airway adjunct as indicated. Place in semi-Fowler's position.	These measures improve lung ventilation and reduce or prevent airway obstruction associated with accumulation of mucus.
Restrict use of hypnotic sedatives or tranquilizers.	In the presence of hypoventilation, respiratory depression and CO_2 narcosis may develop.
Discuss cause of chronic condition, when known, and appropriate interventions and self-care activities.	Promotes participation in therapeutic regimen and may reduce recurrence of disorder.
Collaborative	
Assist with identification and treatment of underlying cause.	Treatment of disorder is directed at improving alveolar ventilation. Multiple team management, including physicians, pulmonologist and respiratory therapists, or neurologists, may be required to address the underlying condition, such as oversedation, brain trauma, COPD, pulmonary edema, aspiration, and promote correction of the acid-base disorder.
Monitor and graph serial ABGs and pulse oximetry readings.	Evaluates therapy needs and effectiveness. *Note:* Pulse oximetry monitoring is used to monitor and show early changes in oxygenation, which can occur before other signs or symptoms are observed.
Administer oxygen as indicated, using appropriate delivery means—endotracheal (ET) intubation with mechanical ventilation, or nasal continuous positive-pressure ventilation or nasal bi-level ventilation.	Prevents or corrects hypoxemia and pulmonary hypertension, and its use prevents the consequences of long-standing hypoxemia.

(continues on page 200)

Increase respiratory rate or tidal volume of ventilator if used.

Increases lung expansion and opens airways to improve ventilation and gas diffusion, preventing respiratory failure.

Assist with ventilatory aids, such as intermittent positive-pressure breathing (IPPB) in conjunction with bronchodilators. Monitor peak flow pressure.

Assists in correction of acidity and mobilization of respiratory secretions.

Maintain hydration (intravenously [IV]/by mouth [PO]) and provide humidification.

Aids in clearing secretions, which improves ventilation, allowing excess CO_2 to be eliminated.

Administer medications, as indicated, for example:

Opioid antagonist, such as naloxone hydrochloride (Narcan) and flumazenil (Romazicon)

Can be useful in reversing the effects of certain opiates and sedative drugs on the respiratory center, stimulating ventilation in presence of drug overdose or sedation, or acidosis resulting from cardiac arrest.

Bronchodilators including beta-agonists, for example, albuterol (Proventil, Ventolin) and salmeterol (Serevent); anticholinergic agents, for example, ipratropium bromide (Atrovent); and methylxanthines, for example, theophylline

Helpful in treating client with acidosis secondary to obstructive lung disease and severe bronchospasm. Theophylline may improve diaphragm muscle contractility and may stimulate the respiratory center.

Electrolytes, as indicated

Respiratory acidosis does not have a great effect on electrolyte levels, although some effects occur on calcium and potassium levels. Acidemia causes an extracellular shift of potassium. Correction of the acidosis may cause a relative serum hypokalemia as potassium shifts back into cells. Potassium imbalance can impair neuromuscular or respiratory function, causing generalized muscle weakness and cardiac dysrhythmias. *Note:* Infusion of sodium bicarbonate is rarely indicated, although it may be considered in cardiopulmonary arrest when pH is less than 7.0.

Provide or refer for pulmonary rehabilitation, as indicated.

Provides restorative and preventative care to reverse respiratory acidosis secondary to underlying conditions, such as bronchial hygiene, breathing retraining, and exercise conditioning. Therapy modalities and length of intervention may vary depending on whether the respiratory acidosis is acute or chronic.

Provide low-carbohydrate, high-fat diet (for example, Pulmocare feedings), if indicated.

Helps reduce CO_2 production and improves respiratory muscle function and metabolic homeostasis.

POTENTIAL CONSIDERATIONS following acute hospitalization (dependent on client's age, physical condition and presence of complications, personal resources, and life responsibilities)
Refer to Potential Considerations relative to underlying cause of acid-base disorder.

RESPIRATORY ALKALOSIS (PRIMARY CARBONIC ACID DEFICIT)

I. **Pathophysiology**—acute or chronic increase in respiratory rate and volume, primarily triggered by hypoxemia or direct stimulation of the central respiratory center of the brain
   a. Acute: $PaCO_2$ is below lower limit of normal, serum pH is alkalemic due to loss of potassium, and phosphate secondary to cellular uptake.
   b. Chronic: $PaCO_2$ is below the lower limit of normal, but pH is normal or near normal because of renal compensation.

II. **Compensatory Mechanisms**—occurs over 2 to 3 days
   a. Decreased respiratory rate (if the body is able to respond to the drop in $PaCO_2$)
   b. Increased renal excretion of bicarbonate
   c. Retention of hydrogen

III. **Etiology**
   a. Alveolar hyperventilation, hypocapnea ($PaCO_2$ less than 35 mm Hg), increased ratio of bicarbonate concentration to $PaCO_2$ (base excess), near-normal or alkaline pH

   b. Most frequently occurring acid-base imbalance in hospitalized clients, with the elderly being at increased risk because of the high incidence of pulmonary disorders and alterations in neurologic status
   c. Conditions or disorders associated with respiratory alkalosis:
      i. Central nervous system (CNS)—such as stroke, meningitis, encephalitis, brain trauma or tumor, pain, hyperventilation, anxiety, psychosis, fever
      ii. Hypoxemia—such as severe anemia, any lung disease that leads to shortness of breath, high altitude
      iii. Drugs—such as salicylates, nicotine, methyxanthines, catecholamines
      iv. Endocrine—such as hyperthyroidism, pregnancy, increased progesterone levels
      v. Stimulation of chest receptors—such as pulmonary embolus, pulmonary edema, aspiration, hemopneumothorax
      vi. Miscellaneous—such as sepsis, liver failure, heat exhaustion, mechanical ventilation (pseudorespiratory alkalosis)

Care Setting

This condition does not occur in isolation, but rather is a complication of a broader problem. Treatment is primarily directed at correcting the underlying disorder causing respiratory alkalosis and is usually found in clients requiring care in a medical-surgical or subacute unit.

Related Concerns

Plans of care specific to predisposing factors, such as:
Anemias—iron deficiency, anemia of chronic disease, pernicious, aplastic, hemolytic, page 493

Cirrhosis of the liver, page 445
Craniocerebral trauma, page 220
Hyperthyroidism (Graves' disease, thyrotoxicosis), page 419
Fluid and electrolyte imbalances, page 903
Heart failure: chronic, page 48
Pneumonia, page 131
Sepsis/septicemia, page 686
Ventilatory assistance (mechanical), page 173

Other Concerns

Metabolic acidosis—primary base bicarbonate deficiency, page 483
Metabolic alkalosis—primary base bicarbonate excess, page 488

Client Assessment Database

Dependent on underlying cause.

DIAGNOSTIC DIVISION MAY REPORT	MAY EXHIBIT
CIRCULATION • History or presence of anemia • Palpitations	• Hypotension • Tachycardia, irregular pulse and dysrhythmias
EGO INTEGRITY	• Extreme anxiety—most common cause of hyperventilation
FOOD/FLUID • Dry mouth • Nausea, vomiting	• Abdominal distention—elevated diaphragm as with ascites, pregnancy • Vomiting
NEUROSENSORY • Headache, tinnitus • Numbness or tingling of face, hands, and toes; circumoral numbness and generalized paresthesia • Lightheadedness, syncope, vertigo, blurred vision	• Confusion, restlessness, obtunded responses, coma • Hyperactive reflexes, positive Chvostek's and Trousseau signs; tetany, seizures • Heightened sensitivity to environmental noise and activity • Muscle weakness, unsteady gait
PAIN/DISCOMFORT • Muscle spasms or cramps • Epigastric pain • Chest tightness	
RESPIRATION • Shortness of breath • History of asthma, pulmonary fibrosis	• Tachypnea; rapid, shallow breathing; hyperventilation—often 40 or more respirations per minute • Intermittent periods of apnea
SAFETY	• Fever
DISCHARGE PLAN CONSIDERATIONS • May require change in treatment or therapy of underlying disease process or condition ⬦ Refer to section at end of plan for postdischarge considerations.	

TEST WHY IT IS DONE	WHAT IT TELLS ME
BLOOD TESTS • *Arterial blood gases (ABGs):* Measure how much oxygen and carbon dioxide is in arterial blood. They also look at the acidity (pH) of the blood. *Normal ABGs at sea level:* • PaO_2: 75 to 100 mm Hg • $PaCO_2$: 35 to 45 mm Hg • pH: 7.35 to 7.45 • SaO_2: 94 to 100% • HCO_3: 22 to 26 mEq/L *Note:* At altitudes of 3,000 feet and above, the oxygen values are lower.	*Arterial pH:* Greater than 7.44 (may be near normal in chronic stage). *HCO_3:* Normal or decreased; less than 25 mEq/L (compensatory mechanism). *$PaCO_2$:* Decreased, less than 36 mm Hg (primary).
• *Electrolytes:* The electrolyte panel is composed of the individual tests for sodium, potassium, chloride, and total carbon dioxide. A related "test" is the anion gap, which is actually a value calculated using the results of an electrolyte panel.	Minor shifts usually occur, for example, serum sodium, potassium, and phosphate decreased due to intracellular shifts; serum chloride increased; and serum calcium decreased.
• *Complete blood count (CBC):* Battery of screening tests which typically includes hemoglobin (Hgb); hematocrit (Hct); red blood cell (RBC) count, morphology, indices, and distribution width index; platelet count and size; white blood cell (WBC) count and differential.	May reveal severe anemia—decreased Hgb and oxygen-carrying capacity; or elevated WBCs (due to, for example, inflammatory process or early sepsis).
OTHER DIAGNOSTIC STUDIES Screening tests as indicated to determine underlying cause: • *Blood cultures:* May identify sepsis—usually gram negative. • *Blood alcohol:* Marked elevation—acute alcoholic intoxication. • *Computed tomography (CT) scan and ventilation/perfusion studies:* May be done to diagnose pulmonary disorders.	

Nursing Priorities

1. Achieve homeostasis.
2. Prevent or minimize complications.
3. Provide information about condition, prognosis, and treatment needs as appropriate.

Discharge Goals

1. Physiological balance restored.
2. Free of complications.
3. Condition, prognosis, and treatment needs understood.
4. Plan in place to meet needs after discharge.

NURSING DIAGNOSIS: **impaired Gas Exchange**

May be related to
Ventilation-perfusion imbalance, such as altered oxygen supply, altered blood flow, altered oxygen-carrying capacity of blood, alveolar-capillary membrane changes

Possibly evidenced by
Dyspnea, tachypnea
Changes in mentation
Hypocapnia, tachycardia
Hypoxia

Desired Outcomes/Evaluation Criteria—Client Will

Electrolyte and Acid-Base Balance (NOC)
Demonstrate improved ventilation and adequate oxygenation of tissue as evidenced by ABGs within client's acceptable limits and absence of symptoms of respiratory distress.
Verbalize understanding of causative factors and appropriate interventions.
Participate in treatment regimen within level of ability or situation.

ACTIONS/INTERVENTIONS	RATIONALE
Acid-Base Management: Respiratory Alkalosis (NIC)	
Independent	
Monitor respiratory rate, depth, and effort; ascertain cause of hyperventilation if possible, for example, anxiety, pain, and improper ventilator settings.	Identifies alterations from usual breathing pattern and influences choice of intervention.
Assess level of awareness and cognition. Note neuromuscular status—strength, tone, reflexes, sensation, and presence of tremors.	Decreased mentation (mild to severe) and tetany or seizures may occur when alkalosis is severe due to shifts in calcium.
Instruct and encourage client to breathe slowly and deeply. Speak in a low, calm tone of voice. Provide safe environment.	May help reassure and calm the agitated client, thereby aiding the reduction of respiratory rate. Assists client to regain control. *Note:* Clients with hyperventilation syndrome as a cause of their respiratory alkalosis may particularly benefit from reassurance and client education in breathing techniques.
Demonstrate appropriate breathing patterns, if appropriate, and assist with respiratory aids, such as rebreathing mask or bag.	Decreasing the rate of respirations can halt the "blowing off" of CO_2, elevating $PaCO_2$ level and normalizing pH.
Provide comfort measures; encourage use of meditation and visualization. Use tepid sponge bath or cool cloths.	Promotes relaxation and reduces stress. Control and reduction of fever reduces potential for seizures and helps reduce respiration rate.
Provide safety and seizure precautions, such as bed in low position, padded side rails, frequent observation.	Changes in mentation and CNS and neuromuscular hyperirritability may result in client harm, especially if tetany or convulsions occur.
Discuss cause of condition, if known, and appropriate interventions and self-care activities.	Promotes participation in therapeutic regimen and may reduce recurrence of disorder.
Collaborative	
Assist with identification and treatment of underlying cause.	Respiratory alkalosis is a complication, not an isolated occurrence and rarely requires emergent treatment (unless pH is greater than 7.5); thus, correction of alkalosis is undertaken by addressing the primary condition, such as hyperventilation of panic attack, organ failure, severe anemia, and drug effect. Because respiratory alkalosis usually occurs in response to some stimulus, treatment is unsuccessful unless the stimulus is controlled.
Monitor and graph serial ABGs and pulse oximetry.	Identifies therapy needs and effectiveness. *Note:* Rapid correction of $PaCO_2$ in individual with chronic respiratory alkalosis (has a lower serum bicarbonate) may cause metabolic acidosis to develop.
Monitor serum potassium and replace, as indicated.	Hypokalemia may occur as potassium is lost via urine or shifted into the cell in exchange for hydrogen in an attempt to correct alkalosis.
Provide sedation and pain medication, as indicated.	Control of pain and sedation may be needed to reduce cause of hyperventilation if client is not responding to conservative measures.
Administer CO_2 (by rebreathing bag or mask) as indicated. Reduce respiratory rate and tidal volume, or add additional dead space (tubing) to mechanical ventilator.	Increasing CO_2 retention may correct carbonic acid deficit, leading to improvement and resolution of alkalotic state.

POTENTIAL CONSIDERATIONS following acute hospitalization (dependent on client's age, physical condition and presence of complications, personal resources, and life responsibilities)
Refer to Potential Considerations relative to underlying cause of acid-base disorder.

CHAPTER 6

Neurological/Sensory Disorders

GLAUCOMA

I. Pathophysiology
a. Irreversible process in which the retinal ganglion cells—nerve cells in front of the optic nerve—die
b. Death of retinal cells and degeneration or atrophy of the optic nerve fibers initially causes loss of peripheral vision, eventually leading to blindness if untreated.

II. Classification
a. Chronic open-angle glaucoma, also called primary open-angle glaucoma (POAG)—most common type
   i. The drainage system becomes clogged, and aqueous humor fluid is unable to drain properly, causing a backup of fluid.
   ii. Develops slowly and may be associated with type 2 diabetes and severe myopia; usually develops in both eyes simultaneously or in one eye, followed by the other within a short period of time.
   iii. No early warning signs; loss of peripheral vision occurs so gradually that substantial optic nerve damage can occur before glaucoma is detected.
   iv. Usually responds well to medication if detected and treated early.
b. Primary narrow-angle (or closed-angle) glaucoma: May be associated with eye trauma, various inflammatory processes, and pupillary dilation after the instillation of mydriatic drops.
c. Acute angle-closure glaucoma: manifested by sudden excruciating pain in or around the eye, blurred vision, and ocular redness.
   i. Constitutes a medical emergency because blindness may ensue suddenly.
   ii. Surgical treatment usually successful and long lasting.

III. Etiology
a. Risk factors: over age 45, diabetes, myopia, long-term steroid use, family history of glaucoma, African American descent (Glaucoma Foundation, 2009)
b. Increased intraocular pressure (IOP) may be a factor in some individuals.
   i. The result of inadequate or obstructed drainage of aqueous humor from the anterior chamber of the eye
   ii. Compresses the nerve or impairs blood supply to the axons of the retinal ganglion
c. Secondary glaucoma can occur as a result of an eye injury—direct trauma to the eye (blow to the head or a direct blow to eye), inflammation, tumor, or can occur in advanced cases of cataract or diabetes.
   i. May be mild or severe
   ii. Treatment depends on whether it is open-angle or angle-closure glaucoma.
d. Pigmentary glaucoma: form of secondary glaucoma in which pigment granules in the back of the iris break into the aqueous humor and clog the drainage canals
   i. Treatment usually includes drug therapy or surgery.
e. Normal-tension glaucoma (NTG)—also known as low-tension or normal-pressure glaucoma—occurs when the optic nerve is damaged even though IOP is not elevated.
   i. Has been linked to systemic heart disease; higher incidence in people of Japanese descent.
   ii. Treatment aimed at keeping eye pressures as low as possible with medication, laser therapy, or filtering surgery.

IV. Statistics
a. Morbidity: Approximately 3 million people in the United States (Brown University, n.d.); estimated 8.7 million physician visits annually (Schappert, 1995); return visits primarily middle-aged and elderly Americans, emphasizing chronic nature of condition (NAMCS, 2007)
b. Cost: Estimated to be greater than $1.5 billion annually to United States government (Brown University, n.d.).

GLOSSARY

Axon: Elongated portion of a neuron that carries information away from the cell body; in the retina, it carries information down the optic nerve.

Glaucoma: A group of eye disorders characterized by progressive optic nerve damage, resulting in loss of vision.

Intraocular pressure (IOP): Hydrostatic pressure created by the vitreous fluid within the eyeball.

Retina: Light-sensitive membrane—innermost layer of the eye—which receives images transmitted through the lens.

Retinal ganglion cell: Neuron located in the inner surface of the retina, which transmits visual information through its axon to the brain.

Care Setting

Glaucoma is treated in a community setting, unless sudden pain and increased IOP requires emergency intervention and close monitoring.

Related Concerns

Psychosocial aspects of care, page 749

Client Assessment Database

DIAGNOSTIC DIVISION MAY REPORT	MAY EXHIBIT
ACTIVITY/REST • Change in usual activities/hobbies due to altered vision	
FOOD/FLUID • Nausea, vomiting (acute glaucoma)	
NEUROSENSORY • Gradual loss of peripheral vision, frequent change of glasses, difficulty adjusting to darkened room, sensitivity to glare, difficulty differentiating between varying shades and brightness, mild headache (chronic glaucoma) • Cloudy or blurred vision, appearance of halos or rainbows around lights, sudden loss of peripheral vision, photophobia, intense pain in the eyebrow area (acute closed-angle glaucoma) • Glasses or treatment change not improving vision • Above symptoms, but painless and gradual onset (chronic closed-angle glaucoma)	• Dilated, fixed, cloudy pupils (acute glaucoma) • Fixed pupil and red, hard eye with cloudy cornea (glaucoma emergency) • Increased tearing • Intumescent cataracts, intraocular hemorrhage (glaucoma secondary to trauma)
PAIN/DISCOMFORT • Mild discomfort or aching, tired eyes (chronic glaucoma) • Sudden or persistent severe pain or pressure in and around eye(s), headache (acute glaucoma)	
SAFETY • History of hemorrhage, trauma, ocular disease, tumor (secondary to trauma) • Difficulty seeing, managing activities	• Inflammatory disease of eye (glaucoma secondary to trauma)
TEACHING/LEARNING • Family history of glaucoma, diabetes, systemic vascular disorders • History of stress, allergies, vasomotor disturbances, such as increased venous pressure, endocrine imbalance, diabetes • History of ocular surgery or cataract removal, steroid use	
DISCHARGE PLAN CONSIDERATIONS • May require assistance with transportation, meal preparation, self-care, homemaker and maintenance tasks. ▶ Refer to section at end of plan for postdischarge considerations.	

TEST WHY IT IS DONE	WHAT IT TELLS ME
• *Ophthalmoscopy:* Assesses internal ocular structures by direct visualization. May be combined with slit-lamp examination for magnification of structures.	Identifies optic nerve damage, corneal and retinal abnormalities, and effects of and general vision deficits associated with glaucoma.
• *Visual acuity tests, such as Snellen and Jayer:* Part of routine eye examination to determine the smallest letters a person can read on a standardized chart or card held 14 to 20 feet away.	Abnormal results indicate eye condition requiring further evaluation of vision impairments.
• *Visual fields test, such as confrontation, tangent screen, and automated or manual perimetry:* Assesses vision when client looks forward while a light passes through peripheral vision fields.	These tests reveal the extent of damage to the optic neurons and demonstrate loss of peripheral vision that may be caused by glaucoma.
• *Fundus photography:* Photographs the optic nerve and other structures at back of eye.	Good early screening tool as it can reveal changes sometimes years in advance of vision loss.
• *Scanning laser polarimetry (SLP):* Uses laser technology to scan the eye and measure corneal and nerve fiber thickness.	Reveals early signs of optic nerve deterioration. A thinner cornea has been associated with an increased risk of POAG (Gordon et al, 2002).
• *Tonometry:* Measures IOP by recording the resistance of the cornea to pressure (indentation) (normal range: 10 to 21 mm Hg).	Pressures consistently greater than 21 mm Hg increase client's risk of glaucoma. In acute angle-closure glaucoma, IOP may be 50 mm Hg or higher. However, open-angle glaucoma can occur even in the absence of IOP (Aref & Schmitt, 2005).
• *Gonioscopy:* Evaluates the anterior chamber structures and the trabecular meshwork and its relationship to the iris. Determines if the drainage angle, where the iris meets the cornea, is open or closed.	Helps differentiate open-angle from angle-closure glaucoma.
• *Corneal pachymetry:* Measures corneal thickness using ultrasound.	A thin cornea may place client at higher risk for developing glaucoma (Brandt et al, n.d.; Van Leeuwen et al, 2006).
• *Provocative tests, such as dark room test, prone test, and mydriatic test:* Tests mirror the physiological conditions that induce pupil dilation.	May be useful in screening for angle-closure glaucoma, but these tests have largely been replaced by gonioscopy (American Optometric Association [AOA], 1994).
• *Ultrasound biomicroscopy (UBM):* Imaging technique that uses high-frequency ultrasound.	Useful for glaucoma entities with a structural component to their etiology.
• *Heidelberg retina tomography (HRT):* Laser-scanning microscope for acquiring and analyzing the posterior segment of the retina.	May be used to identify or monitor glaucoma progression. The retinal nerve fiber layer (RNFL) surrounding the optic nerve thins in glaucoma.
• *Optical coherence tomography (OCT):* Measures RNFL directly as well as corneal thickness.	Monitors glaucoma progression and identifies thinning cornea, which may cause an artificially low reading when the ocular pressure is measured.
• *Glucose tolerance test/fasting blood sugar (FBS):* Determines presence/control of diabetes.	Diabetes and hyperglycemia are sometimes implicated in secondary glaucoma.

Nursing Priorities

1. Prevent further visual deterioration.
2. Promote adaptation to changes in reduced visual acuity.
3. Prevent complications.
4. Provide information about disease process, prognosis, and treatment needs.

Discharge Goals

1. Vision maintained at highest possible level.
2. Client coping with situation in a positive manner.
3. Complications prevented or minimized.
4. Disease process, prognosis, and therapeutic regimen understood.
5. Plan in place to meet needs after discharge.

NURSING DIAGNOSIS: **disturbed visual Sensory Perception**

May be related to
Altered sensory reception: altered status of sense organs—increased IOP, ocular trauma or infection, cataracts
Biochemical imbalances—hyperglycemia/diabetes

Possibly evidenced by
Reported change in sensory acuity—photosensitivity, visual distortions, progressive loss of visual field; measured change in
    sensory acuity

Desired Outcomes/Evaluation Criteria—Client Will

Sensory Function: Vision (NOC)
Maintain current visual field and acuity without further loss.

Risk Control: Visual Impairment (NOC)
Participate in therapeutic regimen.
Follow prescribed medication regimen.

ACTIONS/INTERVENTIONS	RATIONALE
Communication Enhancement: Visual Deficit (NIC)	
Independent	
Ascertain type and degree of visual loss.	Affects choice of interventions and client's future expectations.
Encourage expression of feelings about loss or possibility of loss of vision.	Although early intervention may prevent blindness, client faces the possibility of or may have already experienced partial or complete loss of vision. Although vision loss cannot be restored (even with treatment), further loss can be prevented.
Recommend measures to assist client to manage visual limitations and provide safety, including reducing clutter, arranging furniture out of travel path, turning head to view subjects or objects, correcting for dim light, and problems of night vision.	Reduces safety hazards related to changes in visual fields or loss of vision and papillary accommodation to environmental light.
Elevate head of bed for hospitalized client as indicated.	Aids in reducing acute elevations of IOP.
Medication Administration: Eye (NIC)	
Explain the importance of medication administration as ordered by the physician.	Proper understanding may increase the client's motivation and participation in treatment plan.
Demonstrate and have client or significant other (SO) administer eye drops using correct procedures—placement of drop, counting drops, adhering to schedule, and not missing doses.	Although burdensome, lifelong treatment is needed to control IOP and prevent further loss of vision.
Collaborative	
Assist with administration of medications, as indicated:	
Chronic, open-angle type:	
Miotics, also called cholinergic agonists: for example, pilocarpine (Isopto Carpine, Ocusert, Pilopine HS gel)	These drugs cause pupillary constriction, facilitating the outflow of aqueous humor and lowering IOP. *Note:* Ocusert is a disc (similar to a contact lens) that is placed in the lower eyelid, where it can remain for up to 1 week before being replaced.
Anticholinesterase miotics: for example, demecarium (Humorsol), echothiophate (Phospholine Iodide), and isoflurophate (Floropryl)	These drugs are used for management of glaucoma not controlled with short-acting miotics. *Note:* Because of their potential for serious side effects, some authorities prefer surgery rather than use of the drugs (Glaucoma Research Foundation, n.d.).
Beta-blockers: for example, timolol (Timoptic), betaxolol (Betoptic), levobetaxolol (Betaxon), and carteolol (Ocupress)	These drugs decrease formation of aqueous humor without changing pupil size, vision, or accommodation. *Note:* These drugs may be contraindicated or require close monitoring for systemic effects in the presence of bradycardia or asthma.
Carbonic anhydrase inhibitors: for example, brinzolamide (Azopt) and dorzolamide (Trusopt)	These drugs decrease the amount and rate of production of aqueous humor. *Note:* Systemic adverse effects are common, including mood disturbances, gastrointestinal (GI) upset, and fatigue.
Prostaglandin agonists: for example, bimataprost (Lumigan), Latanaprost (Xalatan), and travaprost (Travatan)	Drugs in this class are commonly prescribed drops for increasing outflow drainage of aqueous humor. *Note:* May be preferred over beta-blockers because of lesser degree of systemic affect; however, may cause more redness of the eye than other drugs.

(continues on page 208)

ACTIONS/INTERVENTIONS (continued)	RATIONALE (continued)
Narrow-angle (angle-closure) type: Miotics (see preceding)	Contract the sphincter muscles of the iris, deepen anterior chamber, and dilate vessels of outflow tract during acute attack or before surgery.
Alpha agonists: for example, apraclonidine (Iopidine) and bromonidine (Alphagan)	These drugs both decrease production and increase drainage of aqueous humor and may be beneficial when client is unresponsive to other medications.
Hyperosmotic agents: for example, mannitol (Osmitrol), glycerin (Ophthalgan, Osmoglyn oral), and isosorbide (Ismotic)	Used to decrease circulating fluid volume, which will decrease production of aqueous humor if other treatments have not been successful.
Provide sedation and analgesics, as necessary.	Acute glaucoma attack is associated with sudden pain, which can precipitate anxiety and agitation, further elevating IOP. Medical management may be required before IOP decreases and pain subsides.
Prepare for surgical intervention as indicated: Laser therapy, such as argon laser trabeculoplasty (ALT), laser cyclophotocoagulation (CPC), or trabeculectomy/trephination with Malento valve implant or aqueous-venous shunt	Surgical treatment may be performed before or after attempts to reduce IOP with medications and include incisional or laser procedures. Filtering operations (laser surgery) are highly successful procedures for reducing IOP by creating an opening between the anterior chamber and the subjunctival spaces so that aqueous humor can bypass the trabecular mesh block. CPC separates ciliary body from the sclera by freezing to facilitate outflow of aqueous humor. *Note:* Apraclonidine (Iopidine) eye drops may be used in conjunction with laser therapy to lessen or prevent postprocedure elevations of IOP. A Malento valve implant or an aqueous venous shunt may be used to correct or prevent scarring over or closure of drainage sac created by trabeculectomy.
Iridotomy	Surgical removal of a portion of the iris facilitates drainage of aqueous humor through a newly created opening in the iris connecting to normal outflow channels. *Note:* Bilateral iridectomy is performed because glaucoma will usually develop in the other eye.
Diathermy or cryosurgery	Destroys the ciliary body and thereby reduces formation of aqueous humor.

NURSING DIAGNOSIS: **Anxiety [specify level]**

May be related to
Physiological factors, change in health status, presence of pain, possibility or reality of loss of vision
Unmet needs
Negative self-talk

Possibly evidenced by
Apprehension, uncertainty
Expressed concern regarding changes in life events

Desired Outcomes/Evaluation Criteria—Client Will

Anxiety Self-Control (NOC)
Appear relaxed and report anxiety is reduced to a manageable level.
Demonstrate positive problem-solving skills.
Use resources effectively.

ACTIONS/INTERVENTIONS	RATIONALE
Anxiety Reduction (NIC) *Independent* Assess anxiety level, degree of pain experienced, suddenness of onset of symptoms, and current knowledge of condition.	These factors affect client's perception of threat to self, potentiate the cycle of anxiety, and may interfere with medical attempts to control IOP.
Provide accurate, honest information. Discuss probability that careful monitoring and treatment can prevent additional loss of vision.	Reduces anxiety related to unknown or future expectations and provides factual basis for making informed choices about treatment.

ACTIONS/INTERVENTIONS (continued)	RATIONALE (continued)
Encourage client to acknowledge concerns and express feelings.	Provides opportunity for client to deal with reality of situation, clarify misconceptions, and problem-solve concerns.
Identify helpful resources.	Provides reassurance that client is not alone in dealing with problems.

NURSING DIAGNOSIS: **deficient Knowledge [Learning Need] regarding condition, prognosis, treatment, and self-care needs**

May be related to
Lack of exposure or unfamiliarity with resources
Lack of recall, information misinterpretation

Possibly evidenced by
Questions, statement of misconception
Inaccurate follow-through of instruction
Development of preventable complications

Desired Outcomes/Evaluation Criteria—Client Will

Knowledge: Illness Care (NOC)
Verbalize understanding of condition, prognosis, and treatment.
Identify relationship of signs and symptoms to the disease process.
Verbalize understanding of treatment needs.
Correctly perform necessary procedures and explain reasons for the actions.

ACTIONS/INTERVENTIONS	RATIONALE
Teaching: Disease Process (NIC) *Independent*	
Review pathology and prognosis of condition and lifelong treatment needs.	Provides opportunity to clarify or dispel misconceptions and present condition as something that is manageable.
Discuss necessity of wearing ID and medical alert bracelet.	Vital to provide information for caregivers in case of emergency to reduce risk of receiving contraindicated drugs such as atropine.
Demonstrate proper technique for administration of eye drops, gels, or discs. Have client or SO perform techniques until accurate with procedures.	Enhances effectiveness of treatment. Provides opportunity for client to show competence and ask questions.
Review importance of maintaining eye medication schedule. Address issues that may keep client from adhering to treatment plan.	This disease can be controlled but not cured, and maintaining a consistent medication regimen is vital to the prevention of blindness. *Note:* When client is not experiencing pain, cooperation with drug regimen and acceptance of lifestyle changes are often difficult to sustain, even if client is aware that blindness can result from failure to treat glaucoma with eye drops. Common factors in compliance with treatment regimen relate to forgetfulness, medication side effects, and financial constraints (Kowing & Kester, 2007).
Identify potential side effects and adverse reactions of treatment, such as decreased appetite, nausea, vomiting, diarrhea, fatigue, "drugged" feeling, decreased libido, impotence, cardiac irregularities, syncope, and heart failure (HF).	Drug side and adverse effects range from uncomfortable to severe or health threatening. Some clients develop sensitivity or allergy to parasympathomimetics, such as pilocarpine, or anticholinesterase drugs. These problems require medical evaluation and possible change in therapeutic regimen.
Encourage client to make necessary changes in lifestyle.	A tranquil lifestyle decreases the emotional response to stress, preventing ocular changes that push the iris forward, which may precipitate an acute attack.
Recommend regular use of sunglasses.	Glaucoma and glaucoma medications can cause eyes to be very light-sensitive. Special-purpose sunglasses that block at least 99% UVB rays and a minimum of 60% UVA rays are optimal for people with eye diseases (Glaucoma Research Foundation, n.d.).
Recommend that exercise and activity restrictions be discussed with healthcare provider.	Exercise restrictions may not be necessary, and regular exercise may be of benefit to the maintenance of normal eye pressures. Although not confirmed by any evidence, heavy lifting, yoga, or other exercises that involve head-down or inverted positions may be harmful.

(continues on page 210)

Discuss dietary considerations, such as adequate fluid, bulk, and fiber intake.

Measures to maintain consistency of stool to avoid constipation and straining during defecation.

Stress importance of routine checkups.

Important to monitor progression or maintenance of disease to allow for early intervention and prevent further loss of vision.

Advise client to immediately report severe eye pain, inflammation, increased photophobia, increased lacrimation, changes in visual field or existence of a veil-like curtain, blurred vision, and flashes of light or particles floating in visual field.

Prompt action may be necessary to prevent further vision loss or other complications, such as detached retina.

Recommend family members be examined regularly for signs of glaucoma.

Hereditary tendency for shallow anterior chambers places family members at increased risk for developing the condition. *Note:* African Americans in every age category should have periodic examinations because of increased incidence and more aggressive course of glaucoma in these individuals.

Identify strategies and resources for socialization, such as support groups, Visually Impaired Society, local library, and transportation services.

Decreased visual acuity may limit client's ability to drive and cause client to withdraw from usual activities.

POTENTIAL CONSIDERATIONS long-term or chronic concerns (dependent on client's age, physical condition and presence of complications, personal resources, and life responsibilities)
- *risk for Trauma*—poor vision
- *impaired Social Interaction*—limited physical mobility (poor vision), inadequate support system
- *ineffective self Health Management*—complexity of therapeutic regimen, economic difficulties, inadequate number and type of cues to action, perceived seriousness (of condition) or benefit (versus side effects)
- *situational low Self-Esteem*—decreased ability to perform activities of daily living (ADLs), loss of independence

---

SEIZURE DISORDERS

I. Pathophysiology
a. Sudden unregulated electrical discharge within the gray matter of the cortex that temporarily interrupts normal brain activity
b. Genetics plays a role in some cases.
c. May be idiopathic or acquired
   i. Idiopathic: In approximately 75% of all seizures, which includes epilepsy, no cause is identified (Fagley, 2007).
   ii. Acquired: Possible causes include acidosis, electrolyte imbalances, hypoglycemia (particularly related to type 1 diabetes), hypoxia, alcohol and drug withdrawal, dehydration, systemic lupus, hypertension, septicemia, tumors, and head trauma (Fagley, 2007).

II. Classification
a. Depends on whether the source of the seizure within the brain is localized (partial or focal onset seizures) or distributed (generalized seizures).
b. In adults, partial seizures are the most common type; can be classified depending on whether consciousness is unaffected (simple-partial seizure) or affected (complex-partial seizure).
   i. Simple (partial motor, partial sensory) seizure may be motor, for example, may manifest as a rhythmic jerking of one hand; sensory, autonomic, or psychic; individual can remember what happens but cannot control what is occurring.
   ii. Complex seizure lasts 30 seconds to 2 minutes and usually begins in temporal or frontal lobe before affecting other areas of the brain; individual appears dazed and confused with or without motor activity being apparent and may be preceded by an aura.

c. Generalized seizures involve loss of consciousness and are classified according to the effect on the body.
   i. Absence seizures (petit mal seizures): brief periods of impaired consciousness lasting up to 20 seconds without aura or postictal phase; there are no convulsions
   ii. Myoclonic: brief, jerky motor movements lasting more than 1 second that often cluster within several minutes
   iii. Clonic: rhythmic, jerky motor movements involving upper and lower extremities, with or without impaired consciousness
   iv. Tonic: sudden tonic extension or flexion of head, trunk, and extremities lasting several seconds
   v. Tonic-clonic (grand mal seizures): all areas of the cortex are involved, with generalized extension of extremities for several seconds, followed by rhythmic clonic movements and a prolonged postictal phase
   vi. Atonic: brief loss of postural tone, often resulting in falls and injury (Cavazos & Lum, 2007)

III. Etiology
a. Major causes in adults include conditions that alter how the brain works or that affect the brain's blood supply (National Institute for Neurological Disorders and Stroke [NINDS], 2008).
   i. Cerebral pathology: traumatic head injury, stroke, infections, hypoxia, expanding brain lesions, and increased intracranial pressure
   ii. Toxic agents: poisons, alcohol, overdoses of prescription or nonprescription drugs, and drugs of abuse (with drugs being the leading cause)

iii. Chemical imbalances: hypoglycemia, hypokalemia, hyponatremia, hypomagnesemia, and acidosis

iv. Fever: acute infections and heatstroke

v. Eclampsia: prenatal hypertension and toxemia of pregnancy

vi. Idiopathic: unknown origin (also known as epilepsy)

b. Risk factors for seizure by adult age group (Franges, 2006)

    i. Young adults: trauma, alcohol withdrawal, illicit drug use; brain tumor; cardiovascular disease

    ii. Adults: brain tumor; cerebrovascular disease, metabolic disorders; alcohol withdrawal

    iii. Older adults: stroke, brain tumor, Alzheimer's-type dementia

IV. Statistics

a. Morbidity: Epilepsy and seizures affect over 3 million Americans of all ages, with 200,000 new cases annually; about 1 in 100 people in the United States have experienced an unprovoked seizure or been diagnosed with epilepsy (NINDS, 2008).

b. Mortality: Most deaths are accidental due to impaired consciousness (Cavazos & Lum, 2007).

c. Cost: Estimated at $12.5 billion in direct and indirect costs annually (Epilepsy Foundation, 1995–2005).

GLOSSARY

Aura: A perceptual disturbance experienced by some people before a seizure in the prodromal phase (see below), often manifesting as the perception of a strange light or an unpleasant smell, but does not necessitate the onset of a seizure. The time span between the appearance of the aura and the onset of a seizure can be a few seconds up to an hour.

Epilepsy: Chronic neurological disorder characterized by recurrent seizures; estimated to affect 2.7 million Americans (Epilepsy Foundation, 1995–2005).

Ictal phase: Considered to be the seizure itself.

Postictal phase: The altered state of consciousness characterized by drowsiness, confusion, nausea, hypertension, headache, and other disorienting symptoms that occurs following a seizure, usually lasting between 5 and 30 minutes, but sometimes longer in the case of larger or more severe seizures.

Prodromal phase: An early symptom indicating the onset of an attack or a disease. Vague changes in emotional reactivity or affective response sometimes preceding aura and lasting minutes to hours, with symptoms such as diminished field of vision, disorientation, aphasia, or photosensitivity.

Seizure: Sudden discharge of electrical activity in the brain.

Care Setting

Seizure disorders are treated in a community setting; however, client with convulsive seizures may require brief inpatient care on a medical or subacute unit for stabilization or for treatment of status epilepticus (a life-threatening emergency).

Related Concerns

Cerebrovascular accident (CVA)/stroke, page 238
Craniocerebral trauma (acute rehabilitative phase), page 220
Psychosocial aspects of care, page 749
Substance dependence/abuse rehabilitation, page 835

Client Assessment Database

DIAGNOSTIC DIVISION MAY REPORT	MAY EXHIBIT
ACTIVITY/REST • Fatigue • General weakness • Limitation of activities, occupation imposed by self, significant other (SO), healthcare provider, or others	• Altered muscle tone, strength • Involuntary movement or contractions of muscles or muscle groups—generalized tonic-clonic seizures
CIRCULATION	• *Ictal:* Hypertension, increased pulse, cyanosis • *Postictal:* Vital signs normal or depressed with decreased pulse and respiration
EGO INTEGRITY • Internal or external stressors related to condition or treatment • Irritability • Fear of death or injury	• Wide range of emotional responses, especially when temporal lobe is involved

(continues on page 212)

DIAGNOSTIC DIVISION **MAY REPORT** (continued)	**MAY EXHIBIT** (continued)
• Sense of helplessness, hopelessness • Social embarrassment and isolation • Changes in relationships	
ELIMINATION • Episodic incontinence	• *Ictal:* Increased bladder pressure and sphincter tone • *Postictal:* Muscles relaxed, resulting in urinary or fecal incontinence
FOOD/FLUID • Food sensitivity • Nausea and vomiting correlating with seizure activity	• Dental or soft-tissue damage—injury during seizure • Gingival hyperplasia—side effect of long-term Dilantin use
NEUROSENSORY • History of headaches, recurring seizure activity, fainting, dizziness • History of head trauma, stroke, cerebral infections • *Prodromal phase:* Vague changes in emotional reactivity or affective response sometimes preceding aura and lasting minutes to hours • Presence of aura • *Postictal:* Weakness, muscle pain, areas of paresthesias or paralysis	Seizure characteristics are as follows: • *Convulsive generalized seizures:* • *Tonic-clonic (grand mal):* Rigidity and jerking, posturing, vocalization, loss of consciousness, dilated pupils, stertorous respiration, excessive salivation (froth), fecal and urinary incontinence, and biting of the tongue may occur and last 2 to 5 minutes • *Tonic phase:* Abrupt increase in muscle tone of torso and face, flexion of arms, extension of legs; lasts seconds • *Clonic phase:* Muscle contraction with relaxation occurring between tonic muscle contractions. Client lies still with flaccid muscles, may have stridorous breathing and excessive salivation. This phase lengthens as tonic muscle activity subsides. • *Postictal:* Client is exhausted, may sleep several hours, then may be weak, confused, and amnesic concerning the episode, with nausea and stiff, sore muscles. • *Partial seizures:* • *Complex (psychomotor/temporal lobe)—Ictal:* Consciousness impaired, with reactions such as dream state, staring, wandering, irritability, hallucinations, hostility, or fear. May display involuntary motor symptoms (lip smacking) and behaviors that appear purposeful but are inappropriate (automatism) and include impaired judgment and, on occasion, antisocial acts; lasts 1 to 3 minutes. • *Postictal:* Absence of memory for these events, mild to moderate confusion • *Simple (focal-motor and Jacksonian):* Often preceded by aura—may report déjà vu or fearful feeling • *Ictal*: May experience no loss of consciousness (unilateral) or lose consciousness (bilateral); convulsive movements and temporary disturbance in part controlled by the brain region involved—frontal lobe (motor dysfunction), parietal (numbness, tingling), occipital (bright, flashing lights), posterotemporal (difficulty speaking). Convulsions may march along limb or side of body in orderly progression. If restrained during seizure, client may exhibit combative and uncooperative behavior; lasts seconds to minutes.

DIAGNOSTIC DIVISION MAY REPORT (continued)	MAY EXHIBIT (continued)
	• *Status epilepticus (SE)—Ictal:* 30 or more minutes of continuous generalized seizure activity or two or more sequential seizures without full recovery of consciousness in between, possibly related to abrupt withdrawal of anticonvulsants and other metabolic phenomena. If absence seizures are the type of seizure activity, SE may go undetected for a period of time because client does not lose consciousness.
PAIN/DISCOMFORT • Headache • *Ictal:* Paroxysmal abdominal pain may occur during some partial or focal seizures without loss of consciousness • *Postictal:* Muscle, back soreness	• Guarding behavior • Alteration in muscle tone • Distraction behavior, restlessness
RESPIRATION	• *Ictal:* Clenched teeth, cyanosis, decreased or rapid respirations; increased mucous secretions • *Postictal:* Apnea
SAFETY • History of accidental falls, injuries, fractures	• Soft-tissue injury, ecchymosis • Decreased general strength and muscle tone
SOCIAL INTERACTION • Problems with interpersonal relationships within family or socially • Limitation or avoidance of social contacts	
TEACHING/LEARNING • Familial history of epilepsy • Drug use or misuse, including alcohol and illicit drugs • Use of herbal supplements, such as aloe, betony, blue cohosh, kava • Increased frequency of episodes, difficulty with learning resulting in failure to improve	
DISCHARGE PLAN CONSIDERATIONS • May require changes in medications, assistance with some homemaker or maintenance tasks relative to issues of safety, and transportation ❱ Refer to section at end of plan for postdischarge considerations.	

Diagnostic Studies

May vary depending upon whether or not the client has a known seizure disorder.

TEST WHY IT IS DONE	WHAT IT TELLS ME
BLOOD TESTS • *Electrolytes:* Substances that will dissociate into ions in solution and acquire the capacity to conduct electricity. Electrolytes include sodium, potassium, chloride, calcium, and phosphate. • *Glucose:* Simple sugar that is a major energy source for all cellular and bodily functions.	Imbalances of sodium, calcium, and magnesium may affect or predispose to seizure activity. Low glucose (hypoglycemia) may precipitate seizure activity.

(continues on page 214)

TEST **WHY IT IS DONE** (continued)	**WHAT IT TELLS ME** (continued)

- *Plasma osmolality levels:* Measure of the concentration of substances, such as sodium, chloride, potassium, and other ions in blood.

Imbalances can both trigger and result from seizures

- *Blood urea nitrogen (BUN):* A waste product in the blood from the breakdown of protein, which is filtered by the kidneys.

Elevated BUN may potentiate seizure activity or may indicate nephrotoxicity related to medication regimen.

- *Liver function tests (LFTs):* Common tests used to evaluate liver function include (and are not limited to) albumin, aluminum phosphide (ALP), alanine aminotransferase (ALT), aspartate aminotransferase (AST), and bilirubin.

May be elevated due to alcohol, drugs, and poisoning; metabolic abnormalities (potentiates seizures); or reflect drug reaction/interaction.

- *Complete blood count (CBC):* Battery of screening tests, which typically includes hemoglobin (Hgb), hematocrit (Hct), red blood cell (RBC) count and morphology, indices, and distribution width index; platelet count and size; white blood cell (WBC) count and differential.

Elevated WBCs may indicate presence of infection—can be a precipitator of SE. Anemia may result from drug therapy.

- *Serum drug levels:* To verify presence and therapeutic levels of antiepileptic drugs (AEDs).

Medication dosage or timing dependent on whether drug is low or elevated.

- *Toxicology screen:* Various tests to determine the type and approximate amount of legal and illegal drugs a person has taken.

May determine potentiating factors, such as alcohol or other drug use.

OTHER DIAGNOSTIC STUDIES

- *Electroencephalogram (EEG):* Recording of the electrical activity of the brain by means of electrodes placed on the surface of the head.

Definitive test for seizure activity, locating area of cerebral dysfunction and measuring brain activity. However, EEGs obtained soon after a suspected seizure often record nonspecific patterns or may be normal. Often, performing an EEG within 24 hours of a seizure is more likely to show an abnormality, and more than one EEG may be necessary to detect seizure activity.

- *Video–EEG monitoring:* Simultaneous use of a video camera and EEG.

May identify exact focus of seizure activity in the brain while providing visual evidence of client symptoms during the attack.

- *Computed tomography (CT) scan:* Uses low radiation x-rays to create a computer-generated, three-dimensional image of the brain.

May reveal such abnormalities as blood clots, cysts, tumors, or scar tissue in the skull or brain related to seizures.

- *Magnetic resonance imaging (MRI) scan:* Uses magnetic fields and computer technology to generate images of the internal anatomy of the brain.

MRI may be used if the cause of seizure is subject to change, such as a benign tumor, which may grow, or a vascular malformation, which could bleed. MRI can also be helpful if the cause of seizure is suspected but indefinite, such as a mild head injury.

- *Positron emission tomography (PET) scan:* Reveals metabolic functions in the brain.

Demonstrates metabolic alterations, such as how much glucose or oxygen is metabolized at site of lesion.

- *Single photon emission computed tomography (SPECT) scan:* Maps cerebral blood flood.

May show local areas of brain dysfunction, which may be especially useful in client with seizure activity when CT and MRI are normal.

- *Magnetic resonance spectroscopy (MRS) scan:* Noninvasive imaging technique that determines the concentration of metabolites within tissues to reveal metabolism and biochemistry of the brain in action.

Locates a potential seizure focus by identifying biochemical changes in the brain tissue where the seizure occurs.

- *Magnetoencephalogram (MEG):* Functional imaging technique that measures magnetic fields generated by the electrical activity of neurons. A map is produced which, when compared with results of MRI, differentiates normal from abnormal brain tissue.

Localizes seizure foci and boundaries of normal tissues to facilitate surgical removal of affected area.

- *Wada's test:* Neuroimaging and neuropsychological testing to examine memory and language functions.

Determines hemispheric dominance in client being evaluated for epilepsy surgery.

Nursing Priorities————————

1. Prevent or control seizure activity.
2. Protect client from injury.
3. Maintain airway and respiratory function.
4. Promote positive self-esteem.
5. Provide information about disease process, prognosis, and treatment needs.

Discharge Goals————————

1. Seizure activity controlled.
2. Complications and injury prevented.
3. Capable, competent self-image displayed.
4. Disease process, prognosis, therapeutic regimen, and limitations understood.
5. Plan in place to meet needs after discharge.

NURSING DIAGNOSIS: **risk for Trauma/Suffocation**

Risk factors may include
Weakness, balancing difficulties
Cognitive limitations, altered consciousness
Loss of large or small muscle coordination
Emotional difficulties

Possibly evidenced by
(Not applicable; presence of signs and symptoms establishes an *actual* diagnosis)

Desired Outcomes/Evaluation Criteria—Client Will

Risk Detection (NOC)
Verbalize understanding of factors that contribute to possibility of trauma or suffocation and take steps to correct situation.

Risk Control (NOC)
Demonstrate behaviors and lifestyle changes to reduce risk factors and protect self from future seizure events and injury.
Modify environment as indicated to enhance safety.
Maintain treatment regimen to control or eliminate seizure activity.

Significant Other [SO]/Caregiver Will

Knowledge: Personal Safety (NOC)
Identify actions or measures to take when seizure activity occurs.

ACTIONS/INTERVENTIONS	RATIONALE
Seizure Precautions (NIC) *Independent*	
Explore with client the various stimuli that may precipitate seizure activity.	Alcohol, various drugs, and other stimuli, such as loss of sleep, flashing lights, and prolonged television viewing, may increase the potential for seizure activity. Client may or may not have control over many precipitating factors, but may benefit from becoming aware of risks.
Discuss seizure warning signs, if appropriate, and usual seizure pattern. Teach SO to recognize warning signs and how to care for client during and after seizure.	Can enable client or SO to protect individual from injury and to recognize changes that require notification of physician and further intervention. Knowing what to do when seizure occurs can prevent injury or complications and decreases SO's feelings of helplessness.
Seizure Management (NIC) In hospitalized client:	
Keep padded side rails up with bed in lowest position, or place bed up against wall, and add floor pad if rails are not available or appropriate.	Minimizes injury should frequent or generalized seizures occur while client is in bed.
Maintain strict bedrest if prodromal signs or aura is experienced. Explain necessity for these actions.	Client may feel restless, need to ambulate or even defecate during aural phase, thereby inadvertently removing self from safe environment and easy observation. Understanding importance of providing for own safety needs may enhance client cooperation.
Stay with client during and after seizure.	Promotes client safety and reduces sense of isolation during event.
Turn head to side and suction airway as indicated. Insert soft bite block per facility protocol, only if jaw relaxed.	Helps maintain airway and reduces risk of oral trauma but should not be "forced" or inserted when teeth are clenched because dental and soft-tissue damage may result. *Note:* Current practice is mixed regarding the use of airways during seizure activity. (Refer to ND: risk for ineffective Airway Clearance/Breathing Pattern, following.)

(continues on page 216)

Cradle head, place on soft area, or assist to floor if out of bed. Do not attempt to restrain.

Gentle guiding of extremities reduces risk of physical injury when client lacks voluntary muscle control. *Note:* If attempt is made to restrain client during seizure, erratic movements may increase, and client may injure self or others.

Perform neurological and vital sign checks after seizure: level of consciousness, orientation, ability to comply with simple commands, ability to speak, memory of incident, weakness or motor deficits, blood pressure (BP), pulse, and respiratory rate.

Documents postictal state and time and completeness of recovery to normal state. May identify additional safety concerns to be addressed.

Reorient client following seizure activity.

Client may be confused, disoriented, and possibly amnesic after the seizure and need help to regain control and alleviate anxiety.

Allow postictal "automatic" behavior without interfering while providing environmental protection.

May display behavior of motor or psychic origin that seems inappropriate or irrelevant for time and place. Attempts to control or prevent activity may result in client becoming aggressive or combative.

Investigate reports of pain.

May be result of repetitive muscle contractions or symptom of injury incurred, requiring further evaluation and intervention.

Observe for SE.

This is a life-threatening emergency that, if left untreated, could cause metabolic acidosis, hyperthermia, hypoglycemia, arrhythmias, hypoxia, increased intracranial pressure, airway obstruction, and respiratory arrest. Immediate intervention is required to control seizure activity and prevent permanent injury or death. *Note:* Although absence seizures may become static, they are not usually life threatening.

Document preseizure activity, presence of aura or unusual behavior, type of seizure activity, such as location and duration of motor activity, loss of consciousness, incontinence, eye activity, respiratory impairment, and cyanosis, and frequency or recurrence. Note whether client fell, expressed vocalizations, drooled, or had automatisms, such as lip smacking, chewing, and picking at clothes.

Helps localize the cerebral area of involvement and may be useful in chronic conditions in helping client and SO prepare for or manage seizure activity.

Collaborative

Administer medications, as indicated, for example:

Long-term drug treatment is required for clients who have recurrent seizures, seizures with an unknown cause, or a cause that can't be reversed. Choice of drug therapy and route of administration depends on seizure type and current severity. Some clients require multiple medications or frequent medication adjustments to control seizure activity. This increases the risk of adverse reactions and problems with adherence.

AEDs, such as first-line drugs, including carbamazepine (Tegretol), ethosuximide (Zarontin), lamotrigine (Lamictal), levetiracetam (Keppra), oxycarbazepine (Trileptal), valproate (Eplim), and valproic divalproex (Depakote)

AEDs include several classes of medications used to decrease the incidence and severity of seizures. AEDs are divided into two categories—first-line and second-line drugs. First-line drugs are prescribed on their own when treatment is started. AEDs treat and/or prevent seizures by raising the seizure threshold, stabilizing nerve cell membranes, reducing the excitability of the neurons, or through direct action on the limbic system, thalamus, and hypothalamus. Goal is optimal suppression of seizure activity with lowest possible dose of drug and with fewest side effects.

Second-line drugs, including hydantoins, such as phenytoin (Dilantin) and fosphenytoin (Cerebyx); benzodizapindes, such as clonazepam (Rivitril) and colobazam (Frisium); barbiturates, such as pentobarbital (Nembutal) and phenobarbital (Luminal); acetazolamide (Diamox), gabapentin (Neurontin), ethotoin (Peganone), and methsuximide (Celotin); miscellaneous drugs, such as piracetam (Nootropil), pregabalin (Lyrica), vigabatrin (Sabril), and zonisamide (Zonegran)

If a first-line drug does not stop seizures from happening, a different first-line drug may be given. Alternatively, a second-line drug may be prescribed alongside the first-line drug when seizures are not adequately controlled by other drugs.

Diazepam (Valium, Diastat rectal gel)

May be used alone or in combination with phenobarbital to suppress status seizure activity. Diastat, a gel, may be administered rectally, even in the home setting, to reduce frequency of seizures and need for additional medical care.

ACTIONS/INTERVENTIONS (continued)	RATIONALE (continued)
Glucose and thiamine	May be given to restore metabolic balance if seizure is induced by hypoglycemia or alcohol.
Monitor and document AED drug levels, corresponding side effects, and frequency of seizure activity.	Blood levels of the various AEDs should be evaluated on a regular basis, such as weekly for a period of time, then monthly, then annually. Blood levels should also be done when breakthrough seizures occur, or any change occurs in the client's status. Standard therapeutic level may not be optimal for individual client if untoward side effects develop or seizures are not controlled.
Monitor CBC, electrolytes, and glucose levels.	Identifies factors that can lower the seizure threshold.
Prepare for aggressive interventions, such as surgery or electrode implantation as indicated.	Vagal nerve stimulator, magnetic beam therapy, or other surgical intervention, such as temporal lobectomy, may be done for intractable seizures or well-localized epileptogenic lesions when client is disabled and at high risk for serious injury. Success has been reported with gamma ray radio-surgery for the treatment of multiple seizure activity that has otherwise been difficult to control.

NURSING DIAGNOSIS: risk for ineffective Airway Clearance/Breathing Pattern

Risk factors may include
Neuromuscular impairment
Tracheobronchial obstruction
Perceptual or cognitive impairment

Possibly evidenced by
(Not applicable; presence of signs and symptoms establishes an *actual* diagnosis)

Desired Outcomes/Evaluation Criteria—Client Will

Respiratory Status: Ventilation (NOC)
Maintain effective respiratory pattern with airway patent and aspiration prevented.

ACTIONS/INTERVENTIONS	RATIONALE
Airway Management (NIC)	
Independent	
Encourage client to empty mouth of dentures or foreign objects if aura occurs and to avoid chewing gum or sucking lozenges if seizures can occur without warning.	Reduces risk of aspiration or foreign bodies lodging in pharynx.
Place in lying position on a flat surface; turn head to side during seizure activity.	Promotes drainage of secretions; prevents tongue from obstructing airway.
Loosen clothing from neck, chest, and abdominal areas.	Facilitates chest expansion, enhancing breathing.
Insert soft airway as indicated per facility protocol and only if jaw is relaxed.	If inserted before jaw is tightened, these devices may prevent biting of tongue and facilitate suctioning and respiratory support if required. Airway adjunct may be indicated after cessation of seizure activity if client is unconscious and unable to maintain safe position of tongue. *Note:* Current opinion is mixed regarding the use of airways during seizure activity.
Suction as needed.	Reduces risk of aspiration or asphyxiation. *Note:* Risk of aspiration is low unless individual has eaten within the last 40 minutes.
Collaborative	
Administer supplemental oxygen or bag ventilation, as needed postictally.	May reduce cerebral hypoxia resulting from decreased circulation and oxygenation secondary to vascular spasm during seizure. *Note:* Artificial ventilation during general seizure activity is of limited or no benefit because it is not possible to move air in and out of lungs during sustained contraction of respiratory musculature. As seizure abates, respiratory function will return unless a secondary problem exists, such as foreign body or aspiration.
Prepare for and assist with intubation, if indicated.	Presence of prolonged apnea postictally may require ventilatory support.

NURSING DIAGNOSIS: Self-Esteem [specify situational or chronic low]

May be related to
Stigma associated with condition
Perception of helplessness

Possibly evidenced by
Verbalization about changed lifestyle
Fear of rejection; negative feelings about body (self-image)
Potential change in perception of role
Change in usual patterns of responsibility
Denial of problem resulting in lack of follow-through or nonparticipation in therapy

Desired Outcomes/Evaluation Criteria—Client Will

Self-Esteem (NOC)
Identify feelings and methods for coping with negative perception of self.
Verbalize increased sense of self-esteem in relation to diagnosis.
Verbalize realistic perception and acceptance of self in changed role or lifestyle.

ACTIONS/INTERVENTIONS	RATIONALE
Self-Esteem Enhancement (NIC)	
Independent	
Discuss feelings about diagnosis and perception of threat to self. Encourage expression of feelings.	Reactions vary among individuals, and previous knowledge or experience with this condition affects acceptance of therapeutic regimen. Verbalization of fears, anger, and concerns about future implications can help client begin to accept and deal with situation.
Identify possible or anticipated public reaction to condition. Encourage client to refrain from concealing problem.	Provides opportunity to problem-solve response, and provides measure of control over situation. Concealment is destructive to self-esteem (potentiates denial), blocking progress in dealing with problem, and may actually increase risk of injury or negative response when seizure does occur.
Explore with client current and past successes and strengths.	Focusing on positive aspects can help alleviate feelings of guilt or self-consciousness and help client begin to accept manageability of condition.
Avoid overprotecting client; encourage activities, providing supervision or monitoring when indicated.	Participation in as many experiences as possible can lessen depression about limitations. Observation or supervision may need to be provided for such activities as gymnastics, climbing, and water sports.
Determine attitudes and capabilities of SO. Help individual realize that client's feelings are normal; however, guilt and blame are not helpful.	Negative expectations from SO may affect client's sense of competency and self-esteem and interfere with support received from SO, limiting potential for optimal management and personal growth.
Stress importance of staff and SO remaining calm during seizure activity.	Anxiety of caregivers is contagious and can be conveyed to the client, increasing or multiplying individual's own negative perceptions of situation and self.
Refer client/SO to support groups, such as Epilepsy Foundation of America, National Association of Epilepsy Centers, and Delta Society's National Service Dog Center.	Provides opportunity to gain information, support, and ideas for dealing with problems from others who share similar experiences. *Note:* Some service dogs have ability to sense or predict seizure activity, allowing client to institute safety measures and increasing independence and personal sense of control.
Discuss referral for psychotherapy with client/SO.	Seizures have a profound effect on personal self-esteem, and client/SO may feel guilt over perceived limitations and public stigma. Counseling can help overcome feelings of inferiority and self-consciousness.

NURSING DIAGNOSIS: deficient Knowledge [Learning Need] regarding condition, prognosis, treatment regimen, self-care, and discharge needs

May be related to
Lack of exposure, unfamiliarity with resources
Information misinterpretation
Lack of recall; cognitive limitation

Possibly evidenced by
Questions, statement of concerns
Increased frequency and lack of control of seizure activity
Lack of follow-through of drug regimen

Desired Outcomes/Evaluation Criteria—Client Will

Knowledge: Illness Care (NOC)
Verbalize understanding of disorder and various stimuli that may increase or potentiate seizure activity.
Adhere to prescribed drug regimen.

Knowledge: Personal Safety (NOC)
Initiate necessary lifestyle and behavior changes as indicated.

ACTIONS/INTERVENTIONS	RATIONALE
Teaching: Disease Process (NIC)	
Independent	
Review pathology and prognosis of condition and lifelong need for treatments as indicated. Discuss client's particular trigger factors, such as flashing lights, hyperventilation, loud noises, video games, and TV viewing, if known.	Provides opportunity to clarify and dispel misconceptions and present condition as something that is manageable within a normal lifestyle.
Review possible effects of female hormonal changes.	Alterations in hormonal levels that occur during menstruation and pregnancy may increase risk of seizure breakthrough.
Discuss significance of maintaining good general health, such as adequate diet; rest; moderate exercise; and avoidance of exhaustion, alcohol, caffeine, and stimulant drugs.	Regularity and moderation in activities may aid in reducing and controlling precipitating factors, enhancing sense of general well-being, and strengthening coping ability and self-esteem. *Note:* Too little sleep or too much alcohol can precipitate seizure activity in some people.
Review importance of good oral hygiene and regular dental care.	Reduces risk of oral infections and gingival hyperplasia.
Encourage client who smokes to refrain from smoking except while supervised.	May cause burns if cigarette is accidentally dropped during aura or seizure activity.
Evaluate need for and provide protective headgear.	Use of helmet may provide added protection for individuals who suffer recurrent and severe seizures.
Identify necessity and promote acceptance of actual limitations; discuss safety measures regarding driving, using mechanical equipment, climbing ladders, swimming, and hobbies.	Reduces risk of injury to self or others, especially if seizures occur without warning.
Discuss local laws or restrictions pertaining to persons with epilepsy or seizure disorder. Encourage awareness but not necessarily acceptance of these policies.	Although legal and civil rights of persons with epilepsy have improved during the past decade, restrictions still exist in some states pertaining to obtaining a driver's license, sterilization, workers' compensation, and required reporting to state agencies.
Teaching: Prescribed Medication (NIC)	
Review medication regimen, necessity of taking drugs as ordered, and not discontinuing therapy without physician supervision. Include directions for missed dose.	Lack of cooperation with medication regimen is a leading cause of seizure breakthrough. Client needs to know risks of status epilepticus resulting from abrupt withdrawal of anticonvulsants. Depending on the drug dose and frequency, client may be instructed to take missed dose if remembered within a predetermined time frame.
Recommend taking drugs with meals if appropriate.	May reduce incidence of gastric irritation, nausea, and vomiting.
Discuss nuisance and adverse side effects of particular drugs, such as drowsiness, fatigue, lethargy, hyperactivity, sleep disturbances, gingival hypertrophy, visual disturbances, nausea or vomiting, rashes, syncope and ataxia, birth defects, and aplastic anemia.	May indicate need for change in dosage or choice of drug therapy. Promotes involvement and participation in decision-making process and awareness of potential long-term effects of drug therapy, and provides opportunity to minimize or prevent complications.

(continues on page 220)

Provide information about potential drug interactions and necessity of notifying other healthcare providers of drug regimen.

Knowledge of anticonvulsant use reduces risk of prescribing drugs that may interact, thus altering seizure threshold or therapeutic effect. For example, phenytoin (Dilantin) potentiates anticoagulant effect of warfarin (Coumadin), whereas isoniazid (INH) and chloramphenicol (Chloromycetin) increase the effect of Dilantin, and some antibiotics, such as erythromycin, can cause elevation of serum level of carbamazepine (Tegretol), possibly to toxic levels.

Review proper use of diazepam rectal gel (Diastat) with client and SO/caregiver as appropriate.

Useful in controlling serial or cluster seizures. Can be administered in any setting and is effective usually within 15 minutes. May reduce dependence on emergency department visits.

Discuss use of over-the-counter (OTC) medications and supplements and herbals.

Anticonvulsant drugs may interact with many other medications and substances. Some medications can decrease the effectiveness of anticonvulsant drugs, or the client may choose a folk remedy or herbal supplement without being aware of its effect.

Encourage client to wear identification tag or bracelet stating the presence of a seizure disorder.

Expedites treatment and diagnosis in emergency situations.

Stress need for routine follow-up care and laboratory testing as indicated; for example, CBC should be monitored biannually and in presence of sore throat or fever and signs of other infection.

Therapeutic needs may change and serious drug side effects such as agranulocytosis or toxicity may develop.

POTENTIAL CONSIDERATIONS following acute hospitalization (dependent on client's age, physical condition and presence of complications, personal resources, and life responsibilities)
- *risk for Injury*—weakness, balancing difficulties, cognitive limitations and altered consciousness, loss of large or small muscle coordination
- *Self-Esteem (specify)*—stigma associated with condition, perception of being out of control, personal vulnerability, negative evaluation of self/capabilities
- *ineffective self Health Management*—social support deficits, perceived benefit (versus side effects of medication), perceived susceptibility (possible long periods of remission)

CRANIOCEREBRAL TRAUMA—ACUTE REHABILITATIVE PHASE

I. Pathophysiology
a. Craniocerebral trauma, also called traumatic brain injury (TBI), acquired brain injury, head injury—Physical injury to the cranium and intracranial structures with varied outcomes, ranging from no apparent (or a temporary neurological) disturbance to permanent impairment of brain function, including persistent vegetative state or even death depending on the extent of the damage
b. TBI may be open or closed and can include brain concussion, contusion, laceration, hemorrhage, or skull fractures.
  i. Concussion: most minor and most common form of head injury
  ii. Intracranial hemorrhage: defined by the region of the brain (intracerebral) or surrounding structures affected, such as subdural, epidural, subarachnoid, brainstem
    1. Intracerebral hemorrhage: may occur along with other brain injuries, particularly contusions, with signs and symptoms dependent on the size and location and may be apparent immediately or develop slowly (Zink, 2005).
    2. Acute subdural hematoma: caused by venous bleeding when bridging veins are torn, occurring in 5% to 25% of all severe head injuries involving a contusion or laceration and often accompanying intracerebral bleeding (Reddy, 2006); signs and symptoms present almost immediately and increase rapidly.
    3. Epidural hematoma: arterial bleeding usually from the middle meningeal artery in the temporal region, typically manifested by a brief loss of consciousness at the time of trauma, then a lucid interval, which may last for several hours; between 30% and 50% of individuals incur neurological deterioration (Reddy, 2006).

II. Etiology
a. Primary injury (Zink, 2005)
  i. Penetrating injury: Object forcibly enters the cranial vault, damaging the protective meningeal layers, cerebral blood vessels, and brain tissue.
  ii. Contact phenomena injury: Object strikes the head, resulting in concussion, cerebral contusion, skull fracture, or intracranial hemorrhage.

iii. Acceleration-deceleration injury: Brain rapidly accelerates and decelerates within the skull, causing the brain to strike the skull, usually in the front and the back of the skull, causing tearing of neuronal tissue and cerebral blood vessels.

iv. Rotational acceleration-deceleration injury: Forces cause the brain to twist within the skull, resulting in torsion and shearing of nerve tissue and blood vessels.

b. Secondary brain injury (Granacher, 2003)

i. Thought to involve inflammation and the natural process of programmed cell death (apoptosis).

ii. Diffuse axonal injury: shearing injury of large nerve fibers (axons covered with myelin) in many areas of the brain, or stretching or shearing of blood vessels from the same forces, producing hemorrhage

iii. Systemic or neurological complications can also cause or exacerbate secondary brain injury—hypotension, hypoxia, hypercapnia, intracranial hypertension, acid-base imbalance, cerebral vasospasm, electrolyte abnormalities, hyperthermia, infection, cerebral ischemia, seizures, and hypoglycemia or hyperglycemia.

c. Leading mechanism for TBI in the United States: (Langlois, 2004)

i. Falls: 28%, highest for children aged 0 to 4 and those aged 75 or older

ii. Motor vehicle-traffic crashes: 20%

iii. Struck by or against: 19%, which includes sports-related injuries

iv. Assaults: 11%, including firearm use

v. Gunshot wounds: most common penetrating injury and most deadly cause of TBI in clients under age 35 (Zink, 2005)

vi. Blasts: leading cause of TBI for active duty military personnel in war zones (Defense and Veterans Brain Injury Center, n.d.)

III. Statistics (Centers for Disease Control and Prevention [CDC], 2006)

a. Morbidity: 1.4 million people sustain a TBI annually in the United States, 1.1 million are treated and released from an emergency department, 235,000 are hospitalized; approximately 2% of the U.S. population currently have a long-term or lifelong need for help to perform activities of daily living as a result of a TBI (Thurman et al, 1999).

b. Mortality: There are 50,000 deaths annually.

c. Cost: Direct medical costs and indirect costs, such as lost productivity of TBI, totaled an estimated $60 billion in the United States in 2000 (Finkelstein, 2006).

GLOSSARY

Amnesia: Loss of memory about recent event or a particular period of time, such as events surrounding injury.

Anomia: Inability to remember names of objects; individual may speak fluently but have to use other words to describe familiar objects.

Aphasia: Loss of ability to communicate or express oneself and to understand language due to brain dysfunction.

Apraxia: Inability to perform complex or skilled movement or use objects properly in the absence of sensory or motor impairments.

Ataxia: Loss of muscle control or coordination, especially with voluntary movement, interfering with an individual's ability to walk, talk, and perform activities of daily living (ADLs).

Closed head injury: Blunt trauma to the brain or brain structures by a direct blow or rapid deceleration, such as striking the windshield of a car, without penetration of the skull.

Cognition: The process of knowing, including awareness of thoughts or perceptions, ability to process information, reasoning, and judgment.

Coma: A state of unconsciousness from which the individual cannot be aroused even with stimulation; completely unresponsive to environment.

Concussion: Injury to brain resulting from impact with an object, such as blow to the head or sudden deceleration, causing temporary loss of normal brain function with or without loss of consciousness.

Contusion: Focal brain injury—bruising of brain tissue and damage to blood vessels due to a blow or rapid deceleration.

Deceleration: Rapid decrease in velocity causing injury when a moving body part hits a stationary object, such as the brain hitting the inside of the skull.

Decerebrate posture: Rigid extension of the arms and legs, pronation of forearms, downward pointing of toes, and backward arching of head in response to noxious stimuli when cerebral control of spinal reflexes is lost, as with severe injury at the level of the brainstem.

Decorticate posture: Muscle rigidity with arms flexed toward chest, fists clenched, and legs extended in response to noxious stimuli and associated with brain injury at or above the upper brainstem.

Dystonia: Involuntary prolonged muscle contractions causing twisting of the body, repetitive movements, and abnormal postures.

Glasgow Coma Scale (GCS): Standardized rating scale used to determine an individual's level of consciousness (LOC) and degree of brain impairment by measuring eye opening and verbal and motor response to stimuli. Scores range from a low of 3 to a high of 15, with score of 12 to 15 suggesting mild brain injury; 9 to 11, moderate injury; and 8 or lower, severe brain injury (CNS, 2006).

Hematoma, intracranial: Collection of blood within the skull caused by ruptured blood vessels, which may be localized in one area of the brain (intracerebral), located above the dura mater (epidural), beneath the dura (subdural), or between the arachnoid membrane and the pia mater (subarachnoid).

Hemiparesis: Weakness or partial paralysis of one side of the body.

(continues on page 222)

Intracranial pressure (ICP): The pressure exerted by cerebrospinal fluid (CSF) within the cranium is normally 8 to 18 mm Hg in a supine adult at rest. An increase in pressure may be due to an increase in CSF or increased pressure within the brain from a lesion or swelling of the brain itself.

Open head injury: Open fracture of the skull as may occur with high-impact crashes, severe assaults with an object, or gunshot or blast injury to the head.

Post-traumatic amnesia (PTA): A state of agitation, confusion, and memory loss following a traumatic brain injury (TBI), which can last a few days to months and is marked by impaired ability to process information accurately and inability to form new memories.

Posturing: Awkward or unnatural posture maintained for a prolonged period of time that may be associated with brain injury, such as decorticate or decerebrate, suggesting a poor prognosis.

Proprioception: Awareness of posture, movement, equilibrium, and relationship of self and limbs to environment.

Quadriparesis: Muscle weakness or lack of control of all four extremities—also called tetraparesis.

Sympathetic storming (also called storming): Exaggerated stress response in individuals with severe TBI (GCS score 3 to 8), with hypothalamic stimulation of the sympathetic nervous system and adrenal glands, thereby causing an increase in circulating corticoids and catecholamines, which results in increased agitation, extreme posturing, hypertension, tachycardia, tachypnea, diaphoresis, and hyperthermia; episodes occur within first 24 hours of injury or in the weeks following injury (Lemke, 2007).

Care Setting

This plan of care focuses on acute care and acute inpatient rehabilitation. Brain injury care for those experiencing moderate to severe trauma progresses along a continuum of care, beginning with acute hospital care and inpatient rehabilitation to subacute and outpatient rehabilitation, as well as home- and community-based services.

Related Concerns

Cerebrovascular accident (CVA)/stroke, page 238
Psychosocial aspects of care, page 749
Seizure disorders, page 210
Surgical intervention, page 782
Thrombophlebitis: deep vein thrombosis, page 111
Total nutritional support: parenteral/enteral feeding, page 469
Upper gastrointestinal/esophageal bleeding, page 306

Client Assessment Database

Data depend on type, location, and severity of injury and may be complicated by additional injury to other vital organs.

DIAGNOSTIC DIVISION MAY REPORT	MAY EXHIBIT
ACTIVITY/REST • Weakness, fatigue • Sleep problems, insomnia • Clumsiness, loss of balance	• Altered consciousness, lethargy • Hemiparesis, quadriparesis • Unsteady gait (ataxia); balance problems • Orthopedic injuries (trauma) • Loss of muscle tone, muscle spasticity
CIRCULATION	• Normal or altered blood pressure (BP) (hypotension or hypertension); prolonged hypertension and arrhythmias can occur as a result of sympathetic storming (Lemke, 2007) • Changes in heart rate, including bradycardia, tachycardia alternating with bradycardia, other dysrhythmias (not usually associated with hemodynamic instability) • Diaphoresis can be severe with storming (Lemke, 2007)
EGO INTEGRITY • Significant other (SO) may report that client's personality changes and behavioral problems are the most difficult disabilities to handle • Problems coping • Difficulty making decisions	• Behavior or personality changes (subtle to dramatic) may include depression, apathy, anxiety, irritability, impulsivity, anger, paranoia, confusion, frustration, agitation, and mood swings

DIAGNOSTIC DIVISION MAY REPORT (continued)	MAY EXHIBIT (continued)
ELIMINATION **FOOD/FLUID** • Nausea • Changes in appetite **HYGIENE** **NEUROSENSORY** • Variable levels of awareness at time of impact, such as feeling dazed, confused, "seeing stars" • Amnesia surrounding trauma events • Visual changes, such as double vision, movement of print or stationary objects such as walls and floor; eye strain and visual fatigue • Changes in thinking ability • Vertigo, problems with balance • Ringing in ears, hearing loss • Tingling, numbness in extremities • Loss of or changes in senses of taste or smell	• Bowel, bladder incontinence or dysfunction • Vomiting, which may be projectile • Swallowing problems—coughing, drooling, dysphagia • Altered bowel sounds • Inability to eat because of altered awareness or consciousness or traumatic injuries • Weight loss due to increased metabolic rate • Problems with bathing, dressing, grooming, feeding, toileting • LOC ranging from lethargy to coma • Pupillary changes—response to light and symmetry; deviation of eyes, inability to follow • Facial asymmetry • Unequal, weak handgrip • Absent or weak deep tendon reflexes • Posturing—decorticate, decerebrate • Seizure activity • Heightened sensitivity to touch and movement—can be painful and/or initiate storming • Apraxia, hemiparesis, quadriparesis • Proprioception • Difficulty with hand-eye coordination • Mental status changes, including altered orientation, alertness or responsiveness, attention, concentration, problem-solving, emotional affect or behavior, and memory. *Note:* The most common impairment among severely head-injured clients is memory loss, characterized by some loss of specific memories and the partial inability to form or store new ones (National Institute for Neurological Disorders and Stroke [NINDS], 2007). • *Vision:* Client may not be able to register what he or she is seeing or may be slow to recognize objects and have difficulty with tracking and hand-eye coordination. • Language and communication problems—difficulty with understanding and producing spoken and written language and with the more subtle aspects of communication, such as body language and emotional, nonverbal signals (NINDS, 2007).
PAIN/DISCOMFORT • Headache of variable intensity and location, usually persistent and long-lasting • Other body pain, especially when brain injury is a component of multiple trauma **RESPIRATION**	• Facial grimacing • Withdrawal response to painful stimulus • Restlessness, moaning • Changes in breathing patterns, such as periods of apnea alternating with hyperventilation • Sustained hyperventilation, which may accompany storming • Noisy respirations, stridor, choking • Rhonchi, wheezes (possible aspiration)

(continues on page 224)

DIAGNOSTIC DIVISION
MAY REPORT (continued)

SAFETY
- History of recent trauma, such as fall, motor vehicle crash, bullet or blast injuries

SOCIAL INTERACTION
- Inability to cope
- Relationship problems and role changes
- Caregiver/SO has difficulty dealing with caregiver burdens and role

TEACHING/LEARNING
- Use of alcohol, other drugs
- Failure to attend to safety issues

DISCHARGE PLAN CONSIDERATIONS
- May require assistance with self-care, ambulation, transportation, food preparation, shopping, treatments, medications, homemaker and maintenance tasks, change in physical layout of home or placement in living facility other than home

▶ Refer to section at end of plan for postdischarge considerations.

MAY EXHIBIT (continued)

- Fractures, dislocations
- Impaired vision, visual field disturbances, abnormal eye movements
- Head or facial lacerations, abrasions, discoloration (raccoon eyes), Battle's sign around ears (trauma signs)
- Drainage from ears or nose—CSF
- Impaired cognition
- Range of motion (ROM) impairment, altered muscle tone, general weakness, incomplete paralysis
- Fever, which may be associated with infection or related to hypermetabolic rate or storming; instability in internal regulation of body temperature
- Behavioral changes indicative of violence to self or others

- Expressive or receptive aphasia, unintelligible speech, repetitive speech, dysarthria, anomia
- Difficulty dealing with environment, interacting with more than one or two individuals at a time

---

Diagnostic Studies

TEST
WHY IT IS DONE

BLOOD TESTS
- *Arterial blood gases (ABGs):* Measures oxygen and carbon dioxide levels and pH.
- *Serum chemistry/electrolytes:* Substances that, in solution, conduct an electric current and are decomposed by their passage. Sodium, potassium, calcium, and magnesium are common electrolytes.
- *Blood glucose:* Monitors for fluctuations in serum glucose levels.

OTHER DIAGNOSTIC STUDIES
- *Computed tomography (CT) scan (with/without contrast):* Uses low radiation x-rays to create a computer-generated, three-dimensional image of the brain.

WHAT IT TELLS ME

Determines presence of ventilation or oxygenation problems that may exacerbate and increase ICP.

May reveal numerous imbalances that contribute to increased ICP and changes in mentation. Increased metabolic rate and diaphoresis can result in elevated sodium (hypernatremia).

Sympathetic storming can result in elevated glucose (hyperglycemia), although hypoglycemia can also occur due to inadequate nutrition.

Screening image of choice in acute brain injury. Identifies space-occupying lesions, hematomas, contusions, hemorrhage, skull fractures, and brain tissue swelling and shift.

Diagnostic Studies (continued)

TEST WHY IT IS DONE (continued)	WHAT IT TELLS ME (continued)
• *Magnetic resonance imaging (MRI):* Uses magnetic fields and computer technology to generate images of the internal anatomy of the brain.	Uses similar to those of CT scan, but more sensitive than CT for detecting cerebral trauma, determining neurological deficits not explained by CT, evaluating prolonged interval of disturbed consciousness, and defining evidence of previous trauma superimposed on acute trauma. *Note:* MRI has limited role in evaluation of acute head injury because of longer procedure time and difficulty obtaining MRI in an acutely injured person.
• *Cerebral angiography:* Invasive imaging procedure used to make detailed x-ray pictures of the blood vessels in the brain.	Demonstrates cerebral circulatory anomalies, such as brain tissue shifts secondary to edema, hemorrhage, and trauma. *Note:* Rarely used in acute head injury, but can be done when subarachnoid or parenchymal hemorrhage is known or suspected.
• *Electroencephalogram (EEG):* Procedure that uses electrodes on the scalp to record electrical activity of the brain.	May reveal presence or development of pathological waves. EEG is not generally indicated in the immediate period of emergency response, evaluation, and treatment of TBI. If the client fails to improve, EEG may help in diagnostic evaluation for seizures, focal or diffuse encephalopathy, or brain death. *Note:* Continuous EEG monitoring can help clinicians evaluate the effectiveness of high-dose barbiturates in achieving suppression of neuronal activity.
• *Skull x-rays:* Determines degree of structural injury and development of complications.	Although largely replaced by CT scan, x-rays can be used to detect changes in bony structure, such as fractures or shifts of midline structures caused by bleeding and brain swelling; also assess degree of foreign body penetration, bone fragments, and so on.
• *Brainstem auditory evoked responses (BAER):* Measures function of central nervous system (CNS), including pathway from brainstem.	Determines levels of cortical and brainstem function.
• *Positron emission tomography (PET) and signal positron emission tomography (SPECT) scans:* Detect changes in metabolic activity in the brain, providing imaging of functioning areas.	May be used for differentiation of type of head injuries. (These procedures are not in widespread clinical use, but are more often used for research.)
• *Lumbar puncture and CSF analysis:* May be performed when CT or MRI is not diagnostic. (Generally contraindicated in acute trauma.)	Determines presence of increased ICP.
• *Toxicology screen:* Detects drugs that may be responsible for or potentiate loss of consciousness.	Findings useful in determining treatment needs.
• *Serum anticonvulsant levels:* May be done to ensure that therapeutic level is adequate to prevent seizure activity.	Results will dictate changes in medication dosage or choice.

Nursing Priorities

1. Maximize cerebral perfusion and function.
2. Prevent or minimize complications.
3. Promote optimal functioning/return to preinjury level.
4. Support coping process and family recovery.
5. Provide information about condition, prognosis, potential complications, treatment plan, and resources.

Discharge Goals

1. Cerebral function improved; neurological deficits resolving or stabilized.
2. Complications prevented or minimized.
3. Activities of daily living (ADLs) met by self or with assistance of other(s).
4. Family acknowledges reality of situation and involved in recovery program.
5. Condition, prognosis, complications, and treatment regimen understood and available resources identified.
6. Plan in place to meet needs after discharge.

NURSING DIAGNOSIS: ineffective cerebral tissue Perfusion

May be related to

Interruption of blood flow by space-occupying lesions (hemorrhage, hematoma), cerebral edema (localized or generalized response to injury, metabolic alterations, drug or alcohol overdose), decreased systemic BP or hypoxia (hypovolemia, cardiac dysrhythmias)

Possibly evidenced by

Altered LOC, memory loss

Changes in motor or sensory responses, restlessness

Changes in vital signs

Desired Outcomes/Evaluation Criteria—Client Will

Neurological Status (NOC)

Maintain usual or improved LOC, cognition, and motor or sensory function.

Demonstrate stable vital signs and absence of signs of increased ICP.

ACTIONS/INTERVENTIONS	RATIONALE
Neurologic Monitoring (NIC) *Independent* Determine factors related to individual situation, cause for coma or decreased cerebral perfusion, and potential for increased ICP.	Influences choice of interventions. Deterioration in neurological signs and symptoms or failure to improve after initial insult may reflect decreased intracranial adaptive capacity, requiring the client be transferred to critical care for monitoring of ICP or surgical intervention.
Monitor and document neurological status frequently and compare with baseline: GCS during first 48 hours	GCS assesses trends and potential for increased ICP and is useful in determining location, extent, and progression or resolution of CN damage. *Note:* The Rancho Los Amigos Scale (or Rancho Levels) may also be used. These levels do not require cooperation from the client and are based on client's response to environmental stimuli and a range of behavioral responses, including no response, confused-agitated, and purposeful-appropriate.
Evaluate eye opening—spontaneous (awake), opens only to painful stimuli, keeps eyes closed (coma)	Determines arousal ability and LOC.
Assess verbal response; note whether client is alert, oriented to person, place, and time, or is confused, uses inappropriate words and phrases that make little sense	Measures appropriateness of speech and content of consciousness. If minimal damage has occurred in the cerebral cortex, client may be aroused by verbal stimuli but may appear drowsy or uncooperative. More extensive damage to the cerebral cortex may be displayed by slow response to commands, lapsing into sleep when not stimulated, disorientation, and stupor. Damage to midbrain, pons, and medulla is manifested by lack of appropriate responses to stimuli.
Assess motor response to simple commands, noting purposeful (obeys command, attempts to push stimulus away) and nonpurposeful (posturing) movement. Note limb movement and document right and left sides separately.	Measures overall awareness and ability to respond to external stimuli and best indicates state of consciousness in the client whose eyes are closed because of trauma or who is aphasic. Consciousness and involuntary movement are integrated if client can both grasp and release the tester's hand or hold up two fingers on command. Purposeful movement can include grimacing or withdrawing from painful stimuli or movements that the client desires, such as sitting up. Other movements (posturing and abnormal flexion of extremities) usually indicate diffuse cortical damage. Absence of spontaneous movement on one side of the body indicates damage to the motor tracts in the opposite cerebral hemisphere.
Monitor vital signs: BP, noting onset of and continuing systolic hypertension and widening pulse pressure; observe for hypotension in multiple trauma client	Normally, autoregulation maintains constant cerebral blood flow despite fluctuations in systemic BP. Loss of autoregulation may follow local or diffuse cerebrovascular damage. Increasing systolic BP accompanied by decreasing diastolic BP (widening pulse pressure) is an ominous sign of increased ICP when accompanied by decreased LOC. Hypovolemia or hypotension associated with multiple trauma may also result in cerebral ischemia and damage.

ACTIONS/INTERVENTIONS (continued)

Heart rate and rhythm, noting bradycardia, alternating bradycardia and tachycardia, and other dysrhythmias

Respirations, noting patterns and rhythm, including periods of apnea after hyperventilation and Cheyne-Stokes respiration

Evaluate pupils, noting size, shape, equality, and light reactivity.

Assess position and movement of eyes, noting whether in midposition or deviated to side or downward. Note loss of doll's eyes or oculocephalic reflex.

Note presence or absence of reflexes—blink, cough, gag, and Babinski.

Cerebral Perfusion Promotion (NIC)

Monitor temperature and regulate environmental temperature, as indicated. Limit use of blankets; administer tepid sponge bath in presence of fever. Wrap extremities in blankets when hypothermia blanket is used.

Monitor intake and output (I&O). Weigh, as indicated. Note skin turgor and status of mucous membranes.

Maintain head and neck in midline or neutral position. Support with small towel rolls and pillows. Avoid placing head on large pillows. Periodically check position and fit of cervical collar or tracheostomy ties when used.

Provide rest periods between care activities and limit duration of procedures.

Decrease extraneous stimuli and provide comfort measures, such as back massage, quiet environment, soft voice, and gentle touch.

Help client avoid or limit coughing, vomiting, and straining at stool or bearing down, when possible. Reposition client slowly; prevent client from bending knees and pushing heels against mattress to move up in bed.

Avoid or limit use of restraints.

Limit number and duration of suctioning passes, for example, two passes less than 10 seconds each. Hyperventilate only when indicated.

Encourage SO to talk to client.

RATIONALE (continued)

Changes in rate (most often bradycardia) and dysrhythmias may develop without impacting hemodynamic stability. However, dysrhythmias can reflect brainstem pressure or injury in the absence of underlying cardiac disease. Tachycardia can reflect hydration status, fever or hyper-metabolic state, and sympathetic storming.

Irregularities can suggest location of cerebral insult, increasing ICP, and need for further intervention, including possible respiratory support. (Refer to ND: risk for ineffective Breathing Pattern following.)

Pupil reactions are regulated by the oculomotor (III) cranial nerve and are useful in determining whether the brainstem is intact. Pupil size and equality is determined by balance between parasympathetic and sympathetic innervation. Response to light reflects combined function of optic (II) and oculomotor (III) cranial nerves.

Position and movement of eyes help localize area of brain involvement. An early sign of increased ICP is impaired abduction of eyes, indicating pressure or injury to the fifth cranial nerve. Loss of doll's eyes indicates deterioration in brainstem function and poor prognosis.

Altered reflexes reflect injury at level of midbrain or brainstem and have direct implications for client safety. Loss of blink reflex suggests damage to the pons and medulla. Absence of cough and gag reflexes reflects damage to medulla. Presence of Babinski reflex indicates injury along pyramidal pathways in the brain.

Fever may reflect damage to hypothalamus. Increased metabolic needs and oxygen consumption occur (especially with fever and shivering), which can further increase ICP.

Useful indicators of total body water, which is an integral part of tissue perfusion. Cerebral trauma and ischemia can result in diabetes insipidus (DI) or syndrome of inappropriate antidiuretic hormone (SIADH). Alterations may lead to hypovolemia or vascular engorgement, either of which can negatively affect cerebral pressure.

Turning head to one side compresses the jugular veins and inhibits cerebral venous drainage, thereby increasing ICP. Tight-fitting collar and ties can also limit jugular venous drainage.

Continual activity can increase ICP and contribute to storming by producing a cumulative stimulant effect.

Provides calming effect, reduces adverse physiological response, and promotes rest to maintain or lower ICP.

These activities increase intrathoracic and intra-abdominal pressures, which can increase ICP.

Mechanical restraints may enhance fight response, increasing ICP. *Note:* Cautious use may be indicated to prevent injury to client when other measures, including medications, are ineffective.

Prevents hypoxia and associated vasoconstriction that can impair cerebral perfusion. *Note:* The use of prophylactic hyperventilation prior to suctioning or as a stand-alone treatment should be avoided, as it can compromise cerebral perfusion. It may be used episodically for brief periods when there is sudden neurological deterioration and ICP is refractory to sedation.

Familiar voices of family and SO appear to have a relaxing effect on many comatose clients, which can reduce ICP.

(continues on page 228)

Investigate increasing restlessness, moaning, and guarding behaviors.

These nonverbal cues may indicate increasing ICP or reflect presence of pain when client is unable to verbalize complaints. Unrelieved pain can in turn aggravate or potentiate increased ICP.

Palpate for bladder distention; maintain patency of urinary drainage if used. Monitor for constipation.

May trigger autonomic responses, potentiating elevation of ICP.

Observe for seizure activity and protect client from injury.

Seizures can occur as a result of cerebral irritation, hypoxia, or increased ICP; additionally, seizures can further elevate ICP, compounding cerebral damage.

Assess for nuchal rigidity, twitching, increased restlessness, irritability, and onset of seizure activity.

Indicative of meningeal irritation, which may occur because of interruption of dura or development of infection during acute or recovery period of brain injury.

Collaborative

Elevate head of bed gradually to 20 to 30 degrees, as tolerated or indicated. Avoid hip flexion greater than 90 degrees.

Promotes venous drainage from head, thereby reducing cerebral congestion and edema, and risk of increased ICP. *Note:* Presence of hypotension can compromise cerebral perfusion pressure, negating beneficial effect of elevating head of bed.

Administer isotonic intravenous (IV) fluids, such as 0.9% sodium chloride, with control device.

Fluids should not be routinely restricted, but should be administered to maintain normal intravascular volume, systemic blood pressure, and cardiac output in order to maintain brain perfusion and decrease risk of cerebral edema and ICP.

Administer supplemental oxygen via appropriate route, such as mechanical ventilator and mask, to maintain appropriate O_2 saturation, as indicated.

Reduces hypoxemia, which is known to increase cerebral vasodilation and blood volume, elevating ICP.

Monitor ABGs or pulse oximetry.

Determines respiratory sufficiency (presence of hypoxia and acidosis) and indicates therapy needs.

Administer medications, as indicated, for example:
  Diuretics, such as mannitol (Osmitrol) and furosemide (Lasix)

Diuretics may be used in acute phase to draw water from brain cells into the intravascular space, reducing cerebral edema and ICP. *Note:* Loop diuretics such as Lasix also reduce production of CSF, which can contribute to increased ICP when cerebral edema impairs CSF circulation. Mannitol usually lowers ICP within a few minutes of IV administration. Individuals being treated with mannitol must receive adequate fluid resuscitation to prevent hypovolemia and hypotension.

  Barbiturates, such as pentobarbital

Barbiturates are the most common class of drugs used to produce deep sedation in the early phase of TBI treatment. The purpose of the therapy is to protect neurons by decreasing the cerebral metabolic rate, altering vascular tone, and inhibiting some of the biochemical intracellular events known to cause secondary brain injury. Because this therapy causes respiratory depression, it should only be used while client is on a ventilator. *Note:* Use of sedatives and opioids for cerebral protection can suppress signs and symptoms of sympathetic storming. The onset of storming episodes frequently coincides with being weaned off these medications. Oral or enteric medications may then be initiated to reduce the adverse effects of sympathetic storming (Zink, 2005).

  Steroids, such as dexamethasone (Decadron) and methyl-prednisolone (Medrol)

May be effective for treating vasogenic edema—decreasing inflammation, reducing tissue edema. *Note:* Use and efficacy of steroids continues to be debated in this condition.

  Anticonvulsant, such as phenytoin (Dilantin)

Dilantin is the drug of choice for treatment and prevention of seizure activity in immediate post-traumatic period to reduce risk of secondary injury from associated increased ICP. Prophylactic anticonvulsive therapy may be continued for an indeterminate period of time.

  Chlorpromazine (Thorazine)

Useful in treating posturing and shivering, which can increase ICP. *Note:* This drug can lower the seizure threshold or precipitate Dilantin toxicity.

  Mild analgesics and sedatives, such as lorazepam (Ativan)

May be indicated to relieve pain and agitation and their negative effects on ICP. Client on ventilator will be sedated and possibly require deep sedation.

ACTIONS/INTERVENTIONS (continued)

Antipyretics, such as acetaminophen (Tylenol)

Initiate cooling measures, as indicated.

Prepare for surgical intervention, such as craniotomy or insertion of ventricular drain or ICP pressure monitor, if indicated, and transfer to higher level of care.

RATIONALE (continued)

Reduces or controls fever and its deleterious effect on cerebral metabolism and oxygen needs and insensible fluid losses.
May be needed to regain or maintain normal core body temperature—hyperthermia exacerbates a hypermetabolic state.
Client may require decompressive craniotomy to remove a section of the skull and make an incision in the dura so that the brain can expand, relieving pressure. Craniotomy may also be performed to remove bone fragments, elevate depressed fractures, evacuate hematoma, control hemorrhage, and debride necrotic tissue. *Note:* Approximately half of severely head-injured clients will need surgery to remove or repair ruptured blood vessels and remove bruised or necrotic brain tissue (NINDS, 2003). One way to monitor ICP is by placing a catheter in one of the brain's lateral ventricles. This device can also be used to drain CSF from the brain, reducing intracranial volume and decreasing ICP. When an intraventricular catheter is in place, draining CSF is the first recommended intervention on the critical pathway for reducing ICP. *Note:* Intracranial pressure monitoring devices are usually placed in conjunction with other cranial surgery procedures, but may be placed in any client with a GCS score less than 9, with an abnormal CT scan. Monitoring of ICP requires more intensive care and complex therapies.

NURSING DIAGNOSIS: **risk for ineffective Breathing Pattern**

Risk factors may include
Neuromuscular impairment—injury to respiratory center of brain
Perception or cognitive impairment
Tracheobronchial obstruction

Possibly evidenced by
(Not applicable; presence of signs and symptoms establishes an *actual* diagnosis)

Desired Outcomes/Evaluation Criteria—Client Will

Respiratory Status: Ventilation (NOC)
Maintain a normal or effective respiratory pattern, free of cyanosis, with ABGs or pulse oximetry within client's acceptable range.

ACTIONS/INTERVENTIONS

Airway Management (NIC)
Independent
Monitor rate, rhythm, and depth of respiration. Note breathing irregularities, for example, apneustic, ataxic, or cluster breathing.

Note competence of gag and swallow reflexes and client's ability to protect own airway. Insert airway adjunct as indicated.

Elevate head of bed as permitted and position on sides, as indicated.
Encourage deep breathing if client is conscious.

RATIONALE

Changes may indicate onset of pulmonary complications, common following brain injury, or indicate location and extent of brain involvement. Slow respiration and periods of apnea (apneustic, ataxic, or cluster breathing patterns) are signs of brainstem injury and warn of impending respiratory arrest.
Ability to mobilize or clear secretions is important to airway maintenance. Loss of swallow or cough reflex may indicate need for artificial airway or intubation. Thickening of pulmonary secretions may occur due to diaphoresis, dehydration, or renal insufficiency. *Note:* Soft nasopharyngeal airways may be preferred to prevent stimulation of the gag reflex caused by hard oropharyngeal airway, which can lead to excessive coughing and increased ICP.
Facilitates lung expansion and ventilation, and reduces risk of airway obstruction by tongue.
Prevents or reduces atelectasis.

(continues on page 230)

ACTIONS/INTERVENTIONS (continued)

Suction with extreme caution, no longer than 10 to 15 seconds. Note character, color, and odor of secretions.

Auscultate breath sounds, noting areas of hypoventilation and presence of adventitious sounds—crackles, rhonchi, and wheezes.

Monitor use of respiratory depressant drugs, such as sedatives.

Collaborative

Monitor and graph serial ABGs and pulse oximetry.

Review chest x-rays.

Administer supplemental oxygen.

Assist with chest physiotherapy when indicated.

RATIONALE (continued)

Suctioning is usually required if client is comatose or immobile and unable to clear own airway. Deep tracheal suctioning should be done with caution because it can cause or aggravate hypoxia, which produces vasoconstriction, adversely affecting cerebral perfusion.

Identifies pulmonary problems such as atelectasis, congestion, and airway obstruction, which may jeopardize cerebral oxygenation or indicate onset of pulmonary infection, a common complication of head injury.

Can increase respiratory embarrassment and complications.

Determines respiratory sufficiency, acid-base balance, and therapy needs.

Reveals ventilatory state and signs of developing complications such as atelectasis and pneumonia.

Maximizes arterial oxygenation and aids in prevention of cerebral hypoxia. If respiratory center is depressed, mechanical ventilation may be required.

Although contraindicated in client with acutely elevated ICP, these measures are often necessary in acute rehabilitation phase to mobilize and clear lung fields and reduce atelectasis or pulmonary complications.

NURSING DIAGNOSIS: **disturbed Sensory Perception [specify]**

May be related to
Altered sensory reception, transmission, and integration—neurological trauma or deficit

Possibly evidenced by
Disorientation to time, place, person
Change in usual response to stimuli
Motor incoordination, alterations in posture, inability to tell position of body parts (proprioception)
Altered communication patterns
Visual and auditory distortions
Poor concentration, altered thought processes or bizarre thinking
Exaggerated emotional responses, change in behavior pattern

Desired Outcomes/Evaluation Criteria—Client Will

Cognition (NOC)
Regain or maintain usual LOC and perceptual functioning.
Acknowledge changes in ability and presence of residual involvement.
Demonstrate behaviors and lifestyle changes to compensate for, or overcome, deficit.

ACTIONS/INTERVENTIONS

RATIONALE

Reality Orientation (NIC)
Independent

Evaluate and continually monitor changes in orientation, ability to speak, mood and affect, sensorium, and thought process.

Assess sensory awareness, including response to touch, hot/cold, dull/sharp, and awareness of motion and location of body parts. Note problems with vision and other senses.

Observe behavioral responses—hostility, crying, inappropriate affect, agitation, and hallucinations. (Refer to ND: disturbed Thought Processes, below.)

Upper cerebral functions are often the first to be affected by altered circulation and oxygenation. Damage may occur at time of initial injury or develop later because of swelling or bleeding. Motor, perceptual, cognitive, and personality changes may develop and persist, with gradual normalization of responses, or changes may remain permanently to some degree.

Information is essential to client safety. All sensory systems may be affected, with changes involving increased or decreased sensitivity or loss of sensation and the ability to perceive and respond appropriately to stimuli.

Individual responses may be variable, but commonalities, such as emotional lability, increased irritability or frustration, apathy, and impulsiveness, exist during recovery from brain injury. Documentation of behavior provides information needed for development of structured rehabilitation.

ACTIONS/INTERVENTIONS (continued)

Document specific changes in abilities, such as focusing and tracking with both eyes, following simple verbal instructions, answering "yes" or "no" to questions, and feeding self with dominant hand.

Eliminate extraneous noise and stimuli, as necessary.

Speak in calm, quiet voice. Use short, simple sentences. Maintain eye contact.

Ascertain and validate client's perceptions and provide feedback. Reorient client frequently to environment, staff, and procedures, especially if vision is impaired.

Provide meaningful stimulation: verbal (talk to client), olfactory (e.g., oil of clove, coffee), tactile (touch, hand holding), and auditory (tapes, television, radio, visitors). Avoid physical or emotional isolation of client.

Provide structured therapies, activities, and environment. Provide written schedule for client to refer to on a regular basis.

Schedule adequate rest and uninterrupted sleep periods.

Use day/night lighting.

Allow adequate time for communication and performance of activities.

Provide for client's safety, such as padded side rails or bed enclosed with safety netting, assistance with ambulation, and protection from hot or sharp objects. Document perceptual deficit and compensatory activities on chart and at bedside.

Identify alternative ways of dealing with perceptual deficits, such as arrange bed, personal articles, and food to take advantage of functional vision; describe where affected body parts are located.

Collaborative

Refer to physical, occupational, speech, and cognitive therapists.

RATIONALE (continued)

Helps localize areas of cerebral dysfunction, and identifies signs of progress toward improved neurological function.

Reduces anxiety, exaggerated emotional responses, and confusion associated with sensory overload.

Client may have limited attention span or understanding during acute and recovery stages, and these measures can help client attend to communication.

Assists client to differentiate reality in the presence of altered perceptions. Cognitive dysfunction and visual deficits potentiate disorientation and anxiety.

Carefully selected sensory input may be useful for coma stimulation as well as for documenting progress during cognitive retraining.

Promotes consistency and reassurance, reducing anxiety associated with the unknown. Promotes sense of control and cognitive retraining.

Reduces fatigue, prevents exhaustion, and improves sleep. *Note:* Absence of rapid eye movement (REM) sleep is known to aggravate sensory perception deficits.

Provides for normal sense of passage of time and sleep-wake pattern.

Reduces frustration associated with altered abilities and delayed response pattern.

Agitation, impaired judgment, poor balance, and sensory deficits increase risk of client injury.

Enables client to progress toward independence, enhancing sense of control, while compensating for neurological deficits.

Interdisciplinary approach can create an integrated treatment plan based on the individual's unique combination of abilities and disabilities with focus on evaluation and functional improvement in physical, cognitive, and perceptual skills.

NURSING DIAGNOSIS: disturbed Thought Processes

May be related to
Physiological changes, psychological conflicts

Possibly evidenced by
Memory deficit or changes in remote, recent, immediate memory
Distractibility, altered attention span and concentration
Disorientation to time, place, person, circumstances, events
Impaired ability to make decisions, problem-solve, reason, abstract, conceptualize
Personality changes; inappropriate social behavior

Desired Outcomes/Evaluation Criteria—Client Will

Distorted Thought Self-Control (NOC)
Maintain or regain usual mentation and reality orientation.
Recognize changes in thinking and behavior.
Participate in therapeutic regimen and cognitive retraining.

ACTIONS/INTERVENTIONS	RATIONALE
Cognitive Stimulation (NIC)	
Independent	
Assess attention span and distractibility. Note level of anxiety.	Attention span and ability to attend or concentrate may be severely shortened, which both causes and potentiates anxiety, affecting thought processes.
Confer with SO to compare past behaviors and preinjury personality with current responses.	Recovery from head injury often includes a prolonged phase of agitation, angry responses, and disordered thought sequences. It is helpful to know about client's past behaviors in order to determine if current behaviors can be attributed solely to the brain injury. *Note:* SOs often have difficulty accepting and dealing with client's aberrant behavior and may require assistance in coping with situation.
Maintain consistency in staff assigned to client to the extent possible.	Provides client with feelings of stability, familiarity, and control of situation.
Present reality concisely and briefly; avoid challenging illogical thinking.	Client may be totally unaware of injury (amnesic) or of extent of injury and therefore deny reality of injury. Structured reality orientation can reduce defensive reactions.
Provide information about injury process in relationship to symptoms. Explain procedures and reinforce explanations given by others.	Loss of internal structure (changes in memory, reasoning, and ability to conceptualize) and fear of the unknown affect processing and retention of information and can compound anxiety, confusion, and disorientation.
Review necessity of recurrent neurological evaluations.	Understanding that assessments are done frequently to prevent or limit complications and that they do not necessarily reflect seriousness of client's condition, may help reduce anxiety.
Reduce provocative stimuli, negative criticism, arguments, and confrontations.	Reduces risk of triggering fight-or-flight response. Aggression, anger, and self-control are common problems in brain-injured clients, who may become violent or physically or verbally abusive.
Listen with regard to client's verbalizations in spite of speech pattern or content.	Conveys interest and worth to individual, enhancing self-esteem and encouraging continued efforts.
Promote socialization within individual limitations.	Reinforcement of positive behaviors, such as appropriate interaction with others, may be helpful in relearning internal structure.
Encourage SO to provide current news and family happenings.	Promotes maintenance of contact with usual events, enhancing reality orientation and normalization of thinking.
Instruct in relaxation techniques. Provide diversional activities.	Can help refocus attention and reduce anxiety to manageable levels.
Maintain realistic expectations of client's ability to control own behavior, comprehend, and remember information.	It is important to maintain an expectation of the ability to improve and progress to a higher level of functioning, to maintain hope, and promote continued work of rehabilitation.
Avoid leaving client alone when agitated or frightened.	Anxiety can lead to loss of control and escalate to panic. Support may provide calming effect, reducing anxiety and risk of injury.
Implement measures to control emotional outbursts or aggressive behavior if needed—speak in a calm voice, tell client to "stop," remove client from the situation, provide distraction, and restrain for brief periods of time, as appropriate.	Client may need help or external control to protect self or others from harm until internal control is regained. Restraints (physical holding, mechanical, and pharmacological) should be used judiciously to avoid escalating violent, irrational behavior.
Inform client and SO that intellectual function, behavior, and emotional functioning will gradually improve, but that some effects may persist for months or even be permanent.	Most brain-injured clients have persistent problems with concentration, memory, and problem-solving. If brain injury was moderate to severe, recovery may be complete or residual effects may remain.
Collaborative	
Refer for neuropsychological evaluation as indicated.	Useful for determining therapeutic interventions for cognitive and neurobehavioral disturbances.
Coordinate participation in cognitive retraining or rehabilitation program, as indicated.	Assists client with learning methods to compensate for disruption of cognitive skills. Addresses problems in concentration, memory, judgment, sequencing, and problem-solving. *Note:* New developments in technology and computer software allow for the creation of interactive sensory-motor virtual reality environments. This provides an opportunity for safe interaction between client and naturalistic environments for the purpose of practicing or establishing effective behavioral responses.
Refer to support groups, such as Brain Injury Association, and social services, visiting nurse, and counseling or therapy, as needed.	Additional long-term assistance may be helpful in supporting and sustaining recovery.

NURSING DIAGNOSIS: impaired physical Mobility

May be related to
Perceptual or cognitive impairment
Decreased strength or endurance
Restrictive therapies, safety precautions—bedrest, immobilization

Possibly evidenced by
Inability to purposefully move within the physical environment, including bed mobility, transfer, ambulation
Impaired coordination, limited ROM, decreased muscle strength or control

Desired Outcomes/Evaluation Criteria—Client Will

Immobility Consequences: Physiological (NOC)
Maintain or increase strength and function of affected or compensatory body part(s).
Regain or maintain optimal position of function, as evidenced by absence of contractures and footdrop.

Mobility (NOC)
Demonstrate techniques or behaviors that enable resumption of activities.
Maintain skin integrity and bladder and bowel function.

ACTIONS/INTERVENTIONS	RATIONALE
Exercise Therapy: Muscle Control (NIC)	
Independent	
Review functional ability and reasons for impairment	Identifies probable functional impairments and influences choice of interventions.
Assess degree of immobility, using a scale to rate dependence (0 to 4).	The client may be completely independent (0), may require minimal assistance or equipment (1), moderate assistance or supervision and teaching (2), extensive assistance or equipment and devices (3), or be completely dependent on caregivers (4). Persons in all categories are at risk for injury, but those in categories 2 to 4 are at greatest risk.
Provide or assist with ROM exercises.	Helps in maintaining movement and functional alignment of joints and extremities.
Instruct and assist client with exercise program and use of mobility aids. Increase activity and participation in self-care as tolerated.	Lengthy convalescence often follows brain injury, and physical reconditioning is an essential part of the program.
Bed Rest Care (NIC)	
Position client to avoid skin and tissue pressure damage. Turn at regular intervals, and make small position changes between turns.	Regular turning more normally distributes body weight and promotes circulation to all areas. If paralysis or limited cognition is present, client should be repositioned frequently.
Provide meticulous skin care, massaging with emollients. Remove wet linen and clothing, and keep bedding free of wrinkles.	Promotes circulation and skin elasticity and reduces risk of skin excoriation.
Maintain functional body alignment—hips, feet, and hands. Monitor for proper placement of devices and signs of pressure from devices.	Use of high-top tennis shoes, "space boots," and T-bar sheepskin devices can help prevent footdrop. Hand splints are variable and designed to prevent hand deformities and promote optimal function. Use of pillows, bedrolls, and sandbags can help prevent abnormal hip rotation.
Support head and trunk, arms and shoulders, and feet and legs when client is in wheelchair or recliner. Pad chair seat with foam or water-filled cushion, and assist client to shift weight at frequent intervals.	Maintains comfortable, safe, and functional posture, and prevents or reduces risk of skin breakdown.
Provide eye care with artificial tears and eye patches, as indicated.	Protects delicate eye tissues from drying. Client may require patches during sleep to protect eyes from trauma if unable to keep eyes closed.
Monitor urinary output. Note color and odor of urine. Assist with bladder retraining when appropriate.	Indwelling catheter used during the acute phase of injury may be needed for an extended period of time before bladder retraining is possible. Once the catheter is removed, several methods of continence control may be tried, such as intermittent catheterization for residual and complete emptying, external catheter, planned intervals on commode, and incontinence pads.
Provide fluids, including 8 oz cranberry juice, within individual tolerance (that is, regarding neurological and cardiac concerns), as indicated.	Once past the acute phase of head injury, and if client has no other contraindicating factors, forcing fluids decreases risk of urinary tract infections and bladder or kidney stone formation. Good hydration provides other positive effects such as normal stool consistency and optimal skin turgor.

(continues on page 234)

Monitor bowel elimination and provide for or assist with a regular bowel routine. Check for impacted stool; use digital stimulation, as indicated. Sit client upright on commode or stool at regular intervals. Add fiber, bulk, and fruit juice to diet, as appropriate.	A regular bowel routine requires simple but diligent measures to prevent complications. Stimulation of the internal rectal sphincter stimulates the bowel to empty automatically if stool is soft enough to do so. Upright position aids evacuation.
Inspect for localized tenderness, redness, skin warmth, muscle tension, or ropy veins in calves of legs. Observe for sudden dyspnea, tachypnea, fever, respiratory distress, and chest pain.	Client is at risk for development of deep vein thrombosis (DVT) and pulmonary embolus (PE), requiring prompt medical evaluation and intervention to prevent serious complications.

Collaborative

Provide flotation mattress and kinetic therapy, as appropriate.	Equalizes tissue pressure, enhances circulation, and helps reduce venous stasis to decrease risk of tissue injury.
Apply and monitor use of sequential compression devices (SCDs) to legs.	SCD may be used to reduce risk of DVT associated with bedrest and limited mobility.

Exercise Therapy: Muscle Control (NIC)

Refer to physical and occupational therapists, as indicated.	Useful in determining individual needs, therapeutic activities, and assistive devices.

NURSING DIAGNOSIS: **risk for Infection**

Risk factors may include
Traumatized tissues, broken skin, invasive procedures
Decreased ciliary action, stasis of body fluids
Nutritional deficits
Suppressed inflammatory response—steroid use
Altered integrity of closed system—CSF leak

Possibly evidenced by
(Not applicable; presence of signs and symptoms establishes an *actual* diagnosis)

Desired Outcomes/Evaluation Criteria—Client Will

Immune Status (NOC)
Maintain normothermia, free of signs of infection.
Achieve timely wound healing when present.

ACTIONS/INTERVENTIONS   **RATIONALE**

Infection Protection (NIC)
Independent

Provide meticulous, clean, or aseptic care; maintain good hand-washing techniques.	First-line defense against nosocomial infections.
Observe areas of impaired skin integrity (wounds, suture lines, invasive line insertion sites), noting drainage characteristics and presence of inflammation.	Early identification of developing infection permits prompt intervention and prevention of further complications.
Monitor temperature routinely. Note presence of chills, diaphoresis, and changes in mentation.	May indicate developing sepsis requiring further evaluation and intervention.
Encourage deep breathing and aggressive pulmonary toilet. Observe sputum characteristics.	Enhances mobilization and clearing of pulmonary secretions to reduce risk of pneumonia and atelectasis. *Note:* Postural drainage should be used with caution if risk of increased ICP exists.
Provide perineal care. Maintain integrity of closed urinary drainage system if used. Encourage adequate fluid intake.	Reduces potential for bacterial growth and ascending infection.
Observe color and clarity of urine. Note presence of foul odor.	Indicators of developing urinary tract infection (UTI) requiring prompt intervention.
Screen and restrict access of visitors or caregivers with upper respiratory infections (URIs).	Reduces exposure of "compromised host."

Collaborative

Obtain specimens, as indicated.	Culture with sensitivities may be done to verify presence of infection and identify causative organism and appropriate treatment choices.

NURSING DIAGNOSIS: **risk for imbalanced Nutrition: Less than Body Requirements**

Risk factors may include

Altered ability to ingest nutrients—decreased LOC

Weakness of muscles required for chewing, swallowing

Hypermetabolic state

Possibly evidenced by

(Not applicable; presence of signs and symptoms establishes an *actual* diagnosis)

Desired Outcomes/Evaluation Criteria—Client Will

Nutritional Status (NOC)

Demonstrate maintenance of desired weight or progressive weight gain toward goal.

Experience no signs of malnutrition, with laboratory values within normal range.

ACTIONS/INTERVENTIONS	RATIONALE
Nutrition Therapy (NIC)	
Independent	
Assess ability to chew, swallow, cough, and handle secretions.	These factors determine choice of feeding options because client must be protected from aspiration.
Auscultate bowel sounds, noting decreased or absent or hyperactive sounds.	Gastrointestinal (GI) functioning is usually preserved in brain-injured clients, so bowel sounds help in determining response to feeding or development of complications, such as ileus.
Weigh, as indicated.	Evaluates effectiveness or need for changes in nutritional therapy.
Provide for feeding safety, such as elevate head of bed while eating or during tube feeding.	Reduces risk of regurgitation and aspiration.
Divide feedings into small amounts and give frequently.	Enhances digestion and client's tolerance of nutrients and can improve client cooperation in eating.
Promote pleasant, relaxing environment, including socialization during meals. Encourage SO to bring in food that client enjoys.	Although the recovering client may require assistance with feeding and use of assistive devices, mealtime socialization with SO or friends can improve intake and normalize the life function of eating.
Check stools, gastric aspirant, and vomitus for blood.	Acute or subacute bleeding may occur (Cushing's ulcer), requiring intervention and alternative method of providing nutrition.
Collaborative	
Consult with dietitian or nutritional support team.	Helps determine the client's requirements for energy and to provide needed nutrients. Careful monitoring of nutrition indicators, such as weight and blood tests, are necessary to prevent problems associated with malnutrition—muscle wasting, pressure sores and decubitus ulcers, renal failure, atelectasis, and pneumonia.
Monitor laboratory studies, for example, prealbumin or albumin, transferrin, amino acid profile, iron, blood urea nitrogen (BUN), nitrogen balance studies, glucose, aspartate aminotransferase (AST) and alanine aminotransferase (ALT), and electrolytes.	Identifies nutritional deficiencies, organ function, and response to nutritional therapy.
Administer feedings by appropriate means—IV, tube feeding, or oral feedings with soft foods and thick liquids. (Refer to CP: Total Nutritional Support: Parenteral/Enteral Feeding.)	Choice of route depends on client needs and capabilities. Tube feedings (nasogastric, jejunostomy) may be required initially, or parenteral route may be indicated in presence of gastric or intestinal pathology. If client is able to swallow, soft foods or semiliquid foods may be more easily managed without aspiration.
Involve speech, occupational, and physical therapists when mechanical problem exists, such as impaired swallow reflexes, wired jaws, contractures of hands, and paralysis.	Individual strategies and devices may be needed to improve ability to eat.

NURSING DIAGNOSIS: interrupted Family Processes

May be related to
Situational transition and crisis
Uncertainty about outcomes, expectations

Possibly evidenced by
Difficulty adapting to change or dealing with traumatic experience constructively
Family not meeting needs of its members
Difficulty accepting or receiving help appropriately
Inability to express or to accept feelings of members

Desired Outcomes/Evaluation Criteria—Client Will

Family Coping (NOC)
Begin to express feelings freely and appropriately.
Identify internal and external resources to deal with the situation.
Direct energies in a purposeful manner to plan for resolution of crisis.
Encourage and allow injured member to progress toward independence.

ACTIONS/INTERVENTIONS	RATIONALE
Family Integrity Promotion (NIC)	
Independent	
Note components of family unit, availability, and involvement of support systems.	Defines family resources and identifies areas of need.
Encourage expression of concerns about seriousness of condition, possibility of death, or incapacitation.	Verbalization of fears gets concerns out in the open and can decrease anxiety and enhance coping with reality.
Listen for expressions of helplessness and hopelessness.	Joy of survival of victim is often quickly replaced by grief and anger at "loss" of the preinjury person and the necessity of dealing with new person that family does not know and may not even like. Prolongation of these feelings may result in depression.
Encourage expression and acknowledgment of feelings. Do not deny or reassure client/SO that everything will be all right.	Because it is not possible to predict the outcome, it is more helpful to assist the person to deal with feelings about what is happening instead of giving false reassurance.
Support family grieving for "loss" of member. Acknowledge normality of wide range of feelings and ongoing nature of process.	Although grief may never be fully resolved and family may vacillate among various stages, understanding that this is typical may help members accept and cope with the situation.
Stress importance of continuous open dialogue between family members.	Provides opportunity to get feelings out in the open. Recognition and awareness promotes resolution of guilt and anger.
Help family recognize needs of all members.	Attention may be so focused on injured member that other members feel isolated or abandoned, which can compromise family growth and unity.
Family Mobilization (NIC)	
Evaluate and discuss family goals and expectations.	Family may believe that if client is going to live, rehabilitation will bring about a cure. Despite accurate information, expectations may be unrealistic. Also, client's early recovery may be rapid, then plateau, resulting in disappointment and frustration.
Reinforce previous explanations about extent of injury, treatment plan, and prognosis. Provide accurate information at current level of understanding and ability to accept.	Client and SO are unable to absorb or recall all information, and blocking can occur because of emotional trauma. As time goes by, reinforcement of information can help reduce misconceptions, fear about the unknown, and future expectations.
Identify individual roles and anticipated and perceived changes.	Responsibilities and roles may have to be partially or completely assumed by others, which can further complicate family coping.
Assess energy direction, whether efforts at problem-solving are purposeful or scattered.	May need assistance to focus energies in an effective way to enhance coping.
Identify and encourage use of previously successful coping behaviors.	Focuses on strengths and reaffirms individual's ability to deal with current crisis.
Demonstrate and encourage use of stress management skills—relaxation techniques, breathing exercises, visualization, and music.	Helps redirect attention toward revitalizing self to enhance coping ability.

ACTIONS/INTERVENTIONS (continued)

Collaborative

Include family in rehabilitation team meetings, care planning, and placement decisions.

Identify community resources, such as visiting nurse, homemaker service, day-care program, respite facility, and legal and financial counselors.

Refer to family therapy and support groups.

RATIONALE (continued)

Facilitates communication, enables family to be an integral part of the rehabilitation, and provides sense of control.

Provides assistance with problems that may arise because of altered role function. Also, as family structure changes over time and client's needs increase with age, additional resources and support are often required.

Cognitive and personality changes are usually very difficult for family to deal with. Decreased impulse control, emotional lability, and inappropriate sexual or aggressive and violent behavior can disrupt family functioning and integrity. Trained therapists and peer role models may assist family to deal with feelings and reality of situation and provide support for decisions that are made.

NURSING DIAGNOSIS: **deficient Knowledge [Learning Need] regarding condition, prognosis, potential complications, treatment, self-care, and discharge needs**

May be related to

Lack of exposure, unfamiliarity with information or resources
Lack of recall, cognitive limitation

Possibly evidenced by

Request for information, statement of misconception
Inaccurate follow-through of instructions

Desired Outcomes/Evaluation Criteria—Client/SO Will

Knowledge: Disease Process (NOC)
Participate in learning process.
Verbalize understanding of condition, prognosis, and potential complications.

Knowledge: Treatment Regimen (NOC)
Verbalize understanding of therapeutic regimen and rationale for actions.
Initiate necessary lifestyle changes and involvement in rehabilitation program.
Correctly perform necessary procedures.

ACTIONS/INTERVENTIONS

Teaching: Disease Process (NIC)
Independent

Evaluate capabilities and readiness to learn for both client and SO.

Review information regarding injury process and aftereffects.

Review and reinforce current therapeutic regimen. Identify ways of continuing program after discharge.

Discuss plans for meeting self-care needs.

Provide written instructions and schedules for activity, medication, and important facts.
Identify signs and symptoms of individual risks, such as delayed CSF leak, post-traumatic seizures, headache, and chronic pain.
Discuss with client/SO development of symptoms, such as reexperiencing traumatic event (flashbacks, intrusive thoughts, repetitive dreams or nightmares); psychic or emotional numbness; and changes in lifestyle, including adoption of self-destructive behaviors.

RATIONALE

Permits presentation of material based on individual needs. *Note:* Client may not be emotionally or mentally capable of assimilating information.
Aids in establishing realistic expectations and promotes understanding of current situation and needs.
Recommended activities, limitations, medications, and therapy needs have been established on the basis of a coordinated interdisciplinary approach, and follow-through is essential to progression of recovery and prevention of complications.
Varying levels of assistance may be required, based on individual situation.
Provides visual reinforcement and reference source after discharge.
Recognizing developing problems provides opportunity for prompt evaluation and intervention to prevent serious complications.
May indicate occurrence or exacerbation of post-trauma response, which can occur months to years after injury, requiring further evaluation and supportive interventions.

(continues on page 238)

Identify community resources, including head injury support groups, social services, rehabilitation facilities, outpatient programs, and home care or visiting nurse.	May be needed to provide assistance with physical care, home management, adjustment to lifestyle changes, and emotional and financial concerns. *Note:* Studies suggest an increased risk of developing Alzheimer's disease and the possibility of acceleration of the aging process in brain injury survivors. SO and families will require continued support to meet these challenges.
Refer for, and reinforce importance of, follow-up care by rehabilitation team.	With diligent work (often for several years with these providers), the client may eventually overcome residual neurological deficits and be able to resume desired and productive lifestyle.

POTENTIAL CONSIDERATIONS following acute hospitalization (dependent on client's age, physical condition and presence of complications, personal resources, and life responsibilities)
- *impaired Memory*—neurological disturbances, anemia, fluid and electrolyte imbalances
- *ineffective Health Maintenance/impaired Home Maintenance*—significant alteration in communication skills, lack of ability to make deliberate or thoughtful judgments, perceptual and cognitive impairments, insufficient finances, unfamiliarity with neighborhood resources, inadequate support systems
- *acute/chronic Pain*—tissue injury and neuronal damage, stress and anxiety
- *chronic Confusion*—head injury

CEREBROVASCULAR ACCIDENT (CVA)/STROKE

I. **Pathophysiology**—Cerebrovascular accident (CVA, "stroke" or "brain attack") is injury or death to parts of the brain caused by an interruption in the blood supply to that area causing disability, such as paralysis or speech impairment.

II. **Types**
   a. Ischemic stroke: Impaired cerebral circulation caused by a partial or complete occlusion of a blood vessel with transient or permanent effects.
      i. Accounts for 80% to 85% of all strokes (Morrison, 2007), with carotid stenosis as the leading cause (Phillips, 2007).
      ii. Subdivided based on the underlying cause.
         1. Large-vessel thrombotic and embolic strokes
         2. Small-vessel thrombotic stroke
         3. Cardioembolic stroke
         4. Other
      iii. Ischemia may be transient and resolve within 24 hours, be reversible with resolution of symptoms over a period of 1 week (reversible ischemic neurological deficit [RIND]), or progress to cerebral infarction with variable effects and degrees of recovery.
   b. Hemorrhagic stroke: result of a vessel wall rupture with bleeding into the brain, compressing brain tissue
      i. Accounts for approximately 15% to 20% of cerebrovascular accidents (Morrison, 2007), with only 20% of patients regaining functional independence (Nassisi, 2008).

III. **Etiology**
   a. Ischemic stroke
      i. Large-vessel thrombotic and embolic strokes result from hypoperfusion, hypertension, and emboli traveling from large arteries to distal branches.
         ii. Small-vessel thrombotic stroke typically stems from plaque, diabetes mellitus, or hypertension.
         iii. Cardioembolic stroke results from atrial fibrillation, valve disease, or ventricular thrombi.
         iv. Other types of ischemic stroke are caused by hyperglycemia and hyperinsulinemia, arterial dissection, arteritis, and drug abuse.
   b. Hemorrhagic stroke
      i. Caused by hemorrhage—subarachnoid or intracerebral—from such conditions as a ruptured aneurysm, arteriovenous malformation (AVM), trauma, infections, tumors, or blood clotting deficiencies.
      ii. Major risk factor: hypertension

IV. **Statistics**
   a. Morbidity: In 2005, prevalence of stroke was estimated at 2.3 million males and 3.4 million females; many of the approximately 5.7 million U.S. stroke survivors have permanent stroke-related disabilities.
   b. Mortality: In 2004, stroke ranked fifth as the cause of death for those aged 45 to 64 years and third for those aged 65 years or older (National Heart, Lung and Blood Institute [NHLBI], 2007), with 150,000 deaths (American Heart Association and American Stroke Association, 2008); hemorrhagic strokes are more severe, and mortality rates are higher than ischemic strokes, with a 30-day mortality rate of 40% to 80% (Nassisi, 2008).
   c. Cost: Estimated direct and indirect cost for 2008 was $65.5 billion (American Heart Association and American Stroke Association, 2008).

GLOSSARY

Agnosia: Impairment of the ability to recognize or comprehend the meaning of various sensory stimuli.

Apraxia: Disorder of voluntary movement consisting of impairment of the performance of skilled or purposeful movements despite physical ability and willingness to move.

Atrial fibrillation: Most common form of irregular heartbeat and a risk factor for embolic ischemic stroke. The condition can cause a pooling of blood in the heart, which can make it easier for clots to form.

Carotid stenosis: Buildup of hardened plaque on the carotid artery wall. This is the leading cause of ischemic stroke.

Cerebral edema: Swelling of the brain.

Contralateral: Refers to the other side. Stroke affecting the *right* side of the brain may cause paralysis, affecting the *left* arm and leg.

Dysarthria: Difficulty in articulating words due to disease of the central nervous system (CNS).

Dysphagia: Difficulty in swallowing.

Embolic stroke: Occurs when a clot is carried into cerebral circulation and causes a localized cerebral infarct.

Embolus: Blood clot that forms in one area of the body and moves to another.

Hemiplegia: One-sided paralysis.

Ipsilateral: Refers to the same side. A stroke on the right side of the brain causes some symptoms on the right side of the body, as opposed to contralateral (the other side).

Thrombosis: Obstruction of a blood vessel by a clot formed at the site of obstruction.

Thrombotic stroke: Type of ischemic stroke usually seen in aging population. It is due to atherosclerosis (plaque buildup), eventually narrowing the lumen of the artery. The symptoms are much more gradual and less dramatic than other strokes due to the slow, ongoing process that produces it. The stroke is "completed" when the condition stabilizes.

Transient ischemic attack (TIA): Temporary lack of adequate blood and oxygen to the brain that causes stroke warning signs but no permanent damage. Generally lasts about 1 minute, but can last up to 5 minutes.

Care Setting

Although the client may initially be cared for in the intensive care unit (ICU) for severe or evolving deficits, this plan of care focuses on the step down from medical unit and subacute and rehabilitation units to the community level.

Related Concerns

Hypertension: severe, page 37

Craniocerebral trauma (acute rehabilitative phase), page 220

Psychosocial aspects of care, page 749

Seizure disorders, page 210

Total nutritional support: parenteral/enteral feeding, page 469

Client Assessment Database

Collected data are determined by location, severity, and duration of pathology.

DIAGNOSTIC DIVISION MAY REPORT	MAY EXHIBIT
ACTIVITY/REST • Difficulty with activity due to weakness, loss of sensation, or paralysis (hemiplegia) • Tires easily • Difficulty resting, pain or muscle twitching	• Altered muscle tone—flaccid or spastic; generalized weakness • One-sided paralysis • Altered level of consciousness (LOC)
CIRCULATORY • History of cardiac disease—myocardial infarction (MI), rheumatic and valvular heart disease, heart failure (HF), bacterial endocarditis, polycythemia	• Arterial hypertension, which is common unless CVA is due to embolism or vascular malformation • Pulse rate may vary due to various factors, such as preexisting heart conditions, medications, effect of stroke on vasomotor center • Dysrhythmias, electrocardiographic (ECG) changes • Bruit in carotid, femoral, or iliac arteries, or abdominal aorta may or may not be present

(continues on page 240)

DIAGNOSTIC DIVISION **MAY REPORT** (continued)	**MAY EXHIBIT** (continued)
EGO INTEGRITY • Feelings of helplessness, hopelessness	• Emotional lability • Exaggerated or inappropriate responses to anger, sadness, happiness • Difficulty expressing self
ELIMINATION	• Change in voiding patterns—incontinence, anuria • Distended abdomen • Distended bladder • May have absent or diminished bowel sounds if neurogenic paralytic ileus present
FOOD/FLUID • History of diabetes, elevated serum lipids (risk factors) • Lack of appetite • Nausea or vomiting during acute event (increased intracranial pressure [ICP]) • Loss of sensation in tongue, cheek, and throat • Dysphagia	• Obesity (risk factor) • Chewing and swallowing problems
NEUROSENSORY • History of TIA, RIND • Dizziness or syncope before stroke or transient during TIA • Severe headache can accompany intracerebral or subarachnoid hemorrhage • Tingling, numbness, and weakness commonly reported during TIAs, found in varying degrees in other types of stroke; involved side seems "dead" • Visual deficits—blurred vision, partial loss of vision (monocular blindness), double vision (diplopia), or other disturbances in visual fields • Sensory loss on contralateral side in extremities and sometimes in ipsilateral side of face • Disturbance in senses of taste, smell	• *Mental status/LOC:* Coma usually presents in the initial stages of hemorrhagic disturbances; consciousness is usually preserved when the etiology is thrombotic in nature • Altered behavior—lethargy, apathy, combativeness • Altered cognitive function—memory, problem-solving, sequencing • *Extremities:* Weakness and paralysis contralateral with all kinds of stroke; unequal hand grasp; diminished deep tendon reflexes (contralateral) • Facial paralysis or paresis (ipsilateral) • *Aphasia:* May be expressive (difficulty producing speech), receptive (difficulty comprehending speech), or global (combination of the two) • Agnosia • Altered body image awareness, neglect or denial of contralateral side of body (unilateral neglect); disturbances in perception • Apraxia • *Pupil size and reaction:* May be unequal; dilated and fixed pupil on the ipsilateral side may be present with hemorrhage or herniation • Nuchal rigidity—common in hemorrhagic stroke • Seizures—common in hemorrhagic stroke
PAIN/DISCOMFORT • Headache of varying intensity	• Guarding, distraction behaviors • Restlessness • Muscle or facial tension
RESPIRATION • Smoking (risk factor)	• Inability to swallow, cough, or protect airway • Labored and irregular respirations • Noisy respirations, rhonchi (aspiration of secretions)

Client Assessment Database (continued)

DIAGNOSTIC DIVISION MAY REPORT (continued)	MAY EXHIBIT (continued)
SAFETY	• Problems with vision • Changes in perception of body spatial orientation (right CVA), neglect • Difficulty seeing objects on left side (right CVA) • Being unaware of affected side • Inability to recognize familiar objects, colors, words, faces • Diminished response to heat and cold, altered body temperature regulation • Swallowing difficulty, inability to meet own nutritional needs • Impaired judgment, little concern for safety, impatience, lack of insight (right CVA)
SOCIAL INTERACTION	• Speech problems • Inability to communicate • Inappropriate behavior
TEACHING/LEARNING • Family history of hypertension, stroke, diabetes • African American heritage (higher risk factor) • Use of oral contraceptives • Smoking, alcohol abuse (risk factors) • Obesity	
DISCHARGE PLAN CONSIDERATIONS • Medication regimen and therapeutic treatments • Assistance with transportation, shopping, food preparation, self-care, and homemaker or maintenance tasks • Changes in physical layout of home • Transition placement before return to home setting	

▶ Refer to section at end of plan for postdischarge considerations.

Diagnostic Studies

TEST WHY IT IS DONE	WHAT IT TELLS ME
• *Blood tests:* Complete blood count (CBC), platelet and clotting studies, erythrocyte sedimentation rate (ESR), metabolic panel, such as renalytes and glucose.	Various laboratory studies may be done to rule out systemic causes of stroke.
• *Computed tomography (CT) scan with or without enhancement:* Demonstrates structural abnormalities and presence of edema, hematoma, ischemia, and infarction.	May not immediately reveal all changes. Ischemic infarction may not be evident for 8 to 12 hours after event. Hemorrhagic events are evident immediately; therefore, emergency CT scan is done prior to administration of thrombolytics. Normal CT scan with a TIA.
• *Magnetic resonance imaging (MRI):* Demonstrates structural abnormalities and presence of edema, hematoma, ischemia, and infarction.	May show evidence of stroke within minutes of occurrence and is especially beneficial for assessing smaller strokes deep within the brain.
• *Positron emission tomography (PET) scan:* Demonstrates adequacy of cerebral blood flow and metabolism.	Abnormal in ischemic event.

(continues on page 242)

TEST WHY IT IS DONE (continued)	WHAT IT TELLS ME (continued)
• *Cerebral angiography:* Procedure that uses x-ray and opaque dye to help identify abnormalities of the blood vessels within the brain.	Helps determine specific cause of stroke, such as hemorrhage or obstructed artery, and pinpoints site of occlusion or rupture.
• *Transcranial Doppler ultrasonography:* Evaluates the velocity of blood flow through major intracranial vessels.	Identifies problems with circulation, such as diminished blood flow or presence of atherosclerotic plaques.
• *Lumbar puncture (LP) with cerebrospinal fluid (CSF) analysis:* Measures intracerebral pressure. Collected fluid analysis assists in diagnosis of cause of CVA.	Pressure is usually normal and CSF is clear in cerebral thrombosis, embolism, and TIA. Pressure elevation and grossly bloody fluid suggest subarachnoid and intracerebral hemorrhage. CSF total protein level may be elevated in cases of thrombosis because of inflammatory process. LP should be performed if septic embolism from bacterial endocarditis is suspected.
• *Stroke scale:* A standardized instrument measuring multiple factors, including LOC, motor and sensory responses, and language, on a numeric scale over time (National Institutes of Health [NIH], 2003).	The higher the score, the more severe the stroke symptoms.
• *X-ray (skull):* Evaluates internal structures of brain.	May show shift of pineal gland to the opposite side from an expanding mass; calcifications of the internal carotid may be visible in cerebral thrombosis; partial calcification of walls of an aneurysm may be noted in subarachnoid hemorrhage.
• *Electrocardiogram (ECG), or echocardiogram:* May be done to rule out cardiac origin as source of embolus.	Twenty percent of strokes are the result of atrial fibrillation or emboli associated with valvular disease, dysrhythmias, or endocarditis (Weir, 2008).

Nursing Priorities

1. Promote adequate cerebral perfusion and oxygenation.
2. Prevent or minimize complications and permanent disabilities.
3. Assist client to gain independence in activities of daily living (ADLs).
4. Support coping process and integration of changes into self-concept.
5. Provide information about disease process, prognosis, and treatment and rehabilitation needs.

Discharge Goals

1. Cerebral function improved and neurological deficits resolving or stabilized.
2. Complications prevented or minimized.
3. ADLs needs met by self or with assistance of other(s).
4. Coping with situation in positive manner and planning for the future.
5. Disease process, prognosis, and therapeutic regimen understood.
6. Plan in place to meet needs after discharge.

NURSING DIAGNOSIS: **ineffective cerebral tissue Perfusion**

May be related to
Interruption of blood flow—occlusive disorder, hemorrhage; cerebral vasospasm, cerebral edema

Possibly evidenced by
Altered LOC; memory loss
Changes in motor or sensory responses; restlessness
Sensory, language, intellectual, and emotional deficits
Changes in vital signs

Desired Outcomes/Evaluation Criteria—Client Will

Neurological Status (NOC)
Maintain usual or improved LOC, cognition, and motor and sensory function.
Demonstrate stable vital signs and absence of signs of increased ICP.
Display no further deterioration or recurrence of deficits.

ACTIONS/INTERVENTIONS	RATIONALE
Cerebral Perfusion Promotion (NIC)	
Independent	
Determine factors related to individual situation, cause for coma, decreased cerebral perfusion, and potential for ICP.	Influences choice of interventions. Deterioration in neurological signs and symptoms or failure to improve after initial insult may reflect decreased intracranial adaptive capacity, which requires that client be admitted to critical care area for monitoring of ICP and for specific therapies geared to maintaining ICP within a specified range. If the stroke is evolving, client can deteriorate quickly and require repeated assessment and progressive treatment. If the stroke is "completed," the neurological deficit is nonprogressive, and treatment is geared toward rehabilitation and preventing recurrence.
Monitor and document neurological status frequently and compare with baseline. (Refer to CP: Craniocerebral Trauma—Acute Rehabilitative Phase, ND: ineffective cerebral tissue Perfusion for complete neurological evaluation.)	Assesses trends in LOC and potential for increased ICP and is useful in determining location, extent, and progression or resolution of CNS damage. May also reveal TIA, which may resolve with no further symptoms or may precede thrombotic CVA.
Monitor vital signs noting:	
Hypertension or hypotension; compare blood pressure (BP) readings in both arms	Fluctuations in pressure may occur because of cerebral pressure or injury in vasomotor area of the brain. Hypertension or hypotension may have been a precipitating factor. Hypotension may follow stroke because of circulatory collapse.
Heart rate and rhythm; auscultate for murmurs	Changes in rate, especially bradycardia, can occur because of the brain damage. Dysrhythmias and murmurs may reflect cardiac disease, which may have precipitated CVA, for example, stroke after MI or from valve dysfunction.
Respirations, noting patterns and rhythm—periods of apnea after hyperventilation, Cheyne-Stokes respiration	Irregularities can suggest location of cerebral insult or increased ICP and need for further intervention, including possible respiratory support. (Refer to CP: Craniocerebral Trauma—Acute Rehabilitative Phase, ND: risk for ineffective Breathing Pattern.)
Evaluate pupils, noting size, shape, equality, and light reactivity.	Pupil reactions are regulated by the oculomotor (III) cranial nerve and are useful in determining whether the brainstem is intact. Pupil size and equality is determined by balance between parasympathetic and sympathetic enervation. Response to light reflects combined function of the optic (II) and oculomotor (III) cranial nerves.
Document changes in vision, such as reports of blurred vision and alterations in visual field or depth perception.	Specific visual alterations reflect area of brain involved, indicate safety concerns, and influence choice of interventions.
Assess higher functions, including speech, if client is alert. (Refer to ND: impaired verbal [and/or written] Communication.)	Changes in cognition and speech content are an indicator of location and degree of cerebral involvement and may indicate increased ICP.
Position with head slightly elevated and in neutral position.	Reduces arterial pressure by promoting venous drainage and may improve cerebral circulation and perfusion.
Maintain bedrest, provide quiet environment, and restrict visitors or activities, as indicated. Provide rest periods between care activities, limiting duration of procedures.	Continual stimulation can increase ICP. Absolute rest and quiet may be needed to prevent recurrence of bleeding, in the case of hemorrhagic stroke.
Prevent straining at stool or holding breath.	Valsalva's maneuver increases ICP and potentiates risk of bleeding.
Assess for nuchal rigidity, twitching, increased restlessness, irritability, and onset of seizure activity.	Indicative of meningeal irritation, especially in hemorrhagic disorders. Seizures may reflect increased ICP or reflect location and severity of cerebral injury, requiring further evaluation and intervention.
Collaborative	
Administer supplemental oxygen, as indicated.	Reduces hypoxemia.
Administer medications, as indicated, for example:	
Intravenous thrombolytics, such as tissue plasminogen activator (tPA), alteplase (Activase), and recombinant prourokinase (Prourokinase)	As the only proven therapy for early acute ischemic stroke, tPA is useful in minimizing the size of the infarcted area by opening blocked vessels that are occluded with clot. Treatment must be started within 3 hours of initial symptoms to improve outcomes. *Note:* These agents are contraindicated in several instances—intracranial hemorrhage as diagnosed by CT scan, recent intracranial surgery, serious head trauma, and uncontrolled hypertension.

(continues on page 244)

Anticoagulants, such as warfarin sodium (Coumadin); low-molecular-weight heparin, for example, enoxaparin (Lovenox) and dalteparin (Fragmin); and direct thrombin inhibitor, such as ximelagatran (Exanta)

May be used to improve cerebral blood flow and prevent further clotting when embolus or thrombosis is the problem.

Antiplatelet agents, such as aspirin (ASA), aspirin with extended-release dipyridamole (Aggrenox), ticlopidine (Ticlid), and clopidogrel (Plavix)

Antiplatelet agents are used following an ischemic stroke or TIA.

Antihypertensives

Preexisting or chronic hypertension requires cautious treatment because aggressive management increases the risk of extension of tissue damage during an evolving stroke. Transient hypertension often occurs during acute stroke and usually resolves without therapeutic intervention.

Peripheral vasodilators, such as cyclandelate (Cyclospasmol), papaverine (Pavabid), and isoxsuprine (Vasodilan)

Used to improve collateral circulation or decrease vasospasm.

Neuroprotective agents, such as calcium channel blockers, excitatory amino acid inhibitors, and gangliosides

These agents are being researched as a means to protect the brain by interrupting the destructive cascade of biochemical events—influx of calcium into cells, release of excitatory neurotransmitters, buildup of lactic acid—to limit ischemic injury.

Phenytoin (Dilantin) and phenobarbital

May be used to control seizures and for sedative action. *Note:* Phenobarbital enhances action of antiepileptics.

Prepare for surgery, as appropriate—carotid endarterectomy, microvascular bypass, and cerebral angioplasty.

May be necessary to resolve hemorrhagic situation and reduce neurological symptoms and risk of recurrent stroke.

Monitor laboratory studies as indicated, such as prothrombin time (PT), activated partial thromboplastin time (aPTT), and Dilantin level.

Provides information about effectiveness and therapeutic level of anticoagulants when used.

NURSING DIAGNOSIS: impaired physical Mobility

May be related to
Neuromuscular involvement: weakness, paresthesia; flaccid, hypotonic paralysis (initially); spastic paralysis
Perceptual or cognitive impairment

Possibly evidenced by
Inability to purposefully move within the physical environment, impaired coordination, limited range of motion (ROM), decreased muscle strength and control

Desired Outcomes/Evaluation Criteria—Client Will

Immobility Consequences: Physiologic (NOC)
Maintain or increase strength and function of affected or compensatory body part.
Maintain optimal position of function as evidenced by absence of contractures and footdrop.
Demonstrate techniques and behaviors that enable resumption of activities.
Maintain skin integrity.

ACTIONS/INTERVENTIONS

RATIONALE

Positioning (NIC)
Independent

Assess functional ability and extent of impairment initially and on a regular basis. Classify according to a 0 to 4 scale. (Refer to CP: Craniocerebral Trauma—Acute Rehabilitative Phase, ND: impaired physical Mobility.)

Identifies strengths and deficiencies and may provide information regarding recovery. Assists in choice of interventions because different techniques are used for flaccid and spastic types of paralysis.

Change positions at least every 2 hours (supine, side lying) and possibly more often if placed on affected side.

Reduces risk of tissue ischemia and injury. Affected side has poorer circulation and reduced sensation and is more predisposed to skin breakdown and pressure ulcers.

Position in prone position once or twice a day if client can tolerate.

Helps maintain functional hip extension; however, may increase anxiety, especially about ability to breathe.

Prop extremities in functional position; use footboard during the period of flaccid paralysis. Maintain neutral position of head.

Prevents contractures and footdrop and facilitates use when or if function returns. Flaccid paralysis may interfere with ability to support head, whereas spastic paralysis may lead to deviation of head to one side.

Use arm sling when client is in upright position, as indicated.

During flaccid paralysis, use of sling may reduce risk of shoulder subluxation and shoulder-hand syndrome.

ACTIONS/INTERVENTIONS (continued)

Evaluate use of and need for positional aids and splints during spastic paralysis:
Place pillow under axilla to abduct arm.
Elevate arm and hand.
Place hard hand-rolls in the palm with fingers and thumb opposed.
Place knee and hip in extended position.
Maintain leg in neutral position with a trochanter roll.
Discontinue use of footboard, when appropriate.

Observe affected side for color, edema, or other signs of compromised circulation.
Inspect skin regularly, particularly over bony prominences. Gently massage any reddened areas and provide aids such as sheepskin pads, as necessary.

Exercise Therapy: Muscle Control (NIC)
Begin active or passive ROM to all extremities (including splinted) on admission. Encourage exercises, such as quadriceps or gluteal exercise, squeezing rubber ball, and extension of fingers and legs and feet.

Assist client to develop sitting balance (such as raise head of bed; assist to sit on edge of bed, having client use the strong arm to support body weight and strong leg to move affected leg; increase sitting time) and standing balance—put flat walking shoes on client, support client's lower back with hands while positioning own knees outside client's knees, and assist in using parallel bars and walker.
Get client up in chair as soon as vital signs are stable except following cerebral hemorrhage.

Pad chair seat with foam or water-filled cushion, and assist client to shift weight at frequent intervals.
Set goals with client/significant other (SO) for increasing participation in activities, exercise, and position changes.
Encourage client to assist with movement and exercises using unaffected extremity to support and move weaker side.

Positioning (NIC)
Collaborative
Provide egg-crate mattress, water bed, flotation device, or specialized bed, such as kinetic, as indicated.

Exercise Therapy: Muscle Control (NIC)
Consult with physical therapist regarding active, resistive exercises and client ambulation.

Assist with electrical stimulation—transcutaneous electrical nerve stimulator (TENS) unit, as indicated.
Administer muscle relaxants and antispasmodics as indicated, such as baclofen (Lioresal) and dantrolene (Dantrium).

RATIONALE (continued)

Flexion contractures occur because flexor muscles are stronger than extensors.
Prevents adduction of shoulder and flexion of elbow.
Promotes venous return and helps prevent edema formation.
Hard cones decrease the stimulation of finger flexion, maintaining finger and thumb in a functional position.
Maintains functional position.
Prevents external hip rotation.
Continued use after change from flaccid to spastic paralysis can cause excessive pressure on the ball of the foot, enhance spasticity, and actually increase plantar flexion.
Edematous tissue is more easily traumatized and heals more slowly.
Pressure points over bony prominences are most at risk for decreased perfusion and ischemia. Circulatory stimulation and padding help prevent skin breakdown and decubitus ulcer development.

Minimizes muscle atrophy, promotes circulation, and helps prevent contractures. Reduces risk of hypercalciuria and osteoporosis if underlying problem is hemorrhage. *Note:* Excessive and imprudent stimulation can predispose to recurrence of bleeding.
Aids in retraining neuronal pathways, enhancing proprioception and motor response.

Helps stabilize BP, restoring vasomotor tone, and promotes maintenance of extremities in a functional position and emptying of bladder and kidneys, reducing risk of urinary stones and infections from stasis. *Note:* If stroke is not completed, activity increases risk of additional bleeding and infarction.
Reduces pressure on the coccyx and prevents skin breakdown.

Promotes sense of expectation of progress and improvement, and provides some sense of control and independence.
May respond as if affected side is no longer part of body and need encouragement and active training to "reincorporate" it as a part of own body.

Promotes even weight distribution, decreasing pressure on bony points and helping to prevent skin breakdown and pressure ulcer formation. Specialized beds help with positioning, enhance circulation, and reduce venous stasis to decrease risk of tissue injury and complications such as orthostatic pneumonia.

Individualized program can be developed to meet particular needs and deal with deficits in balance, coordination, and strength.
May assist with muscle strengthening and increase voluntary muscle control, as well as pain control.
May be required to relieve spasticity in affected extremities.

NURSING DIAGNOSIS: impaired verbal [and/or written] Communication

May be related to

Impaired cerebral circulation; neuromuscular impairment, loss of facial or oral muscle tone and control; generalized weakness and fatigue

Possibly evidenced by

Impaired articulation; soft speech or does not or cannot speak

Inability to modulate speech, find and name words, identify objects; inability to comprehend written or spoken language, global aphasia

Inability to produce written communication, expressive aphasia

Desired Outcomes/Evaluation Criteria—Client Will

Communication (NOC)

Indicate understanding of the communication problems.

Establish method of communication in which needs can be expressed.

Use resources appropriately.

ACTIONS/INTERVENTIONS	RATIONALE
Communication Enhancement: Speech Deficit (NIC)	
Independent	
Assess type and degree of dysfunction, such as receptive aphasia—client does not seem to understand words, or expressive aphasia—client has trouble speaking or making self understood:	Helps determine area and degree of brain involvement and difficulty client has with any or all steps of the communication process. Client may have trouble understanding spoken words (damage to Wernicke's speech area), speaking words correctly (damage to Broca's speech areas), or may experience damage to both areas.
Differentiate aphasia from dysarthria.	Choice of interventions depends on type of impairment. Aphasia is a defect in using and interpreting symbols of language and may involve sensory and/or motor components, such as inability to comprehend written or spoken words or to write, make signs, and speak. A dysarthric person can understand, read, and write language, but has difficulty forming or pronouncing words because of weakness and paralysis of oral musculature, resulting in softly spoken speech.
Listen for errors in conversation and provide feedback.	Client may lose ability to monitor verbal output and be unaware that communication is not sensible. Feedback helps client realize why caregivers are not understanding and responding appropriately and provides opportunity to clarify content and meaning.
Ask client to follow simple commands, such as "Shut your eyes," "Point to the door"; repeat simple words or sentences.	Tests for receptive aphasia.
Point to objects and ask client to name them.	Tests for expressive aphasia—client may recognize item but not be able to name it.
Have client produce simple sounds, such as "sh," "cat."	Identifies dysarthria because motor components of speech (tongue, lip movement, breath control) can affect articulation and may or may not be accompanied by expressive aphasia.
Ask client to write name and/or a short sentence. If unable to write, have client read a short sentence.	Tests for writing disability (agraphia) and deficits in reading comprehension (alexia), which are also part of receptive and expressive aphasia.
Post notice at nurses' station and client's room about speech impairment. Provide special call bell if necessary.	Allays anxiety related to inability to communicate and fear that needs will not be met promptly. Call bell that is activated by minimal pressure is useful when client is unable to use regular call system.
Provide alternative methods of communication, such as writing or felt board and pictures. Provide visual clues—gestures, pictures, "needs" list, and demonstration.	Provides for communication of needs or desires based on individual situation or underlying deficit.
Anticipate and provide for client's needs.	Helpful in decreasing frustration when dependent on others and unable to communicate desires.
Talk directly to client, speaking slowly and distinctly. Use yes/no questions to start, progressing in complexity as client responds.	Reduces confusion and anxiety at having to process and respond to large amount of information at one time. As retraining progresses, advancing complexity of communication stimulates memory and further enhances word and idea association.

ACTIONS/INTERVENTIONS (continued)

Speak with normal volume and avoid talking too fast. Give client ample time to respond. Talk without pressing for a response.

Encourage SO and visitors to persist in efforts to communicate with client, such as reading mail and discussing family happenings even if client is unable to respond appropriately.

Discuss familiar topics—job, family, hobbies, and current events.

Respect client's preinjury capabilities; avoid speaking down to client or making patronizing remarks.

Collaborative
Consult with or refer to speech therapist.

RATIONALE (continued)

Client is not necessarily hearing impaired and raising voice may irritate or anger client. Forcing responses can result in frustration and may cause client to resort to "automatic" speech, such as garbled speech and obscenities.

It is important for family members to continue talking to client to reduce client's isolation, promote establishment of effective communication, and maintain sense of connectedness with family.

Promotes meaningful conversation and provides opportunity to practice skills.

Enables client to feel esteemed because intellectual abilities often remain intact.

Assesses individual verbal capabilities and sensory, motor, and cognitive functioning to identify deficits and therapy needs.

NURSING DIAGNOSIS: disturbed Sensory Perception [specify]

May be related to
Altered sensory reception, transmission, integration—neurological trauma or deficit
Psychological stress—narrowed perceptual fields caused by anxiety

Possibly evidenced by
Disorientation to time, place, person
Change in behavior pattern and usual response to stimuli; exaggerated emotional responses
Poor concentration, altered thought processes, bizarre thinking
Reported or measured change in sensory acuity: hypoparesthesia, altered sense of taste or smell
Inability to tell position of body parts (proprioception)
Inability to recognize or attach meaning to objects (visual agnosia)
Altered communication patterns
Motor incoordination

Desired Outcomes/Evaluation Criteria—Client Will

Cognition (NOC)
Regain and maintain usual LOC and perceptual functioning.
Acknowledge changes in ability and presence of residual involvement.
Demonstrate behaviors to compensate for or overcome deficits.

ACTIONS/INTERVENTIONS

Environmental Management (NIC)
Independent
Review pathology of individual condition.

Observe behavioral responses such as hostility, crying, inappropriate affect, agitation, and hallucination by using Los Ranchos Scale, as appropriate. (Refer to CP: Craniocerebral Trauma—Acute Rehabilitative Phase, ND: disturbed Thought Processes.)

Eliminate extraneous noise and stimuli as necessary.

Speak in calm, quiet voice, using short sentences. Maintain eye contact.

Ascertain and validate client's perceptions. Reorient client frequently to environment, staff, and procedures.

Evaluate for visual deficits. Note loss of visual field, changes in depth perception (horizontal or vertical planes), and presence of diplopia.

RATIONALE

Awareness of type and area of involvement aids in assessing for and anticipating specific deficits and planning care.

Individual responses are variable, but commonalities, such as emotional lability, lowered frustration threshold, apathy, and impulsiveness, may complicate care. Eight-level Los Ranchos Scale aids in documenting progress during initial weeks following insult.

Reduces anxiety and exaggerated emotional responses and confusion associated with sensory overload.

Client may have limited attention span or problems with comprehension. These measures can help client attend to communication.

Assists client to identify inconsistencies in reception and integration of stimuli and may reduce perceptual distortion of reality.

Presence of visual disorders can negatively affect client's ability to perceive environment and relearn motor skills and increases risk of accident and injury.

(continues on page 248)

Approach client from visually intact side. Leave light on; position objects to take advantage of intact visual fields. Patch affected eye or encourage wearing of prism glasses if indicated.

Provides for recognition of the presence of persons or objects; may help with depth perception problems; and prevents client from being startled. Patching may decrease the sensory confusion of double vision, and prism glasses may enhance vision across midline, decreasing neglect of affected side.

Peripheral Sensation Management (NIC)

Assess sensory awareness, such as differentiation of hot and cold, dull or sharp, position of body parts, and muscle and joint sense.

Diminished sensory awareness and impairment of kinesthetic sense negatively affects balance and positioning (proprioception) and appropriateness of movement, which interferes with ambulation, increasing risk of trauma.

Stimulate sense of touch—give client objects to touch and grasp. Have client practice touching walls or other boundaries.

Aids in retraining sensory pathways to integrate reception and interpretation of stimuli. Helps client orient self spatially and strengthens use of affected side.

Protect from temperature extremes; assess environment for hazards. Recommend testing warm water with unaffected hand.

Promotes client safety, reducing risk of injury.

Note inattention to body parts and segments of environment and lack of recognition of familiar objects or persons.

Presence of agnosia (loss of comprehension of auditory, visual, or other sensations, although sensory sphere is intact) may lead to unilateral neglect, inability to recognize environmental cues or meaning of commonplace objects, considerable self-care deficits, and disorientation or bizarre behavior.

Encourage client to watch feet when appropriate and consciously position body parts. Make client aware of all neglected body parts using sensory stimulation to affected side and exercises that bring affected side across midline, reminding person to dress and or care for affected ("blind") side.

Use of visual and tactile stimuli assists in reintegration of affected side and allows client to experience forgotten sensations of normal movement patterns.

NURSING DIAGNOSIS: Self-Care Deficit [specify]

May be related to
Neuromuscular impairment, decreased strength and endurance, loss of muscle control and coordination
Perceptual or cognitive impairment
Pain, discomfort
Depression

Possibly evidenced by
Impaired ability to perform ADLs, such as inability to bring food from receptacle to mouth; inability to wash body part(s) or regulate temperature of water; impaired ability to put on and take off clothing; difficulty completing toileting tasks

Desired Outcomes/Evaluation Criteria—Client Will

Self-Care: Activities of Daily Living (ADLs) (NOC)
Demonstrate techniques and lifestyle changes to meet self-care needs.
Perform self-care activities within level of own ability.
Identify personal and community resources that can provide assistance as needed.

ACTIONS/INTERVENTIONS

RATIONALE

Self-Care Assistance (NIC)
Independent

Assess abilities and level of deficit (0 to 4 scale) for performing ADLs.

Aids in anticipating and planning for meeting individual needs.

Avoid doing things for client that client can do for self, providing assistance as necessary.

These clients may become fearful and dependent, and although assistance is helpful in preventing frustration, it is important for client to do as much as possible for self to maintain self-esteem and promote recovery.

Be aware of impulsive behavior or actions suggestive of impaired judgment.

May indicate need for additional interventions and supervision to promote client safety.

Maintain a supportive, firm attitude. Allow client sufficient time to accomplish tasks.

Clients need empathy and to know caregivers will be consistent in their assistance.

Provide positive feedback for efforts and accomplishments.

Enhances sense of self-worth, promotes independence, and encourages client to continue endeavors.

Create plan for visual deficits that are present, such as the following:
  Place food and utensils on the tray related to client's unaffected side
  Situate the bed so that client's unaffected side is facing the room with the affected side to the wall
  Position furniture against wall, out of travel path

Provide self-help devices, such as button or zipper hook, knife-fork combinations, long-handled brushes, extensions for picking things up from floor, toilet riser, leg bag for catheter, and shower chair. Assist and encourage good grooming and makeup habits.
Encourage SO to allow client to do as much as possible for self.

Assess client's ability to communicate the need to void and ability to use urinal or bedpan. Take client to the bathroom at frequent and scheduled intervals for voiding if appropriate.

Identify previous bowel habits and reestablish normal regimen. Increase bulk in diet. Encourage fluid intake and increased activity.

Collaborative
Administer suppositories and stool softeners.

Consult with rehabilitation team, such as physical or occupational therapist.

Client will be able to see to eat the food.

Will be able to see when getting in or out of bed and observe anyone who comes into the room.
Provides for safety when client is able to move around the room, reducing risk of tripping and falling over furniture.
Enables client to manage for self, enhancing independence and self-esteem; reduces reliance on others for meeting own needs; and enables client to be more socially active.

Reestablishes sense of independence and fosters self-worth and enhances rehabilitation process. *Note:* This may be very difficult and frustrating for the SO/caregiver, depending on degree of disability and time required for client to complete activity.
Client may have neurogenic bladder, be inattentive, or be unable to communicate needs in acute recovery phase, but usually is able to regain independent control of this function as recovery progresses.
Assists in development of retraining program (independence) and aids in preventing constipation and impaction (long-term effects).

May be necessary at first to aid in establishing regular bowel function.
Provides assistance in developing a comprehensive therapy program and identifying special equipment needs that can increase client's participation in self-care.

NURSING DIAGNOSIS: ineffective Coping

May be related to
Situational crises, vulnerability, cognitive perceptual changes

Possibly evidenced by
Inappropriate use of defense mechanisms
Inability to cope or difficulty asking for help
Change in usual communication patterns
Inability to meet basic needs or role expectations
Difficulty problem-solving

Desired Outcomes/Evaluation Criteria—Client Will

Coping (NOC)
Verbalize acceptance of self in situation.
Talk or communicate with SO about situation and changes that have occurred.
Verbalize awareness of own coping abilities.
Meet psychological needs as evidenced by appropriate expression of feelings, identification of options, and use of resources.

Coping Enhancement (NIC)

Independent

Assess extent of altered perception and related degree of disability. Determine Functional Independence Measure score.

Identify meaning of the loss and dysfunction or change to client. Note ability to understand events and provide realistic appraisal of situation.

Determination of individual factors aids in developing plan of care, choice of interventions, and discharge expectations.

Independence is highly valued in American society, but is not as significant in some other cultures. Some clients accept and manage altered function effectively with little adjustment, whereas others have considerable difficulty recognizing and adjusting to deficits. In order to provide meaningful support and appropriate problem-solving, healthcare providers need to understand the meaning of the stroke and limitations to the client.

Determine outside stressors, including family, work, social, and future nursing and healthcare needs.

Helps identify specific needs, provides opportunity to offer information and support and begin problem-solving. Consideration of social factors, in addition to functional status, is important in determining appropriate discharge destination.

Encourage client to express feelings, including hostility or anger, denial, depression, and sense of disconnectedness.

Note whether client refers to affected side as "it" or denies affected side and says it is "dead."

Acknowledge statement of feelings about betrayal of body; remain matter-of-fact about reality that client can still use unaffected side and learn to control affected side. Use words such as weak, affected, and right-left, that incorporate that side as part of the whole body.

Identify previous methods of dealing with life problems. Determine presence and quality of support systems.

Emphasize and provide positive I-messages for small gains either in recovery of function or independence.

Support behaviors or efforts such as increased interest and participation in rehabilitation activities.

Monitor for sleep disturbance, increased difficulty concentrating, statements of inability to cope, lethargy, and withdrawal.

Demonstrates acceptance of and assists client in recognizing and beginning to deal with these feelings.

Suggests rejection of body part or negative feelings about body image and abilities, indicating need for intervention and emotional support.

Helps client see that the nurse accepts both sides as part of the whole individual. Allows client to feel hopeful and begin to accept current situation.

Provides opportunity to use behaviors previously effective, build on past successes, and mobilize resources.

Consolidates gains, helps reduce feelings of anger and helplessness, and conveys sense of progress.

Suggests possible adaptation to changes and understanding about own role in future lifestyle.

May indicate onset of depression (common aftereffect of stroke), which may require further evaluation and intervention.

Collaborative

Refer for neuropsychological evaluation and counseling, if indicated.

May facilitate adaptation to role changes that are necessary for a sense of feeling and being a productive person. *Note:* Depression is common in stroke survivors and may be a direct result of the brain damage or an emotional reaction to sudden-onset disability.

NURSING DIAGNOSIS: **risk for impaired Swallowing**

Risk factors may include

Neuromuscular or perceptual impairment

Possibly evidenced by

(Not applicable; presence of signs and symptoms establishes an *actual* diagnosis)

Desired Outcomes/Evaluation Criteria—Client Will

Swallowing Status (NOC)

Demonstrate feeding methods appropriate to individual situation, with aspiration prevented.

Maintain desired body weight.

ACTIONS/INTERVENTIONS	RATIONALE
Swallowing Therapy (NIC)	
Independent	
Review individual pathology and ability to swallow, noting extent of paralysis, clarity of speech, facial and tongue involvement, ability to protect airway and episodes of coughing or choking; presence of adventitious breath sounds and amount and character of oral secretions. Weigh periodically, as indicated.	Nutritional interventions, including choice of feeding route, are determined by these factors.
Have suction equipment available at bedside, especially during early feeding efforts.	Timely intervention may limit amount and untoward effect of aspiration.
Promote effective swallowing using methods such as the following:	
Schedule activities and medications to provide a minimum of 30 minutes of rest before eating.	Promotes optimal muscle function and helps to limit fatigue.
Provide pleasant environment free of distractions, such as TV.	Promotes relaxation and allows client to focus on task of eating and swallowing.
Assist client with head control or support, and position based on specific dysfunction.	Counteracts hyperextension, aiding in prevention of aspiration and enhancing ability to swallow. Optimal positioning can facilitate intake and reduce risk of aspiration—head back for decreased posterior propulsion of tongue, head turned to weak side for unilateral pharyngeal paralysis, and lying down on either side for reduced pharyngeal contraction.
Place client in upright position during and after feeding, as appropriate.	Uses gravity to facilitate swallowing and reduces risk of aspiration.
Provide oral care based on individual need prior to meal.	Clients with dry mouth require a moisturizing agent, such as artificial saliva or alcohol-free mouthwash, before and after eating; clients with excess saliva will benefit from use of a drying agent, such as lemon or glycerin swabs, before meal and a moisturizing agent afterward.
Season food with herbs, spices, and lemon juice according to client's preference, within dietary restrictions.	Increases salivation, improving bolus formation and swallowing effort.
Serve foods at customary temperature and water always chilled.	Lukewarm temperatures are less likely to stimulate salivation, so foods and fluids should be served cold or warm as appropriate. *Note:* Water is the most difficult to swallow.
Stimulate lips to close or manually open mouth by light pressure on lips or under chin, if needed.	Aids in sensory retraining and promotes muscular control.
Place food of appropriate consistency in unaffected side of mouth.	Provides sensory stimulation (including taste), which may increase salivation and trigger swallowing efforts, enhancing intake. Food consistency is determined by individual deficit. *For example:* Clients with decreased range of tongue motion require thick liquids initially, progressing to thin liquids, whereas clients with delayed pharyngeal swallow will handle thick liquids and thicker foods better. *Note:* Pureed food is not recommended because client may not be able to recognize what is being eaten. Most milk products, peanut butter, syrup, and bananas are avoided because they produce mucus and are sticky.
Touch parts of the cheek with tongue blade or apply ice to weak tongue.	Can improve tongue movement and control necessary for swallowing and inhibits tongue protrusion.
Feed slowly, allowing 30 to 45 minutes for meals.	Feeling rushed can increase stress and level of frustration, may increase risk of aspiration, and may result in client's terminating meal early.
Offer solid foods and liquids at different times.	Prevents client from swallowing food before it is thoroughly chewed. In general, liquids should be offered only after client has finished eating solids.
Limit or avoid use of drinking straw for liquids.	Although use may strengthen facial and swallowing muscles, if client lacks tight lip closure to accommodate straw or if liquid is deposited too far back in mouth, risk of aspiration may be increased.
Encourage SO to bring favorite foods.	Provides familiar tastes and preferences. Stimulates feeding efforts and may enhance swallowing and intake.
Maintain upright position for 45 to 60 minutes after eating.	Helps client manage oral secretions and reduces risk of regurgitation.
Maintain accurate intake and output (I&O); record calorie count.	If swallowing efforts are not sufficient to meet fluid and nutrition needs, alternative methods of feeding must be pursued.

(continues on page 252)

ACTIONS/INTERVENTIONS (continued)

Encourage participation in exercise or activity program.

Collaborative

Review results of radiographic studies, such as video fluoroscopy.

Administer intravenous (IV) fluids and/or tube feedings.

Coordinate multidisciplinary approach to develop treatment plan that meets individual needs.

RATIONALE (continued)

May increase release of endorphins in the brain, promoting a sense of general well-being and increasing appetite.

Aids in determining phase of swallowing difficulties—oral preparatory, oral, pharyngeal, or esophageal phase.

May be necessary for fluid replacement and nutrition if client is unable to take anything orally.

Inclusion of dietitian and speech and occupational therapists can increase effectiveness of long-term plan and significantly reduce risk of silent aspiration.

NURSING DIAGNOSIS: **deficient Knowledge [Learning Need] regarding condition, prognosis, treatment, self-care, and discharge needs**

May be related to
Lack of exposure, unfamiliarity with information resources
Cognitive limitation, information misinterpretation, lack of recall

Possibly evidenced by
Request for information
Statement of misconception
Inaccurate follow-through of instructions
Development of preventable complications

Desired Outcomes/Evaluation Criteria—Client/SO Will

Knowledge: Disease Process (NOC)
Participate in learning process.
Verbalize understanding of condition, prognosis, and potential complications.

Knowledge: Treatment Regimen (NOC)
Verbalize understanding of therapeutic regimen and rationale for actions.
Initiate necessary lifestyle changes.

ACTIONS/INTERVENTIONS

Teaching: Disease Process (NIC)
Independent
Evaluate type and degree of sensory-perceptual involvement.

Include SO and family in discussions and teaching.

Discuss specific pathology and individual potentials.

Identify signs and symptoms requiring further follow-up, such as changes or decline in visual, motor, sensory functions; alteration in mentation or behavioral responses; and severe headache.

Review current restrictions or limitations and discuss planned or potential resumption of activities, including sexual relations.

Review and reinforce current therapeutic regimen, including use of medications to control hypertension, hypercholesterolemia, and diabetes, as indicated and use of aspirin or similar-acting drug, such as ticlopidine (Ticlid) and warfarin sodium (Coumadin). Identify ways of continuing program after discharge.

Provide written instructions and schedules for activity, medication, and important facts.

Encourage client to refer to lists, written communications or notes, and memory book.

Discuss plans for meeting self-care needs.

Refer to discharge planner or home care supervisor and visiting nurse.

RATIONALE

Deficits affect the choice of teaching methods and content and complexity of instruction.

These individuals will be providing support and care and have great impact on client's quality of life.

Aids in establishing realistic expectations and promotes understanding of current situation and needs.

Prompt evaluation and intervention reduces risk of complications and further loss of function.

Promotes understanding, provides hope for future, and creates expectation of resumption of more "normal" life.

Recommended activities, limitations, and medication and therapy needs are established on the basis of a coordinated interdisciplinary approach. Follow-through is essential to progression of recovery and prevention of complications. *Note:* Long-term anticoagulation may be beneficial for clients prone to clot formation; however, these drugs are contraindicated for CVA resulting from hemorrhage.

Provides visual reinforcement and reference source after discharge.

Provides aids to support memory and promotes improvement in cognitive skills.

Varying levels of assistance may be required and need to be planned for based on individual situation.

Home environment may require evaluation and modifications to meet individual needs.

ACTIONS/INTERVENTIONS (continued)

Identify community resources, such as National Stroke Association, American Heart Association's Stroke Connection, stroke support clubs, senior services, Meals on Wheels, adult day care or respite program, and visiting nurse.

Suggest client reduce or limit environmental stimuli, especially during cognitive activities.

Recommend client seek assistance in problem-solving process and validate decisions as indicated.

Identify individual risk factors—hypertension, cardiac dysrhythmias, obesity, smoking, heavy alcohol use, atherosclerosis, poor control of diabetes, and use of oral contraceptives—and discuss necessary lifestyle changes.

Review importance of a balanced diet, low in cholesterol and sodium, if indicated. Discuss role of vitamins and other supplements.

Refer to and reinforce importance of follow-up care by rehabilitation team, such as physical, occupational, speech, and vocational therapists.

RATIONALE (continued)

Enhances coping abilities and promotes home management and adjustment to impairments for both stroke survivors and caregivers. *Note:* Recent innovations include such programs as Menu-Direct, which provides fully prepared meal programs with nutrition-rich foods. Some entrees have soufflé-like consistency to help trigger swallowing response.

Multiple or concomitant stimuli may aggravate confusion and impair mental abilities.

Some clients, especially those with right CVA, may display impaired judgment and impulsive behavior, compromising ability to make sound decisions.

Promotes general well-being and may reduce risk of recurrence. *Note:* Obesity in women has been found to have a high correlation with ischemic stroke.

Improves general health and well-being and provides energy for life activities.

Diligent work may eventually overcome or minimize residual deficits.

NURSING DIAGNOSIS: unilateral Neglect

May be related to
Left hemiplegia from CVA of right hemisphere

Possibly evidenced by
Failure to move eyes, head, limbs, trunk in the neglected hemisphere despite being aware of a stimulus in that space
Appears unaware of positioning of neglected limbs
Lack of safety precautions with regard to the neglected side
Failure to eat food from left side of plate and dress or groom neglected side
Failure to notice people approaching from neglected side

Desired Outcomes/Evaluation Criteria—Client Will

Adaptation to Physical Disability (NOC)
Acknowledge presence of impairment.

Client/Caregiver Will

Identify adaptive or protective measures for individual situation.
Demonstrate behaviors, lifestyle changes necessary to promote physical safety.

ACTIONS/INTERVENTIONS

Unilateral Neglect Management (NIC)
Independent
Reinforce to client the reality of the dysfunction and need to compensate, avoiding participation in client's use of denial.

Instruct client and SO/caregiver in treatment strategies focused on training attention on the neglected side:
  Approach client from unaffected side.
  Encourage client to turn head and eyes to "scan" the environment.
   Discuss affected side while touching, manipulating, and stroking affected side; provide items of varied size, weight, and texture for client to hold.
  Have client look at and handle affected side, bring across midline during care activities.
  Assist client to position affected extremity carefully and to routinely visualize placement or use a mirror to adjust placement.

RATIONALE

Enhances dealing with reality of situation, thus avoiding scenarios (denial) that can limit progress and attainment of goals.

Promotes involvement of all individuals in addressing problem, which may enhance recovery.
Enhances client's awareness and promotes interaction.
Helps client compensate for visual field loss, increasing awareness of environment.
Focuses client's attention on left side, and limb activation treatment provides tactile stimuli to promote use of affected limb in neglected hemisphere.
Encourages client to accept affected limb or side as part of self even though it does not feel like it belongs.
Promotes safety awareness, reducing risk of injury.

(continues on page 254)

ACTIONS/INTERVENTIONS (continued)

Instruct SO/caregiver to monitor alignment of limbs and to inspect skin regularly.

Discuss environmental safety concerns and assist in developing plan to correct risk factors.

Reinforce continuation of prescribed rehabilitation activities and neuropsychological therapies, as indicated.

RATIONALE (continued)

Decreased sensation and positional awareness may result in pressure injuries.

Client may continue to have some ongoing degree of functional impairment, including difficulty with navigating in familiar environments (Barrett & John, 2007).

Maximizes recovery and enhances independence. *Note:* Research indicates that most clients with neglect show early recovery, particularly within the first month, and marked improvement within 3 months (Barrett & John, 2007).

POTENTIAL CONSIDERATIONS following acute hospitalization (dependent on client's age, physical condition and presence of complications, personal resources, and life responsibilities)

- *risk for Injury*—general weakness, visual deficits, balancing difficulties, reduced large and small muscle or hand-eye coordination, cognitive impairment
- *imbalanced Nutrition: Less than Body Requirements*—inability to prepare and ingest food, cognitive limitations, limited financial resources
- *Self-Care Deficit*—decreased strength and endurance, perceptual and cognitive impairment, neuromuscular impairment, muscular pain, depression
- *impaired Home Maintenance*—individual physical limitations, inadequate support systems, insufficient finances, unfamiliarity with neighborhood resources
- *situational low Self-Esteem*—cognitive and perceptual impairment, perceived loss of control in some aspect of life, loss of independent functioning
- *risk for Caregiver Role Strain*—severity of illness and deficits of care receiver, duration of caregiving required, complexity and amount of caregiving task, caregiver isolation, and lack of respite

---

HERNIATED NUCLEUS PULPOSUS (RUPTURED INTERVERTEBRAL DISC)

I. **Pathophysiology**—Occurs when all or part of the gelatinous center of the intervertebral disc (nucleus pulposus) is forced through a weakened part or tear in the disc
   a. Also known as herniated disc (most common term), ruptured disc, slipped disk, or prolapsed intervertebral disc
   b. Symptoms can arise if a disc fragment exerts pressure on a spinal nerve root or the structures collapse because of loss of the cushion normally provided by a healthy nucleus pulposa.

II. **Etiology**
   a. Herniation (either complete or partial) most often occurs in discs of the lumbosacral vertebral areas of L4 to L5 and L5 to S1, as well as the cervical (neck) vertebral areas of C5 to C6 and C6 to C7. Lumbar disc herniation occurs 15 times more often than cervical herniation (Medline plus, 2006).
   b. Disc degeneration is due in part to the aging process but also as a result of sedentary lifestyles with too little (sometimes punctuated by too much) exercise.

   c. Other risk factors include congenital conditions affecting the size of the spinal canal, occupations requiring lifting of heavy objects or repetitive lifting, and accidents or trauma.
   d. Condition affects men and women equally and usually occurs between ages 30 and 50; in older adults, disc herniation occurs more frequently in men—especially those involved in strenuous physical activity (MedlinePlus, 2006).

III. **Statistics**
   a. Morbidity: In 2001, back pain was listed as the leading cause of disability in Americans under age 45 (Edwards et al, 2001); in 2006, low back pain was reported as the most common (27%) source of pain. (National Center for Health Statistics, 2006).
   b. Cost: In 2005, Americans spent $85.9 billion attempting to relieve back and neck pain, which was up from $52.1 billion in 1997 (Brook et al, 2008).

GLOSSARY

Intervertebral disc: The structure in the spine that bears weight and allows motion. It is made of a central portion (nucleus pulposus), which is surrounded by layers of tissue (annulus fibrosis). The disc helps the spine support the body and allows movement between vertebra.

Nucleus pulposus: A semi-gelatinous tissue in the center of an intervertebral disc surrounded and contained by

the annulus fibrosus, which prevents this material from protruding outside the disc space.

Spinal stenosis: Narrowing of the spinal canal as the surrounding tissues enlarge due to the development of bony spurs (osteophytes). Degenerative changes in adjacent ligaments cause loss of elasticity, thereby shortening the spine.

Range of motion (ROM): Flexibility of the joints measured from achievable flexion to extension.

Care Setting

Most disc problems are treated conservatively at the community level, although diagnostics and therapy services may be provided through outpatient facilities. Brief hospitalization is restricted to episodes of severe debilitating pain or neurological deficit.

Related Concerns

Disc surgery, page 262
Psychosocial aspects of care, page 749

Client Assessment Database

Data depend on site, severity, whether acute or chronic, and effects on surrounding structures (including degree of nerve root compression).

DIAGNOSTIC DIVISION MAY REPORT	MAY EXHIBIT
ACTIVITY/REST	
• Inability to perform usual or desired activities	• Atrophy of muscles on the affected side
• History of occupation requiring heavy lifting, sitting, driving for long periods	• Gait disturbances
• Need to sleep on bed board or firm mattress	
• Difficulty falling asleep or staying asleep	
• Decreased ROM of affected extremity or extremities	
ELIMINATION	
• Constipation, difficulty in defecation	
• Urinary incontinence or retention	
EGO INTEGRITY	
• Fear of paralysis	• Anxiety, depression, withdrawal from family or significant other (SO)
• Financial, employment concerns	
NEUROSENSORY	
• Tingling and numbness in legs and feet or hands	• Tenderness or spasm of paravertebral muscles
• Weakness on affected side in extremity or extremities	• Decreased deep tendon reflexes, muscle atrophy (late stage)
	• Muscle weakness
	• Decreased pain perception (sensory)
PAIN/DISCOMFORT	
• Unremitting pain or intermittent episodes of more severe pain	• Pain reproduced by palpation or manipulation of tissues
• Pain knifelike, aggravated by straining, such as coughing, sneezing, bending, lifting, defecation, straight leg raising (lumbar disc)	• Changes in stance, such as leaning away from affected area
• Radiation into head, face, shoulder, shoulder blade area, arms (cervical), buttocks area, legs or feet (lumbar)	• Altered gait, such as walking with a limp or elevated hip on affected side
• Having heard "snapping" sound at time of initial pain or trauma or felt "back giving way"	
• Muscle spasms	
• Limited mobility or forward bending	
SAFETY	
• History of previous back problems	
TEACHING/LEARNING	
• Sedentary or overactive lifestyle	
• Use of herbal supplements for backache, such as ashwaganda, burdock, cayenne, ginger, kava-kava, yarrow	
DISCHARGE PLAN CONSIDERATIONS	
• May require assistance with physical mobility and instrumental activities of daily living (IADLs), such as transportation, self-care, and homemaker and maintenance tasks, and so on	

▶ Refer to section at end of plan for postdischarge considerations.

TEST WHY IT IS DONE	WHAT IT TELLS ME
PROVOCATIVE TESTS • *Discography:* Involves the injection of a contrast material into the nucleus under a given pressure and the assessment of pain response. • *Nerve root blocks:* Involves injection of medication onto or near nerves. The medication that is injected includes local anesthetics, steroids, and opioids.	Determines if, and which, disc is the origin of pain by replicating and then relieving symptoms, particularly in lumbar disc pain. Blocks often provide diagnostic information, helping to determine the source of the pain. Nerve blocks are also used as a treatment, blocking pain pathways, particularly pain that is radiating, such as from the lower back into a leg. The facet joint diagnostic blocking has strong validity, specificity, and sensitivity in the diagnosis of facet joint pain. Sacroiliac joint blocks can also be used to rule out sacroiliac joint involvement, but are less reliable.
ELECTROPHYSIOLOGICAL STUDIES • *Electromyogram (EMG):* Measures the electrical activity of muscles at rest and during contraction. • *Nerve conduction studies (NCS):* Measure how well and how fast the nerves can send electrical signals.	Identifies diseases that damage muscle tissue, nerves, or neuromuscular junctions. Finds the cause of weakness, paralysis, or muscle twitching. *Note:* EMG and NCS are often done together. Can identify damage to the peripheral nervous system, including all the nerves that lead away from the spinal cord and the smaller nerves that branch out from those nerves. Can localize lesion to level of particular spinal nerve root involved in impairment and determine the effect on skeletal muscle. *Note:* EMG and NCS are often done together.
OTHER DIAGNOSTIC STUDIES • *Spinal x-rays:* Detect serious underlying structural and pathological conditions of the vertebrae and spinal cord. • *Magnetic resonance imaging (MRI) scan:* Test that uses magnetic fields to produce two- or three-dimensional images of soft tissues and bones. • *Computed tomography (CT) scan with and without enhancement:* X-ray procedure that combines many x-ray images with the aid of a computer to generate cross-sectional views and, if needed, three-dimensional images of the internal organs and structures of the body. • *Myelogram (also called myelography):* Imaging modality that shows the passage of contrast material in the space around the spinal cord (the subarachnoid space) using fluoroscopy, in which organs can be seen over many seconds. Sometimes performed in conjunction with MRI or used in the client who cannot undergo MRI.	May show degenerative changes in spine or intravertebral space. Can be used to rule out other suspected pathology, such as tumors, osteomyelitis, among others. Diagnostic test of choice for chronic, unremitting back pain due to nerve impingement. Can reveal changes in bone, discs, and soft tissues and can validate disc herniation and surgical considerations. May reveal spinal canal narrowing and disc protrusion. Although rarely performed, the myelogram detects abnormalities of the spinal cord, the spinal canal, the spinal nerve roots, and the blood vessels that supply the spinal cord. Reveals structures causing nerve compression—including narrowing of disc space—and confirms specific location and size of disc herniation and degree of spinal stenosis.

Nursing Priorities

1. Reduce back stress, muscle spasm, and pain.
2. Promote optimal functioning.
3. Support client and SO in rehabilitation process.
4. Provide information concerning condition, prognosis, and treatment needs.

Discharge Goals

1. Pain relieved or manageable.
2. Proper lifting, posture, and exercises demonstrated.
3. Motor function and sensation restored to optimal level.
4. Disease and injury process, prognosis, and therapeutic regimen understood.
5. Plan in place to meet needs after discharge.

NURSING DIAGNOSIS: acute/chronic Pain

May be related to
Physical injury agents: nerve compression, muscle spasm

Possibly evidenced by
Reports of back pain, stiff neck, decreased tolerance for activity
Preoccupation with pain, self or narrowed focus, distraction
Walking with a limp, inability to walk; guarding behavior, leaning toward affected side when standing; altered muscle tone
Facial mask of pain
Changes in sleep patterns; physical or social withdrawal
Autonomic responses (when pain is acute)

Desired Outcomes/Evaluation Criteria—Client Will

Pain Control (NOC)
Report pain is relieved or controlled.
Verbalize methods that provide relief.
Demonstrate use of therapeutic interventions, such as relaxation skills or behavior modification, to relieve pain.

ACTIONS/INTERVENTIONS	RATIONALE
Pain Management (NIC)	
Independent	
Assess client's perceptions of pain, attitude toward pain, and use of specific pain medications	Perception of pain is influenced by age and developmental stage; underlying problem causing the pain; and cognitive, behavioral, and sociocultural factors. Client may have beliefs about medications, and may have high or low tolerance for pain and pain medications.
Perform comprehensive assessment of pain, noting location, duration, precipitating and aggravating factors, and severity using a 0 to 10 scale, or other scales as appropriate. Accept client's description of pain.	Pain assessment helps determine choice of interventions and provides basis for comparison and evaluation of therapy.
Note presence of behaviors associated with pain—changes in vital signs (with acute pain), crying, grimacing, sleep disturbances, withdrawal, or narrowed focus. Evaluate current and past medication use.	Nonverbal evidence of pain. Observations may or may not be congruent with verbal reports, thus indicating need for further evaluation. For instance, the stoic client reporting a 3 on a 10-point pain scale may also be restless, agitated, and sleepless.
Maintain bedrest briefly during acute phase. Place client in semi-Fowler's position with spine, hips, and knees flexed; supine with or without head elevated 10 to 30 degrees; or lateral position.	Bedrest, usually prescribed for a very short time, such as 48 hours, in position of comfort decreases muscle spasm, reduces stress on structures, and facilitates reduction of disc protrusion.
Instruct in logrolling technique for position change if condition requires.	Logrolling reduces flexion, twisting, and strain on back, especially when nerve impingement impairs client's ability to move legs.
Assist with application of brace or corset. Instruct client in how to self-place brace with assistance, then independently.	Braces or corsets are often used briefly during acute phase of ruptured disc or after surgery to provide support and limit flexion or twisting. *Note:* Prolonged use can increase muscle weakness and cause further disc degeneration and nerve impairment.
Limit activity during acute phase as indicated. Provide rest periods. Shorten rest intervals and duration as client improves.	Gradual progression of activities decreases forces of gravity and motion, helping to relieve muscle spasms and reduce edema and stress on structures around affected disc.
Place needed items, such as call bell or phone, within easy reach.	Easy access to commonly used items reduces risk of straining.
Provide comfort measures, such as backrubs, positional and stretching exercises, Therapeutic Touch (TT), and a quiet, calming environment.	Nonpharmacological pain management is an essential nursing function in assisting the client to achieve pain-free periods.
Instruct in and assist with relaxation or visualization techniques, progressive muscle relaxation, and breathing exercises.	These activities refocus attention away from pain, aid in reducing muscle spasms and tension, and promote tissue oxygenation and healing.
Instruct in modification of activities. Encourage correct body mechanics and body posture.	Alleviates stress on muscles and prevents further aggravation of injury.

(continues on page 258)

Evaluate emotional and physical components of individual situation and the impact of current health condition.

Individuals with certain psychological syndromes, such as major depression, somatization disorder, or hypochondriasis, are at increased risk of developing chronic pain syndrome. Any painful condition, such as back pain, can cause or exacerbate emotional responses, such as depression, withdrawal, agitation, and anger.

Provide opportunities to talk with and listen to client concerns.

Client's verbalization of worries can help decrease stress factors associated with illness and hospitalization. Ongoing dialogue provides opportunity to give information and correct misinformation.

Collaborative

Provide orthopedic bed or firm mattress.

Supportive bed reduces back pain associated with spinal misalignment and decreases muscle spasms.

Administer medications, as indicated, for example:

Pain management may be complex and should be geared toward providing consistent and sufficient medication for pain relief while managing side effects.

Nonsteroidal anti-inflammatory drugs (NSAIDs), such as indomethacin (Indocin), ibuprofen (Motrin, Advil), naproxen (Aleve, Anaprox), etodolac (Lodine), diflunisal (Dolobid), and ketoprofen (Orudis)

NSAIDs suppress pain and inflammation, decrease edema and pressure on nerve root(s). *Note:* Epidural or facet joint injection of anti-inflammatory drugs has been found to be helpful in providing short-term pain relief in some clients if other interventions fail to alleviate pain.

Muscle relaxants, such as cyclobenzaprine (Flexeril), baclofen (Lioresal), diazepam (Valium), carisoprodol (Soma), methocarbamol (Robaxin), and metaxalone (Skelaxin)

These medications relax striated muscles, decreasing pain. *Note:* These drugs act centrally on the brain and are likely to cause drowsiness, dizziness, and lightheadedness, especially during initial therapy, raising safety concerns. The nurse must identify and address safety concerns.

Analgesics, such as acetaminophen (Tylenol) with codeine (Tylenol no. 3), hydrocodone (Vicodin, Lortab), oxycodone compound (OxyContin, Roxicet), propoxyphene (Darvon N, Darvocet), butorphanol (Stadol), fentanyl (Duragesic), meperidine (Demerol), and morphine and hydromorphone (Dilaudid)

These medications may be required to relieve moderate to severe pain, usually during periods of exacerbation of symptoms. They must be used with caution for relief of chronic pain because of potential for dependency. When considering the use of these medications, the client's functional abilities must be balanced with quality-of-life needs.

Apply physical supports, such as lumbar brace and cervical collar.

Support of structures decreases muscle stress and spasms as well as reduces pain.

Maintain traction, if indicated.

Traction may occasionally be used to remove weight bearing from affected disc area, thus increasing intravertebral separation and allowing the disc bulge to move away from nerve root.

Consult with physical therapist.

Individualized conservative care program—including hot and cold packs, ultrasound, massage, transcutaneous electrical nerve stimulation (TENS), therapeutic exercises, and pool therapy—can be implemented to relieve muscle spasm and strengthen back, extensor, abdominal, and quadriceps muscles, thus increasing muscular support to lumbar area.

Apply and monitor use and effects of cold or moist hot packs.

Cold packs relieve muscle spasms. Moist hot packs increase circulation to affected muscles. However, prolonged and improper heat application may result in thermal injury to skin.

Reinforce post-myelogram or post-epidural block instructions to the client, such as forcing fluids and positioning appropriately—lying flat or elevating head of bed at 30 degrees, as indicated.

Appropriate positioning decreases the risk of post-procedure headache or spinal fluid leak. Rehydration facilitates replacement of cerebrospinal fluid (CSF) loss.

Assist with the use of TENS unit and other similar devices.

Continuous nerve stimulation by TENS unit reduces or blocks the nerve's ability to transmit pain impulses to the brain.

Refer to rehabilitation and pain management clinic.

Coordinated team efforts may include physical, occupational, and psychological therapy to deal with all aspects of chronic pain and allow client to increase activity and productivity.

Refer for alternative therapies, as appropriate.

Client pain may be amenable to surgery, spinal manipulation, spinal cord stimulation, implantable intrathecal drug administration system, percutaneous lysis of adhesions, and other therapies.

NURSING DIAGNOSIS: impaired physical Mobility

May be related to
Pain and discomfort, muscle spasms
Restrictive therapies, such as bedrest, traction
Neuromuscular impairment

Possibly evidenced by
Reports of pain on movement
Reluctance to attempt or difficulty with purposeful movement
Impaired coordination, limited ROM, decreased muscle strength

Desired Outcomes/Evaluation Criteria—Client Will

Immobility Consequences: Physiological (NOC)
Verbalize understanding of situation, risk factors, and individual treatment regimen.
Be free of complications.
Demonstrate techniques and behaviors that enable resumption of activities.

Mobility (NOC)
Maintain or increase strength and function of affected or compensatory body part.

ACTIONS/INTERVENTIONS	RATIONALE
Bed Rest Care (NIC)	
Independent	
Perform passive ROM exercises and assist with active exercises.	ROM exercises and good body mechanics strengthen abdominal muscles and flexors of spine.
Encourage lower leg and ankle exercises. Evaluate for edema, erythema of lower extremities, and calf pain or tenderness.	These exercises stimulate venous return, decrease venous stasis, and reduce risk of thrombus formation.
Provide good skin care. Gently massage pressure points after each position change. Check skin under brace periodically.	Gentle massage and frequent repositioning reduce the risk of skin irritation and breakdown. Frequent skin assessments and prompt interventions afford early detection of skin breakdown.
Encourage diet high in fiber and adequate fluid intake.	Reduces risk of constipation related to decreased level of activity.
Note emotional and behavioral responses to immobility. Provide diversional activities.	Forced immobility may heighten restlessness and irritability. Diversional activity aids in refocusing attention and enhances coping with actual and perceived limitations.
Exercise Therapy: Ambulation (NIC)	
Provide for safety measures, as indicated by individual situation.	Depending on area of involvement or type of procedure, imprudent activity increases chance of spinal injury. (Refer to CP: Disc Surgery, ND: risk for spinal Trauma.)
Assist with activity, progressive ambulation, and therapeutic exercises.	Activity depends on individual situation. It should begin as early as possible and usually progresses slowly, based on client tolerance.
Demonstrate use of adjunctive devices, such as walker or cane.	Appropriate use of adjunctive devices provides stability and support by compensating for altered muscle tone, strength, balance, and gait.
Collaborative	
Administer pain medication on a regular schedule, or approximately 30 minutes before anticipated painful procedures or activities as indicated.	Client's anticipation of pain can increase muscle tension. Medications can help relax the client, enhance comfort, and improve motivation to increase activity.
Apply antiembolism stockings as indicated.	Promotes venous return, reducing risk of deep vein thrombosis (DVT).

NURSING DIAGNOSIS: Anxiety (specify level)/ineffective Coping

May be related to
Situational crisis
Threat to or change in health status, socioeconomic status, role functioning
Recurrent disorder with continuing pain
Inadequate relaxation, little or no exercise
Inadequate coping methods

Possibly evidenced by
Apprehension, uncertainty, helplessness
Expressed concerns regarding changes in life events

(continues on page 260)

Verbalization of inability to cope
Muscular tension, general irritability, restlessness; insomnia, fatigue
Inability to meet role expectations

Desired Outcomes/Evaluation Criteria—Client Will

Anxiety Self-Control (NOC)
Appear relaxed and report anxiety is reduced to a manageable level.
Identify ineffective coping behaviors and consequences.
Assess the current situation accurately.
Demonstrate effective problem-solving skills.
Develop plan for necessary lifestyle changes.

ACTIONS/INTERVENTIONS	RATIONALE
Coping Enhancement (NIC)	
Independent	
Assess level of anxiety. Determine previous coping strategies. Help client identify strategies to address current perceived or actual problems.	Aids in identifying strengths and skills that may help client deal with current situation and enable others to provide appropriate assistance.
Provide accurate information and honest answers.	Honest answers and accurate information facilitate development of rapport. These enable the client to use own experiences and knowledge to make decisions.
Provide opportunity for expression of concerns, such as possible permanent nerve damage, paralysis, effect on sexual ability, changes in employment, finances, and altered role responsibilities.	Open communication promotes client realization of short- and long-term implications of current condition and can promote coping with situation.
Assess presence of secondary gains that may impede recovery.	Client may unconsciously experience positive reinforcement, such as attention, control of others, and relief from responsibilities. These need to be recognized and addressed positively to promote recovery.
Note behaviors of SO that promote "sick role" for client.	By relieving the client from roles and responsibilities or not allowing the client to perform optimal level of function, the SO may unconsciously enable client to remain dependent.
Collaborative	
Refer to appropriate support groups, social services, financial or vocational counseling, and marital therapy or psychotherapy, as appropriate.	These services provide support for promoting coping and adaptation to life changes.

NURSING DIAGNOSIS: **deficient Knowledge [Learning Need] regarding condition, prognosis, treatment, self-care, and discharge needs**

May be related to
Misinformation, lack of exposure or recall
Information misinterpretation
Unfamiliarity with information resources

Possibly evidenced by
Verbalization of problems, statement of misconception
Inaccurate return demonstration
Development of preventable complications

Desired Outcomes/Evaluation Criteria—Client Will

Knowledge: Disease Process (NOC)
Verbalize understanding of condition, prognosis, and treatment.

Knowledge: Treatment Regimen (NOC)
Initiate necessary lifestyle changes.
Participate in therapeutic regimen.

ACTIONS/INTERVENTIONS	RATIONALE

Teaching: Disease Process (NIC)
Independent

Review disease or injury process and prognosis. Stress activity restrictions or limitations, including avoiding riding in car for long periods, refraining from participation in aggressive sports, and so on.

Knowledge and understanding of the disease, injury, prognosis, and activity limitations help client clarify and accept current lifestyle changes and appropriate modifications. These provide opportunity for client to make informed choices and may enhance cooperation with treatment program and achievement of optimal recovery.

Give information about and instruct in proper body mechanics, back school, ergonomics, and home exercises. Include information about proper posture and body mechanics for standing, sitting, and lifting and use of supportive shoes.

Proper body mechanics reduce the risk of reinjuring back and neck area.

Investigate appropriateness of using pneumatic continuous passive motion (CPM) supports when sitting.

Many individuals with low back pain have difficulty sitting for any length of time. This has a direct negative impact on work and leisure activities. The superficial soft-tissue effects of massage and vibration are usually short lived. CPM slowly moves the spine through the ranges of lordosis on a continuous basis. CPM can be used while sitting, riding in or driving a vehicle, or reclining.

Reduces risk of complications or injury.

Discuss medications and side effects; some medications cause drowsiness (analgesics, muscle relaxants), whereas others can irritate gastric mucosa and aggravate ulcer disease (NSAIDs).

Recommend use of bed boards or firm mattress and small flat pillow under neck. Instruct about sleeping on side with knees flexed, and avoiding prone position.

Bed boards, firm mattress, flat pillows, and positioning provide structural support and prevent hyperextension of the spine. These may decrease muscle strain.

Discuss dietary needs and goals.

Constipation is a complication of opioid analgesic use and immobility. Caloric restrictions promote weight control or reduction and can decrease pressure on the disc when obesity is aggravating back pain.

Instruct client to avoid prolonged heat application, and to alternate heat and cold.

Heat over a long period of time can increase local tissue congestion, and impaired sensitivity to heat can result in thermal injury. Alternating heat and cold during acute pain episodes helps to bring fresh circulation to the area and carry away toxins (heat). Cold applications help reduce nerve pain.

Review use of soft cervical collar.

The soft cervical collar maintains a slight flexion of head. Slight flexion of the head allows maximal opening of intravertebral foramina that may be useful for relieving local pressure in mild to moderate cervical disc disease. *Note:* Hyperextension should be avoided.

Encourage regular medical follow-up.

Medical follow-up monitors progression or resolution of degenerative process. It evaluates effectiveness of pain management and overall treatment regimen. When found ineffective, treatment approaches are modified to improve client

Provide information about what symptoms need to be reported to primary provider, for example, sharp pain, loss of sensation or ability to walk, and change in bowel or bladder control.

Timely reporting of signs and symptoms for further evaluation and prompt management improves client outcomes.

Answer questions about treatment alternatives, such as the following:

Chemonucleolysis

As an alternative to surgery, the enzyme chymopapain or similar proteolytic agent, such as collagenase, may be injected into the disc to dissolve the mucoprotein disc material. Although many clients experience relief, the procedure is not widely done or recommended because of side effects, including allergic reaction to the enzyme, transverse myelitis, and possible paraplegia.

Surgical interventions

Microdiscectomy may be performed to excise fragments of the disc with a comparatively lower risk than more invasive surgery. Percutaneous endoscopic discectomy is another option for minimally invasive approaches for removing disc material. Laminectomy with or without spinal fusion may be performed when conservative treatment is ineffective or when neurological deficits persist. (See CP: Disc Surgery.)

DISC SURGERY

I. Pathophysiology—Laminectomy is the surgical excision of a vertebral posterior arch performed in the presence of a herniated disc for the purpose of relieving pressure on the spinal cord nerve roots and removing a source of pain.

II. Types

a. Open laminectomy is performed under general anesthesia; skin, muscles, and ligaments are cut, bone may be permanently removed.

  i. Procedures include combinations of disc excision, nerve decompression, and bone fusion—with or without spinal instrumentation, such as pedicle screws, plates, rods, fusion cages, bone grafts, or synthetic disc materials.

  ii. Client may be in hospital for several days.

b. Minimally invasive procedures, performed under brief general anesthesia, cause minimal damage to muscles; no bone is removed, and no large incisions are made.

  i. In endoscopic surgery, surgical tools are inserted into a small incision and the herniated disc is removed or remodeled.

  ii. In percutaneous or endoscopic microdiscectomy, disc material is removed through a small puncture in the skin, using a microscope for guidance.

  iii. Damaged discs may be replaced with an artificial disc or interbody cage fusion with the goal of preserving vertebral height and some flexibility and movement (Bitan, 2008; Eidelson, 2002).

  iv. Several other products are currently being tested in the United States, including OP-1—a genetically designed putty—which fuses diseased vertebrae and replaces the conventional bone graft (Food & Drug Administration [FDA], 2004).

  v. Because of an anticipated short recovery period, client may go home on day of surgery.

III. Statistics (Gale, 2007)

a. Morbidity: Approximately 450 cases of herniated disc per 100,000 require surgery; 150,000 cases annually in the United States, with the average age for surgery at 40 to 45 years.

b. Mortality: Rate is between 0.8% and 1%, approximately 1,000 yearly depending on whether a fusion is included with laminectomy and presence of comorbidities.

c. Cost: Average total cost of a lumbar laminectomy is $85,000 or over $12 billion annually in hospital charges.

GLOSSARY

Discectomy: Surgical removal of a herniated disc. Discectomy can be performed in a number of different ways, including open surgery or through less-invasive procedures using microscopes, x-rays, small tools, and lasers.

Laminectomy: Surgical removal of the lamina (back of spinal canal) and spurs inside the canal that are causing spinal nerve compression.

Care Setting

Inpatient or outpatient surgical or orthopedic unit. This plan of care relates to the open surgical procedures where the client experiences a hospital stay.

Related Concerns

Psychosocial aspects of care, page 749
Surgical intervention, page 782

Client Assessment Database

Refer to CP: Herniated Nucleus Pulposus (Ruptured Intervertebral Disc) for data.

TEACHING/LEARNING

Discharge Plan Considerations
• May require assistance with activities of daily living (ADLs), transportation, homemaker or maintenance tasks, vocational counseling, and possible changes in layout of home

▶ Refer to section at end of plan for postdischarge considerations.

Diagnostic Studies

Refer to CP: Herniated Nucleus Pulposus (Ruptured Intervertebral Disc).

Nursing Priorities

1. Maintain tissue perfusion and neurological function.
2. Promote comfort and healing.
3. Prevent or minimize complications.
4. Assist with return to normal mobility.
5. Provide information about condition, prognosis, treatment needs, and limitations.

Discharge Goals

1. Neurological function maintained or improved.
2. Complications prevented.
3. Limited mobility achieved with potential for increasing mobility.
4. Condition, prognosis, therapeutic regimen, and behavior and lifestyle changes are understood.
5. Plan in place to meet needs after discharge.

NURSING DIAGNOSIS: **ineffective tissue Perfusion, [specify]**

May be related to
Diminished or interrupted blood flow—edema of operative site, hematoma formation
Hypovolemia

Possibly evidenced by
Paresthesia or numbness
Decreased range of motion (ROM) or muscle strength

Desired Outcomes/Evaluation Criteria—Client Will

Neurological Status (NOC)
Report or demonstrate normal sensations and movement as appropriate.

ACTIONS/INTERVENTIONS	RATIONALE
Surveillance (NIC)	
Independent	
Check neurological signs periodically and compare with baseline. Assess movement and sensation of hands and arms (cervical) and lower extremities and feet (lumbar).	Although some degree of sensory impairment is usually present, changes in neurological assessments may reflect development or resolution of spinal cord edema or tissue inflammation due to damage to motor nerve roots from surgical manipulation. Assessment findings may also indicate tissue hemorrhage that causes spinal cord compression. Spinal cord compression requires prompt medical evaluation and intervention.
Keep client flat on back for several hours, per protocal.	Pressure to operative site reduces risk of hematoma.
Monitor vital signs. Note skin color, warmth, and capillary refill.	Hypotension, especially postural, with corresponding changes in pulse rate may reflect hypovolemia from blood loss, restriction of oral intake, and nausea and vomiting.

(continues on page 264)

Monitor intake and output (I&O) and wound drains, such as Jackson-Pratt or Hemovac, if used.

Fluid balance indicates circulatory status and replacement needs. Excessive or prolonged blood loss requires evaluation and ongoing assessments to continually determine and provide prompt and appropriate intervention.

Visually check and gently palpate operative site for swelling. Inspect dressing for excess drainage. Test drainage for glucose if cerebrospinal fluid (CSF) leakage is suspected

Changes in contour of operative site suggest hematoma or edema formation. Inspection may reveal frank bleeding or dura leak of CSF, thus requiring prompt intervention. CSF will test positive for glucose.

Assess extremities—particularly lower extremities—for redness, swelling, and pain.

Redness, swelling, and pain in the extremities suggest complications associated with immobility including deep vein thrombosis (DVT).

Collaborative

Administer intravenous (IV) fluids or blood, as indicated.

Fluid replacement depends on the degree of hypovolemia and duration of oozing, bleeding, or leakage of CSF.

Monitor blood counts—hemoglobin (Hgb), hematocrit (Hct), and red blood cells (RBCs).

These laboratory tests help establish fluid status and the need for fluid and blood product replacement. They also indicate effectiveness of fluid resuscitation interventions.

Apply and maintain schedule for wearing anti-embolic hose or sequential compression devices.

Anti-embolic hose, sequential compression devices, and related products reduce the risk for venous stasis in lower extremities.

NURSING DIAGNOSIS: risk for [spinal] Trauma

Risk factors may include
Temporary weakness of vertebral column
Balancing difficulties and changes in muscle coordination

Possibly evidenced by
(Not applicable; presence of signs and symptoms establishes an *actual* diagnosis)

Desired Outcomes/Evaluation Criteria—Client Will

Risk Control (NOC)
Maintain proper alignment of spine.
Recognize need for or seek assistance with activity, as appropriate.

ACTIONS/INTERVENTIONS

RATIONALE

Positioning: Neurologic (NIC)
Independent
Post sign at bedside regarding prescribed position.

Promotes ongoing communication among the members of the healthcare team and reduces risk of inadvertent strain or flexion of operative area.

Provide bed board or firm mattress.
Maintain brace-wearing schedule, as indicated.

Aids in stabilizing back.
Braces may be used to decrease muscle spasm and support the surrounding structures during healing. Establishing a schedule generally enhances client compliance.

Limit activities, as prescribed, when client has had a spinal fusion.

Restricted spinal movement promotes healing of fusion.

Logroll client from side-to-side. Have client fold arms across chest; tighten long back muscles, keeping shoulders and pelvis straight. Use pillows between knees during position change and when on side. Use turning sheet and sufficient personnel when turning, especially on the first postoperative day. Instruct client in these movements as self-care progresses.

Logrolling maintains body alignment. It prevents twisting movements. Twisting movements potentially disrupt alignment, interfering with the overall healing process.

Assist out of bed: logroll to side of bed, splint back, and raise to sitting position. Avoid prolonged sitting. Move to standing position in single smooth motion.

Gradual progression of activity with careful consideration of body alignment protects the surgical area. These maneuvers avoid twisting and flexing of back while arising from bed or chair.

Avoid sudden stretching, twisting, flexing, or jarring of spine.

These precautions reinforce the importance of maintaining body alignment. These movements may cause vertebral collapse, shifting of bone graft, delayed hematoma formation, or subcutaneous wound dehiscence.

ACTIONS/INTERVENTIONS (continued)

Monitor blood pressure (BP). Note reports of dizziness or weakness. Recommend client change position slowly.
Have client wear firm, flat walking shoes when ambulating.

Collaborative

Apply lumbar brace or cervical collar, as appropriate.

Refer to physical therapy. Implement program as outlined.

RATIONALE (continued)

Presence of postural hypotension may result in fainting, falling, and possible injury to surgical site.
Such shoes reduce risk of falls.

Braces or corsets may be used in and out of bed during post-operative phase to support spine and surrounding structures until muscle strength improves. Brace is applied while client is supine in bed. Spinal fusion generally requires a lengthy recuperation period in a corset and collar.
Strengthening exercises may be initiated during the rehabilitative phase to decrease muscle spasm and improve function.

NURSING DIAGNOSIS: risk for ineffective Breathing Pattern/Airway Clearance

Risk factors may include
Tracheal and bronchial obstruction or edema
Decreased lung expansion or pain

Possibly evidenced by
(Not applicable; presence of signs and symptoms establishes an *actual* diagnosis)

Desired Outcomes/Evaluation Criteria—Client Will

Respiratory Status: Ventilation (NOC)
Maintain a normal, effective respiratory pattern free of cyanosis and other signs of hypoxia, with arterial blood gases (ABGs) within acceptable range.

ACTIONS/INTERVENTIONS

Respiratory Monitoring (NIC)
Independent

Inspect for edema of face and neck (cervical laminectomy), especially first 24 to 48 hours after surgery.
Listen for hoarseness. Encourage voice rest.

Auscultate breath sounds. Note presence of wheezes or rhonchi.

Assist with coughing, turning, and deep breathing. Encourage client's use of incentive spirometry or other devices used to aid deep breathing.

Collaborative

Administer supplemental oxygen, if indicated.

Monitor and graph ABGs or pulse oximetry.

RATIONALE

Tracheal edema and compression or nerve injury can compromise respiratory function.
Hoarseness may indicate laryngeal nerve injury or edema of surgical area, which can negatively affect cough and ability to clear airway.
Abnormal breath sounds suggest accumulation of secretions or need to engage in more aggressive therapeutic actions to clear airway.
These maneuvers facilitate movement of secretions and clearing of lungs. They also reduce the risk of such respiratory complications as pneumonia, pulmonary embolus, and others.

Supplemental oxygen may be necessary for periods of respiratory distress or evidence of hypoxia.
Monitors adequacy of breathing and oxygen therapy.

NURSING DIAGNOSIS: acute Pain

May be related to
Physical agent: surgical manipulation, edema, inflammation, or harvesting of bone graft

Possibly evidenced by
Reports of pain
Autonomic responses: diaphoresis, changes in vital signs, pallor
Alteration in muscle tone
Guarding, distraction behaviors or restlessness

Desired Outcomes/Evaluation Criteria—Client Will

Pain Self-Control (NOC)
Report pain is relieved or controlled.
Verbalize methods that provide relief.
Demonstrate use of relaxation skills and diversional activities.

ACTIONS/INTERVENTIONS	RATIONALE

Pain Management (NIC)

Independent

Assess intensity, description, location, radiation of pain, and changes in sensation.

Pain may be mild to severe with radiation to shoulders and occipital area (cervical) or hips and buttocks (lumbar). If bone graft has been taken from the iliac crest, pain may be more severe at the donor site. Numbness or tingling discomfort may reflect return of sensation after nerve root decompression or result from developing edema causing nerve compression.

Instruct in regular use of rating scale, such as 0 to 10.

Standardized tool for rating pain helps in assessment and management of pain.

Review expected manifestations or changes in intensity of pain.

Development or resolution of edema and inflammation during the immediate postoperative phase can affect pressure on various nerves and cause changes in degree of pain. Muscle spasms and improved nerve root sensation intensify pain, especially 3 days after procedure.

Encourage client to assume position of comfort, as indicated. Use logrolling for position change.

Positioning is dictated by physical preference and type of operation; for example, head of bed may be slightly elevated after cervical laminectomy. Readjustment of position aids in relieving muscle fatigue and discomfort. Logrolling avoids tension in the operative areas, maintains straight spinal alignment, and reduces risk of displacing epidural patient-controlled analgesia (PCA) when used.

Provide back rub or massage. Avoid the operative site.

Back rubs and massages relieve or reduce pain by alteration of sensory neurons and muscle relaxation.

Demonstrate and encourage use of relaxation skills, such as deep breathing, visualization, and so on.

Deep breathing and visualization refocus attention, reduce muscle tension, promote sense of well-being, and control or decrease discomfort.

Provide liquid or soft diet; provide room humidifier; and encourage voice rest.

Following anterior cervical laminectomy, such measures reduce discomfort associated with sore throat and difficulty swallowing.

Investigate client reports of return of radicular pain.

Radicular pain suggests complications, such as collapsing of disc space and shifting of bone graft, which require further medical evaluation and intervention. *Note:* Sciatica and muscle spasms often recur after laminectomy, but should resolve within several days or weeks.

Collaborative

Administer analgesics, as indicated, for example:
  Opioids, such as morphine sulfate (MS), codeine, meperidine (Demerol), tramadol (Ultram), oxycodone (Percocet), and hydrocodone (Vicodin, Lortab)

Opioids are used during the first few postoperative days. Nonopioid agents are incorporated as intensity of pain diminishes. *Note:* Opioids may be administered via epidural catheter and PCA.

  Muscle relaxants, such as cyclobenzaprine (Flexeril) and metaxalone (Skelaxin)

Muscle relaxants may be used to relieve muscle spasms resulting from intraoperative nerve irritation.

Instruct client in use of PCA.

PCA gives client control of medication administration (usually opioids) to achieve a more constant level of comfort, which may enhance healing and sense of well-being.

Provide throat sprays, lozenges, or viscous lidocaine (Xylocaine).

Sore throat may be a major complaint following cervical laminectomy.

Apply electrical stimulation, as needed.

May be used to block neural transmission of pain by small diameter nerve fibers.

NURSING DIAGNOSIS: impaired physical Mobility

May be related to
Neuromuscular impairment
Limitations imposed by condition; pain

Possibly evidenced by
Impaired coordination, limited ROM
Reluctance to attempt movement
Decreased muscle strength and control

Desired Outcomes/Evaluation Criteria—Client Will

Knowledge: Personal Safety (NOC)
Demonstrate techniques or behaviors that enable resumption of activities.

Mobility (NOC)
Maintain or increase strength and function of affected body part.

ACTIONS/INTERVENTIONS	RATIONALE
Body Mechanics Promotion (NIC)	
Independent	
Schedule activity or procedures with rest periods. Encourage participation in ADLs within individual limitations.	Activity and rest enhance healing and build muscle strength and endurance. Client participation promotes sense of independence and control.
Provide or assist with passive and active ROM and strengthening exercises, depending on surgical procedure.	Strengthen abdominal muscles and flexors of spine and promote good body mechanics.
Assist with activity or progressive ambulation.	Until healing occurs, activity is limited and advanced slowly according to individual tolerance.
Review proper body mechanics or techniques for participation in activities.	Proper body mechanics reduces the risk of muscle strain, injury, or pain. It also increases client participation and motivation in progressive activity.

Refer to CP: Herniated Nucleus Pulposus (Ruptured Intervertebral Disc), ND: impaired physical Mobility, for futher considerations.

NURSING DIAGNOSIS: Constipation

May be related to
Pain and swelling in surgical area
Immobilization, decreased physical activity
Altered nerve stimulation, ileus
Emotional stress, lack of privacy
Changes and restriction of dietary intake

Possibly evidenced by
Decreased bowel sounds
Increased abdominal girth
Abdominal pain or rectal fullness, nausea
Change in frequency, consistency, and amount of stool

Desired Outcomes/Evaluation Criteria—Client Will

Bowel Elimination (NOC)
Reestablish normal patterns of bowel functioning.
Pass stool of soft or semiformed consistency without straining.

ACTIONS/INTERVENTIONS	RATIONALE
Constipation/Impaction Management (NIC)	
Independent	
Note abdominal distention and auscultate bowel sounds.	Abdominal distention and absence of bowel sounds indicate that bowel is not functioning. Possible cause would be the sudden loss of parasympathetic innervation of the gastrointestinal (GI) system.
Use fracture or child-size bedpan until allowed out of bed.	Careful movement promotes comfort and reduces muscle tension.
Provide privacy.	Promotes psychological comfort.
Encourage early ambulation.	Stimulates peristalsis and thereby facilitates passage of flatus.
Collaborative	
Begin progressive diet, as tolerated.	Solid foods are not started until bowel sounds have returned, flatus has been passed, and danger of ileus formation has abated.
Provide rectal tube, suppositories, and enemas, as needed.	May be necessary to relieve abdominal distention and promote resumption of normal bowel habits.
Administer laxatives or stool softeners, as indicated.	Soften stools, promote normal bowel habits or evacuation, and decrease straining.

NURSING DIAGNOSIS: risk for Urinary Retention

Risk factors may include
Pain and swelling in operative area
Need for remaining flat in bed

Possibly evidenced by
(Not applicable; presence of signs and symptoms establishes an *actual* diagnosis)

Desired Outcomes/Evaluation Criteria—Client Will

Urinary Elimination (NOC)
Empty bladder in sufficient amounts.
Be free of bladder distention, with residuals after voiding within normal limits (WNL).

ACTIONS/INTERVENTIONS	RATIONALE
Urinary Retention Care (NIC)	
Independent	
Observe and record amount and time of voiding.	Determines adequate voiding and bladder function.
Palpate for bladder distention.	May indicate urinary retention.
Force fluids.	Fluid intake helps maintain fluid balance and renal perfusion.
Stimulate bladder emptying by running water, pouring warm water over perineum, or having client put hand in warm water.	These maneuvers relax the urinary sphincter thus stimulating urination.
Collaborative	
Perform ultrasound bladder scan or catheterize for residual after voiding, when indicated. Insert and maintain indwelling catheter as needed.	Helps determine the amount of urine in the bladder. Intermittent or continuous catheterization may be necessary for several days postoperatively until swelling is decreased.

NURSING DIAGNOSIS: deficient Knowledge [Learning Need] regarding condition, prognosis, treatment, self-care, and discharge needs

May be related to
Lack of exposure
Information misinterpretation or lack of recall
Unfamiliarity with information resources

Possibly evidenced by
Request for information, statement of misconception
Inaccurate follow-through of instruction

Desired Outcomes/Evaluation Criteria—Client Will

Knowledge: Disease Process (NOC)
Verbalize understanding of condition, prognosis, and potential complications.
List signs and symptoms requiring medical follow-up.

Knowledge: Treatment Regimen (NOC)
Verbalize understanding of therapeutic regimen.
Initiate necessary lifestyle changes.

ACTIONS/INTERVENTIONS	RATIONALE
Teaching: Disease Process (NIC)	
Independent	
Review particular condition or prognosis.	Individual needs dictate tolerance levels and limitations of activity.
Discuss possibility of unrelieved or renewed pain.	Some pain may continue for several months as activity level increases and scar tissue stretches. Pain relief from surgical procedure could be temporary if other discs in the area have similar amount of degeneration.
Discuss safe and appropriate use of heat, such as warm packs and heating pad.	Increased circulation to the back or surgical area transports nutrients needed for healing to the area and aids in removing pathogens or exudates. Decreases muscle spasms that may result from nerve root irritation during healing process.

ACTIONS/INTERVENTIONS (continued)

Discuss judicious use of cold packs before or after stretching activity, if indicated.

Avoid tub baths per physician recommendation.

Review dietary and fluid needs.

Review or reinforce incisional care.

Identify signs and symptoms requiring notification of health-care provider, such as fever, increased incisional pain, inflammation, wound drainage, and decreased sensation or motor activity in extremities.

Discuss necessity of follow-up care.

Review need for or use of immobilization device, as indicated.

Assess current lifestyle, job, finances, and home and leisure activities.

Listen and communicate regarding alternatives and lifestyle changes. Be sensitive to client's needs.

Note overt and covert expressions of concern about sexuality.

Provide written copy of all instructions.

Identify community resources as indicated, such as social services and rehabilitation and vocational counseling services.

Recommend counseling, sex therapy, and psychotherapy, as appropriate.

Teaching: Prescribed Activity/Exercise (NIC)

Discuss return to activities. Stress importance of increasing activities, as tolerated.

Encourage development of regular exercise program, such as walking and stretching.

Discuss importance of good posture and avoidance of prolonged standing or sitting. Recommend sitting in straight-backed chair with feet on a footstool or flat on the floor.

Stress importance of avoiding activities that increase the flexion of the spine, such as climbing stairs, automobile driving or riding, bending at the waist with knees straight, lifting more than 5 pounds, and engaging in strenuous exercise and sports. Discuss limitations on sexual relations and positions.

Encourage lying-down rest periods, balanced with activity.

Explore limitations and abilities.

RATIONALE (continued)

Cold packs may decrease muscle spasm in some instances more effectively than heat.

Tub baths increase risk of falls and spine twisting or flexing.

Nutrition should be tailored to reduce risk of constipation, reduce obesity, and avoid weight gain, while meeting nutrient requirements to facilitate healing.

Correct incisional care promotes healing and reduces risk of wound infection. *Note:* This information is especially critical for the client's significant other (SO)/caregiver. Clients are usually discharged about 24 hours after surgery.

Prompt evaluation and intervention may prevent complications or permanent injury.

Long-term medical supervision may be needed to manage problems or complications and to reincorporate individual into desired or altered lifestyle and activities.

Correct application and wearing time are important to gaining the most benefit from the brace.

Knowledge of current situation allows nurse to highlight areas for possible intervention, such as referral for occupational or vocational testing and counseling.

Low back pain is a frequent cause of chronic disability. Many clients may have to stop or modify work and have had long-term or chronic pain creating relationship and financial crises. Client may be viewed as being a malingerer, which creates further problems in social and work relationships.

Although client may not ask directly, there may be concerns about the effect of surgery on both the ability to cope with usual role in the family and community and ability to perform sexually.

Printed information serves as useful reference after discharge.

A team effort can be helpful in providing support during recuperative period.

Depression is common in conditions for which a lengthy recuperative time (2 to 9 months) is expected. Therapy may alleviate anxiety, assist client to cope effectively, and enhance healing process. Presence of physical limitations, pain, and depression may negatively affect sexual desire and performance and add additional stress to relationship.

Although the recuperative period may be lengthy, following prescribed activity program promotes muscle and tissue circulation, healing, and strengthening.

Regular exercise promotes healing, strengthens abdominal and erector muscles to provide support to the spinal column, and enhances general physical and emotional well-being.

Proper spine alignment prevents further injuries and stress.

Flexing and twisting of the spine potentially interrupts the healing process and increases risk of injury to spinal cord.

Reduces general and spinal fatigue and assists in the healing and recuperative process.

Placing limitations into perspective with abilities allows client to understand own situation and exercise choice.

Sample clinical pathway follows in Table 6.1.

TABLE 6.1 **Cervical Laminectomy with Fusion. ELOS: 3 Days Orthopedic or Surgical Unit**

ND and Categories of Care	Day 1 Day of Surgery _____	Day 2 POD #1 _____	Day 3 POD #2 _____
ineffective tissue Perfusion, R/T altered blood flow—operative site edema, hematoma formation, hypovolemia	Goals: Maintain proper alignment of cervical spine Display stable/improved sensation in affected limbs	Display expected sensory/motor response Identify appropriate safety measures	
Diagnostic studies		Hb/Hct, RBC Electrolytes	
Additional assessments	VS q1h × 4 then q4h Neurovascular checks UE, q1h × 4 then q4h Dressings/drainage q4h I&O q8h Hemovac (if used) q8h Palpate operative site for swelling, inspect face/neck for edema qh1 × 4	→ qid → qid → → → → q8h	→ → q8h → q8h → bid → D/C → D/C
Medications	IV fluids/blood as indicated	→ D/C or convert to NS lock	
Client education	Purpose/necessity of cervical collar Protocol for position change	Cessation of smoking if indicated	Use of heat Signs/symptoms to be reported to healthcare provider
Additional nursing actions	Position per protocol/HOB elevated 30° Logroll q2h Cervical collar in place BRP w/assistance—tennis shoes—not slippers Fluids as tolerated	→ → Ambulate → → → Advanced diet as tolerated	→ → → → Per self as tolerated →
acute Pain R/T surgical intervention	Report pain controlled	→ Participate in activities to increase comfort	→ Verbalize understanding of therapeutic interventions
Additional assessments	Pain characteristics/change Response to interventions	→ →	→ →
Medications Allergies:_____	Analgesics—PCA or IV Throat spray/lozenges	→ D/C PCA PO analgesics →	→ → D/C
Client education	Orient to unit/room Reporting of pain/effects of interventions Proper use of PCA Recovery/rehabilitation expectations Limitations of movement (e.g., twisting, flexing, pulling) Voice rest (anterior approach)	Relaxation techniques Medication dose, frequency, purpose, side effects	Use of Tens as indicated Signs/symptoms to report to healthcare provider
Additional nursing actions	Provide firm mattress	→	→

| TABLE 6.1 | Cervical Laminectomy with Fusion. ELOS: 3 Days Orthopedic or Surgical Unit (continued) |

ND and Categories of Care	Day 1 Day of Surgery ____	Day 2 POD #1 ____	Day 3 POD #2 ____
	Comfort measures	→	→
impaired physical Mobility R/T musculoskeletal impairment; pain and therapeutic restriction		Reestablish normal bowel/bladder elimination	Verbalize understanding of activity program/ restrictions
			Report plan in place to meet needs postdischarge
Referrals	Social Services	Home Care	
Additional assessments	General muscle tone/strength	→ Ability to perform ADLs independently	→
	Level of functional ability	→	→
	Breath sounds q4h	→ q8h	→
	Bowel sounds q4h	→ q8h	→
	Amount/time of voids	→ D/C	→
		Edema, pain lower extremities, Homans' sign q8h	
Medications		Stool softener	→ /enema if no BM
Client education	Activity level/progression	General wellness—diet, exercise, adequate rest	Activity restrictions, e.g., shower instead of tub bath, no lifting, resumption of work, hobbies, sexual activity
	Bed exercises	Home exercise program	
	Skin care needs	Proper body mechanics	
		Use of assistive devices as required	Provide written copy of instructions
Additional nursing actions	Perform passive and assist with active ROM exercises	→	→
	Encourage participation of ADLs within level of ability	→	→ Per self
	T, C, DB, q2h	→	→ Per self
	Incentive spirometry q4h	→ q4h while awake	→ D/C
	SCD or thigh-high TEDs	→	→
	Skin care per Risk Protocol	→	→

Key: ADLs, activities of daily life; BRP, bathroom privileges; C, cough; D/C, discontinue; DB, deep breath; ELOS, estimated length of stay; Hb/Hct hemoglobin/hematocrit; HOB; I&O, input & output; ND, nursing diagnosis; NS, normal saline; PCA, patient-controlled analgesia; PO, by mouth; POD, postoperative day; q1h, every 1 hour; q4h, every 4 hours; q8h, every 8 hours; qid, 4 times a day; R/T, related to; RBC, red blood cell; ROM, range of motion; T, turn; TEDs, anti-embolism stockings; TENS, transcutaneous electrical nerve stimulator; UE, upper extremities; VS, vital signs.

SPINAL CORD INJURY (ACUTE REHABILITATIVE PHASE)

I. **Pathophysiology**—injury or insult to spinal cord
a. Primary mechanism of injury (Hausman, 2006)
  i. Hyperflexion (sudden acceleration forward) or hyperextension (sudden acceleration forward, followed by sudden deceleration) of neck
  ii. Compression of spine: as with fall from height landing on feet or buttocks, or blow to top of head as in a diving injury
  iii. Rotation injury: Head is rotated beyond normal range.
  iv. Penetrating injuries
    1. Low-velocity, such as knife causing direct and local injury to site
    2. High-velocity, such as bullet or shrapnel causing both direct and indirect damage

b. Secondary mechanism of injury (National Institute for Neurological Disorders and Stroke [NINDS], 2003)
  i. Hemorrhage and vascular insult
  ii. Highly reactive chemicals called oxidants or "free radicals" attack the body's natural defenses and critical cell structures.
  iii. Release of excess neurotransmitters, leading to secondary damage from overexcited nerve cells
  iv. Neurogenic shock with hypoxemia and ischemia
  v. Fluid and electrolyte imbalances
  vi. Damage to axons—Nerve fibers that signal to other cells
  vii. Nerve cells in the spinal cord below the lesion may die, disrupting spinal cord circuits that help control movement and interpret sensory information

(text continues on page 272)

c. Neurological involvement dependent on level of injury, degree of spinal shock, phase, and degree of recovery
   i. *C1 to C3:* Tetraplegia with total loss of muscular and respiratory function
   ii. *C4 to C5:* Tetraplegia with poor pulmonary capacity, complete dependency for activities of daily living (ADLs)
   iii. *C6 to C7:* Tetraplegia with some arm and hand movement allowing some independence in upper body ADLs
   iv. *C7 to T1:* Tetraplegia with limited use of fingers and thumbs, increasing independence
   v. *T2 to L1:* Paraplegia with intact arm function, varying function of intercostal and abdominal muscles, and loss of function below level of injury
   vi. *L1 to L2 or below:* Mixed motor-sensory loss and bowel and bladder dysfunction

II. Classifications
a. Complete: total loss of sensation and voluntary motor function
b. Incomplete: mixed loss of sensation and voluntary motor function

III. Etiology (National Spinal Cord Injury Statistical Center [NSCISC], 2008)
a. Trauma: Leading cause of spinal cord injury (SCI); motor vehicle crashes account for 42% of reported SCI cases since 2005
b. Falls: second most common cause
c. Acts of violence: primarily gunshot wounds

IV. Statistics (NSCISC, 2008)
a. Morbidity: Approximately 12,000 new cases annually and 227,080 to 300,938 individuals living with SCI in 2007; primarily affects young adults (aged 16 to 30); however, since 2005, average age of injury has increased to 39.5 years (may reflect injury to a higher number of persons over 60 and war-related injury statistics); 77.8% are males.
b. Mortality: Rates significantly higher during first year after injury due to pneumonia, pulmonary emboli, sepsis; subsequently, death often related to treatable health problems, such as with cardiovascular and respiratory diseases or diabetes mellitus.
c. Cost: Approching $4 billion annually; in 2005, average first-year expenses for a SCI (all groups) was $198,000 and for quadriplegics with age of injury at age 25, $3 million average lifetime cost.

GLOSSARY

Alignment: Generally refers to objects being in a straight line or being positioned appropriately in relation to each other. After a spinal injury, the vertebrae may become shifted from their normal position, becoming misaligned. Various forms of surgical or nonsurgical treatment may be required to realign the vertebrae.

Allodynia: Pain caused by something that does not normally cause pain; for example, something cold, warm, or a very light touch to the skin can result in pain.

Atelectasis: Incomplete expansion of a portion of the lung or the whole lung secondary to decreased vital capacity and decreased functional residual capacity due to SCI with dysfunction of respiratory muscles.

Autonomic dysreflexia (AD): Potential complication of SCI, an exaggerated response of the nervous system to a specific trigger, such as an overfull bladder, that occurs because the brain is no longer able to control the body's response to the trigger. This response leads to a rapid increase in the body's blood pressure, severe headache, and sweating.

Axon: The long threadlike outgrowth and extension of a nerve cell that carries messages away from the main part of the cell; also referred to as nerve fibers.

Bowel program: The routine that a person uses with regard to emptying his or her bowels.

Cervical vertebrae: The cervical (neck) vertebrae are the upper seven vertebrae in the spinal column, designated C1 through C7 from the top down.

Compression: The act of pressing together, as in a compression fracture, nerve compression, or spinal cord compression.

Flaccid paralysis: Weakness or loss of muscle tone resulting from injury to the nerves innervating the muscles.

Hyperalgesia: An extremely painful response to what is normally only mildly painful.

Hyperextension injury: Occurs when person is struck from behind, or falls striking chin, resulting in a sudden acceleration forward, followed by sudden deceleration.

Hyperflexion injury: Occurs when head is suddenly and forcefully accelerated forward, causing extreme flexion of the neck.

Intercostal muscles: Several groups of muscles that run between the ribs and help form and move the chest wall.

Lumbar vertebrae: The five lumbar vertebrae are situated between the thoracic vertebrae and the sacral vertebrae in the spinal column and are designated as L1 through L5.

Motor: Refers to the activity of the nerves (motor nerves) that send messages away from the brain and spinal cord.

Neurogenic: Starting with or having to do with the nerves or the nervous system, as in neurogenic bladder or bowel, neurogenic shock.

Paralytic ileus: Buildup of pressure in the small intestine that can occur in the early stages after an SCI. Symptoms include absence of normal bowel sounds and visible swelling of the abdomen. It can cause vomiting or force the stomach contents up into the airways.

Paraplegia: Paralysis of the lower part of the body, including the legs.

Phrenic nerve: Nerve that governs movement of the diaphragm during breathing.

Quadriplegia: Complete or incomplete paralysis from the neck downward, affecting all four limbs and the trunk as a result of damage to the spinal cord between C1 and C8. Also called tetraplegia.

Sensory: Relating to sensation, to the perception of a stimulus and the voyage made by incoming (afferent) nerve impulses from the sense organs to the nerve centers.

GLOSSARY (continued)

Spasticity: State of increased tone of a muscle and an increase in the deep tendon reflexes.

Spinal shock: A period of time after an SCI lasting up to 6 weeks when the area around the damaged cord is bruised and swollen. During this time, no messages can pass through the spinal cord below the level of injury, making the loss of function below the injury appear complete. Only when the swelling subsides does the true extent of the damage become clear.

Tetraplegia: Complete or incomplete paralysis from the neck downward, affecting all four limbs and the trunk as a result of damage to the spinal cord between C1 and C8. Also called quadraplegia.

Thoracic vertebrae: The 12 thoracic vertebrae are situated between the cervical (neck) vertebrae and the lumbar vertebrae. The thoracic vertebrae are designated as T1 through T12.

Care Setting

Client is treated in inpatient medical-surgical, subacute, and rehabilitation units.

Related Concerns

Disc surgery, page 262
Fractures, page 632
Pneumonia, page 131
Psychosocial aspects of care, page 749
Thrombophlebitis: deep vein thrombosis, page 111
Total nutritional support: parenteral/enteral feeding, page 469
Upper gastrointestinal/esophageal bleeding, page 306
Ventilatory assistance (mechanical), page 173

Client Assessment Database

Dependent on level of injury.

DIAGNOSTIC DIVISION MAY REPORT	MAY EXHIBIT
ACTIVITY/REST	• Paralysis of muscles—flaccid during spinal shock—at or below level of lesion • Muscle or generalized weakness—cord contusion and compression
CIRCULATION • Palpitations • Dizziness with position changes	• Low blood pressure (BP) • Postural BP changes, orthostatic hypotension • Tachycardia • Chronic bradycardia—lesions T6 and above • Cool, pale extremities • Absence of perspiration in affected area
ELIMINATION	• Bladder and bowel incontinence • Urinary retention • Abdominal distention • Loss of bowel sounds • Melena, coffee-ground emesis or hematemesis
EGO INTEGRITY • Denial, disbelief • Sadness, anger	• Fear • Anxiety • Irritability, restlessness • Withdrawal
FOOD/FLUID	• Abdominal distention • Loss of bowel sounds—paralytic ileus

(continues on page 274)

DIAGNOSTIC DIVISION MAY REPORT (continued)	MAY EXHIBIT (continued)
HYGIENE	• Variable level of dependence in ADLs
NEUROSENSORY • Absence of sensation below area of injury or opposite side sensation • Numbness, tingling, burning, twitching of arms or legs	• Flaccid paralysis—spasticity may develop as spinal shock resolves, depending on area of cord involvement • Loss of sensation—varying degrees may return after spinal shock resolves • Loss of muscle or vasomotor tone and motor function • Loss of or asymmetrical reflexes, including deep tendon reflexes • Changes in pupil reaction, ptosis of upper eyelid • Loss of sweating in affected area
PAIN/DISCOMFORT • Pain or tenderness in muscles • Hyperesthesia immediately above level of injury	• Vertebral tenderness, deformity
RESPIRATION • Shortness of breath, "air hunger," inability to breathe	• Shallow or labored respirations • Increased work of breathing and use of accessory muscles • Poor chest wall expansion • Periods of apnea • Diminished breath sounds, rhonchi • Pallor, cyanosis • Decreased coughing
SAFETY	• Temperature fluctuations, taking on temperature of environment
SEXUALITY • Expressions of concern about return to normal functioning	• Uncontrolled erection (priapism) • Menstrual irregularities
TEACHING/LEARNING	
DISCHARGE PLAN CONSIDERATIONS • Will require varying degrees of assistance with transportation, shopping, food preparation, self-care, finances, medications or treatment, and homemaker and maintenance tasks • May require changes in physical layout of home or placement in a rehabilitative center ▶ Refer to section at end of plan for postdischarge considerations.	

Diagnostic Studies

TEST WHY IT IS DONE	WHAT IT TELLS ME
BLOOD TESTS • *Arterial blood gases (ABGs):* Monitors effectiveness of gas exchange and ventilatory effort.	Abnormalities may be present, depending on level of SCI and limitation of chest expansion and muscle involvement.
OTHER DIAGNOSTIC STUDIES • *Spinal x-rays:* May locate the level and type of bony injury (fracture, dislocation). Determines alignment and reduction after traction or surgery.	Regular lateral x-rays of the neck can usually detect significant cervical injuries. Injury can sometimes be detected using flexion and extension x-rays of the neck if the client is awake and able to move.

Diagnostic Studies (continued)

TEST WHY IT IS DONE (continued)	WHAT IT TELLS ME (continued)
• *Computerized tomography (CT) scan (also known as computerized axial tomography or CAT scan):* Imaging procedure that uses a combination of x-rays and computer technology to produce cross-sectional images of the body.	CT remains the standard for revealing fractures and spinal canal compromise.
• *Magnetic resonance imaging (MRI) scan:* Noninvasive method of obtaining images of internal soft tissue, such as the spinal cord, through the use of powerful magnets and radio waves.	MRI can show bruising and other soft-tissue damage that might not show up in other studies, such as SCI, spinal cord hematoma, hemorrhage or edema, ligament injuries, or other soft-tissue injuries or pathology.
• *Chest x-ray:* Procedure used to evaluate organs and structures within the chest.	Evaluates for lung injury, such as pneumothorax, or complications associated with SCI, such as changes in level of diaphragm reflecting respiratory muscle paralysis, atelectasis, and pneumonia.
• *Pulmonary function studies, such as vital capacity (VC) and tidal volume (VT):* Measures maximum volume of inspiration and expiration.	It is especially important in client with low cervical lesions or thoracic lesions with possible phrenic nerve and intercostal muscle involvement.

Nursing Priorities

1. Maximize respiratory function.
2. Prevent further injury to spinal cord.
3. Promote mobility and independence.
4. Prevent or minimize complications.
5. Support psychological adjustment of client and significant other (SO).
6. Provide information about injury, prognosis and expectations, treatment needs, and possible and preventable complications.

Discharge Goals

1. Ventilatory effort adequate for individual needs.
2. Spinal injury stabilized.
3. Complications prevented or controlled.
4. Self-care needs met by self and with assistance, depending on specific situation.
5. Beginning to cope with current situation and planning for future.
6. Condition, prognosis, therapeutic regimen, and possible complications understood.
7. Plan in place to meet needs after discharge.

NURSING DIAGNOSIS: **risk for ineffective Breathing Pattern**

Risk factors may include
Impairment of innervation of diaphragm (lesions at or above C5)
Complete or mixed loss of intercostal muscle function
Reflex abdominal spasms; gastric distention

Possibly evidenced by
(Not applicable; presence of signs and symptoms establishes an *actual* diagnosis)

Desired Outcomes/Evaluation Criteria—Client Will

Respiratory Status: Ventilation (NOC)
Maintain adequate ventilation as evidenced by absence of respiratory distress and ABGs within acceptable limits and pulse oximetry maintained at 90% or greater.
Demonstrate appropriate behaviors to support respiratory effort.

ACTIONS/INTERVENTIONS	RATIONALE
Respiratory Monitoring (NIC) *Independent* Note client's level of injury when assessing respiratory function. Note presence or absence of spontaneous effort and quality of respirations—labored, using accessory muscles.	C1 to C3 injuries result in complete loss of respiratory function. Injuries at C4 or C5 can result in variable loss of respiratory function, depending on phrenic nerve involvement and diaphragmatic function, but generally cause decreased vital capacity and inspiratory effort. For injuries below C6 or C7, respiratory muscle function is preserved; however, weakness and impairment of intercostal muscles may reduce effectiveness of cough, ability to sigh, and deep breaths.

(continues on page 276)

ACTIONS/INTERVENTIONS (continued)	RATIONALE (continued)
Auscultate breath sounds. Note areas of absent or decreased breath sounds or development of adventitious sounds, such as rhonchi.	Hypoventilation is common and leads to accumulation of secretions, atelectasis, and pneumonia—frequent complications. *Note:* Respiratory complications are among the leading causes of mortality, not only during the acute stage, but also later in life.
Note strength and effectiveness of cough.	Level of injury determines function of intercostal muscles and ability to cough spontaneously and move secretions. High-level paraplegics and all tetraplegics lose the ability to cough and are at greatest risk of developing atelectasis and respiratory failure.
Observe skin color for developing cyanosis or duskiness.	Skin color may reveal impending respiratory failure and need for immediate medical evaluation and intervention.
Assess for abdominal distention and muscle spasm.	Abdominal fullness may impede diaphragmatic excursion, thus reducing lung expansion and further compromising respiratory function.
Monitor and limit visitors, as indicated.	General debilitation and respiratory compromise place client at increased risk for acquiring upper respiratory infections (URIs).
Monitor diaphragmatic movement if phrenic pacemaker is implanted.	Stimulation of phrenic nerve may enhance respiratory effort and decrease dependency on mechanical ventilator.
Elicit concerns or questions regarding mechanical ventilation devices.	Open discussion acknowledges reality of situation. (Refer to CP: Ventilatory Assistance [Mechanical].)
Provide honest answers.	Future respiratory function and support needs will not be totally known until spinal shock resolves and acute rehabilitative phase is completed. Even though respiratory support may be required, alternative devices and techniques may be used to enhance mobility and promote independence.
Maintain client airway: keep head in neutral position, elevate head of bed slightly if tolerated, and use airway adjuncts, as indicated.	Clients with high cervical injury and impaired gag or cough reflex require assistance in preventing aspiration and maintaining patent airway.
Assist client in "taking control" of respirations as indicated. Encourage deep breathing. Focus attention on the steps of breathing.	Breathing may no longer be an involuntary activity but require conscious effort, depending on level of injury or involvement of respiratory muscles.
Assist with coughing, as indicated for level of injury; for example, have client take a deep breath, hold for 2 seconds before coughing, or inhale deeply, then cough at the end of a slow exhalation. Alternatively, assist by placing hands below diaphragm and pushing upward as client exhales ("quad cough").	Assisted coughing facilitates mobilization of respiratory secretions. *Note:* Quad cough procedure is generally reserved for clients with stable injuries once they are in the rehabilitation stage.
Suction as necessary. Monitor pulse oximetry and heart rate during suctioning. Document quality and quantity of secretions.	Suctioning facilitates removal of respiratory secretions. Routine suctioning increases the risk for bradycardia (heart rate less than 60 beats per minute) and hypoxia, especially with tetraplegia.
Reposition and turn periodically. Avoid or limit prone position when indicated.	Repositioning enhances ventilation of all lung segments and mobilizes secretions. It helps reduce the risks of complications such as atelectasis and pneumonia. *Note:* Prone position significantly decreases vital capacity and increases risk of respiratory compromise and failure.
Encourage fluids—at least 1,500 to 2,000 mL/day.	Adequate fluid intake liquefies secretions and promotes mobilization and expectoration.
Collaborative	
Measure and graph: VC, VT, and inspiratory force	Pulmonary function tests determine level of respiratory muscle function. Serial measurements may predict impending respiratory failure (acute injury) or determine level of function after spinal shock phase or while weaning from ventilatory support.
Serial ABGs and pulse oximetry	Documents status of ventilation and oxygenation and identifies respiratory problems, such as hypoventilation, hypoxia, acidosis, among others.
Airway Management (NIC)	
Administer oxygen by appropriate method: nasal prongs, mask, intubation, and ventilator.	Oxygen delivery methods are determined by level of injury, degree of respiratory insufficiency, and respiratory muscle function after spinal shock phase.
Assist with use of respiratory adjuncts, such as incentive spirometer or blow bottles, and aggressive chest physiotherapy, such as chest percussion.	Preventing retained secretions is essential to maximize gas diffusion and to reduce risk of pneumonia.

ACTIONS/INTERVENTIONS (continued)

Refer to or consult with respiratory and physical therapists.

RATIONALE (continued)

Collaboration with respiratory and physical therapists helps identify appropriate therapies that could optimize respiratory function. For example, glossopharyngeal breathing uses muscles of mouth, pharynx, and larynx to swallow air into lungs, thereby increasing VC and chest expansion.

NURSING DIAGNOSIS: risk for [additional spinal] Trauma

Risk factors may include
Temporary weakness and instability of spinal column

Possibly evidenced by
(Not applicable; presence of signs and symptoms establishes an *actual* diagnosis)

Desired Outcomes/Evaluation Criteria—Client Will

Bone Healing (NOC)
Maintain proper alignment of spine without further spinal cord damage.

ACTIONS/INTERVENTIONS

Traction/Immobilization Care (NIC)
Independent

Maintain bedrest and immobilization device(s)—sandbags, traction, halo, hard or soft cervical collars, or brace.

Check external stabilization devices, such as Gardner-Wells tongs or skeletal traction apparatus.

Elevate head of traction frame or bed as indicated. Ensure that traction frames are secured, pulleys are aligned, and weights are hanging free.
Check weights for ordered traction pull (usually 10 to 20 lb).

Reposition at intervals, using adjuncts for turning and support—turn sheets, foam wedges, blanket rolls, and pillows. Use several staff members when turning or logrolling client. Follow special instructions for traction equipment, kinetic bed, and frames once halo is in place.

Collaborative

Assist with preparation and maintain skeletal traction via tongs, calipers, and halo or vest, as indicated.
Prepare for internal stabilization surgery, such as spinal laminectomy or fusion, if indicated.
Administer medications as indicated, such as methylprednisolone (Depo-Medrol).

RATIONALE

Immobilization prevents vertebral column instability and aids healing. *Note:* Traction is used only for cervical spine stabilization.
These devices are used for decompression of spinal fractures and stabilization of vertebral column during the early acute phase of injury to prevent further spinal cord damage.
Creates safe, effective counterbalance to maintain both client's alignment and proper traction pull.

Weight pull depends on client's size and amount of reduction needed to maintain vertebral column alignment.
The use of adjuncts for turning and support maintains proper spinal column alignment and thus reduces the risk of further trauma. *Note:* Grasping the brace or halo vest to turn or reposition client may cause additional injury.

Reduces vertebral fracture and dislocation.

Surgery may be indicated for spinal stabilization, cord decompression, or removal of bony fragments.
Although many experts recommend the use of high-dose cortisone within 8 hours of a nonpenetrating SCI as the standard of care, many national organizations are now changing their recommendations to include this therapy for the improvement of neurological outcome, but are not requiring it, suggesting that its benefits be weighed against the client's potential for developing sepsis.

NURSING DIAGNOSIS: impaired physical Mobility

May be related to
Neuromuscular impairment
Immobilization by traction

Possibly evidenced by
Inability to purposefully move, paralysis
Muscle atrophy, contractures

(continues on page 278)

Desired Outcomes/Evaluation Criteria—Client Will

Immobility Consequences: Physiological (NOC)
Maintain position of function as evidenced by absence of contractures and footdrop.

Neurological Status: Spinal Sensory/Motor Function (NOC)
Increase strength of unaffected and compensatory body parts.
Demonstrate techniques or behaviors that enable resumption of activity.

ACTIONS/INTERVENTIONS	RATIONALE
Bed Rest Care (NIC)	
Independent	
Continually assess motor function, as spinal shock and spinal cord edema resolves, by requesting client to perform certain actions, such as shrug shoulders, spread fingers, and squeeze and release examiner's hands.	Continuous motor function assessment helps determine appropriate interventions for the specific motor impairment.
Provide means to summon help, such as special sensitive call light.	Promotes the client's sense of control and reduces fear of being left alone. *Note:* Ventilator-dependent tetraplegic client may require continuous observation for timely interventions.
Perform or assist with full range of motion (ROM) exercises on all extremities using slow, smooth movements. Include periodic hip hyperextension.	ROM exercises enhance circulation, restore or maintain muscle tone and joint mobility, and prevent disuse contractures and muscle atrophy.
Position arms at 90-degree angle at regular intervals.	Appropriate joint positioning prevents frozen shoulder contractures.
Maintain ankles at 90 degrees with footboard. Use high-top tennis shoes. Place trochanter rolls along thighs when in bed.	These measures prevent external rotation of the hip and footdrop.
Elevate lower extremities at regular intervals when seated. Raise foot of the bed when supine, as appropriate. Assess for edema of ankles and feet	Loss of vascular tone and "muscle action" results in pooling of blood and venous stasis in the lower abdomen and lower extremities, with increased risk of hypotension and thrombus formation. Positioning and frequent assessment is needed to prevent associated complications.
Space periods of rest and activity. Provide uninterrupted rest periods. Encourage client involvement.	Adequate rest and optimal activity prevent fatigue and allows opportunity for maximal efforts and active client participation.
Monitor BP before and after activity in acute phases or until stable. Change position slowly. Use cardiac bed or tilt table, or CircOlectric bed as activity level is advanced.	The loss of sympathetic innervations especially in T6 and higher SCI causes loss of vascular tone, resulting in hypotension and venous pooling. Side-to-side movement or elevation of head can aggravate hypotension and cause syncope.
Reposition periodically even when sitting in chair. Teach client how to use weight-shifting techniques.	Repositioning and weight shifts reduce pressure areas and promote peripheral circulation.
Prepare for weight-bearing activities, such as use of tilt table for upright position and strengthening and conditioning exercises for unaffected body parts.	Early weight bearing reduces osteoporotic changes in long bones and reduces incidence of urinary infections and kidney stones. *Note:* Fifty percent of clients develop heterotopic ossification that can lead to pain and decreased joint flexibility
Encourage use of relaxation techniques.	Relaxation techniques reduce muscle tension and fatigue and may help limit pain of muscle spasms and spasticity.
Inspect skin daily. Observe for pressure areas. Provide meticulous skin care. Teach client to inspect skin surfaces and to use a mirror to look at hard-to-see-areas.	Altered circulation, loss of sensation, and paralysis potentiate pressure sore formation. This is a lifelong consideration. (Refer to ND: risk for impaired Skin Integrity.)
Assist with or encourage pulmonary hygiene by deep breathing, coughing, and suctioning. (Refer to ND: risk for ineffective Breathing Pattern.)	Immobility and bedrest increase the risk of pulmonary infection.
Assess for redness, swelling, and muscle tension of calf tissues. Record calf and thigh measurements, as indicated.	A high percentage of clients with SCI develop thrombi because of altered peripheral circulation, immobilization, and flaccid paralysis.
Investigate sudden onset of dyspnea, cyanosis, and other signs of respiratory distress.	Development of pulmonary emboli may be "silent" because pain perception is altered or deep vein thrombosis (DVT) is not readily recognized.
Collaborative	
Place client in kinetic therapy bed when appropriate.	Kinetic therapy beds effectively immobilize unstable spinal column and improve systemic circulation. They are thought to decrease complications associated with immobility.

ACTIONS/INTERVENTIONS (continued)

Apply anti-embolic hose, leotard, or sequential compression devices (SCDs) to legs, as appropriate.

Consult with physical and occupational therapists and rehabilitation team.

Administer medications, as indicated, for example:
  Vasopressors, such as dobutamine (Dobutrex)

  Muscle relaxants and antispasticity agents, as indicated, such as diazepam (Valium), baclofen (Lioresal), and dantrolene (Dantrium)

  Tizanidine (Zanaflex)

RATIONALE (continued)

These devices limit pooling of blood in lower extremities or abdomen, thus improving vasomotor tone and reducing incidence of thrombus formation and pulmonary emboli.

Collaboration helps in planning and implementing individualized exercise program. The members of the rehabilitation team identify and develop assistive devices to enhance client's function and overall independence.

Vasopressors may be indicated in acute phase to maintain systolic BP greater than 100 mm Hg. The client who requires this level of support will likely be in a critical care unit.

Muscle relaxants and antispasticity agents may be useful after spinal shock phase in limiting or reducing pain. *Note:* Baclofen may be delivered via implanted intrathecal pump on a long-term basis, as appropriate.

Centrally acting α_2-adrenergic agonist reduces spasticity. Short duration of action requires careful dosage monitoring to achieve maximum effect. It may have additive effect with baclofen, but needs to be used with caution because both drugs have similar side effects.

NURSING DIAGNOSIS: disturbed Sensory Perception

May be related to
Destruction of sensory tracts with altered sensory reception, transmission, and integration
Reduced environmental stimuli
Psychological stress—narrowed perceptual fields caused by anxiety

Possibly evidenced by
Measured change in sensory acuity, including position of body parts or proprioception
Change in usual response to stimuli
Motor incoordination
Anxiety, disorientation, bizarre thinking; exaggerated emotional responses

Desired Outcomes/Evaluation Criteria—Client Will

Neurological Status: Spinal Sensory/Motor Function (NOC)
Recognize sensory impairments.

Knowledge: Personal Safety (NOC)
Identify behaviors to compensate for deficits.
Verbalize awareness of sensory needs and potential for deprivation or overload.

ACTIONS/INTERVENTIONS

Peripheral Sensation Management (NIC)
Independent
Assess and document sensory function or deficit, such as by means of touch, pinprick, or heat and cold, progressing from area of deficit to neurologically intact area.

Protect from bodily harm, such as falls, burns, and positioning of arm or objects.

Assist client to recognize and compensate for alterations in sensation.

Explain procedures before and during care while identifying the involved body part.

Provide tactile stimulation by touching the client in intact sensory areas, such as shoulders, face, and head.

Position client to see surroundings and activities. Provide prism glasses when prone on turning frame. Talk to client frequently.

Provide diversional activities, including television, radio, music, and liberal visitation. Use clocks, calendars, pictures, bulletin boards, and so on. Encourage SO and family to discuss general and personal news.

RATIONALE

Changes may not occur during acute phase, but as spinal shock resolves, dermatome charts or anatomic landmarks should document changes, such as, "2 inches above nipple line."

The client may not sense pain or be aware of body position.

Increased attention to alterations in sensation may help reduce anxiety of the unknown and prevent injury.

These measures enhance client perception of "whole" body.

Touching conveys caring and fulfills normal physiological and psychological needs.

These nursing actions provide sensory input, which may be severely limited, especially when client is in prone position.

The activities aid in maintaining reality orientation and provide some sense of normality in daily passage of time.

(continues on page 280)

ACTIONS/INTERVENTIONS (continued)	RATIONALE (continued)
Provide uninterrupted sleep and rest periods.	Adequate sleep and rest reduce sensory overload, enhance orientation and coping abilities, and aid in reestablishing natural sleep patterns.
Note presence of exaggerated emotional responses and altered thought processes, including disorientation and bizarre thinking.	Exaggerated emotional responses and altered thought processes indicate damage to sensory tracts affecting reception or interpretation of stimuli, or psychological stress, requiring further assessment and intervention.

NURSING DIAGNOSIS: acute Pain

May be related to
Physical injury; damage or dysfunction of nervous system
Traction apparatus

Possibly evidenced by
Verbal reports of pain; hyperalgesia immediately above level of injury, burning pain below level of injury (central pain), phantom pain, headaches
Muscle spasm, spasticity
Irritability; restlessness
Self-focusing
Sympathetic mediated responses—temperature, cold, changes of body position, hypersensitivity

Desired Outcomes/Evaluation Criteria—Client Will

Pain Control (NOC)
Identify ways to manage pain.
Demonstrate use of relaxation skills and diversional activities as individually indicated.
Report relief or control of pain and discomfort.

ACTIONS/INTERVENTIONS

RATIONALE

Pain Management (NIC)
Independent

ACTIONS/INTERVENTIONS	RATIONALE
Assess for presence of pain. Help client identify and quantify pain, including, location, type of pain, and intensity on a scale of 0 to 10.	Pain is a frequent problem in the majority of the SCI population and can occur not only above the level of injury but also at or below the level of injury and in both complete and incomplete injuries. An individual with SCI is likely to experience many types of painful sensations at or below the level of injury that can be troublesome to categorize, making effective treatment difficult. Pain can be neuropathic (resulting from abnormal processing of sensory input); can be due to musculoskeletal disorders caused from injury at the time of SCI; or be associated with organ complications such as ulcers or constipation. Pain can also be "segmental," felt at the level of injury in a bandlike pattern (Turner et al, 2001). Client often reports pain above the level of injury, such as chest, back, or headache, possibly from stabilizer apparatus. After resolution of spinal shock phase, client may also report muscle spasms and radicular pain, described as a burning or stabbing pain radiating in a dermatomal pattern—associated with injury to peripheral nerves. Onset of this pain is within days to weeks after SCI and may become chronic.
Evaluate increased irritability, muscle tension, restlessness, and unexplained vital sign changes.	Nonverbal cues indicative of pain or discomfort require timely intervention.
Assist client in identifying precipitating factors.	Burning pain and muscle spasms can be precipitated or aggravated by multiple factors, such as anxiety, tension, external temperature extremes, sitting for long periods, and bladder distention.
Provide comfort measures, such as position changes, massage, ROM exercises, and warm or cold packs, as indicated.	Alternative measures for pain control reduce need for pharmacological agents and provide emotional support.
Encourage use of relaxation techniques, such as guided imagery, visualization, and deep-breathing exercises. Provide diversional activities—television, radio, telephone, and unlimited visitors, as appropriate.	Relaxation and diversional activities refocus attention, promote sense of control, and possibly enhance coping abilities.

ACTIONS/INTERVENTIONS (continued)

Collaborative

Administer medications, as indicated, for example: muscle relaxants, such as dantrolene (Dantrium) and baclofen (Lioresal); analgesics; anti-anxiety agents, such as, alprazalam (Xanax), and diazepam (Valium).

RATIONALE (continued)

These medications relieve muscle spasm and pain associated with spasticity. They also alleviate anxiety and promote rest.

NURSING DIAGNOSIS: Grieving

May be related to
Perceived or actual loss of physiopsychosocial well-being

Possibly evidenced by
Altered communication patterns
Expression of distress, choked feelings, such as denial, guilt, fear, sadness; altered affect
Alterations in sleep patterns

Desired Outcomes/Evaluation Criteria—Client Will

Grief Resolution (NOC)
Express feelings freely and effectively.
Begin to progress through recognized stages of grief, focusing on 1 day at a time.

ACTIONS/INTERVENTIONS	RATIONALE

Grief Work Facilitation (NIC)
Independent

Identify signs of grieving, such as shock, denial, anger, and depression.

Client experiences a wide range of emotional reactions to the injury and its actual and potential impact on life. These stages are not static, and the rate at which client progresses through them is variable.

Shock

Note lack of communication or emotional response and absence of questions.

Shock is the initial reaction associated with overwhelming injury. Primary concern is to maintain life. The client may be too ill to express feelings.

Provide simple, accurate information to client and SO regarding diagnosis and care. Be honest; do not give false reassurance while providing emotional support.

Client's awareness of surroundings and activity may be blocked initially, and attention span may be limited. Little is actually known about the outcome of client's injuries during acute phase, and lack of knowledge may add to frustration and grief of family. Therefore, early focus of emotional support may be directed toward SO.

Encourage expressions of sadness, grief, guilt, and fear among client, SO, and friends.

Acknowledging client and SO feelings and encouraging expression could provide appropriate support.

Incorporate SO into problem-solving and planning for client's care.

Shared clinical decision making with the client and SO establishes therapeutic relationships and provides sense of control of the management of current health situation and the subsequent changes.

Denial

Assist client and SO to verbalize feelings about situation. Avoid judgment about what is expressed.

Important beginning step to deal with what has happened. Helpful in identifying client's coping mechanisms.

Note comments indicating unrealistic outcomes and bargaining with God. Do not confront these comments in early phases of rehabilitation.

Denial may be a useful coping mechanism during the early phases of rehabilitation. Client may accept disability but may deny uncertainty and permanency of limitations.

Focus on present needs—ROM exercises, skin care, and so on.

Attention on "here and now" reduces frustration and hopelessness of uncertain future and may make dealing with today's problems more manageable.

Anger

Identify use of manipulative behavior and reactions to caregivers.

Client may demonstrate manipulative behaviors like spitting, biting, or even pitting caregivers against each other to express anger.

Encourage client to take control when possible—establishing care routines, dietary choices, diversional activities, and so forth.

Encouraging client participation provides a sense of control and responsibility as well as reduces sense of powerlessness.

Accept expressions of anger and hopelessness, such as "let me die." Avoid arguing. Show concern for client.

Nonjudgmental communication of empathy and compassion helps the client regain sense of worth.

(continues on page 282)

Set limits on acting out and unacceptable behaviors when necessary, including abusive language, sexually aggressive or suggestive behavior.

Although it is important to express negative feelings, client and staff need to be protected from violence and embarrassment. Acting out is traumatic for all involved.

Depression

Note loss of interest in living, sleep disturbance, suicidal thoughts, and hopelessness. Listen to, but do not confront, these expressions. Let client know nurse is available for support.

Depression may last for weeks, months, and years. Acceptance and support are critical in facilitating resolution. The client may need psychological counseling.

Arrange visit by individual similarly affected, as appropriate.

Talking with another person who has shared similar feelings and fears and survived may help client reach acceptance of reality of condition and deal with perceived and actual losses.

Collaborative

Consult with and refer to psychiatric nurse, social worker, psychiatrist, and pastor.

Client and SO need assistance to work through feelings of alienation, guilt, and resentment concerning lifestyle and role changes. The family required to make adaptive changes to a member who may be permanently "different" benefits from supportive, long-term assistance and counseling in coping with these changes and the future. Client and SO may suffer great spiritual distress, including feelings of guilt, deprivation of peace, and anger at God, which may interfere with progression through, and resolution of, grief process.

NURSING DIAGNOSIS: situational low Self-Esteem

May be related to
Traumatic injury, situational crisis, forced crisis

Possibly evidenced by
Verbalization of forced change in lifestyle
Fear of rejection or reaction by others
Focus on past strength, function, or appearance
Negative feelings about body
Feelings of helplessness, hopelessness, or powerlessness
Actual change in structure and function
Lack of eye contact
Change in physical capacity to resume role
Confusion about self, purpose, or direction of life

Desired Outcomes/Evaluation Criteria—Client Will

Psychosocial Adjustment: Life Change (NOC)
Verbalize acceptance of self in situation.
Recognize and incorporate changes into self-concept in accurate manner without negating self-esteem.
Develop realistic plans for adapting to role changes and new role.

ACTIONS/INTERVENTIONS

RATIONALE

Self-Esteem Enhancement (NIC)
Independent

Acknowledge difficulty in determining degree of functional incapacity and chance of functional improvement.

During acute phase of injury, long-term effects are unknown, which delays the client's ability to integrate situation into self-concept.

Listen to client's comments and responses to situation.

Active listening provides clues to client's view of self, role changes, needs, and level of acceptance.

Assess dynamics of client and SOs, including client's role in family and cultural factors.

Client's previous role in family unit is disrupted or altered by injury. Role changes add difficulty in integrating self-concept and level of independence.

Encourage SO to treat client as normally as possible, such as discussing home situations and family news.

Involving client in family unit reduces feelings of social isolation, helplessness, and uselessness and provides opportunity for SO to contribute to client's welfare.

ACTIONS/INTERVENTIONS (continued)	RATIONALE (continued)
Provide accurate information. Discuss concerns about prognosis and treatment honestly at client's level of acceptance.	Open discussion of treatment and prognosis may focus on current and immediate needs. Ongoing updates enable assimilation.
Discuss meaning of loss or change with client and SO. Assess interactions between client and SO.	Actual change in body image may be different from that perceived by client. Distortions may be unconsciously reinforced by SO.
Accept client and show concern for individual as a person. Identify and build on client's strengths; give positive reinforcement for progress noted.	Genuine concern and regard for the client as an individual establishes therapeutic atmosphere for self-acceptance and encouragement.
Include client and SO in care, allowing client to make decisions and participate in self-care activities, as possible.	Encouraging client participation in care decision making recognizes that client is still responsible for own life and provides some sense of control over situation. It sets the stage for future lifestyle, pattern, and interaction required in daily care. *Note:* Client may reject all help or may be completely dependent during this phase.
Be alert to sexually oriented jokes, flirting, or aggressive behavior. Elicit concerns, fears, and feelings about current situation and future expectations.	Anxiety develops because of perceived loss and change in masculine or feminine self-image and role. Forced dependency is often devastating, especially in light of change in function and appearance.
Be aware of own feelings and reaction to client's sexual anxiety.	Personal reactions to client's sexual anxiety may be as disruptive as the behavior itself, creating conflicts between client and staff, and can potentially eliminate client's willingness to work through situation and participate in rehabilitation.
Arrange visit by similarly affected person, if client desires and situation allows.	Support groups can provide hope and potential future role model. They can be vital resources during difficulties after discharge.

Collaborative

Refer to counseling or psychotherapy as indicated—psychiatric clinical nurse specialist, psychiatrist, social worker, or sex therapist.	The client may need additional assistance to adjust to change in body image and lifestyle.

NURSING DIAGNOSIS: Bowel Incontinence/Constipation

May be related to
Disruption of innervations to bowel and rectum
Perceptual impairment
Altered dietary and fluid intake
Change in activity level
Medications

Possibly evidenced by
Loss of ability to evacuate bowel voluntarily
Constipation
Gastric dilation, ileus

Desired Outcomes/Evaluation Criteria—Client Will

Bowel Continence (NOC)
Verbalize behaviors and techniques for individual bowel program.
Reestablish satisfactory bowel elimination pattern.

ACTIONS/INTERVENTIONS	RATIONALE

Bowel Management (NIC)
Independent

Auscultate bowel sounds, noting location and characteristics.	Bowel sounds may be absent during spinal shock phase. High tinkling sounds may indicate presence of ileus.
Observe for abdominal distention if bowel sounds are decreased or absent.	Impaired innervation causes paralysis of the bowel (ileus) and bowel distention. *Note:* Overdistention of the bowel is a trigger for AD, once spinal shock subsides. (Refer to ND: risk for Autonomic Dysreflexia.)
Note reports of nausea and onset of vomiting. Check vomitus or gastric secretions (if tube in place) and stools for occult blood.	Gastrointestinal (GI) bleeding may occur in response to injury (Curling's ulcer) or as a side effect of certain therapies—steroids or anticoagulants.

(continues on page 284)

Record frequency, characteristics, and amount of stool.

Recognize signs of fecal impaction—no formed stool for several days, semiliquid stool, restlessness, increased feelings of fullness in or distention of abdomen, presence of nausea, vomiting, and possibly urinary retention.

Establish regular daily bowel program—digital stimulation, prune juice and warm beverage, and use of stool softeners or suppositories at set intervals. Determine a routine of bowel evacuation.

Encourage well-balanced diet that includes bulk and roughage and increased fluid intake at least 1,500 to 2,000 mL/day, including fruit juices.

Observe for incontinence and help client relate incontinence to change in diet or routine.

Restrict intake of caffeinated beverages, such as coffee, tea, colas or energy drinks, if indicated.

Provide meticulous skin care.

Collaborative

Insert and maintain nasogastric (NG) tube and attach to suction if appropriate.

Consult with dietitian or nutritional support team.

Administer medications. as indicated:
Stool softeners, laxatives, suppositories, enemas, such as Therevac-SB

Antacids and histamine H$_2$ antagonists, such as cimetidine (Tagamet) and ranitidine (Zantac)

Assessment of bowel movement helps identify degree of impairment or dysfunction and required level of assistance.

Early intervention is necessary to effectively treat constipation or retained stool and reduce risk of further complications.

A lifelong routine bowel program is necessary to control bowel evacuation. Bowel program is important to the client's physical independence and social acceptance. *Note:* Bowel movements in clients with upper motor neuron damage are generally regulated with suppositories or digital stimulation. Lower motor neurogenic bowel is more difficult to regulate and usually requires manual disimpaction. Incorporating elements of client's usual routine may enhance cooperation and success of program. *Note:* Many clients prefer morning program rather than evening schedule often practiced in acute and rehabilitation setting.

High fiber and fluid intake improve consistency of stool for transit through the bowel. *Note:* Over-the-counter (OTC) fiber products and cereals, prune juice, applesauce, and bran often provide adequate fiber for effective bowel management.

Client can eventually achieve normal routine bowel habits, which enhance independence, self-esteem, and socialization.

Diuretic effect of caffeine can reduce fluid available in the bowel, thus increasing the risk of dry, hard-formed stool.

Loss of sphincter control and innervation in the area potentiates risk of skin irritation and breakdown.

The NG tube may be used initially to reduce gastric distention and prevent vomiting.

Dietary support team aids in creating dietary plan to meet nutritional needs based on digestive and bowel function.

Stool softeners, laxatives, suppositories, and enemas stimulate peristalsis and routine bowel evacuation. Suppositories should be warmed to room temperature and lubricated before insertion. Therevac-SB is a 4-mL enema of docusate and glycerin that may reduce time for bowel care by as much as 1 hour.

Antacids and histamine antagonists neutralize gastric acid to lessen gastric irritation and risk of bleeding.

NURSING DIAGNOSIS: impaired Urinary Elimination

May be related to
Disruption in bladder innervation
Bladder atony
Fecal impaction

Possibly evidenced by
Bladder distention; incontinence or overflow, retention
Urinary tract infections (UTIs)
Bladder, kidney stone formation
Renal dysfunction

Desired Outcomes/Evaluation Criteria—Client Will

Urinary Continence (NOC)
Verbalize understanding of condition.
Maintain balanced intake and output (I&O), with clear, odor-free urine; free of bladder distention or urinary leakage.
Verbalize or demonstrate behaviors and techniques to prevent retention and urinary infection.

ACTIONS/INTERVENTIONS	RATIONALE

Urinary Elimination Management (NIC)
Independent

Assess voiding pattern, including frequency and amount. Compare urine output with fluid intake. Note specific gravity.

Voiding pattern identifies characteristics of bladder function, including effectiveness of bladder emptying, renal function, and fluid balance. *Note:* Urinary complications are a major cause of mortality. Multiple complications can occur when normal innervation to the bladder and urinary sphincter is impaired by urinary incontinence, UTI, upper urinary tract distress, urinary calculi, AD, and bladder cancer (Fonte & Moore, 2008).

Palpate for bladder distention and observe for overflow.

Bladder dysfunction is variable but may include loss of bladder contraction and inability to relax urinary sphincter, resulting in urine retention and reflux incontinence. *Note:* Bladder distention can precipitate AD. (Refer to ND: risk for Autonomic Dysreflexia, following.)

Encourage fluid intake of 1,500 to 2,000 mL/day, including acid ash juices such as cranberry.

Adequate fluid intake helps maintain renal function and reduces risk of infection by decreasing ability of bacteria to adhere to bladder wall (Lynch, 2004; Santillo & Lowe, 2007) and prevents formation of urinary stones. *Note:* Fluid may be restricted for a period during initiation of intermittent catheterization.

Begin bladder retraining per protocol when appropriate, with fluids between certain hours, digital stimulation of trigger area, contraction of abdominal muscles, and so forth.

Timing and type of bladder program depends on type of injury—upper or lower neuron involvement. *Note:* Bladder expression using the Credé maneuver (pushing on the abdomen to forcefully express urine) is included in some programs in an attempt to promote continence and ensure adequate bladder evacuation. Research suggests this maneuver raises intravesical pressures against a closed bladder outlet, raising the risk of vesicoureteral reflux, hernia, rectogenital prolapse, and hemorrhoids (Rigby, 2005).

Observe for changes in urine characteristics—cloudy, bloody, foul odor, and so forth. Test urine with dipstick, as indicated.

Changes in urine characteristics may indicate UTI and increased risk of sepsis. Multistrip dipsticks can provide a quick determination of pH, nitrite, and leukocyte esterase that suggest presence of infection or urinary disease. *Note:* Presence of bacteria in urine is not uncommon if client has indwelling catheter or performs intermittent catheterization. If bacteria are present, the client must be assessed for other signs of developing UTI, and medications may be indicated (Rigby, 2005).

Cleanse perineal area and keep dry. Provide catheter care, as appropriate.

Perineal care decreases risk of skin irritation, breakdown, and development of ascending infection.

Urinary Catheterization (NIC)
Collaborative

Monitor blood urea nitrogen (BUN), creatinine, white blood cell (WBC) count, and urinalysis (UA).

These laboratory tests reflect renal function and identify complications.

Administer vitamin C or urinary antiseptics, such as methenamine mandelate (Mandelamine), as indicated.

These medications maintain acidic environment and prevent bacterial growth.

Refer for further evaluation for bladder and bowel stimulation.

Clinical research is being conducted on the technology of electronic bladder control. The implantable device sends electrical signals to the spinal nerves that control the bladder and bowel.

Keep bladder empty by means of indwelling catheter initially. Determine post-void residuals then consider intermittent catheterization program, as appropriate.

Bladder scans are useful in determining post-void residuals. During the acute phase, an indwelling catheter is used to prevent urinary retention and to monitor urinary output. Intermittent catheterization may be implemented to reduce complications associated with long-term use of indwelling catheters. A suprapubic catheter may also be inserted for long-term management.

Measure residual urine via post-void catheterization, bladder scan, or ultrasound.

Measuring post-void residual is helpful in detecting urinary retention and effectiveness of bladder training program. *Note:* Use of ultrasound is noninvasive and reduces the risk of bladder colonization.

NURSING DIAGNOSIS: risk for Autonomic Dysreflexia

Risk factors may include
Altered nerve function (spinal cord injury at T8 and above)
Bladder, bowel, skin stimulation—tactile, pain, thermal

Possibly evidenced by
(Not applicable; presence of signs and symptoms establishes an *actual* diagnosis)

Desired Outcomes/Evaluation Criteria—Client Will

Symptom Control (NOC)
Recognize signs and symptoms of syndrome.
Identify preventive and corrective measures.

Neurological Status: Autonomic (NOC)
Experience no episodes of dysreflexia.

ACTIONS/INTERVENTIONS	RATIONALE
Dysreflexia Management (NIC)	
Independent	
Identify and monitor precipitating or risk factors, such as bladder or bowel distention or manipulation; bladder spasms, stones, and infection; skin or tissue-pressure areas and prolonged sitting position; and temperature extremes or drafts.	Visceral distention is the most common cause of AD, which is considered an emergency. Treatment of acute episode must be carried out immediately by removing stimulus or treating unresolved symptoms, then interventions must be geared toward prevention.
Observe for signs and symptoms of syndrome—changes in blood pressure, paroxysmal hypertension, tachycardia or bradycardia, autonomic responses, such as sweating, flushing above level of lesion, pallor below injury, chills, goose flesh, piloerection, nasal stuffiness, and severe pounding headache, especially in occiput and frontal regions. Note associated symptoms, such as chest pains, blurred vision, nausea, metallic taste, Horner's syndrome—contraction of pupil, partial ptosis of eyelid, and sometimes loss of sweating over one side of the face.	Early detection and immediate intervention is essential to prevent serious consequences or complications. *Note:* Average systolic BP in tetraplegic client—after spinal shock has resolved—is 120 mm Hg; therefore, readings greater than 140 mm Hg are considered elevated.
Stay with client during episode.	This is a potentially fatal complication. Continuous monitoring and intervention may reduce client's level of anxiety.
Monitor BP frequently (every 3 to 5 minutes) during acute AD. Take action to eliminate stimulus. Continue to monitor BP at intervals after symptoms subside.	Aggressive therapy and removal of stimulus may drop BP rapidly, resulting in a hypotensive crisis, especially in those clients who routinely have low BP. In addition, AD may recur, particularly if stimulus is not eliminated.
Elevate head of bed to 45-degree angle or place client in sitting position.	Elevation of the head of bed lowers BP to prevent intracranial hemorrhage, seizures, or even death. *Note:* Placing the tetraplegic client in sitting position automatically lowers BP.
Correct or eliminate causative stimulus as able, such as bladder, bowel, and skin pressure, including loosening tight leg bands or clothing; removing abdominal binder and elastic stockings; and temperature extremes.	Removing noxious stimulus usually terminates episode and may prevent more serious AD; for example, in the presence of sunburn, topical anesthetic should be applied. Removal of constrictive clothing or restrictive devices also promotes venous pooling to help lower BP. *Note:* Removal of bowel impaction must be delayed until cardiovascular condition is stabilized.
Inform client and SO of warning signals and how to prevent or limit onset of syndrome.	This lifelong problem can be largely controlled by avoiding pressure from overdistention of visceral organs or pressure on the skin.
Collaborative	
Administer medications, as indicated (intravenous [IV], parenteral, oral, or transdermal) and monitor response:	
Diazoxide (Hyperstat) and hydralazine (Apresoline)	These medications reduce BP if severe or sustained hypertension occurs.
Nifedipine (Procardia) and 2% nitroglycerin ointment (Nitrostat)	Sublingual administration usually effective in absence of IV access for diazoxide (Hyperstat), but may require repeat dose in 30 to 60 minutes. These drugs may be used in conjunction with topical nitroglycerin.
Morphine sulfate	Morphine sulfate relaxes smooth muscle to aid in lowering BP and muscle tension.

ACTIONS/INTERVENTIONS (continued)

Miscellaneous other medications, such as phenoxybenza-
mine (Dibenzyline) and mecamylamine (Inversine)

Obtain urinary culture as indicated.

Apply local anesthetic ointment to rectum. Remove impaction
if indicated after symptoms subside.

Prepare client for pelvic or pudendal nerve block or posterior
rhizotomy if indicated.

RATIONALE (continued)

Various medications are being used to alleviate symptoms
associated with AD (Campagnolo, 2006).

UTI is a common trigger for AD.

Ointment blocks further autonomic stimulation and eases later
removal of impaction without aggravating symptoms.

Procedures may be considered if AD does not respond to
other therapies.

NURSING DIAGNOSIS: **risk for impaired Skin/Tissue Integrity**

Risk factors may include

Altered and inadequate peripheral circulation, sensation
Presence of edema, tissue pressure
Altered metabolic state
Immobility, traction apparatus

Possibly evidenced by

(Not applicable; presence of signs and symptoms establishes an *actual* diagnosis)

Desired Outcomes/Evaluation Criteria—Client Will

Risk Control (NOC)

Identify individual risk factors.
Verbalize understanding of treatment needs.
Participate to level of ability to prevent skin breakdown.

ACTIONS/INTERVENTIONS

Skin Surveillance (NIC)

Independent

Inspect all skin areas, noting capillary blanching and refill,
redness, and swelling. Pay particular attention to back of
head, skin under halo frame or vest, and folds where skin
continuously touches.

Observe halo and tong insertion sites. Note swelling, redness,
and drainage.

Encourage continuation of regular exercise program.

Elevate lower extremities periodically, if tolerated.

Avoid or limit injection of medication below the level of injury.

Skin Care: Topical Treatments (NIC)

Massage and lubricate skin with bland lotion or oil. Protect
pressure points by use of elbow or heel pads, lamb's wool,
foam padding, and egg-crate mattress or cushion. Use
skin-hardening agents, such as tincture of benzoin, karaya,
or Sween cream.

Reposition frequently, whether in bed or in sitting position.
Place in prone position periodically.

Wash and dry skin, especially in high-moisture areas such as
perineum. Take care to avoid wetting the lining of brace or
halo vest.

Keep bedclothes dry and free of wrinkles, crumbs, and
creases.

Cleanse halo or tong insertion sites routinely and apply
antibiotic ointment per protocol.

Collaborative

Provide kinetic therapy or alternating-pressure mattress as
indicated.

RATIONALE

Skin is especially prone to breakdown because of changes in
peripheral circulation, inability to sense pressure, immobility, and altered temperature regulation.

These sites are prone to inflammation and infection and provide route for pathological microorganisms to enter cranial
cavity. *Note:* New style of halo frame does not require
screws or pins.

Exercise stimulates circulation that enhances cellular nutrition
and oxygenation.

Elevation of lower extremities enhances venous return and
reduces edema formation.

Areas below the level of injury have reduced circulation and
sensation and are at risk for delayed absorption, local reaction, and tissue necrosis.

Skin care and massage enhance circulation and protect skin
surfaces, thus reducing risk of pressure ulcers. Tetraplegic
and paraplegic clients require lifelong protection from
decubitus ulcer formation, which can cause extensive tissue necrosis and sepsis.

Repositioning improves skin circulation and reduces pressure
on bony prominences.

Clean, dry skin is less prone to excoriation or breakdown.

Preventing excessive moisture and friction reduces skin
irritation.

Halo and tong insertion site care helps prevent local infection
and reduces risk of cranial infection.

Kinetic therapy and alternating pressure mattress improves
systemic and peripheral circulation and reduces pressure
on skin and risk for breakdown.

deficient Knowledge [Learning Need] regarding condition, prognosis, potential complications, treatment, self-care, and discharge needs

May be related to
Lack of exposure or recall
Information misinterpretation
Unfamiliarity with information resources

Possibly evidenced by
Questions, statement of misconception, request for information
Inadequate follow-through of instruction
Inappropriate or exaggerated behaviors—hostile, agitated, apathetic
Development of preventable complication(s)

Desired Outcomes/Evaluation Criteria—Client Will

Knowledge: Disease Process (NOC)
Verbalize understanding of condition, prognosis, and treatment.

Knowledge: Treatment Regimen (NOC)
Correctly perform necessary procedures and explain reasons for the actions.
Initiate necessary lifestyle changes and participate in treatment regimen.

ACTIONS/INTERVENTIONS	RATIONALE
Teaching: Disease Process (NIC) *Independent* Discuss injury process, current prognosis, and future expectations.	Open discussion regarding disease process, current prognosis, and future expectations provides common knowledge base necessary for making informed choices and commitment to the therapeutic regimen. *Note:* Improvement in managing effects of SCI has increased life expectancy of clients to only about 5 years below norm for specific age group. New treatment options, such as ProCord, GM-1, and minocycline, are in clinical trials to determine if they can improve neurological outcomes.
Provide information and demonstrate the following: Positioning and weight shifting	Positioning promotes circulation and reduces tissue pressure and risk of complications.
Use of pillows, supports, and splints	Keeps the spine aligned and prevents or limits contractures, thus improving overall function and independence.
Encourage continued participation in daily exercise and conditioning program.	Daily exercise and conditioning programs reduce spasticity complications and risk of thrombogenesis (common complication), as well as increase mobility, muscle strength, and tone for improving organ and body function. Suggested activities are: (1) squeezing rubber ball and arm exercises enhance upper body strength to increase independence in transfers and wheelchair mobility; (2) tightening and contracting rectum or vaginal muscles improves bladder control; and (3) pushing abdomen up, bearing down, and contracting abdomen strengthen trunk and improve GI function in paraplegic clients.
Identify energy conservation techniques and stress importance of pacing activities, having adequate rest, and avoiding fatigue.	Fatigue is common. It limits client's ability to participate in or manage care, decreases quality of life, and increases feelings of helplessness and hopelessness.
Review drug regimen, noting desired effects and expected side effects, as well as medication interactions.	Medications used to treat spasticity can exacerbate fatigue, necessitating a change in drug choice or dosage. *Note:* Amantadine (Symmetrel) and fluoxetine (Prozac) may be added to decrease sense of fatigue by potentiating the action of dopamine or selectively inhibiting serotonin uptake in the central nervous system (CNS).
Have SO/caregivers participate in client care and demonstrate proper procedures, such as applications of splints, braces, suctioning, positioning, skin care, transfers, bowel and bladder program, checking temperature of bath water, and food.	Participation in client care allows home caregivers to become adept and more comfortable with the care tasks and reduces risk of injury or complications.
Instruct caregiver in techniques to facilitate cough, as appropriate.	Quad coughing is performed to facilitate expectoration of secretions or to move them high enough to be suctioned out.

ACTIONS/INTERVENTIONS (continued)

Recommend applying abdominal binder before arising (tetraplegic) and remind to change position slowly.

Use safety belt and adequate number of people during bed-to-wheelchair transfers.

Instruct in proper skin care, inspecting all skin areas daily, using adequate padding—foam, silicone gel, water pads—in bed and chair, and keeping skin dry. Stress importance of regularly monitoring condition and positioning of support surfaces, such as cushions, mattresses, and overlays.

Discuss necessity of preventing or managing excessive diaphoresis by using tepid bathwater, providing comfortable environment, such as by using fans, and removing excess clothing.

Review nutritional needs, including adequate bulk and roughage. Problem-solve solutions to alterations in muscular strength, tone, and GI function.

Review pain-management strategies. Discuss the potential for future pain management therapies. Recommend avoidance of OTC drugs without approval of healthcare provider.

Discuss ways to identify and manage AD.

Identify symptoms to report immediately to healthcare provider, for example, infection, especially urinary and respiratory; skin breakdown; unresolved AD; and suspected pregnancy.

Stress importance of continuing with rehabilitation team to achieve specific functional goals and continue long-term monitoring of therapy needs.

Evaluate home layout and make recommendations for necessary changes. Identify equipment, medical supply needs, and resources.

Discuss sexual activity and reproductive concerns. Review alternative sexual activities, positions, and spasticity management, as indicated, such as opposing pressure on area of spasm, using pillows for support, regular stretching and ROM exercises, and appropriate medications.

Identify community resources and supports, such as health agencies, visiting nurse, financial counselor, service organizations, and Spinal Cord Injury Foundation.

Coordinate cooperation among community and rehabilitation resources.

Arrange for transmitter or emergency call system.

Plan for alternate caregivers and identify respite services, as needed.

RATIONALE (continued)

Appropriate use of abdominal binders reduces pooling of blood in abdomen and pelvis and minimizes postural hypotension.

Performing transfers with adequate help prevents falls and related injuries to client and caregivers.

Proper skin care reduces skin irritation, thus decreasing incidence of decubitus ulcers. Timely recognition of product fatigue, improper placement, or other misuse can reduce risk of pressure ulcer formation.

Management of excessive diaphoresis promotes cooling as well as reduces skin irritation and possible breakdown.

Adequate nutrition helps meet the energy needs of the client. Bulk and roughage prevent complications like constipation, abdominal distention, and gas formation.

Review of pain management enhances client safety and may improve cooperation with specific regimen. *Note:* Pain often becomes chronic in clients with SCI and may be mechanical, such as overuse syndrome involving joints; radicular, such as injury to peripheral nerves; or central, with burning and aching just below level of injury. Dysesthetic pain, which is distal to site of injury, is extremely disabling and similar to phantom pain. Treatment for these painful conditions may include a team pain-management approach; medications, such as gabapentin (Neurontin), clonazepam (Klonopin), amitriptyline (Elavil); or electrical stimulation.

Prompt and appropriate management of AD hinges on client and caregiver identification of signs and symptoms, prevention of precipitating and risk factors, and timely management. (Refer to ND: risk for Autonomic Dysreflexia.)

Early identification allows intervention to prevent or minimize complications.

No matter what the level of injury, individual may ultimately be able to exercise some independence—manipulating electric wheelchair with mouth stick (C3/C4); being independent for dressing, transfers to bed, car, toilet (C7); or achieving total wheelchair independence (C8 to T4). Over time, new discoveries will continue to modify equipment and therapy needs and increase client's potential.

Physical changes may be required to accommodate client and support equipment. Prior arrangements facilitate the transfer to the home setting.

Concerns about individual sexuality or resumption of activity are frequently an unspoken concern that needs to be addressed. SCI affects all areas of sexual functioning. In addition, choice of contraception is impacted by level of SCI and side effects or adverse complications of specific method. Finally, some female clients may develop AD during intercourse or labor and delivery.

These support resources enhance independence, assist with home management, and provide respite for caregivers.

Various agencies, therapists, and individuals in community may be involved in the long-term care and safety of client. Coordination can ensure that needs are not overlooked and optimal level of rehabilitation is achieved. *Note:* Individuals with SCI are living longer and more injuries are occurring at advanced ages, creating new challenges in care as SCI clients deal with the effects of aging.

Provides reassurance for safety and prompt assistance.

Respite care provides for preventing caregiver strain, illness, and emergencies.

MULTIPLE SCLEROSIS (MS)

I. Pathophysiology
a. Chronic, irregular demyelination of the brain and spinal cord, resulting in varying degrees of cognitive, motor, and sensory dysfunction
b. Often characterized by periods of exacerbations and remissions, but is unrelenting in some individuals.
c. Research suggests that in addition to destruction of myelin sheaths, underlying nerve fibers are also damaged or severed, which may account for the permanent neurological impairment (Lazoff, 2008).

II. Classification (Lubin, 1996)
a. Relapsing-remitting multiple sclerosis (RRMS): periods of dysfunction in which neurological deficits occur in different parts of the body, followed by partial or full recovery, leaving little residual deficit; accounts for the initial course in approximately 85% to 90% of persons with MS
b. Primary-progressive multiple sclerosis (PPMS): Function declines steadily with periods of minimal recovery and increasing disability in about 10% of cases.
c. Secondary-progressive multiple sclerosis (SPMS): After a period of time, RRMS may convert to a secondary progressive pattern characterized by continued progression, with increasing disability in approximately 80% of cases (Hausman, 2006).
d. Progressive-relapsing multiple sclerosis (PRMS): rare form with progressive neurological deficits from onset with clear exacerbations

III. Etiology
a. An autoimmune inflammatory disease, possibly related to viral infection that produces a limited disruption in the blood-brain barrier, thus allowing beta-lymphocyte clones to colonize the central nervous system (CNS).
b. Genetics may play a role in person's susceptibility.
c. Environmental and geographic factors are being investigated.
d. Predominant CNS disorder among young adults, difficult to diagnose, and cannot be diagnosed after only one presentation of symptoms, but rather over time.
e. Individual prognosis variable and unpredictable, thereby presenting complex physical, psychosocial, and rehabilitative issues.

IV. Statistics
a. Morbidity: Approximately 350,000 people in the United States have MS, with 25,000 new cases diagnosed annually (Lazoff, 2008). MS affects women almost three times as often as men (National Institute for Neurological Disorders and Stroke [NINDS], 1996).
b. Mortality: Estimated 2,800 deaths annually, usually due to fulminating MS (rare) or complications of chronic disability, such as pneumonia, pulmonary emboli, or infected decubitus ulcer (Lazoff, 2008); however, average life expectancy is 35 years after onset or approximately 95% of normal.
c. Cost: Because MS is a lifelong, chronic disease—diagnosed primarily in young adults who have an otherwise normal life expectancy—estimates place the annual cost in the United States in the billions of dollars (NINDS, 1996).

GLOSSARY

Ataxia: Incoordination and unsteadiness due to the brain's failure to regulate the body's posture and strength and direction of limb movements.

Babinski's sign: Neurological reflex, which constitutes an important part of the medical examination, based upon what the big toe does when the sole of the foot is stroked. The normal, mature Babinski's reflex is characterized by extension of the great toe and also by fanning of the other toes.

Clonus: Sign of spasticity in which involuntary shaking or jerking of the leg occurs when the toe is placed on the floor with the knee slightly bent.

Contracture: Permanent shortening of the muscles and tendons adjacent to a joint that can result from severe, untreated spasticity and that interferes with normal movement around the affected joint.

Demyelination: Destruction, loss, or removal of the protective myelin sheath coating the axons, resulting in their inability to transmit impulses.

GLOSSARY (continued)

Dysarthria: Poorly articulated speech that results from dysfunction of the muscles controlling speech, usually caused by damage to the central nervous system (CNS) or a peripheral motor nerve. The content and meaning of the spoken words remain normal, however.

Intention tremor: Condition where goal-directed movements produce shaking in the moving body parts, most noticeably in the hands. Tremor is more obvious when performing delicate fine movements than broad sweeping ones.

Neurogenic bladder: Loss of nerve supply to the bladder, which results in an inability to voluntarily control the bladder. It is characterized by a failure to empty, failure to store, or a combination of the two resulting in such symptoms as urinary urgency, frequency, hesitancy, nocturia, and incontinence.

Nystagmus: The jerking to and fro movement of the eyes that occurs when disorder affects the control of eye movement.

Optic neuritis: Inflammation and demyelination of the optic nerve, causing a partial loss of vision.

Paresis: Partial or incomplete paralysis characterized by weakness and reduction in muscular power.

Paresthesia: Abnormal sensations, such as burning, tingling, or a pins and needles feeling.

Scotoma: Blind spot caused by diminished or total lack of function of the retina or optic nerve in a limited area. It may be unnoticed or be seen as a black area in the visual field.

Care Setting

Clients often require community or long-term care with intermittent hospitalization for disease-related exacerbations and complications.

Related Concerns

Extended care, page 801
Pneumonia, page 131
Psychosocial aspects of care, page 749
Sepsis/septicemia, page 686

Client Assessment Database

Symptoms depend on the stage, extent of disease, and areas of neuronal involvement. For example, common signs associated with motor systems of the cerebellum include, and are not limited to, ataxia, diplopia, dizziness, dysphagia, fatigability, and tremors. Signs associated with motor systems of the corticospinal tract include, but are not limited to, Babinski's sign, bladder dysfunction, fatigue, heat sensitivity, paralysis, and trigeminal neuralgia. The following range of symptoms may be present at a given time or over time.

DIAGNOSTIC DIVISIONS MAY REPORT	MAY EXHIBIT
ACTIVITY/REST • Extreme fatigue, reported in about 70% of clients (Lazoff, 2008) • Weakness, exaggerated intolerance to activity, needing to rest after even simple activities such as shaving or showering • Intolerance of temperature extremes, especially heat, such as with summer weather or hot tubs • Limitation in usual activities, employment, hobbies • Numbness, tingling in the extremities • Sleep disturbances, may awaken early or frequently for multiple reasons	• Generalized weakness • Decreased muscle tone or mass • Spasticity • Tremors • Staggering or dragging of feet • Intention tremors or decreased fine motor skills
CIRCULATION • Swelling of feet	• Blue (mottled), puffy extremities • Capillary fragility, especially on face
EGO INTEGRITY • Statements reflecting loss of self-esteem or body image • Expressions of grief • Anxiety or fear of exacerbations, progression of symptoms, pain, disability, rejection, or pity • Keeping illness confidential • Feelings of helplessness, hopelessness, or powerlessness (loss of control) • Personal tragedies, such as divorce, abandonment by significant other (SO) or friends	• Denial or rejection • Mood changes, irritability, restlessness, lethargy, euphoria, depression, or anger

(continues on page 292)

DIAGNOSTIC DIVISIONS MAY REPORT (continued)	MAY EXHIBIT (continued)

ELIMINATION
- Voiding at night
- Urinary or bowel hesitancy or urgency
- Incontinence of varying severity
- Recurrent urinary tract infections (UTIs)

- Loss of urinary or rectal sphincter control
- Kidney stone formation or kidney damage
- Incomplete bladder emptying or retention with overflow

FOOD/FLUID
- Problems getting food to mouth—related to intention tremors of upper extremities
- Difficulty chewing or swallowing due to weak throat muscles
- Sense of food sticking in throat
- Coughing after swallowing
- Hiccups, possibly lasting for extended periods

- Difficulty feeding self
- Weight loss
- Decreased bowel sounds—slowed peristalsis
- Abdominal bloating

HYGIENE
- Use of assistive devices
- Need for individual caregiver

- Difficulty with or dependence in some or all activities of daily living (ADLs)

NEUROSENSORY
- Weakness, nonsymmetrical paralysis of muscles (may affect one, two, or three limbs, usually worse in lower extremities or may be unilateral)
- Paresthesias
- Change in visual acuity (diplopia), scotomas (holes in peripheral vision), or eye pain (optic neuritis)
- Moving head back and forth while watching television, difficulty driving (distorted visual field), blurred vision (difficulty focusing)
- Cognitive changes—attention; comprehension; use of speech; problem-solving; difficulty retrieving or recalling, sorting out information (cerebral involvement)
- Difficulty making decisions
- Communication difficulties, such as coining words
- Seizures

- *Mental status:* Mood swings, depression, euphoria, irritability, apathy, lack of judgment, impairment of short-term memory, disorientation, or confusion
- Scanning speech, slow and hesitant speech, poor articulation
- Partial or total loss of vision in one eye, vision disturbances
- Positional and vibratory senses may be impaired or absent
- Impaired touch, pain sensation
- Facial or trigeminal nerve involvement, nystagmus, diplopia (brainstem involvement)
- Loss of fine or major motor skills
- Changes in muscle tone
- Spastic paresis or total immobility (advanced stages)
- Ataxia, decreased coordination, tremors
- Hyperreflexia, positive Babinski's sign, ankle clonus, absent superficial reflexes (especially abdominal)

PAIN/DISCOMFORT
- Painful muscle cramping, spasms
- Burning pain along nerve pathways
- May be sporadic, intermittent, or constant
- Facial pain
- Dull back pain

- Distraction behaviors (restlessness, moaning), guarding
- Self-focusing

SAFETY
- Fear of falling because of weakness, decreased vision, slowed reflexes, loss of position sense
- History of falls or accidental injuries
- Use of ambulation devices
- Visual impairment
- Suicidal ideation

- Wall, furniture walking

SEXUALITY
- Disturbances in sexual functioning (affected by nerve impairment, fatigue, bowel and bladder control, sense of vulnerability, and effects of medications)

DIAGNOSTIC DIVISIONS MAY REPORT (continued)	MAY EXHIBIT (continued)
• Enhanced or decreased sexual desire • Problems with positioning • Genital anesthesia or hyperesthesia, decreased lubrication (female) • Impotence/nocturnal erections or ejaculatory difficulties (male) • Relationship stresses **SOCIAL INTERACTION** • Feelings of isolation (increased divorce rate and loss of friends) • Difficult time with employment because of excessive fatigue, cognitive dysfunction, physical limitations **TEACHING/LEARNING** • Family history of disease, possibly due to common environmental or inherited factors • Use of prescription and over-the-counter (OTC) medications; forgetting to take medication • Difficulty retaining information • Use of complimentary and alternative products and practices, trying out cures, or doctor shopping **DISCHARGE PLAN CONSIDERATIONS** • May require assistance in ADLs and instrumental activities of daily living (IADLs), depending on individual situation • May eventually need total care or placement in assisted-living or extended-care facility ◗ Refer to section at end of plan for postdischarge considerations.	 • Speech impairment • Lack of social activities and involvement • Withdrawal from interactions with others

Diagnostic Studies

There are no definitive diagnostic tests for MS. However, tests are indicated to support a clinical diagnosis.

TEST WHY IT IS DONE	WHAT IT TELLS ME
DIAGNOSTIC STUDIES • *Magnetic resonance imaging (MRI) scan:* Uses a magnetic field to create detailed images of the brain and spinal cord and to detect lesions in the white matter of the brain. • *Magnetic resonance spectroscopy (MRS):* Provides information about the brain's biochemistry; specifically, it can measure the brain chemical N-acetyl aspartate. • *Magnetization transfer imaging (MTI):* Detects white matter abnormalities before lesions can be seen on standard MRI scans by calculating the amount of "free" water in tissues.	MRI is the mainstay in confirming the diagnosis of MS. It detects presence of characteristic plaques that are due to nerve sheath demyelination Decreased levels of this chemical can indicate nerve damage. Demyelinated tissues and damaged nerves show increased levels of "free" versus "bound" water particles.

(continues on page 294)

TEST **WHY IT IS DONE** (continued)	**WHAT IT TELLS ME** (continued)
• *Diffusion-tensor magnetic resonance imaging (DT-MRI or DTI):* Measures the random motion of water molecules, which are constantly in motion and collide with each other at extremely high speeds. This causes them to spread out, or diffuse. DT-MRI maps this diffusion to produce intricate, three-dimensional images indicating the size and location of demyelinated areas of the brain.	Changes in this process can be measured and correlated with disease progression.
• *Functional MRI (fMRI):* Uses radio waves and a strong magnetic field.	Measures the correlation between physical changes in the brain (such as blood flow) and mental functioning during the performance of cognitive tasks.
• *CT scan with enhancement:* Demonstrates acute brain lesions and ventricular enlargement or thinning.	Differentiates active or relapsing state versus remission as lesions do not enhance in stable disease.
• *Evoked potential tests:* Evoked potentials are electrical signals generated by the nervous system in response to stimuli. In these tests, nerves responsible for each type of function are stimulated electronically, and responses are recorded using electrodes placed over the CNS (brain and spine) and peripheral nerves (median nerve in the wrist, peroneal nerve in the knee).	Visual evoked responses (VER), brainstem auditory evoked responses (BAER), and somatosensory evoked responses (SSER) are abnormal early on in a high percentage of clients with clinically definitive MS or suspected MS.
• *Lumbar puncture:* Needle is inserted between two lower spine (lumbar) vertebrae and cerebrospinal fluid (CSF) is collected and analyzed.	CSF may show elevated levels of IgG (occurs with progressive MS, usually negative in relapsing MS) and IgM. CSF is also tested for presence of antibodies: oligoclonal bands (OCBs), found in more than 85% of clients with MS (Geisser, 2005), and myelin-basic protein (MBP), noted during active demyelination process.

Nursing Priorities

1. Maintain optimal functioning.
2. Assist with or provide for maintenance of ADLs.
3. Support acceptance of changes in body image, self-esteem, and role performance.
4. Provide information about disease process, prognosis, therapeutic needs, and available resources.

Discharge Goals

1. Remain active within limits of individual situation.
2. ADLs are managed by client and caregivers.
3. Changes in self-concept are acknowledged and being dealt with.
4. Disease process, prognosis, and therapeutic regimen are understood and resources identified.
5. Plan in place to meet needs after discharge.

NURSING DIAGNOSIS: Fatigue

May be related to
Decreased energy production, increased energy requirements to perform activities
Psychological and emotional demands
Pain or discomfort
Medication side effects

Possibly evidenced by
Verbalization of overwhelming lack of energy
Inability to maintain usual routines; decreased performance
Impaired ability to concentrate; disinterest in surroundings
Increase in physical complaints

Desired Outcomes/Evaluation Criteria—Client Will

Energy Conservation (NOC)
Identify risk factors and individual actions affecting fatigue.
Identify alternatives to help maintain desired activity level.
Participate in recommended treatment program.
Report improved sense of energy.

ACTIONS/INTERVENTIONS	RATIONALE
Energy Management (NIC)	
Independent	
Note and accept presence of fatigue.	Persistent fatigue is the most commonly reported symptom. Studies indicate that fatigue occurs with expenditure of minimal energy, is more frequent and severe than "normal" fatigue, has a disproportionate impact on ADLs, has a slower recovery time, and may show no direct relationship between fatigue severity and the clinical neurological status.
Identify or review factors affecting ability to be active, such as temperature extremes, inadequate food intake, insomnia, use of medications, or time of day.	Knowledge of these factors provides an opportunity to develop effective measures to maintain or improve mobility.
Accept when client is unable to do activities.	Activity intolerance can vary from moment to moment. Nonjudgmental acceptance of client's evaluation of day-to-day functioning provides opportunity to promote independence and self-esteem.
Determine need for mobility aids, for example, canes, braces, walker, wheelchair, or scooter. Review safety considerations.	Mobility aids can decrease fatigue, enhance independence and comfort, and promote safety.
Schedule ADLs and outside activities in the morning or over time or throughout the course of the day. Investigate use of air conditioning, cooling vest, light-colored clothing, and wide-brimmed hats, if appropriate.	Fatigue commonly worsens when exposed to high temperatures due to weather, environmental heat, exercise, or fever. Some clients report lessening of fatigue with stabilization of body temperature.
Plan care with consistent rest periods between activities. Encourage afternoon nap.	Consistent rest and activity reduces fatigue and aggravation of muscle weakness.
Stress need for stopping exercise or activity before fatigue is exacerbated.	Pushing self beyond individual physical limits can result in excessive or prolonged fatigue and discouragement. In time, client can become very adept at knowing limitations.
Investigate appropriateness of obtaining a service dog.	Service dogs not only can increase client's level of independence, for example, balance and mobility assistance, but also can assist in energy conservation by carrying items in saddlebags, fetching, retrieving, and performing tasks, such as turning lights on and off.
Collaborative	
Recommend participation in support groups that involve fitness, exercise, and other issues related to MS.	Providing support resources can motivate the client to remain at optimal level of activity. Group activities must be carefully selected to meet client's need(s) and prevent discouragement or anxiety.
Administer medications, as indicated, for example: Amantadine (Symmetrel) and pemoline (Cylert)	Amantadine and pemoline help manage fatigue. Common side effects include increased spasticity, insomnia, and paresthesia of hands and feet.
Methylphenidate (Ritalin) and modafinil (Provigil)	CNS stimulants reduce fatigue but may also cause nervousness, restlessness, and insomnia.
Sertraline (Zoloft) and fluoxetine (Prozac)	Antidepressants lift moods and "energize" spirits in clients with depression.
Tricyclic antidepressants, such as amitriptyline (Elavil) and nortriptyline (Pamelor)	Tricyclic antidepressants help treat emotional lability, neurogenic pain, and associated sleep disorders. They help enhance willingness to be more active.
Anticonvulsants, such as carbamazepine (Tegretol), gabapentin (Neurontin), and lamotrigine (Lamictal)	Anticonvulsants treat neurogenic pain and sudden intermittent spasms related to spinal cord irritation.
Steroids, such as prednisone (Deltasone), dexamethasone (Decadron), and methylprednisolone (Solu-Medrol)	Steroids may be used during acute exacerbations to reduce or prevent edema formation at the sclerotic plaques. Long-term therapy seems to have little effect on progression of symptoms.
Antineoplastic agents, such as mitoxantrone (Novantrone)	Antineoplastic agents may be given to reduce neurological disability and frequency of relapses in clients with SPMS (chronic) or worsening RRMS.
Vitamin B	Vitamin B supports nerve cell replication, enhances metabolic functions, and may increase sense of well-being and energy level. (Reports are more anecdotal than research-based).

(continues on page 296)

Immunomodulating agents, such as cyclophosphamide (Cytoxan), azathioprine (Imuran), and methotrexate (Mexate); interferon beta-1a (Avonex, Rebif), interferon beta-1b (Betaseron), glatiramer (Copaxone), and mitoxentrone (Novantrone)

Immunomodulating agents may help treat acute relapses, reduce the frequency of relapse, and promote remission. Current research indicates early treatment with drugs that reduce inflammation and lesion formation may limit permanent damage. Therapy of choice is the use of "A, B, C" drugs: Avonex, Betaseron, and Copaxone. Therapeutic benefits have been reported in clients during all stages of disability with reduction in both steroid use and hospital days. Copaxone chemically resembles a component of myelin and may act as a decoy that diverts immune cells away from myelin target. *Note:* Novantrone may be used if other medications are not effective, but is contraindicated in PPMS.

Prepare for plasma exchange treatment as indicated.

Research suggests that individuals experiencing severe, acute exacerbations not responding to standard high-dose steroid therapy may benefit from a course of plasmapheresis.

NURSING DIAGNOSIS: Self-Care Deficit [specify]

May be related to
Neuromuscular or perceptual impairment; intolerance to activity; decreased strength and endurance; motor impairment, tremors
Pain, discomfort, fatigue
Memory loss
Depression

Possibly evidenced by
Frustration, inability to perform tasks of self-care, poor personal hygiene

Desired Outcomes/Evaluation Criteria—Client Will

Self-Care: Activities of Daily Living (ADLs) (NOC)
Identify individual areas of weakness, needs.
Demonstrate techniques and lifestyle changes to meet self-care needs.
Perform self-care activities within level of own ability.
Identify personal and community resources that provide assistance.

ACTIONS/INTERVENTIONS

RATIONALE

Self-Care Assistance (NIC)
Independent

Determine current activity level or physical condition. Assess degree of functional impairment using a scale of 0 to 4.

Functional assessment provides information to develop plan for rehabilitation. *Note:* Motor symptoms are less likely to improve than sensory ones.

Encourage client to perform at optimal level of function; however, do not rush client.

Encouragement promotes independence and sense of control. It may decrease feelings of helplessness.

Provide assistance with physical limitations. Allow as much autonomy as possible.

Client participation in self-care can ease the frustration over perceived loss of independence.

Encourage client input in planning schedule.

Client's quality of life is enhanced when preferences are considered in daily activities.

Note presence of and accommodate for fatigue.

Fatigue can be very debilitating and greatly impacts ability to participate in ADLs. The subjective nature of reports of fatigue can easily be misinterpreted as manipulative or a form of secondary gain.

Encourage scheduling activities early in the day or during peak energy levels.

Completing ADLs requires high energy expenditure. Poor planning of activities can cause early fatigue, persisting through the rest of the day.

Allow sufficient time to perform task(s). Display patience when movements are slow.

Decreased motor skills and spasticity may interfere with ability to manage simple activities.

Anticipate hygiene and grooming needs. Calmly assist with the care of nails, skin, hair, and mouth and with shaving (use electric razor), as necessary.

The care provider can model matter-of-fact attitude toward assistance with toileting and grooming activities. This facilitates client and SO to accept changing roles and abilities.

Provide assistive devices as indicated: shower chair, elevated toilet seat with arm supports, and others.

Assistive devices reduce fatigue and enhance participation in care.

ACTIONS/INTERVENTIONS (continued)

Frequently reposition the immobile, bed- or chair-bound client. Provide skin care to pressure points, such as sacrum, ankles, and elbows. Position or encourage sleeping in prone position, as tolerated.

Provide massage, active or passive range of motion (ROM), and stretching and toning exercises on a regular schedule. Encourage use of medications, cold packs, splints, and footboards, as indicated.

Provide strategies to promote independent feeding, such as wrapping fork handle with tape, cutting food, and showing how to hold cup with both hands.

Collaborative

Consult with physical and occupational therapists.

Administer medications, as indicated, for example:
Tizanidine (Zanaflex), baclofen (Lioresal), and carbamazepine (Tegretol)

Diazepam (Valium), clonazepam (Klonopin), cyclobenzaprine (Flexeril), gabapentin (Neurontin), and dantrolene (Dantrium)

Meclizine (Antivert) and scopolamine patches (Transderm-Scop)
Prepare for surgical intervention for deep brain stimulation, as appropriate.

RATIONALE (continued)

Repositioning reduces pressure on susceptible areas and prevents skin breakdown. It minimizes flexor spasms at knees and hips.

These maneuvers prevent problems associated with muscle pain, dysfunction, and disuse. They help maintain muscle tone, muscle strength, joint mobility, and proper body alignment. They decrease spasticity and risk of calcium loss from bones.

These strategies promote independence and adequate nutritional intake.

Interdisciplinary consultations provide appropriate interventions that relieve spastic muscles, improve motor functioning, prevent or reduce muscular atrophy and contractures, and promote optimal level of function, independence, and self-worth.

Several drugs are effective for reducing spasticity, promoting muscle relaxation, and inhibiting reflexes at the spinal nerve root level. Tizanidine may have an additive effect with baclofen, but must be used with caution because both drugs have similar side effects. Short duration of action requires careful dosing to maximize therapeutic effect.

A variety of medications are used to manage spasticity. The mechanisms are not well understood, and client responses vary. Therefore, it may take a period of medication trials to discover what provides the most effective relief of muscle spasticity and associated pain. *Note:* Adverse effects include increased muscle weakness, loss of muscle tone, and liver toxicity.

Meclizine and scopolamine patches reduce dizziness, allowing for increased mobility.

Placement of an electrode—similar to a cardiac pacemaker device—in the region of the thalamus provides for small, adjustable electrical impulses to reduce arm tremors and enhance movement without actually destroying brain tissue.

NURSING DIAGNOSIS: low Self-Esteem, (specify situational/chronic)

May be related to
Change in structure and function
Disruption in how client perceives own body
Role reversal; dependence

Possibly evidenced by
Confusion about sense of self, purpose, direction in life
Denial, withdrawal, anger
Negative or self-destructive behavior
Use of ineffective coping methods
Change in self or other's perception of role and physical capacity to resume role

Desired Outcomes/Evaluation Criteria—Client Will

Self-Esteem (NOC)
Verbalize realistic view and acceptance of body.
View self as a capable person.
Participate in and assume responsibility for meeting own needs.
Recognize and incorporate changes in self-concept and role without negating self-esteem.
Develop realistic plans for adapting to role changes.

ACTIONS/INTERVENTIONS	RATIONALE

Self-Esteem Enhancement (NIC)

Independent

Establish or maintain a therapeutic nurse-client relationship. Discuss fears and concerns.	Therapeutic nurse-client relationships convey an attitude of caring and develop a sense of trust between client and caregiver. The client is free to express fears of rejection, loss of previous functioning, changes in appearance, feelings of helplessness, and powerlessness. Open communication promotes a sense of support and well-being.
Note withdrawn behaviors, use of denial, or excessive concern with disease process.	These behaviors serve as initial protective responses. If prolonged, these behaviors may impede effective coping.
Support use of defense mechanisms. Allow the client to deal with the information in own time and way.	Confronting client with reality of situation may result in increased anxiety and lessened ability to cope with actual or perceived changes.
Acknowledge reality of grieving process related to actual or perceived changes. Help client deal realistically with feelings of anger and sadness.	The nature of the disease leads to ongoing losses and life changes. It could potentially block resolution of grieving process.
Review information about course of disease, possibility of remissions, and prognosis.	Information regarding the course of the disease helps empower the client to make decisions regarding daily functioning and healthcare decisions.
Provide accurate verbal and written information about what is happening and discuss with client and SO.	Providing current information facilitates client and SO decision making.
Explain that labile emotions are not unusual. Problem-solve ways to deal with these feelings.	Therapeutic communication relieves anxiety and promotes expression and management of emotions.
Note presence of depression, impaired thought processes, and expression of suicidal ideation; evaluate on a scale of 1 to 10.	Adapting to a long-term, progressively debilitating incurable condition is a difficult emotional adjustment. In addition, cognitive impairment may affect adaptation to life changes. A depressed individual may believe that suicide is the best way to deal with what is happening.
Assess interaction between client and SO. Note changes in relationship.	SO may unconsciously or consciously reinforce negative attitudes and beliefs of client, or issues of secondary gain may interfere with progress and ability to manage situation.
Provide an open environment for client and SO to discuss concerns about sexuality, including management of fatigue, spasticity, arousal, and changes in sensation.	Physical and psychological changes often create stress in the relationship, affect usual roles and expectations, and potentially further impair self-concept.
Discuss use of medications and adjuncts to improve sexual function.	Client and partner may want to explore trial of medications, such as papaverine (Pavabid), dinoprostone (Prostin E$_2$), or other avenues of improving sexual relationship.

Collaborative

Consult with occupational therapist or rehabilitation team.	Identifying assistive devices and equipment enhances level of overall function, participation in activities, and sense of well-being.
Refer to psychiatric clinical nurse specialist, social worker, and psychologist as indicated.	In-depth, supportive counseling may help resolve conflicts and deal with life changes.

NURSING DIAGNOSIS: Powerlessness [specify degree]/Hopelessness

May be related to
Illness-related regimen, unpredictability of disease
Lifestyle of helplessness

Possibly evidenced by
Verbal expressions of having no control or influence over situation
Depression over physical deterioration that occurs despite client compliance with regimen
Nonparticipation in care or decision making when opportunities are provided
Passivity, decreased verbalization and affect
Verbal cues—despondent content, "I can't," sighing
Lack of involvement in care and passively allowing care
Isolating behaviors and social withdrawal

Desired Outcomes/Evaluation Criteria—Client Will

Hope (NOC)
Identify and verbalize feelings.
Use coping mechanisms to counteract feelings of hopelessness.
Identify areas over which individual has control.
Participate, monitor, or control self-care and ADLs.

ACTIONS/INTERVENTIONS	RATIONALE

Hope Instillation (NIC)

Independent

Note behaviors indicative of powerlessness or hopelessness, such as statements of despair, "They don't care" or "It won't make any difference."

Acknowledge reality of situation, at the same time expressing hope for client.

Encourage and assist client to identify activities he or she would like to be involved in, such as volunteer work, within the limits of his or her abilities.

Discuss plans for the future. Suggest visiting alternative care facilities and taking a look at the possibilities for care as condition changes.

Self-Responsibility Facilitation (NIC)

Determine degree of life mastery and locus control.

Assist client to identify factors that are under own control, listing things that can or cannot be controlled.

Encourage client to assume control over as much of own care as possible.

Discuss needs openly, and facilitate actions to meet identified needs.

Incorporate client's daily routine in home care schedule or hospital stay, as possible.

Collaborative

Refer to vocational rehabilitation as indicated.

Identify community resources, such as adult day enrichment program.

These behaviors indicate client's ability to manage life changes.

Although the prognosis may be discouraging, remissions may occur, and because the future cannot be predicted, hope for some quality of life should be expressed and encouraged. Additionally, research is ongoing, and new treatment options may become available.

Staying active and interacting with others helps counteract feelings of helplessness.

Planning promotes sense of control and hope.

Life mastery helps determine success in adjusting to the health condition. The locus of control relates to the ability to manage outcomes related to the disease process. An external locus of control would benefit from positive affirmation.

Knowing and accepting what is beyond individual control can reduce helpless and acting-out behaviors and promote focusing on areas individual can control.

The client can help plan and supervise own care and participate in health decision making.

Open discussion empowers the client. It also helps to deal with manipulative behaviors.

Routines maintain a sense of control, self-determination, and independence.

Vocational rehabilitation assists in development and implementation of a vocational plan that incorporates specific interests and abilities.

Participation in structured activities can reduce sense of isolation and may enhance feeling of self-worth. These resources also provide respite to caregivers.

NURSING DIAGNOSIS: risk for ineffective Coping

Risk factors may include

Physiological changes—cerebral and spinal lesions

Psychological conflicts, anxiety; fear

Impaired judgment, short-term memory loss, confusion, unrealistic perceptions and expectations, emotional lability

Personal vulnerability; inadequate support systems

Multiple life changes

Inadequate coping methods

Possibly evidenced by

(Not applicable; presence of signs and symptoms establishes an *actual* diagnosis)

Desired Outcomes/Evaluation Criteria—Client Will

Coping (NOC)

Recognize relationship between disease process (cerebral lesions) and emotional responses and changes in thinking and behavior.

Verbalize awareness of own capabilities and strengths.

Display effective problem-solving skills.

Demonstrate behaviors and lifestyle changes to prevent or minimize changes in mentation and maintain reality orientation.

ACTIONS/INTERVENTIONS	RATIONALE

Coping Enhancement (NIC)

Independent

Assess current functional capacity and limitations; note presence of distorted thinking processes, labile emotions, and cognitive dissonance. Determine how these affect coping abilities.

Organic or psychological effects may cause client to be easily distracted and to display difficulties with concentration, problem-solving, dealing with what is happening, and being responsible for own care.

Determine client understanding of current situation and previous methods of dealing with life problems.

Client understanding of current health situation provides clues on coping abilities, support system, individual resources, and other needs.

Discuss ability to make decisions, care for children or dependent adults, and handle finances. Identify available options.

Impaired judgment, confusion, and inadequate support systems may interfere with ability to meet own needs and needs of others. Conservatorship, guardianship, or adult protective services may be required until client is able to manage own affairs (if ever).

Maintain an honest, reality-oriented relationship.

Honest, reality-based relationship reduces confusion and minimizes painful, frustrating struggles associated with adaptation to altered environment and lifestyle.

Encourage verbalization of feelings and fears. Accept client statements in a nonjudgmental manner. Note statements reflecting powerlessness and inability to cope. (Refer to ND: Powerlessness/Hopelessness.)

Nonjudgmental approach may diminish client's fear, establish trust, provide opportunities to identify problems, and facilitate the problem-solving process.

Observe nonverbal communication—posture, eye contact, movements, gestures, and use of touch. Correlate with verbal content. Clarify meaning, as appropriate.

Careful assessment of both verbal and nonverbal forms of communication provides insight into client response to the health condition and effective coping strategies.

Provide clues for orientation, such as calendars, clocks, note cards, organizers, and date book.

Memory aids facilitate client orientation and coping.

Encourage client to tape-record important information and listen to the recording periodically.

Repetition puts information in long-term memory, where it is more easily retrieved, and can support decision making and problem-solving process.

Collaborative

Refer to cognitive retraining program.

Improving cognitive abilities can enhance basic thinking skills, including attention span, information processing, learning new skills, insight, judgment, and problem-solving.

Refer to counseling, psychiatric clinical nurse specialist, and psychiatrist, as indicated.

Collaboration with psychiatric services may help resolve issues of self-esteem and regain effective coping skills.

Administer medications, as appropriate, such as amitriptyline (Elavil), bupropion (Wellbutrin), imipramine (Tofranil), trazadone (Desyrel).

These medications improve mood and restful sleep as well as help combat depression and relieve fatigue.

NURSING DIAGNOSIS: compromised/disabled family Coping

May be related to

Situational crisis; temporary family disorganization and role changes

Highly ambivalent family relationship

Prolonged disease and disability progression that exhausts the supportive capacity of SO

Client providing little support in turn for SO

SO with chronically unexpressed feelings of guilt, anxiety, hostility, despair

Possibly evidenced by

Client expresses or confirms concern or complaint about SO response to client's illness

SO withdraws or has limited personal communication with client or displays protective behavior disproportionate to client's abilities or need for autonomy

SO preoccupied with own personal reactions

Intolerance, abandonment

Neglectful care of client

Distortion of reality regarding client's illness

Desired Outcomes/Evaluation Criteria—Family Will

Family Coping (NOC)

Identify or verbalize resources within themselves to deal with the situation.

Express more realistic understanding and expectations of client.

Interact appropriately with client and healthcare providers providing support and assistance as indicated.

Verbalize knowledge and understanding of disability, disease process, and community resources.

ACTIONS/INTERVENTIONS	RATIONALE

Family Involvement Promotion (NIC)
Independent

Note length and severity of illness. Determine client's role in family and how illness has changed the family organization.

Determine SO's understanding of disease process and expectations for the future.

Chronic or unresolved illness, accompanied by changes in role performance and responsibility, often exhausts supportive capacity and coping abilities of SO and family.

Inadequate information or misconception regarding disease process and unrealistic expectations affect ability to cope with current situation. *Note:* A particular area of misconception is the fatigue experienced by clients with MS. Family members may view client's inability to perform activities as manipulative behavior rather than an actual physiological deficit.

Discuss with SO and family members their willingness to be involved in care. Identify other responsibilities and factors impacting participation.

Assess other factors that are affecting abilities of family members to provide needed support, such as own emotional problems and work concerns.

Individuals may not have desire or time to assume responsibility for care. If several family members are available, they may be able to share tasks.

Individual members' preoccupation with own needs and concerns can interfere with providing needed care and support for stresses of long-term illness. Additionally, caregiver(s) may incur decrease or loss of income and risk losing own health insurance if they alter their work hours.

Discuss underlying reasons for client's behaviors.

Helps SO understand and accept and deal with behaviors that may be triggered by emotional or physical effects of MS.

Encourage client and SO to develop and strengthen problem-solving skills to deal with situation.

Family may or may not have handled conflict well before illness. The stress of long-term debilitating condition can create additional problems, including unresolved anger.

Encourage free expression of feelings, including frustration, anger, hostility, and hopelessness.

Individual members may be afraid to express "negative" feelings, believing it will discourage client. Free expression promotes awareness and can help with resolution of feelings and problems (especially when done in a caring manner).

Collaborative

Identify community resources, such as local MS organization, support groups, home care agencies, and respite programs.

Community resources provide information, opportunities to share with others who are experiencing similar difficulties, and potential sources of assistance.

Refer to social worker, financial adviser, psychiatric clinical nurse specialist, and psychiatrist, as appropriate.

Client, SO, and family may need more in-depth assistance from professional sources.

NURSING DIAGNOSIS: impaired Urinary Elimination

May be related to
Neuromuscular impairment, such as spinal cord lesions, neurogenic bladder

Possibly evidenced by
Incontinence, nocturia, frequency
Retention with overflow
Recurrent UTIs

Desired Outcomes/Evaluation Criteria—Client Will

Urinary Continence (NOC)
Verbalize understanding of condition.
Demonstrate behaviors and techniques to prevent or minimize infection.
Empty bladder completely and regularly, voluntarily or by catheter, as appropriate.
Be free of urine leakage between voiding.

ACTIONS/INTERVENTIONS	RATIONALE

Urinary Elimination Management (NIC)
Independent

Note reports of urinary frequency, urgency, burning, incontinence, nocturia, and size and force of urinary stream. Palpate bladder after voiding.

Urinary habits indicate kidney and bladder function and possible UTI. Bladder fullness after voiding indicates inadequate emptying or retention and requires further evaluation and intervention.

(continues on page 302)

ACTIONS/INTERVENTIONS	RATIONALE
Review drug regimen, including prescribed, OTC, and street drug use.	A number of medications, including some antispasmodics, antidepressants, and opioid analgesics; OTC medications with anticholinergic or alpha-agonist properties; or recreational drugs such as cannabis, may interfere with bladder emptying.
Institute bladder training program or timed voiding, as appropriate.	Bladder training program helps restore bladder functioning and reduces incontinence and bladder infection.
Encourage adequate fluid intake, avoiding caffeine and use of aspartame and limiting intake during late evening and at bedtime. Recommend use of cranberry juice and vitamin C.	Sufficient hydration promotes urinary output and aids in preventing infection. *Note:* When client is taking sulfa drugs, sufficient fluids are necessary to ensure adequate excretion of drug, reducing risk of cumulative effects. *Note:* Aspartame, a sugar substitute (e.g., NutraSweet), may cause bladder irritation leading to bladder dysfunction.
Promote continued mobility.	Continued mobility promotes bladder emptying, thus decreases risk of developing UTI.
Recommend good hand-washing and perineal care.	Perineal care reduces skin irritation and risk of ascending infection.
Encourage client to observe for sediment, blood in urine, foul odor, fever, or unexplained increase in MS symptoms, such as spasticity and dysarthria.	Urinary symptoms indicate infection that requires further evaluation and prompt treatment.

Collaborative

ACTIONS/INTERVENTIONS	RATIONALE
Refer to urinary continence specialist, as indicated.	The continence specialist helps develop individual plan of care to meet client's specific needs using the latest techniques and continence products.
Administer medications, as indicated, such as Tolterodine (Detrol), oxybutynin (Ditropan), propantheline (Pro-Banthine), hyoscyamine sulfate (Cytospaz-M), flavoxate (Urispaz).	These medications reduce bladder spasticity and associated urinary symptoms of frequency, urgency, incontinence, and nocturia.
Catheterize, as indicated.	Catheterization may be necessary to relieve or evaluate bladder emptying or urinary retention.
Teach self-catheterization. Instruct in use and care of indwelling catheter.	Self-catheterization helps maintain client autonomy and encourages self-care. Indwelling catheter may be required, depending on client's abilities and degree of urinary problem.
Obtain periodic urinalysis (UA) and urine culture and sensitivity, as indicated.	Monitors kidney and bladder function and identifies presence of UTI. Colony count over 100,000 indicates presence of infection requiring treatment.
Administer anti-infective agents, as necessary, such as nitrofurantoin macrocrystals (Macrodantin), co-trimoxazole (Bactrim, Septra), ciprofloxacin (Cipro), and norfloxacin (Noroxin).	Bacteriostatic agents inhibit bacterial growth and destroy susceptible bacteria. Prompt treatment of infection is necessary to prevent serious complications of ascending urinary infection, sepsis, and shock.

NURSING DIAGNOSIS: **risk for Caregiver Role Strain**

Risk factors may include
Severity of illness of the care receiver, duration of caregiving required, complexity or amount of caregiving tasks
Caregiver is female, spouse
Care receiver exhibits deviant, bizarre behavior
Family and caregiver isolation, lack of respite and recreation

Possibly evidenced by
(Not applicable; presence of signs and symptoms establishes an *actual* diagnosis)

Desired Outcomes/Evaluation Criteria—Caregiver Will

Caregiver Performance: Direct Care (NOC)
Identify individual risk factors and appropriate interventions.
Demonstrate and initiate behaviors or lifestyle changes to prevent development of impaired function.

Caregiver Performance: Indirect Care (NOC)
Use available resources appropriately.
Report satisfaction with plan and support available.

ACTIONS/INTERVENTIONS	RATIONALE
Caregiver Support (NIC)	
Independent	
Note physical and psychosocial condition. Identify client ability to comply with therapeutic regimen.	Careful assessment of physical and psychosocial conditions determines individual needs for planning care and helps identify strengths and needs requiring assistance and accommodation.
Determine caregiver's level of commitment, responsibility, involvement, and anticipated length of care. Use assessment tool, such as Burden Interview, to further determine caregiver's abilities, as appropriate.	Progressive debilitation taxes caregiver and may alter ability to meet client's and own needs. (Refer to ND: compromised/disabled family Coping.)
Discuss caregiver's view of the situation.	Open discussion allows ventilation and clarification of concerns and promotes understanding.
Determine available resources and social support.	Organizations, such as the National MS Society and local support groups, can provide information regarding adequacy of supports and identify needs and possible options.
Facilitate family conference to share information and develop plan for involvement in care activities, as appropriate.	Family conference helps clarify different roles and responsibilities, facilitates coping, and promotes participation and involvement.
Identify additional resources to include financial and legal assistance.	These areas of concern can add to burden of caregiving if not adequately resolved.
Identify adaptive equipment needs, resources for the home, and transportation.	Adaptive devices enhance independence and safety for the client and the caregivers.
Provide information and demonstrate techniques for dealing with acting out, violent, or disoriented behavior.	Information and effective techniques for dealing with such behavior help the caregiver maintain a sense of control and competency and enhances safe care.
Stress importance of self-nurturing, such as pursuing self-development interests, personal needs, hobbies, and social activities.	Taking time for self can lessen risk of burnout or being overwhelmed by situation.
Identify alternate care sources, such as sitter or day-care facility, and senior care services, for example, Meals on Wheels, respite care, and home care agency.	As client's condition worsens, SO may need additional help to maintain client at home.
Assist with short-term and long-term care planning to meet the current and future needs of the recipient of care, including placement in alternative levels of care, extended care, hospice, and so forth.	Short-term and long-term care planning provides ongoing assessment and evaluation of client needs and clinical outcomes and realization of changes in the level of care.
Collaborative	
Refer to supportive services, as indicated.	Medical case manager or social services consultant may be needed to develop ongoing plan to meet changing needs of client and SO/family.

NURSING DIAGNOSIS: deficient Knowledge [Learning Need] regarding condition, prognosis, complications, treatment, and discharge needs

May be related to
Lack of exposure, information misinterpretation
Unfamiliarity with information resources
Cognitive limitation, lack of recall

Possibly evidenced by
Statement of misconception
Request for information
Inaccurate follow-through of instruction; development of preventable complications
Inappropriate or exaggerated behaviors, such as hysterical, hostile, agitated, apathetic

Desired Outcomes/Evaluation Criteria—Client/Caregiver Will

Knowledge: Disease Process
Participate in learning process.
Assume responsibility for own learning and begin to look for information and to ask questions.
Verbalize understanding of condition, disease process, and treatment.
Initiate necessary lifestyle changes.
Participate in prescribed treatment regimen.

ACTIONS/INTERVENTIONS	RATIONALE

Learning Facilitation (NIC)

Independent

Evaluate motivation and readiness to learn of the client, SO, and caregivers.

Motivation and readiness to learn help determine appropriate and pertinent level of information.

Note signs of emotional lability or dissociative states (loss of affect and inappropriate emotional responses).

Client will not process or retain information and has difficulty learning during this time.

Provide information in varied formats based on client perceptual and cognitive abilities and locus of control.

Effective teaching strategies, such as verbal instruction, books, pamphlets, audiovisual materials, and computer problems, are based on understanding the client's attitude toward learning and locus of control.

Encourage active participation of client and SO in learning process, including use of self-paced instruction, as appropriate.

Active participation of client and SO enhances sense of independence and control as well as strengthens compliance with therapeutic regimen.

Teaching: Disease Process (NIC)

Review disease process, prognosis, effects of climate, emotional stress, overexertion, and fatigue.

Clarifies client and SO understanding of current health and living situation.

Identify signs and symptoms that require further evaluation.

Prompt intervention may help limit severity of exacerbation and complications.

Discuss importance of daily routine of rest, exercise, activity, and nutrition. Focus on current capabilities. Instruct in use of appropriate devices to assist with ADLs, such as eating utensils, walking aids, among others.

Discussions on the importance of rest, activity, and nutrition helps reduce fatigue and maintain a level of independence.

Stress importance of weight control.

Excess weight can interfere with balance and motor abilities and make care more difficult.

Review possible problems such as decreased perception of heat and pain, susceptibility to skin breakdown and infections, especially UTIs, and complications.

These effects of demyelination and associated complications may compromise client's safety and precipitate an exacerbation of signs and symptoms.

Identify measures to promote safety and overall health, such as avoiding exposure to individuals with respiratory infections; avoiding hot baths; regular skin monitoring and care; safe transfers to wheelchair, walker, or scooter; and adequate nutrition and hydration.

Review of safety and preventive measures maintains optimal level of function as well as prevents complications.

Discuss increased risk of osteoporosis and review preventive measures—regular exercise; increased intake of calcium and vitamin D; reduced intake of caffeine; cessation of smoking; hormone replacement therapy (HRT) or alternatives, for example, bisphosphonates such as Fosamax; and fall prevention measures such as wearing low-heeled shoes with nonskid soles, use of handrails and grab bars in bathroom and along stairwells, and removal of small area rugs.

These measures reduce the risk for osteoporosis and complications.

Identify bowel elimination concerns. Recommend adequate hydration and intake of fiber; use of stool softeners, bulking agents, suppositories, or possibly mild laxatives; and bowel training program.

Constipation is common. Bowel urgency and accidents may occur as a result of dietary deficiencies or fecal impaction.

Review medications. Recommend avoidance of OTC drugs.

Avoidance of OTC medications reduces likelihood of drug interactions or adverse effects and enhances cooperation with treatment regimen.

Discuss concerns regarding sexual relationships, contraception and reproduction, and effects of pregnancy on the female client. Identify alternative ways to meet individual needs; counsel regarding use of artificial lubrication (females) and provide genitourinary (GU) referral for males regarding available medication and sexual aids.

Pregnancy may be an issue for the young client relative to issues of genetic predisposition and ability to manage pregnancy or parenting. Increased libido is not uncommon and may require adjustments within the existing relationship or in the absence of an acceptable partner. Information about different positions and techniques and other options for sexual fulfillment, such as fondling and cuddling, may enhance personal relationship and feelings of self-worth.

Encourage client to set goals for the future while focusing on the present and what can be done today.

Setting future goals provides opportunity for the client to develop insight and perspective regarding realities of the current situation and uncertainty of the future.

Identify financial concerns.

Loss or change of employment for client or SO impacts income, insurance benefits, and level of independence, requiring additional family or social support.

Refer for vocational rehabilitation, as appropriate.

Assessment of capabilities or job retraining may be indicated due to limitations associated with disease progression.

ACTIONS/INTERVENTIONS (continued)

Recommend contact with local and national MS organizations and other support resources.

RATIONALE (continued)

Ongoing contact such as mailings informs client of programs and services available and can update client's knowledge base. Support groups can provide role modeling and sharing of information and enhance problem-solving ability and individual and family coping.

POTENTIAL CONSIDERATIONS following acute hospitalization (dependent on client's age, physical condition, presence of complications, personal resources, and life responsibilities)
* *risk for Trauma*—weakness, poor vision, balancing difficulties, reduced temperature and tactile sensation, reduced muscle and hand-eye coordination, cognitive or emotional difficulties, insufficient finances to purchase necessary equipment
* *impaired Home Maintenance*—insufficient finances, unfamiliarity with neighborhood resources, inadequate support systems
* *risk for or (actual) Disuse Syndrome*—paralysis and immobilization, severe pain
* *ineffective self Health Management*—economic difficulties, family conflict, social support deficits

CHAPTER 7

Gastrointestinal Disorders

UPPER GASTROINTESTINAL/ESOPHAGEAL BLEEDING

I. Pathophysiology

a. Ulceration and erosion of the mucosa of upper gastrointestinal (GI) organs, including stomach and esophagus, which is indicated by presence of melena, hematemesis, or blood in gastric contents (following lavage)

b. Arises from branches of the celiac artery and superior mesenteric artery

c. Variceal bleeding often arises from esophageal or gastric varices from the coronary vein or short gastric veins in portal hypertension.

II. Etiology

a. Peptic ulcers are localized erosions of the innermost mucosal layer of the digestive tract (Krumberger, 2005).

  i. Duodenal ulcer affects the upper part of the small intestine.

  ii. Gastric ulcer affects the lining of the stomach.

  iii. Common causes of ulcers include infection with *Helicobacter pylori*; alcohol, aspirin, and aspirin-containing medicines; and various other medicines, such as nonsteroidal anti-inflammatory drugs (NSAIDs), used for arthritis.

b. Tear in the mucosa at the gastroesophageal junction (Mallory-Weiss syndrome) can occur as a result of severe vomiting, trauma, or seizures.

c. Hemorrhagic gastritis or stress ulcer can occur as a result of severe physiological stress, such as trauma, burns, surgery, or alcohol abuse (Krumberger, 2005).

d. Esophageal varices is generally associated with alcoholic or post-hepatitis cirrhosis of the liver; approximately 30% of such patients experience hemorrhage (Sartin, 2005).

e. Esophageal or gastric cancer

f. Hiatal hernia, hemophilia, leukemia, and disseminated intravascular coagulation (DIC) are less common causes of upper gastrointestinal bleeding (UGIB).

III. Statistics (Varma & Allen, 2005)

a. Morbidity: Gross bleeding into the GI tract is responsible for about 2% of all emergency medical visits in the United States, with approximately 300,000 hospitalizations annually.

b. Mortality: Rate is approximately 10%.

c. Cost: Estimated at $2.5 million annually in the United States.

GLOSSARY

Esophageal varices: Veins in esophagus and stomach become engorged and fragile due to high blood pressure in the portal vein.

Gastrin: Hormone secreted by the stomach into the gastric venous circulation to stimulate the stomach glands to release gastric acid.

Gastroesophageal reflux disease (GERD): Disorder in which there is recurrent backflow of stomach contents into the esophagus, frequently causing heartburn.

Hematemesis: Bloody vomitus.

Melena: Black, tarry feces due to digestion of blood in stool.

Portal hypertension: Obstruction of portal vein due to hardening of liver from cirrhosis, causing venous blood from intestines and spleen to seek alternate routes to right atrium.

Tarry stool: Stool with high content of blood that has been partially digested, resembling sticky tar with a distinctive blood odor.

Care Setting

Generally, a client with severe, active bleeding is admitted directly to a critical care unit; however, a client may develop GI bleeding on the medical-surgical unit or be admitted there for evaluation or treatment of subacute bleeding.

Related Concerns

Cirrhosis of the liver, page 445
Fluid and electrolyte imbalances, page 903
Psychosocial aspects of care, page 749
Renal failure: acute, page 536
Gastrectomy/gastric resection, page 317

Client Assessment Database

DIAGNOSTIC DIVISION MAY REPORT	MAY EXHIBIT
ACTIVITY/REST • Weakness, fatigue	• Tachycardia • Tachypnea, hyperventilation in response to activity
CIRCULATION • Palpitations • Dizziness with position change	• Hypotension, including postural • Tachycardia, dysrhythmias related to hypovolemia and hypoxemia • Weak and thready peripheral pulse • Capillary refill slow or delayed due to vasoconstriction • *Skin color:* Pallor, cyanosis depending on the amount of blood loss • Skin and mucous membrane moisture exhibiting diaphoresis reflecting shock state, acute pain, and possible emotional reactions
EGO INTEGRITY • Acute or chronic stress factors due to finances, relationship, or employment • Feelings of helplessness	• Signs of anxiety, such as restlessness, pallor, diaphoresis, narrowed focus, trembling, quivering voice
ELIMINATION • Change in usual bowel patterns and characteristics of stool	• Abdominal tenderness, distention • Bowel sounds are often hyperactive during bleeding, hypoactive after bleeding subsides • *Character of stool:* Diarrhea; dark bloody, tarry; constipation may occur due to changes in diet or antacid use • Urine output may be decreased or concentrated
NEUROSENSORY • Fainting, dizziness, lightheadedness, or weakness	• *Mental status:* Level of consciousness (LOC) may be altered, ranging from slight drowsiness, disorientation, and confusion to stupor and coma
PAIN/DISCOMFORT • Pain described as sharp, dull, burning, gnawing, sudden, excruciating (perforation) • Nocturnal pain experienced by many • Vague sensation of discomfort or distress following large meals and relieved by food (acute gastritis) • Left to midepigastric pain that can radiate to the back, often accompanied by vomiting after eating and relieved by antacid (gastric ulcers) • Localized right to midepigastric pain, gnawing, burning, occurring about 2 to 3 hours after meals when stomach is empty and relieved by food or antacids (duodenal ulcers) • Midepigastric pain and burning with regurgitation, seen frequently with chronic GERD • Absence of pain seen frequently with esophageal varices • Elderly more likely to be asymptomatic and present with a decreased appetite and weight loss	• Facial grimacing • Guarding of affected area • Narrowed focus

(continues on page 308)

DIAGNOSTIC DIVISION
MAY REPORT (continued)

SAFETY
- History of previous hospitalizations for GI bleeding or related GI problems, such as peptic or gastric ulcer, gastritis, gastric surgery, irradiation of gastric area
- Recent use of prescription or over-the-counter (OTC) drugs containing acetylsalicylic acid (ASA), steroids, or NSAIDs (NSAIDs are leading cause of drug-induced GI bleeding)
- Chronic use of alcohol or recreational drugs

DISCHARGE PLAN CONSIDERATIONS
- May require changes in therapeutic and medication regimens

- ▶ Refer to section at end of plan for postdischarge considerations.

MAY EXHIBIT (continued)

Diagnostic Studies

TEST
WHY IT IS DONE

WHAT IT TELLS ME

BLOOD TESTS
- *Complete blood count (CBC):* Battery of screening tests that typically includes hemoglobin (Hgb); hematocrit (Hct); red blood cell (RBC) count, morphology, indices, and distribution width index; platelet count and size; white blood cell (WBC) count and differential.

CBC will indicate whether client is anemic (low Hgb) and will also give an idea of the extent of the bleeding (Hgb and Hct) and how chronic it may be. RBC count and platelets may be decreased. WBC count may be elevated, reflecting the body's response to injury. CBC also aids in establishing blood and fluid replacement needs and monitoring effectiveness of therapy. For example, 1 unit of whole blood should raise Hct two to three points. Hct levels may not accurately reflect early or sudden blood loss until 6 to 24 hours after acute bleeding begins.

- *Coagulation profile:* Evaluates ability of blood to clot.

Prolonged in active bleeding. May indicate need for replacement of coagulation factors, such as fresh frozen plasma (FFP). Increased platelets with decreased clotting times may be the body's attempt to restore hemostasis. Severe abnormalities may reveal coagulopathy such as disseminated intravascular coagulation (DIC) as cause of bleeding.

- *Blood urea nitrogen (BUN):* Determines presence of end products of breakdown of blood in GI tract.

Elevated within 24 to 48 hours as blood proteins are broken down in the GI tract and kidney filtration is decreased. BUN greater than 40 with normal creatinine level indicates major bleeding. BUN should return to client's normal level approximately 12 hours after bleeding has ceased.

- *Pepsinogen level:* Precursor of pepsin, which is an enzyme in gastric juice that digests proteins.

Increased by duodenal ulcer; low level suggestive of gastritis.

- *Potassium:* Principle cation in intracellular fluid. It helps regulate the osmotic pressure and acid-base balance.

May initially be depleted because of massive gastric emptying and vomiting or bloody diarrhea. Elevated potassium levels may occur after multiple transfusions of blood or with acute renal impairment

- *Sodium:* Principle cation found in extracellular fluid and in tissue. Sodium regulates osmotic pressure in the cells and fluids, helping to prevent excess loss of water from the tissues.

May be elevated as a hormonal compensation to conserve body fluid.

Diagnostic Studies (continued)

TEST WHY IT IS DONE (continued)	WHAT IT TELLS ME (continued)
• *Arterial blood gases (ABGs):* Assesses gas levels of arterial oxygen (PaO_2), carbon dioxide ($PaCO_2$), and pH.	May reveal initial respiratory alkalosis (elevated $PaCO_2$, compensating for diminished blood flow through lungs). Later, metabolic acidosis develops in response to sluggish liver flow and accumulation of metabolic waste products.
OTHER DIAGNOSTIC STUDIES • *Esophagogastroduodenoscopy (EGD):* Allows direct visualization and therapeutic treatment of abnormal conditions of esophagus, stomach, and duodenum.	Key diagnostic test for upper GI bleeding done to visualize site of bleeding and degree of tissue injury.
• *Capsule endoscopy:* A camera enclosed in a small capsule is swallowed. Images are taken every 2 seconds and transmitted via radio signals to receivers attached to abdomen and then into a receiver worn on a belt.	Can identify lesions, strictures, or bleeding areas in obscure GI bleeding of suspected small-bowel origin.
• *Barium swallow with x-ray:* Visualizes site of bleeding.	May be done after bleeding has ceased for differential diagnosis of cause and site of lesion and presence of structural defects such as strictures.
• *Gastrointestinal nuclear scan:* Scanning of abdomen after injection of a radioactive dye. Radionuclide uptake at sites of bleeding identifies site (not cause) of bleeding.	Test is considered to be more sensitive than EGD, upper GI studies with barium, or angiography in detecting sites of lower GI bleeding or persistent bleeding anywhere in GI tract.
• *Angiography:* Injection of dye into blood vessels followed by x-ray imaging.	GI vasculature may be reviewed if endoscopy is inconclusive or impractical. Demonstrates collateral circulation and possibly bleeding site.
• *H. pylori tests:* Four tests are used: blood antibody test, urea breath test, stool antigen test, and stomach biopsy.	Determines whether an infection with *H. pylori* bacteria may be causing an ulcer or irritation of the stomach lining. *Note:* Fifty to seventy percent of elderly clients with ulcers have been found to have *H. pylori* as an underlying cause. The presence of *H. pylori* increases the risk of peptic ulcer disease 5- to 7-fold, but with the use of NSAIDs, the risk increases 5- to 20-fold.
• *Gastrin analysis:* Gastrin is a hormone secreted in the stomach that stimulates gastric acid secretion.	Elevated level suggests Zollinger-Ellison syndrome or possible presence of multiple poorly healed ulcers.
• *Parietal cell antibodies:* Parietal cells are large cells on the edges of peptic glands of the stomach. They secrete intrinsic factor (needed to absorb vitamin B_{12}) and stomach acid.	Presence suggestive of chronic gastritis.
• *Gastric biopsies:* Small pieces of tissue obtained with biopsy forceps during EGD.	Determines presence of *H. pylori.*
• *Stools:* Determine presence of blood in GI tract.	Testing for blood will be positive.

Nursing Priorities

1. Control hemorrhage.
2. Achieve and maintain hemodynamic stability.
3. Promote stress reduction.
4. Provide information about disease process and prognosis, treatment needs, and potential complications.

Discharge Goals

1. Hemorrhage curtailed.
2. Hemodynamically stable.
3. Anxiety and fear reduced to manageable level.
4. Disease process and prognosis, therapeutic regimen, and potential complications understood.
5. Plan in place to meet needs after discharge.

NURSING DIAGNOSIS: risk for Bleeding

May be related to
Active fluid volume loss—hemorrhage

Possibly evidenced by
(Not applicable; presence of signs and symptoms establishes an *actual* diagnosis)

Desired Outcomes/Evaluation Criteria—Client Will

Blood Loss Severity (NOC)
Be free of signs of bleeding in GI aspirate or stools, with stabilization of Hgb and Hct.

Hydration (NOC)
Demonstrate improved fluid balance as evidenced by individually adequate urinary output with normal specific gravity, stable vital signs, moist mucous membranes, good skin turgor, and prompt capillary refill.

ACTIONS/INTERVENTIONS	RATIONALE
Bleeding Reduction: Gastrointestinal (NIC)	
Independent	
Note color and characteristics of vomitus, nasogastric (NG) tube drainage, and stools.	The first step in managing bleeding is to determine its location. Bright red blood that does not clear signals recent or acute arterial bleeding, perhaps caused by gastric ulceration; dark red blood may be old blood that has been retained in intestine or venous bleeding from varices. Coffee-ground appearance is suggestive of partially digested blood from slowly oozing area. Undigested food indicates obstruction or gastric tumor. In a rapid upper GI bleed, stool color may be red or maroon because of rapid transit time through the GI tract.
Monitor vital signs; compare with client's normal and previous readings. Take blood pressure (BP) in lying, sitting, and standing positions when possible.	Changes in BP and pulse may be used for rough estimate of blood loss; BP less than 90 mm Hg and pulse greater than 110 suggest a 25% decrease in volume, or approximately 1,000 mL. Postural hypotension reflects a decrease in circulating volume. *Note:* Heart rate may not rise above normal until up to 30% of total blood volume is lost.
Note client's individual physiological response to bleeding, such as changes in mentation, weakness, restlessness, anxiety, pallor, diaphoresis, tachypnea, and temperature elevation.	Symptomatology is useful in gauging severity and length of bleeding episode. Worsening of symptoms may reflect continued bleeding, inadequate fluid replacement, and shock.
Measure central venous pressure (CVP) if available.	Reflects circulating volume and cardiac response to bleeding and fluid replacement. CVP values between 5 and 20 cm H₂O usually reflect adequate volume.
Monitor intake and output (I&O) and correlate with weight changes. Measure blood and fluid losses via emesis, gastric suction or lavage, and stools.	Provides guidelines for fluid replacement.
Keep accurate record of subtotals of solutions and blood products during replacement therapy.	Potential exists for overtransfusion of fluids, especially when volume expanders are given before blood transfusions.
Maintain bedrest; prevent vomiting and straining at stool. Schedule activities to provide undisturbed rest periods. Eliminate noxious stimuli.	Activity and vomiting increases intra-abdominal pressure and can predispose to further bleeding.
Elevate head of bed during antacid gavage.	Prevents gastric reflux and aspiration of antacids, which can cause serious pulmonary complications.
Note signs of renewed bleeding after cessation of initial bleed.	Increased abdominal fullness and distention, nausea or renewed vomiting, and bloody diarrhea may indicate return of bleeding.
Observe for secondary bleeding from nose or gums, oozing from puncture sites, or appearance of ecchymotic areas following minimal trauma.	Loss of or inadequate replacement of clotting factors may precipitate development of DIC.
Provide clear or bland fluids when intake is resumed. Avoid caffeinated and carbonated beverages.	More easily digested and reduce risk of added irritation to inflamed tissues. Caffeine and carbonated beverages stimulate hydrochloric acid (HCl) production, possibly potentiating bleeding.
Collaborative	
Prepare for urgent endoscopy.	Indicated within 24 hours of acute UGIB for diagnosis and intervention when client presents with hematemesis, melena, or postural changes in blood pressure.

ACTIONS/INTERVENTIONS (continued)	RATIONALE (continued)
Monitor laboratory studies: Hgb, Hct, RBC count, and BUN/creatinine levels.	Aids in establishing blood replacement needs and monitoring effectiveness of therapy; for example, 1 unit of whole blood should raise Hct two to three points. Levels may initially remain stable because of loss of both plasma and RBCs. *Note:* Levels may not accurately reflect early or sudden blood loss, and low baseline levels may indicate preexisting anemia. BUN greater than 40 with normal creatinine level indicates major bleeding. BUN should return to client's normal level approximately 12 hours after bleeding has ceased.
Administer intravenous (IV) fluids or volume expanders, as indicated:	
0.9% sodium chloride, lactated Ringer's solution	Fluid replacement with isotonic crystalloid solutions depends on degree of hypovolemia and duration (acute or chronic) of bleeding. Other volume expanders, such as albumin, may be infused until type and cross-matching can be completed and blood transfusions begun. The majority of gastric bleeding can be managed without transfusion of blood products. *Note:* Use of lactated Ringer's solution may be contraindicated in presence of hepatic failure because metabolism of lactate is impaired and lactic acidosis may develop.
Fresh whole blood or packed RBCs	Fresh whole blood is indicated only for acute bleeding with severe volume and RBC depletion because stored blood may be deficient in clotting factors. Packed red blood cells (PRCs) are adequate for stable clients with subacute or chronic bleeding to increase oxygen-carrying capability. *Note:* PRCs are preferred for clients with heart failure (HF) to prevent fluid overload.
Platelets	Platelets are given to correct deficits in platelet number and clotting function. Clotting factors and blood components are depleted by two mechanisms: hemorrhagic loss and the clotting process at the site of bleeding.
FFP	FFP is an excellent source for clotting factors. Administered to clients with coagulation deficiencies who are bleeding or about to undergo an invasive procedure.
Insert and maintain large-bore NG tube in acute bleeding.	Provides avenue for removing irritating gastric secretions, blood, and clots; reduces nausea and vomiting; and facilitates diagnostic endoscopy.
Perform gastric lavage with cool or room-temperature saline until aspirate is light pink or clear and free of clots. Simultaneous low-pressure gastric suctioning and continuous saline infusion through the air port of a Salem sump tube may also be used.	Flushes out and breaks up clots and may reduce bleeding by local vasoconstriction. Facilitates visualization by endoscopy to locate bleeding source. *Note:* Research suggests that iced saline is no more effective than room temperature solution in controlling bleeding, and it may actually damage gastric mucosa and lower client's core temperature, which could prolong bleeding by inhibiting platelet function. Controversy also exists as to whether benefit is obtained from any gastric lavage, whether iced or room temperature.
Administer medications, as indicated:	
Proton pump inhibitors (PPIs), such as omeprazole (Prilosec), lansoprazole (Prevacid), robeprazole (Aciphex), pantoprazole (Protonix), and esomeprasole (Nexium)	PPIs have been shown in studies to be most effective after GI bleed to reduce recurrence of bleeding. PPIs (administered orally, by tube, or IV) can suppress acid secretion and have a long duration of action. Used for peptic ulcer disease (PUD) and GERD, or short-term therapy for duodenal ulcers. PPIs can heal duodenal ulcers in 2 to 4 weeks once severe bleeding is controlled. Typically given with antibiotics when *H. pylori* infection is present. Pantoprazole (Protonix), esomeprasole (Nexium), and lansoprazole (Prevacid) are PPIs available for IV administration. *Note:* Contraindicated in clients taking antiretrovirals and lactating females.
Sucralfate (Carafate)	Antiulcer agent that coats the stomach, adheres to the ulcer surface, and reinforces the mucosal barrier. *Note:* Impairs absorption of some drugs, such as theophylline, digoxin, phenytoin, tetracycline, amitriptyline. Contraindicated with heavy metal antagonists.

(continues on page 312)

Misoprostol (Cytotec)	Aids in mucus production and inhibits acid secretions. Used to prevent gastric ulcers associated with NSAID use. *Note:* Contraindicated in pregnancy and lactation.
Antacids: aluminum-based (Amphojel, Basaljel) and magnesium-based (Mylanta, Riopan, Maalox)	Antacids (administered orally or by gavage) may be used to reduce total acid load within the gastric lumen. Effectiveness is greatest for duodenal ulcers. Antacids maintain gastric pH level at 4.5 or higher and reduce risk of recurrence of bleeding. *Note:* Many drugs depend on a stomach pH less than 4 for proper absorption. Check drug reference before administration.
Belladonna and atropine	Anticholinergics may be used to decrease gastric motility, particularly in PUD after acute bleeding has subsided. *Note:* Contraindicated in clients taking potassium chloride supplements.
Octreotide (Sandostatin)	An analog of the hormone somatostatin thought to help control esophageal bleeding by decreasing blood flow to the gut, thereby lowering pressure to the portal system. *Note:* Current guidelines do not recommend use of this drug for nonvariceal GI bleeding.
Vasopressin (Pitressin)	Administration of intra-arterial vasoconstrictors may be needed in severe, prolonged bleeding (varices). *Note:* Effects of Pitressin are systemic, whereas octreotide is more regional.
Vitamin K_1 (AquaMephyton)	Promotes hepatic synthesis of coagulation factors to support clotting. *Note:* Use of sucralfate may decrease absorption of vitamin K.
Antiemetics such as metoclopramide (Reglan), prochlorperazine (Compazine), ondansetron (Zofran), and promethazine (Benadryl)	Alleviate nausea and prevent vomiting. *Note:* Contraindicated in lactating females.
Vitamin B_{12}	In diffuse atrophic gastritis, the intrinsic factor necessary for vitamin B_{12} absorption from the GI tract is not secreted, and individual may develop pernicious anemia.
Anti-infectives, such as tetracycline (Achromycin), metronidazole (Flagyl), amoxicillin (Amoxil), and clarithromycin (Biaxin)	Oral agents may be combined with antacids or histamine blockers to treat infections causing chronic gastritis or peptic ulcers (*H. pylori*).
Assist with and prepare client for GI procedure, such as the following:	
EGD with control of GI bleed, such as:	Hemostasis clips are applied directly to bleeding site, closing bleeding vessel.
Injection therapies	Epinephrine 1:10,000 causes vasoconstriction when injected directly into bleeding site. Volume of this drug also causes tamponade effect.
Variceal ligation	Performed during endoscopy, this banding technique is used often to control hemorrhage and is an effective alternative to sclerotherapy.
Sclerotherapy of esophageal varices with ethanolamine, polidocanol, or combination of sodium tetradecyl, alcohol, and sodium chloride	Performed during endoscopy, injection of an irritating (sclerosing) agent into esophageal varices to create thrombosis of the vein. This is used to stop bleeding and prevent recurrence after initial bleeding is controlled. The percentage of bleeding recurrence is still significant following this therapy in clients with varices.
Electrocoagulation or photocoagulation (laser) therapy	Provides direct coagulation of bleeding sites, such as those due to gastritis, duodenal ulcer, tumor, and esophageal (Mallory-Weiss) tear.
Balloon tamponade	Short-term intervention technique using Sengstaken-Blakemore tubes when medication or sclerotherapy fails to control esophageal bleed.
Surgical intervention	Total or partial gastrectomy, pyloroplasty, and vagotomy may be required to control and prevent future gastric bleeding. Shunt procedures (portacaval, splenorenal, mesocaval, or distal splenorenal) may be performed to divert blood flow and reduce pressure within esophageal vessels when other measures fail.
Radiological interventions	The most frequently used shunt is transjugular intrahepatic portosystemic shunt (TIPS). This controls bleeding in 90% of clients. The principle is the same as a surgically placed shunt for bleeding control.

NURSING DIAGNOSIS: risk for Shock

Risk factors may include
Hypovolemia

Possibly evidenced by
(Not applicable; presence of signs and symptoms establishes an *actual* diagnosis)

Desired Outcomes/Evaluation Criteria—Client Will

Circulation Status (NOC)
Maintain and improve tissue perfusion as evidenced by stabilized vital signs, warm skin, palpable peripheral pulses, ABGs
within client norms, and adequate urine output.

ACTIONS/INTERVENTIONS	RATIONALE
Shock Prevention (NIC)	
Independent	
Investigate changes in level of consciousness and reports of dizziness or headache.	Changes may reflect inadequate cerebral perfusion as a result of reduced arterial blood pressure. *Note:* Changes in sensorium may also reflect elevated ammonia levels or hepatic encephalopathy in client with liver disease.
Investigate reports of chest pain. Note location, quality, duration, and what relieves pain.	May reflect cardiac ischemia related to decreased perfusion. *Note:* Impaired oxygenation status resulting from blood loss can bring on myocardial infarction (MI) in client with cardiac disease.
Auscultate apical pulse. Monitor cardiac rate and rhythm, if continuous electrocardiogram (ECG) available and indicated.	Dysrhythmias and ischemic changes can occur as a result of hypotension, hypoxia, acidosis, electrolyte imbalance, or cooling near the heart if cold saline lavage is used to control bleeding.
Assess skin for coolness; pallor; diaphoresis; delayed capillary refill; and weak, thready peripheral pulses.	Vasoconstriction is a sympathetic response to lowered circulating volume and may occur as a side effect of vasopressin administration.
Note urinary output and specific gravity. Insert Foley catheter to accurately measure urine, as indicated.	Decreased systemic perfusion may cause kidney ischemia and failure, manifested by decreased urine output. Acute tubular necrosis (ATN) may develop if hypovolemic state is prolonged.
Note reports of abdominal pain, especially sudden, severe pain or pain radiating to shoulder.	Pain caused by gastric ulcer is often relieved after acute bleeding because of buffering effects of blood. Continued severe or sudden pain may reflect ischemia due to vasoconstrictive therapy, bleeding into biliary tract (hematobilia), or perforation with onset of peritonitis.
Observe skin for pallor and redness. Massage gently with lotion. Change position frequently.	Compromised peripheral circulation increases risk of skin breakdown as demonstrated by redness over bony prominence that does not blanch when digital pressure applied.
Collaborative	
Monitor ABGs and pulse oximetry.	Identifies hypoxemia and effectiveness of and need for therapy.
Provide supplemental oxygen, if indicated.	Treats hypoxemia and lactic acidosis during acute bleed.
Administer IV fluids, as indicated.	Maintains circulating volume and perfusion. A guideline for fluid replacement is 3 mL of fluid for each 1 mL of blood lost. (Refer to ND: risk for Bleeding.)

NURSING DIAGNOSIS: Fear/Anxiety [specify level]

May be related to
Change in health status, threat of death

Possibly evidenced by
Increased tension, restlessness, irritability, fearfulness
Trembling, tachycardia, diaphoresis
Lack of eye contact, focus on self
Verbalization of specific concern
Withdrawal, panic, or attack behavior

(continues on page 314)

Desired Outcomes/Evaluation Criteria—Client Will

Anxiety Self-Control (NOC)
Discuss fears and concerns recognizing healthy versus unhealthy fears.
Verbalize appropriate range of feelings.
Appear relaxed and report anxiety is reduced to a manageable level.
Demonstrate problem-solving and effective use of resources.

ACTIONS/INTERVENTIONS	RATIONALE
Anxiety Reduction (NIC)	
Independent	
Monitor physiological responses, such as tachypnea, palpitations, dizziness, headache, tingling sensations, and behavioral cues, such as restlessness, irritability, lack of eye contact, and combativeness or attack behavior.	May be indicative of the degree of fear client is experiencing—client may feel out of control of the situation or reach a state of panic. However, symptoms may also be related to physical condition or shock state.
Encourage verbalization of concerns. Assist client in expressing feelings by active listening.	Establishes a therapeutic relationship. Assists client in dealing with feelings, and provides opportunity to clarify misconceptions.
Acknowledge that this is a fearful situation and that others have expressed similar fears.	When client is expressing own fear, the validation that these feelings are normal can help client to feel less isolated.
Provide accurate, concrete information about what is being done, including sensations to expect and usual procedures undertaken.	Involves client in plan of care and decreases unnecessary anxiety about unknowns.
Provide a calm, restful environment.	Removing client from outside stressors promotes relaxation and may enhance coping skills.
Encourage significant other (SO) to stay with client, as able. Respond to call signal promptly. Use touch and eye contact, as appropriate.	Helps reduce fear of going through a frightening experience alone.
Provide opportunity for SO to express feelings and concerns. Encourage SO to project positive, realistic attitude.	Helps SO to deal with own anxiety and fears that can be transmitted to client. Promotes a supportive attitude that can facilitate recovery.
Demonstrate and encourage relaxation techniques such as visualization, deep-breathing exercises, and guided imagery.	Learning ways to relax can be helpful in reducing fear and anxiety. Because client with GI bleeding may be a person who has difficulty relaxing, learning these skills can be important to recovery and prevention of recurrence.
Help client identify and initiate positive coping behaviors used successfully in the past.	Successful behaviors can be fostered in dealing with current fear, enhancing client's sense of self-control and providing reassurance.
Encourage and support client in evaluation of lifestyle.	Changes may be necessary to avoid recurrence of ulcer condition.
Collaborative	
Administer medications, as indicated such as diazepam (Valium), clorazepate (Tranxene), alprazolam (Xanax).	Sedatives and antianxiety agents may be used on occasion to reduce anxiety and promote rest, particularly in client with an ulcer.
Refer to psychiatric clinical nurse specialist, social services, and spiritual advisor.	May need additional assistance during recovery to deal with consequences of emergency situation and adjustments to required and desired changes in lifestyle.

NURSING DIAGNOSIS: **acute/chronic Pain**

May be related to
Chemical burn of gastric mucosa, oral cavity
Physical response, such as reflex muscle spasm in the stomach wall

Possibly evidenced by
Communication of pain descriptors
Abdominal guarding, rigid body posture, facial grimacing
Autonomic responses, such as changes in vital signs in reaction to acute pain

Desired Outcomes/Evaluation Criteria—Client Will

Pain Level (NOC)
Verbalize relief of pain.
Demonstrate relaxed body posture and be able to sleep or rest appropriately.

ACTIONS/INTERVENTIONS	RATIONALE

Pain Management (NIC)

Independent

Note reports of pain, including location, duration, and intensity (0 to 10 scale).

Pain is not always present, but if present, should be compared with client's previous pain symptoms. This comparison may assist in diagnosis of etiology of bleeding and development of complications.

Review factors that aggravate or alleviate pain.

Helpful in establishing diagnosis and treatment needs.

Note nonverbal pain cues such as restlessness, reluctance to move, abdominal guarding, tachycardia, and diaphoresis. Investigate discrepancies between verbal and nonverbal cues.

Nonverbal cues may be both physiological and psychological and may be used in conjunction with verbal cues to evaluate extent and severity of the problem.

Provide small, frequent meals, as indicated for individual client.

Food has an acid-neutralizing effect and dilutes the gastric contents. Small meals prevent distention and the release of gastrin.

Identify and limit foods that create discomfort.

Specific foods that cause distress vary among individuals. Spicy foods, alcohol, and coffee can precipitate dyspepsia.

Assist with active and passive range-of-motion (ROM) exercises.

Reduces joint stiffness, minimizing pain and discomfort.

Provide frequent oral care and comfort measures including back rub and position change.

Halitosis from stagnant oral secretions is unappetizing and can aggravate nausea. Gingivitis and dental problems may arise.

Collaborative

Provide and implement prescribed dietary modifications.

Client may receive nothing by mouth (NPO) initially. When oral intake is allowed, food choices depend on the diagnosis and etiology of the bleeding.

Use regular rather than skim milk, if milk is allowed.

Fat in regular milk may decrease gastric secretions; however, the calcium and protein content (especially in skim milk) increases secretions.

Administer medications, as indicated:

  Analgesics, such as morphine sulfate, ketorolac (Toradol)

Helps relieve acute or severe pain. Morphine also reduces peristaltic activity, and Toradol exerts anti-inflammatory effects.

  Acetaminophen (Tylenol)

Promotes general comfort and rest.

  Antacids

Decrease gastric acidity by absorption or by chemical neutralization. Evaluate choice of antacid in regard to total health picture, such as sodium restriction.

  Anticholinergics, such as belladonna, atropine.

May be given at bedtime to decrease gastric motility, suppress acid production, delay gastric emptying, and alleviate nocturnal pain associated with gastric ulcer.

NURSING DIAGNOSIS: **deficient Knowledge [Learning Need] regarding disease process, prognosis, treatment, self-care, and discharge needs**

May be related to

Lack of information or recall

Unfamiliarity with information resources

Information misinterpretation

Possibly evidenced by

Verbalization of the problem, request for information, statement of misconceptions

Inaccurate follow through of instructions

Development of preventable complications

Desired Outcomes/Evaluation Criteria—Client Will

Knowledge: Disease Process (NOC)

Verbalize understanding of cause of own bleeding episode, if known, and treatment modalities used.

Begin to discuss own role in preventing recurrence.

Knowledge: Treatment Regimen (NOC)

Identify and implement necessary lifestyle changes.

Participate in treatment regimen.

ACTIONS/INTERVENTIONS	RATIONALE

Teaching: Disease Process ⓃⒾⒸ
Independent

Determine client perception of cause of bleeding.

Establishes knowledge base and provides some insight into how the teaching plan needs to be constructed for this individual.

Provide and review information regarding etiology of bleeding, relationship of lifestyle behaviors, and ways to reduce risk and contributing factors. Encourage questions.

Provides knowledge base from which client can make informed choices and decisions about future and control of health problems.

Assist client to identify relationship of food intake and precipitation of and relief from epigastric pain, including avoidance of gastric irritants, such as pepper, caffeine, alcohol, fruit juices, carbonated beverages, and extremely hot, cold, fatty, or spicy foods.

Caffeine stimulates gastric acidity. Alcohol contributes to erosion of gastric mucosa. Although current research indicates that diet does not contribute to the development of PUD, individuals may find that certain foods or fluids increase gastric secretion and pain.

Recommend small, frequent meals or snacks, chewing food slowly, eating at regular time, and avoiding skipping meals.

Frequent eating keeps HCl neutralized and dilutes stomach contents to minimize action of acid on gastric mucosa. Small meals prevent gastric overdistention.

Stress importance of reading labels on OTC drugs and either avoiding products containing aspirin or switching to enteric-coated aspirin. Recommend client discuss alternatives to NSAID use for pain relief.

Aspirin damages the protective mucosa, permitting gastric erosion, ulceration, and bleeding to occur. NSAID use increases the risk of PUD 5 to 20 times.

Review significance of signs and symptoms such as coffee-ground emesis, tarry stools, abdominal distention, and severe epigastric and abdominal pain radiating to shoulder or back.

Prompt medical evaluation and intervention is required to prevent more serious complications, such as perforation and severe bleeding.

Support use of stress-management techniques and avoidance of emotional stress.

Decreases extrinsic stimulation of HCl, reducing risk of recurrence of bleeding.

Review drug regimen, possible side effects, and interaction with other drugs, as appropriate.

Helpful to client understanding of reason for taking drugs and what symptoms are important to report to healthcare provider. *Note:* Aluminum-containing antacids inhibit the intestinal absorption of some drugs and affect scheduling of drug intake. Some men may incur impotence when using prescription-strength cimetidine (Tagamet). Alternative drug choices are PPIs and histamine H_2 blockers.

Encourage client to inform all healthcare providers of bleeding history.

May affect drug choices and concomitant prescriptions. Misoprostol (Cytotec) can be given with NSAIDs to inhibit gastric acid secretion and reduce risk of gastric irritability and lesions resulting from NSAID therapy.

Discuss importance of cessation of smoking. Refer to support groups and healthcare provider for assistance, as client desires, with treatments such as nicotine replacement gums or antismoking drugs.

Ulcer healing may be delayed in people who smoke, particularly in those who use cimetidine (Tagamet). Smoking stimulates gastric acidity and is associated with increased risk of peptic ulcer development and recurrence. *Note:* Many support services are available to the client who wants to stop smoking.

Refer to support groups or counseling for lifestyle and behavior changes and reduction of associated risk factors.

Alcohol users have a higher incidence of gastritis and esophageal varices.

POTENTIAL CONSIDERATIONS following acute hospitalization (dependent on client's age, physical condition and presence of complications, personal resources, and life responsibilities)
• *ineffective self Health Management*—decisional conflicts such as use of NSAIDs for arthritic and chronic pain condition, perceived benefits, including cessation of smoking and economic difficulties, particularly with the cost of medication

GASTRECTOMY/GASTRIC RESECTION

I. Indications and Procedures

a. Cancer

    i. Adenocarcinoma—most frequent diagnosis

    ii. Generally requires open technique and abdominal incision

    iii. Laparoscopic gastrectomy may be performed in early stage gastric cancers or when surgery is intended only for palliation of pain and symptomatic relief rather than cure.

    iv. Type of resection depends on whether the location of the gastric erosion is proximal or distal.

b. Ulcers

    i. Gastrectomy (usually partial) is performed for treatment of severe peptic ulcer where disease does not respond satisfactorily to medical therapy, for presence of bleeding or perforated ulcer, or for pyloric obstruction.

    ii. Antrectomy is usual procedure of choice for severe ulcer disease.

    iii. Antrectomy may be combined with other surgical procedures, such as a vagotomy, in presence of duodenal ulcers.

II. Statistics

a. Morbidity: An estimated 21,500 Americans will be diagnosed with gastric cancer in 2008, and two-thirds are over the age of 66 (National Cancer Institute [NCI], 2008).

b. Mortality: Operative mortality rate in gastric cancer is as low as 1% to 3% (Layke & Lopez, 2004).

GLOSSARY

Adenocarcinoma: Cancer that begins in the epithelial cells, which line certain internal organs (including stomach) and have secretory properties.

Afferent loop syndrome: Complication following gastrectomy, characterized by abdominal bloating and pain after eating, frequently followed by nausea and vomiting. This is treated by surgical correction.

Antrectomy: Limited form of gastrectomy where the antrum, or lower portion of the stomach preceding the pylorus, is removed.

Distal: Refers to a part of the body that is farther away from the center of the body than another part.

Feeding tubes: Identified according to the anatomic location in which they enter the alimentary tract—nasogastric (NG), orogastric (OG), nasointestinal (NI), or jejunal.

Gastric resection: Operation to remove all or part of the stomach.

Paralytic (adynamic) ileus: Loss of intestinal motility persisting more than 3 days postoperative, leading to abdominal distention with absent or hypoactive bowel sounds, nausea, vomiting, and obstipation or constipation.

Proximal: Toward the center of the body or closer to the top of an organ rather than being farther away.

Pyloric obstruction: Blockage at the exit of the stomach.

Subtotal gastrectomy (also called partial gastrectomy): Removal of up to three-quarters of the stomach.

Total gastrectomy: Removal of the entire stomach.

Vagotomy: Vagus nerve is surgically severed to reduce acid production in the stomach.

Care Setting

The client is admitted to inpatient or same day outpatient surgical unit. The procedure may be done as an open procedure or via laparoscope.

Related Concerns

Cancer, page 846

Pancreatitis, page 458

Peritonitis, page 349

Psychosocial aspects of care, page 749

Surgical intervention, page 782

Total nutritional support: parenteral/enteral feeding, page 469

Upper gastrointestinal/esophageal bleeding, page 306

Data depend on the underlying condition necessitating surgery. (Refer to CP: Upper Gastrointestinal/Esophageal Bleeding.)

DIAGNOSTIC DIVISION

DISCHARGE PLAN CONSIDERATIONS:
- Assistance with administration of enteral feedings or total parenteral nutrition (TPN), if required
- Acquisition of supplies

⬧ Refer to section at end of plan for postdischarge considerations.

Nursing Priorities

1. Promote healing and adequate nutritional intake.
2. Prevent complications.
3. Provide information about surgical procedure, prognosis, treatment needs, and concerns.

Discharge Goals

1. Nutritional intake adequate for individual needs.
2. Complications prevented or minimized.
3. Surgical procedure, prognosis, therapeutic regimen, and long-term needs understood.
4. Plan in place to meet needs after discharge.

In addition to nursing diagnoses identified in this care plan, refer to CP: Surgical Intervention for nursing interventions related to general surgery.

NURSING DIAGNOSIS: **risk for imbalanced Nutrition: Less than Body Requirements**

Risk factors may include
Restriction of fluids and food
Change in digestive process, absorption of nutrients

Possibly evidenced by
(Not applicable; presence of signs and symptoms establishes an *actual* diagnosis)

Desired Outcomes/Evaluation Criteria—Client Will

Nutritional Status (NOC)
Maintain stable weight and demonstrate progressive weight gain toward goal with normalization of laboratory values. Be free of signs of malnutrition.

ACTIONS/INTERVENTIONS	RATIONALE
Nutrition Therapy (NIC)	
Independent	
Maintain patency of NG, OG, or NI tube when used. Be aware of feeding tube placement—enterostomal or jejunostomal. Notify physician if tube becomes dislodged.	Intestinal tubes are inserted to provide rest for gastrointestinal (GI) tract during acute postoperative phase until return of normal GI function. These are attached to suction. Feeding tubes may be inserted at time of surgery or later and are used to provide enteral feedings once gut is functional. *Note:* Although several methods have been used to identify tube placement at the bedside, such as aspiration of gastric contents, measurement of trypsin, pH, and pepsin levels, abdominal radiographs may be necessary to confirm location of tube, and the physician/surgeon may need to reposition the tube endoscopically to prevent injury to the operative area.
Note character and amount of gastric drainage.	Drainage may be bloody for first few hours and then should clear or turn greenish gold. Continued or recurrent bleeding suggest complications and should be reported to physician.

ACTIONS/INTERVENTIONS (continued)

Caution client to limit the intake of ice chips.

Provide oral hygiene on a regular, frequent basis, including petroleum jelly for lips.

Auscultate for resumption of bowel sounds and note passage of flatus.

Monitor tolerance to fluid and food intake when resumed, noting abdominal distention, reports of increased pain or cramping, and nausea and vomiting.

Note admission weight and compare with subsequent readings.

Collaborative

Collaborate with nutritional team and dietitian, as indicated.

Administer intravenous (IV) fluids, parenteral or enteral nutrition, as indicated.

Monitor laboratory studies: hemoglobin/hematocrit (Hgb/Hct), electrolytes, and total protein and prealbumin.

Progress diet as tolerated, advancing from liquids to soft, formula run through a blender and bland diet with small feedings offered several times per day.

Caution client to avoid drinking fluids during mealtimes.

Administer medications, as indicated:
  Anticholinergics and antispasmodics, such as atropine and propantheline (Pro-Banthine)
  Fat-soluble vitamin supplements, including vitamin B_{12} and calcium

  Iron preparations
  Protein supplements
  Pancreatic enzymes and bile salts
  Medium-chain triglycerides (MCT)

RATIONALE (continued)

Excessive intake of ice produces nausea and can wash out electrolytes via the NG tube.

Prevents discomfort of dry mouth and cracked lips caused by fluid restriction and the NG tube.

Peristalsis can be expected to return about the third postoperative day, signaling readiness to resume oral intake.

Complications such as paralytic ileus, obstruction, delayed gastric emptying, or gastric dilation, may occur. Even if the above complications do not occur, "dumping syndrome" is a fairly common aftereffect of stomach surgery. Symptoms include bloating, nausea, weakness, sweating, and rapid heartbeat 30 to 60 minutes after a meal. (Refer to ND: deficient Knowledge [Learning Need], below.)

Provides information about adequacy of dietary intake and determination of nutritional needs.

Aids in determining number of calories and types of nutrients for meeting client's nutritional needs.

Meets fluid and nutritional needs until oral intake can be resumed. *Note:* Early enteral feedings have been found to stimulate gut immunological function and can assist in maintaining gut structure and function. TPN is usually reserved for clients who are critically ill at the time of surgery or those with total gastrectomy. (Refer to CP: Total Nutritional Support: Parenteral/Enteral Feeding for additional interventions.)

Indicators of fluid and nutritional needs and effectiveness of therapy. Detects developing complications.

After NG or feeding tube is removed, intake is advanced gradually to prevent gastric irritation and distention.

Client will quickly feel full when eating even small amounts of food. Adding fluid to meals reduces the nutrients client is able to eat.

May be given to manage dumping syndrome, enhancing digestion and absorption of nutrients.

Depending on the type and extent of gastric surgery performed, absorption of nutrients, vitamins, and minerals may be impaired to a significant degree. For example, removal of the stomach prevents absorption of vitamin B_{12} (owing to loss of intrinsic factor) and can lead to pernicious anemia. Rapid emptying of the stomach reduces absorption of calcium.

Corrects iron deficiency anemia.

Additional protein may be helpful for tissue repair and healing.

Enhance digestive process.

Promote absorption of fats and fat-soluble vitamins to prevent malabsorption problems.

NURSING DIAGNOSIS: **deficient Knowledge [Learning Need] regarding procedure, prognosis, treatment, self-care, and discharge needs**

May be related to
Lack of exposure, recall
Information misinterpretation
Unfamiliarity with information resources

Possibly evidenced by
Questions, statement of misconception
Inaccurate follow-through of instruction
Development of preventable complications

(continues on page 320)

deficient Knowledge [Learning Need] regarding procedure, prognosis, treatment, self-care, and discharge needs (continued)

Desired Outcomes/Evaluation Criteria—Client Will

Knowledge: Disease Process (NOC)
Verbalize understanding of procedure, disease process, and prognosis.
Verbalize understanding of functional changes.

Knowledge: Treatment Regimen (NOC)
Identify necessary interventions and behaviors to maintain appropriate weight.
Correctly perform necessary procedures, explaining reasons for actions.

ACTIONS/INTERVENTIONS	RATIONALE
Teaching: Disease Process (NIC)	
Independent	
Review surgical procedure and long-term expectations.	Provides knowledge base from which informed choices can be made. Recovery following gastric surgery is often slower than may be anticipated with similar types of surgery. Improved strength and partial normalization of dietary pattern may not be evident for at least 3 months, and full return to usual intake (three "normal" meals a day) may take up to 12 months. This prolonged convalescence may be difficult for the client and significant other (SO) to deal with, especially if he or she has not been adequately prepared.
Discuss and identify stress situations and how to avoid them. Investigate job-related issues.	Stress and stress reactions can alter gastric motility, interfering with optimal digestion, especially if client has been very ill in conjunction with the surgery. *Note:* Client may require vocational counseling if change in employment is indicated.
Review dietary needs and regimen, such as low-carbohydrate, low-fat, high-protein, and importance of maintaining vitamin and mineral supplementation.	May prevent deficiencies, enhance healing, and promote cooperation with therapy. *Note:* Low-fat diet may be required to reduce risk of alkaline reflux gastritis. Vitamin and mineral supplementation is necessary after gastrectomy to correct certain deficiencies, especially vitamin B_{12}, iron, and folate. Vitamin D and calcium are also needed to prevent and treat the bone problems that often occur. Such problems include softening and bending of the bones, which can produce pain and osteoporosis (Helwick, 2002).
Discuss the importance of eating small, frequent meals slowly and in a relaxed atmosphere; resting after meals; avoiding extremely hot or cold food; restricting high-fiber foods, caffeine, milk products, alcohol, and excess sugars and salt; and taking fluids between meals rather than with food.	These measures can be helpful in avoiding gastric distention or irritation and stress on surgical repair, dumping syndrome, and reactive hypoglycemia. *Note:* Ice-cold fluids or foods can cause gastric spasms.
Instruct in avoiding certain fibrous foods, and discuss the necessity of chewing food well.	Client may have impaired ability to digest such foods as citrus skins or seeds, which can collect, forming a mass (phytobezoar formation) that is not excreted.
Recommend foods containing pectin: citrus fruits, bananas, apples, yellow vegetables, and beans.	Increased intake of these foods may reduce incidence of dumping syndrome
Identify foods that can cause gastric irritation and increase gastric acid: chocolate, spicy foods, whole grains, and raw vegetables.	Limiting or avoiding these foods reduces risk of gastric bleeding and recurrent ulcer formation in some individuals.
Identify symptoms that may indicate dumping syndrome, such as weakness, profuse perspiration, epigastric fullness, nausea or vomiting, abdominal cramping, faintness, flushing, explosive diarrhea, and palpitations occurring within 15 minutes to 1 hour after eating.	Can cause severe discomfort or even shock and reduces absorption of nutrients. Usually self-limiting (1 to 3 weeks after surgery) but can become chronic.
Discuss signs of hypoglycemia and corrective interventions, such as ingesting cheese and crackers and orange or grape juice.	Awareness helps clients take actions to prevent progression of symptoms.
Suggest client weigh self on a regular basis.	Change in dietary pattern—early satiety due to change in stomach size—and efforts to avoid dumping syndrome may cause client to limit intake, causing weight loss.
Review medication purpose, dosage, schedule, and possible side effects.	Understanding therapeutic needs can reduce risk of complications. Anticholinergics or pectin powder may be given to reduce incidence of dumping syndrome; antacids or histamine antagonists reduce gastric irritation.

ACTIONS/INTERVENTIONS (continued)

Caution client to read labels and avoid products containing aspirin or Motrin.

Discuss reasons and importance of cessation of smoking. Offer referral for assistance if client is interested in smoking cessation.

Identify signs and symptoms requiring medical evaluation, such as persistent nausea, vomiting or abdominal fullness, weight loss, diarrhea, foul-smelling fatty or tarry stools, bloody or coffee-ground vomitus, and presence of bile and fever. Instruct client to report changes in pain characteristics.

Emphasize importance of regular checkups with healthcare provider.

RATIONALE (continued)

Can cause gastric irritation and bleeding.

Smoking stimulates gastric acid production, relaxes lower esophageal sphincter, and may cause vasoconstriction, compromising mucous membranes and increasing risk of gastric and esophageal irritation and ulceration.

Prompt recognition and intervention may prevent serious consequences or potential complications such as pancreatitis, peritonitis, and afferent loop syndrome.

Necessary to detect developing complications—anemia, problems with nutrition, and recurrence of disease.

POTENTIAL CONSIDERATIONS following acute hospitalization (dependent on client's age, physical condition, presence of complications, personal resources, and life responsibilities)

• *risk for imbalanced Nutrition: Less than Body Requirements*—change in digestive process and absorption of nutrients, early satiety, gastric irritation

• *Fatigue*—decreased energy production, states of discomfort, increased energy requirements to perform activities of daily living (ADLs)

INFLAMMATORY BOWEL DISEASE (IBD): ULCERATIVE COLITIS, CROHN'S DISEASE

I. Pathophysiolgy—Abnormal response of the immune system, leading to chronic inflammation of various portions of the alimentary tract

II. Classifications

  a. Ulcerative colitis (UC)

    i. Usually starts in rectum and distal portions of the colon, possibly spreading upward to involve the sigmoid and descending colon or the entire colon

    ii. Intermittent, with acute exacerbation and long remissions; however, 30% to 40% of individuals have continuous symptoms.

    iii. Cure is effected only by total removal of colon and rectum and rectal mucosa.

  b. Crohn's disease

    i. Found in any portion of the alimentary tract from the mouth to the anus, most commonly in the small intestine or terminal ileum

    ii. Slowly progressive chronic disease with intermittent acute episodes

    iii. Five types of Crohn's disease (A.D.A.M. Encyclopedia, 2007)

      1. Ileocolitis, the most common form, affects the lowest part of the small intestine and the large intestine.

      2. Ileitis affects the ileum.

      3. Gastroduodenal Crohn's disease causes inflammation in the stomach and first part of the small intestine (duodenum).

      4. Jejunoileitis causes spotty patches of inflammation in the top half of the small intestine or jejunum.

      5. Crohn's granulomatous colitis only affects the large intestine.

    iv. No known cure

III. Etiology (National Digestive Diseases Information Clearinghouse [NDDIC], 2007)

  a. Unknown, but may result from a complex interplay between genetic and environmental factors

  b. Inability to downregulate immune responses, and consequently, the mucosal immune system remains chronically activated and the intestine chronically inflamed (Hanauer, 2006)

  c. Additional risk factors include smoking (in Crohn's disease) and use of nonsteroidal anti-inflammatory drugs (NSAIDs) or isotretinion (Acutane).

  d. Periods of remission are interspersed with episodes of acute inflammation, characterized by frequent episodes of diarrhea, abdominal pain, fever, and weight loss.

  e. Extraintestinal manifestations (EMs) include systemic inflammation affecting most of the body's organ systems—internal organs, eyes, blood, skin, and musculoskeletal system.

IV. Statistics (National Women's Health Information Center, 2005)

  a. Morbidity: More than 1 million people in the United States are affected, with 30,000 new cases annually; higher incidence in late adolescence, with onset often between ages 15 and 35; men and women equally affected.

  b. Mortality: Rare, although life expectancy may be reduced in certain populations, such as older age at onset and development of pancolitis (Loftus, 2003).

  c. Cost: Estimated at $100 billion for nonadherence to long-term medical therapy for UC (Kane, 2006).

Alimentary tract: Organs comprising the pharynx, esophagus, stomach, small intestine, and large intestine, all of which are involved in digestion and absorption.

Borborygmus: Loud, rumbling bowel sounds caused by peristalsis.

Erythema nodosum: Inflammatory process with raised, tender, red nodules located under the skin, which are 1 to 5 cm in size.

Ileoanal anastomosis, or pull-through operation: Removes the colon and the inside of the rectum, leaving the outer muscles of the rectum. The surgeon then attaches the ileum to the inside of the rectum and the anus, creating a pouch in which waste is stored and passed through the anus in the usual manner.

Ileostomy: Creates a small opening in the abdomen, called a stoma, and attaches the end of the small intestine, called the ileum, to it. Waste travels through the small intestine and exits the body through the stoma. A pouch is worn over the opening to collect waste, and the client empties the pouch as needed.

Peristalsis: Progressive, involuntary rippling motion of muscles in the digestive tract.

Pyoderma gangrenosum: Inflammatory, purulent, pinpoint necrotic papules that can progress to deep ulcers.

Steatorrhea: Foul-smelling and fatty stools seen in some malabsorption syndromes.

Stomatitis: Inflammation or ulceration of the mouth including the lips, tongue, and mucous membranes.

Care Setting

Care is usually handled at the community level; however, severe exacerbations requiring advanced pain control, nutrition, and rehydration may necessitate short stay in acute care medical unit.

Related Concerns

Fluid and electrolyte imbalances, page 903

Peritonitis, page 349

Psychosocial aspects of care, page 749

Total nutritional support: parenteral/enteral feeding, page 469

Client Assessment Database (Ulcerative Colitis)

DIAGNOSTIC DIVISION MAY REPORT	MAY EXHIBIT
ACTIVITY/REST • Weakness, fatigue, malaise, exhaustion • Insomnia, not sleeping through the night because of diarrhea • Feeling restless • Restriction of activities or work due to effects of disease process	
CIRCULATION	• Tachycardia—response to fever, dehydration, inflammatory process, and pain • *Blood pressure:* Hypotension, including postural changes • Bruising, ecchymotic areas—insufficient vitamin K intake
EGO INTEGRITY • Anxiety, apprehension, emotional upsets, such as feelings of helplessness, hopelessness • Acute or chronic stress factors, such as family and job-related, expense of treatment	• Withdrawal, narrowed focus • Depression
ELIMINATION • Stool texture varying from soft-formed to mushy or watery • Unpredictable, intermittent, frequent, uncontrollable episodes of bloody diarrhea (as many as 10 to 30 stools per day) • Sense of urgency and cramping (tenesmus) • Passing blood, pus, or mucus with or without passing feces • Rectal bleeding • Intermittent constipation	• Diminished or hyperactive bowel sounds, absence of peristalsis or presence of visible peristaltic waves

Client Assessment Database (Ulcerative Colitis) (continued)

DIAGNOSTIC DIVISION MAY REPORT (continued)	MAY EXHIBIT (continued)

FOOD/FLUID
- Anorexia
- Nausea, vomiting
- Weight loss (not common, but can occur as a result of decreased intake)
- Dietary intolerances and sensitivities, such as with raw fruits or vegetables, dairy products, fatty foods

- Decreased subcutaneous fat and muscle mass
- Weakness, poor muscle tone and skin turgor
- Mucous membranes pale; sore, dry, inflamed buccal cavity; cracking of tongue due to dehydration or malnutrition

HYGIENE
- Inability to maintain self-care

- Stomatitis reflecting vitamin deficiency

PAIN/DISCOMFORT
- Mild abdominal cramping to severe pain and tenderness in lower-left quadrant; may be relieved with defecation
- Migratory joint pain, tenderness (arthritis)
- Eye pain, sensitivity to light (photophobia)

- Abdominal tenderness, distension, rigidity

SAFETY
- History of systemic lupus erythematosus (SLE), hemolytic anemia, vasculitis
- Arthritis—worsening of symptoms with exacerbations in bowel disease
- Temperature elevation 104°F to 105°F (40°C to 40.6°C) (acute exacerbation)
- Blurred vision
- Allergies to foods—release of histamine into bowel has an inflammatory effect

- Skin lesions may be present, such as erythema nodosum on arms, face; pyoderma gangrenosum on trunk, legs, ankles

SEXUALITY
- Reduced frequency, avoidance of sexual activity

SOCIAL INTERACTION
- Relationship or role problems related to condition
- Inability to be socially active

TEACHING/LEARNING
- Family history of inflammatory bowel disease (IBD), immune disorders; increased prevalence in Jewish population
- Use of multiple medications or over-the-counter (OTC) medications for bowel health and use of herbal remedies, such as peppermint, psyllium, chamomile

DISCHARGE PLAN CONSIDERATIONS
- Assistance with dietary requirements, medication regimen, psychological support

▸ Refer to section at end of plan for postdischarge considerations.

| TEST
WHY IT IS DONE	WHAT IT TELLS ME
BLOOD TESTS	
• *Complete blood count (CBC):* Battery of screening tests that typically includes hemoglobin (Hgb); hematocrit (Hct); red blood cell (RBC) count, morphology, indices, and distribution width index; platelet count and size; white blood cell (WBC) count and differential.	May show hyperchromic anemia (active disease generally present because of blood loss and iron deficiency); leukocytosis may occur, especially in fulminating or complicated cases and in clients on steroid therapy. Platelets may be increased (thrombocytosis) as a result of inflammatory process.
• *Erythrocyte sedimentation rate (ESR):* Measures inflammation in the body.	Elevated in acute inflammation according to severity of disease.
• *Serum iron levels:* Measures the level of iron in the liquid part of client's blood.	Lowered because of blood loss, poor dietary intake, or malabsorption.
• *Prothrombin time (PT):* One of several tests for blood for clotting; used to identify a bleeding disorder.	Prolonged in severe cases from altered factors VII and X caused by vitamin K deficiency.
• *Electrolytes:* Charged minerals that, in solution, conduct an electric current to transport nutrients and wastes across cell membranes, regulate fluid balance, and help maintain pH level.	Decreased levels of potassium, magnesium, and zinc because of malabsorption; common in severe disease.
• *Prealbumin/albumin/total proteins:* Measurement of level of proteins in plasma to determine nutritional status.	Decreased because of loss of plasma proteins, disturbed liver function, and decreased dietary intake.
OTHER DIAGNOSTIC STUDIES	
• *Endoscopic examinations (proctosigmoidoscopy or colonoscopy):* Gold standard for diagnosing UC, especially when biopsy is included.	Identifies inflamed and lacerated tissues, deep ulcerations, adhesions, and changes in luminal wall; rules out bowel obstruction.
• *Stool specimens:* Examination of feces are used in initial diagnosis and in following disease progression.	Mainly composed of mucus, blood, pus, and intestinal organisms, especially *Entamoeba histolytica* (active stage). Fecal leukocytes and RBCs indicate inflammation of gastrointestinal (GI) tract. Stool that is positive for bacterial pathogens, ova, and parasites or *Clostridium* indicates infection. Stool positive for fat indicates malabsorption.
• *Rectal biopsy and cytology:* Biopsy removes a small piece of rectal (anal) tissue for examination. Cytology is a study of the cells.	Neoplastic changes can be detected as well as characteristic inflammatory infiltrates, called crypt abscesses.
• *Barium enema (also called lower GI series):* X-ray of the rectum, colon, and lower part of the small intestine. Barium is given rectally to coat the lining of the colon so that abnormal areas will show up on the x-ray.	May be performed after visual examination, although rarely done during acute, relapsing stage because it can exacerbate condition.
• *Magnetic resonance imaging (MRI), computed tomography (CT) scan, and ultrasound:* Various scans may be done to detect pathology.	May reveal intestinal abscesses, masses, strictures, or fistulas (possible complications of UC).

Client Assessment Database (Crohn's Disease)

| DIAGNOSTIC DIVISION
MAY REPORT	MAY EXHIBIT
ACTIVITY/REST	
• Weakness, fatigue, malaise, exhaustion	
• Feelings of restlessness	
• Restriction of activities or work due to effects of disease process	
EGO INTEGRITY	
• Anxiety, apprehension, emotional upsets, feelings of helplessness, hopelessness	• Withdrawal, narrowed focus, depression
• Acute or chronic stress factors, such as family and job-related, expense of treatment	

DIAGNOSTIC DIVISION MAY REPORT (continued)	MAY EXHIBIT (continued)

ELIMINATION
- Unpredictable, intermittent, frequent, uncontrollable episodes of nonbloody diarrhea; soft or semiliquid with flatus
- Foul-smelling, fatty stools
- History of renal stones (increased oxalates in the urine)

- Hyperactive bowel sounds with gurgling, splashing sound
- Visible peristalsis

FOOD/FLUID
- Anorexia; nausea, vomiting
- Weight loss; failure to grow
- Dietary intolerance, sensitivity, such as to dairy products or fatty foods

- Decreased subcutaneous fat and muscle mass
- Weakness, poor muscle tone and skin turgor
- Mucous membranes pale

HYGIENE
- Inability to maintain self-care

PAIN/DISCOMFORT
- Tender abdomen with cramping pain in lower right quadrant (inflammation involving all layers of bowel wall and possibly the mesentery); pain in midlower abdomen (jejunal involvement)
- Referred tenderness to periumbilical region
- Perineal tenderness, pain
- Migratory joint pain, tenderness (arthritis)
- Eye pain, sensitivity to light (photophobia)

- Abdominal tenderness, distension

SAFETY
- History of arthritis, SLE, hemolytic anemia, vasculitis
- Temperature elevation—low-grade fever
- Blurred vision

- Skin lesions may present: erythema nodosum on face, arms; pyoderma gangrenosum on trunk, legs, ankles; perineal lesions, anorectal fistulas
- Ankylosing spondylitis
- Uveitis, conjunctivitis or iritis
- Clotting disorders

SOCIAL INTERACTION
- Relationship or role problems related to condition; inability to be active socially

TEACHING/LEARNING
- Family history of IBD, immune disorders, cultural factor—increased prevalence in Jewish population, northern European, and Anglo-Saxon derivation
- Use of multiple medications or OTC medications for bowel health and use of herbal remedies, such as aloe, chamomile, flax, garlic, boswellia, echinacea, goldenseal

DISCHARGE PLAN CONSIDERATIONS
- Assistance with dietary requirements, medication regimen, psychological support

▶ Refer to section at end of plan for postdischarge considerations.

TEST WHY IT IS DONE	WHAT IT TELLS ME
BLOOD TESTS • *Complete Blood Count CBC:* Battery of screening tests that typically includes Hgb; Hct; RBC count, morphology, indices, and distribution width index; platelet count and size; WBC count and differential.	Anemia (low Hgb and hypochromic, occasionally macrocytic RBCs) may occur because of blood loss from the mucosa and iron deficiency. WBCs are usually increased.
• *ESR and C-reactive protein (CRP):* Measure amount of inflammation in the body.	Increased in client with active inflammation.
• *Prealbumin/albumin/total proteins:* Measurement of level of protein in plasma to determine nutritional status.	Decreased because of loss of intestinal proteins.
• *Serum iron-binding capacity, folic acid:* Helps to determine nutritional status and diagnose cause of anemia.	Decreased because of chronic infection or secondary to blood loss. Alterations may occur because of poor vitamin B$_{12}$ absorption.
• *Blood clotting studies:* Measurement of coagulation time to determine bleeding disorders.	
• *Electrolytes:* Charged minerals that, in solution, conduct an electric current to transport nutrients and wastes across cell membranes, regulate fluid balance, and help maintain pH level.	Potassium, calcium, and magnesium may be decreased due to malabsorption. Sodium may be increased if kidney dysfunction is present.
OTHER DIAGNOSTIC STUDIES • *Endoscopic examination—esophagogastroduodenoscopy, sigmoidoscopy, or colonoscopy with biopsy:* Gold standard for diagnosis, especially when biopsy included.	Identifies inflamed and lacerated tissues, deep ulcerations, adhesions, changes in luminal wall; rules out bowel obstruction. Any granuloma in the biopsy confirms diagnosis of Crohn's disease.
• *Barium swallow or barium enema:* Radiographic studies of the upper GI tract or rectum, colon, and lower part of the small intestine. Barium is given orally or rectally to coat the lining of the GI tract so that abnormal areas will show up on the x-ray.	Barium swallow may demonstrate luminal narrowing in the terminal ileum, stiffening of the bowel wall, mucosal irritability, or ulceration. Fistulas are common and are usually found in the terminal ileum, but may be present in segments throughout the GI tract.
• *MRI, CT scan, and ultrasound:* Various scans may be done to detect pathology.	May reveal kidney stones, gallstones, or other diseases of the liver and biliary system (possible complications of Crohn's disease).
• *Stool examination:* Examination of feces are used in initial diagnosis and in following disease progression.	Stool may be positive for occult blood (mucosal erosion); WBCs may be increased, indicating infection; steatorrhea and bile salts may be noted.
• *Urine oxalate:* Increased excretion may reflect malabsorption in distal small intestine.	Very high levels of urinary oxalate are a result of a lack of intestinal calcium, chronic diarrhea, and low urinary calcium (can cause kidney stones).

Nursing Priorities

1. Control diarrhea and promote optimal bowel function.
2. Minimize or prevent complications.
3. Promote optimal nutrition.
4. Minimize mental and emotional stress.
5. Provide information about disease process, treatment needs, and long-term aspects and potential complications of recurrent disease.

Discharge Goals

1. Bowel function stabilized.
2. Complications prevented or controlled.
3. Dealing positively with condition.
4. Disease process, prognosis, therapeutic regimen, and potential complications understood.
5. Plan in place to meet needs after discharge.

NURSING DIAGNOSIS: **Diarrhea**

May be related to
Inflammation, irritation, or malabsorption of the bowel
Presence of toxins
Segmental narrowing of the lumen

Possibly evidenced by
Increased bowel sounds, peristalsis
Frequent, and often severe, watery stools (acute phase)
Changes in stool color
Abdominal pain; urgency, cramping

Desired Outcomes/Evaluation Criteria—Client Will

Bowel Elimination (NOC)
Report reduction in frequency of stools and return to more normal stool consistency.
Identify and avoid contributing factors.

ACTIONS/INTERVENTIONS	RATIONALE
Diarrhea Management (NIC)	
Independent	
Observe and record stool frequency, characteristics, amount, and precipitating factors.	Helps differentiate individual disease and assesses severity of episode.
Promote bedrest and provide bedside commode.	Rest decreases intestinal motility and reduces the metabolic rate when infection or hemorrhage is a complication. Urge to defecate may occur without warning and be uncontrollable, thus increasing risk of incontinence and falls if facilities are not close at hand.
Remove stool promptly. Provide room deodorizers.	Reduces noxious odors to avoid undue client embarrassment.
Identify foods and fluids that precipitate diarrhea, such as raw vegetables and fruits, whole-grain cereals, condiments, carbonated drinks, and milk products.	Avoiding intestinal irritants promotes intestinal rest.
Restart oral fluid intake gradually. Offer clear liquids hourly and avoid cold fluids.	Provides colon rest by omitting or decreasing the stimulus of foods and fluids. Gradual resumption of liquids may prevent cramping and recurrence of diarrhea; however, cold fluids can increase intestinal motility.
Provide opportunity to vent frustrations related to disease process.	Presence of disease with unknown cause that is difficult to cure and that may require surgical intervention can lead to stress reactions that may aggravate condition.
Observe for fever, tachycardia, lethargy, leukocytosis, decreased serum protein, anxiety, and prostration.	May signify that toxic megacolon or perforation and peritonitis are imminent or have occurred, necessitating immediate medical intervention.
Collaborative	
Administer medications, as indicated:	
Antidiarrheals, such as diphenoxylate (Lomotil), loperamide (Imodium), and anodyne suppositories	Decreases GI motility or propulsion (peristalsis) and diminishes digestive secretions to relieve cramping and diarrhea. *Note:* Use with caution in UC because they may precipitate toxic megacolon.
Anti-inflammatories, such as mesalamine (Pentasa, Asacol); mesalamine-containing drugs, for example, sulfasalazine (Azulfidine); and aminosalicylates, drugs that contain 5-aminosalicyclic acid (5-ASA), such as olsalazine (Dipentum) and balsalazide (Calazal)	Most people with mild or moderate ulcerative colitis are treated first with the group of drugs containing mesalamine, a substance that helps control inflammation. Sulfasalazine is the most commonly used of these drugs. Clients who do not benefit from it or who cannot tolerate it may receive 5-ASA agents, which are given orally, through an enema, or in a suppository, depending on the location of the inflammation in the colon. This class of drugs is also used in cases of relapse.
Steroids, such as adrenocorticotropic hormone (ACTH), hydrocortisone (Cortenema, Cortifoam), prednisolone (Delta-Cortef), and prednisone (Deltasone)	Decreases acute inflammatory process. Steroid enemas (Cortenema) may be given in mild to moderate disease to aid absorption of the drug—possibly with atropine sulfate or belladonna suppository. Current research suggests an 8-week course of time-release steroids may effect remission in Crohn's disease; however, steroids are contraindicated if intra-abdominal abscesses are suspected.

(continues on page 328)

ACTIONS/INTERVENTIONS (continued)

Immune system suppressors, also called immunomodulators, such as azathioprine (Imuran), 6-mercaptopurine (Purinethol), methotrexate (Mexate), and cyclosporine (Sandimmune)

Tissue necrosis factor (TNF) blocker, such as infliximab (Remicade)

Anti-infectives, such as metronidazole (Flagyl) and ciprofloxacin (Cipro)

Prepare for surgical intervention, such as colectomy, proctocolectomy, or ileostomy.

RATIONALE (continued)

Immunosuppressant may be given to block inflammatory response, decrease steroid requirements, and promote healing of fistulas.

This drug is the first of a group of medications that blocks the body's inflammation response. Approved for the treatment of moderate to severe Crohn's disease that does not respond to standard therapies (mesalamine substances, corticosteroids, immunosuppressive agents) and for the treatment of open, draining fistulas.

Used to treat bacterial overgrowth in the small intestine caused by stricture, fistulas, or prior surgery. May be part of a long-term treatment regimen.

May be necessary if perforation or bowel obstruction occurs or disease is unresponsive to medical treatment. *Note:* About 25% to 40 % of UC clients and 66% to 75% of clients with Crohn's disease will eventually have their colons removed (NDDIC, 2007). Surgery is performed to relieve symptoms that do not respond to medical therapy or to correct complications such as blockage, perforation, abscess, or bleeding in the intestine. Surgery to remove part of the intestine can help people with Crohn's disease, but it is not a cure. Surgery to remove the colon and rectum (proctocolectomy) is followed by ileostomy, or ileoanal anastomsis.

NURSING DIAGNOSIS: risk for deficient Fluid Volume

Risk factors may include
Excessive losses through normal routes—severe frequent diarrhea, vomiting
Hypermetabolic state—inflammation, fever
Restricted intake—nausea, anorexia

Possibly evidenced by
(Not applicable; presence of signs and symptoms establishes an *actual* diagnosis)

Desired Outcomes/Evaluation Criteria—Client Will

Hydration (NOC)
Maintain adequate fluid volume as evidenced by moist mucous membranes, good skin turgor, and capillary refill; stable vital signs; and balanced intake and output (I&O) with urine of normal concentration and amount.

ACTIONS/INTERVENTIONS

RATIONALE

Fluid/Electrolyte Management (NIC)
Independent

Monitor I&O. Note number, character, and amount of stools; estimate insensible fluid losses (e.g., diaphoresis). Measure urine specific gravity and observe for oliguria.

Assess vital signs (blood pressure [BP], pulse, temperature).

Observe for excessively dry skin and mucous membranes, decreased skin turgor, and slowed capillary refill.

Weigh daily.

Provides information about overall fluid balance, renal function, and bowel disease control, as well as guidelines for fluid replacement.

Hypotension (including postural), tachycardia, and fever can indicate response to and effect of fluid loss.

Indicates excessive fluid loss and resultant dehydration.

Indicator of overall fluid and nutritional status.

NURSING DIAGNOSIS: imbalanced Nutrition: Less than Body Requirements

May be related to
Altered absorption of nutrients
Hypermetabolic state
Medically restricted intake; fear that eating may cause diarrhea

NURSING DIAGNOSIS: **imbalanced Nutrition: Less than Body Requirements** (continued)

Possibly evidenced by
Weight loss, decreased subcutaneous fat and muscle mass, poor muscle tone
Hyperactive bowel sounds, steatorrhea
Pale conjunctiva and mucous membranes
Aversion to eating

Desired Outcomes/Evaluation Criteria—Client Will

Nutritional Status (NOC)
Demonstrate stable weight or progressive gain toward goal with normalization of laboratory values and absence of signs of malnutrition.

ACTIONS/INTERVENTIONS	RATIONALE
Nutrition Therapy (NIC)	
Independent	
Assess weight, age, body mass, strength, and activity and rest levels. Ascertain stage of disease process and its effects on client's nutritional status.	Provides comparative baseline.
Inspect oral mucosa.	May reveal ulcerations and/or provide information about the integrity of the entire GI tract, affecting ability to eat and absorb nutrients.
Evaluate client's appetite.	Appetite may be suppressed because of altered taste, early satiety, meal-related cramping, diarrhea, or a combination of these factors.
Weigh frequently.	Provides information about dietary needs and effectiveness of therapy.
Encourage bedrest or limited activity during acute phase of illness.	Decreasing metabolic needs aids in preventing caloric depletion and conserves energy.
Recommend rest before meals.	Quiets peristalsis and increases available energy for eating.
Provide oral hygiene.	A clean mouth can enhance the taste of food.
Serve foods in well-ventilated, pleasant surroundings, with unhurried atmosphere and congenial company.	Pleasant environment aids in reducing stress and is more conducive to eating.
Avoid or limit foods that might cause or exacerbate abdominal cramping and flatulence—milk products, foods high in fiber or fat, alcohol, caffeinated beverages, chocolate, peppermint, tomatoes, and orange juice.	Individual tolerance varies, depending on stage of disease and area of bowel affected.
Record intake and changes in symptomatology.	Useful in identifying specific deficiencies and determining GI response to foods.
Promote client participation in dietary planning as possible.	Provides sense of control for client and opportunity to select foods desired and enjoyed, which may increase intake.
Encourage client to verbalize feelings concerning resumption of diet.	Hesitation to eat may be the result of fear that food will cause exacerbation of symptoms.
Collaborative	
Keep client nothing-by-mouth (NPO) status, as indicated.	Resting the bowel decreases peristalsis and diarrhea, limiting malabsorption and loss of nutrients. *Note:* Client with toxic colitis is NPO and placed on parenteral nutrition.
Resume or advance diet as indicated—clear liquids progressing to bland, low residue, and then high-protein, high-calorie, caffeine-free, nonspicy, and low-fiber, as indicated.	Allows the intestinal tract to readjust to the digestive process. Protein is necessary for tissue healing integrity. Low bulk decreases peristaltic response to meal. *Note:* Dietary measures depend on client's condition, for example, if disease is mild, client may do well on low-residue, low-fat diet high in protein and calories with lactose restriction. In moderate disease, elemental enteral products may be given to provide nutrition without overstimulating the bowel.
Provide nutritional support, for example:	
Enteral feedings, such as Ultra Clear Plus via nasogastric (NG) tube, percutaneous endoscopic gastrostomy (PEG), or J-tube	Many clinical studies have shown early enteral feeding is beneficial in reducing the effects of malabsorption and providing essential nutrients. Although elemental enteral solutions cannot provide all needed nutrients, they can prevent gut atrophy.
Intravenous total parenteral nutrition (TPN)	This regimen rests the GI tract completely while providing essential nutrients. Short-term TPN is indicated during periods of disease exacerbation when bowel rest is needed. (Refer to CP: Total Nutritional Support: Parenteral/Enteral Feeding.)

(continues on page 330)

ACTIONS/INTERVENTIONS (continued)

Administer medications as indicated, for example:
  Belladonna alkaloids (Donnatal), butabarbital sodium with belladonna (Butibel); propantheline bromide (Pro-Banthi-ine)

  Iron (ImFeD/injectable)

  Vitamin B$_{12}$ (Crystamine, Rubesol)

  Folic acid (Folvite)

  Vitamin C (Ascorbicap)

RATIONALE (continued)

Anticholinergics given 15 to 30 minutes before eating provide relief from cramping pain and diarrhea, decreasing gastric motility and enhancing time for absorption of nutrients.
Prevents and treats anemia. Oral route for iron supplement is ineffective because of intestinal alterations that severely reduce absorption.
Malabsorption of vitamin B$_{12}$ results from significant loss of functional ileum. Replacement of vitamin B$_{12}$ reverses bone marrow depression caused by prolonged inflammatory process, promoting RBC production and correction of anemia.
Folate deficiency is common in presence of Crohn's disease because of decreased intake or absorption and effect of drug therapy sulfasalazine (Azulfidine).
Promotes tissue regeneration and healing.

NURSING DIAGNOSIS: Anxiety [specify level]

May be related to
Physiological factors and sympathetic stimulation (inflammatory process)
Perceived or actual threat to self-concept
Threat to, or change in, health status, socioeconomic status, role functioning, interaction patterns

Possibly evidenced by
Exacerbation of acute stage of disease
Increased tension, distress, apprehension
Expressed concern regarding changes in life
Somatic complaints
Focus on self

Desired Outcomes/Evaluation Criteria—Client Will

Anxiety Control (NOC)
Appear relaxed and report anxiety reduced to a manageable level.
Verbalize awareness of feelings of anxiety and healthy ways to deal with them.

ACTIONS/INTERVENTIONS

Anxiety Reduction (NIC)
Independent
Note behavioral clues—restlessness, irritability, withdrawal, lack of eye contact, and demanding behavior.

Encourage verbalization of feelings. Provide feedback.

Acknowledge that the anxiety and problems are similar to those expressed by others. Active-listen client's concerns.
Provide accurate, concrete information about what is being done, such as reason for bedrest, restriction of oral intake, and procedures.
Provide a calm, restful environment.

Encourage staff/SO to project caring, concerned attitude.

Help client identify and initiate positive coping behaviors used in the past.
Assist client to learn new coping mechanisms, such as stress management techniques and organizational skills.

Collaborative
Administer medications, as indicated, for example, sedatives, such as barbiturates and phenobarbital (Luminal); anti-anxiety agents, such as diazepam (Valium) and alprazolam (Xanax).

RATIONALE

Indicators of degree of anxiety or stress, for example, client may feel out of control at home or work managing personal problems. Stress may develop as a result of physical symptoms of condition and the reaction of others.
Establishes a therapeutic relationship. Assists client/significant other (SO) in identifying problems causing stress. Client with severe diarrhea may hesitate to ask for help for fear of becoming a burden to the staff.
Validation that feelings are normal can help reduce stress/isolation and belief that "I am the only one."
Involving client in plan of care provides sense of control and helps decrease anxiety.

Removing client from outside stressors promotes relaxation and helps reduce anxiety.
A supportive manner can help client feel less stressed, allowing energy to be directed toward healing and recovery.
Successful behaviors can be fostered in dealing with current problems or stress, enhancing client's sense of self-control.
Learning new ways to cope can be helpful in reducing stress and anxiety, enhancing disease control.

May be used to reduce anxiety and to facilitate rest, particularly in the client with UC.

ACTIONS/INTERVENTIONS (continued)	RATIONALE (continued)
Refer to psychiatric clinical nurse specialist, social services, or spiritual advisor.	May require additional assistance in regaining control and coping with acute episodes or exacerbations, as well as learning to deal with the chronicity and consequences of the disease and therapeutic regimen.

NURSING DIAGNOSIS: acute Pain

May be related to
Hyperperistalsis, prolonged diarrhea, skin and tissue irritation, perirectal excoriation, fissures, fistulas

Possibly evidenced by
Reports of colicky, cramping abdominal pain; referred pain
Guarding or distraction behaviors, restlessness
Facial mask of pain; self-focusing

Desired Outcomes/Evaluation Criteria—Client Will

Pain Level (NOC)
Report pain is relieved or controlled.
Appear relaxed and able to sleep and rest appropriately.

ACTIONS/INTERVENTIONS	RATIONALE
Pain Management (NIC)	
Independent	
Encourage client to report pain.	May try to tolerate pain rather than request analgesics.
Assess reports of abdominal cramping or pain, noting location, duration, and intensity (such as 0–10 scale). Investigate and report changes in pain characteristics.	Colicky intermittent pain occurs with Crohn's disease. Predefecation pain frequently occurs in UC with urgency, which may be severe and continuous. Changes in pain characteristics may indicate spread of disease or developing complications, such as bladder fistula, perforation, and toxic megacolon.
Note nonverbal cues, such as restlessness, reluctance to move, abdominal guarding, withdrawal, and depression. Investigate discrepancies between verbal and nonverbal cues.	Body language or nonverbal cues may be both physiological and psychological and may be used in conjunction with verbal cues to determine extent and severity of the problem.
Review factors that aggravate or alleviate pain.	May pinpoint precipitating or aggravating factors (e.g., stressful events, food intolerance) or identify developing complications.
Encourage client to assume position of comfort, such as knees flexed.	Reduces abdominal tension and promotes sense of control.
Provide comfort measures (e.g., back rub, reposition) and diversional activities.	Promotes relaxation, refocuses attention, and may enhance coping abilities.
Cleanse rectal area with mild soap and water (or wipes) after each stool and provide skin care with a moisture barrier ointment (e.g., A&D ointment, Sweem ointment, karaya gel, Desitin, petroleum jelly, zinc oxide, dimethicone).	Protects skin from bowel acids, preventing excoriation.
Provide sitz bath, as appropriate.	Enhances cleanliness and comfort in the presence of perianal irritation and fissures.
Observe for ischiorectal and perianal fistulas.	Fistulas may develop from erosion and weakening of intestinal bowel wall.
Observe and record abdominal distension, increased temperature, and decreased BP.	May indicate developing intestinal obstruction from inflammation, edema, and scarring.
Collaborative	
Implement prescribed dietary modifications, for example, commence with liquids and increase to solid foods as tolerated.	Complete bowel rest can reduce pain and cramping.
Administer medications as indicated, for example:	
Analgesics	Pain varies from mild to severe and necessitates management to facilitate adequate rest and recovery. *Note:* Opiates should be used with caution because they may precipitate toxic megacolon.
Anticholinergics	Relieve spasms of GI tract and resultant colicky pain.
Anodyne suppositories	Relax rectal muscle, decreasing painful spasms.

NURSING DIAGNOSIS: ineffective Coping

May be related to
Multiple stressors, repeated over period of time; situational crisis
Unpredictable nature of disease process
Personal vulnerability; inadequate coping method; lack of support systems
Severe pain
Lack of sleep, rest

Possibly evidenced by
Verbalization of inability to cope, discouragement, anxiety
Preoccupation with physical self, chronic worry, emotional tension, poor self-esteem
Depression and dependency

Desired Outcomes/Evaluation Criteria—Client Will

Coping (NOC)
Assess the current situation accurately.
Identify ineffective coping behaviors and consequences.
Acknowledge own coping abilities.
Demonstrate necessary lifestyle changes to limit or prevent recurrent episodes.

ACTIONS/INTERVENTIONS	RATIONALE
Coping Enhancement (NIC)	
Independent	
Assess client's/SO's understanding and previous methods of dealing with disease process.	Enables the nurse to deal more realistically with current problems. Anxiety and other problems may have interfered with previous health teaching and client learning.
Determine outside stressors, such as family, relationships, and social or work environment.	Stress can alter autonomic nervous response, affecting the immune system and contributing to exacerbation of disease. Even the goal of independence in the dependent client can be an added stressor.
Provide opportunity for client to discuss how illness has affected relationships, including sexual concerns.	Stressors of illness affect all areas of life, and client may have difficulty coping with feelings of fatigue and pain in relation to relationship and sexual needs.
Help client identify individually effective coping skills.	Use of previously successful behaviors can help client deal with current situation and plan for the future.
Provide emotional support:	
Active-listen in a nonjudgmental manner.	Aids in communication and understanding client's viewpoint. Adds to client's feelings of self-worth.
Maintain nonjudgmental body language when caring for client.	Prevents reinforcing client's feelings of being a burden, for example, frequent need to empty bedpan or commode.
Assign same staff as much as possible.	Provides a more therapeutic environment and lessens the stress of constant adjustments.
Provide uninterrupted sleep or rest periods.	Exhaustion brought on by the disease tends to magnify problems, interfering with ability to cope.
Encourage use of stress management skills, such as relaxation techniques, visualization, guided imagery, and deep-breathing exercises.	Refocuses attention, promotes relaxation, and enhances coping abilities.
Collaborative	
Include client/SO in team conferences to develop individualized program.	Promotes continuity of care and enables client/SO to feel a part of the plan, imparting a sense of control and increasing cooperation with therapeutic regimen.
Administer medications as indicated, for example, anti-anxiety agents, such as lorazepam (Ativan) and alprazolam (Xanax).	Aids in psychological and physical rest. Conserves energy and may strengthen coping abilities.
Refer to resources, as indicated, such as local support group, social worker, psychiatric clinical nurse specialist, or spiritual advisor.	Additional support and counseling can assist client/SO in dealing with specific stress or problem areas.

NURSING DIAGNOSIS: **deficient Knowledge, [Learning Need] regarding condition, prognosis, treatment, self-care, and discharge needs**

May be related to
Information misinterpretation, lack of recall
Unfamiliarity with resources

Possibly evidenced by
Questions, request for information, statements of misconceptions
Inaccurate follow-through of instructions
Development of preventable complications or exacerbations

Desired Outcomes/Evaluation Criteria—Client Will

Knowledge: Disease Process (NOC)
Verbalize understanding of disease processes and possible complications.
Identify stress situations and specific action(s) to deal with them.

Knowledge: Treatment Regimen (NOC)
Verbalize understanding of therapeutic regimen.
Participate in treatment regimen.
Initiate necessary lifestyle changes.

ACTIONS/INTERVENTIONS	RATIONALE
Teaching: Disease Process (NIC) *Independent*	
Determine client's perception of disease process.	Establishes knowledge base and provides some insight into individual learning needs.
Review disease process, cause and effect relationship of factors that precipitate symptoms, and identify ways to reduce contributing factors. Encourage questions.	Precipitating or aggravating factors are individual; therefore, client needs to be aware of what foods, fluids, and lifestyle factors can precipitate symptoms. Accurate knowledge base provides opportunity for client to make informed decisions or choices about future and control of chronic disease. Although most clients know about their own disease process, they may have outdated information or misconceptions.
Review medications, purpose, frequency, dosage, and possible side effects.	Promotes understanding and may enhance cooperation with regimen.
Remind client to observe for side effects of steroids (such as ulcers, facial edema, and muscle weakness) if used on a long-term basis.	Steroids may be used to control inflammation and to effect a remission of the disease; however, drug may lower resistance to infection and cause fluid retention.
Stress importance of good skin care, including proper hand-washing techniques and perineal skin care.	Reduces spread of bacteria and risk of skin irritation or breakdown and infection.
Recommend cessation of smoking.	Can increase intestinal motility, aggravating symptoms.
Emphasize need for long-term follow-up and periodic reevaluation.	Clients with IBD are at increased risk for colon/rectal cancer, and regular diagnostic evaluations may be required.
Identify appropriate community resources, such as Crohn's and Colitis Foundation of America (CCFA), United Ostomy Association of America, home healthcare providers and visiting nurse services, dietitian, and social services.	Client may benefit from the services of these agencies in coping with chronicity of the disease and evaluating treatment options.

POTENTIAL CONSIDERATIONS following acute hospitalization (dependent on client's age, physical condition and presence of complications, personal resources, and life responsibilities)

- *acute Pain*—hyperperistalsis, prolonged diarrhea, skin and tissue irritation, perirectal excoriation, fissures, fistulas
- *ineffective Coping*—multiple stressors, repeated over period of time; unpredictable nature of disease process; personal vulnerability; severe pain; situational crisis
- *risk for Infection*—traumatized tissue, change in pH of secretions, altered peristalsis, suppressed inflammatory response, chronic disease, malnutrition
- *ineffective self Health Management*—complexity of therapeutic regimen, perceived benefit, powerlessness

333

FECAL DIVERSIONS: POSTOPERATIVE CARE OF ILEOSTOMY AND COLOSTOMY

I. Procedures—incontinent diversions (primary focus of this plan of care), laporoscopic colectomy, and continent diversions, such as the Kock pouch and the ileoanal reservoir

a. Ileostomy

    i. Performed when the entire colon, rectum, and anus must be removed, in which case the ileostomy is permanent; or, a temporary ileostomy can be done to provide complete bowel rest in conditions, such as with chronic colitis and in some trauma cases.

    ii. Most frequently performed for complications of inflammatory bowel disease—Crohn's disease and ulcerative colitis—including intestinal perforation or intestinal stricture causing obstruction, abscess, or massive hemmorhage (Clark, 2005; Boehmke, 2006).

    iii. May also be done because of intestinal trauma, polyps, cancer, or complications from cancer (Clark, 2005).

b. Colostomy may be performed at several locations: the ascending, transverse, descending, or sigmoid colon.

    i. Ascending colostomy is positioned in the upper right side of the abdomen.

    ii. Transverse colostomy is positioned in the mid-to-right upper abdomen.

        1. Performed for diverticulitis, bowel obstruction, trauma, or cancer of the descending or sigmoid colon

        2. Usually temporary, but can be permanent when the lower portion of the colon must be removed or permanently rested

    iii. Descending/sigmoid colostomy is positioned in the lower left side of the abdomen.

        1. Most common permanent stoma with opening in the lower end of the colon

        2. Performed for cancer of rectum or sigmoid colon as well as for diverticulitis, bowel obstruction, trauma, and paralysis (Clark, 2004)

II. Etiology—dependent on underlying pathology requiring procedure

III. Statistics

a. Morbidity: An estimated 75,000 to 100,000 individuals undergo ostomy surgery annually (Ringhofer, 2005); approximately 500,000 Americans have some type of stoma (Turnbull, 2003).

b. Mortality: Uncommon depending on age, reason for procedure (such as Crohn's disease versus penetrating trauma or cancer), and comorbidities.

GLOSSARY

Anus: Terminal part of the rectum.

Colon: Part of the intestine that stores digested food and absorbs water. Also referred to as the large intestine or the large bowel.

Colostomy: Surgical opening to bring a portion of the large intestine through the abdominal wall to form a stoma.

Ileostomy: Opening that is surgically constructed in the ileum with the intestine brought through the abdominal wall to form a stoma.

Ileum: Lowest part or end of the small intestine.

Irrigation: Enema that is brought through the stoma, used by some colostomates, to regulate the passage of stool.

Peristalsis: Progressive waves of motion, which occur without voluntary control, to push contents through the intestine.

Pouching system: Device worn over the stoma, which acts as a reservoir for the stool that empties out of the stoma. There are many different pouching system options.

Prolapse: A "falling out" in which the stoma becomes longer.

Rectum: Lowest portion of the large intestine.

Skin barrier: Solid square or round piece of adhesive material that is used to protect the skin from stool.

Stenosis: Narrowing or tightness of the stoma, which may cause obstruction.

Stoma: Opening at the end of the colon or ileum, which is brought through the surface of the skin. It often protrudes like a nipple and is $3/4$ to $1 3/4$ inches in diameter. It is usually pink to red in color.

Care Settings

Care is handled in an inpatient acute care surgical unit.

Related Concerns

Cancer, page 846

Fluid and electrolyte imbalances, page 903

Inflammatory bowel disease (IBD): ulcerative colitis, Crohn's disease, page 321

Psychosocial aspects of care, page 749

Surgical intervention, page 782

Total nutritional support: parenteral/enteral feeding, page 469

Client Assessment Database

Data depend on the underlying problem, duration, and severity (e.g., obstruction, perforation, inflammation, congenital defects).

DIAGNOSTIC DIVISION MAY REPORT	MAY EXHIBIT

TEACHING/LEARNING
• *Discharge plan considerations*
  • Assistance with dietary concerns
  • Management of ostomy
  • Acquisition of supplies
 	
▸ Refer to section at end of plan for postdischarge considerations.	

Nursing Priorities

1. Assist client/significant other (SO) in psychosocial adjustment.
2. Prevent complications.
3. Support independence in self-care.
4. Provide information about procedure, prognosis, treatment needs, potential complications, and community resources.

Discharge Goals

1. Adjusting to perceived or actual changes.
2. Complications prevented or minimized.
3. Self-care needs met by self or with assistance depending on specific situation.
4. Procedure, prognosis, therapeutic regimen, and potential complications understood and sources of support identified.
5. Plan in place to meet needs after discharge.

NURSING DIAGNOSIS: risk for impaired Skin Integrity

Risk factors may include
Absence of sphincter at stoma
Character and flow of effluent and flatus from stoma
Reaction to product or chemicals; improper fitting or care of appliance/skin

Possibly evidenced by
(Not applicable; presence of signs and symptoms establishes an *actual* diagnosis)

Desired Outcomes/Evaluation Criteria—Client Will

Ostomy Self-Care (NOC)
Maintain skin integrity around stoma.
Identify individual risk factors.
Demonstrate behaviors or techniques to promote healing and/or prevent skin breakdown.

ACTIONS/INTERVENTIONS

Ostomy Care (NIC)
Independent
Inspect stoma and peristomal skin area with each pouch change. Note irritation, bruises (dark, bluish color), and rashes.

RATIONALE

Monitors healing process and effectiveness of appliances. Identifies areas of concern and need for further evaluation and intervention. Early identification of stomal ischemia or infection (from changes in normal bowel flora) provides for timely interventions to prevent serious complications. Stoma should be red and moist. Ulcerated areas on stoma may be from a pouch opening that is too small or a faceplate that cuts into stoma. In clients with an ileostomy, the effluent is rich in enzymes, increasing the likelihood of skin irritation. In clients with a colostomy, skin care is not as great a concern because the enzymes are no longer present in the effluent.

(continues on page 336)

Clean with warm water and pat dry. Use soap only if area is covered with sticky stool. If paste has collected on the skin, let it dry, and then peel it off.

Maintaining a clean and dry area helps prevent skin breakdown, and increases adherence of appliances.

Measure stoma periodically—at least weekly for first 6 weeks, then once a month for 6 months. Measure both width and length of stoma.

As postoperative edema resolves, the stoma shrinks and the size of the appliance must be altered to ensure proper fit, so that effluent is collected as it flows from the ostomy and contact with the skin is prevented.

Verify that the opening on the adhesive backing of the pouch is no more than 1/16 to 1/8 inch (2–3 mm) larger than the base of the stoma, with adequate adhesive barrier to apply pouch.

Prevents trauma to the stoma tissue and protects the peristomal skin. Adequate adhesive area prevents the skin barrier wafer from being too tight. *Note:* Too tight a fit may cause stomal edema or stenosis.

Use a transparent, odor-proof drainable pouch.

A transparent appliance during the first 4 to 6 weeks allows easy observation of stoma without necessity of removing pouch and irritating skin.

Apply appropriate skin barrier—hydrocolloid wafer, karaya gum, extended-wear skin barrier, or similar products.

Protects skin from pouch adhesive, enhances adhesiveness of pouch, and facilitates removal of pouch when necessary. *Note:* Sigmoid colostomy may not require an appliance if elimination is regulated through irrigation.

Empty, rinse, and cleanse ostomy pouch on a routine basis, using appropriate equipment.

Frequent changes of the adhesive barrier wafer are irritating to the skin and should be avoided. Emptying and rinsing the pouch with the proper solution removes bacteria and odor-causing stool and flatus.

Support surrounding skin when gently removing appliance. Apply adhesive removers as indicated, and then wash thoroughly.

Prevents tissue irritation and destruction associated with "pulling" pouch off.

Investigate reports of burning, itching, or blistering around stoma.

Indicative of effluent leakage with peristomal irritation, or possibly *Candida* infection, requiring intervention.

Evaluate adhesive product and appliance fit on ongoing basis.

Provides opportunity for problem solving. Determines need for further intervention.

Collaborative

Consult with certified wound, ostomy, continence (WOC) nurse.

Helpful in choosing products appropriate for client's particular rehabilitation needs, including type of ostomy, physical and mental status, abilities to handle self-care, and financial resources.

Apply corticosteroid aerosol spray and prescribed antifungal powder or other product, as indicated.

Assists in healing if peristomal irritation persists and fungal infection develops. *Note:* These products can have potent side effects and should be used sparingly.

NURSING DIAGNOSIS: disturbed Body Image

May be related to
Biophysical—presence of stoma, loss of control of bowel elimination
Psychosocial—altered body structure
Disease process—cancer, colitis, and associated treatment regimen

Possibly evidenced by
Verbalization of change in body image, fear of rejection or reaction of others, and negative feelings about body
Actual change in structure and/or function—ostomy
Not touching or looking at stoma, refusal to participate in care

Desired Outcomes/Evaluation Criteria—Client Will

Body Image (NOC)
Verbalize acceptance of self in situation, incorporating change into self-concept without negating self-esteem.
Demonstrate beginning acceptance by viewing and touching stoma and participating in self-care.
Verbalize feelings about stoma and illness; begin to deal constructively with situation.

ACTIONS/INTERVENTIONS

RATIONALE

Body Image Enhancement (NIC)
Independent

Ascertain whether support and counseling were initiated when the possibility and/or necessity of ostomy was first discussed.

Provides information about client's/SO's level of knowledge and anxiety about individual situation.

ACTIONS/INTERVENTIONS (continued)	RATIONALE (continued)
Encourage client/SO to verbalize feelings regarding the ostomy. Acknowledge normality of feelings of anger, depression, and grief over loss. Discuss daily "ups and downs" that can occur.	Helps client realize that feelings are not unusual and that feeling guilty about them is not necessary or helpful. Client needs to recognize feelings before they can be dealt with effectively.
Review reason for surgery and future expectations.	Client may find it easier to deal with an ostomy done to correct long-term disease than for traumatic injury, even if ostomy is only temporary. Also, client who will be undergoing a second procedure to convert ostomy to a continent or anal reservoir, may possibly encounter less severe self-image problems because body function eventually will be "more normal."
Note behaviors of withdrawal, increased dependency, manipulation, or noninvolvement in care.	Suggestive of problems in adjustment that may require further evaluation and more extensive therapy.
Provide opportunities for client/SO to view and touch stoma, using the moment to point out positive signs of healing, normal appearance, and so forth. Remind client that it will take time to adjust, both physically and emotionally.	Although integration of stoma into body image can take months or even years, looking at the stoma and hearing comments made in a normal, matter-of-fact manner can help client with this acceptance. Touching stoma reassures client/SO that it is not fragile and that slight movements of stoma actually reflect normal peristalsis.
Provide opportunity for client to deal with ostomy through participation in self-care.	Independence in self-care helps improve self-confidence and acceptance of situation.
Plan care activities with client.	Promotes sense of control and gives message that client can handle situation, enhancing self-concept.
Maintain positive approach during care activities, avoiding expressions of disdain or revulsion. Do not take angry expressions of client/SO personally.	Assists client/SO to accept body changes and feel good about self. Anger is most often directed at the situation and lack of control or powerlessness individual has over what has happened—not with the individual caregiver.
Ascertain client's desire to visit with a person with an ostomy. Make arrangements for visit, if desired.	A person who is living with an ostomy can be a good support system and role model. Shared experiences helps reinforce teaching and facilitates acceptance of change as client realizes "life does go on" and can be relatively normal.

NURSING DIAGNOSIS: acute Pain

May be related to
Physical factors—disruption of skin or tissues (incisions, drains)
Biological factors—activity of disease process (cancer, trauma)
Psychological factors—fear, anxiety

Possibly evidenced by
Reports of pain, self-focusing
Guarding and distraction behaviors, restlessness
Autonomic responses—changes in vital signs

Desired Outcomes/Evaluation Criteria—Client Will

Pain Level (NOC)
Verbalize that pain is relieved or controlled.
Appear relaxed and able to sleep or rest appropriately.

Pain Control (NOC)
Demonstrate use of relaxation skills and general comfort measures, as indicated for individual situation.

ACTIONS/INTERVENTIONS	RATIONALE
Pain Management (NIC)	
Independent	
Assess pain, noting location, characteristics, and intensity (such as 0–10 scale).	Helps evaluate degree of discomfort and effectiveness of analgesia or may reveal developing complications. Because abdominal pain usually subsides gradually by the third or fourth postoperative day, continued or increasing pain may reflect delayed healing or peristomal skin irritation. *Note:* Pain in anal area associated with abdominal-perineal resection may persist for months.
Encourage client to verbalize concerns. Active-listen these concerns, and provide support by acceptance, remaining with client, and giving appropriate information.	Reduction of anxiety and fear can promote relaxation and comfort.

(continues on page 338)

ACTIONS/INTERVENTIONS (continued)	RATIONALE (continued)
Provide comfort measures, such as mouth care, back rub, and repositioning. Assure client that position change will not injure stoma.	Prevents drying of oral mucosa and associated discomfort. Reduces muscle tension, promotes relaxation, and may enhance coping abilities.
Encourage use of relaxation techniques such as guided imagery and visualization. Provide diversional activities.	Helps client rest more effectively and refocuses attention, thereby reducing pain and discomfort.
Assist with range-of-motion exercises and encourage early ambulation. Avoid prolonged sitting position.	Reduces muscle and joint stiffness. Ambulation returns organs to normal position and promotes return of usual level of functioning. *Note:* Presence of edema, packing, and drains (if perineal resection has been done) increases discomfort and creates a sense of needing to defecate. Ambulation and frequent position changes reduce perineal pressure.
Investigate and report abdominal muscle rigidity, involuntary guarding, and rebound tenderness.	Suggestive of peritoneal inflammation, which requires prompt medical intervention.

Collaborative

Administer medication, such as opioids, analgesics, and patient-controlled analgesia (PCA), as indicated.	Relieves pain, enhances comfort, and promotes rest. PCA may be more beneficial, especially following anal-perineal repair.
Provide sitz baths.	Relieves local discomfort, reduces edema, and promotes healing of perineal wound.
Apply and monitor effects of transcutaneous electrical nerve stimulator unit.	Cutaneous stimulation may be used to block transmission of pain stimulus.

NURSING DIAGNOSIS: impaired Skin/Tissue Integrity

May be related to
Invasion of body structure, such as with perineal resection
Stasis of secretions or drainage
Altered circulation, edema; malnutrition

Possibly evidenced by
Disruption of skin and tissue—presence of incision and sutures, drains

Desired Outcomes/Evaluation Criteria—Client Will

Wound Healing: Primary Intention (NOC)
Achieve timely wound healing free of signs of infection.

ACTIONS/INTERVENTIONS	RATIONALE

Wound Care (NIC)
Independent

Observe wounds, noting characteristics of drainage.	Postoperative hemorrhage is most likely to occur during the first 48 hours, whereas infection may develop at any time. Depending on type of wound closure, complete healing may take 6 to 8 months.
Change dressings as needed.	Large amounts of serous drainage require that dressings be changed frequently to reduce skin irritation and potential for infection.
Encourage side-lying position with head elevated. Avoid prolonged sitting.	Promotes drainage from perineal wound/drains, reducing risk of pooling. Prolonged sitting increases perineal pressure, reducing circulation to wound, and may delay healing.

Collaborative

Irrigate wound as indicated, using normal saline (NS), diluted hydrogen peroxide, or antibiotic solution.	May be required to treat preoperative inflammation, infection, or intraoperative contamination.
Provide sitz baths.	Promotes cleanliness and facilitates healing, especially after packing is removed—usually day 3 to 5.

NURSING DIAGNOSIS: risk for deficient Fluid Volume

Risk factors may include
Excessive losses through normal routes—preoperative emesis and diarrhea; high-volume ileostomy output
Losses through abnormal routes—nasogastric (NG) or intestinal tube, perineal wound drainage tubes
Medically restricted intake
Altered absorption of fluid—loss of colon function
Hypermetabolic states—inflammation, healing process

NURSING DIAGNOSIS: **risk for deficient Fluid Volume** (continued)

Possibly evidenced by
(Not applicable; presence of signs and symptoms establishes an *actual* diagnosis)

Desired Outcomes/Evaluation Criteria—Client Will

Hydration (NOC)
Maintain adequate hydration as evidenced by moist mucous membranes, good skin turgor and capillary refill, stable vital signs, and individually appropriate urinary output.

ACTIONS/INTERVENTIONS	RATIONALE
Fluid/Electrolyte Management (NIC)	
Independent	
Monitor intake and output (I&O) carefully and measure liquid stool. Weigh regularly.	Provides direct indicators of fluid balance. Greatest fluid losses occur with ileostomy, but they generally do not exceed 500 to 800 mL/day.
Monitor vital signs, noting postural hypotension and tachycardia. Evaluate skin turgor, capillary refill, and mucous membranes.	Reflects hydration status and possible need for fluid replacement.
Limit intake of ice chips during period of gastric intubation.	Ice chips can stimulate gastric secretions and wash out electrolytes.
Collaborative	
Monitor laboratory results, such as Hct and electrolytes.	Detects homeostasis or imbalance and aids in determining replacement needs.
Administer intravenous (IV) fluid and electrolytes as indicated.	May be necessary to maintain adequate tissue perfusion and organ function.

NURSING DIAGNOSIS: **risk for Imbalanced Nutrition: Less than Body Requirements**

Risk factors may include
Prolonged anorexia, altered intake preoperatively
Hypermetabolic state—preoperative inflammatory disease; healing process
Presence of diarrhea; altered absorption
Restriction of bulk and residue-containing foods

Possibly evidenced by
(Not applicable; presence of signs and symptoms establishes an *actual* diagnosis)

Desired Outcomes/Evaluation Criteria—Client Will

Nutritional Status (NOC)
Maintain weight or demonstrate progressive weight gain toward goal with normalization of laboratory values and be free of signs of malnutrition.
Plan diet to meet nutritional needs and limit gastrointestinal (GI) disturbances.

ACTIONS/INTERVENTIONS	RATIONALE
Nutrition Therapy (NIC)	
Independent	
Obtain a thorough nutritional assessment.	Identifies deficiencies and needs to aid in choice of interventions.
Auscultate bowel sounds.	Return of intestinal function indicates readiness to resume oral intake.
Resume solid foods slowly.	Reduces incidence of abdominal cramps and nausea.
Identify odor-causing foods, for instance, cabbage, fish, and beans, and temporarily restrict from diet. Gradually reintroduce one food at a time.	Sensitivity to certain foods is not uncommon following intestinal surgery. Client can experiment with food several times before determining whether it is creating a problem.
Recommend client increase use of yogurt, buttermilk, and acidophilus preparations.	May help prevent gas and decrease odor formation.
Suggest client with ileostomy limit prunes, dates, stewed apricots, strawberries, grapes, bananas, cabbage family, and beans, and avoid foods high in cellulose, such as peanuts.	These products increase ileal effluent. Digestion of cellulose requires colonic bacteria that are no longer present.

(continues on page 340)

ACTIONS/INTERVENTIONS (continued)	RATIONALE (continued)
Discuss mechanics of swallowed air as a factor in the formation of flatus and some ways client can exercise control. Discuss use of a pouch with a filter to help with the management of gas.	Drinking through a straw, snoring, anxiety, smoking, ill-fitting dentures, and gulping down food increase the production of flatus. Too much flatus not only necessitates frequent emptying, but also can cause leakage from too much pressure within the pouch.
Collaborative	
Consult with dietitian and nutrition specialist.	Helpful in assessing client's nutritional needs in light of changes in digestion and intestinal function, including absorption of vitamins and minerals.
Advance diet from liquids to low-residue food when oral intake is resumed.	Low-residue diet may be maintained during first 6 to 8 weeks to provide adequate time for intestinal healing.
Administer enteral or parenteral feedings when indicated.	In the presence of severe debilitation or intolerance of oral intake, parenteral or enteral feedings may be given to supply needed components for healing and prevention of catabolic state. (Refer to CP: Total Nutritional Support: Parenteral/Enteral Feeding.)

NURSING DIAGNOSIS: **Sleep Deprivation**

May be related to
External factors—necessity of ostomy care, excessive flatus or ostomy effluent
Internal factors—psychological stress, fear of leakage of pouch or injury to stoma

Possibly evidenced by
Verbalizations of interrupted sleep, not feeling well-rested
Changes in behavior—irritability, listlessness or lethargy

Desired Outcomes/Evaluation Criteria—Client Will

Sleep (NOC)
Sleep or rest between disturbances.
Report increased sense of well-being and feeling rested.

ACTIONS/INTERVENTIONS	RATIONALE
Sleep Enhancement (NIC)	
Independent	
Explain necessity to monitor intestinal function in early postoperative period.	Client is more apt to be tolerant of disturbances by staff if he or she understands the reasons for, and importance of, care.
Provide adequate pouching system. Empty pouch before retiring and, if necessary, on an agreed-upon schedule.	Excessive flatus or effluent can occur despite interventions. Emptying on a regular schedule minimizes threat of leakage.
Let client know that stoma will not be injured when sleeping.	Client will be able to rest better if feeling secure about stoma and ostomy function.
Restrict intake of caffeine-containing foods and fluids.	Caffeine may delay client's falling asleep and interfere with REM (rapid eye movement) sleep, resulting in client not feeling well-rested.
Support continuation of usual bedtime rituals.	Promotes relaxation and readiness for sleep.
Collaborative	
Determine cause of excessive flatus or effluent and possible actions, such as conferring with dietitian regarding restriction of foods if diet-related.	Identification of cause enables institution of corrective measures that may promote sleep or rest.
Administer analgesics or sedatives at bedtime, as indicated.	Pain can interfere with client's ability to fall, or remain, asleep. Timely medication can enhance rest or sleep during initial postoperative period. *Note:* Pain pathways in the brain lie near the sleep center and may contribute to wakefulness.

NURSING DIAGNOSIS: risk for Constipation/Diarrhea

Risk factors may include
Placement of ostomy in descending or sigmoid colon
Inadequate diet or fluid intake

Possibly evidenced by
(Not applicable; presence of signs and symptoms establishes an *actual* diagnosis)

Desired Outcomes/Evaluation Criteria—Client Will

Bowel Elimination (NOC)
Establish an elimination pattern suitable to physical needs and lifestyle with effluent of appropriate amount and consistency.

ACTIONS/INTERVENTIONS	RATIONALE
Bowel Management (NIC)	
Independent	
Investigate delayed onset or absence of effluent. Auscultate bowel sounds.	Postoperative paralytic or adynamic ileus usually resolves within 48 to 72 hours, and ileostomy should begin draining within 12 to 24 hours. Delay may indicate persistent ileus or stomal obstruction, which may occur postoperatively because of edema, improperly fitting pouch (too tight), prolapse, or stenosis of the stoma.
Inform client with an ileostomy that initially the effluent is liquid. If constipation occurs, it should be reported to enterostomal nurse or physician.	Although the small intestine eventually begins to take on water-absorbing functions to permit a more semisolid, pasty discharge or absence of output may indicate an obstruction. Absence of stool requires emergency medical attention.
Review dietary pattern and amount and type of fluid intake.	Adequate intake of fiber and roughage provides bulk, and fluid is an important factor in determining the consistency of the stool.
Review physiology of the colon and discuss irrigation management of sigmoid ostomy, if indicated.	This knowledge helps client understand individual care needs. *Note:* Irrigation is usually not appropriate in the first 3 to 6 months after surgery.
Ascertain client's previous bowel habits and lifestyle.	Assists in formulation of a timely and effective irrigation schedule for client with a colostomy, if appropriate.
Demonstrate use of irrigation equipment per institution policy or under guidance of physician or certified WOC nurse.	Irrigations may be done on a daily basis if appropriate, although there are differing views on this practice. Many believe cleaning the bowel on a regular basis is helpful. Others believe that this interferes with normal functioning. Most authorities agree that occasional irrigation is useful for emptying the bowel to avoid leakage when special events are planned.
Instruct client in the use of closed-end pouch or a patch, dressing or adhesive strip when irrigation is successful and the sigmoid colostomy effluent becomes more manageable, with stool expelled every 24 hours.	Enables client to feel more comfortable socially and is less expensive than regular ostomy pouches.
Involve client in care of the ostomy on an increasing basis.	Rehabilitation can be facilitated by encouraging client independence and control.

NURSING DIAGNOSIS: risk for Sexual Dysfunction

Risk factors may include
Altered body structure and function, radical resection or treatment procedures
Vulnerability, psychological concern about response of significant other (SO)
Disruption of sexual response pattern, such as erectile difficulty

Possibly evidenced by
(Not applicable; presence of signs and symptoms establishes an *actual* diagnosis)

Desired Outcomes/Evaluation Criteria—Client Will

Sexual Functioning (NOC)
Verbalize understanding of relationship of physical condition to sexual problems.
Identify satisfying and acceptable sexual practices and explore alternative methods.
Resume sexual relationship as appropriate.

ACTIONS/INTERVENTIONS	RATIONALE

Sexual Counseling (NIC)

Independent

Determine client's and SO's sexual relationship before the disease or surgery and whether they anticipate problems related to presence of ostomy.

Identifies future expectations and desires. Mutilation and loss of privacy and control of a bodily function can affect client's view of personal sexuality. When coupled with the fear of rejection by SO, the desired level of intimacy can be greatly impaired. Sexual needs are very basic, and client will be rehabilitated more successfully when a satisfying sexual relationship is continued or developed as desired.

Review with client and SO sexual functioning in relation to own situation.

Understanding if nerve damage has altered normal sexual functioning (e.g., erection) helps client and SO to understand the need for exploring alternative methods of satisfaction.

Reinforce information given by the physician. Encourage questions. Provide additional information as needed.

Reiteration of data previously given assists client and SO to hear and process the knowledge again, moving toward acceptance of individual limitations or restrictions and prognosis, such as that it may take up to 2 years to regain potency after a radical procedure or that a penile prosthesis may be necessary.

Discuss likelihood of resumption of sexual activity in approximately 6 weeks after discharge, beginning slowly and progressing, such as cuddling and caressing until both partners are comfortable with body image and function changes. Include alternative methods of stimulation, as appropriate.

Knowing what to expect in progress of recovery helps client avoid performance anxiety and reduce risk of "failure." If the couple is willing to try new ideas, this can assist with adjustment and may help to achieve sexual fulfillment.

Encourage dialogue between partners. Suggest wearing pouch cover, T-shirt, short nightgown, or special underwear designed for sexual contact.

Disguising ostomy appliance may aid in reducing feelings of self-consciousness and embarrassment during sexual activity.

Stress awareness of factors that might be distracting—unpleasant odors and pouch leakage. Encourage use of sense of humor.

Promotes resolution of solvable problems. Laughter can help individuals deal more effectively with difficult situation and promote positive sexual experience.

Problem-solve alternative positions for coitus.

Minimizing awkwardness of appliance and physical discomfort can enhance satisfaction.

Discuss and role play possible interactions or approaches when dealing with new sexual partners.

Rehearsal is helpful in dealing with actual situations when they arise, preventing self-consciousness about "different" body image.

Provide birth control information as appropriate and stress that impotence does not necessarily mean client is sterile.

Confusion may exist that can lead to an unwanted pregnancy.

Collaborative

Arrange meeting with an ostomy visitor, if appropriate.

Sharing of how these problems have been resolved by others can be helpful and reduce sense of isolation.

Refer to counseling or sex therapy, as indicated.

If problems persist longer than several months after surgery, a trained therapist may be required to facilitate communication between client and SO.

NURSING DIAGNOSIS: **deficient Knowledge [Learning Need] regarding condition, prognosis, treatment, self-care, and discharge needs**

May be related to
Lack of exposure, recall; information misinterpretation
Unfamiliarity with information resources

Possibly evidenced by
Questions; statement of misconception, misinformation
Inaccurate follow-through of instruction, performance of ostomy care
Inappropriate or exaggerated behaviors—hostile, agitated, apathetic, withdrawal

Desired Outcomes/Evaluation Criteria—Client Will

Knowledge: Ostomy Care (NOC)
Verbalize understanding of condition, disease process, prognosis, and potential complications.
Verbalize understanding of therapeutic needs.
Correctly perform necessary procedures and explain reasons for the action.
Initiate necessary lifestyle changes.

ACTIONS/INTERVENTIONS	RATIONALE

Learning Facilitation (NIC)
Independent

Evaluate client's emotional, cognitive, and physical capabilities.

These factors affect client's ability to master care tasks and willingness to assume responsibility for ostomy care.

Include written and picture (photo, video, Internet) learning resources.

Provides reference for obtaining support, equipment, and additional information after discharge to support client efforts for independence in self-care.

Teaching: Disease Process (NIC)

Review anatomy, physiology, and implications of surgical intervention. Discuss future expectations, including anticipated changes in character of effluent.

Provides knowledge base from which client can make informed choices and offers an opportunity to clarify misconceptions regarding individual situation. (Temporary ileostomy may be converted to ileoanal reservoir at a future date; ileostomy and ascending colostomy cannot be regulated by diet, irrigations, or medications.)

Instruct client/SO in stomal care. Allot time for return demonstrations and provide positive feedback for efforts.

Promotes positive management and reduces risk of improper ostomy care and development of complications.

Recommend increased fluid intake during warm weather months.

Loss of normal colon function of conserving water and electrolytes can lead to dehydration and constipation.

Discuss possible need to decrease salt intake.

Salt can increase ileal output, potentiating risk of dehydration and increasing frequency of ostomy care needs and client's inconvenience.

Identify symptoms of electrolyte depletion, such as anorexia, abdominal muscle cramps, feelings of faintness or cold in arms and legs, general fatigue or weakness, bloating, and decreased sensations in extremities.

Loss of colon function altering fluid and electrolyte absorption may result in sodium and potassium deficits requiring dietary correction with foods and fluids high in sodium—bouillon and Gatorade—or potassium—orange juice, prunes, tomatoes, bananas, and Gatorade.

Discuss need for periodic evaluation and administration of supplemental vitamins and minerals, as appropriate.

Depending on portion and amount of bowel resected, lack of absorption may cause deficiencies.

Stress importance of chewing food well, adequate intake of fluids with and following meals, only moderate use of high-fiber foods, and avoidance of cellulose.

Reduces risk of bowel obstruction in client with ileostomy.

Review foods that are, or may be, a source of flatus, such as carbonated drinks, beer, beans, cabbage, onions, fish, and highly seasoned foods; or odor, such as onions, cabbage, eggs, fish, and beans.

These foods may be restricted or eliminated, based on individual reaction, for better ostomy control, or it may be necessary to empty the pouch more frequently if these foods are ingested.

Identify foods associated with diarrhea, such as green beans, broccoli, and highly seasoned foods.

Promotes more even effluent and better control of evacuations.

Recommend foods used to manage constipation, such as bran, celery, and raw fruits, and discuss importance of increased fluid intake.

Proper management can prevent or minimize problems of constipation.

Discuss resumption of presurgery level of activity. Suggest emptying the ostomy appliance before leaving home and carrying fresh supplies. Recommend resources for obtaining attractive appliances and decorative cummerbunds as appropriate.

With a little planning, client should be able to manage same degree of activity as previously enjoyed and in some cases increase activity level. A cummerbund can provide both physical and psychological support when client is involved in activities such as tennis and swimming.

Talk about the possibility of sleep disturbance, anorexia, and loss of interest in usual activities.

"Homecoming depression" may occur, lasting for months after surgery, requiring patience, support, and ongoing evaluation as client adjusts to living with a stoma.

Explain necessity of notifying healthcare providers and pharmacists of type of ostomy and avoidance of sustained-release medications for client with ileostomy.

Presence of ostomy may alter rate and extent of absorption of oral medications and increase risk of drug-related complications such as diarrhea, constipation, or peristomal excoriation. Liquid, chewable, or injectable forms of medication are preferred for clients with ileostomy to maximize absorption of drug.

Counsel client concerning medication use and problems associated with altered bowel function. Refer to pharmacist for teaching or advice, as appropriate.

Client with an ostomy has two key problems: altered disintegration and absorption of oral drugs and unusual or pronounced adverse effects. Some of the medications that client may respond to differently include laxatives, salicylates, H_2-receptor antagonists, antibiotics, and diuretics.

Discuss effect of medications on effluent, that is, changes in color, odor, and consistency of stool, and need to observe for drug residue indicating incomplete absorption.

Understanding decreases anxiety regarding intestinal function and enhances independence in self-care.

Stress necessity of close monitoring of chronic health conditions requiring routine oral medications.

Monitoring of clinical symptoms and serum blood levels is indicated because of altered drug absorption, requiring periodic dosage adjustments.

(continues on page 344)

Identify community resources, such as United Ostomy Association of America, the Crohn's and Colitis Foundation of America, Ostomy Rehabilitation Program, local ostomy support group, certified WOC nurse, visiting nurse, and pharmacy and medical supply house.

Continued support after discharge is essential to facilitate the recovery process and client's independence in care. WOC nurse can be very helpful in solving appliance problems, identifying alternatives to meet individual client needs.

POTENTIAL CONSIDERATIONS following acute hospitalization (dependent on client's age, physical condition and presence of complications, personal resources, and life responsibilities)
- *risk for impaired Skin Integrity*—absence of sphincter at stoma, character and flow of effluent and flatus from stoma
- *ineffective Coping*—situational crises, vulnerability
- *impaired Social Interaction*—self-concept disturbance, concern for loss of control of bodily functions

---

APPENDECTOMY

I. Pathophysiology—Events occur so rapidly that process takes about 1 to 3 days.
  a. Appendix becomes blocked by feces, a foreign object, or tumor.
  b. Obstruction, along with continued secretion of mucus, causes the wall of the appendix to become distended.
  c. Blood supply to the wall of the appendix is reduced, causing ischemia and accumulation of toxins.
  d. Wall of the appendix starts to break down, and normal bacteria found in the gut attacks the decaying appendix.
  e. Leads to necrosis and perforation of the appendix.

II. Staging—Usually has three stages (Santacroce & Ochoa, 2006).
  a. Edematous stage
    i. Individual may experience spon-taneous recovery from inflammation at this stage or it may progress.
    ii. Peritoneal fold attaching the appendix to the ileum (mesoappendix) often becomes inflamed.
  b. Purulent stage
    i. Spontaneous remission rarely occurs.
    ii. Can progress to perforation and rupture
    iii. Peritonitis possible

  c. Gangrenous stage
    i. Spontaneous regression never occurs.
    ii. Peritonitis present

III. Etiology
  a. Obstruction of appendix lumen causes it to become vulnerable to invasion of bacteria normally found in the gut.
  b. Peak incidence in individuals in their late teens and early 20s; occurs more commonly in men than in women.

IV. Procedures—Inflamed appendix may be surgically removed using an open incision or using a laparoscopic approach with laser.
  a. Presence of multiple adhesions, retroperitoneal positioning of the appendix, or the likelihood of rupture necessitates an open or traditional procedure.
  b. Laparoscopic procedure results in significantly less postoperative pain, lower wound infection rate, and faster return to normal activities.

V. Statistics
  a. Morbidity: Approximately 250,000 cases are reported annually in the United States.
  b. Mortality: In 2002, 480 deaths occurred related to diseases of the appendix in the United States (National Vital Statistics and Records [NVSR], 2005).

GLOSSARY

Abcess: Collection of pus in any part of the body that is surrounded by inflammation and infection.

Appendix: A small out-pouching from the beginning of the ascending colon. Formally called the vermiform appendix because it was thought to be wormlike.

Erythema: Redness of tissues.

McBurney's point: Name given to the point over the right side of the abdomen that is one-third of the distance from the anterior superior iliac spine to the umbilicus.

Peritonitis: Inflammation of the peritoneum, the tissue layer of cells lining the inner wall of the abdomen and pelvis.

Rebound tenderness: Pain felt when a hand pressing on the abdomen is suddenly released; a symptom of peritoneal inflammation.

Umbilicus: Belly button, navel.

Care Setting

Although many of the interventions included here are appropriate for the short-stay client, this plan of care addresses the traditional appendectomy care provided on a surgical unit, after being diagnosed in the emergency department (ED).

Related Concerns

Peritonitis, page 349
Psychosocial aspects of care, page 749
Surgical intervention, page 782

Client Assessment Database (Preoperative)

DIAGNOSTIC DIVISION MAY REPORT	MAY EXHIBIT
ACTIVITY/REST • Malaise	
CIRCULATION	• Tachycardia
ELIMINATION • Constipation of recent onset • Diarrhea (occasional)	• Abdominal distention, tenderness • Rebound tenderness, rigidity • Decreased or absent bowel sounds
FOOD/FLUID • Anorexia • Nausea, vomiting nearly always follows onset of pain	
PAIN/DISCOMFORT • Abdominal pain around the umbilicus, which may have a gradual onset and become increasingly severe • Pain may localize in right lower quadrant (RLQ) • Pain aggravated by walking, sneezing, coughing, or deep breathing • Increasingly severe, generalized pain or the sudden cessation of severe pain suggests perforation or infarction of the appendix	• Guarding behavior; lying on side or back with knees flexed • Palpation may elicit pain in RLQ, at McBurney's point • Increased RLQ pain with extension of right leg and upright position • Rebound tenderness on left side
RESPIRATION	
SAFETY	• Tachypnea; shallow respirations • Fever, usually low-grade
TEACHING/LEARNING • History of other conditions associated with abdominal pain, such as Crohn's disease, irritable bowel syndrome, peptic ulcer, painful ovulation, that may require differentiation from current pain problem • May occur at any age	
DISCHARGE PLAN CONSIDERATIONS • May need brief assistance with transportation and homemaker tasks ▮ Refer to section at end of plan for postdischarge considerations.	

TEST WHY IT IS DONE	WHAT IT TELLS ME
BLOOD TESTS • *Complete blood count (CBC):* Battery of screening tests that typically includes hemoglobin (Hgb); hematocrit (Hct); red blood cell (RBC) count, morphology, indices, and distribution width index; platelet count and size; and white blood cell (WBC) count and differential.	WBCs are often elevated above 12,000/mm³; neutrophil count often elevated to greater than 75%.
• *C-reactive protein (CRP):* Protein produced by the liver when bacterial infections occur and rapidly increases within the first 12 hours.	CRP levels greater than 1 mg/dL are commonly reported in client with appendicitis. Very high levels of CRP (greater than 3mg/dL) in this client can indicate gangrenous evolution of the disease. However, CRP normalization occurs 12 hours after onset of symptoms.
OTHER DIAGNOSTIC STUDIES • *Abdominal computed tomography (CT) scan, also called CAT scan:* X-ray procedure that uses a computer to produce a detailed picture of a cross-section of the abdomen.	Gold standard test for differentiation of appendicitis from other causes of abdominal pain, such as perforating ulcer, cholecystitis, and reproductive organ infections, or to localize drainable abscesses.
• *Ultrasonography:* Technique for imaging internal structures of the body by measuring and recording the reflection of pulsed or continuous high-frequency sound waves.	Method for quickly scanning abdomen. May be done as screening test as a normal appendix does not visualize.
• *Abdominal x-rays:* Nonsensitive and nonspecific in diagnosing appendicitis.	May reveal hardened bit of fecal material in appendix (fecalith) and localized ileus.

Nursing Priorities

1. Prevent complications.
2. Promote comfort.
3. Provide information about surgical procedure, prognosis, treatment needs, and potential complications.

Discharge Goals

1. Complications prevented or minimized.
2. Pain alleviated or controlled.
3. Surgical procedure, prognosis, therapeutic regimen, and possible complications understood.
4. Plan in place to meet needs after discharge.

NURSING DIAGNOSIS: **risk for Infection**

Risk factors may include
Inadequate primary defenses, perforation or rupture of the appendix, peritonitis, abscess formation
Invasive procedures, surgical incision

Possibly evidenced by
(Not applicable; presence of signs and symptoms establishes an *actual* diagnosis)

Desired Outcomes/Evaluation Criteria—Client Will

Wound Healing: Primary Intention (NOC)
Achieve timely wound healing, free of signs of infection and inflammation, purulent drainage, erythema, and fever.

ACTIONS/INTERVENTIONS	RATIONALE
Infection Control (NIC) *Independent* Practice and instruct in good hand-washing and aseptic wound care. Encourage and provide perineal care.	Reduces risk of spread of bacteria.
Inspect incision and dressings. Note characteristics of drainage from wound or drains (if inserted) and presence of erythema.	Provides for early detection of developing infectious process and monitors resolution of preexisting peritonitis.

ACTIONS/INTERVENTIONS (continued)

Monitor vital signs. Note onset of fever, chills, diaphoresis, changes in mentation, and reports of increasing abdominal pain.

Obtain drainage specimens, if indicated.

Collaborative

Administer antibiotics, as appropriate.

Prepare for and assist with incision and drainage (I&D) if indicated.

RATIONALE (continued)

Suggestive of presence of infection, developing sepsis, abscess, and peritonitis.

Gram's stain, culture, and sensitivity testing is useful in identifying causative organism and choice of therapy.

Antibiotics given before appendectomy are primarily for prophylaxis of wound infection and are not usually continued postoperatively. Therapeutic antibiotics are administered if the appendix is ruptured or abscessed, or peritonitis has developed.

May be necessary to drain contents of localized abscess.

NURSING DIAGNOSIS: risk for deficient Fluid Volume

Risk factors may include
Preoperative vomiting, postoperative restrictions—nothing by mouth (NPO)
Hypermetabolic state—fever, healing process
Inflammation of peritoneum with sequestration of fluid

Possibly evidenced by
(Not applicable; presence of signs and symptoms establishes an *actual* diagnosis)

Desired Outcomes/Evaluation Criteria—Client Will

Hydration (NOC)
Maintain adequate fluid balance as evidenced by moist mucous membranes, good skin turgor, stable vital signs, and individually adequate urinary output.

ACTIONS/INTERVENTIONS

Fluid Monitoring (NIC)
Independent
Monitor blood pressure (BP) and pulse.

Inspect mucous membranes; assess skin turgor and capillary refill.

Monitor intake and output (I&O); note urine color and concentration and specific gravity.

Auscultate bowel sounds. Note passing of flatus and bowel movement.

Provide clear liquids in small amounts when oral intake is resumed, and progress diet as tolerated.

Give frequent mouth care with special attention to protection of the lips.

Collaborative
Maintain nasogastric (NG) and intestinal suction, as indicated.

Administer intravenous (IV) fluids and electrolytes.

RATIONALE

Variations help identify fluctuating intravascular volumes or changes in vital signs associated with immune response to inflammation.

Indicators of adequacy of peripheral circulation and cellular hydration.

Decreasing output of concentrated urine with increasing specific gravity suggests dehydration and need for increased fluids.

Indicators of return of peristalsis and readiness to begin oral intake. *Note:* This may not occur in the hospital if client has had a laparoscopic procedure and been discharged in less than 24 hours.

Reduces risk of gastric irritation and vomiting to minimize fluid loss.

Dehydration results in drying and painful cracking of the lips and mouth.

Although not frequently needed, an NG tube may be inserted preoperatively and maintained in immediate postoperative phase to decompress the bowel, promote intestinal rest, and prevent vomiting.

The peritoneum reacts to irritation and infection by producing large amounts of intestinal fluid, pulling fluid from the vascular space and possibly reducing the circulating blood volume, resulting in dehydration and relative electrolyte imbalances.

May be related to
Distention of intestinal tissues by inflammation
Presence of surgical incision

Possibly evidenced by
Reports of pain
Facial grimacing, muscle guarding, distraction behaviors
Autonomic responses

Desired Outcomes/Evaluation Criteria—Client Will

Pain Level (NOC)
Report pain is relieved or controlled.
Appear relaxed, able to sleep and rest appropriately.

ACTIONS/INTERVENTIONS	RATIONALE
Pain Management (NIC)	
Independent	
Assess pain, noting location, characteristics, and severity (0 to 10 scale). Investigate and report changes in pain, as appropriate.	Useful in monitoring effectiveness of medication and progression of healing. Changes in characteristics of pain may indicate developing abscess or peritonitis, requiring prompt medical evaluation and intervention.
Provide accurate, honest information to client/ significant other (SO).	Being informed about progress of situation provides emotional support, helping to decrease anxiety.
Keep at rest in semi-Fowler's position.	Gravity localizes inflammatory exudate into lower abdomen or pelvis, relieving abdominal tension, which is accentuated by supine position.
Encourage early ambulation.	Promotes normalization of organ function; stimulates peristalsis and passing of flatus, reducing abdominal discomfort.
Provide diversional activities.	Refocuses attention, promotes relaxation, and may enhance coping abilities.
Collaborative	
Keep NPO and maintain NG suction initially.	Decreases discomfort of early intestinal peristalsis and gastric irritation or vomiting.
Administer analgesics, as indicated.	Relief of pain facilitates cooperation with other therapeutic interventions, such as ambulation and pulmonary toilet.
Place ice bag on abdomen periodically during initial 24 to 48 hours, as appropriate.	Soothes and relieves pain through desensitization of nerve endings. *Note:* Do not use heat because it may cause tissue congestion and increase edema formation.

NURSING DIAGNOSIS: **deficient Knowledge [Learning Need] regarding condition, prognosis, treatment, self-care, and discharge needs**

May be related to
Lack of exposure or recall; information misinterpretation
Unfamiliarity with information resources

Possibly evidenced by
Questions; request for information; verbalization of problem, concerns
Statement of misconception
Inaccurate follow-through of instruction
Development of preventable complications

Desired Outcomes/Evaluation Criteria—Client Will

Knowledge: Illness Care (NOC)
Verbalize understanding of disease process and potential complications.
Verbalize understanding of therapeutic needs.
Participate in treatment regimen.

ACTIONS/INTERVENTIONS	RATIONALE

Teaching: Disease Process (NIC)
Independent

Identify symptoms requiring medical evaluation—increasing pain, edema and erythema of wound, presence of drainage, and fever.

Review postoperative activity restrictions—heavy lifting, exercise, sexual activity, sports, and driving.

Encourage progressive activities as tolerated with periodic rest periods.

Recommend use of mild laxative or stool softeners as necessary and avoidance of enemas.

Discuss care of incision, including dressing changes, bathing restrictions, and return to physician for suture and staple removal.

Prompt intervention reduces risk of serious complications, such as delayed wound healing and peritonitis.

Provides information for client to plan for return to usual routines without untoward incidents.
Prevents fatigue, promotes healing and feeling of well-being, and facilitates resumption of normal activities.
Assists with return to usual bowel function; prevents undue straining for defecation.
Understanding promotes cooperation with therapeutic regimen, enhancing healing and recovery process.

POTENTIAL CONSIDERATIONS following acute hospitalization (dependent on client's age, physical condition, presence of complications, personal resources, and life responsibilities)
• *risk for ineffective self Health Management*—perceived seriousness or susceptibility, perceived benefit, demands made on individual (family, work)

PERITONITIS

I. Pathophysiology
  a. Inflammation of the serosal membrane that lines the abdominal cavity and its viscera
  b. Intra-abdominal infection may be localized or generalized, with or without abscess formation.

II. Classification
  a. Categorized as primary, secondary, or tertiary
    i. Primary, or bacterial peritonitis, is rare, with the peritoneum spontaneously infected via the blood and lymphatic circulation.
    ii. Secondary peritonitis is related to a pathological process in a visceral organ.
    iii. Tertiary peritonitis is a persistent or recurrent infection after adequate initial therapy.
  b. Can be acute or chronic in nature

III. Etiology
  a. Infectious agents
    i. Most common pathogens include gram-negative organisms, such as *Escherichia coli* and *Klebsiella pneumoniae*, and gram-positive organisms, such as *Streptococcus*.
    ii. Resistant and unusual organisms, such as *Enterococcus*, *Candida*, and *Enterobacter*, are found in a significant proportion of tertiary cases.
  b. Other sources of inflammation
    i. Primary peritonitis: chronic liver disease with ascites formation most common cause, use of peritoneum for dialysis

    ii. Secondary peritonitis: rupture or perforation of internal organ or instillation of irritating substance causing chemical irritation
      1. Gastrointestinal (GI) tract: ruptured appendix, perforated gastric or duodenal ulcer; cholecystitis with stone perforation; perforated colon caused by diverticulitis or cancer; pancreatitis, ulcerative colitis, and Crohn's disease
      2. Ovaries and uterus: pelvic inflammatory disease, ovarian cyst
      3. Traumatic injuries: blunt and penetrating trauma
      4. Iatrogenic trauma to GI tract, such as during endoscopic procedures; inadvertent bowel injury or anastomosis dehiscence; instrumentation such as occurs with peritoneal dialysis or percutaneous stent placement (Peralta et al, 2006)

IV. Statistics (Peralta et al, 2006)
  a. Morbidity: As many as 70% of survivors of primary peritonitis have a recurrent episode within 1 year; dialysis-related secondary peritonitis rate is approximately 1 in 24 patient-treatment months (Kean et al, 2000).
  b. Mortality: Approximately 10% to 30% in primary peritonitis, dependent on early versus delayed therapy, and 50% with recurrent episode; in secondary peritonitis rate of less than 5% with simple abscesses increasing to greater than 30% to 50% in severe infections, 50% to 70% in tertiary peritonitis.

Ascites: Accumulation of serous fluid in the peritoneal cavity.

Borborygmus: Intermittent loud, rushing bowel sounds.

Peritoneum: Serous membrane that lines the abdominal cavity and covers the visceral organs.

Peritonitis: Inflammation of the peritoneum that may be generalized throughout the peritoneum, affecting the visceral and parietal surfaces of the abdominal cavity, or localized in one area as an abscess.

Postural hypotension: A drop in blood pressure (hypotension) due to a change in body position (posture) when a person moves to a more vertical position.

Rebound tenderness (also known as Blumberg sign): Pressing a hand on the abdomen elicits less pain than releasing the hand abruptly, which will aggravate the pain, as the peritoneum snaps back into place.

Viscera: Internal organs enclosed within the abdominal cavity.

Care Setting

The client is admitted to an inpatient acute medical or surgical unit.

Related Concerns

Appendectomy, page 344

Inflammatory bowel disease (IBD): ulcerative colitis, Crohn's disease, page 321

Pancreatitis, page 458

Psychosocial aspects of care, page 749

Peritoneal dialysis (PD), page 570

Sepsis/septicemia, page 686

Surgical intervention, page 782

Total nutritional support: parenteral/enteral feeding, page 469

Upper gastrointestinal/esophageal bleeding, page 306

Client Assessment Database

DIAGNOSTIC DIVISION MAY REPORT	MAY EXHIBIT
CIRCULATION	• Tachycardia, diaphoresis, pallor, hypotension (signs of shock) • Tissue edema
ELIMINATION • Inability to pass stool or flatus • Occasional diarrhea	• Hiccups • Decreased urinary output, dark color • Decreased or absent bowel sounds (ileus) • Intermittent loud, rushing bowel sounds • Abdominal rigidity, distention, rebound tenderness; hyperresonance or tympani (ileus) • Loss of dullness over liver (free air in abdomen)
FOOD/FLUIDS • Loss of appetite • Nausea, vomiting • Thirst	• Hypoactive bowel sounds (generalized ileus) • Projectile vomiting • Dry mucous membranes, swollen tongue, poor skin turgor
PAIN/DISCOMFORT • Sudden, severe, or persistent severe abdominal pain • Pain may be generalized, localized, referred to shoulder, intensified by movement	• Abdominal distention, rigidity, rebound tenderness • Distraction behaviors, restlessness, self-focus • Muscle guarding of abdomen, flexion of knees • Lying in rigid position, almost unmoving (Movious, 2006)
RESPIRATION	• Shallow respirations • Tachypnea

Client Assessment Database (continued)

DIAGNOSTIC DIVISION MAY REPORT (continued)	MAY EXHIBIT (continued)
SAFETY	• Fever—usually greater than 101°F (38°C), although hypothermia may be present with severe sepsis • Chills
SEXUALITY • History of pelvic organ inflammation (salpingitis), puerperal infection, septic abortion, retroperitoneal abscess	
TEACHING/LEARNING • History of recent trauma with abdominal penetration, such as gunshot or stab wound or blunt trauma to the abdomen, bladder perforation or ruptured gallbladder, perforated carcinoma of the stomach, perforated gastric or duodenal ulcer, gangrenous obstruction of the bowel, perforation of diverticulum, ulcerative colitis (UC), regional ileitis, strangulated hernia	
DISCHARGE PLAN CONSIDERATIONS • Assistance with homemaker and maintenance tasks ◗ Refer to section at end of plan for postdischarge considerations.	

Diagnostic Studies

TEST WHY IT IS DONE	WHAT IT TELLS ME
BLOOD TESTS • *Complete blood count (CBC):* Battery of screening tests that typically includes hemoglobin (Hgb); hematocrit (Hct); red blood cell (RBC) count, morphology, indices, and distribution width index; platelet count and size; white blood cell (WBC) count and differential.	WBCs are elevated—sometimes more than 20,000—except in elderly or immunocompromised client or client with certain infections, such as fungal or cytomegalovirus, who may demonstrate leukopenia. RBCs, Hgb, and Hct may be increased, indicating hemoconcentration secondary to extracellular fluid loss into the peritoneal cavity.
• *Serum protein/albumin:* Visceral proteins considered to be markers for fluid and nutrition status.	May be decreased because of fluid shifts, lack of food intake, and nothing by mouth (NPO) status.
• *Serum amylase and lipase:* Enzymes produced by the pancreas, which aid in digestion of starches and fats.	Usually elevated when pancreatitis is cause.
• *Serum electrolytes:* Substances that dissociate into ions in solution and acquire the capacity to conduct electricity. Common electrolytes include sodium, potassium, chloride, calcium, and phosphate. Provides baseline data and can be used to evaluate and monitor fluid and electrolyte balance.	Water and electrolytes are lost in vomitus and drainage from the gastrointestinal tubes, and the client cannot take anything by mouth. Large quantities of body fluids and electrolytes collect in the peritoneal cavity instead of circulating normally throughout the body, increasing the problems of water and electrolyte imbalance.
• *Arterial blood gases (ABGs):* Evaluates arterial blood levels of oxygen (PaO_2), carbon dioxide ($PaCO_2$), and pH.	Respiratory alkalosis and metabolic acidosis may be noted.
• *Cultures:* Specimens may be taken from blood, exudate, or secretions; ascites fluid; or peritoneal dialysate to evaluate source and causative organism (aerobic and anaerobic).	Causative organisms, including *E. coli* or streptococci, are often cultured. Rarely, pneumococcus is the cause. Sensitivities may also be done to identify effective antimicrobial agent. Gram's stain and aerobic and anaerobic cultures can show multiple organisms.

(continues on page 352)

TEST WHY IT IS DONE (continued)	WHAT IT TELLS ME (continued)
OTHER DIAGNOSTIC STUDIES • *Computed tomography (CT) scan (abdominal/pelvic):* X-ray procedure that uses a computer to produce a detailed picture of a cross-section of the body.	Gold standard for diagnosis of peritonitis, peritoneal abscess, and related visceral pathology.
• *Ultrasound scan (abdominal/pelvic):* Scan that uses sound waves to produce an electronic image of the organs of the pelvis.	Can often diagnose cause of peritonitis, such as cholecystitis, perihepatic abscess, pancreatitis, ruptured appendix, ovarian abscess, or diverticulitis. Ultrasonography can also detect increased amounts of ascites and peritoneal fluid.
• *Abdominal x-ray:* Identifies pathology within the abdomen.	May reveal gas distention of bowel or ileus. When perforated viscera is the cause, free air will be found in the abdomen.
• *Chest x-ray:* Identifies signs of perforated viscera.	Presence of free air causes elevation of the diaphragm.
• *Peritoneal tap or lavage (paracentesis):* Puncture of the wall of a cavity with a needle in order to draw off excess fluid or to obtain a sample for analysis.	Peritoneal fluid samples generally demonstrate low pH and glucose or elevated protein and lactate dehydrogenase (LDH) levels and may contain blood, pus and exudate, amylase, bile, and creatinine.

Nursing Priorities

1. Control infection.
2. Restore and/or maintain circulating volume.
3. Promote comfort.
4. Maintain nutrition.
5. Provide information about disease process, possible complications, and treatment needs.

Discharge Goals

1. Infection resolved.
2. Complications prevented or minimized.
3. Pain relieved.
4. Disease process, potential complications, and therapeutic regimen understood.
5. Plan in place to meet needs after discharge.

NURSING DIAGNOSIS: **risk for Infection [septicemia]**

Risk factors may include
Inadequate primary defenses—broken skin, traumatized tissue, altered peristalsis
Inadequate secondary defenses—immunosuppression
Invasive procedures

Possibly evidenced by
(Not applicable; presence of signs and symptoms establishes an *actual* diagnosis)

Desired Outcomes/Evaluation Criteria—Client Will

Infection Status (NOC)
Achieve timely healing, be free of purulent drainage or erythema, and be afebrile.

Risk Control (NOC)
Verbalize understanding of the individual causative or risk factor(s).

ACTIONS/INTERVENTIONS	RATIONALE
Infection Control (NIC) *Independent* Note individual risk factors: abdominal trauma, acute appendicitis, and peritoneal dialysis.	Influences choice of interventions.
Assess vital signs frequently, noting unresolved or progressing hypotension, decreased pulse pressure, tachycardia, fever, and tachypnea.	Signs of impending septic shock. Circulating endotoxins eventually produce vasodilation, shift of fluid from circulation, and a low cardiac output state. *Note:* These clients frequently are critically ill and medical or postsurgical intensive care is required. (Refer to CP: Sepsis/Septicemia.)
Note changes in mental status, such as new onset confusion and stupor.	Hypoxemia, hypotension, and acidosis can cause deteriorating mental status.

ACTIONS/INTERVENTIONS (continued)

Note skin color, temperature, and moisture.

Monitor urine output.

Maintain strict aseptic technique in caring for abdominal drains, incisions or open wounds, dressings, and invasive sites. Cleanse with appropriate solution.

Perform and model good hand-washing technique. Monitor staff and client compliance with hand washing.

Observe drainage from wounds or drains.

Maintain sterile technique when catheterizing client, provide catheter care, and encourage perineal cleansing on a routine basis.

Monitor or restrict visitors and staff, as appropriate. Provide protective isolation if indicated.

Collaborative

Obtain specimens for culture and monitor results of serial blood, urine, and wound cultures.

Assist with peritoneal aspiration, if indicated.

Administer antimicrobials, for example cephalosporins, such as, cefizoxime (Cefizox), cefotaxime (Claforan), ceftriaxone (Rocephin); extended spectrum penicillins, such as piperacillin/tazobactam (Zosyn); fluoroquinolones, such as ciprofloxacin (Cipro), alatrovafloxacin (Trovan); antifungals, such as metronidazole (Flagyl); aminoglycosides, such as gentamicin (Garamycin), tobrimycin (Tobi), amikacin (Amikin).

Prepare for surgical intervention, as indicated:

Open incision, laparoscopic débridement and lavage

Ostomy procedure

RATIONALE (continued)

Warm, flushed, dry skin is early sign of septicemia. Later manifestations include cool, clammy, pale skin and cyanosis as shock becomes refractory.

Oliguria develops as a result of decreased renal perfusion, circulating toxins, and effects of antibiotics.

Prevents access or limits spread of infecting organisms and cross-contamination.

Reduces risk of cross-contamination and spread of infection.

Provides information about status of infection.

Prevents access and limits bacterial growth in urinary tract.

Reduces risk of exposure to, or acquisition of, secondary infection in immunosuppressed client.

Culture identifies causative microorganisms and helps in assessing effectiveness of antimicrobial regimen.

May be done to remove fluid and to identify infecting organisms so appropriate antibiotic therapy can be instituted.

Therapy is systemic and directed at the particular identified organism(s), such as anaerobic bacteria, fungus, and gram-negative bacilli. Optimal duration of antimicrobial therapy depends on the underlying pathology, severity of infection, and speed and effectiveness of source control. Antimicrobials may be administered by intravenous (IV) or by intraoperative lavage.

Surgery may be treatment of choice and curative in acute, localized peritonitis; for example, to drain localized abscess; remove peritoneal exudates, ruptured appendix or gallbladder; plicate perforated ulcer; or resect bowel. Intraoperative lavage may be used to remove necrotic debris and treat inflammation that is poorly localized or diffuse. Multiple additional operations may be needed to control source of infection, drain abscesses, or clean out necrotic material. In this instance, the abdominal closure is temporary, using various dressings, mesh coverings, and Velcro-like skin-closure devices, thus providing ready access to affected area while also preventing contamination from the outside. Later surgical procedures may also be required for permanent closure or repair of abdominal wall. *Note:* If peritonitis is diffuse, medical management is necessary before or in place of surgical treatment.

Temporary colostomy procedure may be performed if the colon is source of infection, such as in ruptured diverticulum, to facilitate treatment of the infection and bowel healing.

NURSING DIAGNOSIS: deficient [mixed] Fluid Volume

May be related to

Fluid shifts from extracellular, intravascular, and interstitial compartments into intestines and/or peritoneal space

Vomiting; medically restricted intake; nasogastric (NG) or intestinal aspiration

Fever, hypermetabolic state

Possibly evidenced by

Dry mucous membranes, poor skin turgor, delayed capillary refill, weak peripheral pulses

Diminished urinary output; dark, concentrated urine

Hypotension; tachycardia

Desired Outcomes/Evaluation Criteria—Client Will

Fluid Balance (NOC)

Demonstrate improved fluid balance as evidenced by adequate urinary output with normal specific gravity, stable vital signs, moist mucous membranes, good skin turgor, prompt capillary refill, and weight within acceptable range.

ACTIONS/INTERVENTIONS	RATIONALE

Fluid/Electrolyte Management (NIC)

Independent

Monitor vital signs, noting presence of hypotension (including postural changes), tachycardia, tachypnea, and fever. Measure central venous pressure (CVP) if available.

Aids in evaluating degree of fluid deficit, effectiveness of fluid replacement therapy, and response to medications.

Maintain accurate intake and output (I&O) and correlate with daily weights. Include measured and estimated losses, such as with gastric suction, drains, dressings, Hemovacs, diaphoresis, and abdominal girth for third spacing of fluid.

Reflects overall hydration status. Urine output may be diminished because of hypovolemia and decreased renal perfusion, but weight may still increase, reflecting tissue edema or ascites accumulation (third spacing). Gastric suction losses may be large, and a great deal of fluid can be sequestered in the bowel and peritoneal space (ascites).

Measure urine specific gravity.

Reflects hydration status and changes in renal function, which may warn of developing acute renal failure in response to hypovolemia and effect of toxins. *Note:* Many antibiotics also have nephrotoxic effects that may further affect kidney function and urine output.

Observe skin and mucous membrane dryness and turgor. Note peripheral and sacral edema.

Hypovolemia, fluid shifts, and nutritional deficits contribute to poor skin turgor and taut edematous tissues.

Eliminate noxious sights or smells from environment. Limit intake of ice chips.

Reduces gastric stimulation and vomiting response. *Note:* Excessive use of ice chips during gastric aspiration can increase gastric washout of electrolytes.

Change position frequently, provide frequent skin care, and maintain dry, wrinkle-free bedding.

Edematous tissue with compromised circulation is prone to breakdown.

Collaborative

Monitor laboratory studies: Hgb/Hct, electrolytes, protein, albumin, BUN, and creatinine (Cr).

Provides information about hydration and organ function. Significant consequences to systemic function are possible as a result of fluid shifts, hypovolemia, hypoxemia, circulating toxins, and necrotic tissue products.

Administer plasma, blood, fluids, electrolytes, and diuretics, as indicated.

Replenishes and maintains circulating volume and electrolyte balance. Colloids, such as plasma or blood, help move water back into intravascular compartment by increasing osmotic pressure gradient. Diuretics may be used to assist in excretion of toxins and to enhance renal function.

Maintain NPO status with NG or intestinal aspiration.

Reduces vomiting caused by hyperactivity of bowel; manages stomach and intestinal fluids.

NURSING DIAGNOSIS: acute Pain

May be related to
Chemical irritation of the parietal peritoneum (toxins)
Trauma to tissues
Accumulation of fluid in abdominal and peritoneal cavity (abdominal distention)

Possibly evidenced by
Verbalizations of pain
Muscle guarding, rebound tenderness
Facial mask of pain, self-focus
Distraction behavior, autonomic or emotional responses (anxiety)

Desired Outcomes/Evaluation Criteria—Client Will

Pain Control (NOC)
Report pain is relieved or controlled.
Demonstrate use of relaxation skills or other methods to promote comfort.

ACTIONS/INTERVENTIONS	RATIONALE

Pain Management (NIC)

Independent

Investigate pain reports, noting location, duration, intensity (0 to 10 scale), and characteristics such as dull, sharp, or constant.

Changes in location or intensity are not uncommon but may reflect developing complications. Pain tends to become constant, more intense, and diffuse over the entire abdomen as inflammatory process accelerates; pain may localize if an abscess develops.

ACTIONS/INTERVENTIONS (continued)

Maintain semi-Fowler's position as indicated.

Move client slowly and deliberately, splinting painful area.

Provide comfort measures, such as massage, back rubs, and deep breathing. Instruct in relaxation and visualization exercises. Provide diversional activities.

Provide frequent oral care. Remove noxious environmental stimuli.

Collaborative

Administer medications, as indicated, for example:
Analgesics and opioids

Antiemetics, such as hydroxyzine (Vistaril)

Antipyretics, such as acetaminophen (Tylenol)

RATIONALE (continued)

Facilitates fluid and wound drainage by gravity, reducing diaphragmatic irritation and abdominal tension, thereby reducing pain.

Reduces muscle tension and guarding, which may help minimize pain of movement.

Promotes relaxation and may enhance client's coping abilities by refocusing attention.

Reduces nausea and vomiting, which can increase intra-abdominal pressure and pain.

Reduces metabolic rate and intestinal irritation from circulating and local toxins, which aid in pain relief and promote healing. *Note:* Pain is usually severe and may require opioid pain control.

Reduces the nausea and vomiting that can increase abdominal pain.

Reduces discomfort associated with fever.

NURSING DIAGNOSIS: **risk for imbalanced Nutrition: Less than Body Requirements**

Risk factors may include
Nausea, vomiting, intestinal dysfunction
Metabolic abnormalities, increased metabolic needs

Possibly evidenced by
(Not applicable; presence of signs and symptoms establishes an *actual* diagnosis)

Desired Outcomes/Evaluation Criteria—Client Will

Nutritional Status (NOC)
Maintain usual weight and positive nitrogen balance.

ACTIONS/INTERVENTIONS

Nutrition Management (NIC)
Independent
Auscultate bowel sounds, noting absent and hyperactive sounds.

Monitor NG tube output. Note presence of vomiting and diarrhea.

Measure abdominal girth.

Assess abdomen frequently for return to softness, reappearance of normal bowel sounds, and passage of flatus.
Weigh regularly.

Collaborative
Monitor BUN, protein, prealbumin or albumin, glucose, and nitrogen balance, as indicated.
Administer enteral or parenteral feedings, as indicated.

Advance diet as tolerated—clear liquids to soft food.

RATIONALE

Although bowel sounds are frequently absent, inflammation of the intestine may be accompanied by intestinal hyperactivity, diminished water absorption, and diarrhea.

Large amounts of gastric aspirant, or severe vomiting and diarrhea suggest bowel obstruction, requiring further evaluation.

Provides quantitative evidence of changes in intestinal distention and accumulation of ascitic fluid.

Indicates return of normal bowel function and ability to resume oral intake.

Initial losses or gains reflect changes in hydration, but sustained losses suggest nutritional deficit.

Reflects organ function and nutritional status and needs.

Enteral feedings, even at low volumes, have been shown to maintain gut mucosal integrity and to reduce the incidence of infectious complications, making the choice of enteral feedings preferable over parenteral solutions whenever possible. (Refer to CP: Total Nutritional Support: Enteral/Parenteral Feedings.)

Client may have some degree of gut dysfunction for quite some time, making it necessary for careful progression of diet when oral intake is resumed.

NURSING DIAGNOSIS: Anxiety [specify level]/Fear

May be related to
Situational crisis
Threat of death, change in health status
Physiological factors, hypermetabolic state

Possibly evidenced by
Increased tension, helplessness
Apprehension, uncertainty, worry, sense of impending doom
Sympathetic stimulation; restlessness, focus on self

Desired Outcomes/Evaluation Criteria—Client Will

Anxiety Self-Control (NOC)
Verbalize awareness of feelings and healthy ways to deal with them.
Report anxiety is reduced to a manageable level.
Appear relaxed.

ACTIONS/INTERVENTIONS	RATIONALE
Anxiety Reduction (NIC)	
Independent	
Evaluate anxiety level, noting client's perception of situation and verbal and nonverbal responses. Encourage free expression of emotions.	Apprehension may be escalated by severe pain, severity of illness, urgency of diagnostic procedures, and possibility of surgery.
Review physiological factors present, such as sepsis or toxins related to infection, medications, and metabolic imbalances.	These factors are present in seriously ill client and can cause or contribute to anxiety.
Provide ongoing information regarding disease process and anticipated treatment.	Knowing what to expect can reduce anxiety for both client and significant other (SO). Also, ongoing review helps to identify those factors adding to anxiety that could be changed—client getting more uninterrupted sleep or adding or deleting medications.
Provide presence. Acknowledge anxiety and fear. Do not deny or reassure client that everything will be all right. Be accurate and factual in providing information. Correct misconceptions about disease process and possible treatments.	Affirms client's value as a human being in need of assistance in dealing with a serious health threat; helps client and SO identify and deal with reality.
Schedule adequate rest and uninterrupted periods for sleep.	Limits fatigue, conserves energy, and can enhance coping ability.
Provide comfort measures: family presence, quiet environment, soft music, back rub, and Therapeutic Touch (TT).	Promotes relaxation and enhances ability to deal with situation.

Refer to CP: Psychosocial Aspects for Care, for additional interventions.

NURSING DIAGNOSIS: deficient Knowledge [Learning Need] regarding condition, prognosis, treatment, self-care, and discharge needs

May be related to
Lack of exposure, recall
Information misinterpretation
Unfamiliarity with information resources

Possibly evidenced by
Questions, request for information
Statement of misconception
Inaccurate follow-through of instruction

Desired Outcomes/Evaluation Criteria—Client Will

Knowledge: Disease Process (NOC)
Verbalize understanding of disease process and potential complications.
Identify relationship of signs and symptoms to the disease process and correlate symptoms with causative factors.

Knowledge: Treatment Regimen (NOC)
Verbalize understanding of therapeutic needs.
Correctly perform necessary procedures and explain reasons for actions.

ACTIONS/INTERVENTIONS	RATIONALE

Teaching: Disease Process (NIC)
Independent
Review underlying disease process and recovery expectations.

Identify signs and symptoms requiring medical evaluation, such as recurrent abdominal pain or distention, vomiting, fever, chills, or presence of purulent drainage, swelling, and erythema of surgical incision (if present).
Discuss medication regimen, schedule, and possible side effects.

Recommend gradual resumption of usual activities, allowing for adequate rest.
Review activity limitations, such as avoiding heavy lifting.

Demonstrate sterile or clean dressing change as appropriate. Have client/SO demonstrate ability to manage these procedures.

Emphasize importance of medical follow-up care.

Refer to community resources, as needed or desired, such as visiting nurse, home healthcare, and durable medical equipment suppliers.

Provides knowledge base from which client can make informed choices.
Early recognition and treatment of developing complications may prevent more serious illness or injury.

Antibiotics may be continued for varying periods of time after discharge depending on extent of the infection and length of stay in acute care facility.
Prevents fatigue and enhances feeling of well-being.

Reduces chance of undue intra-abdominal pressure and muscle tension.
Client/SO may have a long period of home management of surgical wound(s), depending on extent of infection and treatment. Slow recovery time is often associated with such a complex condition.
Necessary to monitor resolution of infection and effectiveness of therapeutic interventions.
Supports transition to home, promotes self-care, and increases likelihood of successful outcome.

POTENTIAL CONSIDERATIONS following acute hospitalization (dependent on client's age, physical condition, presence of complications, personal resources, and life responsibilities)
• *Fatigue*—decreased metabolic energy production, increased energy requirements to perform activities of daily living (ADLs), states of discomfort
• *acute Pain*—chemical irritation of the peritoneum, prolonged healing process

CHOLECYSTITIS WITH CHOLELITHIASIS

I. Pathophysiology—An acute or chronic inflammation of the gallbladder associated with obstruction by gallstones
  a. Common bile duct stones are formed in the bile duct (primary) or formed in and transported from the gallbladder (secondary).
  b. Cholelithiasis is usually asymptomatic.
  c. Cholecystitis can result if stone becomes lodged in one of the ducts.
II. Etiology
  a. Stones most often develop in and obstruct the common bile duct or the cystic duct; also found in the hepatic, small bile, and pancreatic ducts.
    i. Ninety percent of cases involve stones in the cystic duct (calculous cholecystitis), whereas the other 10% involve cholecystitis without stones (acalculous cholecystitis) (Gladden & Migala, 2007).
    ii. Stones are made up of cholesterol, calcium bilirubinate, or a mixture caused by changes in the bile composition.

  b. Bile cultures are positive for bacteria in 50% to 75% of cases; however, bacterial proliferation may be a result or consequence of cholecystitis, but not the precipitating factor (Gladden & Migala, 2007).
  c. Other causes include stasis of bile or bacterial infection or ischemia of the gallbladder.
  d. Failure to remove impacted stone can lead to bile stasis or bacteremia and septicemia causing cholangitis—a medical emergency.
III. Statistics (Gladden & Migala, 2007)
  a. Morbidity: Gallstones are two to three times more frequent in females than in males; perforation occurs in 10% to 15% of cases, and 25% to 30% of clients either require surgery or develop complications.
  b. Mortality: An estimated 10,000 deaths occur annually; about 7,000 deaths are a result of gallstone complications, such as acute pancreatitis. With calculous cholecystitis, there is an expected 4% mortality rate; with acalculous cholecystitis, a 10% to 50% mortality rate.

Biliary colic: Typically constant and slowly progressive pain that is usually located in the epigastrium or right upper quadrant; most common presenting symptom in cholelithiasis.

Cholangitis: Inflammation of the common bile duct due to an impacted stone obstructing bile drainage, which can lead to bacteremia and septicemia.

Cholecystitis: Inflammation of the gallbladder.

Cholelithiasis: Stones in the gallbladder.

Clay-colored stool: Reflects absence of bile in stool due to infection of liver or blockage of bile flow out of the liver.

Dyspepsia: Feeling of fullness and bloating after eating; also involves belching, heartburn, nausea, and sometimes vomiting.

Eructation: Belching.

Gallstones: Generally the result of cholesterol precipitating out of bile (cholesterol stones) or of free bilirubin combining with calcium to create bile pigment stones.

Hematemesis: Bloody vomitus.

Jaundice: Yellow tinge to skin and sclera in eyes due to bile absorption into circulatory system.

Lithotripsy: Use of high-energy shock waves to fragment and disintegrate gallstones.

Melena: Black, tarry feces due to presence of digested blood in stool.

Murphy's sign: Inability to take in a breath due to pain when examiner's hand is pressing on gallbladder.

Sonographic Murphy's sign: Pain when the ultrasound probe is pushed directly on the gallbladder.

Steatorrhea: Fatty stools.

Care Setting

Severe acute attacks may require brief hospitalization on a medical unit. This plan of care deals with the acutely ill, hospitalized client. Surgery is usually performed after symptoms have subsided, but during the hospitalization, for acute illness. (Refer to CP: Cholecystectomy.)

Related Concerns

Cholecystectomy, page 364

Fluid and electrolyte imbalances, page 903

Psychosocial aspects of care, page 749

Total nutritional support: parenteral/enteral feeding, page 469

Client Assessment Database

DIAGNOSTIC DIVISION MAY REPORT	MAY EXHIBIT
ACTIVITY/REST • Fatigue	• Restlessness
CIRCULATION	• Tachycardia • Diaphoresis • Hypotension, if septic
ELIMINATION • Change in color of urine and stools	• Abdominal distention • Palpable mass in right upper quadrant (RUQ) • Dark, concentrated urine • Clay-colored stool, or steatorrhea
FOOD/FLUID • Anorexia, nausea, and vomiting • Intolerance of fatty and "gas-forming" foods, recurrent regurgitation, heartburn, indigestion, flatulence, dyspepsia • Belching	• Obesity or recent weight loss • Normal to hypoactive bowel sounds
PAIN/DISCOMFORT • Severe epigastric and right upper abdominal pain, may radiate to midback, right shoulder and scapula, or to front of chest • Pain increases with movement • Midepigastric colicky pain associated with eating, especially after meals rich in fats	• Rebound tenderness, muscle guarding, or abdominal rigidity when RUQ is palpated • Positive Murphy's sign

Client Assessment Database (continued)

DIAGNOSTIC DIVISION MAY REPORT (continued)	MAY EXHIBIT (continued)
• Episodes of severe or ongoing pain starting suddenly, sometimes at night, with episodes of constant pain typically lasting 1 to 5 hours • Recurring episodes of similar pain	
RESPIRATION	• Increased respiratory rate • Splinted respiration marked by short, shallow breathing
SAFETY	• Low-grade fever • High fever and chills indicating septic complications • Jaundice with dry, itching skin (pruritus) • Bleeding tendencies caused by vitamin K deficiency
TEACHING/LEARNING • Familial tendency for gallstones • Recent pregnancy and delivery; history of diabetes mellitus (DM), inflammatory bowel disease (IBD), blood dyscrasias	
DISCHARGE PLAN CONSIDERATIONS • May require support with dietary changes and weight reduction ◗ Refer to section at end of plan for postdischarge considerations.	

Diagnostic Studies

TEST WHY IT IS DONE	WHAT IT TELLS ME
• *Complete blood count (CBC):* Assesses relationship of red blood cells to fluid volume, or viscosity, and may indicate risk factors, such as anemia, blood loss, or hypercoagulability.	Moderately elevated white blood cell (WBC) count (leukocytosis) may be present in acute cholecystitis. A normal WBC count does not rule out cholecystitis. The hematocrit (Hct) rises when the number of red blood cells (RBCs) increases or when the plasma volume is reduced, as in dehydration from nausea and vomiting, or blood loss from any point in the digestive tract.
• *Alkaline phosphatase (ALP):* An enzyme related to the bile ducts.	Elevated level is observed in 25% of clients with cholecystitis (Gladden & Migala, 2007).
• *Alanine aminotransferase (ALT) and aspartate aminotransferase (AST):* Enzymes primarily found in the liver.	ALT and AST may both be elevated in cholecystitis or with common bile duct obstruction.
• *Bilirubin:* A yellowish pigment produced from the breakdown of hemoglobin (Hgb) and RBCs.	The two different tests of bilirubin (total and direct) are often evaluated together if a person has jaundice. Jaundice is an indication that the bile duct is blocked and bile is accumulating in the bloodstream. Jaundice may be noted in approximately 15% of patients (Gladden & Migala, 2007).
• *Amylase:* An enzyme produced in the pancreas.	Cholecystitis can elevate this enzyme due to the close proximity of the liver to the pancreas.
• *Prothrombin levels:* Evaluates the ability of the blood to clot properly.	Reduced when obstruction to the flow of bile into the intestine decreases absorption of vitamin K.
• *Total protein:* Measures albumin and all other proteins in blood, including antibodies made to help fight off infection.	Inadequate production of albumin from liver disease results in a low protein count.

(continues on page 360)

TEST WHY IT IS DONE (continued)	WHAT IT TELLS ME (continued)
OTHER DIAGNOSTIC STUDIES • *Abdominal radiographs (multipositional):* X-rays of the abdomen.	Calcified gallstones are present in 10% to 15% of cases; x-rays can also visualize calcification of the gallbladder wall (Gladden & Migala, 2007).
• *Abdominal/biliary system ultrasound:* Most common screening test, also identifies abnormalities of surrounding tissues.	Right upper abdominal ultrasound is 90% to 95% sensitive for cholecystitis and 98% sensitive and specific for simple cholelithiasis. Sonographic Murphy's sign is 86% to 92% sensitive. May also reveal dilated common bile duct or dilated ducts in the liver (Gladden & Migala, 2007).
• *Computed tomography (CT) scan:* X-ray procedure that uses a computer to produce a detailed picture of a cross-section of the body.	Demonstrates dilated bile ducts, gallbladder, tumors, abscesses, perforation, and other complications.
• *Endoscopic retrograde cholangiopancreatography (ERCP):* Endoscopic procedure that allows direct visualization of the anatomy and may be used therapeutically to remove stones.	Visualizes biliary tree by cannulation of the common bile duct through the duodenum. Allows endoscopic removal of 90% of stones. Allows stenting of common bile ducts that are damaged, inflamed, or strictured. Larger stones can be reduced in size by mechanical lithotripsy during ERCP.
• *Hepatoiminodiacetic acid (HIDA) scan:* Radioisotope injected intravenously (IV) that allows diagnosis of acute cholecystitis.	HIDA scan has been found to be up to 95% accurate in diagnosing acute cholecystitis, although scanning can miss stones due to loops of bowel obstructing view (Gladden & Migala, 2007).
• *Magnetic resonance cholangiopancreatography (MRCP):* An application of magnetic resonance imaging to the hepatobiliary and pancreatic system.	Provides images of biliary tree and pancreatic ducts without use of contrast dye.
• *Oral cholecystography (OCG):* Preferred method of visualizing general appearance and function of gallbladder, including presence of filling defects, structural defects, and stones in ducts.	Assesses structure and function of ducts and detects remaining stones after lithotripsy or cholecystectomy as well as surgical complications.
• *Percutaneous transhepatic cholangiography (PTC):* Diagnostic test used to visualize the anatomy of the biliary tract. A contrast medium is injected into a bile duct in the liver, after which x-rays are taken.	May be done to visualize the biliary tree in cases where ERCP has been unsuccessful.

Nursing Priorities

1. Relieve pain and promote rest.
2. Maintain fluid and electrolyte balance.
3. Prevent complications.
4. Provide information about disease process, prognosis, and treatment needs.

Discharge Goals

1. Pain relieved.
2. Homeostasis achieved.
3. Complications prevented and minimized.
4. Disease process, prognosis, and therapeutic regimen understood.
5. Plan in place to meet needs after discharge.

NURSING DIAGNOSIS: acute Pain

May be related to
Biological injuring agents: obstruction or ductal spasm, inflammatory process, tissue ischemia and necrosis

Possibly evidenced by
Reports of pain, biliary colic
Facial mask of pain; guarding behavior
Autonomic responses including changes in blood pressure (BP), pulse
Self-focusing; narrowed focus

Desired Outcomes/Evaluation Criteria—Client Will

Pain Control (NOC)
Report pain is relieved or controlled.
Demonstrate use of relaxation skills and diversional activities as indicated for individual situation.

ACTIONS/INTERVENTIONS	RATIONALE
Pain Management (NIC)	
Independent	
Observe and document location, severity (0 to 10 scale), and character of pain, such as steady, intermittent, or colicky.	Assists in differentiating cause of pain and provides information about disease progression or resolution, development of complications, and effectiveness of interventions.
Note response to medication, and report to physician if pain is not being relieved.	Severe pain not relieved by routine measures may indicate developing complications and the need for further intervention.
Promote bedrest, allowing client to assume position of comfort.	Bedrest in low-Fowler's position reduces intra-abdominal pressure; however, client will naturally assume least painful position.
Use soft cotton linens; calamine lotion; oil bath; and cool, moist compresses, as indicated.	Reduces irritation and dryness of the skin and itching sensation.
Control environmental temperature.	Cool surroundings aid in minimizing dermal discomfort.
Encourage use of relaxation techniques such as guided imagery, visualization, and deep-breathing exercises. Provide diversional activities.	Promotes rest, redirects attention, and may enhance coping.
Make time to listen to and maintain frequent contact with client.	Helpful in alleviating anxiety and refocusing attention, which can relieve pain.
Collaborative	
Maintain nothing by mouth (NPO) status; insert and maintain nasogastric (NG) suction, as indicated.	Removes gastric secretions that stimulate release of cholecystokinin and gallbladder contractions.
Administer medications, as indicated, for example:	
Anticholinergics, such as dicyclomine (Bentyl), clyco-pyrrolate (Robinul), and propantheline (Pro-Banthine)	Antispasmodics and anticholinergics are thought to decrease gallbladder and biliary tree tone, which decreases pain.
Sedatives, such as phenobarbital	Promote rest and relax smooth muscle, relieving pain.
Opioids, such as meperidine (Demerol) and hydrocodone with acetaminphen (Vicodin, Lortab)	When pain is unrelieved by medications such as dicyclomine, opioids may be given to reduce severe pain.
Antiemetics, such as ondansetron (Zofran), prochlorperazine (Compazine), and promethazine (Phenergan)	Relieves nausea and vomiting.
Antibiotics, either single agent or anti-infective combinations	To treat infectious process, reducing inflammation and potential for systemic complications. Treatment for acute cholecystitis usually requires single-agent therapy, but for more serious infections, combination drug treatment has increased broad-spectrum coverage.
Oral dissolution therapy, such as ursodeoxycholic acid (Urso, Actigall)	Although a rarely chosen option for mainstream treatment of cholecystitis with cholelithiasis, oral dissolution is possible. It can dissolve some stones less than 5 mm in size. However, the therapy takes 6 to 12 months and stones often recur.
Prepare for procedures, such as the following:	
Endoscopic sphincterotomy plus extraction of stones during ERCP	Procedure done to widen the mouth of the common bile duct where it empties into the duodenum. The procedure may be done to assist in retrieving stones from the common duct by means of a tiny basket or balloon on the end of the endoscope. Stones must be smaller than 15 mm. Larger stones may be crushed with a mechanical lithotripter inserted through the endoscope.
Extracorporeal shock wave lithotripsy (ESWL)	Shock wave treatment is a little-used therapy due to high recurrence of stones. It may be indicated in a client with mild to moderate symptoms, with a single cholesterol stone (0.5 mm or larger), or in client without biliary tract obstruction. *Note:* This procedure is contraindicated in clients with pacemakers or implantable defibrillators.
Laparoscopic or open surgical intervention	Cholecystectomy may be indicated because of the size of stones, degree of tissue involvement, or presence of necrosis or sepsis. (Refer to CP: Cholecystectomy.)

NURSING DIAGNOSIS: risk for deficient Fluid Volume

Risk factors may include
Excessive losses through gastric suction; vomiting, distention, and gastric hypermotility
Medically restricted intake
Altered clotting process

(continues on page 362)

Possibly evidenced by
(Not applicable; presence of signs and symptoms establishes an *actual* diagnosis)

Desired Outcomes/Evaluation Criteria—Client Will

Hydration (NOC)
Demonstrate adequate fluid balance evidenced by stable vital signs, moist mucous membranes, good skin turgor, capillary refill, individually appropriate urinary output, and absence of vomiting.

ACTIONS/INTERVENTIONS	RATIONALE

Fluid/Electrolyte Management (NIC)
Independent

Maintain accurate record of intake and output (I&O), noting output less than intake and increased urine specific gravity. Assess skin and mucous membranes, peripheral pulses, and capillary refill.	Provides information about fluid status and circulating volume and replacement needs.
Monitor for signs and symptoms of increased or continued nausea or vomiting, abdominal cramps, weakness, twitching, seizures, irregular heart rate, paresthesia, hypoactive or absent bowel sounds, and depressed respirations.	Prolonged vomiting, gastric aspiration, and restricted oral intake can lead to deficits in sodium, potassium, and chloride.
Eliminate noxious sights and smells from environment.	Reduces stimulation of vomiting center.
Perform frequent oral hygiene with alcohol-free mouthwash; apply lubricants.	Decreases dryness of oral mucous membranes and reduces risk of oral bleeding.
Assess for unusual bleeding: oozing from injection sites, epistaxis, bleeding gums, ecchymosis, petechiae, hematemesis, and melena.	Prothrombin is reduced and coagulation time prolonged when bile flow is obstructed, increasing risk of bleeding or hemorrhage.
Use small-gauge needles for injections and apply firm pressure for longer than usual after venipuncture.	Reduces trauma, risk of bleeding, and hematoma formation.

Collaborative

Keep client NPO as necessary.	Decreases gastrointestinal (GI) secretions and hypermotility.
Insert NG tube, connect to suction, and maintain patency, as indicated.	Provides rest for GI tract and relief of vomiting.
Administer antiemetics, such as promethazine (Phenergan), prochlorperazine (Compazine), or ondansetron (Zofran).	Helpful in reducing nausea and vomiting often associated with cholecystitis and, particularly, common bile duct obstruction.
Review laboratory studies such as Hgb/Hct, electrolytes, arterial blood gases (ABGs) (pH), and clotting times.	Aids in evaluating circulating volume, identifies deficits, and influences choice of intervention for replacement or correction.
Administer IV fluids, electrolytes, and vitamin K.	Maintains circulating volume and corrects imbalances. Vitamin K provides replacement of factors necessary for the clotting process.

NURSING DIAGNOSIS: **risk for imbalanced Nutrition: Less than Body Requirements**

Risk factors may include
Self-imposed or prescribed dietary restrictions, nausea and vomiting, dyspepsia, pain
Loss of nutrients; impaired fat digestion due to obstruction of bile flow

Possibly evidenced by
(Not applicable; presence of signs and symptoms establishes an *actual* diagnosis)

Desired Outcomes/Evaluation Criteria—Client Will

Nutritional Status (NOC)
Report relief of nausea and vomiting.
Demonstrate progression toward desired weight gain or maintain weight as individually appropriate.

ACTIONS/INTERVENTIONS	RATIONALE

Nutrition Management (NIC)
Independent

Estimate or calculate caloric intake. Keep comments about appetite to a minimum.	Identifies nutritional deficiencies and needs. Focusing on problem creates a negative atmosphere and may interfere with intake.

ACTIONS/INTERVENTIONS (continued)	RATIONALE (continued)
Weigh, as indicated.	Monitors effectiveness of dietary plan.
Consult with client about likes and dislikes, foods that cause distress, and preferred meal schedule.	Involving client in planning enables client to have a sense of control and encourages eating.
Provide a pleasant atmosphere at mealtime; remove noxious stimuli.	Useful in promoting appetite and reducing nausea.
Provide oral hygiene before meals.	A clean mouth enhances appetite.
Offer effervescent drinks with meals if tolerated.	May lessen nausea and relieve gas. *Note:* May be contraindicated if beverage causes gas formation with subsequent gastric discomfort.
Assess for abdominal distention, frequent belching, guarding, and reluctance to move.	Nonverbal signs of discomfort associated with impaired digestion, gas pain.
Ambulate and increase activity, as tolerated.	Helpful in expulsion of flatus and reduction of abdominal distention. Contributes to overall recovery and sense of well-being and decreases possibility of secondary problems related to immobility such as pneumonia and thrombophlebitis.

Collaborative

Consult with dietitian and nutritional support team, as indicated.	Useful in establishing individual nutritional needs and most appropriate route.
Begin low-fat liquid diet after NG tube is removed.	Limiting fat content reduces stimulation of gallbladder and pain associated with incomplete fat digestion and is helpful in preventing recurrence.
Advance diet as tolerated, usually low-fat, nonspicy, high-fiber. Restrict gas-producing foods such as onions, cabbage, and popcorn, and foods and fluids high in fat such as butter, fried foods, and nuts.	Meets nutritional requirements while minimizing stimulation of the gallbladder.
Monitor laboratory studies: blood urea nitrogen (BUN), prealbumin, albumin, total protein, and transferrin levels.	Provides information about nutritional deficits and effectiveness of therapy.
Provide parenteral or enteral feedings as needed.	Alternative feeding may be required depending on degree of disability and gallbladder involvement and need for prolonged gastric rest.

NURSING DIAGNOSIS: **deficient Knowledge [Learning Need] regarding condition, prognosis, treatment, self-care, and discharge needs**

May be related to
Lack of knowledge or recall
Information misinterpretation
Unfamiliarity with information resources

Possibly evidenced by
Questions, request for information
Statement of misconception
Inaccurate follow-through of instruction
Development of preventable complications

Desired Outcomes/Evaluation Criteria—Client Will

Knowledge: Illness Care (NOC)
Verbalize understanding of disease process, prognosis, and potential complications.
Verbalize understanding of therapeutic needs.
Initiate necessary lifestyle changes and participate in treatment regimen.

ACTIONS/INTERVENTIONS	RATIONALE
Teaching: Disease Process (NIC)	
Independent	
Provide explanations of and reasons for test procedures and preparation needed.	Information can decrease anxiety, thereby reducing sympathetic stimulation.
Review disease process and prognosis. Discuss hospitalization and prospective treatment as indicated. Encourage questions and expression of concerns.	Provides knowledge base from which client can make informed choices. Effective communication and support at this time can diminish anxiety and promote healing.

(continues on page 364)

Review drug regimen if chemical stone dissolution is chosen, along with possible side effects.

Gallstones often recur, necessitating long-term therapy. Development of diarrhea and cramps during chenodiol (Chenix) therapy may be dose-related and correctable. *Note:* Women of childbearing age should be counseled regarding birth control to prevent pregnancy and risk of fetal hepatic damage.

Discuss weight reduction programs, if indicated.

Obesity is a risk factor associated with cholecystitis, and weight loss is beneficial in medical management of chronic condition.

Instruct client to avoid food and fluids high in fats such as whole milk, ice cream, butter, fried foods, nuts, gravies, and pork; and gas producers such as cabbage, beans, onions, carbonated beverages, or gastric irritants such as spicy foods, caffeine, and citrus.

May prevent recurrence of and limit severity of gallbladder attacks.

Review signs and symptoms requiring medical intervention, such as recurrent fever; persistent nausea and vomiting; pain; jaundice of skin or eyes; itching; dark urine; clay-colored stools; blood in urine, stools, or vomitus; or bleeding from mucous membranes.

Indicative of progression of disease process and development of complications requiring further intervention.

Recommend resting in semi-Fowler's position after meals.

Promotes flow of bile and general relaxation during initial digestive process.

Suggest client limit gum chewing, sucking on drinking straw, hard candy, or smoking.

Promotes gas formation, which can increase gastric distention and discomfort.

Discuss avoidance of aspirin-containing products, forceful blowing of nose, straining for bowel movement, and contact sports. Recommend use of soft toothbrush and electric razor.

Reduces risk of bleeding related to changes in coagulation time, mucosal irritation, and trauma.

POTENTIAL CONSIDERATIONS following acute hospitalization (dependent on client's age, physical condition and presence of complications, personal resources, and life responsibilities)
• *acute Pain*—recurrence of obstruction or ductal spasm, inflammation, tissue ischemia

---

CHOLECYSTECTOMY

I. **Indications**—For the treatment of symptomatic gallstones, infection of the gallbladder or biliary ducts, calcified gallbladder, or cancer or trauma

II. **Procedures**
  a. Laparoscopic cholecystectomy: for removal of gallstones; performed using video endoscopy, with instruments inserted through small abdominal incisions
  b. Open cholecystectomy: for multiple or large gallstones, common bile duct stones, history of previous surgeries with scarring, or unsuccessful laparoscopic cholecystectomy

III. **Statistics** (Heuman et al, 2006)
  a. Morbidity: On an annual basis, approximately 500,000 Americans develop symptoms or complications of gallstones, requiring cholecystectomy.
  b. Mortality: Several hundred deaths (annually) are attributed to complications of cholecystectomy.

GLOSSARY

Adventitious sounds: Abnormal breath sounds heard when listening to the chest, which may include crackles (rales), rhonchi, or wheezes.

Cholecystitis: Inflammation of the gallbladder.

Cholelithiasis: Stones in the gallbladder.

Gallstones: Solid masses made of cholesterol or bilirubin that form in the gallbladder or bile ducts; majority of gallstones in clients (in United States) are composed of cholesterol, resulting from cholesterol precipitating out of bile; bile pigment stones are a result of free bilirubin combining with calcium (Sartin, 2005a).

Hematemesis: Vomiting of blood.

Jaundice: Yellow tinge to skin and sclera in eyes due to bile absorption into circulatory system.

Melena: Black, tarry feces due to digestion of blood in stool.

T-tube: Drain tube inserted into cystic duct at the point of surgical closure and exiting through stab wound in skin to allow bile to drain.

Care Setting

This procedure is usually done on a short-stay basis; however, in the presence of suspected complications such as empyema, gangrene, or perforation, an inpatient stay on a surgical unit is indicated.

Related Concerns

Cholecystitis with cholelithiasis, page 357
Pancreatitis, page 458
Peritonitis, page 349
Psychosocial aspects of care, page 749
Surgical intervention, page 782

Client Assessment Database (Preoperative)

Refer to CP: Cholecystitis with Cholelithiasis.

DIAGNOSTIC DIVISION

TEACHING/LEARNING
• *Discharge plan considerations:* May require assistance with wound care, supplies, and homemaker tasks

⬧ Refer to section at end of plan for postdischarge considerations.

Diagnostic Studies

Refer to CP: Cholecystitis with Cholelithiasis.

Nursing Priorities

1. Promote respiratory function.
2. Prevent complications.
3. Provide information about disease, procedure(s), prognosis, and treatment needs.

Discharge Goals

1. Ventilation and oxygenation adequate for individual needs.
2. Complications prevented or minimized.
3. Disease process, surgical procedure, prognosis, and therapeutic regimen understood.
4. Plan in place to meet needs after discharge.

NURSING DIAGNOSIS: ineffective Breathing Pattern

May be related to
Pain
Muscular impairment
Decreased energy and fatigue

Possibly evidenced by
Tachypnea, respiratory depth changes, reduced vital capacity
Holding breath, reluctance to cough

Desired Outcomes/Evaluation Criteria—Client Will

Respiratory Status: Ventilation (NOC)
Establish effective breathing pattern.
Experience no signs of respiratory compromise or complications.

ACTIONS/INTERVENTIONS	RATIONALE
Respiratory Monitoring (NIC)	
Independent	
Observe respiratory rate and depth.	Shallow breathing, splinting with respirations, and holding breath may result in hypoventilation and atelectasis.
Auscultate breath sounds.	Areas of decreased or absent breath sounds suggest atelectasis, whereas adventitious sounds reflect congestion.

(continues on page 366)

ACTIONS/INTERVENTIONS (continued)

Assist client to turn, cough, and deep-breathe periodically. Demonstrate how to splint incision. Instruct in effective breathing techniques.

Elevate head of bed; maintain low-Fowler's position. Support abdomen when coughing or ambulating.

Collaborative

Assist with respiratory treatments, such as incentive spirometer.

Administer analgesics regularly or continuously by patient-controlled analgesia (PCA), such as morphine sulfate, hydromorphone (Dilaudid), and ketorolac (Toradol).

RATIONALE (continued)

Promotes ventilation of all lung segments and mobilization and expectoration of secretions.

Facilitates lung expansion. Splinting provides incisional support and decreases muscle tension to promote cooperation with therapeutic regimen.

Maximizes expansion of lungs to prevent or resolve atelectasis.

Facilitates movement and effective coughing, deep breathing, and activity.

> **NURSING DIAGNOSIS:** **risk for deficient Fluid Volume**
>
> **Risk factors may include**
> Losses from nasogastric (NG) aspiration, vomiting
> Medically restricted intake
> Altered coagulation, such as reduced prothrombin, prolonged coagulation time
>
> **Possibly evidenced by**
> (Not applicable; presence of signs and symptoms establishes an *actual* diagnosis)
>
> ### Desired Outcomes/Evaluation Criteria—Client Will
>
> **Hydration** (NOC)
> Display adequate fluid balance as evidenced by stable vital signs, moist mucous membranes, good skin turgor, capillary refill, and individually appropriate urinary output.

ACTIONS/INTERVENTIONS

Fluid/Electrolyte Management (NIC)
Independent

Monitor intake and output (I&O), including drainage from NG tube, T-tube, and wound. Weigh client periodically.

Monitor vital signs. Assess mucous membranes, skin turgor, peripheral pulses, and capillary refill.

Observe for signs of bleeding, such as hematemesis, melena, petechiae, ecchymosis, epistaxis, and oozing from incision and injection sites.

Use small-gauge needles for injections, and apply firm pressure for longer than usual after venipuncture.

Have client use soft toothbrush or cotton or sponge swabs and alcohol-free mouthwash instead of a toothbrush, if bleeding is a problem.

Collaborative

Monitor laboratory studies, such as complete blood count (CBC), electrolytes, prothrombin and clotting time, and amylase.

Administer the following, as indicated:
  Intravenous (IV) fluids, blood products, and vitamin K

  Electrolytes (such as potassium, sodium, and chloride)

RATIONALE

Provides information about replacement needs and organ function. Initially, 200 to 1,000 mL of bile drainage per 24 hours may be expected via the T-tube, decreasing as more bile enters the intestine. Continuing large amounts of bile drainage may be an indication of unresolved obstruction or, occasionally, a biliary fistula. *Note:* Sudden cessation of drainage may indicate blockage of tube.

Indicators of adequacy of circulating volume and perfusion.

Prothrombin is reduced and coagulation time prolonged when bile flow is obstructed, increasing risk of bleeding or hemorrhage.

Reduces trauma and risk of bleeding or hematoma formation.

Avoids trauma and bleeding of the gums. Alcohol can be drying and cause irritation to mucosa.

Provides information about circulating volume, electrolyte balance, and adequacy of clotting factors. The hematocrit (Hct) rises when plasma volume is reduced, as in dehydration from vomiting. Falling hemoglobin (Hgb) and Hct may reflect bleeding as a complication of obstructed bile flow, surgical procedure, or preexisting bleeding disorder. Elevated white blood cells (WBCs) can indicate inflammation from surgery, peritonitis, or pancreatitis or other infection. Damage to the pancreas is indicated by elevated levels of amylase.

Maintains adequate circulating volume and aids in replacement of clotting factors.

Imbalances resulting from excessive gastric or surgical fluid losses may require replacement via oral and parenteral routes.

NURSING DIAGNOSIS: impaired Skin/Tissue Integrity

May be related to
Chemical substance—bile, stasis of secretions
Altered nutritional state (obesity) or metabolic state
Invasion of body structure—T-tube punctures or incision

Possibly evidenced by
Disruption of skin or subcutaneous tissues

Desired Outcomes/Evaluation Criteria—Client Will

Wound Healing: Primary/Secondary Intention (NOC)
Achieve timely wound healing without complications.
Demonstrate behaviors to promote healing and prevent skin breakdown.

ACTIONS/INTERVENTIONS	RATIONALE
Wound Care (NIC)	
Independent	
Observe the color and character of NG and T-tube drainage.	Initially, drainage may contain blood and blood-stained fluid, normally changing to greenish-brown (bile color) after the first several hours.
Maintain T-tube in closed collection system.	Prevents skin irritation and reduces risk of contamination.
Check the T-tube and incisional drains; make sure they are free flowing.	T-tube may remain in common bile duct for 7 to 10 days to remove retained tiny stones and gravel. Incision site drains are used to remove any accumulated fluid and bile. Correct positioning prevents backup of the bile in the operative area.
Anchor drainage tube, allowing sufficient tubing to permit free turning and avoid kinks and twists.	Avoids dislodging tube and occlusion of the lumen.
Change dressings often initially, then as needed. Clean the skin with soap and water. Use sterile petroleum jelly gauze, zinc oxide, or karaya powder around the incision.	Keeps the skin around the incision clean and provides a barrier to protect skin from excoriation from bile leaking outside of T-tube.
Apply Montgomery straps for client who had open cholecystectomy.	Facilitates frequent dressing changes and minimizes skin trauma.
Use a disposable ostomy bag over a stab wound drain.	Ostomy appliance may be used to collect heavy drainage for more accurate measurement of output and protection of the skin.
Place client in low- or semi-Fowler's position.	Facilitates drainage of bile.
Monitor puncture sites (three to five) if endoscopic procedure is done.	These areas may bleed, or staples and Steri-Strips may loosen at puncture wound sites.
Observe for hiccups, abdominal distention, or other signs of peritonitis such as rigid abdomen, fever, and severe right upper quadrant (RUQ) abdominal pain suggesting pancreatitis.	Dislodgment of the T-tube can result in diaphragmatic irritation or more serious complications if bile drains into abdomen or pancreatic duct is obstructed.
Observe skin for itching, sclera for jaundice, and urine for change in color to dark brown.	May indicate obstruction of bile flow from retained gallstone.
Note color and consistency of stools.	Clay-colored stools result when bile is not present in the intestines.
Investigate reports of increased or unrelenting RUQ pain, development of fever and tachycardia, and leakage of bile drainage around tube or from wound.	Signs suggestive of abscess or fistula formation, requiring medical intervention.
Collaborative	
Administer antibiotics, as indicated.	Necessary for treatment of abscess or infection.
Clamp the T-tube per schedule.	Tests the patency of the common bile duct before tube is removed.
Prepare for surgical interventions, as indicated.	Drainage of blocked duct or fistulectomy may be required to treat abscess or repair fistula. Bile duct injury will require stenting of duct or surgical repair if stenting not successful.
Monitor laboratory studies, for instance WBC count.	Leukocytosis reflects inflammatory process, for example, abscess formation or development of peritonitis or pancreatitis.

deficient Knowledge [Learning Need] regarding condition, prognosis, treatment, self-care, and discharge needs

May be related to
Lack of exposure, information misinterpretation
Unfamiliarity with information resources
Lack of recall

Possibly evidenced by
Questions, statement of misconception
Request for information
Inaccurate follow-through of instructions

Desired Outcomes/Evaluation Criteria—Client Will

Knowledge: Illness Care (NOC)
Verbalize understanding of disease process, surgical procedure and prognosis, and potential complications.
Verbalize understanding of therapeutic needs.
Correctly perform necessary procedures and explain reasons for the actions.
Initiate necessary lifestyle changes and participate in therapeutic regimen.

ACTIONS/INTERVENTIONS	RATIONALE
Teaching: Disease Process (NIC) *Independent* Review disease process, surgical procedure, and prognosis.	Provides knowledge base on which client can make informed choices.
Demonstrate care of incisions and dressings and drains.	Promotes independence in care and reduces risk of complications, such as infection and biliary obstruction.
Instruct in periodic drainage of T-tube collection bag and recording of output.	Reduces risk of reflux, strain on tube, and appliance seal. Provides information about resolution of ductal edema and return of ductal function for appropriate timing of T-tube removal.
Emphasize importance of maintaining low-fat diet, eating frequent small meals, and gradual reintroduction of foods and fluids containing fats over a 4- to 6-month period.	During initial 6 months after surgery, low-fat diet limits need for bile and reduces discomfort associated with inadequate digestion of fats.
Discuss use of medication such as dehydrocholic acid (Decholin).	Oral replacement of bile salts may be required in certain clients to facilitate digestion and treat malabsorption of fats.
Discuss avoiding or limiting use of alcoholic beverages.	Minimizes risk of pancreatic involvement.
Inform client that loose stools may occur for several months.	Intestines require time to adjust to stimulus of continuous output of bile.
Advise client to note and avoid foods that seem to aggravate the diarrhea.	Although radical dietary changes are not usually necessary, certain restrictions may be helpful, such as fats in small amounts. After a period of adjustment, client usually will not have problems with most foods.
Identify signs and symptoms requiring notification of healthcare provider, such as dark urine, jaundiced sclera and skin, clay-colored stools, excessive stools, or recurrent heartburn and bloating.	Indicators of obstruction of bile flow or altered digestion, requiring further evaluation and intervention.
Review activity limitations, depending on individual situation.	Resumption of usual activities is normally accomplished within 4 to 6 weeks.

POTENTIAL CONSIDERATIONS following acute hospitalization (dependent on client's age, physical condition, presence of complications, personal resources, and life responsibilities)
• *Diarrhea*—continuous excretion of bile into bowel, changes in digestive process
• *risk for Infection*—invasive procedure (discharge with T-tube in place)

CHAPTER 8

Metabolic and Endocrine Disorders

EATING DISORDERS: ANOREXIA NERVOSA/BULIMIA NERVOSA

I. **Pathophysiology:** Eating disorders encompass a spectrum of psychological problems that involve insufficient or excessive food intake, resulting in significant health problems across the life span.
   a. Anorexia nervosa (AN)
      i. Serious, chronic illness of starvation associated with a severe disturbance of body image and a morbid fear of obesity
      ii. Constellation of factors involved include an individual's genetic makeup, personality, and psychological and emotional challenges
      iii. Divided into early, mild, or established stages
   b. Bulimia nervosa (BN)
      i. Chronic cycle involving binge eating and purging
      ii. Characterized by binges of overeating, which may be extreme, followed by self-induced vomiting, purging, and misuse of laxatives, diuretics, or enemas; may also involve nonpurging behaviors such as excessive exercise and fasting
      iii. Fear of gaining weight motivates purging or compensatory behaviors
      iv. Often seen in persons of normal weight, but may be seen in overweight clients
   c. Binge eating disorder (BED)
      i. Characterized by binge eating without inappropriate compensatory behaviors such as purging or fasting
      ii. Ingestion of large amounts of food with a sense of loss of control; frequent dieting without weight loss

II. **Etiology** (Murphy, 2007)
   a. The hypothalamus, which regulates appetite by signaling hunger and satiety, may not release balanced amounts of neurotransmitters, such as serotonin or pancreatic polypeptides.
   b. Occurs in either sex and in people of any race, age, or social stratum
   c. Both AN and BN can be present in the same individual.
   d. Risk factors
      i. Personal characteristics: low self-esteem and feelings of helplessness
      ii. Social factors: popular cultural preferences, media images, peer pressure, occupational expectations, for example, model, dancer, athlete

   iii. Family structure: theory suggests that girls who live in families that highly value perfection are at a greater risk for developing an eating disorder.
   iv. Presence of psychiatric comorbidities: anxiety, depression, addictive behavior, or impulse control disorders
   v. Genetics

III. **Statistics**
   a. AN, BN, BED
      i. Morbidity: Estimated to affect 8 million Americans (7 million females, 1 million males); only 1 in 10 individuals with an eating disorder receive treatment (South Carolina Department of Mental Health [SCDMH], 2006); incidence increasing in middle-aged women (Pryor, 2007).
      ii. Mortality: Eating disorders have the highest mortality rate of any mental illness; without treatment, up to 20% of people with serious eating disorders die, the highest mortality rate for any mental illness (Murphy, 2007).
      iii. Cost: More than $3.8 billion was spent annually in the United States in 2001 (PsychCentral, 2004).
   b. AN
      i. Morbidity: More common in girls and women, although approximately 10% to 15% of cases occur in males (Bernstein, 2008); only about 50% of those affected will recover, with best results occurring if treatment is begun within the first 6 months of onset and supportive parents and family are present (Speranza, 2007).
      ii. Mortality: Ranges from 10% to 20% and often related to length of illness (Speranza, 2007).
   c. BN
      i. Morbidity: Most common in white (more than 95%) adolescents (more than 75%) and young adults, affecting primarily adolescent girls (6%) and college-aged women (5%); lifetime prevalence about 3% (National Institute of Mental Health, 2007).
      ii. Mortality: Up to 3% eventually die of complications from the disease; leading cause of death is suicide, which is more common in persons with BN than those with AN (Moreno & Judd, 2008).

Abnormal involuntary movement scale (AIMS): System used to assess abnormal involuntary movements, such as hand tremors or rhythmic movements of the tongue and jaw, which may result from the long-term administration of psychotropic drugs.

Electroconvulsive therapy (ECT): Use of an electric shock to produce convulsions and thereby treat drug-resistant psychiatric disorders, such as some cases of major depression, bipolar disorder, suicidal ideation, and schizophrenia.

Family therapy: Focuses on the interdependent relationships within the family as a whole.

Margination: Adhesion of leukocytes to the walls of blood vessels during early stage of inflammatory process.

Obsessive-compulsive disorder (OCD): Chronic anxiety disorder most commonly characterized by obsessive, distressing, intrusive thoughts and related compulsions.

Osteopenia: Decrease in the amount of bone density.

Recovery environment: The individual in treatment and the supportive family members work together to create an environment in which all feel safe to express their feelings without judgment, criticism, or guilt.

Refeeding syndrome: Serious complication of electrolyte imbalance and cardiopulmonary compromise, which occurs with rapid increase of nutritional intake or total parenteral nutrition (TPN).

Total parenteral nutrition (TPN): Nutritional therapy specifically designed to prevent or correct protein-calorie malnutrition, which is administered via an enteral or parenteral route.

Care Setting

Acute care is provided through inpatient stay on a medical or behavioral unit and for correction of severe nutritional deficits and electrolyte imbalances or initial psychiatric stabilization. Long-term care is provided in an outpatient or day treatment program (partial hospitalization) or in the community.

Related Concerns

Dysrhythmias, page 88

Fluid and electrolyte imbalances, page 903

Metabolic alkalosis—primary base bicarbonate excess, page 488

Total nutritional support: parenteral/enteral feeding, page 469

Psychosocial aspects of care, page 749

Client Assessment Database

DIAGNOSTIC DIVISION MAY REPORT	MAY EXHIBIT
ACTIVITY/REST • Disturbed sleep patterns—early-morning insomnia, fatigue • Feeling "hyper" or anxious • Increased activity, avid exerciser, participation in high-energy sports • Employment in positions or professions that emphasize and require strict weight control, such as gymnasts, jockeys, models, dancers, skaters, actors, wrestlers, flight attendants, and others for whom thinness is emphasized and overly rewarded (Mehler & Anderson, 1999)	• Periods of hyperactivity, constant vigorous exercising (AN)
CIRCULATION • Feeling cold even when room is warm	• Low blood pressure (BP), orthostatic changes in BP or heart rate • Cold hands and feet • Tachycardia, bradycardia, dysrhythmias

Client Assessment Database (continued)

DIAGNOSTIC DIVISION MAY REPORT (continued)	MAY EXHIBIT (continued)
EGO INTEGRITY • Lack of control over eating, for example, cannot stop eating or cannot control what or how much is eaten (BN) • Feeling disgusted with self, depressed or very guilty because of overeating • Distorted or unrealistic body image; reports self as fat regardless of weight (denial), and sees thin body as fat • Persistent overconcern with body shape and weight • Unrealistic pleasure in weight loss, while denying oneself pleasure in other areas • High self-expectations • Stress factors—family move, divorce, onset of puberty • Suppression of angry feelings	• Emotional states of depression, withdrawal, anger, anxiety, pessimistic outlook • Psychiatric illness, such as depression, anxiety, bipolar disorder, OCD
ELIMINATION • Diarrhea or constipation • Laxative and diuretic abuse	
FOOD/FLUID • Constant hunger or denial of hunger; normal or exaggerated appetite that rarely vanishes until late in the disorder (AN) • Intense fear of gaining weight (females); may have prior history of being overweight (particularly males) • Preoccupation with food, such as calorie counting, gourmet cooking • Recurrent episodes of binge eating, a feeling of lack of control over behavior during eating binges, a minimum average of two binge-eating episodes a week for at least 3 months (BN) • Regularly engages in self-induced vomiting either independently or as a complication of anorexia, or strict dieting or fasting	• Weight loss and maintenance of body weight 15% or more below that expected; refusal to maintain body weight over minimal norm for age and height (AN) • Weight may be normal or slightly above or below normal (BN) • No medical illness evident to account for weight loss • Cachectic appearance, skin may be dry, yellowish, pale, with poor turgor (AN) • Preoccupation with food—calorie counting, hiding food, cutting food into small pieces, rearranging food on plate • Irrational thinking about eating, food, and weight • Swollen salivary glands; sore, inflamed buccal cavity; continuous sore throat (BN) • Vomiting, bloody vomitus (may indicate esophageal tearing—Mallory-Weiss syndrome) • Excessive gum chewing
HYGIENE	• Increased hair growth on body (lanugo), hair loss (axillary, pubic), hair is dull, not shiny • Brittle nails • Erosion of tooth enamel, gums in poor condition, ulcerations of mucosa • Enlarged salivary glands; dry mouth; reddened, dry, cracked lips
NEUROSENSORY	• Appropriate affect (except in regard to body and eating) or depressive affect • *Mental changes:* Apathy, confusion, memory impairment brought on by malnutrition or starvation • Hysterical or obsessive personality style; absence of other psychiatric illness or thought disorder—although a significant number may show evidence of an affective disorder
PAIN/DISCOMFORT • Headaches • Sore throat or mouth • Generalized vague complaints • Vague abdominal pain and distress, bloating	

(continues on page 372)

DIAGNOSTIC DIVISION MAY REPORT (continued)	MAY EXHIBIT (continued)

SAFETY

- Body temperature below normal
- Recurrent infectious processes (indicative of depressed immune system)
- Eczema and other skin problems, abrasions and calluses may be noted on back of hands from sticking finger down throat to induce vomiting (BN)

SEXUALITY

- Absence of at least three consecutive menstrual cycles due to decreased levels of estrogen in response to malnutrition (AN)
- Promiscuity or loss of sexual interest
- History of sexual abuse
- Homosexual or bisexual orientation—higher percentage in male clients than in general population

- Breast atrophy
- Amenorrhea related to hypothalamic function

SOCIAL INTERACTION

- Middle-class or upper-class family background
- History of being a quiet, cooperative child
- Problems of control issues in relationships, difficult communications with others, especially authority figures
- Poor communication within family of origin
- Engagement in power struggles
- An emotional crisis of some sort, such as divorce, the onset of puberty, or an unwanted family move
- Altered relationships or problems with relationships, withdrawal from friends and social contacts
- Abusive family relationships
- Sense of helplessness
- History of legal difficulties— shoplifting, drug use

- Passive father, dominant mother
- Family members closely fused
- Togetherness prized
- Personal boundaries not respected

TEACHING/LEARNING

- Family history of higher than normal incidence of depression
- Other family members with eating disorders (genetic predisposition)
- Health beliefs and practice—certain foods have "too many" calories, use of "health" foods, and so forth
- Substance abuse
- Use of herbal or over-the-counter (OTC) preparations to control weight gain, such as bitter orange, green tea extract, guarana rhodiola, laxatives (bisacodyl, cascara, senna), high-fiber supplements
- Use of prescription diet medications—Meridia, phenteramine, Xenical (often obtained without prescription via Internet)

DISCHARGE PLAN CONSIDERATIONS

- Assistance with maintenance of treatment plan

▶ Refer to section at end of plan for postdischarge considerations.

TEST WHY IT IS DONE	WHAT IT TELLS ME
BLOOD TESTS	
• *Complete blood count (CBC):* Battery of screening tests that typically include hemoglobin (Hgb); hematocrit (Hct); red blood cell (RBC) count, morphology, indices, and distribution width index; platelet count and size; white blood cell (WBC) count and differential.	Determines presence of anemia (not due to blood loss). WBCs are reduced (leukopenia) due to margination; lymphocytes are increased (lymphocytosis). Platelets show significantly less than normal activity (thrombocytopenia) by the enzyme monoamine oxidase, which is thought to be a marker for depression. Hgb may be elevated in extreme dehydration.
• *Electrolytes:* Provides baseline data and can be used to evaluate and monitor fluid and electrolyte balance.	Imbalances may include decreased potassium, sodium, chloride, and magnesium. Hypokalemia and hypochloremic metabolic alkalosis are observed with vomiting; acidosis is present in cases of laxative abuse (BN). Hyponatremia may be a result of excess water intake (AN).
• *Erythrocyte sedimentation rate (ESR):* Helps exclude unrecognized chronic medical conditions.	Tends to be low in presence of eating disorders.
• *Albumin or prealbumin:* Transport proteins in plasma and assist in maintaining oncotic pressure within the vascular bed.	Serum protein and albumin are often normal in AN because, although the amount of food is restricted, it often contains high-quality proteins.
• *Amylase:* Digestive enzyme primarily located in pancreas and salivary glands.	Elevated in up to 30% of clients in presence of repeated vomiting; reflects hypersecretion of the salivary glands.
• *Aspartate aminotransferase/alanine aminotransferase (AST/ALT), aluminum phosphide (ALP), total bilirubin, and direct bilirubin:* Liver function tests to determine associated impairment or damage and gallbladder involvement.	Liver function studies may be minimally elevated (AN). In BN, liver function tests are usually normal, although amylase may be elevated because of vomiting (Moreno & Judd, 2008).
• *Cholesterol, high-density lipoprotein (HDL), low-density lipoprotein (LDL), and triglycerides:* Types of lipids.	Dramatic elevations in cholesterol are observed in cases of starvation. This elevation may be secondary to (1) decrease in triiodothyronine (T_3) levels, (2) low cholesterol-binding globulin, and (3) leakage of intrahepatic cholesterol.
ENDOCRINE TESTS	
• *T_3, thyroxine (T_4), and thyroid-stimulating hormone (TSH):* Thyroid function tests.	T_4 levels are usually normal; however, circulating T_3 levels may be low. TSH response to thyrotropin-releasing hormone (TRH) is abnormal in AN reflecting euthyroid sick syndrome.
• *Pituitary function:* Propranolol-glucagon stimulation test studies the response of human growth hormone (hGH).	Depressed in anorexia. Gonadotropic hypofunction is noted.
• *Cortisol:* Hormone involved in a variety of different bodily functions, including the immune system, regulation of blood sugar, liver function, and response to stress.	May be elevated.
• *Dexamethasone suppression test (DST):* Evaluates hypothalamic-pituitary function.	Dexamethasone resistance indicates cortisol suppression, suggesting malnutrition or depression (positive in BN).
• *Luteinizing hormone (LH) secretions test:* Produced by the anterior lobe of the pituitary gland that stimulates ovulation and the development of the corpus luteum in females and the production of testosterone by the interstitial cells of the testis in males.	Pattern often resembles those of prepubertal girls.
• *Estrogen:* Hormone secreted by the ovaries that affects many aspects of the female body, including menstrual cycle and sexual maturation and functioning.	Decreased.
• *Serum glucose:* Glucose serves as the main source of energy for the body.	In AN, hypoglycemia is often present because of lack of carbohydrates in the diet or low glycogen levels in the liver.
OTHER DIAGNOSTIC STUDIES	
• *Urinalysis and renal function:* To evaluate hydration status and organ integrity.	Ketones in the urine represent starvation. Elevated specific gravity may indicate water loading to gain weight before weigh in. Blood urea nitrogen (BUN) may be normal or elevated if severe dehydration is present.

(continues on page 374)

TEST **WHY IT IS DONE** (continued)	**WHAT IT TELLS ME** (continued)
• *Urine drug screen:* Rules out substance abuse.	May reveal comorbidity or presence of emetine, which is a by-product of ipecac use.
• *Fecal occult blood:* Identifies associated gastrointestinal (GI) complications.	Positive result may indicate esophagitis, gastritis, or repeated colon irritation from laxative use.
• *Electrocardiogram (ECG):* Record of the electrical activity of the heart.	Abnormal tracing with low-voltage, T-wave inversion, prolonged QT interval, bradycardia, and dysrhythmias may be present reflecting electrolyte imbalances.
• *Chest x-ray or computed tomography (CT) scan:* Determine presence of associated complications.	May reveal rib fractures associated with repeated vomiting in presence of hypocalcemia or evidence of osteopenia. Changes reflecting emphysema (AN) may resolve with refeeding and weight gain. Heart size may be decreased.
• *Dual energy absorptiometry (DEXA) scan:* Measures bone density and is used to assess risk for fracture.	May reveal osteoporosis.
• *Genetic testing:* Determines familial risk factor that may contribute to disturbance in appetite regulation.	Gene for agouti-related protein, which may affect body mass index (BMI), fat mass, and percent of body fat, has been found to be higher in anorexic clients than in the general population.

Nursing Priorities

1. Obtain client's cooperation in treatment.
2. Reestablish adequate, appropriate nutritional intake.
3. Correct fluid and electrolyte imbalance.
4. Assist client to develop realistic body image and improve self-esteem.
5. Provide support and involve significant other (SO), if available, in treatment program.
6. Coordinate total treatment program with other disciplines.
7. Provide information about disease, prognosis, and treatment to client and SO.

Discharge Goals

1. Adequate nutrition and fluid intake maintained.
2. Maladaptive coping behaviors and stressors that precipitate anxiety recognized.
3. Adaptive coping strategies and techniques for anxiety reduction and self-control implemented.
4. Self-esteem increased.
5. Disease process, prognosis, and treatment regimen understood.
6. Plan in place to meet needs after discharge.

NURSING DIAGNOSIS: **imbalanced Nutrition: Less than Body Requirements**

May be related to
Inadequate food intake, self-induced vomiting
Chronic, excessive laxative use

Possibly evidenced by
Body weight 15% or more below expected, or may be within normal range or overweight (bulimia)
Pale conjunctiva and mucous membranes, poor skin turgor and muscle tone, edema
Excessive loss of hair, increased growth of hair on body (lanugo)
Amenorrhea
Hypothermia
Bradycardia, cardiac irregularities, hypotension

Desired Outcomes/Evaluation Criteria—Client Will

Knowledge: Diet (NOC)
Verbalize understanding of nutritional needs.

Nutritional Status (NOC)
Establish a dietary pattern with caloric intake adequate to regain or maintain appropriate weight.
Demonstrate weight gain toward individually expected range.

ACTIONS/INTERVENTIONS	RATIONALE

Eating Disorders Management (NIC)

Independent

Establish a minimum weight goal and daily nutritional requirements.

Provides comparative baseline for effectiveness of therapy. *Note:* Malnutrition is a mood-altering condition, leading to depression and affecting cognitive function and decision making. Improved nutritional status enhances thinking ability, allowing initiation of psychological work.

Contract with client regarding commitment to therapeutic program and meeting specific dietary needs and goals.

When client agrees to a contract, individual success is enhanced.

Use a consistent approach. Sit with client while eating; present and remove food without persuasion or comment. Promote pleasant environment and record intake.

Client detects urgency and may react to pressure. Any comment that might be seen as coercion provides focus on food. When staff responds in a consistent manner, client can begin to trust staff responses. The single area in which client has exercised power and control is food and eating, and she or he may experience guilt or rebellion if forced to eat. Structuring meals and decreasing discussions about food will decrease power struggles with client and avoid manipulative games.

Provide small, frequent, and nutritionally dense meals and supplemental snacks, as appropriate.

Gastric dilation may occur if refeeding is too rapid following a period of starvation dieting. Client may feel bloated for weeks while body adjusts to increased food intake. *Note:* Client at risk for developing refeeding syndrome.

Make selective menu available, and allow client to control choices as much as possible.

Client who gains confidence in self and feels in control of environment is more likely to eat preferred foods.

Be alert to choices of low-calorie foods and beverages, hoarding food, and disposing of food in various places, such as pockets or wastebaskets.

Client will try to avoid taking in what is viewed as excessive calories and may go to great lengths to avoid eating.

Maintain a regular weighing schedule, such as Monday and Friday before breakfast in same attire, and graph results.

Provides accurate ongoing record of weight loss or gain. Also diminishes obsessing about changes in weight.

Weigh with back to scale, depending on program protocols.

Although some programs prefer that client does not see the results of the weighing, this can force the issue of trust in client who usually does not trust others.

Avoid room checks and other control devices whenever possible.

External control reinforces feelings of powerlessness and therefore is usually not helpful.

Provide one-to-one supervision and have client with bulimia remain in the day room area or in sight with no bathroom privileges for a specified period, such as 2 to 3 hours, following eating if contracting is unsuccessful.

Prevents vomiting during or immediately after eating. Client may desire food and eating, but use a binge-purge syndrome to control weight. *Note:* Some clients purge for the first time in response to establishment of a weight-gain program.

Monitor exercise program and set limits on physical activities. Chart activity and level of work—pacing and so on.

Moderate exercise helps in maintaining muscle tone and combating depression; however, client may exercise excessively to burn calories.

Maintain matter-of-fact, nonjudgmental attitude if giving tube feedings, parenteral fluids, and so on.

Perception of punishment is counterproductive to client's self-confidence and faith in own ability to control destiny.

Be alert to possibility of client disconnecting feeding tube and emptying enteral or parenteral fluids if used. Check measurements, and tape tubing snugly.

Sabotage behavior is common in attempt to prevent weight gain.

Monitor for signs of refeeding syndrome reflecting fluid and electrolyte disorders, increased cardiac workload, and oxygen consumption.

Refeeding syndrome and congestive heart failure can occur because of too rapid an increase in oral intake. Heart size diminishes because of malnutriton and may have a difficult time compensating for an increase in circulating volume.

Collaborative

Provide nutritional therapy within a hospital treatment program, as indicated when condition is life-threatening.

Cure of the underlying problem cannot happen without improved nutritional status. Hospitalization provides a controlled environment in which food intake, vomiting, elimination, medications, and activities can be monitored. It also separates client from SO, who may be a contributing factor, and provides exposure to others with the same problem, creating an atmosphere for sharing.

Involve client in setting up and carrying out program of behavior modification. Provide reward for weight gain as individually determined; ignore loss.

Provides structured eating situation while allowing client some control in choices. Behavior modification may be effective in mild cases or for short-term weight gain.

Provide diet and snacks with substitutions of preferred foods when available.

Having a variety of foods available enables client to have a choice of potentially enjoyable foods.

(continues on page 376)

ACTIONS/INTERVENTIONS (continued)

Administer nutritional diet by prescribed means—regular food with supplements, high-calorie liquid diet, or tube feedings if needed.

Run through a blender anything left on the tray after a given period of time and tube-feed, if indicated.

Administer enteral or parenteral nutrition, as appropriate.

Avoid giving laxatives.

Administer medication, as indicated, for example:
  Vitamins, minerals, electrolytes

  Serotonin and histamine antagonist, such as cyproheptadine (Periactin)

  Selective serotonin reuptake inhibitors (SSRIs), such as fluoxetine (Prozac) and other antidepressants, such as tricyclics, for example, amitriptyline (Elavil) and imipramine (Tofranil); dopamine reuptake blocker, such as bupropion (Wellbutrin); 5-HT2 blocker, such as trazadone (Desryel)

  Monoamine oxidase inhibitors (MAOIs), such as phenelzine (Nardil) and tranylcypromine sulfate (Parnate)
  Antipsychotic drugs, such as risperadone (Risperdal), olanzapine (Zyprexa), chlorpromazine (Thorazine), and lithium (Eskalith, Lithane, Lithobid)

Perform AIMS (Abnormal Involuntary Movement Scale) after initiation of, and periodically during, treatment with antipsychotic medications.
Monitor electrolytes, as indicated.

Prepare for or assist with electroconvulsive therapy (ECT), if indicated. Discuss reasons for use and help client understand this is not punishment.

RATIONALE (continued)

When caloric intake is insufficient to sustain metabolic needs, nutritional support can be used to prevent malnutrition and death while therapy is continuing. High-calorie liquid feedings may be given as medication, at preset times separate from meals, or as an alternative means of increasing caloric intake.

This method of feeding may be used as part of a behavior modification program to provide total intake of needed calories.

TPN, or hyperalimentation, may be required for life-threatening situations; however, enteral feedings are preferred because they preserve GI function and reduce atrophy of the gut.

Use is counterproductive because they may be used by client to rid body of food or calories.

In AN, medication is usually limited to use in managing medical complications, such as calcium and vitamin D for osteopenia (which can be severe), potassium, magnesium, and phosphorus. Restoring electrolytes before refeeding decreases the risk of refeeding syndrome.

May be used for client with severe anorexia and no binging and purging. A serotonin and histamine antagonist that may be used in high doses to stimulate the appetite, decrease preoccupation with food, and combat depression. Does not appear to have serious side effects, although decreased mental alertness may occur.

Various antidepressants may be used to lift depression, stimulate appetite, and stabilize AN. Many of these same drugs are also found to be useful in reducing binge-purge cycles in BN. *Note:* Use must be closely monitored because of potential side effects, although side effects from SSRIs are less significant than those associated with tricyclics.

May be used to treat depression when other drug therapy is ineffective; decreases urge to binge in BN.

Newer antipsychotic drugs, such as Risperdal or Zyprexa, are being used to manage eating disorders, especially in presence of dual disorder, such as with bulimia and bipolar disorder. These drugs can reduce tension, anxiety, and nervousness and increase cooperation with psychotherapeutic program. However, some antipsychotic drugs are used only when absolutely necessary for severely delusional, overactive, hospitalized client as a last resort (e.g., Thorazine). Possibility of extrapyramidal side effects is a concern.

Provides baseline and monitors for the development of extrapyramidal side effects, indicating need for change in therapy.

Refeeding syndrome may develop with rapid decrease in potassium, magnesium, and phosphate levels.

In rare and difficult cases in which malnutrition is severe or life threatening, a short-term ECT series may enable client to begin eating and become accessible to psychotherapy.

NURSING DIAGNOSIS: [actual/] risk for deficient Fluid Volume

May be related to
Inadequate intake of food and liquids
Consistent self-induced vomiting
Chronic, excessive laxative or diuretic use

Possibly evidenced by (actual)
Dry skin and mucous membranes, decreased skin turgor
Increased pulse rate, body temperature, decreased BP
Output greater than input (diuretic use); concentrated urine and decreased urine output (dehydration)
Weakness
Change in mental state
Hemoconcentration, altered electrolyte balance

Desired Outcomes/Evaluation Criteria—Client Will

Hydration (NOC)
Maintain and demonstrate improved fluid balance, as evidenced by adequate urine output, stable vital signs, moist mucous membranes, and good skin turgor.

Risk Control (NOC)
Verbalize understanding of causative factors and behaviors necessary to correct fluid deficit.

ACTIONS/INTERVENTIONS	RATIONALE
Fluid/Electrolyte Management (NIC)	
Independent	
Monitor vital signs, capillary refill, status of mucous membranes, and skin turgor.	Indicators of adequacy of circulating volume. Orthostatic hypotension may occur with risk of falls and injury following sudden changes in position.
Monitor amount and types of fluid intake. Measure urine output accurately.	Client may abstain from all intake, with resulting dehydration, or substitute fluids for caloric intake, disturbing electrolyte balance.
Discuss strategies to stop vomiting and laxative or diuretic use.	Helping client deal with the feelings that lead to vomiting and laxative or diuretic use will prevent continued fluid loss. *Note:* Client with bulimia has learned that vomiting provides a release of anxiety.
Identify actions necessary to regain or maintain optimal fluid balance, such as specific fluid intake schedule.	Involving client in plan to correct fluid imbalances improves chances for success.
Collaborative	
Review electrolyte and renal function test results.	Fluid and electrolyte shifts or depressed renal function can adversely affect client's recovery and may require additional intervention.
Administer intravenous (IV) fluids and electrolytes, as indicated.	Used to correct fluid and electrolyte imbalances and prevent cardiac dysrhythmias.

NURSING DIAGNOSIS: disturbed Thought Processes

May be related to
Severe malnutrition, electrolyte imbalance
Psychological conflicts—sense of low self-worth, perceived lack of control

Possibly evidenced by
Impaired ability to make decisions, problem-solve
Non–reality-based verbalizations
Ideas of reference
Altered sleep patterns—may go to bed late (stay up to binge and purge) and get up early
Altered attention span, distractibility
Perceptual disturbances with failure to recognize hunger, fatigue, anxiety, and depression

Desired Outcomes/Evaluation Criteria—Client Will

Distorted Thought Control (NOC)
Verbalize understanding of causative factors and awareness of impairment.
Demonstrate behaviors to change or prevent malnutrition.
Display improved ability to make decisions and problem-solve.

ACTIONS/INTERVENTIONS	RATIONALE

Delusion Management (NIC)
Independent

Be aware of client's distorted thinking ability.	Allows caregiver to have more realistic expectations of client and provide appropriate information and support.
Listen to but avoid challenging irrational or illogical thinking. Present reality concisely and briefly.	It is difficult to respond logically when thinking ability is physiologically impaired. Client needs to hear reality, but challenging client leads to distrust and frustration. *Note:* Even though client may gain weight, she or he may continue to struggle with attitudes and behaviors typical of eating disorders, major depression, and substance dependence.
Adhere strictly to nutritional regimen.	Improved nutrition is essential to improved brain functioning. (Refer to ND: imbalanced Nutrition: Less than Body Requirements.)

Collaborative

Review electrolyte and renal function tests.	Imbalances negatively affect cerebral functioning and require correction before therapeutic interventions can begin.

NURSING DIAGNOSIS: **disturbed Body Image/chronic low Self-Esteem**

May be related to
Morbid fear of obesity, perceived loss of control in some aspect of life
Personal vulnerability; unmet dependency needs
Dysfunctional family system
Continual negative evaluation of self

Possibly evidenced by
Distorted body image—views self as fat even in the presence of normal body weight or severe emaciation
Expresses little concern, uses denial as a defense mechanism, and feels powerless to prevent or make changes
Expressions of shame, guilt
Overly conforming, dependent on others' opinions

Desired Outcomes/Evaluation Criteria—Client Will

Body Image (NOC)
Establish a more realistic body image.

Self-Esteem (NOC)
Acknowledge self as an individual.
Accept responsibility for own actions.

ACTIONS/INTERVENTIONS	RATIONALE

Body Image Enhancement (NIC)
Independent

Have client draw picture of self.	Provides opportunity to discuss client's perception of self and body image, and realities of individual situation.
Involve in personal development program, preferably in a group setting. Provide information about proper application of makeup and grooming.	Learning about methods to enhance personal appearance may be helpful to long-range sense of self-esteem and image. Feedback from others can promote feelings of self-worth.
Recommend consultation with an image consultant.	Positive image enhances sense of self-esteem.
Suggest disposing of "thin" clothes as weight gain occurs.	Provides incentive to at least maintain and not lose weight. Not seeing "thin" clothes removes visual reminder of thinner self.
Assist client to confront changes associated with puberty and sexual fears. Provide sex education as necessary.	Major physical and psychological changes in adolescence can contribute to development of eating disorders. Feelings of powerlessness and loss of control of feelings, in particular sexual sensations, can lead to an unconscious desire to desexualize self. Client often believes that these fears can be overcome by taking control of bodily appearance, development, and function.

ACTIONS/INTERVENTIONS (continued)

RATIONALE (continued)

Self-Esteem Enhancement (NIC)

Establish a therapeutic nurse-client relationship.

Promote self-concept without moral judgment.

State rules clearly regarding weighing schedule, remaining in sight during medication and eating times, and consequences of not following the rules. Without undue comment, be consistent in carrying out rules.

Confront denial and respond with reality when client makes unrealistic statements such as "I'm gaining weight, so there's nothing really wrong with me."

Be aware of own reaction to client's behavior. Avoid arguing.

Assist client to assume control in areas other than dieting and weight loss, such as management of own daily activities and work and leisure choices.

Help client formulate goals for self not related to eating and create a manageable plan for reaching those goals, one at a time, progressing from simple to more complex.

Note client's withdrawal from or discomfort in social settings.

Encourage client to take charge of own life in a more healthful way by making own decisions and accepting self as she or he is at this moment.

Let client know that it is acceptable to be different from family, particularly mother.

Encourage client to express anger and acknowledge when it is verbalized.

Assist client to learn strategies other than eating for dealing with feelings. Have client keep a diary of feelings, particularly when thinking about food.

Assess feelings of helplessness and hopelessness.

Be alert to suicidal ideation and behavior.

Collaborative

Use cognitive-behavioral or interpersonal psychotherapy approach rather than interpretive therapy.

Involve in group therapy.

Within a helping relationship, client can begin to trust and try out new thinking and behaviors.

Client sees self as weak willed even though part of person may feel sense of power and control, for example, through dieting and weight loss.

Consistency is important in establishing trust. As part of the behavior modification program, client knows risks involved in not following established rules (e.g., decrease in privileges). Failure to follow rules is viewed as client's choice and accepted by staff in matter-of-fact manner so as not to provide reinforcement for the undesirable behavior.

Client may be denying the psychological aspects of own situation and is often expressing a sense of inadequacy and depression.

Feelings of disgust, hostility, and infuriation are not uncommon when caring for these clients. Prognosis often remains poor even with a gain in weight because other problems may remain. Many clients continue to see themselves as fat, and there is also a high incidence of affective disorders, social phobias, obsessive-compulsive symptoms, drug abuse, and psychosexual dysfunction. Nurse needs to deal with own feelings so they do not interfere with care of client.

Feelings of personal ineffectiveness, low self-esteem, and perfectionism are often part of the problem. Client feels helpless to change and requires assistance to problem-solve methods of control in life situations.

Client needs to recognize ability to control other areas in life and may need to learn problem-solving skills to achieve this control. Setting realistic goals fosters success.

May indicate feelings of isolation and fear of rejection and judgment by others. Avoidance of social situations and contact with others can compound feelings of worthlessness.

Client often does not know what she or he may want for self. Parents, generally mother, often make decisions for client. Client may also believe she or he has to be the best in everything and holds self responsible for being perfect.

Developing a sense of identity separate from family and maintaining sense of control in other ways beside dieting and weight loss is a desirable goal of therapy and program.

Important to know that anger is part of self and as such is acceptable. Expressing anger may need to be taught to client because anger is generally considered unacceptable in the family, and therefore client does not express it.

Feelings are the underlying issue, and client often uses food instead of dealing with feelings appropriately. Client needs to learn to recognize feelings and how to express them clearly.

Lack of control is a common and underlying problem for this client and may be accompanied by more serious emotional disorders.

Intense anxiety and panic about weight gain, depression, and hopeless feelings may lead to suicidal attempts, particularly if client is impulsive.

Although both therapies have similar results, cognitive-behavioral seems to work more quickly. Interaction between individuals is more helpful for client to discover feelings, impulses, and needs from within own self. Client has not learned this internal control as a child and may not be able to interpret or attach meaning to behavior.

Provides an opportunity to talk about feelings and try out new behaviors.

(continues on page 380)

Refer to occupational and recreational therapy.

Can develop interest and skills to fill time that has been occupied by obsession with eating. Involvement in recreational activities encourages social interactions with others and promotes fun and relaxation.

Encourage participation in directed activities such as group hiking, bicycle tours, and wilderness adventures, such as the Outward Bound Program.

Although exercise is often used negatively by these clients, participation in these directed activities provides an opportunity to learn self-reliance, enhance self-esteem, and realize that food is the fuel required by the body to do its work.

Refer to therapist trained in dealing with sexuality, as indicated.

May need professional assistance to deal with sexuality issues and accept self as a sexual adult.

NURSING DIAGNOSIS: impaired Parenting

May be related to
Issues of control in family
Situational or maturational crises
History of inadequate coping methods

Possibly evidenced by
Dissonance among family members
Family developmental tasks not being met
Focus on "identified client" (IP)
Family needs not being met
Family member(s) acting as enablers for IP
Ill-defined family rules, function, and roles

Desired Outcomes/Evaluation Criteria—Family Will

Parenting (NOC)
Demonstrate individual involvement in problem-solving process directed at encouraging client toward independence.
Express feelings freely and appropriately.
Demonstrate more autonomous coping behaviors with individual family boundaries more clearly defined.
Recognize and resolve conflict appropriately with the individuals involved.

ACTIONS/INTERVENTIONS

RATIONALE

Family Therapy (NIC)
Independent
Identify patterns of interaction. Encourage each family member to speak for self. Prevent two members discussing a third without that member's participation.

Helpful information for planning interventions. The enmeshed, overinvolved family members often speak for each other and need to learn to be responsible for their own words and actions.

Discourage members from asking for approval from each other. Be alert to verbal or nonverbal checking with others for approval. Acknowledge competent actions of client.

Each individual needs to develop own internal sense of self-esteem. Individual often is living up to others' (family's) expectations rather than making own choices. Acknowledgment provides recognition of self in positive ways.

Listen with regard when client speaks.

Sets an example and provides a sense of competence and self-worth in that client has been heard and attended to.

Encourage individuals not to answer to everything.

Reinforces individualization and return to privacy.

Communicate message of separation—that it is acceptable for family members to be different from each other.

Individuation needs reinforcement. Such a message confronts rigidity and opens options for different behaviors.

Encourage and allow expression of feelings, such as crying or anger by individuals.

Often these families have not allowed free expression of feelings and need help and permission to learn and accept this.

Prevent intrusion in dyads by other members of the family.

Inappropriate interventions in family subsystems prevent individuals from working out problems successfully.

Reinforce importance of parents as a couple who have rights of their own.

The focus on the child with anorexia is very intense and often is the only area around which the couple interacts. The couple needs to explore their own relationship and restore the balance within relationship to help prevent its disintegration.

Prevent client from intervening in conflicts between parents. Assist parents in identifying and solving their marital differences.

Triangulation occurs in which a parent-child coalition exists. Sometimes the child is openly pressed to ally self with one parent against the other. The symptom (anorexia) is the regulator in the family system, and the parents deny their own conflicts.

ACTIONS/INTERVENTIONS (continued)	RATIONALE (continued)
Be aware and confront sabotage behavior on the part of family members.	Feelings of blame, shame, and helplessness may lead to unconscious behavior designed to maintain the status quo.
Collaborative	
Refer to community resources, such as:	
Parents' groups, Parent Effectiveness classes	May help reduce overprotectiveness, and support and facilitate the process of dealing with unresolved conflicts and change.
Family therapy groups	Eating disorders are not caused by families but are a family problem. Family therapy groups provide a forum for families to talk about their concerns and misconceptions, learning from others. As family members gain knowledge, they can use it to learn new skills of communication and encouragement, instead of using emotion (Gorham, 2005).
Individual family therapy, as indicated	Individual family therapy focuses on developing a recovery environment in which family members work together to create a safe environment.

NURSING DIAGNOSIS: risk for impaired Skin Integrity

Risk factors may include
Altered nutritional and metabolic state, edema
Dehydration, cachectic changes—skeletal prominence

Possibly evidenced by
(Not applicable; presence of signs and symptoms establishes an *actual* diagnosis)

Desired Outcomes/Evaluation Criteria—Client Will

Risk Control (NOC)
Verbalize understanding of causative factors and absence of itching.
Identify and demonstrate behaviors to maintain soft, supple, intact skin.

ACTIONS/INTERVENTIONS	RATIONALE
Skin Surveillance (NIC)	
Independent	
Observe for reddened, blanched, and excoriated areas.	Indicators of increased risk of breakdown, requiring more intensive treatment.
Encourage bathing every other day instead of daily if this is an area of concern.	Frequent baths contribute to dryness of the skin.
Use skin cream twice a day and after bathing.	Lubricates skin and decreases itching.
Massage skin gently, especially over bony prominences.	Improves circulation to the skin and enhances skin tone.
Discuss importance of frequent position changes and need for remaining active.	Enhances circulation and perfusion to skin by preventing prolonged pressure on tissues.
Emphasize importance of adequate nutrition and fluid intake. (Refer to ND: imbalanced Nutrition: Less than Body Requirements.)	Improved nutrition and hydration will improve skin condition.

NURSING DIAGNOSIS: deficient Knowledge [Learning Need] regarding condition, prognosis, treatment, self-care, and discharge needs

May be related to
Lack of exposure to or unfamiliarity with information about condition
Learned maladaptive coping skills

Possibly evidenced by
Verbalization of misconception of relationship of current situation and behaviors
Preoccupation with extreme fear of obesity and distortion of own body image
Refusal to eat, binging and purging, abuse of laxatives and diuretics, excessive exercising
Verbalization of need for new information
Expressions of desire to learn more adaptive ways of coping with stressors

(continues on page 382)

Desired Outcomes/Evaluation Criteria—Client Will

Knowledge: Illness Care (NOC)
Verbalize awareness of and plan for lifestyle changes to maintain normal weight.
Identify relationship of signs and symptoms such as weight loss and tooth decay, to behaviors of not eating or binging-purging.
Assume responsibility for own learning.
Seek out sources and resources to assist with making identified changes.

ACTIONS/INTERVENTIONS	RATIONALE
Learning Facilitation (NIC)	
Independent	
Determine level of knowledge and readiness to learn.	Learning is easier when it begins where the learner is.
Note blocks to learning, including physical, intellectual, and emotional issues.	Malnutrition, family problems, drug abuse, affective disorders, and obsessive-compulsive symptoms can be blocks to learning requiring resolution before effective learning can occur.
Teaching: Disease Process (NIC)	
Discuss familial tendencies and genetic risk for eating disorder.	Recent research supports the findings suggesting that anorexia and bulimia are disorders that occur in families; for example, this client is more likely to have an immediate family member or even a more distant relative with either disorder. The disease may be inheritable with single or multiple genes combined with environmental factors and traits such as perfectionism, maturity fears, and low self-esteem.
Provide written information for client and SOs.	Helpful as reminder of and reinforcement for learning.
Discuss consequences of behavior and potential for recovery and relapse.	Sudden death can occur because of electrolyte imbalances and suppression of the immune system. Liver damage may result from protein deficiency, or gastric rupture may follow binge eating and vomiting.
Review dietary needs, answering questions as indicated. Encourage inclusion of high-fiber foods and adequate fluid intake.	Client and family may need assistance with planning for new way of eating. Constipation may occur when laxative use is curtailed.
Encourage the use of relaxation and other stress-management techniques, such as visualization, guided imagery, and biofeedback.	New ways of coping with feelings of anxiety and fear help client manage these feelings in more effective ways, assisting in giving up maladaptive behaviors of not eating or binging-purging.
Assist with establishing a sensible exercise program. Caution regarding overexercise.	Exercise can assist with developing a positive body image and combats depression—release of endorphins in the brain enhances sense of well-being. However, client may use excessive exercise as a way to control weight.
Discuss need for information about sex and sexuality.	Because avoidance of own sexuality is an issue for this client, realistic information can be helpful in beginning to deal with self as a sexual being.
Refer to National Association of Anorexia Nervosa and Associated Disorders, Overeaters Anonymous, and other local resources, as appropriate.	May be a helpful source of support and information for client and SO.

POTENTIAL CONSIDERATIONS following acute hospitalization (dependent on client's age, physical condition and presence of complications, personal resources, and life responsibilities)
• *risk for imbalanced Nutrition: Less than Body Requirements*—inadequate food intake, self-induced vomiting, history of chronic laxative use
• *ineffective self Health Management*—complexity of therapeutic regimen, perceived seriousness and benefits, mistrust of regimen and healthcare personnel, excessive demands made on individual, family conflict

Sample clinical pathway follows in Table 8.1.

TABLE 8.1 Sample Pathway: Eating Disorders Program. ELOS: 28 Days Behavioral Unit

ND and Categories of Care	Time Dimension	Goals/Actions	Time Dimension	Goals/Actions	Time Dimension	Goals/Actions
imbalanced Nutrition: Less than Body Requirements R/T inadequate intake, self-induced vomiting, laxative use	Ongoing	Gain 3 lb/wk as indicated	Day 2–28	Consume at least 75% of food provided at each meal	Day 15–28	Demonstrate ability to select foods to meet at least 80% of nutritional needs
risk for deficient Fluid Volume R/T inadequate intake, self-induced vomiting, laxative use	Ongoing	Be free of S/S of dehydration	Day 2–28	Ingest at least 1,500 mL fluid/day	Day 22–28	Refrain from self-induced vomiting
	Ongoing	Display balanced I&O	Day 3	Vital signs WNL	Day 28	Be free of S/S of malnutrition, with all laboratory results WNL
Referral Diagnostic studies	Day 1 & prn Day 1	Dietitian Electrolytes, CBC, BUN/Cr, lipid profile, glucose, plasma proteins, thyroid function UA	Day 14	Repeat selected studies		
Additional assessments	Day 1–2 Day 1 Day 1–28	ECG, as indicated Vital signs/I&O q shift Weight Types of amount of food/fluid intake Behavior/purging following meals Level of activity	Day 3–7 Day 7, 14	q AM 7:30 a.m./same clothes	Day 8–28	As indicated
Medications Allergies:	Day 1–28	Appetite stimulant Tricyclic antidepressant Vitamin supplement				
Client education	Day 1 & prn	Orient to unit and schedule Behavior modification program Minimum weight goal and initial nutritional needs	Day 7–14	Principles of nutrition; foods for maintenance of wellness	Day 21–28	Incorporating nutritional plan into lifestyle and home setting

(continues on page 384)

TABLE 8.1 Sample Pathway: Eating Disorders Program. ELOS: 28 Days Behavioral Unit (continued)

ND and Categories of Care	Time Dimension	Goals/Actions	Time Dimension	Goals/Actions	Time Dimension	Goals/Actions
Additional nursing actions	Day 1–3	Assist client with formulation of behavioral contract and monitoring of cooperation	Day 7–28	Involve mother/SO as appropriate in nutritional counseling and planning for future		
	Day 1–7	Administer tube feeding or food that has been ground in a blender as indicated				
	Day 1–21	Bathroom locked for 1 hr following meals				
	Day 1–28	Provide social setting for meals				
ineffective Denial R/T presence of overwhelming anxiety-producing feelings, learned response pattern, personal/family value system	Ongoing	Participate in behavior modification program and adhere to unit policies	Day 8–28	Attend and contribute to group sessions	Day 18–28	Verbalize acceptance of reality that eating behaviors are maladaptive
	Day 2–28	Cooperate with therapy to restore nutritional well-being	Day 14	Develop trusting relationship with at least one staff member on each shift	Day 28	Demonstrate ability to cope more adaptively Identify ways to gain control in life situation Refrain from use of manipulation of others to achieve control Plan in place to meet needs after discharge
Referrals	Day 5 (or when physical condition stable)	Psychologist, social worker, psycho-dramatist	Day 8–28	Group psychotherapy sessions	Day 25	Community resource contact person(s)
Additional assessments	Day 1/ongoing	Degree and stage of denial	Day 5–7	Readiness to participate in group sessions		
	Day 1–17	Perception of situation	Day 7–28	Congruence between verbalizations and behaviors (insight)		
		Ability to trust	Day 8–28	Degree/quality of involvement in group sessions		

Client education	Day 1 and prn	Use of manipulation to achieve control Privileges and responsibilities of behavior modification Consequences of behaviors	Day 3/ongoing	Eating disorder and consequences of eating behavior	Day 21	Role of support group/community resources
Additional nursing actions	Day 1/ongoing	Encourage expression of feelings	Day 5–28	Promote involvement in unit activities	Day 21–28	Involve family as appropriate in long-range planning for meeting individual needs
		Avoid agreeing with inaccurate statements/perceptions Provide positive feedback for desired insight and behaviors Set limits on maladaptive behavior	Day 8–28	Support interactions with family members Encourage interactions in group sessions		
disturbed Body Image/chronic low Self-Esteem R/T perceived loss of control, unmet dependency needs, personal vulnerability, negative evaluation of self	Day 7	Acknowledge that attention will not be given to discussion of body image and food	Day 21	Acknowledge misperception of body image as fat Verbalize positive self-attributes	Day 28	Demonstrate realistic body image and self-awareness Verbalize acceptance of self, including "imperfections" Acknowledge self as sexual being
Referrals	Day 1 (or when physical condition stable)	Therapists: occupational, recreational, music, art	Day 14	Image consultant	Day 28	Therapist to address issue of sexuality postdischarge as indicated
Additional assessments	Day 1–7	Suicidal ideation or behaviors	Day 8	Individual strengths and weaknesses		
	Day 3	Sexual history including abuse	Day 8–28	Congruency of feelings and perceptions with actions		
	Day 3–28	Perception of body image Family patterns of interaction				

(continues on page 386)

TABLE 8.1 Sample Pathway: Eating Disorders Program. ELOS: 28 Days Behavioral Unit (continued)

ND and Categories of Care	Time Dimension	Goals/Actions	Time Dimension	Goals/Actions	Time Dimension	Goals/Actions
Client education	Day 1–28	Responsibility for self in family setting	Day 8–10	General wellness needs	Day 21–28	Sex education reflecting individual sexuality and needs
	Day 7–28	Clarify misconceptions of body image	Day 8–28	Human behavior and interactions with family and others		
			Day 14	Personal appearance and grooming		
			Day 14–28	Alternative coping strategies for dealing with feelings		
Additional nursing actions	Day 1	Develop therapeutic relationship	Day 7	Compare actual measurement of client's body with client's perceptions	Day 14–28	Have client keep diary of feelings, especially when thinking of food
	Day 1–28	Provide positive feedback for participation and independent decision making	Day 7–9	Assist with planning to meet individual goals		Role-play new behaviors for dealing with feelings and conflicts
		Confront sabotage behavior by family members	Day 8–28	Involve in physical activity/exercise program		
	Day 3–5	Encourage control in areas other than diet				
	Day 4–6	Support development of goals not related to eating				

Key: BUN/Cr, blood urea nitrogen/creatinine; CBC, complete blood count; ECG, electrocardiogram; ELOS, estimated length of stay; I&O, intake and output; ND, nursing diagnosis; prn, as needed; q, every; q AM, every morning; R/T, related to; SO, significant other; SS, signs and symptoms; UA, urinalysis; WNL, within normal limits.

EATING DISORDERS: OBESITY

I. Pathophysiology

a. A chronic excess accumulation of body fat, at least 20% over average desired weight for age, sex, and height, or a body mass index (BMI) greater than 30 for persons of either sex

b. Negatively impacts all body systems and increases risk of multiple physical and psychological pathologies, including hypertension, heart disease, diabetes, arthritis, depression and anxiety disorders, difficulty maintaining personal relationships, prejudice and discrimination, and limited access to public conveniences

II. Etiology

a. Causes are multiple, complex, and cannot be attributed simply to a disorder of willpower or the result of insufficient exercise

  i. Variations in metabolism, body fat distribution, and appetite regulation can be attributed to genetic factors (Farooqi & O'Rahilly, 2007).

  ii. Physiological factors

    1. Lesions in the hypothalamus—appetite and satiety centers

    2. Hypothyroidism—may interfere with basal metabolism

    3. Diabetes mellitus—decreased insulin production or utilization

    4. Cushing's disease—increased cortisone production

  iii. Environmental influences, behavioral and societal issues: includes availability of high-fat, calorie-dense conve-nience foods, large portions, and sedentary lifestyle

  iv. Psychosocial influences: possibility of unresolved dependency needs with individual fixed in the oral stage of pychosexual development, with food believed to be a coping mechanism for dealing with life's problems

b. Most likely influenced by multiple factors as demonstrated by the Transactional Model of Stress/Adaptation (Townsend, 2006)

III. Statistics

a. Morbidity: Approximately 34%, over 72 million of Americans, are termed as being obese in 2006 (Centers for Disease Control and Prevention [CDC], 2007).

b. Mortality: An estimated 112,000 premature deaths are associated with obesity (BMI less than or equal to 30) annually (CDC, 2005a).

c. Cost: In 2000, more than $117 billion was spent to manage obesity in the United States (CDC, 2005a); approximately $52 billion are direct costs of healthcare, with $33 billion spent on weight-loss products and services annually (Uwaifo & Arioglu, 2006).

GLOSSARY

Anthropometric measurements: Body measurements, including height, weight, body mass index (BMI), waist-to-hip ratio, and percentage of body fat.

Appestat: Control mechanism in the brain that signals either hunger or fullness.

Body mass index (BMI): Number calculated from an individual's weight and height, measured in kilograms divided by height in square meters, correlating to direct measures of body fat.

Circadian rhythm: Internal body clock that regulates the 24-hour cycle of biological processes including sleep, wakefulness, and hunger.

Cushing's syndrome: Endocrine (hormonal) disorder resulting from excessive exposure to or production of the hormone cortisol.

Endomorphic body type: Descriptive of a type of body that is soft and round or pear-shaped with disposition of fat predominately in the abdomen, hips, thighs, and buttocks.

Energy balance: Weight is balanced by the amount of energy calories obtained from food equating to the energy the body uses.

Hyperlipidemia: Elevated high levels of total cholesterol and triglycerides, normal or elevated low-density lipoprotein (LDL, "bad cholesterol"), and low high-density lipoprotein (HDL, "good cholesterol").

Obesity: Having a high amount of extra body fat, with BMI greater than 30.

Overweight: Having extra body weight from muscle, bone, fat, and/or water, with BMI between 25 and 29.9.

Pickwickian syndrome: Extreme obesity along with shallow breathing, sleep apnea, excessive sleepiness, and heart failure.

Polycythemia: Excess number of red blood cells in circulating blood, which can contribute to blood clots.

Transactional model of stress/adaptation: Begins with the precipitating event, leading to predisposing factors, cognitive appraisal, primary and secondary responses, and quality of individual's response, resulting in adaptive (effective) or maladaptive (refusal to eat and other ineffective behaviors).

Yo-yo dieting: Repeatedly losing weight by dieting and subsequently regaining it.

Care Setting

Community level unless morbid obesity requires brief inpatient stay.

Related Concerns

Cerebrovascular accident (CVA)/stroke, page 238

Cholecystitis with cholelithiasis, page 357

Cirrhosis of the liver, page 445

Diabetes mellitus/diabetic ketoacidosis, page 405

Heart failure: chronic, page 48

Hypertension: severe, page 37

Myocardial infarction, page 74

Obesity: bariatric surgery—gastric partitioning/gastroplasty, gastric bypass, page 396

Psychosocial aspects of care, page 749

Thrombophlebitis: deep vein thrombosis, page 111

Client Assessment Database

DIAGNOSTIC DIVISION MAY REPORT	MAY EXHIBIT
ACTIVITY/REST • Fatigue, constant drowsiness • Inability or lack of desire to be active or engage in regular exercise, sedentary lifestyle • Dyspnea with exertion • Relying on cars, instead of walking • Environmental problems such as lack of sidewalks, safe places to walk • Work schedules that leave little time for exercise	• Increased heart rate or respirations with activity
CIRCULATION	• Hypertension • Edema
EGO INTEGRITY • Cultural and lifestyle factors affecting food choices • Weight may or may not be perceived as a problem • Eating relieves unpleasant feelings—loneliness, frustration, boredom • Perception of body image as undesirable • Significant other's (SO's) resistance to weight loss (may sabotage client's efforts)	• Reluctant to engage in social activities
FOOD/FLUID • Normal and excessive ingestion of food • Experimentation with numerous types of diets (yo-yo dieting) with varied or short-lived results • History of recurrent weight loss and gain	• Weight disproportionate to height • Endomorphic body type • Failure to adjust food intake to diminishing requirements—change in lifestyle from active to sedentary, aging
PAIN/DISCOMFORT • Pain or discomfort on weight-bearing joints or spine	• Difficulty with movement, negotiating stairs, long walks
RESPIRATION • Dyspnea	• Cyanosis, respiratory distress if Pickwickian syndrome is present
SEXUALITY • Menstrual disturbances, amenorrhea • Problems with relationships • Menopause • Pregnancy(ies)	• Hormone regulation problems, such as polycystic ovarian syndrome

Client Assessment Database (continued)

DIAGNOSTIC DIVISION
MAY REPORT (continued)

TEACHING/LEARNING
- Problem may be lifelong or related to life event
- Family history of obesity
- Concomitant health problems may include hypertension, diabetes, gallbladder and cardiovascular disease, hypothyroidism

DISCHARGE PLAN CONSIDERATIONS
- May require support with therapeutic regimen; home modifications, assistive devices and equipment

▶ Refer to section at end of plan for postdischarge considerations.

MAY EXHIBIT (continued)

Diagnostic Studies

TEST
WHY IT IS DONE

BLOOD TESTS (MAY INCLUDE, NOT LIMITED TO THE FOLLOWING)
- *Lipid profile:* total cholesterol, triglycerides, and HDL and LDL: Fats circulating in the blood.

- *Endocrine function (thyroid, pituitary, growth hormone, pancreas, etc.):* Determines which gland(s) are involved and may determine the cause of obesity. May involve measuring hormone levels and their metabolites in the blood and urine.

OTHER DIAGNOSTIC TESTS
- *Anthropometric measurements (including and not limited to the following):* Tests are used to determine client's current status and nutritional needs and to monitor effectiveness of interventions.
- *BMI:* Estimate of body composition that correlates an individual's weight and height to lean body mass.

- *Waist circumference (WC):* Common measure used to assess abdominal fat content.

- *Urine test:* May be used for differential diagnosis.

WHAT IT TELLS ME

Obesity is often associated with hyperlipidemia, which is defined as high total cholesterol, elevated triglycerides, normal or elevated LDL, and low HDL.

The goal of testing is to identify the hormone(s) that are being under- or overproduced, which may be negatively affecting client's weight. Examples of conditions may include hypothyroidism, hypopituitarism, hypogonadism, hyperglycemia and hyperinsulinemia, and elevated cortisol.

Various means of testing may be employed, depending on availability of equipment and money, to measure physical characteristics such as weight and distribution and percentage of fat to lean muscle.

The World Health Organization (WHO) criteria for obesity are based on BMI. Under these guidelines, for adults, grade 1 overweight is a BMI of 25 to 29.9. Grade 2 overweight (commonly called obesity) is a BMI of 30 to 39.9. Grade 3 overweight (commonly called severe or morbid obesity) is a BMI greater than or equal to 40. A BMI greater than 50 is termed super obese (Uwaifo & Arioglu, 2006).

According to the National Institutes of Health, a high WC is associated with an increased risk for type 2 diabetes, hypertension, and cardiovascular disease when the BMI is also elevated. Risk is considered extremely high in men with WC greater than 40 inches and in women with WC greater than 35 inches (National Heart Lung and Blood Institute [NHLBI], 2008).

A 24-hour urinary free cortisol test may be performed when Cushing's syndrome or other endocrine states associated with elevated cortisol are clinically suspected.

Nursing Priorities

1. Assist client to identify a workable method of weight control, incorporating healthful foods and activity.
2. Promote improved self-concept, including body image and self esteem.
3. Encourage health practices to provide for weight control throughout life.

Discharge Goals

1. Healthy patterns for eating and weight control identified.
2. Weight loss toward desired goal established.
3. Positive perception of self verbalized.
4. Plans developed for future weight control.
5. Plan in place to meet needs after discharge.

NURSING DIAGNOSIS: **imbalanced Nutrition: More than Body Requirements**

May be related to
Food intake that exceeds body needs
Psychosocial factors
Socioeconomic status

Possibly evidenced by
Weight of 20% or more over optimum body weight; excess body fat by skinfold or other measurements
Reported or observed dysfunctional eating patterns, intake more than body requirements

Desired Outcomes/Evaluation Criteria—Client Will

Knowledge: Diet (NOC)
Identify inappropriate behaviors and consequences associated with overeating or weight gain.
Demonstrate appropriate change in lifestyle and behaviors, including eating patterns and food quantity and quality, and involvement in individual exercise program.

Nutritional Status (NOC)
Display weight loss with optimal maintenance of health.

ACTIONS/INTERVENTIONS	RATIONALE
Weight Reduction Assistance (NIC)	
Independent	
Review individual cause for obesity—organic or nonorganic.	Identifies and influences choice of some interventions.
Ascertain previous dieting history. Determine which diets and strategies have been used, results, and individual frustrations and factors interfering with success.	Client may have tried multiple diets, with little lasting change in body weight and feel negatively about embarking on another plan.
Implement and review daily food diary, for example, total caloric intake, types and amounts of food, and eating habits and associated feelings.	Provides the opportunity for the individual to focus on a realistic picture of the amount of food ingested and corresponding eating habits and feelings. Identifies patterns requiring change and a base on which to tailor the dietary program.
Determine client's motivation for weight loss, for instance, health issues, own satisfaction, and to gain approval from others. Discuss client's and SO's view of self, including what being fat does for the client. Notice occurrence of negative feedback from SO(s).	Helps to clarify client's motivation and potential for success in weight reduction. Client's family and cultural practices greatly influence client's self-view regarding food and body image. Feedback from family may reveal control issues impacting motivation for change.
Formulate an eating plan with the client, using knowledge of individual's height, body build, age, gender, and individual patterns of eating, as well as energy and nutrient requirements.	An important factor in the success of any weight loss program is adherence to a sound nutritional plan. Although there is little basis for recommending one commercial diet plan over another, a good reducing diet should contain foods from all basic food groups, with a focus on low-fat intake and adequate protein intake to prevent loss of lean muscle mass. It is helpful to keep the plan as similar to client's usual eating pattern as possible. A plan developed with and agreed to by the client is more likely to be successful.
Emphasize the importance of avoiding fad diets.	Elimination of needed components can lead to metabolic imbalances; for example, excessive reduction of carbohydrates can lead to fatigue, headache, instability, weakness, and metabolic acidosis (ketosis), thus interfering with effectiveness of weight-loss program.
Discuss need to give self permission to include desired or craved food items in dietary plan.	Denying self by excluding favorite foods results in a sense of deprivation and feelings of guilt and failure when individual "succumbs to temptation." These feelings can sabotage weight loss.

ACTIONS/INTERVENTIONS (continued)

Be alert to binge eating and develop strategies for dealing with these episodes, such as substituting other actions for eating.

Identify realistic incremental goals for weekly weight loss.

Weigh periodically as individually indicated, and obtain appropriate body measurements.

Determine current activity level and exercise program. Factor in caloric needs.

Develop an appetite re-education plan with client.

Emphasize the importance of avoiding tension at mealtimes and not eating too quickly.

Encourage client to eat only at a designated eating place and to avoid standing while eating.

Discuss restriction of salt intake and diuretic drugs if used.

Reassess caloric requirements every 2 to 4 weeks; provide additional support when plateaus occur.

Collaborative

Perform comprehensive nutritional assessment to determine calorie, nutrient, and vitamin and supplement requirements for individual.

Provide medications, as indicated, for example:
  Appetite-suppressant drugs, such as diethylpropion (Tenuate), mazindol (Sanorex), and sibutramine (Meridia)

  Hormonal therapy, such as thyroid (Euthroid) and levothyroxine (Synthroid)

  Orlistat (Xenical)

  Vitamin and mineral supplements

Hospitalize for fasting regimen or stabilization of medical problems, when indicated.

Prepare for bariatric surgical interventions, such as gastric banding or bypass, as indicated.

RATIONALE (continued)

The client who binges experiences guilt about it, which is also counterproductive because negative feelings may sabotage further weight loss efforts.

Reasonable weight loss of 1 to 2 lb/week results in longer-lasting effects. Excessive or rapid loss may result in fatigue and irritability and ultimately lead to failure in meeting goals for weight loss. Motivation is more easily sustained by meeting "stair-step" goals.

Provides information about effectiveness of therapeutic regimen and visual evidence of success of client's efforts. During hospitalization for controlled fasting, daily weighing may be required. Weekly weighing is more appropriate after discharge.

Exercise promotes weight loss by reducing appetite and enhancing sense of well-being and accomplishment.

Signals of hunger and fullness often are not recognized, have become distorted, or are ignored.

Reducing tension provides a more relaxed eating atmosphere and encourages more leisurely eating patterns. This is important because a period of time is required for the appestat mechanism to know the stomach is full.

Techniques that modify behavior may be helpful in avoiding diet failure.

Water retention may be a problem because of increased fluid intake and fat metabolism.

Changes in weight and exercise necessitate changes in plan. As weight is lost, changes in metabolism occur, resulting in plateaus when weight remains stable for periods of time. This can create distrust and lead to accusations of "cheating" on caloric intake, which are not helpful. Client may need additional support at this time.

Intake can be calculated by several different formulas, but weight reduction is based on the basal caloric requirement for 24 hours depending on client's sex, age, current or desired weight, and length of time estimated to achieve desired weight. *Note:* Standard tables are subject to error when applied to individual situations, and circadian rhythms and lifestyle patterns need to be considered.

May be used with caution and supervision at the beginning of a weight-loss program to support client during stress of behavioral changes. They are effective for only a few weeks and may cause problems of dependence in some people.

May be necessary when hypothyroidism is present. However, when no deficiency is present, replacement therapy is not helpful and may actually be harmful.

Lipase inhibitor blocks absorption of dietary fat. Facilitates weight loss and maintenance when used in conjunction with a reduced-calorie diet. Also reduces risk of regaining after weight loss.

Obese individuals have large fuel reserves but are often deficient in vitamins and minerals. *Note:* Use of Xenical inhibits absorption of water-soluble vitamins and beta-carotene. Vitamin supplement should be given at least 2 hours before or after Xenical.

Aggressive therapy and support may be necessary to initiate weight loss, although fasting is not generally a treatment of choice. Client can be monitored more effectively in a controlled setting to minimize complications such as orthostatic hypotension, anemia, and cardiac irregularities.

These interventions may be necessary to help the client lose weight when obesity is life-threatening. (Refer to CP: Obesity: Bariatric Surgery.)

NURSING DIAGNOSIS: sedentary Lifestyle

May be related to
Lack of interest, motivation, resources
Lack of training or knowledge of specific exercise needs
Safety concerns or fear of injury

Possibly evidenced by
Physical deconditioning
Daily routine lacking in physical exercise

Desired Outcomes/Evaluation Criteria—Client Will

Knowledge: Prescribed Activity (NOC)
Verbalize understanding of importance of regular exercise to weight loss and general well-being.
Identify necessary precautions and safety concerns and self-monitoring techniques.
Formulate realistic exercise program with gradual increase in activity.

ACTIONS/INTERVENTIONS	RATIONALE
Exercise Promotion (NIC)	
Independent	
Review necessity for and benefits of regular exercise.	Exercise promotes weight loss by reducing appetite, increasing energy, toning muscles, and enhancing cardiac fitness and sense of well-being and accomplishment.
Determine current activity level and plan progressive exercise program tailored to the individual's physical condition, goals, and choice.	Commitment on the part of the client enables the setting of more realistic goals and adherence to the plan.
Identify perceived and actual barriers to exercise.	Lack of resources, including proper apparel such as supportive shoes and comfortable clothing, a safe place to walk, or facility membership for water aerobics, reduces the likelihood of individual adhering to specific program. In addition, fear of discrimination or ridicule by others may limit client's willingness to exercise in public.
Discuss appropriate warm-up exercises, cool-down activities, and specific techniques to avoid injury.	Preventing muscle injuries allows client to stay active. Time spent recuperating from exercise-induced injuries may result in relapse to sedentary habits.
Determine optimal exercise heart rate. Demonstrate proper technique to monitor pulse and discuss signs and symptoms requiring modification of activity.	Promotes safety as client exercises to tolerance, not peer pressure.
Identify alternatives to chosen activity program to accommodate weather, travel, and so forth.	Promotes continuation of program.
Discuss use of mechanical devices or equipment for weight reduction.	Fat loss occurs on a generalized overall basis, and there is no evidence that spot reducing or mechanical devices aid in weight loss in specific areas; however, specific types of exercise or equipment may be useful in toning specific body parts.
Recommend keeping a graph of activity as exercise program advances.	Provides visual record of progress and positive reinforcement for efforts.
Suggest client identify an exercise buddy.	Provides support and companionship, increasing likelihood of adherence to program.
Encourage involvement in social activities that are not centered on food—bike ride or nature hike, attending musical event, and group sporting activities.	Provides opportunity for pleasure and relaxation not associated with food.
Collaborative	
Involve physical therapist or exercise physiologist in developing progressive program.	Facilitates development of an appropriate program of activities that are geared to obese individual and considers impact of client's weight on ability to perform specific activities and safety concerns.

NURSING DIAGNOSIS: disturbed Body Image/chronic low Self-Esteem

May be related to

Biophysical factors—changes in health status

Psychosocial factors—client's view of self; changes in body image, personal identity

Family or subculture encouragement of overeating—slimness is valued in this society, and mixed messages are received when thinness is stressed

Perceived failure at ability to control weight

Control, sex, and love issues

Possibly evidenced by

Verbalization of negative feelings about body—mental image often does not match physical reality

Fear of rejection or reaction by others

Feelings of hopelessness, powerlessness

Preoccupation with change—attempts to lose weight

Lack of follow-through with diet plan

Verbalization of powerlessness to change eating habits

Desired Outcomes/Evaluation Criteria—Client Will

Body Image (NOC)

Verbalize a more realistic self-image.

Demonstrate some acceptance of self as is rather than an idealized image.

Self-Esteem (NOC)

Seek information and actively pursue appropriate weight loss.

Acknowledge self as an individual who has responsibility for self.

ACTIONS/INTERVENTIONS	RATIONALE
Body Image Enhancement (NIC)	
Independent	
Determine client's view of being fat and what it does for the individual.	Mental image includes our ideal and is usually not up-to-date. Fat and compulsive eating behaviors may have deep-rooted psychological implications, such as compensation for lack of love and nurturing or a defense against intimacy. In addition, chronically obese client may report long-term discrimination in family, social, and professional settings. She or he may experience mixed feelings of fear and shame or compensate for psychological trauma by developing a strong or "big" personality.
Promote open communication, avoiding criticism or judgment about client's behavior.	Supports client's own responsibility for weight loss, enhances sense of control, and promotes willingness to discuss difficulties and setbacks and to problem-solve. *Note:* Distrust and accusations of "cheating" on caloric intake are not helpful.
Outline and clearly state responsibilities of client and nurse.	It is helpful for each individual to understand area of own responsibility in the program so that misunderstandings do not arise.
Graph weight on a weekly basis.	Provides ongoing visual evidence of weight changes, reinforcing reality.
Ensure availability of properly sized equipment, including gowns; blood pressure cuff; wider and strong wheelchair, bed, commode, and transfer devices, when providing inpatient care.	Healthcare providers have a moral and legal obligation to meet the client's needs for comfort and safety.
Encourage client to use imagery to visualize self at desired weight and to practice handling of new behaviors.	Mental rehearsal is very useful in helping the client plan for and deal with anticipated change in self-image or occasions that may arise, such as family gatherings or special dinners, where constant decisions about eating many foods will occur.
Provide information about the use of makeup, hairstyles, and ways of dressing to maximize figure assets.	Enhances feelings of self-esteem and promotes improved body image.
Encourage buying clothes instead of food treats as a reward for weight loss and life successes.	Properly fitting clothes enhance the body image as small losses are made and the individual feels more positive. Waiting until the desired weight loss is reached can become discouraging.
Suggest the client dispose of "fat clothes" as weight loss occurs.	Removes the "safety valve" of having clothes available "in case" the weight is regained. Retaining fat clothes can convey the message that the weight loss will not occur or be maintained.

(continues on page 394)

ACTIONS/INTERVENTIONS (continued)	RATIONALE (continued)
Be alert to myths the client and SO may have about weight and weight loss.	Beliefs about what an ideal body looks like or unconscious motivations can sabotage efforts to lose weight. Some of these include the feminine thought of "If I become thin, men will view me as a sexual object"; the masculine counterpart, "I don't trust myself to stay in control of my sexual feelings"; as well as issues of strength, power, or the "good cook" image.
Help staff be aware of and deal with own feelings when caring for client.	Judgmental attitudes, feelings of disgust, anger, and weariness can interfere with care and be transmitted to client, reinforcing negative self-concept and image.
Self-Esteem Enhancement (NIC)	
Identify basic sense of self-esteem and image client has of existential, physical, and psychological self. Determine locus of control.	Provides insight into view of self as fat and own ability to control weight. Information necessary to determine individual needs and treatment plan.
Determine client perception of threat to self.	Client's perception of what problem weight poses is more important than what the threat really is and needs to be dealt with before reality can be addressed.
Provide privacy during care activities.	Individual knows size makes it hard to care for her or him and usually is sensitive and self-conscious about body.
Have client recall coping patterns related to food in family of origin and explore how these may affect current situation.	Parents act as role models for the child. Maladaptive coping patterns, such as overeating, are learned within the family system and are supported through positive reinforcement. Food may be substituted by the parent for affection and love, and eating is associated with a feeling of satisfaction, becoming the primary defense.
Determine relationship history and possibility of sexual abuse.	May contribute to current issues of self-esteem and patterns of coping.
Identify client's motivation for weight loss and assist with goal setting.	The individual may harbor repressed feeling of hostility, which may be expressed inward on the self. Because of a poor self-concept, the person often has difficulty with relationships. *Note:* When losing weight for someone else, the client is less likely to be successful or maintain weight loss.
Assist client to identify feelings that lead to compulsive eating. Encourage journaling.	People often eat because of depression, anger, and guilt. Awareness of emotions that lead to overeating can be the first step in changing behavior.
Develop strategies for doing something beside eating for dealing with these feelings, such as talking with a friend.	Replacing eating with other activities helps retrain old patterns and establish new ways to deal with feelings.
Collaborative	
Refer to community support and/or therapy group.	Support groups can provide companionship, enhance motivation, decrease loneliness and social ostracism, and give practical solutions to common problems. Group therapy can be helpful in dealing with underlying psychological concerns.

NURSING DIAGNOSIS: impaired Social Interaction

May be related to
Verbalized or observed discomfort in social situations
Self-concept disturbance

Possibly evidenced by
Reluctance to participate in social gatherings
Verbalization of a sense of discomfort with others

Desired Outcomes/Evaluation Criteria—Client Will

Social Involvement (NOC)
Verbalize awareness of feelings that lead to poor social interactions.
Become involved in achieving positive changes in social behaviors and interpersonal relationships.

ACTIONS/INTERVENTIONS	RATIONALE
Socialization Enhancement (NIC)	
Independent	
Review family patterns of relating and social behaviors.	Social interaction is primarily learned within the family of origin. When inadequate patterns are identified, actions for change can be instituted.
Encourage client to express feelings and perceptions of problems.	Helps identify and clarify reasons for difficulties in interacting with others, such as feeling unloved or unlovable and insecure about sexuality.
Assess client's use of coping skills and defense mechanisms.	May have coping skills that will be useful in the process of weight loss. Defense mechanisms used to protect the individual may contribute to feelings of aloneness or isolation.
Have client list behaviors that cause discomfort.	Identifies specific concerns and suggests actions that can be taken to effect change.
Involve in role playing new ways to deal with identified behaviors or situations.	Practicing these new behaviors enables the individual to become comfortable with them in a safe situation.
Discuss negative self-concepts and self-talk, such as, "No one wants to be with a fat person," "Who would be interested in talking to me?"	May be impeding positive social interactions.
Encourage use of positive self-talk such as telling oneself "I am OK," or "I can enjoy social activities and do not need to be controlled by what others think or say."	Positive strategies enhance feelings of comfort and support efforts for change.
Collaborative	
Refer for ongoing family or individual therapy, as indicated.	Client benefits from involvement of SO to provide support and encouragement.

NURSING DIAGNOSIS: deficient Knowledge [Learning Need] regarding condition, prognosis, treatment, self-care, and discharge needs

May be related to
Lack of or misinterpretation of information
Lack of interest in learning, lack of recall
Inaccurate or incomplete information presented

Possibly evidenced by
Statements of lack of, or request for, information about obesity and nutritional requirements
Verbalization of problem with weight reduction
Inadequate follow-through with previous diet and exercise instructions

Desired Outcomes/Evaluation Criteria—Client Will

Knowledge: Diet (NOC)
Verbalize understanding of need for lifestyle changes to maintain or control weight.
Establish individual goal and plan for attaining that goal.
Begin to look for information about nutrition and ways to control weight.

ACTIONS/INTERVENTIONS	RATIONALE
Teaching: Prescribed Diet (NIC)	
Independent	
Determine level of nutritional knowledge and what client believes is most urgent need.	Necessary to know what additional information to provide. When client's views are listened to, trust is enhanced.
Identify individual long-term goals for health, such as lowering blood pressure, controlling serum lipid and glucose levels.	A high relapse rate at 5-year follow-up suggests obesity cannot be reliably reversed. Shifting the focus from initial weight loss and percentage of body fat to overall management of wellness may enhance rehabilitation.
Provide information about ways to maintain satisfactory food intake in settings away from home.	"Smart" eating when dining out or when traveling helps individual manage weight while still enjoying social outlets.
Identify other sources of information—books, tapes, community classes, and groups.	Using different avenues of accessing information furthers client's learning. Involvement with others who are also losing weight can provide support.

(continues on page 396)

ACTIONS/INTERVENTIONS (continued)	RATIONALE (continued)
Emphasize necessity of continued follow-up care or counseling, especially when plateaus occur.	As weight is lost, changes in metabolism occur, interfering with further loss by creating a plateau as the body activates a survival mechanism, attempting to prevent "starvation." This requires new strategies and aggressive support to continue weight loss.
Discuss use of medications; advise client to discuss with physician and pharmacist any additions to regimen such as over-the-counter (OTC) medications, antibiotics, and herbal supplements.	Obesity can alter the pharmacokinetic properties of medications. Changes in dosages may be needed based on the degree to which drugs are absorbed, resulting in subtherapeutic or toxic drug levels, or dangerous side effects and interactions that might occur.
Instruct client about risk of deep vein thrombosis (DVT) and self-care including ankle exercises, walking to limit of ability, and reporting any unusual discomfort in legs.	The very obese client is at higher risk for DVT and pulmonary embolism than the general population because of immobility, stasis, and polycythemia related to chronic respiratory insufficiency.
Discuss necessity of good skin care, especially in skin folds, such as abdomen, breasts, groin, perineal areas, during hot weather and times of immobility or following exercise.	Client is at risk for developing pressure ulcers and can be prone to yeast infections. Frequent skin care such as cleansing and drying the tissues, and using antifungal creams in skin folds, as appropriate, can prevent skin breakdown.
Identify alternative ways to "reward" self and family for accomplishments or to provide solace.	Reduces likelihood of relying on food to deal with feelings.

> **POTENTIAL CONSIDERATIONS** following acute hospitalization (dependent on client's age, physical condition and presence of complications, personal resources, and life responsibilities in addition to above nursing diagnoses)
> • *ineffective self Health Management*—complexity of therapeutic regimen, perceived seriousness and benefits, mistrust of regimen or healthcare personnel, excessive demands made on individual, family conflict

OBESITY: BARIATRIC SURGERY—GASTRIC PARTITIONING/GASTROPLASTY, GASTRIC BYPASS

I. Indications
a. Weight and health of extremely obese persons can be favorably changed by bariatric surgery (National Institutes of Health [NIH], 2008).
b. Improvement in comorbid conditions associated with morbid obesity—glucose intolerance and diabetes, hypertension, hyperlipidemia, and sleep apnea

II. Procedures
a. Open approaches with abdominal incisions or by laparoscopy
b. Extremely obese individuals, or those with previous abdominal surgery or complicating medical problems, may require open approach.
c. Three types of surgical procedures are offered.
   i. Restrictive
   1. Small pouch with a restricted outlet is created across the stomach just distal to the gastroesophageal junction; a small opening remains through which food passes into lower stomach.
   2. Reduces the amount of food the stomach can hold to 15 to 30 mL and slows passage of food through the stomach, resulting in a feeling of fullness

3. Most common procedures include stapling or banding of the stomach.
   a. Vertical banded gastroplasty (VBG): permits normal digestion of food, decreasing risk of anemia or vitamin deficiencies as compared with gastric bypass
   b. Laparoscopic adjustable gastric banding (LAGB): allows band adjustments depending on client's weight loss and appetite; it is considered by some to be the safest procedure (Salemeh, 2006)
   c. Gastric sleeve (GS): restricts food intake without decreasing absorption of food, with most of the stomach removed; sensations of hunger may be reduced through decreased production of the hormone, ghrelin (Weight-Control Information Network [WIN], 2008)
   ii. Malabsorptive
   1. Biliopancreatic diversion (BPD): excludes most of the small intestine from the digestive tract so that fewer calories and nutrients are absorbed
   2. Produces significant weight loss

iii. Combined restrictive and malabsorptive
1. Roux-en-Y gastric bypass: partial bypass of the small intestine results in fewer calories being absorbed
2. Greater weight loss is achieved.

III. **Complications** (Beauchamp-Johnson, 2006; Bouldin et al, 2006; Salemeh, 2006; Trus et al, 2005)

a. Anastomotic leak: occurs at gastrojejunostomy or jejunostomy site; can result in peritonitis, sepsis, and death

b. Intestinal obstruction: associated with stenosis at anastomosis sites

c. Wound complications: laparoscopic procedures associated with higher risk of infection (1.5%) and hernias (1.8%) than open procedures

d. Nutritional complications: risk for iron, calcium, thiamine, folate, and vitamin B_{12} deficiencies can occur early or late and are long term

IV. **Statistics**

a. Morbidity: Between 2002 and 2004, frequency of procedure increased threefold (from previous 3-year period) to over 106,000 bariatric procedures, with ages ranging from 18 to 64; women outnumbered men 5:1 (U.S. Department of Health and Human Services [USDHHS], 2006).

b. Mortality: Laparoscopic banding procedures account for less than 1%; gastric bypass account for 1% to 2%; mortality rates are higher in the "super obese," those individuals who have a body mass index (BMI) greater than 50, and in those who have undergone BPD due to long-term complications (Bouldin et al, 2006; NIH, 2008; Salemeh, 2006; Trus et al, 2005).

c. Cost: Average cost is $20,000 to $25,000 per uncomplicated procedure (NIH, 2008); $948 million in hospital costs for bariatric surgery in 2002 (Encinosa et al, 2005).

GLOSSARY

Biliopancreatic diversion (BPD): Removal of the lower portion of the stomach, creating a gastric sleeve (GS) with the small pouch that remains, which is connected directly to the small intestine, completely bypassing the duodenum and upper small intestine.

Body mass index (BMI): Uses individual's weight in kilograms divided by height in meters squared to produce a unit of measure for classifying body composition.

Gastric sleeve (GS): Usually performed as the first stage of biliopancreatic bypass with duodenal switch for clients who may be at high risk for complications from more extensive types of surgery.

Ghrelin: Hormone produced primarily in the stomach (and also the pancreas), impacting sensation of hunger, stimulating appetite, and increasing fat storage.

Laparoscopic adjustable gastric banding (LAGB): Implantation of an inflatable silicon band around uppermost part of the stomach.

Roux-en-Y gastric bypass: Combines gastric restriction, by creating a small pouch similar in size to the adjustable gastric band, and malabsorption, with food bypassing 90% of the stomach, the duodenum, and a portion of the jejunum.

Vertical banded gastroplasty (VBG): Rows of staples placed vertically in the strongest sidewall of the stomach and insertion of a polypropylene band around the outlet of the resulting pouch.

Care Setting

Care is provided in an inpatient acute surgical unit.

Related Concerns

Eating disorders: obesity, page 387
Peritonitis, page 349
Psychosocial aspects of care, page 749
Surgical intervention, page 782
Thrombophlebitis: deep vein thrombosis, page 111

Refer to Endocrine Disorders: Obesity Database for additional assessment information.

DIAGNOSTIC DIVISION MAY REPORT	MAY EXHIBIT
ACTIVITY/REST • Difficulty sleeping • Exertional discomfort, inability to participate in desired activity or sports	
EGO INTEGRITY • Motivated to lose weight for oneself (or for gratification of others) • Fear or anxiety about procedure and ability to deal with post-operative adjustments • History of psychiatric illness or treatment	• Anxiety, depression
ELIMINATION • Urinary stress incontinence	
FOOD/FLUID • History of yo-yo dieting, years of failed dieting; weight fluctuations; dysfunctional eating patterns	• Weight exceeding ideal body weight by 100 lb, or BMI more than 40 (morbid obesity), or BMI of 25 to 40 with comorbid conditions, such as diabetes, sleep apnea, or heart disease (Beauchamp-Johnson, 2006)
HYGIENE • Difficulty with dressing, bathing, or self-care activities	
PAIN/DISCOMFORT • Incisional pain	• Guarding behavior • Positioning to avoid pain • Facial mask, grimacing • Restlessness, moaning, irritability
TEACHING/LEARNING • Presence of chronic conditions—hypertension, diabetes, heart failure, arthritis, sleep apnea, Pickwickian syndrome, infertility • Learning about lifelong healthy eating and physical activity habits, medical follow-up, and vitamin and mineral supplementation	
DISCHARGE PLAN CONSIDERATIONS • May require support with therapeutic regimen and weight loss, assistance with self-care, homemaker and maintenance tasks ▶ Refer to section at end of plan for postdischarge considerations.	

Diagnostic Studies

Studies depend on individual situation and are used to rule out underlying disease and provide a preoperative workup, including psychiatric evaluation.

Nursing Priorities

1. Support respiratory function.
2. Prevent or minimize complications.
3. Provide appropriate nutritional intake.
4. Provide information regarding surgical procedure, postoperative expectations, and treatment needs.

Discharge Goals

1. Ventilation and oxygenation adequate for individual needs.
2. Complications prevented or controlled.
3. Nutritional intake modified for specific procedure.
4. Procedure, prognosis, and therapeutic regimen understood.
5. Plan in place to meet needs after discharge.

NURSING DIAGNOSIS: **ineffective Breathing Pattern**

May be related to
Decreased lung expansion
Pain, anxiety
Decreased energy, fatigue
Tracheobronchial obstruction

Possibly evidenced by
Shortness of breath, dyspnea
Tachypnea, respiratory depth changes, reduced vital capacity
Wheezes, rhonchi
Abnormal arterial blood gases (ABGs)

Desired Outcomes/Evaluation Criteria—Client Will

Respiratory Status: Ventilation (NOC)
Maintain adequate ventilation.
Experience no cyanosis or other signs of hypoxia, with ABGs within acceptable range.

ACTIONS/INTERVENTIONS	RATIONALE
Ventilation Assistance (NIC)	
Independent	
Monitor respiratory rate and depth. Auscultate breath sounds. Investigate presence of pallor and cyanosis, increased restlessness, or confusion.	Respirations may be shallow because of incisional pain, analgesia, immobility, and obesity itself, causing hypoventilation and potentiating risk of atelectasis and hypoxia. *Note:* Many anesthetic agents are fat soluble, so the postoperative "resedation" and the potential for respiratory complications are increased.
Elevate head of bed 30 to 45 degrees.	Encourages optimal diaphragmatic excursion and lung expansion and minimizes pressure of abdominal contents on the thoracic cavity. *Note:* When kept recumbent, obese clients are at high risk for severe hypoventilation postoperatively.
Encourage deep-breathing exercises. Assist with coughing and splint incision.	Promotes maximal lung expansion and aids in clearing airways, thus reducing risk of atelectasis and pneumonia. *Note:* Use of abdominal binder—properly fitted and placed at least 2 inches below the xiphoid process—can encourage deep breathing.
Turn periodically and ambulate as early as possible.	Promotes aeration of all segments of the lung, mobilizing and aiding movement of secretions. *Note:* If client was a good candidate for bariatric surgery, she or he was probably relatively healthy before operation and is usually able to turn self, walk, and transfer to chair within 8 hours of surgery.
Pad side rails and teach client to use them as armrests.	Using the side rail as an armrest allows for greater chest expansion.
Use small pillow under head, when indicated.	Many obese clients have large, thick necks, and use of large, fluffy pillows may obstruct the airway.
Collaborative	
Administer supplemental oxygen.	Maximizes available O$_2$ for exchange and reduces work of breathing.
Assist in use of blow bottle or incentive spirometer.	Enhances lung expansion; reduces potential for atelectasis.
Monitor ABGs or pulse oximetry, as indicated.	Reflects ventilation, oxygenation, and acid-base status. Used as a basis for evaluating need for and effectiveness of respiratory therapies.
Monitor patient-controlled analgesia (PCA) and administer analgesics, as appropriate.	Maintenance of comfort level enhances participation in respiratory therapy and promotes increased lung expansion. *Note:* For the first 48 hours after the procedure, intravenous (IV) PCA is the method of choice. Oral medications are usually the next level of pain management.

NURSING DIAGNOSIS: risk for ineffective tissue Perfusion [specify]

Risk factors may include
Diminished blood flow, hypovolemia
Decreased hemoglobin concentration in the blood
Impaired oxygen transport
Interruption of venous blood flow (thrombosis)

Possibly evidenced by
(Not applicable; presence of signs and symptoms establishes an *actual* diagnosis)

Desired Outcomes/Evaluation Criteria—Client Will

Circulation Status (NOC)
Maintain perfusion as individually appropriate—skin warm and dry, peripheral pulses present and strong, and vital signs within acceptable range.

Risk Control (NOC)
Identify causative or risk factors.
Demonstrate behaviors to improve or maintain circulation.

ACTIONS/INTERVENTIONS	RATIONALE
Surveillance (NIC)	
Independent	
Monitor vital signs, palpate peripheral pulses routinely, and evaluate capillary refill and changes in mentation. Note 24-hour fluid balance.	Indicators of circulatory adequacy. (Refer to ND: risk for deficient Fluid Volume, below.)
Encourage frequent range-of-motion (ROM) exercises for legs and ankles. Maintain schedule of sequential compression devices (SCD) on lower extremities when used.	Stimulates circulation in the lower extremities, reduces high-risk complications associated with venous stasis, such as DVT and pulmonary embolus (PE).
Assess for redness, edema, and discomfort in calf.	Indicators of thrombus formation, but warning signs may not always be present in obese individuals.
Encourage early ambulation; discourage sitting and dangling legs at the bedside.	Sitting constricts venous flow, whereas walking encourages venous return.
Provide adequate and appropriate equipment, including trapeze for turning, transfer device, walker, and wheelchair, and sufficient staff for handling client.	Helpful in dealing with obese client for moving and ambulating. Reduces risk of traumatic injury to both client and caregivers.
Evaluate for complications, such as rigid abdomen, nonincisional abdominal pain, fever, tachycardia, and low blood pressure.	Although rare, client can develop abdominal complications, such as abdominal compartment syndrome, sepsis or septic shock secondary to anastomotic leak or wound infection, requiring intensive interventions or return to surgery.
Collaborative	
Administer heparin therapy, as indicated.	May be used prophylactically to reduce risk of thrombus formation or to treat thromboemboli.
Monitor hemoglobin (Hgb), hematocrit (Hct), and coagulation studies, such as prothrombin time (PT) and International Normalized Ratio (INR).	Provides information about circulatory volume and alterations in coagulation and indicates therapy needs and effectiveness.

NURSING DIAGNOSIS: risk for deficient Fluid Volume

Risk factors may include
Excessive gastric losses—nasogastric suction, diarrhea
Reduced intake

Possibly evidenced by
(Not applicable; presence of signs and symptoms establishes an *actual* diagnosis)

Desired Outcomes/Evaluation Criteria—Client Will

Hydration (NOC)
Maintain adequate fluid volume with balanced intake and output (I&O) and be free of signs reflecting dehydration.

ACTIONS/INTERVENTIONS	RATIONALE

Fluid/Electrolyte Management (NIC)
Independent

Assess vital signs, noting changes in blood pressure (BP), such as orthostatic hypotension, tachycardia, and fever. Assess skin turgor, capillary refill, and moisture of mucous membranes.

Monitor I&O, measuring nasogastric (NG) suction losses.

Evaluate muscle strength and tone. Observe for muscle tremors.

Establish individual needs and replacement schedule.

Encourage increased oral intake when able.

Collaborative

Administer IV fluids, as indicated.

Monitor electrolyte levels and replace, as indicated.

Indicators of dehydration and hypovolemia and adequacy of current fluid replacement. *Note:* Adequately-sized cuff must be used to ensure factual measurement of BP. If cuff is too small, reading will be falsely elevated.

Changes in gastric capacity and intestinal motility and nausea greatly influence intake and fluid needs, increasing risk of dehydration.

Large gastric losses may result in decreased magnesium and calcium, leading to neuromuscular weakness and tetany.

Determined by amount of measured losses and estimated insensible losses and dependent on gastric capacity.

Permits discontinuation of invasive fluid support measures and contributes to return of normal bowel functioning.

Replaces fluid losses and restores fluid balance in immediate postoperative phase until client is able to take sufficient oral fluids.

Use of NG tube, vomiting, or onset of diarrhea can deplete electrolytes, affecting organ function.

NURSING DIAGNOSIS: **risk for imbalanced Nutrition: Less than Body Requirements**

Risk factors may include
Decreased intake, dietary restrictions, early satiety
Increased metabolic rate and healing
Malabsorption of nutrients and impaired absorption of vitamins

Possibly evidenced by
(Not applicable; presence of signs and symptoms establishes an *actual* diagnosis)

Desired Outcomes/Evaluation Criteria—Client Will

Knowledge: Diet (NOC)
Identify individual nutritional needs.

Nutritional Status (NOC)
Display behaviors to maintain adequate nutritional intake.
Demonstrate appropriate weight loss with normalization of laboratory values.

ACTIONS/INTERVENTIONS	RATIONALE

Weight Reduction Assistance (NIC)
Independent

Establish hourly intake schedule. Measure and provide food and fluids in amount specified.

Instruct in how to eat slowly. Take small bites, using a baby spoon. Chew food thoroughly. Take 3 to 60 minutes to eat meal, then refrain from eating until next scheduled mealtime.

Avoid taking fluids with meals and for 30 minutes before or after meals. Encourage almost constant sipping of fluids between scheduled eating times.

Avoid high-calorie fluids—milkshakes, sodas, and alcoholic beverages.

Emphasize importance of recognizing satiety and stopping intake.

Require that client sit up to drink and eat.

Determine foods that are gas forming and eliminate them from diet.

After gastric restriction procedures, stomach capacity is reduced to approximately 30 to 50 mL, necessitating frequent, small feedings. Ultimately, management of optimal nutrition depends on reducing the amount of food passing through the gastrointestinal (GI) system at one time.

Increases satiety and reduces risk of overeating.

Although fluids are a necessary part of the client's intake, the stomach is too small to hold food and fluids at the same time.

These can sabotage weight loss.

Overeating may cause nausea and vomiting, as well as having the potential to damage surgical anastomosis.

Reduces possibility of aspiration.

May cause nausea and bloating, interfering with digestion and causing client to restrict nutritional intake.

(continues on page 402)

ACTIONS/INTERVENTIONS (continued)	RATIONALE (continued)
Discuss food preferences with client and include those foods in puréed diet when possible.	May enhance intake and promote sense of participation and control.
Weigh on regular schedule.	Monitors losses and aids in assessing nutritional needs and effectiveness of therapy.
Collaborative	
Refer to dietitian or multidisciplinary team.	Provides assistance in planning a diet that meets client's nutritional needs as well as offering individualized treatment and support. *Note:* Because quantity is strictly limited, foods should be nutrient dense, low in fat and sugars, and high in protein (Beauchamp-Johnson, 2006).
Administer vitamin supplements (may use chewable vitamins) and vitamin B_{12} injections, folate, and calcium, as indicated.	Because absorption is impaired, supplements will be needed for life to prevent complications associated with vitamin deficiencies. Increased intestinal motility following bypass procedure lowers calcium level and increases absorption of oxalates, which can lead to urinary stone formation.

NURSING DIAGNOSIS: [actual/] risk for impaired Skin Integrity

May be related to
Trauma, surgery, difficulty in approximation of suture line of fatty tissue
Reduced vascularity, altered circulation
Altered nutritional state—obesity

Possibly evidenced by (actual)
Disruption of skin surface, altered healing

Desired Outcomes/Evaluation Criteria—Client Will

Wound Healing: Primary Intention (NOC)
Display timely wound healing without complications.
Demonstrate behaviors that reduce tension on suture line.

Tissue Integrity: Skin and Mucous Membranes (NOC)
Display intact skin free of signs of pressure or breakdown.

ACTIONS/INTERVENTIONS	RATIONALE
Wound Care (NIC)	
Independent	
Support and instruct client in incisional support when turning, coughing, deep breathing, and ambulating.	Reduces possibility of dehiscence and incisional hernia.
Observe incisions periodically, noting approximation of wound edges, hematoma formation and resolution, and presence of bleeding and drainage.	Verifies status of healing, provides for early detection of developing complications requiring prompt evaluation and influencing choice of interventions.
Provide routine incisional care, being careful to keep dressing dry and sterile. Assess and maintain patency of drains.	Promotes healing. Accumulation of serosanguineous drainage in subcutaneous layers increases tension on suture line, may delay wound healing, and serves as a medium for bacterial growth.
Pressure Management (NIC)	
Encourage frequent positional change, inspect pressure points, and massage gently, as indicated. Apply transparent skin barrier to elbows and heels, if indicated.	Reduces pressure on skin, promoting peripheral circulation and reducing risk of skin breakdown. Skin barrier reduces risk of shearing injury.
Provide meticulous skin care, pay particular attention to skin folds common in the very obese client.	Moisture or excoriation enhances growth of bacteria that can lead to postoperative infection.
Collaborative	
Provide foam, water, or air mattress, as indicated.	Reduces skin pressure and enhances circulation.

NURSING DIAGNOSIS: risk for Infection

Risk factors may include
Inadequate primary defenses—broken or traumatized tissues, decreased ciliary action, stasis of body fluids
Invasive procedures

Possibly evidenced by
(Not applicable; presence of signs and symptoms establishes an *actual* diagnosis)

Desired Outcomes/Evaluation Criteria—Client Will

Immobility Consequences: Physiological (NOC)
Be free of nosocomial infection.

Wound Healing: Primary Intention (NOC)
Achieve timely wound healing free of signs of local or generalized infectious process.

ACTIONS/INTERVENTIONS	RATIONALE
Infection Protection (NIC)	
Independent	
Emphasize and model proper hand-washing technique.	Prevents spread of bacteria and cross-contamination.
Maintain aseptic technique in dressing changes and invasive procedures.	Reduces risk of nosocomial infection.
Inspect surgical incisions and invasive line sites for erythema and purulent drainage.	Early detection of developing infection provides for prevention of more serious complications.
Encourage frequent position changes, deep breathing, coughing, and use of respiratory adjuncts, such as incentive spirometer.	Promotes mobilization of secretions, reducing risk of pneumonia.
Provide routine catheter care; encourage good perineal care. Remove catheter as early as possible.	Prevents ascending bladder infections.
Encourage client to drink acid-ash juices, such as cranberry.	Maintains urine acidity and prevents bacteria from adhering to the bladder wall to retard bacterial growth.
Observe for reports of abdominal pain, especially after third postoperative day, elevated temperature, and increased white blood cell (WBC) count.	Suggests possibility of developing peritonitis.
Collaborative	
Apply topical antimicrobials or antibiotics, as indicated.	Reduces bacterial or fungal colonization on skin; prevents infection in the wound.
Administer IV antibiotics, as indicated.	A prophylactic antibiotic regimen is usually standard in these clients to reduce risk of perioperative contamination and peritonitis.
Obtain specimen of purulent drainage or sputum for culture and sensitivity.	Identifies infectious agent; aids in choice of appropriate therapy.

NURSING DIAGNOSIS: Diarrhea

May be related to
Rapid transit of food through shortened small intestine
Changes in dietary fiber and bulk
Inflammation, irritation, and malabsorption of bowel

Possibly evidenced by
Loose, liquid stools, increased frequency
Increased and hyperactive bowel sounds

Desired Outcomes/Evaluation Criteria—Client Will

Treatment Behavior: Illness or Injury (NOC)
Verbalize understanding of causative factors and rationale of treatment regimen.
Follow through with treatment recommendations.

Bowel Elimination (NOC)
Regain near-normal bowel function.

Diarrhea Management (NIC)
Independent

Observe and record stool frequency, characteristics, and amount.

Diarrhea often develops after resumption of diet because of shortened transit time through the GI tract and dumping syndrome. This condition is usually self-limiting, but can cause discomfort and social difficulties when persistent.

Encourage diet high in fiber and bulk within dietary limitations, with moderate fluid intake as diet resumes.

Increases consistency of the effluent. Although fluid is necessary for optimal body function, excessive amounts contribute to diarrhea.

Restrict fat intake, as indicated.

Low-fat diet reduces risk of steatorrhea and limits laxative effect of decreased fat absorption.

Observe for signs of dumping syndrome such as instant diarrhea, sweating, nausea, and weakness after eating.

Rapid emptying of food from the stomach may result in gastric distress and alter bowel function.

Assist with frequent perianal care, using ointments as indicated. Provide whirlpool bath.

Anal irritation, excoriation, and pruritus occur because of diarrhea. The client often cannot reach the area for proper cleansing and may be embarrassed to ask for help.

Collaborative

Administer medications such as diphenoxylate with atropine (Lomotil), as indicated.

Antidiarrheals may be necessary to control frequency of stools until body adjusts to changes in function brought about by surgery.

Monitor serum electrolytes.

Large gastric losses potentiate the risk of electrolyte imbalance, which can lead to more serious or life-threatening complications.

NURSING DIAGNOSIS: **deficient Knowledge [Learning Need] regarding condition, prognosis, treatment, self-care, and discharge needs**

May be related to
Lack of exposure, unfamiliarity with resources
Information misinterpretation
Lack of recall

Possibly evidenced by
Questions, request for information
Statement of misconceptions
Inaccurate follow-through of instructions
Development of preventable complications

Desired Outcomes/Evaluation Criteria—Client Will

Knowledge: Disease Process (NOC)
Verbalize understanding of surgical procedure, potential complications, and postoperative expectations.

Knowledge: Treatment Regimen (NOC)
Verbalize understanding of therapeutic needs and rationale for actions.
Initiate necessary lifestyle changes and participate in treatment regimen.

Teaching: Disease Process (NIC)
Independent

Review specific surgical procedure and postoperative expectations.

Provides knowledge base from which informed choices can be made and goals formulated. Initial weight loss is rapid, with client often losing half of the total weight loss during the first 6 months. Weight loss then gradually stabilizes over a 2-year period.

Address concerns about altered body size and image.

Anticipation of problems can be helpful in dealing with situations that arise. (Refer to CP: Eating Disorders: Obesity, ND: disturbed Body Image/chronic low Self-Esteem.)

Review medication regimen, dosage, and side effects.

Knowledge may enhance client's involvement with therapeutic regimen. *Note:* As client loses weight, the dosages of many medications may need to be recalculated because body fat alters the pharmacokinetics of many medications (Beauchamp-Johnson, 2006).

ACTIONS/INTERVENTIONS (continued)

Recommend avoidance of alcohol.

Discuss responsibility for self-care with client and significant other (SO).

Emphasize importance of regular medical follow-up, including laboratory studies, and discuss possible health problems.

Encourage progressive exercise and activity program balanced with adequate rest periods.

Review proper eating habits, for example, eat small amounts of food slowly and chew well and sit at table in calm, relaxed environment; eat only at prescribed times, avoid between-meal snacking, and do not "make up" skipped feedings.

Identify signs of hypokalemia, for example, diarrhea, muscle cramps, weakness of lower extremities, weak or irregular pulse, and dizziness with position changes.

Discuss symptoms that may indicate dumping syndrome: weakness, profuse perspiration, nausea, vomiting, faintness, flushing, and epigastric discomfort or palpitations occurring during or immediately following meals. Problem-solve solutions.

Review symptoms requiring medical evaluation including persistent nausea or vomiting, abdominal distention or tenderness, change in pattern of bowel elimination, fever, purulent wound drainage, excessive weight loss, plateauing, or weight gain.

Refer to bariatric postoperative program or community support groups.

RATIONALE (continued)

High caloric count contributes to slowed weight loss as well as liver and pancreatic dysfunction.

Full involvement in weight loss program is important for successful outcome after procedure.

Periodic assessment and evaluation, for example, over 3 to 12 months, promotes early recognition of such complications as liver dysfunction, malnutrition, electrolyte imbalances, and kidney stones, which may develop following bypass procedure.

Promotes weight loss, enhances muscle tone, and minimizes postoperative complications while preventing undue fatigue.

Focuses attention on eating, increasing awareness of intake and feelings of satiety.

Increasing dietary intake of potassium (e.g., milk, coffee, potatoes, carrots, bananas, oranges) may correct deficit, preventing serious respiratory or cardiac complications.

Generally occurring in early postoperative period (1 to 3 weeks), syndrome is usually self-limiting, but may become chronic and require medical intervention.

Early recognition of developing complications allows for prompt intervention, preventing serious outcome.

Involvement with others who have dealt with same problems enhances coping; may promote cooperation with therapeutic regimen and long-term positive recovery.

POTENTIAL CONSIDERATIONS following acute hospitalization (dependent on client's age, physical condition and presence of complications, personal resources, and life responsibilities)
- *risk for imbalanced Nutrition: More than Body Requirements*—dysfunctional eating patterns, observed use of food as reward or comfort measure, history of morbid obesity

Refer to Potential Considerations in Surgical Intervention plan of care.

DIABETES MELLITUS/DIABETIC KETOACIDOSIS

I. Pathology
  a. Diabetes mellitus (DM) is a chronic metabolic disorder in which the body cannot metabolize carbohydrates, fats, and proteins because of a lack of, or ineffective use of, the hormone insulin.

  b. Diabetic ketoacidosis (DKA) is a life-threatening emergency caused by a relative or absolute deficiency of insulin.

II. Classification
  a. Three primary types that are different disease entities but share the symptoms and complications of hyperglycemia

  b. Type 1, type 2, and impaired glucose tolerance or pre-diabetes—formerly known as "borderline diabetes"

III. Etiology
  a. Conditions or situations known to exacerbate glucose and insulin imbalance

    i. Previously undiagnosed or newly diagnosed type 1 diabetes

    ii. Food intake in excess of available insulin

    iii. Adolescence and puberty

    iv. Exercise in uncontrolled diabetes

    v. Stress associated with illness, infection, trauma, or emotional distress

  b. Type 1 diabetes (American Diabetes Association [ADA], 2004a)

(text continues on page 406)

i. An autoimmune disease possibly triggered by genetic and environmental factors, such as with virus, toxin, stress
   1. Destroys beta-cells in the pancreas
   2. When 80% to 90% of the beta cells are destroyed, overt symptoms occur.
ii. Totally insulin-deficient; clients require exogenous insulin to survive (Peeples & Seley, 2007).
iii. Characteristics
   1. Usually occurs before 30 years of age, but can occur at any age
   2. Peak incidence occurs during puberty
   3. Abrupt onset of signs and symptoms of hyperglycemia
   4. Prone to ketoacidosis
c. Type 2 diabetes (ADA, 2004a)
   i. Involves a decreased ability to use the insulin produced in the pancreas (Peeples & Seley, 2007)
      1. Decreased insulin secretion in response to glucose levels
      2. Insulin resistance blocking cells from absorbing glucose
      3. Excess production of glucose because of defective insulin secretory response
   ii. Accounts for 90% to 95% of all diabetes in the United States

iii. Characteristics
   1. Usually occurs after 30 years of age, but is now occurring in children and adolescents.
   2. Increased prevalence in some ethnic groups—African Americans, Hispanic/Latino, Native Americans, Asian Americans, and Pacific Islanders
   3. Strong genetic predisposition
   4. Frequently obese
   5. Not prone to ketoacidosis until late in course or with prolonged hyperglycemia
d. Associated with many complications, including heart disease and stroke, high blood pressure, blindness, kidney and nervous system disease, amputations, and complications of pregnancy

IV. Statistics
a. Morbidity: More than 20.8 million Americans diagnosed with either type 1 or type 2 diabetes; affects 20% of people over the age of 65 years; approximately 1.5 million new cases of diabetes diagnosed in 2005 (National Diabetes Information Clearinghouse [NDIC], 2007).
b. Mortality: In 2002, diabetes was reported to be the sixth leading cause of death (NDIC, 2007).
c. Cost: In 2007, the total cost (direct and indirect) of diabetes in the United States was estimated to be $174 billion (ADA, 2007).

GLOSSARY

Acetone: Chemical formed in the blood when the body uses fat instead of glucose for energy. Acetone passes through the body into the urine. Someone with high levels of acetone can have breath that smells fruity and is called "acetone breath."

Beta cells: Cells that make insulin found in areas of the pancreas called the Islets of Langerhans.

Blood glucose: The main sugar that the body makes from food. Glucose is carried through the bloodstream to provide energy to all of the body's living cells.

Dawn phenomenon: An abrupt increase in fasting levels of serum glucose concentrations between the hours of 5 a.m. and 9 a.m., without preceding hypoglycemia, especially in diabetic patients receiving insulin therapy.

Diabetic neuropathy: Family of nerve disorders caused by diabetes, causing numbness, pain, and weakness in the hands, arms, feet, and legs. About half of all diabetics have some form of neuropathy.

Gastroparesis: Delayed emptying of food and secretions from the stomach to the small bowel due to autonomic neuropathy.

Hyperglycemia: High blood glucose.

Hypoglycemia: Low blood glucose.

Insulin: Hormone produced by the pancreas that helps the body use blood glucose for energy. A person lacking this hormone is dependent on supplemental, outside (exogenous) sources.

Insulin resistance: Body is unable to use the insulin that it makes because of cell-receptor defect resulting in inability of cells to absorb glucose.

Ketoacidosis: Condition in which very high blood sugar levels along with a very low level of insulin result in a dangerous accumulation of ketones in the blood and urine. Coma or death can result if condition is not treated.

Ketones: Chemical substances produced when the body breaks down fat for energy. When ketones build up in the body over a long period of time, serious illness or coma can result.

Kussmaul respirations: Abnormal respiratory pattern characterized by rapid, deep breathing, often seen in client with metabolic acidosis.

Lactic acidosis: The buildup of lactic acid in the body. Cells make lactic acid when they use glucose for energy. If too much lactic acid stays in the body, the balance tips and the person begins to feel ill. Lactic acidosis may be caused by diabetic ketoacidosis or liver or kidney disease.

Metabolic acidosis: A pH imbalance in which the body has accumulated too much acid and does not have enough bicarbonate to effectively neutralize the effects of the acid. It can be brought on by a lack of insulin, a starvation diet, a gastrointestinal (GI) disorder, or a major organ dysfunction. For a person with diabetes, this can lead to diabetic ketoacidosis.

Paresthesias: Sensation of numbness or tingling, indicating nerve irritation, which may be due to diabetic neuropathy.

Somogyi effect: A swing to a high level of glucose in the blood from an extremely low level, usually occurs after an untreated insulin reaction during the night. The swing is caused by the release of stress hormones to counter low glucose levels.

Care Settings

DM is managed in the community setting. Diabetic ketoacidosis (DKA) may be encountered in any setting, with mild DKA managed at the community level; however severe metabolic imbalance requires inpatient acute care on a medical unit.

Related Concerns

Amputation, page 646
Fluid and electrolyte imbalances, page 903
Metabolic acidosis—primary base bicarbonate deficiency, page 483
Psychosocial aspects of care, page 749

Client Assessment Database

Data depend on the severity and duration of metabolic imbalance, length and stage of diabetic process, and effects on other organ function.

DIAGNOSTIC DIVISION MAY REPORT	MAY EXHIBIT
ACTIVITY/REST • Sleep and rest disturbances • Weakness, fatigue, difficulty walking and moving • Muscle cramps, decreased muscle strength	• Tachycardia and tachypnea at rest or with activity • Lethargy, disorientation, coma • Decreased muscle strength and tone
CIRCULATION • History of hypertension; acute myocardial infarction (MI), claudication, numbness, tingling of extremities (long-term effects) • Leg ulcers, slow healing	• Tachycardia • Postural blood pressure (BP) changes; hypertension • Decreased and absent pulses • Dysrhythmias • Crackles; jugular vein distention (JVD) —if heart failure present • Hot, dry, flushed skin; sunken eyeballs—if dehydration is severe
EGO INTEGRITY • Life stressors, including financial concerns related to condition	• Anxiety, irritability
ELIMINATION • Change in usual voiding pattern • Excessive urination (polyuria) • Nocturia • Pain and burning, difficulty voiding (infection neurogenic bladder) • Recent and recurrent urinary tract infections (UTIs) • Abdominal tenderness, bloating, diarrhea	• Pale, yellow, dilute urine • Polyuria may progress to oliguria and anuria if severe hypovolemia occurs • Cloudy, odorous urine (infection) • Abdomen firm, distended • Bowel sounds diminished or hyperactive (diarrhea)
FOOD/FLUID • Loss of appetite, nausea and vomiting • Not following prescribed diet, increased intake of glucose and carbohydrates • Weight loss over a period of days or weeks • Thirst • Use of medications exacerbating dehydration, such as diuretics	• Dry and cracked skin, poor skin turgor • Abdominal rigidity and distention • Halitosis and sweet, fruity breath odor
NEUROSENSORY • Fainting spells, dizziness • Headaches • Tingling, numbness, weakness in muscles • Visual disturbances	• Confusion, disorientation • Drowsiness, lethargy, stupor and coma (later stages) • Deep tendon reflexes (DTRs) may be decreased • Seizure activity (late stages of DKA or hypoglycemia)
PAIN/DISCOMFORT • Abdominal bloating and pain	• Facial grimacing with abdominal palpation, guarding

(continues on page 408)

DIAGNOSTIC DIVISION
MAY REPORT (continued)

RESPIRATION
- Air hunger (late stages of DKA)
- Cough, with and without purulent sputum (infection)

SAFETY
- Dry, itching skin, skin ulcerations
- Paresthesia (diabetic neuropathy)

SEXUALITY
- Vaginal discharge (prone to infection)
- Problems with impotence (men), orgasmic difficulty (women)

TEACHING/LEARNING
- Familial risk factors, such as diabetes mellitus, heart disease, stroke, hypertension
- Slow and delayed healing
- Use of drugs, such as steroids, thiazide diuretics, phenytoin (Dilantin), and phenobarbital (can increase glucose levels)
- May or may not be taking diabetic medications as ordered

DISCHARGE PLAN CONSIDERATIONS
- May need assistance with dietary regimen, glucose monitoring, medication administration, and supplies, self-care

▶ Refer to section at end of plan for postdischarge considerations.

MAY EXHIBIT (continued)

- Tachypnea
- Kussmaul's respiration (metabolic acidosis)
- Rhonchi, wheezes
- Yellow or green sputum (infection)

- Fever, diaphoresis
- Skin breakdown, lesions and ulcerations
- Decreased general strength and range of motion (ROM)
- Weakness and paralysis of muscles, including respiratory musculature—if potassium levels are markedly decreased

Diagnostic Studies

TEST WHY IT IS DONE	WHAT IT TELLS ME
BLOOD TESTS • *Serum glucose:* The gold standard for diagnosing diabetes is an elevated blood sugar level after an overnight fast. A value above 140 mg/dL on at least two occasions typically means a person has diabetes. Normal fasting sugar levels run between 70 and 110 mg/dL.	DKA is defined as glucose greater than 250 mg/dL in association with an arterial pH of less than 7.30 or serum bicarbonate of less than 15 mEq/L and ketonemia (serum ketones).
• *Fatty acids:* Types of naturally occurring and synthetic lipid compounds.	When insulin levels are too low or there is not enough glucose to use for energy, the body burns fatty acids for energy. The body then makes ketone bodies, waste products that cause the acid level in the blood to become too high. This in turn may lead to ketoacidosis.
• *Serum osmolality:* Measures the concentration of particles found in the fluid part of blood to help evaluate the body's water balance. Normal calculated values range from 280 to 303 mOsm/K.	Osmolality increases with dehydration and decreases with overhydration. In DKA, osmolality is elevated.
• *Glucogon:* Hormone that raises the blood glucose level.	Elevated level is associated with conditions that produce (1) actual hypoglycemia; (2) relative lack of glucose, such as trauma or infection; or (3) lack of insulin. Therefore, glucagon may be elevated with severe DKA despite hyperglycemia.

Diagnostic Studies (continued)

TEST / WHY IT IS DONE (continued)	WHAT IT TELLS ME (continued)
• **Hemoglobin A_{1C} (HgbA$_{1C}$):** Test that determines how much glucose has been sticking to part of the Hgb during the past 3 to 4 months, with the previous 2 weeks most heavily weighted. Recommended level is 7%.	Currently, the gold standard for measuring glycemic control. Useful in differentiating inadequate control versus incident-related DKA, such as current upper respiratory infection. A result greater than 8% represents average blood glucose of 200 mg/dL or greater and signals a need for changes in treatment.
• **Serum insulin:** Peptide hormone that enables the body to metabolize and use glucose.	May be decreased or absent (type 1) or normal to high (type 2), indicating insulin insufficiency or improper use (endogenous and exogenous). Insulin resistance may develop secondary to formation of antibodies.
• **Electrolytes:**	
• **Sodium:** The body's most abundant extracellular ion plays a key role in maintaining fluid balance and neuromuscular conduction or transmission of impulses.	May be normal, elevated, or decreased.
• **Potassium:** Major cation of the intracellular fluid needed to regulate intracellular osmotic pressure and water balance; also regulates neuromuscular excitability and aids in maintenance of acid-base balance, synthesis of protein, and metabolism of carbohydrates.	Normal, or falsely elevated, reflecting cellular shifts, then markedly decreased.
• **Phosphorus:** Essential mineral required for energy production—utilization of carbohydrates and fats and synthesis of protein—and activation of various enzymes and hormones.	Frequently decreased.
• **Arterial blood gases (ABGs):** Assessment of ABG levels of oxygen (PaO$_2$), carbon dioxide (PaCO$_2$), bicarbonate (HCO$_3^-$), and pH.	Usually reflect low pH and decreased HCO$_3^-$ (metabolic acidosis) with compensatory respiratory alkalosis.
• **Complete blood count (CBC):** Battery of screening tests, which typically includes Hgb; hematocrit (Hct); red blood cell (RBC) count, morphology, indices, and distribution width index; platelet count and size; white blood cell (WBC) count and differential.	Hct may be elevated reflecting dehydration; reduced WBCs or leukocytosis suggests hemoconcentration, response to stress or infection.
• **Serum amylase:** Digestive enzyme produced by the pancreas, which breaks down carbohydrates and starches.	May be elevated, indicating acute pancreatitis as cause of DKA.
OTHER DIAGNOSTIC STUDIES:	
• **Urine:** Urine glucose correlates poorly with blood glucose, being dependent on renal glucose threshold (150 to 300 mg/dL) and should be used only if measuring of blood glucose is not possible or as a confirmatory test. Ketones should be self-monitored during febrile illness or when DKA symptoms are present.	In DKA, urine tests are positive for glucose and ketones. Specific gravity and osmolality may be elevated if dehydration is present.
• **Cultures and sensitivities:** Specimens may include urine, sputum, or wound drainage.	May reveal source of infection and identify effective antimicrobial agent.

Nursing Priorities

1. Restore fluid and electrolyte and acid-base balance.
2. Correct or reverse metabolic abnormalities.
3. Identify and assist with management of underlying cause or disease process.
4. Prevent complications.
5. Provide information about disease process, prognosis, self-care, and treatment needs.

Discharge Goals

1. Homeostasis achieved.
2. Causative and precipitating factors corrected or controlled.
3. Complications prevented or minimized.
4. Disease process, prognosis, self-care needs, and therapeutic regimen understood.
5. Plan in place to meet needs after discharge.

NURSING DIAGNOSIS: deficient Fluid Volume [specify]

May be related to
Osmotic diuresis from hyperglycemia
Excessive gastric losses—diarrhea, vomiting
Restricted intake—nausea, confusion

Possibly evidenced by
Increased urinary output, dilute urine
Weakness, thirst, sudden weight loss
Dry skin and mucous membranes, poor skin turgor
Hypotension, tachycardia, delayed capillary refill

Desired Outcomes/Evaluation Criteria—Client Will

Fluid Balance (NOC)
Demonstrate adequate hydration as evidenced by stable vital signs, palpable peripheral pulses, good skin turgor and capillary refill, individually appropriate urinary output, and electrolyte levels within normal range.

ACTIONS/INTERVENTIONS	RATIONALE
Fluid/Electrolyte Management (NIC)	
Independent	
Obtain history from client and significant other (SO) related to duration and intensity of symptoms, such as vomiting and excessive urination.	Helps estimate total volume depletion. Symptoms may have been present for varying amounts of time—hours to days. Presence of infectious process results in fever and hypermetabolic state, increasing insensible fluid losses.
Monitor vital signs:	
Note orthostatic BP changes	Hypovolemia may be manifested by hypotension and tachycardia. Estimates of severity of hypovolemia may be made when client's systolic BP drops more than 10 mm Hg from a recumbent to a sitting or standing position. *Note:* Cardiac neuropathy may block reflexes that normally increase heart rate.
Respiratory pattern, such as Kussmaul's respirations, acetone breath	Lungs remove carbonic acid through respirations, producing a compensatory respiratory alkalosis or ketoacidosis. Acetone breath is due to breakdown of acetoacetic acid and should diminish as ketosis is corrected.
Respiratory rate and quality; use of accessory muscles, periods of apnea, and appearance of cyanosis	Correction of hyperglycemia and acidosis will cause the respiratory rate and pattern to approach normal. In contrast, increased work of breathing—shallow, rapid respirations—and presence of cyanosis may indicate respiratory fatigue and that client is losing ability to compensate for acidosis.
Temperature, skin color, and moisture	Although fever, chills, and diaphoresis are common with infectious process, fever with flushed, dry skin may reflect dehydration. *Note:* Although fever is a common precipitating factor for DKA, clients may be normothermic or hypothermic because of peripheral vasodilation.
Assess peripheral pulses, capillary refill, skin turgor, and mucous membranes.	Indicators of level of hydration and adequacy of circulating volume.
Monitor intake and output (I&O); note urine specific gravity.	Provides ongoing estimate of volume replacement needs, kidney function, and effectiveness of therapy.
Weigh daily.	Provides the best assessment of current fluid status and adequacy of fluid replacement.
Maintain fluid intake of at least 2,500 mL/day within cardiac tolerance when oral intake is resumed.	Maintains hydration and circulating volume.
Promote comfortable environment. Cover client with light sheets.	Avoids overheating, which could promote further fluid loss.
Investigate changes in mentation and sensorium.	Changes in mentation can be due to abnormally high or low glucose, electrolyte abnormalities, acidosis, decreased cerebral perfusion, or developing hypoxia. Regardless of the cause, impaired consciousness can predispose client to aspiration.
Collaborative	
Administer fluids, as indicated:	
Isotonic (0.9%) or lactated Ringer's solution without additives	Type and amount of fluid depends on degree of deficit and individual client response. *Note:* Client with DKA is often severely dehydrated and commonly needs 5 to 10 L of isotonic saline, 2 to 3 L within first 2 hours of treatment.

ACTIONS/INTERVENTIONS (continued)	RATIONALE (continued)
Albumin, plasma, dextran	Plasma expanders may occasionally be needed if the deficit is life threatening and BP does not normalize with rehydration efforts.
Insert and maintain indwelling urinary catheter.	Provides for accurate and ongoing measurement of urinary output, especially if autonomic neuropathies result in neurogenic bladder with urinary retention and overflow incontinence. May be removed when client is stable to reduce risk of infection.
Monitor laboratory studies, such as the following:	
Hct	Assesses level of hydration; Hct is often elevated because of hemoconcentration associated with osmotic diuresis.
Blood urea nigrogen (BUN)/creatinine (Cr)	Elevated values may reflect cellular breakdown from dehydration or signal the onset of renal failure.
Serum osmolality	Elevated because of hyperglycemia and dehydration.
Sodium	May be decreased, reflecting shift of fluids from the intracellular compartment as with osmotic diuresis. High sodium values reflect severe fluid loss and dehydration or sodium reabsorption in response to aldosterone secretion.
Potassium	Initially, hyperkalemia occurs in response to metabolic acidosis, but as this potassium is lost in the urine, the absolute potassium level in the body is depleted. As insulin is replaced and acidosis is corrected, serum potassium deficit becomes apparent.
Administer potassium and other electrolytes intravenously (IV) or by oral route, as indicated.	Potassium should be added to the IV as soon as urinary flow is adequate, to prevent hypokalemia. *Note:* Potassium phosphate may be drug of choice when IV fluids contain sodium chloride in order to prevent chloride overload. Phosphate concentrations tend to decrease with insulin therapy.
Administer bicarbonate, if indicated, for example, if pH is less than 7.1.	Not routinely necessary and given with caution to help correct acidosis in the presence of hypotension or shock, lactic acidosis, or severe hyperkalemia.
Insert nasogastric (NG) tube and attach to suction, as indicated.	Decompresses stomach and may relieve vomiting.

NURSING DIAGNOSIS: unstable blood Glucose Level

May be related to

Lack of diabetes management or adherence to diabetes action plan; inadequate blood glucose monitoring or medication management

Insulin deficiency—decreased uptake or utilization of glucose by the tissues resulting in increased protein and fat metabolism

Weight gain or loss

Rapid growth periods or pregnancy

Change in physical health status

Hypermetabolic state—release of stress hormones, such as epinephrine, cortisol, and growth hormone

Infectious process

Possibly evidenced by

Increased urinary output, dilute urine

Reported inadequate food intake, lack of interest in food

Weakness, fatigue, poor muscle tone

Altered level of consciousness (LOC)

Increased ketones

Desired Outcomes/Evaluation Criteria—Client Will

Blood Glucose Level (NOC)

Maintain glucose in satisfactory range.

Diabetes Self-Management (NOC)

Acknowledge factors that lead to unstable glucose and DKA.

Verbalize understanding of body and energy needs.

Verbalize plan for modifying factors to prevent or minimize complications.

ACTIONS/INTERVENTIONS	RATIONALE

Hyperglycemia Management (NIC)

Independent

Determine individual factors that may have contributed to current situation. Note client's age, developmental level, and awareness of needs.

Occasionally client with unknown diabetes will present with DKA, especially a young person with some type of precipitating infection. However, many times DKA is precipitated by failure of diabetes management, possibly related to dietary factors, activity, or medications. Because DKA presents more frequently in the young client with type 1 diabetes, there may be a failure to account for developmental changes, such as an adolescent growth spurt or pregnancy.

Perform fingerstick glucose testing. Ascertain whether client and SO(s) are adept at blood monitoring and are testing according to plan.

All available glucose monitors will provide satisfactory readings if properly used and maintained and routinely calibrated. *Note:* Unstable blood glucose is often associated with failure to perform testing on a regular schedule.

For client on insulin:

Review type(s) of insulin used, such as rapid, short-acting, intermediate, long-acting, premixed, and the delivery method—subcutaneous, inhaled, or pump. Note times when short-acting and long-acting insulins are administered.

These factors affect timing of effects and provide clues to potential timing of glucose instability.

Check injection sites.

Insulin absorption can vary from day to day in healthy sites and is less absorbable in lypohypertrophic (lumpy) tissues.

Review client's dietary program and usual pattern; compare with recent intake.

Identifies deficits and deviations from therapeutic plan, which may precipitate unstable glucose and uncontrolled hyperglycemia.

Weigh daily or as indicated.

Assesses adequacy of nutritional intake—both absorption and utilization. *Note:* Eating disorders are a contributing factor in 20% of recurrent DKA in young clients.

Auscultate bowel sounds. Note reports of abdominal pain and bloating, nausea, or vomiting. Maintain nothing by mouth (NPO) status, as indicated.

Hyperglycemia and fluid and electrolyte disturbances decrease gastric motility and function resulting in gastroparesis, affecting choice of interventions. *Note:* Long-term difficulties with gastroparesis and poor intestinal motility suggest autonomic neuropathies affecting the GI tract and requiring symptomatic treatment.

Provide liquids containing nutrients and electrolytes as soon as client can tolerate oral fluids; progress to more solid food as tolerated.

Oral route is preferred when client is alert and bowel function is restored.

Identify food preferences, including ethnic and cultural needs.

Incorporating as many of the client's food preferences into the meal plan as possible increases cooperation with dietary guidelines after discharge.

Include SO in meal planning, as indicated.

Promotes sense of involvement; provides information for SO to understand nutritional needs of client. *Note:* Various methods available for dietary planning include carbohydrate counting, exchange list, point system, or preselected menus.

Observe for signs of hypoglycemia—changes in LOC, cool and clammy skin, rapid pulse, hunger, irritability, anxiety, headache, lightheadedness, and shakiness.

Once carbohydrate metabolism resumes, blood glucose level will fall, and as insulin is being adjusted, hypoglycemia may occur. If client is comatose, hypoglycemia may occur without notable change in LOC. This potentially life-threatening emergency should be assessed and treated quickly per protocol. *Note:* Type 1 diabetics of long standing may not display usual signs of hypoglycemia because normal response to low blood sugar may be diminished.

Collaborative

Monitor laboratory studies, such as serum glucose, acetone, pH, and HCO_3^-.

Blood glucose will decrease slowly with controlled fluid replacement and insulin therapy. With the administration of optimal insulin dosages, glucose can then enter the cells and be used for energy. When this happens, acetone levels decrease and acidosis is corrected.

ACTIONS/INTERVENTIONS (continued)

Administer rapid-acting insulin, such as regular (Humulin R), lispro (Humalog), or aspart (Novalog) by intermittent or continuous IV method, for example, IV bolus followed by a continuous drip via pump of approximately 5 to 10 units/hour so that glucose is reduced by 50 to 75 mg/dL/hour.

Administer glucose solutions, for example, 5% dextrose and half-normal saline.

Consult with nutritionist or dietitian for resumption of oral intake.

Provide diet of approximately 60% carbohydrates, 20% proteins, and 20% fats in designated number of meals and snacks.

RATIONALE (continued)

Rapid-acting insulin is used in hyperglycemic crisis. The IV route is the initial route of choice because absorption from subcutaneous tissues may be erratic. Many believe the continuous method is the optimal way to facilitate transition to carbohydrate metabolism and reduce incidence of hypoglycemia. *Note:* Intermediate insulin, such as NPH, Humulin N, Lente, and long-acting insulin, such as Ultralente, protamine zinc insulin (PZI), and glargine (Lantus), may be part of the client's usual or added insulin, but are not part of crisis hyperglycemic treatment.

Glucose solutions may be added after insulin and fluids have brought the blood glucose to approximately 400 mg/dL. As carbohydrate metabolism approaches normal, care must be taken to avoid hypoglycemia.

Useful in calculating and adjusting diet to meet client's specific needs; answer questions and assist client and SO in developing meal plans.

Complex carbohydrates help to maintain more stable glucose levels, reduce serum cholesterol levels, and promote satiation. Food intake is scheduled according to specific insulin characteristics, such as peak effect, and individual client response. *Note:* A snack of complex carbohydrates at bedtime is especially important if insulin is given in divided doses to prevent hypoglycemia during sleep and potential Somogyi response.

NURSING DIAGNOSIS: risk for Infection, [sepsis]

Risk factors may include
High glucose levels, decreased leukocyte function, alterations in circulation
Preexisting respiratory infection or UTI

Possibly evidenced by
(Not applicable; presence of signs and symptoms establishes an *actual* diagnosis)

Desired Outcomes/Evaluation Criteria—Client Will

Knowledge: Infection Control (NOC)
Identify interventions to prevent or reduce risk of infection.
Demonstrate techniques and lifestyle changes to prevent development of infection.

ACTIONS/INTERVENTIONS

Infection Control (NIC)
Independent
Observe for signs of infection and inflammation—fever, flushed appearance, wound drainage, purulent sputum, and cloudy urine.
Promote good hand washing by staff and client.
Maintain aseptic technique for IV insertion procedure, administration of medications, and providing site care. Rotate IV sites, as indicated.
Provide catheter and perineal care. Teach the female client to clean from front to back after elimination.

Provide conscientious skin care, gently massage bony areas, keep the skin dry, and keep linens dry and wrinkle-free.
Inspect client's feet, noting presence of ulcers or infected ingrown toenails, or other problems requiring medical or nursing intervention.
Auscultate breath sounds.

RATIONALE

Client may be admitted with infection, which could have precipitated the ketoacidotic state, or may develop a nosocomial infection.
Reduces risk of cross-contamination.
High glucose in the blood creates an excellent medium for bacterial growth.

Minimizes risk of UTI. Comatose client may be at particular risk if urinary retention occurred before hospitalization. *Note:* Elderly female diabetic clients are especially prone to UTIs and vaginal yeast infections. Many UTIs are asymptomatic, possibly related to neurogenic bladder.
Peripheral circulation may be impaired, placing client at increased risk for skin irritation and breakdown and infection.
Foot injuries and impaired circulation are associated with many complications in diabetics, including cellulitis and amputations. *Note:* Cellulitis can precipitate episode of DKA.
Rhonchi indicate accumulation of secretions possibly related to pneumonia or bronchitis that may have precipitated the DKA.

(continues on page 414)

ACTIONS/INTERVENTIONS (continued)

Place in semi-Fowler's position.
Reposition and encourage coughing and deep breathing if client is alert and cooperative. Otherwise, suction airway, using sterile technique, as needed.
Provide tissues and trash bag in a convenient location for sputum and other secretions. Instruct client in proper handling of secretions.
Encourage and assist with oral hygiene.
Encourage adequate dietary and fluid intake (at least 2,500 mL/day if not contraindicated by cardiac or renal dysfunction), including 8 oz of cranberry juice per day, as appropriate.

Collaborative
Obtain specimens for culture and sensitivities, as indicated.

Administer antibiotics, as appropriate.

RATIONALE (continued)

Facilitates lung expansion and reduces risk of aspiration.
Aids in ventilating all lung areas and mobilizing secretions. Prevents stasis of secretions with increased risk of infection.
Minimizes spread of infection.

Reduces risk of oral and gum disease.
Decreases susceptibility to infection. Increased urinary flow prevents stasis and aids in maintaining urine acidity, reducing bacteria growth and flushing organisms out of system. *Note:* Use of cranberry juice can help prevent bacteria from adhering to the bladder wall, reducing the risk of recurrent UTI.

Identifies organism(s) so that most appropriate drug therapy can be instituted.
Early treatment may help prevent sepsis.

NURSING DIAGNOSIS: **risk for disturbed Sensory Perception, (specify)**

Risk factors may include
Endogenous chemical alteration: glucose and insulin and electrolyte imbalance

Possibly evidenced by
(Not applicable; presence of signs and symptoms establishes an *actual* diagnosis)

Desired Outcomes/Evaluation Criteria—Client Will

Neurological Status (NOC)
Maintain usual level of mentation.
Recognize and compensate for existing sensory impairments.

ACTIONS/INTERVENTIONS

Neurological Monitoring (NIC)
Independent
Monitor vital signs and mental status.

Address client by name; reorient as needed to place, person, time, and situation. Give short explanations, speaking slowly and enunciating clearly.
Schedule nursing time to provide for uninterrupted rest periods.
Keep client's routine as consistent as possible. Encourage participation in activities of daily living (ADLs) as able.
Protect client from injury—avoid or limit use of restraints as able, place bed in low position—when cognition is impaired. Pad bed rails if client is prone to seizures.
Evaluate visual acuity, as indicated.

Investigate reports of hyperesthesia, pain, or sensory loss in the feet and legs. Look for ulcers, reddened areas, pressure points, and loss of pedal pulses.

Provide bed cradle. Keep hands and feet warm, avoiding exposure to cool drafts, hot water, or heating pad.

RATIONALE

Provides a baseline from which to compare abnormal findings, for instance, fever may affect mentation.
Decreases confusion and helps maintain contact with reality.

Promotes restful sleep, reduces fatigue, and may improve cognition.
Helps keep client in touch with reality and maintain orientation to the environment.
Disoriented client is prone to injury, especially at night, and precautions need to be taken as indicated. Seizure precautions reduce risk of physical injury.
Retinal edema or detachment, hemorrhage, presence of cataracts, or temporary paralysis of extraocular muscles may impair vision, requiring corrective therapy or supportive care.
Peripheral neuropathies may result in severe discomfort and absent or distorted tactile sensation, potentiating risk of dermal injury and impaired balance. *Note:* Mononeuropathy affects a single nerve (most often femoral or cranial), causing sudden pain and loss of motor and sensory function along affected nerve path.
Reduces discomfort and potential for dermal injury. *Note:* Sudden development of cold hands and feet may reflect hypoglycemia, suggesting need to evaluate serum glucose level.

ACTIONS/INTERVENTIONS (continued)	RATIONALE (continued)
Assist with ambulation or position changes.	Promotes client safety, especially when sense of balance is affected.
Collaborative Carry out prescribed regimen for correcting DKA, as indicated.	Alteration in thought processes and potential for seizure activity is usually alleviated once hyperosmolar state is corrected.
Monitor laboratory values, such as blood glucose, serum osmolality, Hgb/Hct, and BUN/Cr.	Imbalances can impair mentation. *Note:* If fluid is replaced too quickly, water intoxication can occur—sodium concentration falls, water enters brain cells, and confusion, disorientation, or coma may develop.

NURSING DIAGNOSIS: Fatigue

May be related to
Decreased metabolic energy production
Altered body chemistry—insufficient insulin
Increased energy demands—hypermetabolic state, infection

Possibly evidenced by
Overwhelming lack of energy, inability to maintain usual routines, decreased performance, being accident-prone
Impaired ability to concentrate, listlessness, disinterest in surroundings

Desired Outcomes/Evaluation Criteria—Client Will

Endurance (NOC)
Verbalize increase in energy level.
Display improved ability to participate in desired activities.

ACTIONS/INTERVENTIONS	RATIONALE
Energy Management (NIC) *Independent*	
Discuss with client the need for activity. Plan schedule with client and identify activities that lead to fatigue.	Education may provide motivation to increase activity level even though client may feel too weak initially.
Alternate activity with periods of rest and uninterrupted sleep.	Prevents excessive fatigue.
Monitor pulse, respiratory rate, and BP before and after activity.	Indicates physiological levels of tolerance.
Discuss ways of conserving energy while bathing, transferring, and so on.	Client will be able to accomplish more with a decreased expenditure of energy.
Increase client participation in ADLs, as tolerated.	Increases confidence level, self-esteem and tolerance level. *Note:* Elderly clients may experience a "lag effect" in which exercise may precipitate hypoglycemia as late as 24 hours after exercising, leading to extensive fatigue and muscle tremors.

NURSING DIAGNOSIS: Powerlessness

May be related to
Long-term, progressive illness that is not curable
Dependence on others

Possibly evidenced by
Reluctance to express true feelings, expressions of having no control or influence over situation
Apathy, withdrawal, anger
Does not monitor progress, nonparticipation in care or decision making
Depression over physical deterioration or complications despite client cooperation with regimen

Desired Outcomes/Evaluation Criteria—Client Will

Health Beliefs: Perceived Control (NOC)
Acknowledge feelings of helplessness.
Identify healthy ways to deal with feelings.
Assist in planning own care and independently take responsibility for self-care activities.

ACTIONS/INTERVENTIONS	RATIONALE

Self-Responsibility Facilitation (NIC)
Independent

Encourage client and SO to express feelings about hospitalization and disease in general.	Identifies concerns and facilitates problem-solving.
Acknowledge normality of feelings.	Recognition that these reactions are normal can help client problem-solve and seek help as needed. Diabetic control is a full-time job that serves as a constant reminder of both presence of condition and threat to client's health and life.
Assess how client has handled problems in the past; identify locus of control.	Knowledge of individual's style helps determine needs for treatment goals. Client whose locus of control is internal usually looks at ways to gain control over own treatment program. Client who operates with an external locus of control wants to be cared for by others and may project blame for circumstances onto external factors.
Provide opportunity for SO to express concerns and discuss ways in which he or she can be helpful to client.	Enhances sense of being involved and gives SO a chance to problem-solve solutions to help client prevent recurrence.
Ascertain expectations and goals of client and SO.	Unrealistic expectations and pressure from others or self may result in feelings of frustration or loss of control and may impair coping abilities. *Note:* Even with rigid adherence to medical regimen, complications and setbacks may occur.
Determine whether a change in relationship with SO has occurred.	Constant energy and thought required for diabetic control often shifts the focus of a relationship. Development of psychological concerns and visceral neuropathies affecting self-concept, especially sexual role function, may add further stress.
Encourage client to make decisions related to care, such as ambulation, time for activities, and so forth.	Communicates to client that some control can be exercised over care.
Support participation in self-care and give positive feedback for efforts.	Promotes feeling of control over situation.

NURSING DIAGNOSIS: **deficient Knowledge [Learning Need] regarding disease, prognosis, treatment, self-care, and discharge needs**

May be related to
Lack of exposure or recall, information misinterpretation
Unfamiliarity with information resources

Possibly evidenced by
Questions or request for information, verbalization of the problem
Inaccurate follow-through of instructions, development of preventable complications

Desired Outcomes/Evaluation Criteria—Client Will

Knowledge: Diabetes Management (NOC)
Verbalize understanding of disease process and potential complications.
Identify relationship of signs and symptoms to the disease process and correlate symptoms with causative factors.
Correctly perform necessary procedures and explain reasons for the actions.
Initiate necessary lifestyle changes and participate in treatment regimen.

ACTIONS/INTERVENTIONS	RATIONALE

Learning Facilitation (NIC)
Independent

Create an environment of trust by listening to concerns and being available.	Rapport and respect need to be established before client will be willing to take part in the learning process.
Work with client in setting mutual goals for learning.	Participation in the planning promotes enthusiasm and cooperation with the principles learned.
Select a variety of teaching strategies, such as demonstrating needed skills and having client do return demonstration, incorporating new skills into the hospital routine.	Use of different means of accessing information promotes information retention.

ACTIONS/INTERVENTIONS (continued)

RATIONALE (continued)

Teaching: Disease Process (NIC)

Discuss essential elements, such as the following:

Explain the normal blood glucose range and how it compares with client's level, the type of diabetes the client has, and the relationship between insulin deficiency and a high glucose level

Provides knowledge base from which client can make informed lifestyle choices.

Reasons for the ketoacidotic episode

Knowledge of the precipitating factors may help avoid recurrences.

Acute and chronic complications of the disease, including visual disturbances, neurosensory and cardiovascular changes, renal impairment, and hypertension

Awareness helps client be more consistent with care and may prevent or delay onset of complications.

Demonstrate fingerstick testing, or similar procedure, such as palm or armstick, or continuous glucose monitoring system (GlucoWatch), and have client and SO return demonstration until proficient. Instruct client to check urine ketones if glucose is higher than 250 mg/dL.

Self-monitoring of blood glucose four or more times a day allows flexibility in self-care, promotes tighter control of serum levels, such as 60 to 130 mg/dL before meals and after meal peak level of less than 180 mg/dL, and may prevent or delay development of long-term complications (ADA, 2007). *Note:* Various new devices have been released or are in testing. Some use a laser perforator instead of a sharp lancet, others are bloodless. In addition to glucose levels, several devices can measure glycosylated albumin or fructosamine in the home, providing a measure of blood glucose control over the past 7 to 10 days.

Discuss dietary plan, limiting intake of sugar, fat, salt, and alcohol; eating complex carbohydrates, especially those high in fiber such as fruits, vegetables, whole grains; and ways to deal with meals outside the home.

Medical nutrition therapy for diabetes encourages client to make meal choices based on individual unique needs and preferences. Awareness of importance of dietary control aids client in planning meals, and sticking to regimen. Fiber can slow glucose absorption, decreasing fluctuations in serum levels, but may cause GI discomfort, increase flatus, and affect vitamin and mineral absorption.

Review medication regimen, including onset, peak, and duration of prescribed insulin, as applicable, with client and SO.

Understanding all aspects of drug usage promotes proper use. Dose algorithms are created, taking into account drug dosages established during inpatient evaluation, usual amount and schedule of physical activity, and meal plan. Including SO provides additional support and resource for client.

Review client's type of basal insulin—lente, NPH, ultralente, glargine (Lantus)—and bolus insulin—regular, lispro, aspart (Novolog)—as indicated. Review self-administration of insulin, either injection or pump, and care of equipment. Have client demonstrate procedure: drawing up and injecting insulin, insulin pen technique, or use of continuous pump.

Verifies understanding and correctness of procedure. Identifies potential problems, such as vision, memory, and so on, so that alternative solutions can be found for insulin administration. *Note:* If multiple daily injections are required, combinations of rapid-acting plus short-acting, intermediate, and long-acting insulin are used. If the pump method is used, client programs his or her own basal and bolus settings. Only rapid-acting insulin, Humalog or Novolog, is administered, with a basal dose throughout the day and bolus doses before meals and as needed. An insulin pump more closely mimics normal pancreatic activity because the basal rate may be changed relative to client's activity level, presence of stressors and infection, and menstrual cycle.

Discuss timing of insulin injection and mealtime.

One of the many inconveniences people with diabetes cope with is having to decide at least 30 to 60 minutes in advance when they are going to have a meal for the timely administration of regular human injections. Insulin lispro (Humalog) or aspart (Novolog) may be helpful because it works best when taken within 15 minutes of eating. With the onset twice as fast as regular human insulin and a duration approximately half as long, Humalog and Novolog closely mimic pancreatic activity. However, hypoglycemia may develop more rapidly and be more severe than with use of regular insulin. A blood glucose level below 80 mg/dL indicates that insulin should be injected after eating rather than before the meal.

Review individual's target blood glucose levels.

Although this range varies per person, the ideal range for the adult diabetic is considered to be 80 to 120 mg/dL. *Note:* Clients with an insulin pump may maintain blood glucose levels between 120 mg/dL and 200 mg/dL with no urinary ketones.

(continues on page 418)

Emphasize importance and necessity of maintaining diary of glucose testing, medication dose and time, dietary intake, activity, feelings, sensations, and life events.

Aids in creating overall picture of client situation to achieve better disease control and promotes self-care and independence.

Discuss factors that play a part in diabetic control such as aerobic versus isometric exercise, stress, surgery, and illness. Review "sick day" rules.

This information promotes diabetic control and can greatly reduce the occurrence of ketoacidosis. *Note:* Aerobic exercise such as walking and swimming promotes effective use of insulin, lowering glucose levels, and strengthens the cardiovascular system. A "sick day" management plan helps maintain equilibrium during illness, minor surgery, severe emotional stress, exogenous steroids (as with spinal or joint injections or any oral treatment for asthma and arthritis), or any condition that might send glucose spiraling upward.

Review effects of smoking on insulin use. Encourage cessation of smoking.

Nicotine constricts the small blood vessels, and insulin absorption is delayed for as long as these vessels remain constricted.

Establish regular exercise or activity schedule and identify corresponding insulin concerns.

Exercise times should not coincide with the peak action of insulin. A snack should be ingested before or during exercise as needed, and rotation of injection sites should avoid the muscle group that will be used in the activity (for instance, abdominal site is preferred over thigh or arm before jogging or swimming) to prevent accelerated uptake of insulin.

Identify the symptoms of hypoglycemia—weakness, dizziness, lethargy, hunger, irritability, diaphoresis, pallor, tachycardia, tremors, headache, and changes in mentation—and explain causes.

May promote early detection and treatment, preventing or limiting occurrence. However, approximately 30% of insulin-dependent clients are asymptomatic when hypoglycemic. *Note:* Early-morning hyperglycemia may reflect the "dawn phenomenon," indicating need for additional insulin, or the Somogyi effect, requiring a decrease in medication dosage and/or change in diet such as bedtime or hour of sleep (HS) snack. Testing serum levels at 3 a.m. aids in identifying the specific problem.

Instruct SO in emergency use of glucagon.

Given for treatment of severe hypoglycemia when client is unable to take oral carbohydrates. Prompt intervention may prevent more serious complications.

Instruct in importance of routine daily examination of the feet and proper foot care. Demonstrate ways to examine feet, inspect shoes for fit, and care for toenails, calluses, and corns. Encourage use of natural fiber stockings.

Prevents or delays complications associated with peripheral neuropathies and circulatory impairment, especially cellulitis, gangrene, and amputation. *Note:* Studies show that approximately 15% of all clients with diabetes will develop a foot or leg ulcer during the course of the disease. Also, 50% of all nontraumatic lower extremity amputations occur in people with diabetes. Prevention is therefore critical.

Stress importance of regular eye examinations, especially for clients who have had type 1 diabetes for 5 years or more.

Changes in vision may be gradual and are more pronounced in persons with poorly controlled DM and BP. Problems include changes in visual acuity and may progress to retinopathy and blindness. *Note:* Retinopathy is the most frequent cause of new blindness among adults 20 to 74 years of age.

Arrange for vision aids when needed, such as magnifying sleeve for insulin syringe, prefilled insulin pens, large-print instructions, and one-touch or talking glucose meters.

Adaptive aids have been developed in recent years to help the visually impaired manage their own DM more effectively.

Discuss sexual functioning and answer questions client and SO may have.

Impotence may be first symptom of onset of DM. *Note:* Counseling and use of penile prosthesis may be of benefit.

Emphasize importance of using medical alert ID device.

Can promote quick entry into the health system and appropriate care with fewer resultant complications in the event of an emergency.

Recommend reading product labels and avoidance of over-the-counter (OTC) drugs without prior discussion with healthcare provider.

These products may contain sugars and interact with prescribed medications.

Discuss importance of follow-up care.

Helps maintain tighter control of disease process and may prevent exacerbations of DM, retarding development of systemic complications.

ACTIONS/INTERVENTIONS (continued)

Review signs and symptoms requiring medical evaluation—fever, cold, or flu symptoms; cloudy, odorous urine; painful urination; delayed healing of cuts or sores; sensory changes with pain or tingling of lower extremities; changes in blood sugar level; and presence of ketones in urine.

Identify community resources such as the American Diabetic Association, Internet resources and online diabetes bulletin boards, visiting nurse, weight loss or smoking cessation clinics, contact person, or diabetic instructor.

RATIONALE (continued)

Prompt intervention may prevent development of more serious or life-threatening complications.

Continued support is usually necessary to sustain lifestyle changes and promote well-being.

POTENTIAL CONSIDERATIONS following acute hospitalization (dependent on client's age, physical condition and presence of complications, personal resources, and life responsibilities)

- *risk for unstable blood Glucose*—lack of acceptance of diagnosis, inadequate blood glucose monitoring, activity level, stress
- *ineffective self Health Management*—complexity of therapeutic regimen, economic concerns, perceived susceptibility (recurrence of problem)
- *disturbed peripheral/visual Sensory Perception*—endogenous chemical alternations (elevated glucose level)

HYPERTHYROIDISM (GRAVES' DISEASE, THYROTOXICOSIS)

I. Pathophysiology: failure of a complex feedback mechanism resulting in excessive secretion or release of thyroid hormone

II. Etiology

  a. Metabolic imbalance resulting from overproduction of the thyroid hormones triiodothyronine (T_3) and thyroxine (T_4)

  b. Thyrotoxic crisis or thyroid storm—untreated or inadequately treated severe hyperthyroidism creating a life-threatening emergency

  c. Varied causation

    i. Autoimmune

      1. Toxic diffuse goiter or Graves' disease: most common cause, accounting for 80% of hyperthyroidism diagnoses (Fisher, 2002)

      2. Hashimoto thyroiditis

      3. Subacute and "silent" thyroiditis

    ii. Toxic multinodular goiter (TMG): second most common cause of hyperthyroidism (Fisher, 2002; Schraga, 2008)

    iii. Thyroid or pituitary tumors

    iv. Drug-induced: iodine, excessive thyroid hormone replacement, certain other drugs, such as amiodarone

    v. Bacterial or viral infections

    vi. Pregnancy: hyperemesis gravidarum, toxemia, molar pregnancy

    vii. Iatrogenic: manipulation of thyroid gland during surgery

III. Statistics (Schraga, 2008)

  a. Morbidity: Occurs in about 1% of U.S. population, with more than 3 million diagnosed with Graves' disease; approximately 1% to 2% of individuals with hyperthyroidism progress to thyroid storm.

  b. Mortality: Adult mortality rate from thyroid storm is approximately 10% to 20%, but may be as high as 75% in hospitalized individuals due to comorbidities.

GLOSSARY

Ablation: Removal or excision, usually carried out surgically, but may be done chemically with radioactive iodine.

Autoimmune disease: Illness that occurs when the body tissues are attacked by its own immune system.

Diaphoresis: Excessive sweating; may be associated with exercise or with emotional, physical, and mental stress.

Endocrine gland: Gland that releases a chemical messenger, known as a hormone, directly into the bloodstream, which will affect other parts of the body. The thyroid is an endocrine gland.

Euthyroid: Situation where thyroid-stimulating hormone (TSH) test values are in the normal range, and the thyroid is neither hyperthyroid nor hypothyroid.

Exophthalmos: Abnormal bulging of the eye, with resulting inability to close lid.

Extraocular muscles: The six muscles that control the movements of the eye. The actions of the extraocular muscles depend on the position of the eye at the time of muscle contraction.

Goiter: Enlargement of the thyroid gland.

Inotropic support: Substance that influences the contractility of heart cells.

Nodule: A small solid collection of tissue that is palpable.

Plasmapheresis: The process of separating certain cells, such as excess antibodies, from the plasma in the blood by a machine; only the cells are returned to the person.

(text continues on page 420)

Pretibial myxedema: A skin condition associated with Graves' disease characterized by swollen, itchy patches of skin on the front of the lower legs or shins.

Radioactive iodine (RAI): An isotope of the chemical element iodine that is radioactive. Used in diagnostic tests as well as in radiotherapy of a hyperactive thyroid gland, most often due to Graves' disease.

Subtotal thyroidectomy: Surgical removal of five-sixths of the gland, leaving enough of the gland to produce normal amounts of thyroid hormone.

Thyroid storm (thyrotoxicosis): A rarely encountered manifestation of hyperthyroidism that may be precipitated by surgical or chemical ablation of the thyroid; medication overdosage; and toxemia of pregnancy, surgery, and trauma. It constitutes a medical emergency.

Tremor: Abnormal repetitive shaking movement of the body due to varied causes, including thyroid disease.

Care Setting

Most people with classic hyperthyroidism rarely need hospitalization. Critically ill clients and those with extreme manifestations of thyrotoxicosis, plus a significant concurrent illness, require inpatient acute care on a medical unit.

Related Concerns

Heart failure: chronic, page 48

Psychosocial aspects of care, page 749

Thyroidectomy, page 429

Client Assessment Database

Data depend on the severity and duration of hormone imbalance and involvement of other organs.

DIAGNOSTIC DIVISION MAY REPORT	MAY EXHIBIT
ACTIVITY/REST	
• Nervousness, increased irritability	• Muscle atrophy
• Insomnia	
• Muscle weakness	
• Incoordination	
• Extreme fatigue	
CIRCULATION	
• Palpitations	• Dysrhythmias—atrial fibrillation, gallop rhythm
• Chest pain (angina)	• Tachycardia at rest
	• Murmurs
	• Elevated blood pressure (BP) with widened pulse pressure
	• Circulatory collapse, shock (thyrotoxic crisis)
ELIMINATION	
• Urinating in large amounts	
• Stool changes; diarrhea	
EGO INTEGRITY	
• Recent stressful experience—emotional and physical	• Emotional lability—mild euphoria to delirium
	• Anxiety and depression
FOOD/FLUID	
• Recent and sudden weight loss	• Enlarged thyroid, goiter
• Increased appetite, large meals, frequent meals, thirst	• Diaphoresis (may be profuse with thyrotoxicosis)
• Nausea and vomiting	• Nonpitting edema, especially in front of the shinbone
NEUROSENSORY	
	• Rapid and hoarse speech
	• Mental status and behavior alterations—confusion, disorientation, nervousness, irritability, delirium, frank psychosis, stupor, coma
	• Fine tremor in hands; purposeless, quick, jerky movements of body parts
	• Hyperactive deep tendon reflexes (DTRs)
	• Paralysis (thyrotoxic hypokalemia)

Client Assessment Database (continued)

DIAGNOSTIC DIVISION MAY REPORT (continued)	MAY EXHIBIT (continued)
PAIN/DISCOMFORT • Eye pain, sensitivity to light	
RESPIRATION • Difficulty breathing	• Increased respiratory rate, tachypnea • *Breath sounds:* crackles, wheezes (pulmonary edema associated with thyrotoxic crisis)
SAFETY • Heat intolerance, excessive sweating • Itching skin • Allergy to iodine (may be used in testing)	• Elevated temperature • Skin smooth, warm, and flushed • Exophthalmos, lid retraction, conjunctival irritation, tearing • Pruritic, erythematous lesions—often in pretibial area—that become brawny
SEXUALITY • Decreased libido • Hypomenorrhea, amenorrhea • Impotence	
TEACHING/LEARNING • Family history of thyroid problems • History of hypothyroidism, thyroid hormone replacement therapy or antithyroid therapy, premature withdrawal of antithyroid drugs, recent partial thyroidectomy • History of insulin-induced hypoglycemia, cardiac disorders or surgery, recent illness (pneumonia), trauma; x-ray contrast studies	
DISCHARGE PLAN CONSIDERATIONS • May require assistance with treatment regimen, self-care activities, homemaker and maintenance tasks ▶ Refer to section at end of plan for postdischarge considerations.	

Diagnostic Studies

TEST WHY IT IS DONE	WHAT IT TELLS ME
BLOOD TESTS • *Thyroid Function Tests:*	
• *TSH:* Measures the amount of TSH in the blood; it is done first to evaluate thyroid function.	TSH is suppressed in hyperthyroidism (except when etiology is a TSH-secreting pituitary tumor or pituitary resistant to thyroid hormone).
• *Tyyroxine (T_4):* Produced by the thyroid gland when the pituitary gland releases TSH. Free T_4 can be measured directly (FT_4) or calculated by index (FTI). Total T_4 measures both bound and free T_4. Free T_4 affects tissue function, whereas bound T_4 does not.	Total T_4, FT_4, and FTI are elevated in hyperthyroidism.
• *Triiodothyronine (T_3):* Small amount produced directly by thyroid gland. Most T_3 is made by other tissues that convert T_4 into T_3. T_4 has a greater effect on metabolism than T_3 even though T_3 is normally present in lower amounts than T_4. Total T_3 measures both bound and free T_3 (FT_3).	Both T_3 and T_4 are increased in hyperthyroidism; however, T_3 appears to be the more accurate diagnostic indicator of hyperthyroidism than T_4. T_3 becomes abnormal earlier than T_4 and returns to normal later than T_4 in hyperthyroidism.

(continues on page 422)

TEST WHY IT IS DONE (continued)	WHAT IT TELLS ME (continued)
• *Triiodothyronine uptake (T_3U):* An indirect measurement of the amount of the protein thyroxine-binding globulin (TBG) that can bind T_3 and T_4.	A high T_4 value combined with a high T_3U value usually confirms the presence of hyperthyroidism.
OTHER DIAGNOSTIC STUDIES • *Radioactive iodine uptake (RAIU) scanning:* Measures both thyroid function and thyroid size. During this procedure, the amount of iodine "taken up" by the thyroid is measured, and images are taken. A gamma camera scan operating in a fixed position views the entire thyroid gland at once. A computerized rectilinear thyroid (CRT) scan uses computer technology to enhance thyroid nodules.	RAIU testing shows whether the entire thyroid gland is overactive, or if only portions of the thyroid are overactive as in Graves' disease. Hot spots represent areas of increased hormone production, as in nodular hyperthryoidism. Cold spots, or particularly weak energy spots, represent poorly functioning or nonfunctioning areas of the thyroid gland.
• *Thyroid ultrasound:* Uses high-frequency sound waves to obtain an image of the thyroid gland, obtain accurate measurements, and identify nodules. Also aids in performing thyroid needle biopsy by improving accuracy if the nodule cannot be felt easily on examination.	Differentiates a "solid" nodule from a fluid-filled cyst; however, it does not differentiate as to whether a nodule is benign or malignant. Determines if a nodule is getting smaller or is growing larger during treatment.
• *Needle or open biopsy:* May be done to determine cause of thyroid nodules.	Differentiates malignant from benign nodules.
• *Electrocardiogram (ECG):* Provides a record of the electrical activity of the heart.	May show tachycardia and other dysrthymias, such as atrial fibrillation (AF). Enlarged heart and AF often are seen in elderly clients.

Nursing Priorities

1. Reduce metabolic demands and support cardiovascular function.
2. Provide psychological support.
3. Prevent complications.
4. Provide information about disease process, prognosis, and therapy needs.

Discharge Goals

1. Homeostasis achieved.
2. Current situation being dealt with effectively.
3. Complications prevented and minimized.
4. Disease process, prognosis, and therapeutic regimen understood.
5. Plan in place to meet needs after discharge.

NURSING DIAGNOSIS: risk for decreased Cardiac Output

Risk factors may include
Uncontrolled hyperthyroidism, hypermetabolic state
Increasing cardiac workload
Changes in venous return and systemic vascular resistance (SVR)
Alterations in rate, rhythm, conduction

Possibly evidenced by
(Not applicable; presence of signs and symptoms establishes an *actual* diagnosis)

Desired Outcomes/Evaluation Criteria—Client Will

Circulatory Status (NOC)
Maintain adequate cardiac output for tissue needs as evidenced by stable vital signs, palpable peripheral pulses, good capillary refill, usual mentation, and absence of dysrhythmias.

ACTIONS/INTERVENTIONS	RATIONALE
Hemodynamic Regulation (NIC)	
Independent	
Monitor BP lying, sitting, and standing, if able. Note widened pulse pressure.	General and orthostatic hypotension may occur as a result of excessive peripheral vasodilation and decreased circulating volume. Widened pulse pressure reflects compensatory increase in stroke volume and decreased SVR.
Monitor central venous pressure (CVP), if available.	Provides more direct measure of circulating volume and cardiac function.
Investigate reports of chest pain and angina.	May reflect increased myocardial oxygen demands and ischemia.
Assess pulse and heart rate while client is sleeping.	Provides a more accurate assessment of tachycardia.
Auscultate heart sounds, noting extra heart sounds and development of gallops and systolic murmurs.	Prominent S_1 and murmurs are associated with forceful cardiac output of hypermetabolic state; development of S_3 may warn of impending cardiac failure.
Monitor ECG, noting rate and rhythm. Document dysrhythmias.	Tachycardia greater than normally expected, with fever and increased circulatory demand, may reflect direct myocardial stimulation by thyroid hormone. Dysrhythmias often occur and may compromise cardiac function and output.
Auscultate breath sounds, noting adventitious sounds such as crackles.	Early sign of pulmonary congestion, reflecting developing cardiac failure.
Monitor temperature, provide cool environment, limit bed linens and clothes, and administer tepid sponge baths.	Fever, which may exceed 104°F (40.0°C), can occur as a result of excessive hormone levels increasing diuresis and dehydration, causing increased peripheral vasodilation, venous pooling, and hypotension.
Observe for signs and symptoms of severe thirst, dry mucous membranes, weak and thready pulse, poor capillary refill, decreased urinary output, and hypotension.	Rapid dehydration can occur, which reduces circulating volume and compromises cardiac output.
Record intake and output (I&O). Note urine specific gravity.	Significant fluid losses through vomiting, diarrhea, diuresis, or diaphoresis can lead to profound dehydration, concentrated urine, and weight loss.
Weigh daily. Encourage chair rest and bedrest; limit nonessential activity.	Activity increases metabolic and circulatory demands, which may potentiate cardiac failure.
Note history of asthma and bronchoconstrictive disease, sinus bradycardia and heart blocks, advanced heart failure (HF), or current pregnancy.	Presence and potential recurrence of these conditions affects choice of therapy; for example, use of beta-adrenergic blocking agents is contraindicated.
Observe for adverse side effects of adrenergic antagonists, such as severe decrease in pulse and BP, signs of vascular congestion and HF, and cardiac arrest.	Indicates need for reduction and discontinuation of therapy.
Collaborative	
Administer intravenous (IV) fluids, as indicated.	Rapid fluid replacement may be necessary to improve circulating volume, but must be balanced against signs of cardiac failure and need for inotropic support.
Administer medications, as indicated, such as:	
Beta-blockers, for example, propranolol (Inderal), atenolol (Tenormin), nadolol (Corgard), and pindolol (Visken)	Beta-blockers are the mainstay of symptomatic therapy for thyrotoxicosis, such as tachycardia, tremors, and nervousness. Propranolol has been used with the greatest success due to the additional benefit of inhibition of peripheral conversion of T_4 to T_3 (Schraga, 2008).
Thyroid hormone antagonists, for example, propylthiouracil (PTU) and methimazole (Tapazole)	Antithyroid drugs block thyroid hormone synthesis and inhibit conversion of T_4 to T_3. May be definitive long-term treatment or used to prepare client for surgery, but effect is slow and will not relieve thyroid storm. *Note:* Once PTU therapy is begun, abrupt withdrawal may precipitate thyroid crisis.
Oral strong iodine solution (Lugol's solution) or supersaturated potassium iodide (SSKI)	Acts to prevent release of thyroid hormone into circulation by increasing the amount of thyroid hormone stored within the gland. May interfere with radioactive iodine (RAI) treatment and may exacerbate the disease in some people. May be used as surgical preparation to decrease size and vascularity of the gland or to treat thyroid storm. *Note:* Should be started 1 to 3 hours after initiation of antithyroid drug therapy to minimize hormone formation from the iodine.

(continues on page 424)

423

RAI (Na^{131}I or Na^{125}I) following NRC regulations for radio-pharmaceutical substances

RAI therapy is the treatment of choice for almost all clients with Graves' disease because it destroys abnormally functioning gland tissue. Peak results take 6 to 12 weeks, and several treatments may be necessary; however, a single dose controls hyperthyroidism in about 90% of clients. *Note:* This therapy is contraindicated during pregnancy. Also, people preparing or administering the dose must have their own thyroid burden measured, and contaminated supplies and equipment must be monitored and stored until decayed.

Corticosteroids, for example, dexamethasone (Decadron)

Provides glucocorticol support, decreases hyperthermia, relieves relative adrenal insufficiency, inhibits calcium absorption, and reduces peripheral conversion of T_4 to T_3. *Note:* May be given before thyroidectomy and discontinued after surgery.

Digoxin (Lanoxin)

May be required in clients with HF before beta-adrenergic blocking therapy can be considered and safely initiated.

Furosemide (Lasix)

Diuresis may be necessary if HF occurs. *Note:* It also may be effective in reducing calcium level if neuromuscular function is impaired.

Potassium (KCl, K-Lyte)

Increased losses of K^+ through intestinal and renal routes may result in dysrhythmias if not corrected.

Acetaminophen (Tylenol)

Drug of choice to reduce temperature and associated metabolic demands. Aspirin is contraindicated because it actually increases level of circulating thyroid hormones by blocking binding of T_3 and T_4 with thyroid-binding proteins.

Sedatives and barbiturates

Promote rest, thereby reducing metabolic demands and cardiac workload.

Muscle relaxants

Reduce shivering associated with hyperthermia, which can further increase metabolic demands.

Monitor laboratory and diagnostic studies, as indicated:
Serum potassium

Hypokalemia resulting from intestinal losses, altered intake, or diuretic therapy may cause dysrhythmias and compromise cardiac function and output. *Note:* In the presence of thyrotoxic paralysis (primarily occurring in Asian men), close monitoring and cautious replacement are indicated because rebound hyperkalemia can occur as condition abates, releasing potassium from the cells.

Serum calcium

Elevation may alter cardiac contractility.

Sputum culture

Pulmonary infection is most frequent precipitating factor of crisis.

Serial ECGs

May demonstrate effects of electrolyte imbalance or ischemic changes reflecting inadequate myocardial oxygen supply in presence of increased metabolic demands.

Chest x-rays

Cardiac enlargement may occur in response to increased circulatory demands. Pulmonary congestion may be noted with cardiac decompensation.

Provide supplemental oxygen (O_2), as indicated.

May be necessary to support increased metabolic demands and O_2 consumption.

Provide hypothermia blanket, as indicated.

Occasionally used to lower uncontrolled hyperthermia (104°F [40.0°C] and higher) to reduce metabolic demands, O_2 consumption, and cardiac workload.

Administer transfusions; assist with plasmapheresis, hemoperfusion, and dialysis as appropriate.

May be done to achieve rapid depletion of extrathyroidal hormone pool in desperately ill and comatose client.

Prepare for surgical or chemical ablation therapy.

RAI is usually the treatment of choice for hyperthyroidism, with the purpose of reversing the overactivity; this is referred to as radioactive iodine ablation, or chemical ablation. Subtotal thyroidectomy may be performed once euthyroid state is achieved, may be performed for thyroid cancer, or for individuals who are intolerant of antithyroid medications or who refuse RAI therapy (American Association of Clinical Endocrinologists [AACE], 2006).

NURSING DIAGNOSIS: Fatigue

May be related to
Hypermetabolic state with increased energy requirements
Irritability of central nervous system (CNS), altered body chemistry

Possibly evidenced by
Verbalization of overwhelming lack of energy to maintain usual routine, decreased performance
Emotional lability and irritability; nervousness, tension
Jittery behavior
Impaired ability to concentrate

Desired Outcomes/Evaluation Criteria—Client Will

Endurance (NOC)
Verbalize increase in level of energy.
Display improved ability to participate in desired activities.

ACTIONS/INTERVENTIONS	RATIONALE
Energy Management (NIC)	
Independent	
Monitor vital signs, noting pulse rate at rest and when active.	Pulse is typically elevated, and even at rest tachycardia up to 160 beats per minute may be noted.
Note development of tachypnea, dyspnea, pallor, and cyanosis.	O₂ demand and consumption are increased in hypermetabolic state, potentiating risk of hypoxia with activity.
Provide quiet environment, cool room, decreased sensory stimuli, soothing colors, and quiet music.	Reduces stimuli that may aggravate agitation, hyperactivity, and insomnia.
Encourage client to restrict activity and rest in bed as much as possible.	Helps counteract effects of increased metabolism.
Provide comfort measures—judicious touch and massage and cool showers.	May decrease nervous energy, promoting relaxation.
Provide for calming diversional activities—reading, radio, and television.	Allows for use of nervous energy in a constructive manner, serves as a distraction, and may reduce anxiety.
Avoid topics that irritate or upset client. Discuss ways to respond to these feelings.	Increased irritability of the CNS may cause client to be easily excited, agitated, and prone to emotional outbursts.
Discuss with SO reasons for fatigue and emotional lability.	Understanding that the behavior is physically based may enhance coping with current situation and encourage SO to respond positively and provide support for client.
Collaborative	
Administer medications, as indicated, such as sedatives and anti-anxiety agents.	May be prescribed to help combat nervousness, hyperactivity, and insomnia.

NURSING DIAGNOSIS: risk for imbalanced Nutrition: Less than Body Requirements

Risk factors may include
Increased metabolism with increased appetite and intake with loss of weight
Nausea and vomiting, diarrhea
Relative insulin insufficiency, hyperglycemia

Possibly evidenced by
(Not applicable; presence of signs and symptoms establishes an *actual* diagnosis)

Desired Outcomes/Evaluation Criteria—Client Will

Nutritional Status (NOC)
Demonstrate stable weight with normal laboratory values and be free of signs of malnutrition.

ACTIONS/INTERVENTIONS	RATIONALE

Nutrition Therapy (NIC)

Independent

Monitor daily food intake. Weigh daily and report losses.

Encourage client to eat and increase number of meals and snacks, using high-calorie foods that are easily digested.

Avoid foods that increase peristalsis, such as tea, coffee, fibrous and highly seasoned foods, and fluids that cause diarrhea—apple and prune juice.

Collaborative

Consult with dietitian to provide diet high in calories, protein, carbohydrates, and vitamins.

Administer medications, as indicated, such as glucose and vitamin B complex.

—

Continued weight loss in face of adequate caloric intake may indicate failure of antithyroid therapy.

Aids in keeping caloric intake high enough to keep up with rapid expenditure of calories caused by hypermetabolic state.

Increased motility of gastrointestinal (GI) tract may result in diarrhea and impair absorption of needed nutrients.

May need assistance to ensure adequate intake of nutrients, identify appropriate supplements.

Given to meet energy requirements and prevent or correct hypoglycemia.

NURSING DIAGNOSIS: **Anxiety [specify level]**

May be related to

Physiological factors: hypermetabolic state (CNS stimulation), pseudocatecholamine effect of thyroid hormones

Possibly evidenced by

Increased feelings of apprehension, shakiness, loss of control, panic
Changes in cognition, distortion of environmental stimuli
Extraneous movements, restlessness, tremors

Desired Outcomes/Evaluation Criteria—Client Will

Anxiety Self-Control (NOC)
Appear relaxed.
Report anxiety reduced to a manageable level.
Identify healthy ways to deal with feelings.

ACTIONS/INTERVENTIONS	RATIONALE

Anxiety Reduction (NIC)

Independent

Observe behavior indicative of level of anxiety.

Monitor physical responses, noting palpitations, repetitive movements, hyperventilation, and insomnia.

Stay with client, maintaining calm manner. Acknowledge fear and allow client's behavior to belong to client.

Describe and explain procedures, surrounding environment, or sounds that may be heard by client.

Speak in brief statements, using simple words.

Reduce external stimuli. Place in quiet room; provide soft, soothing music; reduce bright lights; and reduce number of persons interacting with client.

Discuss with client and SO reasons for emotional lability and psychotic reaction. (Refer to ND: risk for disturbed Thought Processes, below.)

Reinforce expectation that emotional control should return as drug therapy progresses.

—

Mild anxiety may be displayed by irritability and insomnia. Severe anxiety progressing to panic state may produce feelings of impending doom, terror, inability to speak or move, shouting, and swearing.

Increased number of beta-adrenergic receptor sites, coupled with effects of excess thyroid hormones, produces clinical manifestations of catecholamine excess even when normal levels of norepinephrine and epinephrine exist.

Affirms to client and SO that although client feels out of control, environment is safe. Avoiding personal responses to inappropriate remarks or actions prevents conflicts and overreaction to stressful situation and client behavior.

Provides accurate information, which reduces distortions and misinterpretations that can contribute to anxiety and fear reactions.

Attention span may be shortened and concentration reduced, limiting ability to assimilate information.

Creates a therapeutic environment, shows recognition that unit activity and personnel may increase client's anxiety.

Understanding that behavior is physically based enhances acceptance of situation and encourages different responses and approaches.

Provides information and reassures client that the situation is temporary and will improve with treatment.

ACTIONS/INTERVENTIONS (continued)	RATIONALE (continued)
Collaborative	
Administer anti-anxiety agents or sedatives and monitor effects.	May be used in conjunction with medical regimen to reduce effects of hyperthyroid secretion.
Refer to support systems, as needed, including counseling, social services, and pastoral care.	Ongoing therapy support may be desired and required by client and SO if crisis precipitates lifestyle alterations.

NURSING DIAGNOSIS: risk for disturbed Thought Processes

Risk factors may include
Physiological changes: increased CNS stimulation and accelerated mental activity
Altered sleep patterns

Possibly evidenced by
(Not applicable; presence of signs and symptoms establishes an *actual* diagnosis)

Desired Outcomes/Evaluation Criteria—Client Will

Distorted Thought Self-Control (NOC)
Maintain usual reality orientation.
Recognize changes in thinking and behavior and causative factors.

ACTIONS/INTERVENTIONS	RATIONALE
Delirium Management (NIC)	
Independent	
Assess thinking processes, such as memory; attention span; and orientation to person, place, time, and situation.	Determines extent of interference with sensory processing.
Note changes in behavior.	May be hypervigilant, restless, extremely sensitive, or crying, or may develop frank psychosis.
Assess level of anxiety. (Refer to ND: Anxiety.)	Anxiety may alter thought processes and ability to think clearly.
Provide quiet environment: decreased stimuli, cool room, and dim lights. Limit procedures and personnel.	Reduction of external stimuli may decrease hyperactivity and hyperreflexia, CNS irritability, and auditory and visual hallucinations.
Reorient to person, place, time, and situation, as indicated.	Helps establish and maintain awareness of reality and environment.
Present reality concisely and briefly without challenging illogical thinking.	Limits defensive reaction.
Provide clock, calendar, and room with outside window; alter level of lighting to simulate day and night.	Promotes continual orientation cues to assist client in maintaining sense of normalcy.
Encourage visits by family and SO. Provide support as needed.	Aids in maintaining socialization and orientation. *Note:* Client's agitation and psychotic behavior may precipitate family quarrels and conflicts.
Provide safety measures, such as padded side rails, close supervision, or use of soft restraints as last resort, as necessary.	Prevents injury to client who may be hallucinating and disoriented.
Collaborative	
Administer medication, as indicated, such as sedatives and anti-anxiety agents and antipsychotic drugs.	Promotes relaxation and reduces CNS hyperactivity and agitation to enhance thinking ability.

NURSING DIAGNOSIS: risk for impaired Tissue Integrity

Risk factors may include
Alterations of protective mechanisms of eye—impaired closure of eyelid.

Possibly evidenced by
(Not applicable; presence of signs and symptoms establishes an *actual* diagnosis)

Desired Outcomes/Evaluation Criteria—Client Will

Tissue Integrity: Skin and Mucous Membranes (NOC)
Maintain moist eye membranes, free of ulcerations.

Risk Control (NOC)
Identify measures to provide protection for eyes and prevent complications.

ACTIONS/INTERVENTIONS	RATIONALE

Surveillance (NIC)

Independent

Encourage use of dark glasses when awake and taping the eyelids shut during sleep, as needed.

Elevate the head of the bed and restrict salt intake, if indicated.

Instruct client in extraocular muscle exercises, if appropriate.

Provide opportunity for client to discuss feelings about altered appearance and measures to enhance self-image.

Collaborative

Administer medications, as indicated, for example:
  Methylcellulose drops and artificial tears
  Adrenocorticotropic hormone (ACTH) and prednisone

  Antithyroid drugs

  Diuretics
Prepare for surgery, as indicated.

RATIONALE (right column)

Protects exposed cornea if client is unable to close eyelids completely because of edema and fibrosis of fat pads.

Decreases tissue edema when appropriate.

Improves circulation and maintains mobility of the eyelids.

Protruding eyes may be viewed as unattractive. Appearance can be enhanced with proper use of makeup, overall grooming, and use of shaded glasses.

Lubricates the eyes, reducing risk of lesion formation.

Given to decrease rapidly progressive and marked inflammation (AACE, 2006).

May decrease signs and symptoms or prevent worsening of the condition.

Can decrease edema in mild involvement.

Eyelids may need to be sutured shut temporarily to protect the corneas until edema resolves (rare), or increasing space within sinus cavity and adjusting musculature may return eye to a more normal position (AACE, 2006).

NURSING DIAGNOSIS: **deficient Knowledge [Learning Need] regarding condition, prognosis, treatment, self-care, and discharge needs**

May be related to

Lack of exposure or recall

Information misinterpretation

Unfamiliarity with information resources

Possibly evidenced by

Questions, request for information, statement of misconception

Inaccurate follow-through of instructions and development of preventable complications

Desired Outcomes/Evaluation Criteria—Client Will

Knowledge: Illness Care (NOC)

Verbalize understanding of disease process and potential complications.

Identify relationship of signs and symptoms to the disease process and correlate symptoms with causative factors.

Verbalize understanding of therapeutic needs.

Participate in treatment regimen.

Initiate necessary lifestyle changes.

ACTIONS/INTERVENTIONS	RATIONALE

Teaching: Disease Process (NIC)

Independent

Review disease process and future expectations.

Provide information appropriate to individual situation.

Identify stressors and discuss precipitators to thyroid crises—personal, social, and job concerns; infection; and pregnancy.

Provide information about signs and symptoms of hypothyroidism and the need for continuing follow-up care.

Discuss drug therapy, including need for adhering to regimen and expected therapeutic and side effects.

**RATIONALE **

Provides knowledge base from which client can make informed choices.

Severity of condition, cause, age, and concurrent complications determine course of treatment.

Psychogenic factors are often of prime importance in the occurrence and exacerbation of this disease.

Client who has been treated for hyperthyroidism needs to be aware of possible development of hypothyroidism, which can occur immediately after treatment or as long as 5 years later.

Antithyroid medication, either as primary therapy or in preparation for thyroidectomy, requires adherence to a medical regimen over an extended period to inhibit hormone production. Agranulocytosis is the most serious side effect that can occur, and alternative drugs may be given if problems arise.

ACTIONS/INTERVENTIONS (continued)

Identify signs and symptoms requiring medical evaluation, such as fever, sore throat, and skin eruptions.

Explain need to check with physician and pharmacist before taking other prescribed or over-the-counter (OTC) drugs.

Emphasize importance of planned rest periods.

Review need for nutritious diet and periodic review of nutrient needs; avoid caffeine, red and yellow food dyes, and artificial preservatives.

Stress necessity of continued medical follow-up.

RATIONALE (continued)

Early identification of toxic reactions (thiourea therapy) and prompt intervention are important in preventing development of agranulocytosis.

Antithyroid medications can affect or be affected by numerous other medications, requiring monitoring of medication levels, side effects, and interactions.

Prevents undue fatigue and reduces metabolic demands. As euthyroid state is achieved, stamina and activity level will increase.

Provides adequate nutrients to support hypermetabolic state. As hormonal imbalance is corrected, diet will need to be readjusted to prevent excessive weight gain. Irritants and stimulants should be limited to avoid cumulative systemic effects.

Required to monitor effectiveness of therapy and for prevention of potentially fatal complications.

POTENTIAL CONSIDERATIONS following acute hospitalization (dependent on client's age, physical condition and presence of complications, personal resources, and life responsibilities)
- *Fatigue*—hypermetabolic state diminishing body energy reserves, prolonged recovery
- *risk for imbalanced Nutrition: More than Body Requirements*—change in basal metabolic rate (BMR) and metabolic needs

THYROIDECTOMY

I. **Indications**: thyroid cancer, hyperthyroidism, large goiters constricting tissues or structures in the neck
II. **Procedures**
  a. May be done as an open, minimally invasive, or endoscopic procedure
  b. Video-assisted, minimally invasive surgical technique that markedly shortens incision length to typically around 1 in. versus 3 in. with traditional surgical procedure
  c. Totally endoscopic procedure that involves the creation of an invisible incision—using special instrumentation and technique—with part or all of the thyroid gland removed through small puncture sites in the underarm area and avoiding a neck incision.
  d. Total thyroidectomy: Entire gland and surrounding lymph nodes are removed.
    i. Performed in cases of malignancy or when there is a high risk of developing multiple sites of thyroid cancer
    ii. Presence of numerous separate nodules
    iii. Enlarged thyroid makes breathing and swallowing difficult
  e. Lobectomy: Lobe is removed with or without the isthmus between the lobes.
    i. Done to remove single nodule or multiple nodules in a single lobe
  f. Subtotal thyroidectomy: Up to five-sixths of the gland is removed.
    i. Performed when antithyroid drugs do not correct hyperthyroidism or RAI therapy is contraindicated
    ii. Procedure of choice for hyperthyroidism, with 95% cure rate
III. **Statistics** (Fallon, 2003)
  a. Frequency of procedure: In 2001, approximately 34,500 cases performed in United States.
  b. Morbidity: 12% to 50% of individuals develop hypothyroidism within first year.
  c. Mortality: Essentially zero for procedure, or about the level associated with general surgery (Kaplan & Angelos, 2006); in thyroid storm (rare complication) 20% to 30%.

GLOSSARY

Chvostek's sign: Spasm of facial muscles when facial nerve is tapped, reflecting severe hypocalcemia.
Laryngeal stridor: Harsh sound occurring during inspiration when air passes through a constricted airway.
Parathyroidectomy: Excision of one or both parathyroid glands that regulate use of calcium and phosphorus in the body, which is usually an inadvertent complication during thyroidectomy.

Tetany: Intermittent tonic spasms of the extremities associated with hypocalcemia and hyperphosphatemia.
Trousseau's sign: Muscle spasm and paresthesia of the hand and wrist with compression of upper arm, as with application of tourniquet or blood pressure (BP) cuff, indicative of latent tetany and severe hypocalcemia.

Care Setting

Care is given in an inpatient acute surgical unit.

Related Concerns

Cancer, page 846
Hyperthyroidism (Graves' disease, thyrotoxicosis), page 419
Psychosocial aspects of care, page 749
Surgical intervention, page 782

Client Assessment Database

Refer to CP: Hyperthyroidism (Graves' disease, Thyrotoxicosis) for assessment information.

DIAGNOSTIC DIVISION MAY REPORT	MAY EXHIBIT
TEACHING/LEARNING • *Discharge Plan Considerations:* May need assistance with self-care and other activities of daily living (ADLs), transportation ◗ Refer to section at end of plan for postdischarge considerations.	

Nursing Priorities

1. Reverse and manage hyperthyroid state preoperatively.
2. Prevent complications.
3. Relieve pain.
4. Provide information about surgical procedure, prognosis, and treatment needs.

Discharge Goals

1. Complications prevented and minimized.
2. Pain alleviated.
3. Surgical procedure and prognosis and therapeutic regimen understood.
4. Plan in place to meet needs after discharge.

NURSING DIAGNOSIS: risk for ineffective Airway Clearance

Risk factors may include
Tracheal obstruction; swelling, bleeding, laryngeal spasms.

Possibly evidenced by
(Not applicable; presence of signs and symptoms establishes an *actual* diagnosis)

Desired Outcomes/Evaluation Criteria—Client Will

Respiratory Status: Airway Patency (NOC)
Maintain patent airway, with aspiration prevented.

ACTIONS/INTERVENTIONS	RATIONALE
Airway Management (NIC) *Independent* Monitor respiratory rate, depth, and work of breathing.	Respirations may remain somewhat rapid because of hyperthyroid state, but development of respiratory distress is indicative of tracheal compression from edema or hemorrhage.
Auscultate breath sounds, noting presence of rhonchi.	Rhonchi may indicate airway obstruction and accumulation of copious thick secretions.
Assess for dyspnea, stridor, "crowing," and cyanosis. Note quality of voice.	Indicators of tracheal obstruction or laryngeal spasm, requiring prompt evaluation and intervention.
Keep head of bed elevated 30 to 45 degrees. Caution client to avoid bending neck; support head with pillows in the immediate postoperative period.	Enhances breathing and reduces likelihood of tension on surgical wound.
Assist with repositioning, deep breathing exercises, and coughing, as indicated.	Maintains clear airway and ventilation. Although "routine" coughing is not encouraged and may be painful, it may be necessary to clear secretions.
Ascertain that suction equipment is functioning and available. Suction mouth and trachea, as indicated, noting color and characteristics of sputum.	Edema and pain may impair client's ability to clear own airway.

ACTIONS/INTERVENTIONS (continued)	RATIONALE (continued)
Check dressing frequently, especially posterior portion.	If bleeding occurs, anterior dressing may appear dry because blood pools dependently. *Note:* Highest risk of bleeding is first postoperative 2 hours, but risk continues up to 24 hours.
Investigate reports of difficulty swallowing and drooling of oral secretions.	May indicate edema and sequestered bleeding in tissues surrounding operative site.
Keep tracheostomy tray at bedside.	Compromised airway may create a life-threatening situation requiring emergency procedure.
Collaborative	
Provide steam inhalation; humidify room air.	Reduces discomfort of sore throat and tissue edema and promotes expectoration of secretions.
Assist with and prepare for procedures, such as: Tracheostomy	Although rare, tracheostomy may be necessary to obtain airway if obstructed by edema of glottis or hemorrhage.
Return to surgery	May require ligation of bleeding vessels.

NURSING DIAGNOSIS: impaired verbal Communication

May be related to
Vocal cord injury, laryngeal nerve damage
Tissue edema; pain and discomfort

Possibly evidenced by
Impaired articulation, does not or cannot speak; use of nonverbal cues such as gestures

Desired Outcomes/Evaluation Criteria—Client Will

Communication (NOC)
Establish method of communication in which needs can be understood.

ACTIONS/INTERVENTIONS	RATIONALE
Communication Enhancement: Speech Deficit (NIC) *Independent*	
Assess speech periodically and encourage voice rest.	Hoarseness and sore throat may occur secondary to tissue edema or surgical damage to recurrent laryngeal nerve and may last several days. Permanent nerve damage can occur (rare) that causes paralysis of vocal cords and or compression of the trachea.
Keep communication simple. Ask yes and no questions.	Reduces demand for response; promotes voice rest.
Provide alternative methods of communication as appropriate—slate board, letter and picture board. Place intravenous (IV) line to minimize interference with written communication.	Facilitates expression of needs.
Anticipate needs as much as possible. Visit client frequently.	Reduces anxiety and client's need to communicate.
Post notice of client's voice limitations at central station and answer call light promptly.	Prevents client from straining voice to make needs known and summon assistance.
Maintain quiet environment.	Enhances ability to hear whispered communication and reduces necessity for client to raise and strain voice to be heard.

NURSING DIAGNOSIS: risk for Injury, [tetany, thyroid storm]

Risk factors may include
Chemical imbalance, such as with hypocalcemia, increased release of thyroid hormones, excessive central nervous system (CNS) stimulation

Possibly evidenced by
(Not applicable; presence of signs and symptoms establishes an *actual* diagnosis)

Desired Outcomes/Evaluation Criteria—Client Will

Physical Injury Severity (NOC)
Demonstrate absence of injury with complications minimized or controlled.

ACTIONS/INTERVENTIONS	RATIONALE

Surveillance (NIC)

Independent

Monitor vital signs, noting elevated temperature, tachycardia (140 to 200 beats/minute), dysrhythmias, respiratory distress, and cyanosis—developing pulmonary edema or heart failure (HF).

Manipulation of gland during subtotal thyroidectomy may result in increased hormone release, causing thyroid storm.

Evaluate reflexes periodically. Observe for neuromuscular irritability—twitching, numbness, paresthesias, positive Chvostek's and Trousseau's signs, and seizure activity.

Hypocalcemia with tetany (usually transient) may occur 1 to 7 days postoperatively and indicates hypoparathyroidism, which can occur because of inadvertent trauma to and partial to total removal of parathyroid gland(s) during surgery.

Keep side rails raised and padded, bed in low position, and airway at bedside. Avoid use of restraints.

Reduces potential for injury if seizures occur. (Refer to CP: Seizure Disorders, ND: risk for Trauma/Suffocation.)

Collaborative

Monitor serum calcium levels.

Clients with levels less than 7.5 mg/100 mL generally require replacement therapy.

Administer medications, as indicated, for example:
IV calcium (gluconate or chloride)

Corrects deficiency, which is usually temporary but may be permanent. *Note:* Use with caution in clients taking digoxin because calcium increases cardiac sensitivity to digoxin, potentiating risk of toxicity.

Phosphate-binding agents

Helpful in lowering elevated phosphorus levels associated with hypocalcemia.

Sedatives

Promotes rest, reducing exogenous stimulation.

Anticonvulsants

Controls seizure activity associated with thyroid storm until corrective therapy is successful.

NURSING DIAGNOSIS: acute Pain

May be related to
Surgical interruption and manipulation of tissues and muscles
Postoperative edema

Possibly evidenced by
Reports of pain
Narrowed focus, guarding behavior, restlessness
Autonomic responses

Desired Outcomes/Evaluation Criteria—Client Will

Pain Control (NOC)
Report pain is relieved and controlled.
Demonstrate use of relaxation skills and diversional activities appropriate to situation.

ACTIONS/INTERVENTIONS	RATIONALE

Pain Management (NIC)

Independent

Assess verbal reports and nonverbal cues of pain, noting location, intensity (0 to 10 scale), and duration.

Useful in evaluating pain, choice of interventions, and effectiveness of therapy.

Place in semi-Fowler's position and support head and neck in neutral position with sandbags or small pillows as required in immediate postoperative phase. Instruct client to use hands to support neck during movement and to avoid hyperextension of neck.

Prevents hyperextension of the neck and protects integrity of the suture line. Movement restriction is imposed for only a few hours postoperatively to prevent stress on the suture line and reduce muscle tension. Gentle flexing and stretching is then permitted according to pain tolerance to help prevent neck soreness.

Keep call light and frequently needed items within easy reach.

Limits stretching and muscle strain in operative area.

Give cool liquids or soft foods, such as ice cream or popsicles.

Although both may be soothing to sore throat, soft foods may be better tolerated than liquids if client experiences difficulty swallowing.

Encourage client to use relaxation techniques, such as guided imagery, soft music, and progressive relaxation.

Helps refocus attention and assists client to manage pain and discomfort more effectively.

Collaborative

Administer analgesics and throat sprays and lozenges, as necessary.

Reduces pain and discomfort; enhances rest.

Provide ice collar, if indicated.

Reduces tissue edema and decreases perception of pain.

NURSING DIAGNOSIS: **deficient Knowledge [Learning Need] regarding condition, prognosis, treatment, self-care, and discharge needs**

May be related to
Lack of exposure and recall; misinterpretation
Unfamiliarity with information resources

Possibly evidenced by
Questions, request for information, statement of misconception
Inaccurate follow-through of instructions and development of preventable complications

Desired Outcomes/Evaluation Criteria—Client Will

Knowledge: Disease Process (NOC)
Verbalize understanding of surgical procedure and prognosis and potential complications.

Knowledge: Treatment Regimen (NOC)
Verbalize understanding of therapeutic needs.
Participate in treatment regimen.
Initiate necessary lifestyle changes.

ACTIONS/INTERVENTIONS	RATIONALE
Teaching: Disease Process (NIC) *Independent* Review surgical procedure and future expectations.	Provides knowledge base from which client can make informed decisions.
Discuss need for well-balanced, nutritious diet and, when appropriate, inclusion of iodized salt.	Promotes healing and helps client regain and maintain appropriate weight. Use of iodized salt is often sufficient to meet iodine needs unless salt is restricted for other healthcare problems, such as with HF.
Recommend avoidance of goitrogenic foods—excessive ingestion of seafood, soybeans, and turnips.	Contraindicated after partial thyroidectomy because these foods inhibit thyroid activity.
Identify foods high in calcium, such as dairy products, and vitamin D, such as fortified dairy products, egg yolks, and liver.	Maximizes supply and absorption of calcium if parathyroid function is impaired.
Encourage progressive general exercise program.	In clients with subtotal thyroidectomy, exercise can stimulate the thyroid gland and production of hormones, facilitating recovery of general well-being.
Review postoperative exercises to be instituted after incision heals—flexion, extension, rotation, and lateral movement of head and neck.	Regular range-of-motion (ROM) exercises strengthen neck muscles and enhance circulation and healing process.
Review importance of rest and relaxation, avoiding stressful situations and emotional outbursts.	Effects of hyperthyroidism usually subside completely, but it takes some time for the body to recover.
Instruct in incisional care—cleansing and dressing application.	Enables client to provide competent self-care. *Note:* Neck incisions heal rapidly and are watertight within 24 to 36 hours.
Recommend the use of loose-fitting scarves to cover scar, avoiding the use of jewelry.	Covers the incision without aggravating healing or precipitating infections of suture line.
Apply moisturizers or vitamin E cream after sutures have been removed.	Softens tissues and may help minimize scarring.
Discuss possibility of change in voice.	Normal surgical area swelling and vocal cord dysfunction can cause changes in pitch and quality of voice, which may be temporary or permanent.
Review drug therapy and the necessity of continuing even when feeling well.	If thyroid hormone replacement is needed because of surgical removal of gland, client needs to understand rationale for replacement therapy and consequences of failure to routinely take medication.
Identify signs and symptoms requiring medical evaluation: fever, chills, continued and purulent wound drainage, erythema, gaps in wound edges, sudden weight loss, intolerance to heat, nausea and vomiting, diarrhea, insomnia, weight gain, fatigue, intolerance to cold, constipation, and drowsiness.	Early recognition of developing complications, such as infection, hyperthyroidism, or hypothyroidism, may prevent progression to life-threatening situation.
Stress necessity of continued medical follow-up.	Provides opportunity for evaluating effectiveness of therapy and prevention of complications.

HEPATITIS

I. Pathophysiology
a. Causes widespread damage to liver cells (hepatocytes) either directly or indirectly from inflammation or autoimmune response
b. May be acute or chronic
   i. Acute: Swelling of hepatocytes reduces ability to detoxify drugs; produce clotting factors, plasma proteins, bile, and glycogen; and store fat-soluble vitamins.
   ii. Chronic: inflammation and necrosis of liver of more than 6 months' duration

II. Etiology
a. Infectious causes: viral, bacterial, fungal, or parasitic
   i. Viruses are designated by letters A through G, with several terms used interchangeably, for example, hepatitis B is known as HBV or HepB; types A through D are endemic in the United States and transmitted by blood and other body fluids, sexual or close contact with infected person, and fecal contamination of food and water.
   ii. Other viruses: cytomegalovirus (CMV), Epstein-Barr virus (EBV), *Mycobacterium avium* complex (MAC), herpes simplex, varicella-zoster, toxoplasmosis, and histoplasmosis
b. Noninfectious causes: physical or toxic chemical agents, autoimmune
   i. Toxic agents: carbon tetrachloride, vinyl chloride; alcohol, cocaine, acetaminophen, isoniazid, anabolic steroids, methyldopa, erythromycin; poisonous mushrooms
   ii. Autoimmune: no identifiable etiology; two types, with type 1 most common form in North America

III. Statistics
a. Morbidity: HAV, HBV, and HCV cause more than 90% of cases of acute viral hepatitis in the United States (Buggs & Kim, 2006).
   i. The Centers for Disease Control and Prevention (CDC) reported 7,653 acute clinical cases of HAV in 2003, with the estimate of actual clinical cases at 33,000 and estimated number of new infections in the United States at 61,000 (Gilroy & Mukherjee, 2006).
   ii. About 1.25 million people are chronic HBV carriers, and the disease causes about 5,000 deaths each year (Mukherjee, 2005); 22,000 pregnant women in the United States are infected with HBV and can transmit the virus to their newborns.
   iii. HCV is a leading cause of chronic hepatitis and cirrhosis worldwide; studies have shown that almost 30% of persons with human immunodeficiency virus (HIV) infection also have hepatitis (Baker, 2007).
b. Mortality: Approximately 100 Americans die from HAV, and another 5,000 die from cirrhosis and 1,000 from liver cancer due to HBV infections (Buggs & Kim, 2006); chronic liver disease associated with persistent hepatitis virus infection accounts for an estimated 16,000 deaths per year—70% from HCV, 20% from HBV, and 10% from combined infection with HCV and HBV (Gilroy & Mukherjee, 2006); fatality rate for hepatits E is 4% (Schwartz et al, 2006).
c. Cost: Annual cost associated with HAV is estimated at $200 million in the United States (Hepatitis Foundation International [HFI], 2003).

GLOSSARY

Acute hepatitis: Often self-limiting, although approximately 5% to 10% of clients with HBV and 80% to 85% of clients with HCV progress to a chronic state (Buggs & Kim, 2006).

Anorexia: Loss of appetite as result of disease.

Ascites: Buildup of fluid in the abdomen due to a number of conditions, including severe liver disease.

Asterixis: Involuntary jerking movements of hands and feet associated with hepatic encephalopathy.

Autoimmune: Persistent inflammation and necrosis with hypergammaglobulinemia and autoantibodies without other common causes of hepatitis.

Biological response modifiers (BMRs): Substances that stimulate the body's response to infection and disease.

Chronic hepatitis: Persistent inflammation and necrosis lasting more than 6 months, commonly due to hepatitis B, C, or D virus.

Ecchymosis: Skin discoloration consisting of a large, irregularly formed hemorrhagic area, with colors changing from blue-black to greenish-brown or yellow; commonly called a bruise.

Fulminant hepatitis: Occurs suddenly and with great intensity or severity, progressing to encephalopathy within 8 weeks of onset and death if liver transplant is not performed.

Hepatic encephalopathy: Brain dysfunction directly due to the liver dysfunction most often seen in advanced cirrhosis. Encephalopathy may cause disturbances of consciousness and progress to coma.

Hepatocyte: Parenchymal liver cell.

Jaundice: Yellow staining of the skin and sclerae (and sometimes other tissues and body fluids) by abnormally high blood levels of the bile pigment bilirubin.

Melena: Bloody stools.
Palmar erythema: Redness of the palms of the hands caused by dilation and congestion of capillaries.
Pruritus: Severe itching of the skin.
Right upper quadrant (RUQ): Anatomic location of the liver.
Spider angiomas: Abnormal collection of blood vessels near the surface of the skin, which can occur anywhere but are most common on the face and trunk.

Splenomegaly: Enlarged spleen.
Toxic hepatitis: Liver inflammation often due to common drugs used to treat disease or chemicals found in the workplace.
Urticaria: Vascular reaction of the skin marked by transient appearance of slightly elevated patches, which are more red or pale than the surrounding skin and often are accompanied by severe itching; may also be called hives.

Care Setting

Care can frequently be provided in the outpatient setting or at the community level. In states of acute hepatic inflammation, brief inpatient acute care on a medical unit may be required to monitor and treat hepatic failure or hepatic encephalopathy.

Related Concerns

Alcohol: acute withdrawal, page 819
Cirrhosis of the liver, page 445
Psychosocial aspects of care, page 749
Renal dialysis—general considerations, page 560
Substance dependence/abuse rehabilitation, page 835
Total nutritional support: parenteral/enteral feeding, page 469

Client Assessment Database

Data depend on the cause (type of hepatitis) and severity of liver involvement and damage.

DIAGNOSTIC DIVISION MAY REPORT	MAY EXHIBIT
ACTIVITY/REST • Fatigue • Weakness, general malaise, muscle aches	
CIRCULATION	• Bradycardia—in severe hyperbilirubinemia • Jaundiced sclera, skin, mucous membranes
ELIMINATION • Dark urine, clay-colored stools • Diarrhea, constipation	
FOOD/FLUID • Loss of appetite, weight loss • Weight gain—edema, ascites • Nausea, vomiting	• Ascites • Abdominal distention due to liver enlargement
NEUROSENSORY	• Irritability, drowsiness, lethargy • Asterixis
PAIN/DISCOMFORT • Abdominal cramping, RUQ tenderness • Joint pain • Headache	• Muscle guarding, restlessness
SAFETY • Blood transfusions or organ transplant received prior to viral screening tests • Tattoos (possible equipment source) • Itching (pruritus)	• Fever—usually low grade • Urticaria, maculopapular lesions, irregular patches of erythema • Spider angiomas, palmar erythema, gynecomastia in men (sometimes present in alcoholic hepatitis) • Splenomegaly, posterior cervical node enlargement

(continues on page 436)

DIAGNOSTIC DIVISION MAY REPORT (continued)	MAY EXHIBIT (continued)

SEXUALITY
- Lifestyle or behaviors increasing risk of exposure—unprotected sexual intercourse with infected person

TEACHING/LEARNING
- History of known or possible exposure to virus, bacteria, or toxins—from contaminated food, water, needles, surgical equipment or blood; carriers (symptomatic or asymptomatic); recent surgical procedure with halothane anesthesia, exposure to toxic chemicals, such as carbon tetrachloride, vinyl chloride
- History of known or possible exposure to hepatotoxic prescription, such as sulfonamides, phenothiazines, isoniazid, or over-the-counter (OTC) drug use, such as acetaminophen
- Use of herbal supplements associated with hepatotoxicity, such as chaparral, Jin Bu Huan, germander, comfrey, mistletoe, skullcap, margosa oil, pennyroyal
- Use of street injection drugs or alcohol
- Travel to or immigration from China, Africa, Southeast Asia, Middle East (HBV and HCV are endemic in these areas)
- Concurrent diabetes, heart failure (HF), malignancy, or renal disease

DISCHARGE PLAN CONSIDERATIONS
- May require assistance with homemaking, maintenance tasks, shopping, transportation

▶ Refer to section at end of plan for postdischarge considerations.

Diagnostic Studies

TEST WHY IT IS DONE	WHAT IT TELLS ME
BLOOD TESTS	
• *Hepatitis A, B, C, D, E viral panels (antibody/antigen tests):* Detect antibodies to the various viruses.	HAV—active infection or recovery from a prior infection. HBV—recovery from prior infection or immunity from HBV vaccine; chronic HBV or HBV carrier. HCV—chronic carrier. HDV—active only when found along with HBV. HEV—indicate prior infection (rare in United States).
• *Liver enzymes/isoenzymes:* Of limited value in differentiating viral from nonviral hepatitis.	Abnormal—may be 4 to 10 times normal values.
• *Alanine aminotransferase (ALT):* Considered best liver enzyme test for detecting hepatitis.	Elevation usually occurs before other symptoms, such as jaundice, are noted.
• *Alkaline phosphatase (ALP):* Liver enzyme test for detecting hepatitis.	Usually only slightly elevated unless severe biliary obstruction is present.

Diagnostic Studies (continued)

TEST / WHY IT IS DONE (continued)	WHAT IT TELLS ME (continued)
• *Complete blood count (CBC):* Battery of screening tests that typically includes hemoglobin (Hgb); hematocrit (Hct); red blood cell (RBC) count, morphology, indices, and distribution width index; platelet count and size; white blood cell (WBC) count and differential—the percentage of each of the five types of mature WBCs: neutrophils, lymphocytes (B cells and T cells), monocytes, eosinophils, and basophils.	RBCs are decreased because of shortened life span of RBCs—liver enzyme alterations or hemorrhage. WBCs may be abnormally low (leukopenia) or high (leukocytosis); monocytes may be increased (monocytosis), and lymphocytes may be increased and atypical in appearance.
• *Serum albumin:* Measures the main body protein manufactured by the liver.	Level is decreased.
• *Prothrombin time (PT):* One of several clotting factors that is produced by the liver. Evaluates the body's ability to produce a clot in a reasonable amount of time.	May be prolonged—liver dysfunction.
• *Serum bilirubin:* Yellow-red substance that results from the breakdown of Hgb, a normal process of the liver, then excreted via the intestines.	High level indicates the liver is incapable of adequately removing bilirubin in a timely manner due to blockage of bile ducts or liver disease, such as acute hepatitis. Accumulation of bilirubin is responsible for jaundice of the skin and mucous membranes.

OTHER DIAGNOSTIC TESTS
The following tests may be done in differentiating hepatitis from gallbladder disorders, biliary obstruction, or liver abscesses.

• *Liver scan:* May be indicated for differential diagnosis, to identify underlying chronic liver disease, or for evaluating organ function.	Helps estimate the severity of parenchymal damage.
• *Liver biopsy:* Considered if diagnosis is uncertain or if clinical course is atypical or unduly prolonged.	Provides initial assessment of disease severity in client with chronic HBV or chronic HVC.
• *Urinalysis:* Checks the urine for bilirubin for the nonjaundiced client with suspected viral hepatitis.	Elevated bilirubin levels and proteinuria and hematuria may occur.
• *Stool:* Bile gives the stool its normal brown color.	Clay-colored stools indicate lack of normal bile excretion into the intestine.

Nursing Priorities
1. Reduce demands on liver while promoting physical well-being.
2. Prevent complications.
3. Enhance self-concept and acceptance of situation.
4. Provide information about disease process, prognosis, and treatment needs.

Discharge Goals
1. Basic self-care needs are met.
2. Complications prevented or minimized.
3. Dealing with reality of current situation.
4. Disease process, prognosis, transmission, and therapeutic regimen understood.
5. Plan in place to meet needs after discharge.

NURSING DIAGNOSIS: impaired Liver Function

May be related to
Viral infection, such as viruses A, B, C, D
HIV coinfection
Hepatotoxic medications—acetaminophen, statins
Substance abuse—alcohol, cocaine
Exposure to environmental toxins

Possibly evidenced by
Presence of virus or antibodies, abnormal liver function tests
Presence of jaundice, hepatic enlargement

(continues on page 438)

Desired Outcomes/Evaluation Criteria—Client Will

Treatment Behavior: Illness or Injury (NOC)
Demonstrate behaviors or lifestyle changes to limit effects of condition.
Be free of signs of liver failure as evidenced by liver function studies within normal limits (WNL) and absence of jaundice, hepatic enlargement, or altered mental status.

ACTIONS/INTERVENTIONS	RATIONALE
Infection Control/Substance Use Treatment (NIC)	
Independent	
Determine presence of condition(s), as listed above. Note whether problem is acute—viral hepatitis or acetaminophen overdose—or chronic—long-standing alcoholic hepatitis.	Influences choice of interventions.
Review medications—sulfonamides, phenothiazines, isoniazid—for hepatotoxic drugs or OTC drug use such as acetaminophen.	May require changes in usual medication regimen and client education about hepatic effects of OTC drugs.
Ascertain if client works in high-risk occupation; for example, performs tasks that involve contact with blood, blood-contaminated body fluids, other body fluids, or sharps or needles.	Helps in identifying source of infection—occupational high risk for exposure to HBV and HCV.
Assess for exposure to contaminated food or untreated drinking water or for evidence of poor sanitation practices by food-service workers, if source is known.	Helps in identifying source of infection—risk for exposure to enteric viruses, such as HAV and HEV.
Collaborative	
Review results of laboratory tests, such as hepatitis viral titers, liver function, and other diagnostic studies.	Identifies cause of hepatitis, influences choice of interventions, and monitors response to therapies.
Assist with treatment of underlying condition.	Supports organ function and minimizes liver damage and risk of organ failure. For chronic HBV and HCV infections, in particular, the goals of therapy are to reduce liver inflammation and fibrosis and to prevent progression to cirrhosis and the associated complications (Buggs & Kim, 2006).
Administer medications, as indicated, for example:	The particular or combination of medication used depends on the type of infection.
Antivirals, such as, amantidine (Symmetrel), famciclovir (Famvir), and entecavir (Baraclude)	Inhibit viral reproduction.
Lamivudine (Epivir), adefovir dipivoxil (Hepsera), tenofovin (Viread), and telbivudine (Tyzeka)	Help reduce viral load and treat chronic active HBV. Alternative choice for individuals unable or unwilling to use interferon; or, in the presence of impaired immune function such as coinfection with HIV (Mukherjee, 2005). *Note:* Long-term therapy required because the virus begins to replicate when drug is terminated.
BMRs, such as interferon alpha-2a (Roferon A) and interferon alpha-2b (Intron A)	Reduce viral load and treat symptoms of HCV; may lead to temporary improvement in liver function. Also used in HDV. *Note:* Interferons have been found to induce remission in 25% to 50% of clients with chronic HBV and in 40% of those with chronic HCV (Buggs & Kim, 2006).
Pegylated interferons, such as peginterferon alpha-2a (Pegasys) and peginterferon alpha-2b (Peg-Intron)	These BMRs have largely replaced standard interferons in the treatment of HCV.
Ribavirin (Rebetol, Copegus)	Used in conjunction with interferon or peginterferon to improve the effectiveness of these drugs (Buggs & Kim, 2006), especially in removing the higher HCV RNA loads associated with HIV coinfection (Baker, 2007). Combination therapy has a lower relapse rate than monotherapy (National Institute of Diabetes and Digestive and Kidney Disorders [NIDDK], 2006). *Note:* These treatments lead to improvement, not cure, of the disease.
Anti-infectives appropriate to causative agents, such as, gram-negative, anaerobic bacteria, fungus, or secondary infectious process	Treat bacterial hepatitis or prevent/limit secondary infections.

ACTIONS/INTERVENTIONS (continued)	RATIONALE (continued)
Steroid therapy, such as prednisone (Deltasone), alone or in combination with azathioprine (Imuran)	Steroids may be contraindicated because they can increase risk of relapse or development of chronic hepatitis in clients with viral hepatitis; however, anti-inflammatory effect may be useful in chronic active hepatitis, especially idiopathic, to reduce nausea and vomiting and to enable client to retain food and fluids. A brief course may also be useful in cholestatic HAV to shorten the illness (Buggs & Kim, 2006). Steroids may decrease serum aminotransferase and bilirubin levels, but they do not affect liver necrosis or regeneration. Combination therapy has fewer steroid-related side effects.
Administer antidote or assist with procedures as indicated, such as lavage, catharsis, or hyperventilation, depending on route of exposure.	Removal of causative agent in toxic hepatitis may limit degree of tissue involvement and damage.
Refer to specialist or liver treatment center for consideration of other treatment options, for example, transplantation, as indicated.	Currently, almost one-half of all liver transplants in the United States are performed for end-stage HCV. However, reinfection of the transplanted liver by the virus usually occurs and may require a second transplant (HFI, 2003).

NURSING DIAGNOSIS: Fatigue

May be related to
Decreased metabolic energy production
States of discomfort
Altered body chemistry—changes in liver function, effect on target organs

Possibly evidenced by
Reports of lack of energy, inability to maintain usual routines
Decreased performance
Increase in physical complaints

Desired Outcomes/Evaluation Criteria—Client Will

Endurance (NOC)
Report improved sense of energy.
Perform activities of daily living (ADLs) and participate in desired activities at level of ability.

ACTIONS/INTERVENTIONS	RATIONALE
Energy Management (NIC)	
Independent	
Encourage bedrest and chair (recliner) rest during toxic state. Provide quiet environment and limit visitors as needed.	Promotes rest and relaxation. Available energy is used for healing. Activity and an upright position are believed to decrease hepatic blood flow, which prevents optimal circulation to the liver cells.
Recommend changing position frequently. Model and instruct caregiver in good skin care.	Promotes optimal respiratory function and minimizes pressure areas to reduce risk of tissue breakdown.
Do necessary tasks quickly and at one time, as tolerated.	Allows for extended periods of uninterrupted rest.
Determine and prioritize role responsibilities, alternative providers and possible community resources available, such as Meals on Wheels and homemaker and housekeeper services.	Promotes problem-solving of most pressing needs of individual and family.
Identify energy-conserving techniques, such as sitting to shower and brush teeth, planning steps of activity so that all needed materials are at hand, and scheduling rest periods.	Helps minimize fatigue, allowing client to accomplish more and feel better about self.
Increase activity as tolerated. Demonstrate and perform range-of-motion (ROM) exercises.	Prolonged bedrest can be debilitating. This can be offset by limited activity alternating with rest periods.
Encourage and instruct in stress management techniques, such as progressive relaxation, visualization, and guided imagery, as desired. Discuss appropriate diversional activities, such as radio, TV, and reading.	Promotes relaxation and conserves energy, redirects attention, and may enhance coping.
Monitor for recurrence of anorexia and liver tenderness and enlargement.	Indicates lack of resolution or exacerbation of the disease, requiring further rest and change in therapeutic regimen.

(continues on page 440)

ACTIONS/INTERVENTIONS (continued)

Collaborative

Administer medications, as indicated, for example, sedatives and anti-anxiety agents, such as diazepam (Valium) and lorazepam (Ativan).

Monitor serial liver enzyme levels.

RATIONALE (continued)

Assists in managing required rest. *Note:* Use of certain medications such as prochlorperazine (Compazine) and chlorpromazine (Thorazine) is contraindicated because of hepatotoxic effects.

Aids in determining appropriate levels of activity because premature increase in activity potentiates risk of relapse.

NURSING DIAGNOSIS: imbalanced Nutrition: Less than Body Requirements

May be related to

Insufficient intake to meet metabolic demands—anorexia, nausea, vomiting

Altered absorption and metabolism of ingested foods—reduced peristalsis (visceral reflexes), bile stasis

Increased caloric needs, hypermetabolic state

Possibly evidenced by

Aversion to eating, lack of interest in food; altered taste sensation

Abdominal pain, cramping

Loss of weight, poor muscle tone

Desired Outcomes/Evaluation Criteria—Client Will

Treatment Behavior: Illness or Injury (NOC)

Initiate behaviors and lifestyle changes to regain or maintain appropriate weight.

Nutritional Status (NOC)

Demonstrate progressive weight gain toward goal with normalization of laboratory values and no signs of malnutrition.

ACTIONS/INTERVENTIONS

Weight Gain Assistance (NIC)

Independent

Monitor dietary intake and calorie count. Provide meals in several small feedings and offer largest meal at breakfast.

Encourage mouth care before meals.

Recommend eating in upright position.

Encourage intake of fruit juices, carbonated beverages, and hard candy throughout the day.

Collaborative

Consult with dietitian or nutritional support team to provide diet according to client's needs, with fat and protein intake as tolerated.

Monitor serum glucose, as indicated.

Administer medications, as indicated, for example:

Antiemetics, such as metoclopramide (Reglan) and trimethobenzamide (Tigan)

Antiulcer agents and antacids, such as lansoprazole (Prevacid), esomeprazole (Nexium), and magnesium hydroxide/aluminum hydroxide (Maalox, Mylanta)

Vitamins, such as B complex, C, and other dietary supplements, as indicated

Provide supplemental feedings, enteral or parenteral nutrition if needed.

RATIONALE

Large meals are difficult to manage when client is anorexic. Anorexia may also worsen during the day, making intake of food difficult later in the day.

Eliminating unpleasant taste may enhance appetite.

Reduces sensation of abdominal fullness and may enhance intake.

These supply extra calories and may be more easily digested and tolerated than other fluids and foods.

Useful in formulating dietary program to meet individual needs. Fat metabolism varies according to bile production and excretion and may necessitate restriction of fat intake if diarrhea develops. If tolerated, a normal or increased protein intake helps with liver regeneration. Protein restriction may be indicated in severe disease, such as fulminating hepatitis, because the accumulation of the end products of protein metabolism can potentiate hepatic encephalopathy.

Hyperglycemia or hypoglycemia may develop, necessitating dietary changes or insulin administration. Fingerstick monitoring may be done by client on a regular schedule to determine therapy needs.

Given before meals these drugs may reduce nausea and increase food tolerance. *Note:* Prochlorperazine (Compazine) is contraindicated in hepatic disease.

Counteracts gastric acidity, reducing irritation and risk of bleeding.

Corrects deficiencies and aids in the healing process.

May be necessary to meet nutrient requirements if marked deficits are present and intestinal symptoms are prolonged.

NURSING DIAGNOSIS: **risk for deficient Fluid Volume/Bleeding**

Risk factors may include
Excessive losses through vomiting and diarrhea, third-space shift
Altered clotting process

Possibly evidenced by
(Not applicable; presence of signs and symptoms establishes an *actual* diagnosis)

Desired Outcomes/Evaluation Criteria—Client Will

Hydration (NOC)
Maintain adequate hydration, as evidenced by stable vital signs, good skin turgor, capillary refill, strong peripheral pulses, and individually appropriate urinary output.

Coagulation Status (NOC)
Be free of signs of hemorrhage with clotting times WNL.

ACTIONS/INTERVENTIONS	RATIONALE
Fluid/Electrolyte Management (NIC)	
Independent	
Monitor intake and output (I&O) and compare with periodic weight. Note enteric losses, such as vomiting and diarrhea.	Provides information about replacement needs and effects of therapy. *Note:* Diarrhea may be due to transient flulike response to viral infection or may represent a more serious problem of obstructed portal blood flow with vascular congestion in the gastrointestinal (GI) tract. Or, it may be the intended result of medication use, such as neomycin or lactulose, to decrease serum ammonia levels in the presence of hepatic encephalopathy.
Assess vital signs, peripheral pulses, capillary refill, skin turgor, and mucous membranes.	Indicators of circulating volume and perfusion.
Bleeding Precautions (NIC)	
Check for ascites for edema formation. Measure abdominal girth, as indicated.	Useful in monitoring progression and resolution of fluid shifts associated with edema and ascites.
Use small-gauge needles for injections, applying pressure for longer than usual after venipuncture.	Reduces possibility of bleeding into tissues.
Have client use cotton or sponge swabs and alcohol-free mouthwash instead of toothbrush.	Avoids trauma and bleeding of the gums. *Note:* Alcohol-based mouthwash may be irritating to dry mucosa.
Observe for signs of bleeding—hematuria and melena, ecchymosis, and oozing from gums or puncture sites.	Prothrombin levels are reduced and coagulation times prolonged when vitamin K absorption is altered in GI tract, and synthesis of prothrombin is decreased in affected liver.
Fluid/Electrolyte Management (NIC)	
Collaborative	
Monitor periodic laboratory values, such as Hgb/Hct, sodium, albumin, and clotting times.	Reflects hydration status and identifies sodium retention and protein deficits, which may lead to edema formation. Deficits in clotting potentiate risk of bleeding.
Administer antidiarrheal agents, such as diphenoxylate with atropine (Lomotil).	Reduces fluid and electrolyte loss from GI tract.
Provide intravenous (IV) fluids (usually glucose) and electrolytes:	Provides fluid and electrolyte replacement in acute toxic state.
Protein hydrolysates	Correction of albumin and protein deficits can aid in return of fluid from tissues to the circulatory system. May follow albumin administration with an IV diuretic to pull fluids from interstitial space into intravascular space to reduce ascites.
Bleeding Precautions (NIC)	
Administer medications, as indicated, for example:	
Vitamin K	Because absorption is altered, supplementation may prevent coagulation problems, which may occur if clotting factors are decreased.
Antacids or H$_2$-receptor antagonists, such as lansoprazole (Prevacid) and cimetidine (Tagamet).	Neutralizes or reduces gastric secretions to lower risk of gastric irritation and bleeding.
Infuse fresh-frozen plasma (FFP), as indicated.	May be required to replace clotting factors in the presence of coagulation defects.

NURSING DIAGNOSIS: situational low Self-Esteem

May be related to
Annoying, debilitating symptoms; confinement or isolation; length of illness and recovery period

Possibly evidenced by
Verbalization of change in lifestyle, fear of rejection or reaction of others, negative feelings about body, feelings of helplessness
Depression, lack of follow-through, self-destructive behavior

Desired Outcomes/Evaluation Criteria—Client Will

Self-Esteem (NOC)
Verbalize feelings.
Identify methods for coping with negative perception of self.
Verbalize acceptance of self in situation, including length of recovery and need for isolation.
Acknowledge self as worthwhile; be responsible for self.

ACTIONS/INTERVENTIONS	RATIONALE
Self-Esteem Enhancement (NIC)	
Independent	
Contract with client regarding time for listening. Encourage discussion of feelings and concerns.	Establishing time enhances trusting relationship. Providing opportunity to express feelings allows client to feel more in control of the situation. Verbalization can decrease anxiety and depression and facilitate positive coping behaviors. Client may need to express feelings about being ill, length and cost of illness, possibility of infecting others, and (in severe illness) fear of death. May have concerns regarding the stigma of the disease.
Avoid making moral judgments regarding lifestyle, such as alcohol use, drug abuse, and sexual practices.	Client may already feel upset or angry and condemn self; judgments from others will further damage self-esteem.
Discuss recovery expectations.	Recovery period may be prolonged (months), potentiating family and situational stress and necessitating need for planning, support, and follow-up.
Assess effect of illness on economic factors of client and significant other (SO).	Financial problems may exist because of loss of client's role functioning in the family and prolonged recovery.
Offer diversional activities based on energy level.	Enables client to use time and energy in constructive ways that enhance self-esteem and minimize anxiety and depression.
Suggest client wear bright reds or blues and blacks instead of yellows or greens.	Enhances appearance because yellow skin tones are intensified by yellow and green colors. *Note:* Jaundice usually peaks within 1 to 2 weeks, then gradually resolves over 2 to 4 weeks.
Collaborative	
Make appropriate referrals for help as needed, such as community case manager, social services, and other community agencies.	Can facilitate problem-solving and help involved individuals cope more effectively with situation.

NURSING DIAGNOSIS: risk for Infection [secondary/spread]

Risk factors may include
Inadequate secondary defenses—leukopenia, suppressed inflammatory response
Immunosuppression
Malnutrition
Insufficient knowledge to avoid exposure to pathogens

Possibly evidenced by
(Not applicable; presence of signs and symptoms establishes an *actual* diagnosis)

Desired Outcomes/Evaluation Criteria—Client Will

Risk Control (NOC)
Verbalize understanding of individual causative and risk factor(s).
Demonstrate techniques and initiate lifestyle changes to avoid reinfection and transmission to others.

ACTIONS/INTERVENTIONS	RATIONALE

Infection Control (NIC)

Independent

Establish isolation techniques for enteric and respiratory infections according to infection guidelines and policy. Model and emphasize need for effective hand washing.

Prevents transmission of viral disease to others. Thorough hand washing is effective in preventing virus transmission. HAV and HEV are transmitted by oral-fecal route and contaminated water, milk, and food, especially inadequately cooked shellfish. Types A, B, C, and D are transmitted by contaminated blood or blood products; needle punctures; open wounds; and contact with saliva, urine, stool, and semen. Incidence of both HBV and HCV has increased among healthcare providers and high-risk clients. *Note:* Toxic and alcoholic types of hepatitis are not communicable and do not require special measures or isolation.

Stress need to monitor and restrict visitors, as indicated.

Client exposure to infectious processes, especially respiratory, potentiates risk of secondary complications.

Explain isolation procedures to client and SO.

Understanding reasons for safeguarding themselves and others can lessen feelings of isolation and stigmatization. Isolation may last 2 to 3 weeks from onset of illness, depending on type and duration of symptoms.

Collaborative

Administer anti-infective medications, as appropriate.

Used to treat or limit secondary infections

NURSING DIAGNOSIS: **risk for impaired Skin/Tissue Integrity**

Risk factors may include
Chemical substance—bile salt accumulation in the tissues

Possibly evidenced by
(Not applicable; presence of signs and symptoms establishes an *actual* diagnosis)

Desired Outcomes/Evaluation Criteria—Client Will

Tissue Integrity: Skin and Mucous Membranes (NOC)
Display intact skin and tissues free of excoriation.
Report absence or decrease of pruritus and scratching.

ACTIONS/INTERVENTIONS	RATIONALE

Skin Surveillance (NIC)

Independent

Encourage use of cool showers and baking soda or starch baths. Avoid use of alkaline soaps. Apply calamine lotion, as indicated.

Prevents excessive dryness of skin. Provides relief from itching associated with accumulation of bile salts in jaundiced skin.

Provide diversional activities.

Aids in refocusing attention and reducing tendency to scratch.

Suggest use of knuckles if desire to scratch is uncontrollable. Keep fingernails cut short and apply gloves on comatose client or during hours of sleep. Recommend wearing loose-fitting clothing. Provide soft cotton linens.

Reduces potential for dermal injury.

Provide a soothing massage at bedtime.

May be helpful in promoting sleep by reducing skin irritation.

Observe skin for areas of redness and breakdown.

Early detection of problem areas allows for additional intervention to prevent complications and promote healing.

Avoid comments regarding client's appearance.

Minimizes psychological stress associated with skin changes.

Collaborative

Administer medications, as indicated, for example:
Antihistamines, such as diphenhydramine (Benadryl) and azatadine (Optimine)

Relieves itching. *Note:* Use cautiously in severe hepatic disease.

Antilipemic, such as cholestyramine (Questran)

May be used to bind bile acids in the intestine and prevent their absorption. Note side effects of nausea and constipation.

443

deficient Knowledge [Learning Need] regarding condition, prognosis, treatment, self-care, and discharge Needs

May be related to
Lack of exposure or recall, information misinterpretation
Unfamiliarity with resources

Possibly evidenced by
Questions or statements of misconception, request for information
Inaccurate follow-through of instructions, development of preventable complications

Desired Outcomes/Evaluation Criteria—Client Will

Knowledge: Illness Care (NOC)
Verbalize understanding of disease process, prognosis, and potential complications.
Identify relationship of signs and symptoms to the disease and correlate symptoms with causative factors.
Verbalize understanding of therapeutic needs.
Initiate necessary lifestyle changes and participate in treatment regimen.

ACTIONS/INTERVENTIONS	RATIONALE
Teaching: Disease Process (NIC) *Independent* Assess level of understanding of the disease process, prognosis, and possible treatment options.	Identifies areas of lack of knowledge or misinformation and provides opportunity to give additional information as necessary. *Note:* Liver transplantation may be needed in the presence of fulminating disease with liver failure.
Provide specific information regarding prevention and transmission of disease: for example, contacts may require gamma globulin; personal items should not be shared; and observe strict hand washing and sanitizing of clothes, dishes, and toilet facilities while liver enzymes are elevated. Avoid intimate contact, such as kissing and sexual contact, and exposure to infections, especially respiratory infections.	Needs vary with type of hepatitis, causative agent, and individual situation.
Plan resumption of activity, as tolerated, with adequate periods of rest. Discuss restriction of heavy lifting, strenuous exercise, and contact sports.	It is not necessary to wait until serum bilirubin levels return to normal, which may take as long as 2 months, to resume activity. Strenuous activity needs to be limited until the liver returns to normal size. When client begins to feel better, he or she needs to understand the importance of continued adequate rest in preventing relapse or recurrence.
Help client identify appropriate diversional activities.	Enjoyable activities promote rest and help client avoid focusing on prolonged convalescence.
Encourage continuation of balanced diet.	Promotes general well-being and enhances energy for healing process and tissue regeneration.
Identify ways to maintain usual bowel function, such as adequate intake of fluids and dietary roughage and moderate exercise to tolerance.	Decreased level of activity, changes in food and fluid intake, and slowed bowel motility may result in constipation.
Discuss the side effects and dangers of taking OTC and certain prescribed drugs that are known to have adverse effects on the liver. Advise client to notify pharmacists and all future healthcare providers of diagnosis.	Some drugs are toxic to the liver; many others are metabolized by the liver and should be avoided in severe liver diseases because they may cause cumulative toxic effects or chronic hepatitis.
Discuss restrictions on donating blood.	Prevents spread of infectious disease. Most state laws prevent accepting as donors those who have a history of any type of hepatitis.
Emphasize importance of follow-up physical examination and laboratory evaluation.	Disease process may take several months to resolve. If symptoms persist longer than 6 months, liver biopsy may be required to verify presence of chronic hepatitis.
Discuss need for immunizations.	Recovery from hepatitis A and B results in protective antibodies in the client, so he or she will not get those strains again. There is currently no vaccine available against HCV. However, people should be vaccinated against HAV and HBV. Guidelines include everyone under the age of 18 years, individuals exposed to blood and body fluids or sharing a household with an infected person, people traveling to areas where infection rates are known to be high, men who have sex with men, illicit injection drug users, and persons receiving hemodialysis or who have clotting disorders or liver disease.

ACTIONS/INTERVENTIONS (continued)

Give information regarding availability of gamma globulin, immune serum globulin (ISG), hepatitis immune globulin (H-BIG), HBV vaccine (Recombivax HB, Engerix-B) through health department or family physician.

Review necessity of avoidance of alcohol, illicit drugs, and tobacco.

Refer to community resources and drug and alcohol treatment program, as indicated.

RATIONALE (continued)

Immune globulins may be effective in preventing viral hepatitis in those who have been exposed, depending on type of hepatitis and period of incubation.

These substances increase hepatic irritation, and interfere with recovery.

May need additional assistance to withdraw from substance and maintain abstinence to avoid further liver damage.

POTENTIAL CONSIDERATIONS following acute hospitalization (dependent on client's age, physical condition and presence of complications, personal resources, and life responsibilities)

- *Fatigue*—generalized weakness, decreased strength and endurance, pain, imposed activity restrictions, depression
- *impaired Home Maintenance*—prolonged recovery and chronic condition, insufficient finances, inadequate support systems, unfamiliarity with neighborhood resources
- *imbalanced Nutrition: Less than Body Requirements*—insufficient intake to meet metabolic demands: anorexia, nausea and vomiting; altered absorption and metabolism of ingested foods; increased calorie needs and hypermetabolic state
- *risk for Infection*—inadequate secondary defenses; malnutrition; insufficient knowledge to avoid exposure to pathogens
- *risk for impaired Liver Function*—viral infection, comorbidities, continued drug or alcohol use, tissue necrosis

CIRRHOSIS OF THE LIVER

I. Pathophysiology (Murphy, 2006)
a. Alteration in structure and degenerative changes resulting from buildup of diffuse bands of fibrotic connective tissue causing widespread destruction of hepatic cells, impairing liver function, and impeding blood flow through the liver
b. Compensated cirrhosis: Liver function may continue for some time, even with significant scarring, but metabolic abnormalities can occur, such as coagulation defects and malnutrition.
c. Decompensated cirrhosis: progression of failure with significant complications, such as portal hypertension with bleeding varices, ascites, peritonitis, hepatorenal syndrome, and encephalopathy

II. Etiology
a. Rate of progression of fibrosis to cirrhosis varies for unknown reasons.
b. Multiple causation (Wolf, 2007)
  i. Hepatitis C (26%), B, and D (15%)
  ii. Alcoholic liver disease (21%)
  iii. Cholestatic diseases: biliary atresia, primary biliary cirrhosis, cystic fibrosis, primary sclerosing cholangitis

  iv. Miscellaneous liver disorders, including autoimmune, Wilson's disease, alpha$_1$-antitrypsin deficiency, hemochromatosis
  v. Injury from trauma, drugs, or other environmental toxins

III. Treatment
a. Goals are to slow the progression of the disease and alleviate the symptoms.
b. Liver transplantation is currently the only life-saving procedure for end-stage disease.

IV. Statistics
a. Morbidity: In 2005, 112,000 hospitalizations for chronic liver disease or cirrhosis; approximately 17,000 individuals awaiting liver transplant (Scientific Registry of Transplant Recipients [SRTR], 2007).
b. Mortality: Approximately 35,000 deaths annually due to chronic liver disease and cirrhosis (Wolf, 2007); in 2005, cirrhosis and other liver disorders were listed as the 12th leading cause of death in the United States (Hsiang-Ching, 2008).

GLOSSARY

Ascites: Buildup of fluid in the abdomen, due to a number of conditions including severe liver disease.
Asterixis: Involuntary jerking movements of hands and feet associated with hepatic encephalopathy.
Ecchymosis: Skin discoloration consisting of a large, irregularly formed hemorrhagic area with colors

changing from blue-black to greenish-brown or yellow; commonly referred to as a bruise.
Fetor hepaticus: Particularly foul-smelling breath, which frequently precedes hepatic coma.
Hematemesis: Bloody vomitus.

(text continues on page 446)

Hepatic encephalopathy: Brain dysfunction directly due to liver dysfunction seen in advanced cirrhosis, resulting in disturbances of consciousness and progressing to coma.

Hepatomegaly: Enlarged liver.

Hepatorenal syndrome: Represents a continuum of kidney dysfunction observed in individuals with cirrhosis caused by the vasoconstriction of large and small renal arteries.

Jaundice: Yellow staining of the skin and sclerae (and sometimes other tissues and body fluids) because of abnormally high blood levels of bilirubin.

Melena: Bloody stools.

Oliguria: Urinary output less than 400 mL/day.

Palmar erythema: Redness of the palms of the hands caused by dilation and congestion of capillaries.

Peritoneovenous shunt: Surgically implanted device for continuous draining of ascitic fluid into the venous system. Fluid is removed via a pressure-sensitive one-way valve. It is connected to a tube under the subcutaneous tissue of the chest wall to the neck, where it enters the internal jugular vein and terminates in the superior vena cava.

Petechiae: Tiny red dots on the skin caused by minute hemorrhage, indicating low platelet count or other blood disorder.

Spider angiomas: Abnormal collection of blood vessels near the surface of the skin; can occur anywhere, but are most common on the face and trunk.

Splenomegaly: Enlarged spleen.

Telangiectasis: Visibly dilated blood vessel on the skin or mucosal surface.

Care Setting

Client may be hospitalized on a medical unit during initial or recurrent acute episodes with potentially life-threatening complications. Otherwise, this condition is managed at the community, outpatient level.

Related Concerns

Alcohol: acute withdrawal, page 819

Substance dependence/abuse rehabilitation, page 835

Fluid and electrolyte imbalances, page 903

Psychosocial aspects of care, page 749

Renal dialysis—general considerations, page 560

Renal failure: acute, page 536

Total nutritional support: parenteral/enteral feeding, page 469

Upper gastrointestinal/esophageal bleeding, page 306

Client Assessment Database

Data depend on underlying cause of the condition.

DIAGNOSTIC DIVISION MAY REPORT	MAY EXHIBIT
ACTIVITY/REST • Weakness • Fatigue, exhaustion	• Lethargy • Decreased muscle mass and tone
CIRCULATION • History of or recent onset of heart failure (HF), pericarditis, rheumatic heart disease, or cancer, causing liver impairment leading to failure • Easy bruising, nosebleeds, bleeding gums	• Hypertension or hypotension (fluid shifts) • Dysrhythmias, extra heart sounds—S_3, S_4 • Jugular vein distention (JVD), distended abdominal veins, spider angiomas, collateral circulation • Ecchymosis, petechiae • Anemia, leukopenia, thromboctyopenia, coagulation disorders, splenomegaly
ELIMINATION • Flatulence • Diarrhea or constipation • Gradual abdominal enlargement	• Abdominal distention (hepatomegaly, splenomegaly, ascites) • Decreased or absent bowel sounds • Clay-colored stools, melena • Hemorrhoidal varices • Dark, concentrated urine; oliguria (hepatorenal syndrome, failure)

Client Assessment Database (continued)

DIAGNOSTIC DIVISION MAY REPORT (continued)	MAY EXHIBIT (continued)
FOOD/FLUID • Anorexia • Food intolerance, ingestion • Nausea, vomiting • Hematemesis	• Weight loss or gain (fluid) • Tissue wasting, delayed wound healing • Edema generalized in tissues • Dry skin, poor turgor • Halitosis or fetor hepaticus, bleeding gums • Hypoalbuminemia
NEUROSENSORY • Significant other (SO)/family may report personality changes, depressed mentation	• Changes in mentation, confusion, hallucinations, coma • Slowed, slurred speech • Asterixis
PAIN/DISCOMFORT • Abdominal tenderness and right upper quandrant (RUQ) pain • Severe itching • Pins-and-needles sensation, burning pain in extremities (peripheral neuropathy)	• Guarding or distraction behaviors • Self-focus
RESPIRATION • Dyspnea	• Tachypnea, shallow respiration, adventitious breath sounds • Limited thoracic expansion because of ascites • Hypoxia
SAFETY • Itching, dryness of the skin (pruritus)	• Fever—more common in alcoholic cirrhosis • Jaundiced skin and sclera • Spider angiomas, telangiectasis • Palmar erythema • Confusion progressing to delirium and coma (hepatic encephalopathy) • Unsteady or shaky, jerking movements
SEXUALITY • Menstrual disorders (women) • Impotence (men)	• Testicular atrophy, gynecomastia, loss of hair—chest, underarm, pubic
TEACHING/LEARNING • History of long-term alcohol or injection drug use or abuse, alcoholic liver disease, use of drugs affecting liver function • History of biliary system disease, hepatitis, exposure to toxins, liver trauma	
DISCHARGE PLAN CONSIDERATIONS • May need assistance with self-care and other activities of daily living (ADLs), homemaking and maintenance tasks ▸ Refer to section at end of plan for postdischarge considerations.	

Diagnostic Studies

TEST WHY IT IS DONE	WHAT IT TELLS ME
BLOOD TESTS • *Serum bilirubin (total and indirect unconjugated):* Bilirubin results from the breakdown of hemoglobin.	Elevated because of cellular disruption, or biliary obstruction, causing jaundice.

(continues on page 448)

TEST WHY IT IS DONE (continued)	WHAT IT TELLS ME (continued)

- *Liver enzymes:*
  - *Aspartate aminotransferase/alanine aminotransferase (AST/ALT), lactate dehydrogenase (LDH), and isoenzymes (LDH$_5$):* Detects liver damage.

  Increased because of cellular damage and release of enzymes. Most specific indicator of hepatitis as cause (Murphy, 2006).

  - *Alkaline phosphatase (ALP) and isoenzyme (APL$_1$):* Enzyme found in high concentration in the liver cells forming the bile ducts as well as in other tissues. APL$_1$ is more specific to the liver and helpful in determining type and extent of cirrhosis.

  Elevated in biliary obstruction.

- *Gamma glutamyl transpeptidase (GGTP):* Screens for liver disease and alcohol abuse.

  Level is elevated.

- *Serum albumin:* Protein of the highest concentration in plasma. Transports substances, such as bilirubin, calcium, progesterone, and drugs, and regulates osmotic pressure of blood, keeping fluid from leaking out into the tissues.

  Because albumin is made by the liver, decreased serum albumin may result from liver disease. Decreased albumin may also be explained by malnutrition or a low-protein diet.

- *Immunoglobulin (Ig) A, G, and M:* Proteins found in blood or other bodily fluids used by the immune system to identify and neutralize foreign objects, such as bacteria and viruses.

  Levels are increased.

- *Complete blood count (CBC):* Battery of screening tests, which typically includes hemoglobin (Hgb); hematocrit (Hct); red blood cell (RBC) count, morphology, indices, and distribution width index; platelet count and size; white blood cell (WBC) count and differential.

  Hb, Hct, and RBCs may be decreased because of bleeding and RBC destruction. Anemia is seen with hypersplenism and iron deficiency. Leukopenia may be present as a result of hypersplenism.

- *Bleeding/clotting:*
  - *Prothrombin time (PT):* Measures length of time required for blood sample to clot.

  Prolonged because of decreased production of clotting proteins and fat-soluble vitamin K deficiency, leading to easy bleeding.

  - *Fibrinogen and other clotting factors:* Used to monitor the progression of liver disease over time.

  Decreased; chronically low levels seen in end-stage liver disease.

- *Blood urea nitrogen (BUN):* Urea is the end product of protein metabolism formed in the liver from amino acids and from ammonia compounds.

  Elevation indicates breakdown of blood proteins and possible kidney dysfunction because of diuretic use in treatment of ascites.

- *Serum ammonia:* Product of breakdown of protein, which is normally converted to urea and excreted.

  Elevated because of inability to convert ammonia to urea.

- *Serum glucose:* One of the simple sugars in the blood, which serves as primary energy source for cells.

  Low blood glucose (hypoglycemia) suggests impaired synthesis of glycogen from glucose (glycogenesis).

- *Electrolytes:* Substances that dissociate into ions in solution and acquire the capacity to conduct electricity. Common electrolytes include sodium, potassium, chloride, calcium, and phosphate.

  Low potassium (hypokalemia) may reflect increased aldosterone, although various imbalances may occur. Low calcium (hypocalcemia) may occur because of impaired absorption of vitamin D.

- *Nutrient studies:* Evaluate nutritional status.

  Deficiency of vitamins A, B$_{12}$, C, and K; folic acid; and iron may be noted.

- *Viral tests:* Determine if cirrhosis is caused by viral hepatitis.

  Hepatitis B, C, or D may be present.

OTHER DIAGNOSTIC STUDIES

- *Abdominal ultrasonography with Doppler:* Diagnostic technique that uses sound waves to produce an image of internal body structures.

  May be first assessment performed in individual with suspected liver disease to detect ascites and enlarged liver and spleen. It can also identify biliary duct obstruction or bile stones. Nodularity, irregularity, and atrophy are ultrasonographic hallmarks of cirrhosis. In advanced disease, the gross liver appears small and multinodular, ascites may be detected, and Doppler flow can be significantly decreased in the portal circulation.

- *Liver biopsy:* Biopsy can be performed via percutaneous, transjugular, laparoscopic, open operative, or computed tomography (CT)-guided fine-needle approaches. Samples are obtained for microscopic evaluation.

  Detects fatty infiltrates, fibrosis, destruction of hepatic tissues, tumors (primary or metastatic), and associated ascites.

TEST WHY IT IS DONE (continued)	WHAT IT TELLS ME (continued)
• *Percutaneous transhepatic cholangiography (PTHC):* X-ray procedure where dye is injected directly into the drainage system of the liver. If necessary, a catheter may be inserted to allow the bile to drain into a collection bag outside the body or into the small intestine.	Shows whether there is a blockage in the liver or the bile ducts that drain it. May be done to differentiate causes of jaundice or to perform biliary drainage.
• *Hepatobiliary iminodiacetic acid (HIDA) scan:* The client is given a radioactive tracer intravenously (IV) that is excreted by the liver into bile ducts.	Identifies blockages in the biliary system.
• *Urine and stool urobilinogen:* Serves as guide for differentiating liver disease, hemolytic disease, and biliary obstruction.	May or may not be present.

Nursing Priorities

1. Maintain adequate nutrition.
2. Prevent complications.
3. Enhance self-concept and acceptance of situation.
4. Provide information about disease process, prognosis, potential complications, and treatment needs.

Discharge Goals

1. Nutritional intake adequate for individual needs.
2. Complications prevented or minimized.
3. Deals effectively with current reality.
4. Disease process, prognosis, potential complications, and therapeutic regimen understood.
5. Plan in place to meet needs after discharge.

NURSING DIAGNOSIS: imbalanced Nutrition: Less than Body Requirements

May be related to
Inadequate diet; inability to process, digest nutrients
Anorexia, nausea, vomiting, indigestion, early satiety (ascites)
Abnormal bowel function

Possibly evidenced by
Weight loss
Changes in bowel sounds and function
Poor muscle tone, muscle wasting; fatigue
Imbalances in nutritional studies

Desired Outcomes/Evaluation Criteria—Client Will

Nutritional Status (NOC)
Demonstrate progressive weight gain toward goal with client-appropriate normalization of laboratory values.
Experience no further signs of malnutrition.

ACTIONS/INTERVENTIONS	RATIONALE
Nutrition Therapy (NIC) *Independent* Evaluate client's risk for malnutrition.	Eighty-five percent to 90% of the blood that leaves the stomach and intestines carries nutrients to the liver where they are converted into substances the body can use. The client with liver dysfunction often has malnutrition because of inadequate dietary intake due to poor food choices or preference for alcohol rather than food and may currently have malabsorption syndrome due to inability to process or digest nutrients, anorexia, nausea or vomiting, indigestion, or early satiety associated with ascites. Because of the decreased secretion of bile into the gut, client may have difficulty absorbing fat and fat-soluble vitamins A, D, E, and K. These deficiencies can lead to such complications as decreased vision in the dark, due to vitamin A deficiency; bone disease, due to vitamin D deficiency; neurological impairment, due to vitamin E deficiency; and decreased production of clotting proteins in the liver, due to vitamin K deficiency (Brettler, 2003).

(continues on page 450)

Determine interest in eating and ability to chew, swallow, and taste. Discuss eating habits, including food preferences, intolerances, or aversions. Note availability and use of support systems.

Factors that affect ingestion and digestion of nutrients.

Determine dietary intake and perform calorie count if client is eating.

Provides information about intake, needs, and deficiencies. Client with cirrhosis requires a balanced protein diet providing 2,000 to 3,000 calories per day to permit liver cell regeneration.

Weigh, as indicated. Compare changes in fluid status and recent weight history.

It may be difficult to use weight as a direct indicator of nutritional status in view of edema and ascites. *Note:* Undigested fat that passes into the large intestine can cause diarrhea and lead to weight loss (Brettler, 2003).

Assist or encourage client to eat; explain reasons for the types of diet. Feed client if tiring easily, or have SO assist client. Consider preferences in food choices.

Improved nutrition is vital to recovery. Client may eat better if family is involved and preferred foods are included as much as possible. Client and family must understand protein intake limitations and how best to meet needs and desires within limitations.

Encourage client to eat all meals and supplementary feedings.

Client may demonstrate loss of interest in food because of nausea, generalized weakness, and fatigue—which is often first reported symptom and seen in approximately 70% of clients with cirrhosis (Taylor, 2008).

Recommend or provide small, frequent meals.

Poor tolerance to larger meals may be due to increased intra-abdominal pressure or ascites.

Limit such high-salt foods as canned soups and vegetables, processed meats, and condiments. Provide salt substitutes if allowed, avoiding those containing ammonia.

Salt limitations can help manage fluid complications in cirrhosis, including ascites or tissue edema. Salt substitutes enhance the flavor of food and aid in increasing appetite; ammonia potentiates risk of encephalopathy.

Restrict intake of caffeine and gas-producing or spicy and excessively hot or cold foods.

Aids in reducing gastric irritation, diarrhea, and abdominal discomfort that may impair oral intake and digestion.

Encourage or provide frequent mouth care, especially before meals.

Client is prone to sore and bleeding gums and bad taste in mouth, which contributes to anorexia.

Provide assistance with activities as needed. Promote undisturbed rest periods, especially before meals.

Conserving energy reduces metabolic demands on the liver and promotes cellular regeneration.

Recommend cessation of smoking.

Reduces excessive gastric stimulation and risk of irritation and bleeding.

Collaborative

Monitor nutritional laboratory studies: serum glucose, prealbumin or albumin, total protein, and ammonia.

Glucose may be decreased because of impaired glycogenesis, depleted glycogen stores, or inadequate intake. Protein may be low because of impaired metabolism, decreased hepatic synthesis, or loss into peritoneal cavity (ascites). Protein-calorie malnutrition contributes to further development of fatty liver and deterioration of function. Elevation of ammonia level may require restriction of protein intake to prevent serious complications.

Maintain nothing by mouth (NPO) status, when indicated.

Gastrointestinal (GI) rest may be required in acutely ill clients to reduce demands on the liver and production of ammonia and urea in the GI tract. When this is the case, nutrition must be supplied by another method—enteral or parenteral feedings.

Determine nutritional and caloric needs using appropriate methods, such as total energy expenditure (TEE), body mass index (BMI), Harris-Benedict equation, or indirect calorimetry test, as indicated.

Identifies energy requirements and deficits. Skinfold measurements and indirect calorimetry are useful in assessing changes in muscle mass, energy expenditure, and subcutaneous fat reserves.

Consult with dietitian or nutritionist to provide diet that is high in calories and simple carbohydrates, low in fat, and low to moderate in protein. Limit sodium, as necessary. Provide liquid supplements, as indicated.

Because client's intake is usually limited, high-calorie foods are desired. Carbohydrates supply readily available energy. Fats are poorly absorbed because of liver dysfunction and may contribute to abdominal discomfort. Proteins are needed to improve serum protein levels, reducing edema and promoting liver cell regeneration. However, protein can also elevate ammonia levels and must be restricted if ammonia level is elevated or if client has clinical signs of hepatic encephalopathy. In addition, these individuals may tolerate vegetable protein better than meat protein.

Provide enteral tube feedings or total parenteral nutrition (TPN), if indicated.

May be required to supplement diet or to provide nutrients when client is too nauseated or anorexic to eat or when esophageal varices interfere with oral intake. (Refer to CP: Total Nutritional Support: Parenteral/Enteral Feedings.)

ACTIONS/INTERVENTIONS (continued)

Administer medications, as indicated, for example:
  Vitamin supplements (especially fat-soluble vitamins A, D, E, K) and B vitamins (thiamine, iron, folic acid)
  Zinc sulfate
  Digestive enzymes, such as pancrelipase (Niokase) and lactulose
  Antiemetics, such as trimethobenzamide (Tigan)

RATIONALE (continued)

Replacement required because of the inability of the liver to process or store vitamins.
Improves sense of taste and may enhance appetite.
May be tried to promote digestion of fats and reduce incidence of steatorrhea and diarrhea.
Used with caution to reduce nausea and vomiting and enhance oral intake.

NURSING DIAGNOSIS: **excess Fluid Volume**

May be related to
Compromised regulatory mechanism—syndrome of inappropriate antidiuretic hormone (SIADH), decreased plasma proteins, malnutrition
Excess sodium and fluid intake

Possibly evidenced by
Edema, anasarca, weight gain
Intake greater than output, oliguria, changes in urine specific gravity
Dyspnea, adventitious breath sounds, pleural effusion
Blood pressure (BP) changes, altered central venous pressure (CVP)
JVD, positive hepatojugular reflex
Altered electrolyte levels
Change in mental status

Desired Outcomes/Evaluation Criteria—Client Will

Fluid Balance (NOC)
Demonstrate stabilized fluid volume, with balanced intake and output (I&O), stable weight, vital signs within client's normal range, and absence of edema.

ACTIONS/INTERVENTIONS

RATIONALE

Fluid/Electrolyte Management (NIC)
Independent

Measure I&O, noting positive balance—intake in excess of output. Weigh daily, and note gain more than 0.5 kg/day.

Reflects circulating volume status, developing or resolving fluid shifts, and response to therapy. Positive fluid balance and weight gain often reflects continuing fluid retention. *Note:* Decreased circulating volume and fluid shifts can directly affect renal function and urine output, resulting in hepatorenal syndrome.

Monitor BP and CVP, if available. Note JVD and abdominal vein distention.

BP elevations are usually associated with fluid volume excess but may not occur because of fluid shifts out of the vascular space. JVD and presence of distended abdominal veins are associated with vascular congestion.

Assess respiratory status, noting increased respiratory rate and dyspnea.

Indicative of pulmonary congestion or edema.

Auscultate lungs, noting diminished or absent breath sounds and developing adventitious sounds—crackles.

Increasing pulmonary congestion may result in consolidation, impaired gas exchange, and complications, such as pulmonary edema.

Monitor for cardiac dysrhythmias. Auscultate heart sounds, noting development of S_3/S_4 gallop rhythm.

May be caused by HF, decreased coronary arterial perfusion, or electrolyte imbalance.

Assess degree of peripheral and dependent edema.

Fluids shift into tissues as a result of sodium and water retention, decreased albumin, and increased antidiuretic hormone (ADH).

Measure abdominal girth.

Reflects accumulation of fluid or ascites resulting from loss of plasma proteins and fluid into peritoneal space. *Note:* Excessive fluid accumulation can reduce circulating volume, resulting in hypotension and dehydration.

Encourage bedrest when ascites is present.

May promote recumbency-induced diuresis.

Provide frequent mouth care and occasional ice chips, particularly if NPO; schedule fluid intake around the clock.

Decreases sensation of thirst, especially when fluid intake is restricted.

(continues on page 452)

ACTIONS/INTERVENTIONS (continued)

Collaborative

Monitor serum albumin and electrolytes, particularly potassium and sodium.

Monitor serial chest x-rays.

Restrict sodium and fluids, as indicated.

Administer salt-free albumin and plasma expanders, as indicated.

Administer medications, as indicated, for example:
 Diuretics, such as spironolactone (Aldactone) and furosemide (Lasix)

 Potassium

 Positive inotropic drugs and arterial vasodilators

RATIONALE (continued)

Decreased serum albumin affects plasma colloid osmotic pressure, resulting in edema formation. Reduced renal blood flow, accompanied by elevated ADH and aldosterone levels and the use of diuretics to reduce total body water, may cause various electrolyte shifts and imbalances.

Vascular congestion, pulmonary edema, and pleural effusions frequently occur.

Sodium may be restricted to minimize fluid retention in extravascular spaces. Fluid restriction may be necessary to correct dilutional hyponatremia.

Albumin may be given to increase the colloid osmotic pressure in the vascular compartment, thereby increasing effective circulating volume and decreasing formation of ascites.

Used with caution to control edema and ascites, block effect of aldosterone, and increase water excretion while sparing potassium when conservative therapy with bedrest and sodium restriction do not alleviate problem. Diuretic given in coordination with albumin administration may enhance fluid removal.

Serum and cellular potassium are usually depleted because of liver disease and urinary losses.

Given to increase cardiac output and improve renal blood flow and function, thereby reducing excess fluid.

NURSING DIAGNOSIS: **risk for impaired Skin Integrity**

Risk factors may include

Altered circulation and metabolic state
Accumulation of bile salts in skin
Poor skin turgor, skeletal prominence, presence of edema, ascites

Possibly evidenced by

(Not applicable; presence of signs and symptoms establishes an *actual* diagnosis)

Desired Outcomes/Evaluation Criteria—Client Will

Risk Control (NOC)

Maintain skin integrity.
Identify individual risk factors and demonstrate behaviors or techniques to prevent skin breakdown.

ACTIONS/INTERVENTIONS

Skin Surveillance (NIC)
Independent

Discuss itching with client, addressing areas involved and time of day when client is most uncomfortable.

Inspect skin surfaces and pressure points routinely. Gently massage bony prominences or areas of continued stress. Use emollient lotions and limit use of soap for bathing.

Encourage and assist with repositioning on a regular schedule, while in bed or chair, and active or passive range-of-motion (ROM) exercises, as appropriate.

Recommend elevating lower extremities.

Keep linens dry and free of wrinkles.

Suggest clipping fingernails short and provide mittens or gloves, if indicated.

RATIONALE

Pruritus affects about two-thirds of clients with primary biliary cirrhosis; the cause is unknown. The itching often worsens during the evening and improves during the day. It typically begins in the palms and soles, and then spreads to the rest of the body. Prolonged, repeated scratching can result in excoriations and thickening and darkening of the skin (Heathcote, 2000).

Edematous tissues are more prone to breakdown and to the formation of decubitus ulcers. Ascites may stretch the skin to the point of tearing in severe cirrhosis.

Repositioning reduces pressure on edematous tissues to improve circulation. Exercises enhance circulation and improve or maintain joint mobility.

Enhances venous return and reduces edema formation in extremities.

Moisture aggravates pruritus and increases risk of skin breakdown.

Prevents client from inadvertently injuring the skin, especially while sleeping.

ACTIONS/INTERVENTIONS (continued)	RATIONALE (continued)
Encourage, or provide, perineal care following urination and bowel movement.	Prevents skin excoriation breakdown from bile salts.
Collaborative	
Use alternating pressure mattress, egg-crate or foam mattress, waterbed, or sheepskins, as indicated.	Reduces dermal pressure, increases circulation, and diminishes risk of tissue ischemia and breakdown.
Apply calamine lotion and provide baking soda baths.	May be soothing and provide relief of itching.
Administer medications, such as cholestyramine (Questran), colestipol (Colestid), hydroxyzine (Atarax), and dronabinol (Marinol), if indicated.	Although the cause of pruritus is unknown, it may be associated with jaundice or bile salts in skin and may respond to these treatments.

NURSING DIAGNOSIS: risk for ineffective Breathing Pattern

Risk factors may include
Intra-abdominal fluid collection (ascites)
Decreased lung expansion, accumulated secretions
Decreased energy, fatigue

Possibly evidenced by
(Not applicable; presence of signs and symptoms establishes an *actual* diagnosis)

Desired Outcomes/Evaluation Criteria—Client Will

Respiratory Status: Ventilation (NOC)
Maintain effective respiratory pattern and be free of dyspnea and cyanosis, with arterial blood gases (ABGs) and vital capacity within acceptable range.

ACTIONS/INTERVENTIONS	RATIONALE
Ventilation Assistance (NIC)	
Independent	
Monitor respiratory rate, depth, and effort.	Rapid, shallow respirations or dyspnea may be present because of hypoxia or fluid accumulation in abdomen.
Auscultate breath sounds, noting crackles, wheezes, and rhonchi.	Indicates developing complications—presence of adventitious sounds reflects accumulation of fluid while diminished sounds suggest atelectasis—increasing risk of pulmonary infection.
Investigate changes in level of consciousness (LOC).	Changes in mentation may reflect hypoxemia and respiratory failure, which often accompany hepatic coma.
Keep head of bed elevated. Position client on side.	Facilitates breathing by reducing pressure on the diaphragm and minimizes risk of aspiration of secretions.
Encourage frequent repositioning, deep-breathing exercises, and coughing, as appropriate.	Aids in lung expansion and mobilizing secretions.
Monitor temperature. Note presence of chills, increased coughing, and changes in color or character of sputum.	Indicative of onset of infection, such as pneumonia.
Collaborative	
Monitor serial ABGs, pulse oximetry, vital capacity measurements, and chest x-rays.	Reveals changes in respiratory status and developing pulmonary complications.
Provide supplemental oxygen (O$_2$) as indicated.	May be necessary to treat or prevent hypoxia. If respirations or oxygenation are inadequate, mechanical ventilation may be required.
Demonstrate and assist with respiratory adjuncts, such as incentive spirometer.	Reduces incidence of atelectasis and enhances mobilization of secretions.
Prepare for and assist with acute care procedures, such as: Paracentesis	Occasionally done to remove ascites fluid to relieve abdominal pressure when respiratory embarrassment is not corrected by other measures.
Peritoneovenous shunt	Surgical implant of a catheter to return accumulated fluid in the abdominal cavity to systemic circulation via the vena cava; provides long-term relief of ascites and improvement in respiratory function.

NURSING DIAGNOSIS: risk for Bleeding

Risk factors may include

Abnormal blood profile; altered clotting factors—decreased production of prothrombin, fibrinogen, and factors VIII, IX, and X; impaired vitamin K absorption; and release of thromboplastin

Portal hypertension, development of esophageal varices

Possibly evidenced by

(Not applicable; presence of signs and symptoms establishes an *actual* diagnosis)

Desired Outcomes/Evaluation Criteria—Client Will

Coagulation Status (NOC)

Maintain homeostasis with absence of bleeding.

Risk Control (NOC)

Demonstrate behaviors to reduce risk of bleeding.

ACTIONS/INTERVENTIONS	RATIONALE
Bleeding Precautions (NIC)	
Independent	
Assess for signs and symptoms of GI bleeding; for instance, check all secretions for frank or occult blood. Observe color and consistency of stools, nasogastric (NG) drainage, or vomitus.	The GI tract—esophagus and rectum—is the most usual source of bleeding because of its mucosal fragility and alterations in homeostasis associated with cirrhosis.
Observe for presence of petechiae, ecchymosis, and bleeding from one or more sites.	Subacute disseminated intravascular coagulation (DIC) may develop secondary to altered clotting factors.
Monitor pulse, BP, and CVP, if available.	An increased pulse with decreased BP and CVP may indicate loss of circulating blood volume, requiring further evaluation.
Note changes in mentation and LOC.	Changes may indicate decreased cerebral perfusion secondary to hypovolemia or hypoxemia.
Avoid rectal temperature; be gentle with GI tube insertions.	Rectal and esophageal vessels are most vulnerable to rupture.
Encourage use of soft toothbrush and electric razor, avoiding straining for stool, forceful nose blowing, and so forth.	In the presence of clotting factor disturbances, minimal trauma can cause mucosal bleeding.
Use small needles for injections. Apply pressure to small bleeding or venipuncture sites for longer than usual.	Minimizes damage to tissues, reducing risk of bleeding and hematoma.
Recommend avoidance of aspirin-containing products.	Prolongs coagulation, potentiating risk of hemorrhage.
Collaborative	
Monitor Hgb and Hct, platelets, and clotting factors.	Indicators of anemia, active bleeding, or impending complications, such as DIC.
Administer medications, as indicated, for example: Supplemental vitamins, such as vitamins K, D, and C	Promotes prothrombin synthesis and coagulation, if liver is functional. Vitamin C deficiencies increase susceptibility of GI system to irritation and bleeding.
Stool softeners	Prevents straining for stool with resultant increase in intra-abdominal pressure and risk of bleeding hemorrhoidal varices, especially when client has portal hypertension.
Provide gastric lavage with cool saline solution or water, as indicated.	In presence of acute bleeding, evacuation of blood from GI tract may reduce ammonia production and risk of hepatic encephalopathy. (Refer to CP: Upper Gastrointestinal/Esophageal Bleeding.)
Assist with insertion and maintenance of intestinal or esophageal tube, such as Sengstaken-Blakemore tube.	Temporarily controls bleeding of esophageal varices by balloon tamponade when control by other means, such as lavage, and hemodynamic stability cannot be achieved.
Prepare for procedures, such as direct ligation or banding of varices, esophagogastric resection, transjugular intrahepatic portosystemic shunt (TIPS), and splenorenal-portacaval anastomosis.	May be needed to control active hemorrhage or to decrease portal and collateral blood vessel pressure to minimize risk of recurrence of bleeding. TIPS is a nonsurgical procedure to relieve portal hypertension and decompress varices by creating a shunt between the systemic and portal venous systems to redirect portal blood flow.

NURSING DIAGNOSIS: risk for acute Confusion

Risk factors may include
Alcohol abuse
Inability of liver to detoxify certain enzymes and drugs

Possibly evidenced by
(Not applicable; presence of signs and symptoms establishes an *actual* diagnosis)

Desired Outcomes/Evaluation Criteria—Client Will

Cognition (NOC)
Maintain usual level of mentation and reality orientation.
Initiate behaviors or lifestyle changes to prevent or minimize recurrence of problem.

ACTIONS/INTERVENTIONS	RATIONALE
Reality Orientation (NIC)	
Independent	
Observe for changes in behavior and mentation: lethargy, confusion, drowsiness, slowing or slurring of speech, and irritability. Arouse client at intervals, as indicated.	Ongoing assessment of behavior and mental status is important because of fluctuating nature of hepatic encephalopathy or impending hepatic coma.
Review current medication regimen.	Adverse drug reactions or interactions may potentiate or exacerbate confusion.
Evaluate sleep and rest schedule.	Difficulty falling asleep or staying asleep leads to sleep deprivation, exacerbating cognition problems and fatigue.
Note development or presence of asterixis, fetor hepaticus, and seizure activity.	Suggests elevating serum ammonia levels and increased risk of progression to encephalopathy.
Consult with SO about client's usual behavior and mentation.	Provides baseline for comparison of current status.
Have client write name periodically and keep this record for comparison. Report deterioration of ability. Have client do simple arithmetic computations.	Easy test of neurological status and muscle coordination.
Reorient to time, place, person, and situation, as needed.	Assists in maintaining reality orientation, reducing confusion and anxiety.
Maintain a pleasant, quiet environment and approach in a slow, calm manner. Encourage uninterrupted rest periods.	Reduces excessive stimulation and sensory overload, promotes relaxation, and may enhance coping.
Provide continuity of care. If possible, assign same nurse over a period of time.	Familiarity provides reassurance, aids in reducing anxiety, and provides a more accurate documentation of subtle changes.
Reduce provocative stimuli and confrontation. Refrain from forcing activities. Assess potential for violent behavior.	Avoids triggering agitated, violent responses; promotes client safety.
Discuss current situation and future expectations.	Client and SO may be reassured that intellectual as well as emotional function may improve as liver involvement resolves.
Maintain bedrest and assist with self-care activities.	Reduces metabolic demands on liver, prevents fatigue, and promotes healing, lowering risk of ammonia buildup.
Identify and provide for safety needs, such as supervision during smoking, bed in low position, side rails up, and pad, if necessary. Provide close supervision.	Reduces risk of injury when confusion, seizures, or violent behavior occurs.
Investigate temperature elevations. Monitor for signs of infection.	Infection may precipitate hepatic encephalopathy caused by tissue catabolism and release of nitrogen.
Recommend avoidance of narcotics or sedatives, anti-anxiety agents, and limiting or restricting use of medications metabolized by the liver.	Certain drugs are toxic to the liver, whereas other drugs may not be metabolized because of cirrhosis, causing cumulative effects that affect mentation, mask signs of developing encephalopathy, or precipitate coma.
Collaborative	
Monitor laboratory studies, such as ammonia, electrolytes, pH, blood urea nitrogen (BUN), glucose, and CBC with differential.	Elevated ammonia levels, hypokalemia, metabolic alkalosis, hypoglycemia, anemia, and infection can precipitate or potentiate development of hepatic coma.
Eliminate or restrict protein in diet. Provide glucose supplements and adequate hydration.	Ammonia is responsible for mental changes in hepatic encephalopathy. Dietary changes may result in constipation, which also increases bacterial action and formation of ammonia. Glucose provides a source of energy, reducing need for protein catabolism.
Administer medications, as indicated, for example:	
Ursodeoxycholic acid (urosodiol, UDCA, Actigall)	Major medication used to slow the progression of the disease; may delay need for transplantation.

(continues on page 456)

Immunosuppressive agents, such as corticosteroids (Prednisolone, DeltaCortef), methotrexate (Rheumatrex/Folex), and cyclosporine (Sandimmune/Neoral); anti-inflammatory agents, such as colchicines	These agents may inhibit immune reactions that mediate inflammatory processes and progression of the disease.
Electrolytes	Corrects imbalances and may improve cerebral function and metabolism of ammonia.
Stool softeners, colonic purges such as magnesium sulfate, enemas, and lactulose	Removes protein and blood from intestines. Acidifying the intestine produces diarrhea and decreases production of nitrogenous substances, reducing risk or severity of encephalopathy. *Note:* Long-term use of lactulose may be required for clients with hepatic encephalopathy to reduce ammonia on a daily or regular basis.
Bactericidal agents, such as neomycin (Mycifradin) and kanamycin (Kantrex)	Destroys intestinal bacteria, reducing production of ammonia, to prevent encephalopathy.
Administer supplemental O_2.	Mentation is affected by O_2 concentration and utilization in the brain.
Assist with procedures as indicated, such as dialysis, plasma-pheresis, or extracorporeal liver perfusion.	May be used to reduce serum ammonia levels if encephalopathy develops or other measures are not successful.

NURSING DIAGNOSIS: **Self-Esteem [specify]/disturbed Body Image**

May be related to
Biophysical changes, altered physical appearance
Uncertainty of prognosis, changes in role function
Personal vulnerability
Self-destructive behavior—alcohol-induced disease

Possibly evidenced by
Verbalization of change or restriction in lifestyle
Fear of rejection or reaction by others
Negative feelings about body and abilities
Feelings of helplessness, hopelessness, or powerlessness

Desired Outcomes/Evaluation Criteria—Client Will

Self-Esteem (NOC)
Verbalize understanding of changes and acceptance of self in the present situation.
Identify feelings and methods for coping with negative perception of self.

ACTIONS/INTERVENTIONS

RATIONALE

Self-Esteem Enhancement (NIC)
Independent

Discuss situation and encourage verbalization of fears and concerns. Explain relationship between nature of disease and symptoms.	Client is very sensitive to body changes and may also experience feelings of guilt when cause is related to alcohol or other drug use.
Support and encourage client; provide care with a positive, friendly attitude.	Caregivers sometimes allow judgmental feelings to affect the care of client and need to make every effort to help client feel valued as a person.
Encourage family/SO to verbalize feelings, visit freely, and participate in care.	Family/SO may feel guilty about client's condition and may be fearful of impending death. They need nonjudgmental emotional support and free access to client. Participation in care helps them feel useful and promotes trust between staff, client, and family/SO.
Assist client/SO to cope with change in appearance; suggest clothing that does not emphasize altered appearance, such as use of red, blue, or black clothing.	Client may present unattractive appearance as a result of jaundice, ascites, and ecchymotic areas. Providing support can enhance self-esteem and promote client's sense of control.

Collaborative

Refer to support services, such as counselors, psychiatric resources, social service, clergy, and alcohol treatment program.	Increased vulnerability and concerns associated with this illness may require services of additional professional resources.

deficient Knowledge [Learning Need] regarding condition, prognosis, treatment, self-care, and discharge needs

May be related to

Lack of exposure or recall; information misinterpretation

Unfamiliarity with information resources

Possibly evidenced by

Questions, request for information, statement of misconception

Inaccurate follow-through of instructions, development of preventable complications

Desired Outcomes/Evaluation Criteria—Client Will

Knowledge: Illness Care (NOC)

Verbalize understanding of disease process, prognosis, and potential complications.

Correlate symptoms with causative factors.

Knowledge: Health Behaviors (NOC)

Identify and initiate necessary lifestyle changes.

Actively participate in care.

ACTIONS/INTERVENTIONS	RATIONALE
Teaching: Disease Process (NIC)	
Independent	
Review disease process and future expectations.	Provides knowledge base from which client can make informed choices.
Emphasize importance of avoiding alcohol. Give information about medical and community services available to aid in alcohol rehabilitation, if indicated.	Alcohol is one of the leading causes for the development of cirrhosis.
Inform client of altered effects of medications with cirrhosis and the importance of using only drugs prescribed or cleared by a healthcare provider who is familiar with client's history.	Some drugs are hepatotoxic, especially opioids, sedatives, and hypnotics. In addition, the damaged liver has a reduced ability to metabolize all drugs, potentiating cumulative effect and aggravation of bleeding tendencies.
Review procedure for maintaining function of peritoneovenous shunt when present.	Several types of shunts are available, so it is important that client and SO understand care needed for client's shunt. For example, Denver shunt requires client to periodically pump the chamber to maintain patency of the device, and client with a LeVeen shunt may wear an abdominal binder or engage in a Valsalva's maneuver to maintain shunt function.
Assist client with identifying support person(s).	Because of length of recovery, potential for relapses, and slow convalescence, support systems are extremely important in maintaining behavior modifications.
Emphasize the importance of good nutrition. Recommend avoidance of high-protein and salty foods, onions, and strong cheeses. Provide written dietary instructions.	Proper dietary maintenance and avoidance of foods high in sodium and protein aid in remission of symptoms and help prevent ammonia buildup and further liver damage. Written instructions are helpful for client to refer to at home.
Stress necessity of follow-up care and adherence to therapeutic regimen.	Chronic nature of disease has potential for life-threatening complications. Provides opportunity for evaluation of effectiveness of regimen, including patency of shunt if used.
Discuss sodium and salt substitute restrictions and necessity of reading labels on food, OTC drugs, and herbal agents.	Minimizes ascites and edema formation. Overuse of substitutes may result in other electrolyte imbalances. Food, OTC medications, and personal care products, including antacids and some mouthwashes, may contain sodium or alcohol and may be toxic to the liver or be primarily metabolized by the liver.
Encourage scheduling activities with adequate rest periods.	Adequate rest decreases metabolic demands on the body and increases energy available for tissue regeneration.
Promote diversional activities that are enjoyable to client.	Prevents boredom, facilitates rest, and minimizes anxiety and depression.
Recommend avoidance of persons with infections, especially upper respiratory infections.	Decreased resistance, altered nutritional status, and impaired immune responses potentiate risk of infection.
Instruct client and SO of signs and symptoms that warrant notification of healthcare provider, such as increased abdominal girth, rapid weight loss or gain, increased peripheral edema, increased dyspnea, fever, blood in stool or urine, excess bleeding of any kind, and jaundice.	Prompt reporting of symptoms provides opportunity to treat complications before they become life-threatening. *Note:* Client may be evaluated for additional medical or surgical interventions, including liver transplantation.

(continues on page 458)

Instruct SO to notify healthcare providers of any confusion, untidiness, night wandering, tremors, or personality change.

Changes reflecting deterioration in mental status may be apparent to SO, although insidious changes may be noted by others with less frequent contact with client.

POTENTIAL CONSIDERATIONS following acute hospitalization (dependent on client's age, physical condition and presence of complications, personal resources, and life responsibilities)

- *Fatigue*—decreased metabolic energy production, states of discomfort, altered body chemistry, such as changes in liver function, effect on target organs, alcohol withdrawal
- *imbalanced Nutrition: Less than Body Requirements*—inadequate diet, inability to process and digest nutrients, anorexia, nausea and vomiting, indigestion, early satiety (ascites), abnormal bowel function
- *risk for ineffective self Health Management*—perceived benefit, social support deficit, economic difficulties.
- *dysfunctional Family Processes*—abuse of alcohol, resistance to treatment, inadequate coping and lack of problem-solving skills, addictive personality and codependency
- *risk for Caregiver Role Strain*—addiction or codependency; family dysfunction before caregiving situation; presence of situational stressors, such as economic vulnerability, hospitalization, changes in employment

---

PANCREATITIS

I. Pathophysiology

a. Inflammation of pancreas with premature activation of pancreatic enzymes resulting in localized damage to the pancreas, autodigestion, and fibrosis of the pancreas

b. Leads to wide range of metabolic consequences and life-threatening complications, such as hypovolemia, shock, acute renal failure, diabetes, acute respiratory distress syndrome (ARDS), and multiorgan failure

II. Types

a. Acute
   i. Sudden inflammation occurs over a short period of time.
   ii. Severity ranges from mild abdominal discomfort to a life-threatening illness.
   iii. Can result in bleeding into the gland, serious tissue damage, infection, and cyst formation
   iv. Release of enzymes and toxins into bloodstream can damage other vital organs, including the heart, lungs, and kidneys.

b. Chronic
   i. Commonly follows acute episode when inflammation is ongoing
   ii. Development may be delayed, as in alcohol abuse.

III. Etiology

a. Acute
   i. Biliary tract disease, such as obstruction by gallstones, is most common cause—about 40% (Gardner et al, 2008).
   ii. Alcohol abuse—approximately 35% (Gardner et al, 2008)
   iii. Trauma: blunt or penetrating
   iv. Procedures: endoscopic or surgical
   v. Viral infections: mumps, mononucleosis, varicella
   vi. Bacterial infections: *Mycoplasma pneumoniae*, salmonellosis, tuberculosis
   vii. Drugs: sulfonamides, glucocorticoids, thiazide diuretics, nonsteroidal anti-inflammatory drugs (NSAIDs)
   viii. Unknown cause—about 10% to 15% of cases

b. Chronic (Obideen & Yashke, 2008)
   i. Intraductal obstruction: alcohol abuse, stones, or tumors
   ii. Alcohol abuse—about 60% of cases
   iii. Direct toxins and toxic metabolites
   iv. Recurrent acute pancreatitis that heals with fibrosis
   v. Ischemia from obstruction and fibrosis exacerbates or perpetuates disease, rather than in initiating disease
   vi. Autoimmune disorders: primary biliary cirrhosis, renal tubular acidosis

IV. Statistics

a. Morbidity: An estimated 87,000 individuals are diagnosed with chronic pancreatitis annually in the United States (Obideen & Yashke, 2008); more than 220,000 were estimated to be hospitalized for acute pancreatitis in 2007 (Gardner et al, 2008).

b. Mortality: Rate is less than 1% for mild acute pancreatitis, but can approach 10% to 30% for severe acute pancreatitis (Lie, 2007); biliary pancreatitis associated with higher mortality rate than alcoholic pancreatitis; in presence of necrosis without organ failure, mortality rate is near zero, but with organ failure rate is approximately 30% (Gardner et al, 2008).

c. Cost: More than $2 billion is spent annually in the United States (Fagenholz, 2007).

GLOSSARY

Atelectasis: Collapse of lung tissue affecting all or part of the lung.

Chyme: Thick liquid made of partially digested food and stomach juices that is made in the stomach and moves into the small intestine for further digestion.

Coagulopathy: Defect in the blood-clotting mechanisms.

Cullen's sign: Blue-black bruising around the umbilicus area, indicative of intraperitoneal hemorrhage.

Disseminated intravascular coagulopathy: Pathological process where the blood starts to coagulate throughout the whole body. This depletes the body of platelets and coagulation factors, which results in a paradoxical situation in which there is a high risk for simultaneous catastrophic thromboembolism and massive hemorrhage.

Endocrine function: Pertains to hormones and the glands that make and secrete them into the bloodstream where they travel to distant organs. The Islets of Langerhans produce and secrete insulin.

Exocrine function: Refers to glands that secrete their products into ducts. Pancreatic enzymes are produced in the pancreas, accumulate in the intralobular ducts, and empty into the main pancreatic duct, which drains into the duodenum when needed for digestion.

Hemorrhagic pancreatitis: Hemorrhage caused by digestion of vessel walls by pancreatic enzymes.

Ileus: Partial or complete blockage of the small and/or large intestine.

Interstitial edema: Abnormally large fluid volume in tissues between the body's cells (interstitial spaces).

Pancreas: Gland located in the upper, posterior abdomen responsible for insulin production and the manufacture and secretion of digestive enzymes leading to carbohydrate, fat, and protein metabolism.

Pancreatic pseudocyst: Collection of tissue, fluid, debris, pancreatic enzymes, and blood. The fluid is usually pancreatic juice that has leaked out of a damaged pancreatic duct.

Peristalsis: Pattern of smooth muscle contractions that propels food and fluid through the esophagus and intestines.

Pleural effusion: An abnormal accumulation of fluid in the pleural space around the lungs.

Steatorrhea: Symptom in which fecal matter is frothy or foul-smelling and floats because of a high fat content.

Systemic inflammatory response syndrome (SIRS): Inflammation of the whole body (the "system") without a proven source of infection. It is a medical emergency.

Care Setting

The client is treated in an inpatient acute medical unit or intensive care unit (ICU) for initial incident or exacerbations with serious complications; otherwise, condition is managed at the community level.

Related Concerns

Alcohol: acute withdrawal, page 819

Substance dependence/abuse rehabilitation, page 835

Diabetes mellitus/diabetic ketoacidosis, page 405

Peritonitis, page 349

Psychosocial aspects of care, page 749

Renal failure: acute, page 536

Sepsis/septicemia, page 686

Total nutritional support: parenteral/enteral feeding, page 469

Client Assessment Database

DIAGNOSTIC DIVISION MAY REPORT	MAY EXHIBIT
ACTIVITY/REST • Malaise, fatigue	• Agitation, restlessness, apprehension
CIRCULATION	• Hypertension (acute pain) • Hypotension and tachycardia accompany hypovolemic shock or sepsis or SIRS • Generalized edema • Ascites • Skin pale, mottled areas; flushing may be present in acute stage from systemic inflammation; jaundiced (inflammation or obstruction of common duct); Cullen's sign from accumulation of blood (hemorrhagic pancreatitis)

(continues on page 460)

DIAGNOSTIC DIVISION MAY REPORT (continued)	MAY EXHIBIT (continued)

ELIMINATION
- Diarrhea
- Absence of bowel movements
- Abdominal bloating
- Dark and decreased urine

- *Bowel sounds:* May be decreased or absent—reduced peristalsis or ileus
- Dark amber or brown, foamy urine (bile)
- Steatorrhea
- Scanty urine (oliguria) progressing to absence of urine (anuria), which may be a compensatory response to hypovolemia

FOOD/FLUID
- Food intolerance, loss of appetite
- Frequent or persistent vomiting, retching, dry heaves
- Weight loss

- Diffuse abdominal tenderness to palpation
- Abdominal rigidity, distention
- Hypoactive bowel sounds

NEUROSENSORY

- Confusion, agitation
- Coarse tremors of extremities from hypocalcemia

PAIN/DISCOMFORT
- Unrelenting severe deep abdominal pain, usually located in the epigastrium and periumbilical regions, but may radiate to the back (acute pancreatitis)
- Onset may be sudden and may follow an episode of heavy drinking or a large meal
- Poorly localized, dull, cramping, burning, deep, or aching abdominal pain may be reported with long-term or chronic pancreatitis
- Radiation to chest and back
- May increase in supine position

- Abdominal guarding; may curl up on left side with both arms over abdomen and knees and hips flexed
- Abdominal rigidity

RESPIRATION

- Tachypnea with or without dyspnea
- Decreased depth of respiration with splinting or guarding actions
- Bibasilar crackles—associated with pleural effusion

SAFETY

- Fever
- Agitation, confusion

SEXUALITY
- Current pregnancy (third trimester) with shifting of abdominal contents and compression of biliary tract

TEACHING/LEARNING
- Family history of pancreatitis
- Signs and symptoms of hyperglycemic crisis
- History of cholelithiasis with partial or complete common bile duct obstruction, gastritis, duodenal ulcer, duodenitis, diverticulitis, Crohn's disease, recent abdominal surgery (such as procedures on the pancreas, biliary tract, stomach, or duodenum), external abdominal trauma
- Excessive alcohol intake (90% of cases)
- Use of medications—salicylates, pentamidine, antihypertensives, opiates, thiazides, steroids, some antibiotics, estrogens
- Infectious diseases—mumps, hepatitis B, Coxsackie viral infection

Client Assessment Database (continued)

DIAGNOSTIC DIVISION MAY REPORT (continued)	MAY EXHIBIT (continued)

DISCHARGE PLAN CONSIDERATIONS
- May require assistance with dietary program and activities of daily living (ADLs) at home

▶ Refer to section at end of plan for postdischarge considerations.

Diagnostic Studies

TEST WHY IT IS DONE	WHAT IT TELLS ME
BLOOD TESTS	
• *Serum amylase:* Common biochemical marker for acute pancreatitis.	Increased because of obstruction of normal outflow of pancreatic enzymes. May be five or more times the normal level in acute pancreatitis, and then fall back within normal ranges because serum half-life is short. Levels are elevated in chronic pancreatitis, but not as high as in acute phase, and may return to near normal levels in late stage of chronic disease.
• *Serum lipase:* More specific to the pancreas than amylase and has a longer half-life.	Elevates along with amylase, but stays elevated longer. Levels are elevated to a lesser degree in chronic pancreatitis, and return to normal levels in late stage of chronic disease.
• *Serum bilirubin:* Substance formed when red blood cells (RBCs) break down and are excreted by the liver.	Elevation is common (may be caused by alcoholic liver disease or compression of common bile duct). Excessive bilirubin causes jaundice and may be excreted in urine and stools.
• *Alkaline phosphatase:* Enzyme concentrated in liver and biliary tract.	Usually elevated if pancreatitis is accompanied by biliary disease.
• *C-reactive protein (CRP):* An acute-phase reactant protein produced in the liver.	A CRP value greater than or equal to 10 mg/dL strongly indicates severe pancreatitis and SIRS.
• *Serum albumin:* Most abundant plasma protein transports substances such as bilirubin, calcium, progesterone, and drugs, and creates oncotic pressure to keep fluid from leaking out into the tissues.	May be decreased because of increased capillary permeability and movment of fluid into extracellular space.
• *Serum calcium:* Chemical element necessary for the normal function of the heart, nerves, and bones.	Hypocalcemia occurs early on because of the release of fatty acids combining with calcium, rendering it unusable to the body.
• *Potassium:* Electrolyte needed to regulate water balance, levels of acidity, and blood pressure.	Hypokalemia may occur because of gastric losses; hyperkalemia may develop secondary to tissue necrosis, acidosis, and renal insufficiency.
• *Magnesium:* Essential mineral needed for protein, bone, and fatty acid formation, making new cells, activating B vitamins, relaxing muscles, clotting of blood, and producing and using insulin.	Diuretic therapy, chronic alcoholism, cirrhosis, and pancreatitis can all cause excessive magnesium loss, as can losses from the gastrointestinal (GI) tract through nasogastric suctioning, fistula drainage, and diarrhea (Astle, 2005).
• *Triglycerides:* One of the many fats formed by the union of glycerol and fatty acids and may indicate cause of condition.	High triglyceride levels are often indicative of high levels of insulin. Levels may exceed 1,700 mg/dL and may be causative agent in acute pancreatitis.
• *Complete blood count (CBC):* Battery of screening tests that typically includes hemoglobin (Hgb); hematocrit (Hct); RBC count, morphology, indices, and distribution width index; platelet count and size; white blood cell (WBC) count and differential.	WBC count of 10,000 to 25,000 is present in 80% of clients with acute pancreatitis. Hgb may be lower because of bleeding. Hct may be elevated because of hemoconcentration associated with vomiting, hypovolemia, or from effusion of fluid into pancreas or retroperitoneal area.
• *Serum glucose:* One of the simple sugars in the blood.	Transient elevations of more than 200 mg/dL are common, especially during initial or acute attacks. Sustained hyperglycemia reflects widespread pancreatic cell damage and necrosis and is a poor prognostic sign.

(continues on page 462)

TEST WHY IT IS DONE (continued)	WHAT IT TELLS ME (continued)
• *Partial thromboplastin time (PTT):* Tests length of time for blood sample to clot to identify bleeding or clotting problems.	Prolonged if coagulopathy develops because of liver involvement and fat necrosis.
• *Immunoglobulin (Ig) G4:* Used to assist in differentiating etiology of disease and possible treatment.	Elevations may reflect autoimmune response as cause of acute episode.
OTHER DIAGNOSTIC TESTS	
• *Ultrasound of abdomen:* Technique that uses sound waves to produce an image of internal body structures.	Most useful initial test to determine etiology of pancreatitis and to identify pancreatic inflammation, abscesses, pseudocysts, or obstruction of biliary tract by gallstones.
• *Computed tomography (CT) scan:* X-ray procedure that uses a computer to produce a detailed picture of a cross-section of the body to look for complications of pancreatitis and determine treatment options.	Can identify complications of pancreatic disease, such as fluid around the pancreas, abscess, or pancreatic pseudocyst. Most accurate in chronic disease state.
• *Magnetic resonance cholangiopancreatography (MRCP):* Imaging technique that uses magnetic resonance imaging (MRI) to visualize the biliary and pancreatic ducts.	May identify suspected biliary and pancreatic duct obstruction as a cause for pancreatitis.
• *Endoscopic retrograde cholangiopancreatography (ERCP):* Test that combines endoscopy with x-rays to provide the most accurate view of the pancreatic and bile ducts.	Used to diagnose fistulas, obstructive biliary disease, and pancreatic ductal system abnormalities, such as strictures or calcifications.
• *Endoscopic ultrasonography (EUS):* May be the most accurate test for imaging the pancreas.	Obtains a more detailed image than ERCP because the high-frequency transducer can be introduced adjacent to the pancreas. Reveals presence of stones, ductal dilatation, cysts, and so on.
• *CT-guided needle aspiration:* Procedure that uses special x-rays to show a mass while the radiologist advances a needle to remove fluid from a cyst or group of cells.	Performed in order to determine whether infection is present or if pseudocyst develops that requires aspiration. Also may be used to differentiate infected necrosis from sterile necrosis in patients with severe necrotizing pancreatitis.
• *Abdominal x-ray:* Anteroposterior (AP) and oblique views help identify pathology and complications.	May show dilated loop of small bowel adjacent to pancreas or other intra-abdominal precipitator of pancreatitis, presence of free intraperitoneal air caused by perforation or abscess formation, or presence of pancreatic calcifications common in chronic alcoholic, hereditary, or tropical pancreatitis.
• *Chest x-ray:* Identifies associated respiratory complications.	May demonstrate diffuse, pulmonary infiltrates. Client may demonstrate signs and symptoms of hypoxemia requiring respiratory support and mechanical ventilation.
• *Upper GI series:* X-rays of the esophagus, stomach, and small intestine (upper GI tract) taken after the client drinks a solution containing barium.	Frequently exhibits pancreatic enlargement and inflammation.
• *Urinalysis:* May reveal developing complications.	Glucose, myoglobin, blood, and protein may be present.
• *Urine amylase:* Used for differential diagnosis of pancreatis and pseudocyst of pancrease.	Can increase dramatically within 2 to 3 days after onset of attack. *Note:* Elevated serum amylase levels with normal or low urine levels may indicate decreased renal function.
• *Stool tests:* Measures the levels of elastase, an enzyme found in fluids produced by the pancreas.	Elastase breaks down proteins and may be passed in stool when digestion is impaired. In addition, increased fat content may be found in stool, indicative of insufficient digestion of fats and protein.

Nursing Priorities

1. Control pain and promote comfort.
2. Prevent and treat fluid and electrolyte imbalance.
3. Reduce pancreatic stimulation while maintaining adequate nutrition.
4. Prevent complications.
5. Provide information about disease process, prognosis, and treatment needs.

Discharge Goals

1. Pain relieved or controlled.
2. Hemodynamically stable.
3. Complications prevented or minimized.
4. Disease process, prognosis, potential complications, and therapeutic regimen understood.
5. Plan in place to meet needs after discharge.

NURSING DIAGNOSIS: acute Pain

May be related to
Obstruction of pancreatic, biliary ducts
Chemical contamination of peritoneal surfaces by pancreatic exudate, autodigestion of pancreas
Extension of inflammation to the retroperitoneal nerve plexus

Possibly evidenced by
Reports of pain
Self-focusing, grimacing, distraction or guarding behaviors
Autonomic responses, alteration in muscle tone

Desired Outcomes/Evaluation Criteria—Client Will

Pain Control (NOC)
Report pain is relieved or controlled.
Follow prescribed therapeutic regimen.
Demonstrate use of methods that provide relief.

ACTIONS/INTERVENTIONS	RATIONALE
Pain Management (NIC)	
Independent	
Investigate verbal reports of pain, noting specific location and intensity (0 to 10 scale). Note factors that aggravate and relieve pain.	Pain is often diffuse, severe, and unrelenting in acute or hemorrhagic pancreatitis. Severe pain is often the major symptom in client with chronic pancreatitis. Isolated pain in the right upper quadrant (RUQ) reflects involvement of the head of the pancreas. Pain in the left upper quadrant (LUQ) suggests involvement of the pancreatic tail. Localized pain may indicate development of pseudocysts or abscesses.
Maintain bedrest during acute attack and provide quiet, restful environment.	Decreases stimulation of pancreatic secretions, thereby reducing pain.
Promote position of comfort, such as on one side with knees flexed or sitting up and leaning forward.	Reduces abdominal pressure and tension, providing some measure of comfort and pain relief. *Note:* Supine position often increases pain.
Provide alternative comfort measures including repositioning and back rub, and quiet diversional activities such as TV or radio. Encourage relaxation techniques, such as guided imagery and visualization.	Promotes relaxation and enables client to refocus attention; may enhance coping.
Keep environment free of food odors.	Sensory stimulation can activate pancreatic enzymes, increasing pain.
Administer intravenous (IV) analgesics in timely manner, and in smaller, more frequent doses, during acute episode. Consider use of patient-controlled analgesia (PCA), if appropriate.	Severe or prolonged pain can aggravate shock and is more difficult to relieve, requiring larger doses of medication, which can mask underlying problems and complications and may contribute to respiratory depression.
Maintain meticulous skin care, especially in presence of draining abdominal wall fistulas.	Pancreatic enzymes can digest the skin and tissues of the abdominal wall, creating abscesses and ulceration.
Collaborative	
Administer medication, as indicated, for example:	
Opioid analgesics, such as meperidine (Demerol), morphine sulfate, and tramadol (Ultram)	Meperidine is usually effective in relieving pain and may be preferred over morphine, which may have a side effect of biliary-pancreatic spasms. Paravertebral block has been used to achieve prolonged pain control. *Note:* Pain in clients who have recurrent or chronic pancreatitis episodes may be more difficult to manage because they may develop tolerance to normal doses of the opioids given for pain control.
Sedatives such as diazepam (Valium) and antispasmodics such as atropine	Potentiate action of opioid to promote rest and to reduce ductal spasm, thereby reducing metabolic needs and enzyme secretions.
Histamine blockers, such as lansoprazole (Prevacid), cimetidine (Tagamet), ranitidine (Zantac), and famotidine (Pepcid)	Decreasing production of hydrochloric acid inhibits pancreatic enzyme activity and associated pain.
Withhold food and fluid, as indicated.	Client should be kept nothing by mouth (NPO) status until pain and nausea subside to limit or reduce release of pancreatic enzymes and resultant pain.

(continues on page 464)

ACTIONS/INTERVENTIONS (continued)

Maintain gastric suction when used.

Prepare for surgical intervention, if indicated.

RATIONALE (continued)

Nasogastric (NG) tube may be used for client with ileus or protracted vomiting to prevent accumulation of gastric secretions and pancreatic enzyme activity.

Surgical exploration may be required in presence of intractable pain or complications involving the biliary tract, such as pancreatic abscess or pseudocyst. *Note:* Surgery is not performed during acute stage, unless it would actually cure the problem, such as removing stone causing biliary tract obstruction.

NURSING DIAGNOSIS: **risk for deficient Fluid Volume/Bleeding**

Risk factors may include
Excessive losses—vomiting, gastric suctioning
Increase in size of vascular bed (vasodilation effects of kinins)
Third-space fluid transudation, ascites formation
Alteration of clotting process, hemorrhage

Possibly evidenced by
(Not applicable; presence of signs and symptoms establishes an *actual* diagnosis)

Desired Outcomes/Evaluation Criteria—Client Will

Hydration (NOC)
Maintain adequate hydration as evidenced by stable vital signs, good skin turgor, prompt capillary refill, strong peripheral pulses, and individually appropriate urinary output.

ACTIONS/INTERVENTIONS

Fluid/Electrolyte Management (NIC)
Independent

Auscultate heart sounds; note rate and rhythm. Monitor and document rhythm and changes.

Monitor blood pressure (BP), noting trends. Measure central venous pressure (CVP), if available.

Investigate changes in sensorium: confusion and slowed responses.

Measure intake and output (I&O), including vomiting or gastric aspirate, and diarrhea. Calculate 24-hour fluid balance.
Note decrease in urine output (less than 400 mL/24 hours).

Record color and character of gastric drainage, measure pH, and note presence of occult blood.
Weigh, as indicated; correlate with calculated fluid balance.

Note poor skin turgor, dry skin and mucous membranes, or reports of thirst.

RATIONALE

Cardiac changes and dysrhythmias may reflect hypovolemia or electrolyte imbalance, commonly hypokalemia and hypocalcemia. Hyperkalemia may occur related to tissue necrosis, acidosis, and renal insufficiency and may precipitate lethal dysrhythmias if uncorrected. *Note:* Cardiovascular complications are common in severe pancreatitis and include myocardial infarction (MI), pericarditis, and pericardial effusion with or without tamponade.

Fluid sequestration with shifts into third space, bleeding, and release of vasodilators (kinins) and cardiac depressant factor triggered by pancreatic ischemia may result in profound hypotension. Reduced cardiac output and poor organ perfusion can precipitate widespread systemic complications. Systemic infection (septic shock) is also possible, exacerbating hypovolemic status.

Changes may be related to hypovolemia, hypoxia, electrolyte imbalance, or impending delirium tremens (in client with acute pancreatitis secondary to excessive alcohol intake). Severe pancreatic disease may cause toxic psychosis.

Indicators of replacement needs and effectiveness of therapy.

Oliguria may occur, signaling renal impairment or acute tubular necrosis (ATN), related to increase in renal vascular resistance or altered renal blood flow.

Risk of gastric hemorrhage is high.

Weight loss may suggest hypovolemia; however, edema, fluid retention, and ascites may be reflected by increased or stable weight, even in the presence of muscle wasting.

Further physiological indicators of dehydration.

ACTIONS/INTERVENTIONS (continued)	RATIONALE (continued)
Observe and record peripheral and dependent edema. Measure abdominal girth if ascites present.	Edema and fluid shifts occur as a result of increased vascular permeability, sodium retention, and decreased colloid osmotic pressure in the intravascular compartment.
Inspect skin for petechiae, hematomas, and unusual wound or venipuncture bleeding. Note hematuria, mucous membrane bleeding, and bloody gastric contents.	Disseminated intravascular coagulation (DIC) may be initiated by release of active pancreatic proteases into the circulation. The most frequently affected organs are the kidneys, skin, and lungs.
Observe and report coarse muscle tremors, twitching, and positive Chvostek's or Trousseau's sign.	These are symptoms of calcium imbalance. Calcium binds with free fats in the intestine and is lost by excretion in the stool.
Collaborative	
Administer fluid replacement, as indicated, such as saline solutions, albumin, blood and blood products, and dextran.	Choice of replacement solution may be less important than rapidity and adequacy of volume restoration. Saline solutions and albumin may be used to promote mobilization of fluid back into vascular space. Low-molecular-weight dextran is sometimes used to reduce risk of renal dysfunction and pulmonary edema associated with pancreatitis.
Monitor laboratory studies—Hgb/Hct, protein, albumin, electrolytes, blood urea nitrogen (BUN), creatinine, urine osmolality, sodium and potassium, and coagulation studies.	Identifies deficits, replacement needs, and developing complications.
Replace electrolytes—sodium, potassium, chloride, and calcium, as indicated.	Decreased oral intake and excessive losses greatly affect electrolyte and acid-base balance, which is necessary to maintain optimal cellular and organ function.
Prepare for and assist with peritoneal lavage or hemoperitoneal dialysis.	Removes toxins and pancreatic enzymes and may allow for more rapid correction of metabolic abnormalities in severe acute pancreatitis.

NURSING DIAGNOSIS: imbalanced Nutrition: Less than Body Requirements

May be related to
Vomiting, decreased oral intake; prescribed dietary restrictions
Loss of digestive enzymes (related to pancreatic outflow obstruction, necrosis, or autodigestion)

Possibly evidenced by
Reported inadequate food intake
Aversion to eating, reported altered taste sensation, lack of interest in food
Weight loss
Poor muscle tone

Desired Outcomes/Evaluation Criteria—Client Will

Nutritional Status (NOC)
Demonstrate progressive weight gain toward goal with normalization of laboratory values.
Experience no signs of malnutrition.

Knowledge: Diet (NOC)
Demonstrate behaviors or lifestyle changes to regain and maintain appropriate weight.

ACTIONS/INTERVENTIONS	RATIONALE
Nutrition Management (NIC)	
Independent	
Assess abdomen, noting presence and character of bowel sounds, abdominal distention, and reports of nausea.	Gastric distention and intestinal atony are frequently present, resulting in reduced or absent bowel sounds. Return of bowel sounds and relief of symptoms signal readiness for discontinuation of NG.
Provide frequent oral care.	Decreases vomiting stimulus and soothes inflamed, dry mucous membranes associated with dehydration and mouth breathing when NG tube is in place.

(continues on page 466)

ACTIONS/INTERVENTIONS (continued)

Assist client in selecting food and fluids that meet nutritional needs and restrictions when diet is resumed.

Observe color, consistency, and amount of stools. Note frothy consistency and foul odor.

Maintain NPO status and gastric suctioning during acute phase.

Resume oral intake with liquids and advance diet slowly to provide high-protein, high-carbohydrate diet, when indicated.

Collaborative
Provide medium-chain triglycerides (MCTs), such as Portagen.

Administer enteral or parenteral feedings, as indicated.

Administer medications, as indicated, for example:
Vitamins, such as A, D, E, and K

Replacement enzymes, such as pancreatin (Dizymes) and pancrelipase (Protilase, Cotazym)

RATIONALE (continued)

Previous dietary habits may be unsatisfactory in meeting current needs for tissue regeneration and healing. Use of gastric stimulants, such as caffeine, alcohol, cigarettes, or gas-producing foods, or ingestion of large meals may result in excessive stimulation of the pancreas and recurrence of symptoms.

Steatorrhea may develop from incomplete digestion of fats.

Prevents stimulation and release of pancreatic enzymes (secretin) when chyme and hydrochloric acid enter the duodenum.

Oral feedings given too early in the course of illness may exacerbate symptoms.

MCTs are elements of enteral feeding that provide supplemental calories or nutrients that do not require pancreatic enzymes for digestion and absorption.

Enteral feedings may be preferred to prevent gut atrophy when tolerated; however, IV administration of calories, lipids, and amino acids should be instituted before nitrogen depletion is advanced. (Refer to CP: Total Nutritional Support: Parenteral/Enteral Feedings.)

Replacement required because fat metabolism is altered, reducing absorption and storage of fat-soluble vitamins.

Used in chronic pancreatitis to correct deficiencies to promote digestion and absorption of nutrients.

NURSING DIAGNOSIS: **risk for unstable blood Glucose Level**

Risk factors may include
Decreased insulin production, increased glucagon release
Physical health status, stress

Possibly evidenced by
(Not applicable; presence of signs and symptoms establishes an *actual* diagnosis)

Desired Outcomes/Evaluation Criteria—Client Will

Hyperglycemia Management (NOC)
Maintain glucose in satisfactory range.

ACTIONS/INTERVENTIONS

Hyperglycemia Management (NIC)
Independent
Note signs of increased thirst and urination or changes in mentation and visual acuity.

Perform and monitor results of bedside fingerstick glucose testing and dipstick testing of urine for sugar and acetone (ketones).

Collaborative
Monitor serum glucose, as indicated.

Provide insulin, as appropriate.

Advance diet as tolerated and based on specific nutritional needs.

RATIONALE

May warn of developing hyperglycemia associated with increased release of glucagon (damage to alpha cells) or decreased release of insulin (damage to beta cells).

Early detection of inadequate glucose utilization may prevent development of hyperglycemic crisis. IV insulin may be required to control serum glucose within normal ranges.

Indicator of insulin needs because hyperglycemia is frequently present, although not usually in levels high enough to produce ketoacidosis.

Corrects persistent hyperglycemia caused by injury to cells and increased release of glucocorticoids. Insulin therapy is usually short-term unless permanent damage to pancreas occurs.

Loss of pancreatic function or reduced insulin production may require initiation of a diabetic diet.

NURSING DIAGNOSIS: risk for Infection, [sepsis]

Risk factors may include
Inadequate primary defenses: stasis of body fluids, altered peristalsis, change in pH of secretions
Immunosuppression
Nutritional deficiencies
Tissue destruction, chronic disease

Possibly evidenced by
(Not applicable; presence of signs and symptoms establishes an *actual* diagnosis)

Desired Outcomes/Evaluation Criteria—Client Will

Immune Status (NOC)
Achieve timely healing; be free of signs of infection.
Be afebrile.

Risk Control (NOC)
Participate in activities to reduce risk of infection.

ACTIONS/INTERVENTIONS	RATIONALE
Infection Protection (NIC)	
Independent	
Use strict aseptic technique when changing surgical dressings or working with IV lines, indwelling catheters, tubes, or drains. Change soiled dressings promptly.	Limits sources of infection, which can lead to sepsis in a compromised client.
Model and emphasize importance of good hand washing.	Reduces risk of cross-contamination.
Observe rate and characteristics of respirations and breath sounds. Note occurrence of cough and sputum production.	Pulmonary complications of pancreatitis include atelectasis, pleural effusion, pneumonia, and ARDS. Fluid accumulation and limited mobility predisposes client to respiratory infections and atelectasis. Accumulation of ascites fluid may cause elevated diaphragm and shallow abdominal breathing.
Encourage frequent position changes, deep breathing, and coughing. Assist with ambulation as soon as stable.	Enhances ventilation of all lung segments and promotes mobilization of secretions.
Observe for signs of infection, such as the following:	
Fever and respiratory distress in conjunction with jaundice	Cholestatic jaundice and decreased pulmonary function may be first sign of sepsis or ARDS.
Increased abdominal pain, rigidity and rebound tenderness, diminished or absent bowel sounds	Suggestive of peritonitis.
Increased abdominal pain and tenderness, recurrent fever (higher than 101°F [38.3°C]), leukocytosis, hypotension, tachycardia, and chills	Abscesses can occur 2 weeks or more after the onset of pancreatitis and should be suspected whenever client is deteriorating despite supportive measures.
Collaborative	
Obtain culture specimens, such as blood, wound, urine, sputum, or pancreatic aspirate.	Identifies presence of infection and causative organism.
Administer anti-infective therapies as indicated, such as imipenem/cilastatin (Primaxin), metronidazole (Flagyl), and levofloxacin (Levaquin); cephalosporins, such as cefoxitin sodium (Mefoxin); and aminoglycosides, such as gentamicin (Garamycin) and tobramycin (Nebcin).	Broad-spectrum anti-infectives are generally recommended for pancreatitis sepsis; however, therapy will be based on the specific organisms cultured.
Prepare for surgical intervention, as necessary.	Abscesses may be surgically drained with resection of necrotic tissue. Sump tubes may be inserted for antibiotic irrigation and drainage of pancreatic debris. Pseudocysts (persisting for several weeks) may be drained because of the risk and incidence of infection and rupture.

NURSING DIAGNOSIS: risk for ineffective Breathing Pattern/impaired Gas Exchange

May be related to
Pain, with splinting of respirations; upper abdominal distention and elevated diaphragm; pleural effusion
Alveolar or capillary membrane changes—interstitial edema, pulmonary congestion

Possibly evidenced by
(Not applicable; presence of signs and symptoms establishes an *actual* diagnosis)

Desired Outcomes/Evaluation Criteria—Client Will

Respiratory Status: Ventilation (NOC)
Maintain adequate ventilation with respiratory rate and rhythm normal for client, breath sounds clear, and free of dyspnea or shortness of breath.

Respiratory Status: Gas Exchange (NOC)
Display arterial blood gases (ABGs) within client's normal range.

ACTIONS/INTERVENTIONS	RATIONALE
Respiratory Monitoring (NIC)	
Independent	
Evaluate respiratory rate and depth. Note respiratory effort; for example, presence of dyspnea, use of accessory muscles, and nasal flaring.	Client responses are variable. Rate and effort may be increased by pain, accumulation of secretions, or abdominal distention. Respiratory depression can occur with use of opioid analgesics. Early recognition and treatment of abnormal ventilation may prevent complications.
Auscultate breath sounds. Note areas of diminished or absent breath sounds and presence of adventitious sounds, such as rhonchi or crackles.	Loss of active breath sounds in an area of previous ventilation may reflect atelectasis. Crackles or rhonchi may be indicative of fluid accumulation due to interstitial edema, pulmonary congestion, or infection.
Encourage client participation and responsibility for deep-breathing exercises, use of adjuncts, and coughing, as indicated. Reposition frequently.	Stimulates respiratory function and lung expansion. Effective in preventing and resolving pulmonary congestion.
Reinforce splinting of abdomen with pillows during deep breathing or coughing.	May enhance effectiveness of cough effort.
Note increasing restlessness, confusion, and lethargy.	May indicate impaired gas exchange and possible ARDS, requiring prompt evaluation and intervention.
Collaborative	
Monitor and graph serial ABGs and pulse oximetry, and review chest x-ray reports.	Decreasing oxygen level or saturation and increasing $PaCO_2$ and changes in chest x-rays suggest developing complications requiring further evaluation and treatment.
Administer supplemental oxygen O_2, if indicated.	Increases available O_2 for tissue and organ function. *Note:* Inability to maintain adequate oxygenation indicates need for more aggressive therapy or mechanical ventilation. (Refer to CP: Ventilation Assistance [Mechanical].)

NURSING DIAGNOSIS: deficient Knowledge [Learning Need] regarding condition, prognosis, treatment, self-care, and discharge needs

May be related to
Lack of exposure or recall
Information misinterpretation, unfamiliarity with information resources

Possibly evidenced by
Questions, request for information, statement of misconception
Inaccurate follow-through of instructions, development of preventable complications

Desired Outcomes/Evaluation Criteria—Client Will

Knowledge: Illness Care (NOC)
Verbalize understanding of condition, disease process, and potential complications.
Verbalize understanding of therapeutic needs.
Correctly perform necessary procedures and explain reasons for the actions.
Initiate necessary lifestyle changes and participate in treatment regimen.

ACTIONS/INTERVENTIONS	RATIONALE

Teaching: Disease Process (NIC)

Independent

Review specific cause of current episode and prognosis. Discuss other causative and associated factors such as excessive alcohol intake, gallbladder disease, duodenal ulcer, and some drugs—oral contraceptives, thiazide diuretics, glucocorticoids, and sulfonamides.

Explore availability of treatment programs for chemical dependency, if indicated.

Emphasize the importance of follow-up care, and review symptoms that need to be reported immediately to physician, such as recurrence of pain, persistent fever, nausea and vomiting, abdominal distention, frothy or foul-smelling stools, and general intolerance of food.

Review importance of initially continuing bland, low-fat diet with frequent small feedings and restricted caffeine, and gradual resumption of a normal diet within individual tolerance.

Instruct in use of pancreatic enzyme replacements and bile salt therapy as indicated, avoiding concomitant ingestion of hot foods or fluids.

Recommend cessation of smoking. Refer for medical and support interventions, if client desires.

Discuss signs and symptoms of diabetes mellitus: polydipsia, polyuria, weakness, and weight loss.

Provides knowledge base on which client can make informed choices. Avoidance may help limit damage and prevent development of a chronic condition.

Alcohol abuse is currently the most common cause of recurrence of chronic pancreatitis. Usage of other drugs, whether prescribed or illicit, is increasing as a factor. *Note:* Pain of pancreatitis can be severe and prolonged and may lead to narcotic dependence. It may benefit from referral to a pain clinic.

Prolonged recovery period requires close monitoring to prevent recurrence and complications, such as infection and pancreatic pseudocysts.

Understanding the purpose of the diet in maximizing the use of available enzymes while avoiding overstimulation of the pancreas may enhance client involvement in self-monitoring of dietary needs and responses to foods.

If permanent damage to the pancreas has occurred, exocrine deficiencies will occur, requiring long-term replacement. Hot foods or fluids can inactivate enzymes.

Nicotine stimulates gastric secretions and unnecessary pancreatic activity.

Damage to the beta cells may result in a temporary or permanent alteration of insulin production.

POTENTIAL CONSIDERATIONS following acute hospitalization (dependent on client's age, physical condition and presence of complications, personal resources, and life responsibilities)

- *imbalanced Nutrition: Less than Body Requirements*—preexisting malnutrition, prescribed dietary restrictions, persistent nausea and vomiting, imbalances in digestive enzymes
- *risk for unstable blood Glucose Level*—lack of acceptance of diagnosis; deficient knowledge of disease management; medication management
- *acute/chronic Pain*—chemical irritation of peritoneal surfaces by pancreatic enzymes, spasms of biliary ducts, general inflammatory process
- *dysfunctional Family Processes*—abuse of alcohol, resistance to treatment, inadequate coping and lack of problem-solving skills, addictive personality, codependency
- *ineffective self Health Management*—complexity of therapeutic regimen, economic difficulties, mistrust of regimen, perceived benefit, social support deficits

TOTAL NUTRITIONAL SUPPORT: PARENTERAL/ENTERAL FEEDING

I. Pathophysiology: Malnutrition is a disorder of body composition in which nutritional intake is less than required and results in reduced organ function, abnormalities in blood chemistry, reduced body mass, and worsened clinical outcomes.

   a. Nutritional status is affected by multiple factors, including eating behaviors, disease states, economics, and environment.

   b. In the acutely or chronically ill client, the impact of malnutrition includes muscle mass loss, progressive weakness, potential for infection, poor healing, and a higher rate of systemic complications.

   c. When oral intake is inadequate or not possible, specifically designed nutritional therapy can be administered via an enteral or parenteral route to prevent or correct protein-calorie malnutrition.

II. Clinical Indication for Feeding

   a. Preexisting nutritional deprivation; unplanned or unexplained loss of 10% in body weight

   b. Anticipated or actual inadequate energy intake by mouth, such as inability to consume food or drink orally for 7 days or more, based on individual nutritional status

(text continues on page 470)

c. Critically ill individuals, because of their increased metabolic demands and limited nutritional reserve, commonly require nutritional support.

d. The Joint Commission for Accreditation of Healthcare Organizations (JCAHO) recognizes the negative impact of malnutrition in hospitals and long-term care institutions and has, in turn, made nutritional assessment, support, and ongoing reassessment an essential part of accreditation requirements (JCAHO, 1997).

III. Etiology of Malnutrition

a. Can exist in persons who are underfed or overfed, occurring in both extremely thin and obese individuals

b. May result from an inadequate or unbalanced diet, digestive difficulties, absorption problems, or other medical conditions

   i. Acute conditions, such as surgery, severe burns, infections, and trauma, that drastically increase short-term nutritional requirements

   ii. Chronic diseases associated with nutrient loss, nutrient demand, and with malabsorption, such as celiac disease, cystic fibrosis, pancreatic insufficiency, pernicious anemia

   iii. Conditions and treatments associated with malnutrition through decreased intake, such as depressed appetite, difficulty swallowing, and nausea associated with both cancer and chemotherapy, as well as with HIV/AIDS and its drug therapies

c. Certain age groups, such as elderly clients, require fewer calories but continue to require adequate nutritional support because they are often less able to absorb nutrients, due in part to decreased stomach acid production, and are more likely to have one or more chronic ailments that may affect their nutritional status.

IV. Routes for Feeding

a. Enteral nutrition

   i. Gastrointestinal (GI) intubation is preferred for clients with functional GI tract, but who are unable to consume an adequate nutritional intake or for whom oral intake is contraindicated or impossible.

   ii. Feeding may be done via flexible catheter (such as nasogastric [NG], orogastric tube) or enterostomy (such as gastrostomy, duodenostomy, or jejunostomy tube).

   iii. Feeding may be short-term for supplementation of oral intake or long-term to provide for all of client's nutrition.

b. Parenteral nutrition

   i. May be chosen because of altered metabolic states or when mechanical or functional abnormalities of the GI tract prevent enteral feeding

   ii. Goals are to improve the client's nutritional status; establish and maintain a positive nitrogen balance; improve or maintain muscle strength and mass; promote weight gain; and encourage the healing process through infusion of amino acids, fat, carbohydrates, trace elements, vitamins, and electrolytes, as indicated.

   iii. The average adult requires approximately 1,500 calories per day in order to maintain energy stores.

   iv. Nutritional support is provided via an intravenous (IV) route, either centrally or peripherally.

     1. Central: Formula is concentrated hyperosmolar and must be infused via a central vein (subclavian or jugular) into the superior vena cava or peripherally inserted central catheter (PICC), inserted into the arm and passed into a major blood vessel.

     2. Peripheral: Formula is similar, but less concentrated than central formula and is infused via a peripheral vein.

GLOSSARY

Basal metabolic rate (BMR): Number of calories the body burns at rest to maintain normal body functions.

Bitot's spots: Triangular, shiny, gray spots on the conjunctiva seen in vitamin A deficiency.

Cachexia: Profound and marked state of general ill health and malnutrition.

Catabolism: Metabolic breakdown of complex molecules into simpler ones, often resulting in a release of energy.

Harris-Benedict equation: Formula that uses BMR and then applies an activity factor to determine total daily energy expenditure (calories).

Ideal body weight (IBW): Calculation for men: 106 lbs for first 5 feet plus 6 lbs for each additional inch of height. Women: 100 lbs for first 5 feet plus 5 lbs for each additional inch of height.

Indirect caliometry: Estimation of energy expenditure via the measurement of oxygen consumption and carbon dioxide production.

Malabsorption: Inability of the body to use one or more available nutrients.

Protein calorie malnutrition (PCM), also called protein energy malnutrition (PEM): Severe deficiency of protein plus inadequate caloric intake to meet energy needs.

Total energy expenditure (TEE): Amount of energy spent, on average, in a typical day measured in calories (k/day).

Care Setting

Client may be treated in any setting, including community or home care.

Related Concerns

Acquired immunodeficiency syndrome (AIDS), page 709

Anemias, page 493

Burns: thermal, chemical, and electrical—acute and convalescent phases, page 667

Cancer, page 846

Cirrhosis of the liver, page 445

Chronic obstructive pulmonary disease (COPD) and asthma, page 120

Diabetes mellitus/diabetic ketoacidosis, page 405

Eating disorders: anorexia nervosa/bulimia nervosa, page 369

Eating disorders: obesity, page 387

Fluid and electrolyte imbalances, page 903

Fractures, page 632

Inflammatory bowel disease (IBD): ulcerative colitis, Crohn's disease, page 321

Obesity: bariatric surgery—gastric partitioning/gastroplasty, gastris bypass, page 396

Pancreatitis, page 458

Psychosocial aspects of care, page 749

Renal failure: chronic, page 548

Surgical intervention, page 782

Client Assessment Database

Clinical signs listed here depend on the degree and duration of malnutrition and include observations indicative of vitamin, mineral, protein, and calorie deficiencies.

DIAGNOSTIC DIVISIONS MAY REPORT	MAY EXHIBIT
ACTIVITY/REST	• Muscle wasting—temporal, intercostal, gastrocnemius, dorsum of hand • Thin extremities • Flaccid muscles • Decreased activity tolerance
CIRCULATION	• Tachycardia, bradycardia • Diaphoresis, • Pallor, cyanosis
ELIMINATION • Diarrhea or constipation, flatulence associated with food intake	• Abdominal distention, increased girth, ascites • Abdominal tenderness on palpation • Stools may be loose, hard-formed, fatty, or clay-colored
FOOD/FLUID • Recent weight loss or weight loss of 10% or more of body weight within previous 6 months • Unplanned weight loss of more than 20 lbs in the last 3 months • Problems with chewing, swallowing, choking, or saliva production • Changes in the taste of food • Anorexia • Nausea, vomiting • Inadequate oral intake (nothing by mouth [NPO]) status for 7 to 10 days	• Actual measured weight as compared with usual, or weight is less than 90% of IBW for height, sex, and age • Actual weight equal to or greater than 120% of IBW • A distorted actual body mass weight may occur because of the presence of edema, ascites, organomegaly, tumor bulk • Bowel sounds diminished, hyperactive, or absent • Thyroid, parotid enlargement • Lips and mucous membranes dry, cracked, red, swollen • Tongue may be smooth, pale, slick, coated; color often magenta, beefy red; lingual papillae atrophy or swelling

(continues on page 472)

DIAGNOSTIC DIVISIONS MAY REPORT (continued)	MAY EXHIBIT (continued)

<table>
<tr><td></td><td>• Gums swollen, bleeding
• Dentition may be poor, such as lack of teeth, multiple cavities, denture problems</td></tr>
<tr><td>NEUROSENSORY</td><td>• Lethargy, apathy, listlessness, irritability, disorientation
• Gag and swallow reflex may be decreased or absent
• Loss of balance and coordination</td></tr>
<tr><td>RESPIRATION</td><td>• Increased respiratory rate; respiratory distress
• Dyspnea, increased sputum production
• Breath sounds, crackles (protein deficiency-related fluid shifts)</td></tr>
<tr><td>SAFETY
• Recent course of radiation therapy (radiation enteritis)</td><td>• Hair may be fragile, coarse, lackluster, falling out (alopecia); decreased pigmentation may be present
• Skin dry, scaly, tented; "flaky paint" dermatosis; edematous
• Draining or unhealed wounds; pressure sores
• Ecchymosis; perifollicular petechiae
• Subcutaneous fat loss
• Eyes sunken, dull, dry, with pale conjunctiva; Bitot's spots or scleral icterus
• Nails may be brittle, thin, flattened, ridged, spoon-shaped</td></tr>
</table>

SEXUALITY
• Loss of libido
• Amenorrhea

TEACHING/LEARNING
• History or presence of conditions causing protracted protein and caloric losses—malabsorption or short-gut syndrome, diarrhea, acute pancreatitis, renal dialysis, fistulas, draining wounds, thermal injuries, problems with chewing or swallowing (such as due to stroke or Parkinson's disease)
• Presence of factors known to alter nutritional requirements and increase energy demands—single or multiorgan failure, sepsis, fever, AIDS, cancer, trauma, extensive burns, use of steroids, antitumor agents, immunosuppressants
• Use of treatments that greatly alter intake and medications that cause untoward drug and nutrient interactions—laxatives, anticonvulsants, diuretics, antacids, opioids, immunosuppressants, radiation, high-dose chemotherapy
• Illness of psychiatric origin—anorexia nervosa or bulimia
• Educational and social factors—lack of nutrition knowledge or kitchen facilities, reduced or limited financial resources

DISCHARGE PLAN CONSIDERATIONS
• May require assistance with solution preparation, therapy supplies, and maintenance of feeding device for home nutritional care

⬦ Refer to section at end of plan for postdischarge considerations.

Diagnostic Studies

TEST WHY IT IS DONE	WHAT IT TELLS ME
• *Anthropometrics:* Techniques that deal with the measurement of the size, weight, and proportions of the human body.	
• *Weight:* What people are expected to weigh based on age, sex, and height.	A malnourished person could weigh less or more than their IBW. Weight may be inaccurate because of factors such as edema or ascites.
• *Body mass index (BMI):* Calculates body composition.	Measures ratios of lean-to-fat body weight. Classifications include underweight (less than 18.5), normal weight (18.5 to 24.9), overweight (25 to 29.9), and obese (greater than 30).
• *Skin-fold measurement:* Estimates subcutaneous body fat by measuring skinfold thickness using calipers. Measurements can use from three to nine different standard anatomical sites around the body.	Fat reserves less than in the 10th percentile suggest advanced depletion; levels less than the 30th percentile suggest mild-to-moderate depletion.

BLOOD TESTS

• *Visceral proteins:* Nonmuscular proteins useful in monitoring nutritional status.	Deficits suggest malnutrition.
• *Serum albumin:* Protein deficiency results in decreased synthesis of albumin.	An albumin level of less than 3 g/day often indicates malnutrition. However, overhydration and dehydration affect its concentration, and its long half-life makes it unreliable as a nutrition marker, especially in acute depletion or repletion. It is more accurate in chronic protein deficiency states (Mears, 2005).
• *Serum transferrin:* An iron-transport protein more sensitive to changes in visceral protein stores than albumin; also, its shorter half-life and smaller blood pool makes it a more accurate early marker for protein depletion.	Level of less than 150 mg/dL is considered severe depletion.
• *Prealbumin (PAB) also called transthyretin and thyroxine transport protein:* Excellent sensitivity to nutritional status. PAB has a shorter half-life than albumin, and levels respond quickly to nutritional therapy, making it a more sensitive indicator of improvement and change in protein status.	Levels of less than 17 mg/dL are noted with end-stage liver disease; it is affected by inflammation, infection, and trauma (Mears, 2005).
• *Retinol-binding protein (RBP):* Carrier protein of vitamin A.	Concentration falls during protein and calorie deprivation and rises rapidly with supplementation (Mears, 2005).
• *C-reactive protein (CRP):* Acute inflammation phase protein.	Increases dramatically during systemic inflammation and catabolism, while visceral proteins fall. CRP values return to normal once the body starts to synthesize proteins, such as PAB.
• *Total lymphocyte count:* Indicator of the status of the immune system.	Less than 1,500 cells/mm³ indicates leukopenia and results from decreased generation of T cells, which are very sensitive to malnutrition. Less than 800 cells/mm³ indicates severe depletion. Levels are also altered by severe stress, renal failure, cancer, infection, and administration of corticosteroids.
• *Tests of micronutrients:* Trace elements required for body to produce enzymes, hormones, and substances required for growth and development.	
• *Potassium:* Electrolyte needed to regulate water balance, levels of acidity, and blood pressure.	Deficiency occurs with inadequate intake and with loss of potassium-containing fluids—urine, diarrhea, vomiting, fistula drainage, and continuous NG suctioning. Potassium is also lost from cells during muscle wasting and is excreted by the kidneys.
• *Sodium:* The body's most abundant extracellular ion plays a key role in maintaining fluid balance—where sodium goes, water will follow.	Levels depend on state of hydration and presence of active loss as may exist in excessive diuresis, GI suctioning, and burns.
• *Phosphorus:* Essential mineral required for normal function of nerves and muscles and bone formation.	May be decreased, reflecting inadequate intake or increased cellular uptake; may be elevated in renal failure.

(continues on page 474)

TEST WHY IT IS DONE (continued)	WHAT IT TELLS ME (continued)
• *Magnesium:* Essential mineral needed for protein, bone, and fatty acid formation; making new cells; activating B vitamins; relaxing muscles; clotting of blood; and producing and using insulin.	Deficiency is common in alcoholics, chronic vomiting, and diarrhea; may be elevated in renal failure.
• *Calcium:* Chemical element necessary for the normal function of the heart, muscles, nerves, and bone formation.	Levels are decreased with conditions associated with hypoalbuminemia, such as renal failure (majority of calcium is bound to albumin). Absorption is decreased by fat malabsorption and low-protein diet.
• *Zinc:* Essential mineral for normal growth, bone development, enzyme activity and metabolism, and wound healing.	Deficiency is seen in alcoholic cirrhosis or may be secondary to hypoalbuminemia and GI losses (diarrhea).
• *Tests reflecting protein (nitrogen) loss:*	
• *Nitrogen balance studies:* Nitrogen excretion via urine, stool, and insensible losses often exceeds nitrogen intake in the acutely ill, reflecting catabolic response to stress and use of endogenous protein stores for energy production (gluconeogenesis).	Blood urea nitrogen (BUN) may be severely decreased because of chronic malnutrition and depletion of skeletal protein stores.
• *24-hour creatinine (Cr) excretion:* Because Cr is concentrated in muscle mass, there is a correlation between lean body mass and 24-hour Cr excretion. Actual values are compared with ideal values based on height and weight times 100.	Cr height index of 60% to 80% indicates moderate depletion; less than 60% indicates severe depletion.
OTHER DIAGNOSTIC STUDIES	
• *Chest x-ray:* Procedure used to evaluate organs and structures within the chest for symptoms of disease.	May be normal or show evidence of pleural effusion; small heart silhouette.
• *Electrocardiogram (ECG):* A record of the electrical activity of the heart that provides important information concerning the spread of electricity to the different parts of the heart.	May be normal or demonstrate low voltage, dysrhythmias, and patterns reflective of electrolyte imbalances.

Nursing Priorities

1. Promote consistent intake of adequate calorie and protein requirements.
2. Prevent complications.
3. Minimize energy losses and needs.
4. Provide information about condition, prognosis, and treatment needs.

Discharge Goals

1. Nutritional intake adequate for individual needs.
2. Complications prevented or minimized.
3. Fatigue alleviated.
4. Condition, prognosis, and therapeutic regimen understood.
5. Plan in place to meet needs after discharge.

NURSING DIAGNOSIS: **imbalanced Nutrition: Less than Body Requirements**

May be related to
Conditions that interfere with nutrient intake or increase nutrient need or metabolic demand—cancer and associated treatments, anorexia, surgical procedures, dysphagia, or decreased level of consciousness

Possibly evidenced by
Body weight 10% or more under ideal
Decreased subcutaneous fat or muscle mass, poor muscle tone
Changes in gastric motility and stool characteristics

Desired Outcomes/Evaluation Criteria—Client Will

Nutritional Status NOC
Demonstrate stable weight or progressive weight gain toward goal, with normalization of laboratory values and no signs of malnutrition.

Nutrition Therapy (NIC)
Independent
General

Assess nutritional status continually during daily nursing care, noting energy level; condition of skin, nails, hair, oral cavity; and desire to eat.

Weigh daily and compare with admission weight.

Document oral intake by use of 24-hour recall, food history, and calorie counts, as appropriate.

Ensure accurate collection of specimens (urine and stool) for nitrogen balance studies.

Administer nutritional solutions at prescribed rate via infusion control device, as needed. Adjust rate to deliver prescribed hourly intake. Do not increase rate to "catch up" if infusion slows.

Be familiar with electrolyte content of nutritional solutions.

Schedule activities with adequate rest periods. Promote relaxation techniques.

Total Parenteral Nutrition (TPN) Administration (NIC)

Observe appropriate "hang" time of parenteral solutions per protocol.

Monitor fingerstick glucose per protocol, such as four times per day (JCAHO, 1997; Moghissi, 2009) during initiation of therapy.

Enteral Tube Feeding (NIC)

Assess GI function and tolerance to enteral feedings, knowing type of tube used, such as NG or small bowel. Note bowel sounds, reports of nausea and abdominal discomfort, presence of diarrhea or constipation, development of weakness, lightheadedness, diaphoresis, tachycardia, and abdominal cramping.

Check gastric residuals if bolus feedings are done and as otherwise indicated. Hold feeding and return aspirate per protocol for type and rate of feeding used if residual is greater than predetermined level.

Maintain patency of enteral feeding tubes by flushing with 20 mL warm water before and after feeding and as indicated, such as between multiple doses of medications or when checking gastric residuals.

Transitional

Emphasize importance of transition to oral feedings as appropriate.

Assess gag reflex, ability to chew or swallow, and motor skills when progressing to transitional feedings.

Provides the opportunity to observe deviations from normal client baseline and influences choice of interventions.

Establishes baseline, aids in monitoring effectiveness of therapeutic regimen, and alerts nurse to inappropriate trends in weight loss or gain.

Identifies imbalance between estimated nutritional requirements and actual intake.

Inaccurate collection can alter test results, leading to improper interpretation of client's current status and needs.

Nutritional support prescriptions are based on individually estimated caloric and protein requirements. A consistent rate of nutrient administration ensures proper utilization with fewer side effects, such as hyperglycemia or dumping syndrome. *Note:* Continuous and cyclic infusions of enteral formulas are generally better tolerated than bolus feedings and result in improved absorption.

Metabolic complications of nutritional support often result from a lack of appreciation of changes that can occur because of refeeding—hyperglycemia, hyperosmolar nonketotic coma (HHNC), and electrolyte imbalances.

Conserves energy and reduces calorie needs. (Refer to ND: Fatigue.)

Effectiveness of IV vitamins diminishes and solution degrades after 24 hours.

High glucose content of solutions may lead to pancreatic fatigue, requiring use of supplemental insulin to prevent hyperglycemic complications. *Note:* Fingerstick determination of glucose level is more accurate than urine testing because of variations in renal glucose threshold.

Because protein turnover of the GI mucosa occurs approximately every 3 days, the GI tract is at great risk for early dysfunction and atrophy from disease and malnutrition. Intolerance of formula or presence of dumping syndrome may require alteration of rate of administration, concentration or type of formula, or possibly change to parenteral administration. *Note:* Use of postpyloric feeding tube eliminates need for active bowel sounds as a criterion for tolerance.

Delayed gastric emptying can be caused by a specific disease process, such as paralytic ileus, surgery, shock; by drug therapy, especially opioids; or the protein and fat content of the individual formula. *Note:* Replacement of gastric aspirate reduces loss of gastric acid and electrolytes.

Enteral formulas contain protein that can clog feeding tubes (more likely with small-bore or silicone than with polyurethane tubes), necessitating removal or replacement of tube. *Note:* Cranberry juice or colas are not recommended because they may actually cause an obstruction by promoting formula coagulation. Pancrelipase, a pancreatic enzyme, may be effective in clearing tubing of persistent clog.

Although client may have little interest in food or desire to eat, transition to oral feedings is preferred in view of potential side effects and complications of nutritional support therapy.

May require additional interventions, such as retraining by dysphagia expert or speech therapist, or long-term nutritional support.

(continues on page 476)

ACTIONS/INTERVENTIONS (continued)

Provide self-help utensils as indicated, such as plate guard, utensils with built-up handles, and lidded cups.

Create optimal environment, such as removing noxious stimuli, bedpans, and soiled linens. Provide cheerful, attractive tray or table, soft music, and companionship.

Allow adequate time for chewing, swallowing, and savoring food; provide socialization and feeding assistance, as indicated.

Offer small, frequent feedings; incorporate client's likes and dislikes in meal planning as much as possible, and include "home foods," as appropriate.

Provide calorie-containing beverages when oral intake is possible, such as juices, Jell-O water, and dietary supplements (Boost, Sustacal, Ensure); add Polycase to beverages or water.

Collaborative

Refer to nutritional team and registered dietitian.

Determine nutritional and caloric needs, using appropriate method, such as TEE, BMI, Harris-Benedict equation, and indirect calorimetry test, as indicated.

Enteral Tube Feeding/TPN Administration (NIC)

Assist with insertion and confirm proper placement of feeding tube as appropriate, such as using chest x-ray for central venous catheter or aspiration of green gastric fluid or golden small bowel contents from feeding tube, before administration of solutions. Check pH (0 to 5) of aspirated stomach contents.

Administer dextrose-electrolyte or dextrose–amino acid and lipid emulsions (3-in-1) solutions, as indicated.

Coinfuse lipid emulsions if 3-in-1 solutions are not used.

Administer medications, as indicated, for example:
Multivitamin preparations

Insulin

RATIONALE (continued)

Clients with neuromuscular deficits, such as those due to stroke or brain injury, may require use of special aids developed to facilitate feeding.

Encourages client's attempts to eat, reduces anorexia, and introduces some of the social pleasures usually associated with mealtime.

Clients need encouragement and assistance to overcome underlying problems such as anorexia, fatigue, and muscular weakness.

May enhance client's desire for food and amount of intake.

Maximizes calorie intake when oral intake is limited or restricted.

Aids in identification of nutrient deficits and specific need for parenteral or enteral nutritional intervention.

Several methods are available to provide an estimation of calorie and protein needs. TEE is based on resting and activity energy expenditure and thermic effect of food. BMI estimates caloric needs according to energy requirements per kilogram of body weight. Harris-Benedict provides a reasonable estimate of resting energy expenditure in kilocalories per day. Indirect calorimetry test measures oxygen (O_2) consumption at basal or resting metabolic rate to aid in estimating calorie and protein requirements. *Note:* Although any of these tests may accurately determine individual needs, a standard formula for projecting energy requirements in the ill client is to provide 30 kcal/kg for weight maintenance, 25 kcal/kg for weight loss, or 35 kcal/kg for weight gain.

Reduces risk of feeding-induced complications, including pneumothorax or hemothorax, hydrothorax, air embolus, arterial puncture with central venous line, or aspiration from NG tube.

Solutions provide calories, essential amino acids, and micronutrients, usually combined with lipids for complete nutrition known as total nutrient admixtures (TNA). Solutions are modified to meet specific needs, such as lower protein in renal and liver failure or higher fat in respiratory failure. *Note:* 3-in-1 solution bags are larger (2 to 3 L) and can infuse over a 24-hour period, eliminating the need for frequent bag changes and reducing line manipulation and risk of contamination.

Useful in meeting excessive caloric requirements (e.g., due to burns) or as a source of essential fatty acids during long-term hyperalimentation. *Note:* Lipid solutions may be contraindicated in clients with alterations in fat metabolism or in the presence of pancreatitis, liver damage, anemia, coagulation disorders, or pulmonary disease.

Water-soluble vitamins are added to parenteral solutions. Other vitamins may be given for identified deficiencies.

High glucose content of solutions may require exogenous insulin for metabolism, especially in presence of pancreatic insufficiency or disease. *Note:* Now insulin is usually added directly to parenteral solution.

ACTIONS/INTERVENTIONS (continued)

Diphenoxylate with atropine (Lomotil), camphorated tincture of opium (paregoric), and metoclopramide (Reglan)

Monitor laboratory studies: serum glucose, electrolytes, transferrin, prealbumin, albumin, total protein, phosphate, BUN/Cr, liver enzymes, complete blood count (CBC), and arterial blood gases (ABGs)

RATIONALE (continued)

GI side effects of enteral feeding may need to be controlled with antidiarrheal agents (Lomotil/paregoric) or peristaltic stimulants (Reglan) if more conservative measures such as alteration of rate or strength or type of formula are not successful.

Serum chemistries, blood counts, and lipid profiles are performed before initiation of therapy, providing a baseline for comparison with repeat studies to determine therapy needs and monitor for complications. Untoward metabolic effects of TPN include hypokalemia, hyponatremia and fluid retention, hyperglycemia, hypophosphatemia, increased CO_2 production resulting in respiratory compromise, elevation of liver function tests, and renal dysfunction.

NURSING DIAGNOSIS: risk for Infection

Risk factors may include

Invasive procedures—insertion of venous catheter, surgically placed gastrostomy or jejunostomy feeding tube
Malnutrition, chronic disease
Environmental exposure—access devices in place for extended periods; improper preparation and handling or contamination of the feeding solution

Possibly evidenced by

(Not applicable; presence of signs and symptoms establishes an *actual* diagnosis)

Desired Outcomes/Evaluation Criteria—Client Will

Immune Status (NOC)
Experience no fever or chills.
Demonstrate clean catheter insertion sites, free of drainage and erythema or edema.

ACTIONS/INTERVENTIONS

Infection Protection (NIC)
Independent
Stress and model proper hand-washing technique.
Maintain sterile technique for invasive procedures. Provide routine site care, as appropriate.
Encourage frequent position changes and being out of bed or ambulation, as tolerated.
Screen visitors and care providers for infectious processes, especially upper respiratory infection (URI).
Monitor and assist with respiratory exercises and use of adjuncts, such as incentive spirometer. Auscultate lungs for adventitious sounds.

Assess vital signs, including temperature, per protocol.

Total Parenteral Nutrition (TPN) Administration (NIC)
Maintain an optimal aseptic environment during bedside insertion of central venous catheters and during changes of TPN bottles and administration tubing.
Secure external portion of catheter and administration tubing to dressing with tape. Note intactness of skin suture.

Maintain a sterile occlusive dressing over catheter insertion site. Perform central or peripheral venous catheter dressing care per protocol.

RATIONALE

Reduces risk of cross-contamination.
Prevents entry of bacteria, reducing risk of nosocomial infections.
Limits stasis of body fluids, promotes optimal functioning of organ systems and GI tract.
Reduces risk of transmission of viruses that are difficult to treat.

Promotes deep breathing to clear airways and reduce risk of pneumonia. Presence of wheezes suggests retained secretions and potential complications requiring intervention.
A rise in pulse and temperature may provide warning of infectious process unless client's immune system is too compromised to respond.

Catheter-related sepsis may result from entry of pathogenic microorganisms through skin insertion tract or from touch contamination during manipulations of TPN system.
Manipulation of catheter in and out of insertion site can result in tissue trauma or coring and potentiate entry of skin organisms into catheter tract.
Protects catheter insertion sites from potential sources of contamination. *Note:* Central venous catheter sites can easily become contaminated from tracheotomy or endotracheal secretions, or from wounds of the head, neck, and chest.

(continues on page 478)

ACTIONS/INTERVENTIONS (continued)

Inspect insertion site of catheter for erythema, induration, drainage, and tenderness.

Refrigerate premixed solutions before use; observe a 24-hour hang time for amino acid or total nutrient admixtures solutions and a 12-hour hang time for IV fat emulsions.
Monitor urinary output and serum glucose levels.

Enteral Tube Feeding (NIC)

Keep manipulations of enteral feeding system to a minimum and wash hands before opening system. Handle the system as little as possible.
Alternate nares for tube placement in long-term NG feedings.

Provide daily and as needed site care to abdominally placed feeding tubes.

Refrigerate reconstituted enteral formulas before use; observe a hang time of 4 to 8 hours; discard unused formula after 24 hours.

Infection Protection (NIC)
Collaborative

Aseptically prepare parenteral solutions or enteral formulas for administration. When possible, use prepackaged sterile enteral feeding formula.

Notify physician if signs of infection are present. Follow protocol for obtaining appropriate culture specimens of blood and solutions, and change bottle and tubing, as indicated.
Administer antibiotics, as indicated.

RATIONALE (continued)

The catheter is a potential irritant to the surrounding skin and subcutaneous skin tract, and extended use may result in insertion site irritation and infection.
TPN solutions and fat emulsions have been shown to support the growth of a variety of pathogenic organisms once contaminated.
A rise in temperature or loss of glucose tolerance (glycosuria, hyperglycemia) is an early indication of possible catheter-related sepsis.

Touch contamination of formula is caused by caregiver administration technique.

Reduces risk of trauma and infection of paranasal tissue, especially important in facial trauma or burns.
GI secretions leaking through or around gastrostomy or jejunostomy tube tracts can cause skin breakdown severe enough to require removal of the feeding tube.
Enteral formulas easily support bacterial growth due to high concentration of glucose and lipids and can be contaminated from several sources, including when preparation is mixed or poured or via frequent aspiration of gastric or small bowel contents, use of open system, and use of blue dye.

TPN solutions should be prepared under a laminar flow hood in the pharmacy. Enteral formulas should be mixed in a clean environment in the dietary or pharmacy department. *Note:* Additives to TPN solutions, as a rule, should not be made on the unit because of the potential for contamination and drug incompatibilities.
Necessary to identify source of infection and initiate appropriate therapy. May require removal of TPN line and culture of catheter tip.

May be given prophylactically or for specifically identified organism.

NURSING DIAGNOSIS: risk for Injury [multifactor]

Risk factors may include
External environment—catheter-related complications such as air emboli and septic thrombophlebitis
Internal factors—effects of therapy, drug interactions

Possibly evidenced by
(Not applicable; presence of signs and symptoms establishes an *actual* diagnosis)

Desired Outcomes/Evaluation Criteria—Client Will

Risk Control (NOC)
Be free of complications associated with nutritional support.
Modify environment and correct hazards to enhance safety for in-home therapy.

ACTIONS/INTERVENTIONS

RATIONALE

Surveillance (NIC)
Independent
Parenteral

Maintain a closed central IV system using Luer-Lok connections and taping of all connections.
Administer appropriate TPN solution via peripheral or central venous route, including peripherally inserted central catheter (PICC) lines and tunneled catheters.

Inadvertent disconnection of central IV system can result in lethal air emboli.
Solutions containing high concentrations of dextrose more than 10% must be delivered via a central vein because they result in chemical phlebitis when delivered through small peripheral veins.

ACTIONS/INTERVENTIONS (continued)	**RATIONALE** (continued)
Monitor for potential drug and nutrient interactions.	Various interactions are possible, such as digoxin in conjunction with diuretic therapy, which can cause hypomagnesemia; hypokalemia may result from chronic use of laxatives, mineralocorticoid steroids, diuretics, or amphotericin.
Assess catheter for signs of displacement out of central venous position: extended length of catheter on skin surface, leaking of IV solution onto dressing, client complaints of neck arm pain, tenderness at catheter site, or swelling of extremity on side of catheter insertion.	Central venous catheter tip may slip out of superior vena cava and migrate into smaller innominate and jugular veins, causing a chemical thrombophlebitis. Incidence of subclavian or superior vena cava thrombosis is increased with extended use of central venous catheters.
Inspect peripheral TPN catheter site routinely and change sites at least every other day or per protocol.	Peripheral TPN solutions, although less hyperosmolar, can still irritate small veins and cause phlebitis. Peripheral venous access is often limited in malnourished clients, but site should still be changed if signs of irritation develop.
Investigate reports of severe chest pain or coughing in clients with central line. Turn client to left side in Trendelenburg position, if indicated, and notify physician.	Suggests presence of air embolus requiring immediate intervention to displace air into apex of heart away from the pulmonary artery.
Maintain an occlusive dressing on catheter insertion sites for 24 hours after subclavian catheter is removed.	Extended catheter use may result in development of catheter skin tract. Once the catheter is removed, air embolus is still a potential risk until skin tract has sealed.
Enteral Assess gastrostomy or jejunostomy tube sites for evidence of malposition.	Indwelling and mushroom catheters are still used for feeding tubes inserted via the abdomen. Migration of the catheter balloon can result in duodenal or jejunal obstruction. Improperly sutured gastrostomy tubes may easily fall out.
Collaborative Review chest x-ray, as indicated.	Central parenteral line placement is routinely confirmed by x-ray.
Consult with pharmacist in regard to site and time of delivery of drugs that might have action adversely affected by enteral formula.	Absorption of vitamin D is impaired by administration of mineral oil, which inhibits micelle formation of bile salts, and by neomycin, which inactivates bile salts. Aluminum-containing antacids bind with the phosphorus in the feeding solution, potentiating hypophosphatemia.

NURSING DIAGNOSIS: risk for Aspiration

Risk factors may include
Presence of GI tube, bolus tube feedings, medication administration
Increased intragastric pressure, delayed gastric emptying

Possibly evidenced by
(Not applicable; presence of signs and symptoms establishes an *actual* diagnosis)

Desired Outcomes/Evaluation Criteria—Client Will

Aspiration Prevention (NOC)
Maintain clear airway, free of signs of aspiration.

ACTIONS/INTERVENTIONS	**RATIONALE**
Aspiration Precautions (NIC) *Independent* Confirm placement of nasoenteral feeding tubes. Determine feeding tube position in stomach by x-ray, confirm pH of 0 to 5 for the gastric fluid withdrawn through tube, or auscultate injected air before intermittent feedings. Observe for ability to speak and cough.	Malplacement of nasoenteral feeding tubes may result in aspiration of enteral formula. Clients at particular risk include those who are intubated or obtunded and those who have had a cerebrovascular accident (CVA) or surgery of the head, neck, and upper GI system. *Note:* The reliability of the pH method is reduced if antacids or certain other medications have been given orally or via NG in the past 4 hours. In addition, when using auscultatory method to assess tube placement, air sounds can be transmitted to the epigastrium even if the tube is malpositioned in lung or proximal jejunum.

(continues on page 480)

479

Maintain aspiration precautions during enteral feedings, such as the following:

Keep head of bed elevated at 30 to 45 degrees during feeding and for at least 1 hour after feeding.

Reduces risk of regurgitation or gastric reflux.

Inflate tracheostomy cuff during and for 1 hour after intermittent feeding. Interrupt continuous feeding when client is in prone position.

Aspiration of enteral formulas is highly irritating to the lung parenchyma and may result in pneumonia and respiratory compromise.

Add blue food coloring to enteral formula, as indicated.

Helps identify aspiration of enteral formula and tracheal esophageal fistula, if discovered in sputum or lung secretions. *Note:* Avoid use of methylene blue dye, which may cause false-positive guiac test when assessing for GI bleeding.

Monitor gastric residuals between or before bolus feedings (as previously noted in ND: imbalanced Nutrition: Less than Body Requirements).

Presence of large gastric residuals may potentiate an incompetent esophageal sphincter, leading to vomiting and aspiration.

Note characteristics of sputum and tracheal aspirate. Investigate development of dyspnea, cough, tachypnea, and cyanosis. Auscultate breath sounds.

Presence of formula in tracheal secretions or signs and symptoms reflecting respiratory distress suggests aspiration.

Note indicators of NG tube intolerance, such as absence of gag reflex, high risk of aspiration, and frequent removal of NG feeding tubes.

May require consideration of surgically placed feeding tube, percutaneous endoscopic gastrostomy (PEG), or jejunostomy for client safety and consistency of enteral formula delivery.

Collaborative

Review abdominal x-ray if performed.

Confirmation of placement of gastric feeding tube should be obtained by x-ray. *Note:* Injection of air boluses is no longer recommended.

NURSING DIAGNOSIS: **risk for imbalanced Fluid Volume**

Risk factors may include

Active loss or failure of regulatory mechanisms specific to underlying disease process or trauma; complications of nutrition therapy—high-glucose solutions, hyperglycemia (hyperosmolar nonketotic coma and severe dehydration)

Inability to obtain or ingest fluids

Possibly evidenced by

(Not applicable; presence of signs and symptoms establishes an *actual* diagnosis)

Desired Outcomes/Evaluation Criteria—Client Will

Fluid Balance (NOC)

Display moist skin, moist mucous membranes, stable vital signs, and individually adequate urinary output; be free of edema and excessive weight loss or inappropriate gain.

ACTIONS/INTERVENTIONS

RATIONALE

Fluid Management (NIC)

Independent

Assess for clinical signs of dehydration such as thirst, dry skin and mucous membranes, hypotension, or fluid excess, including peripheral edema, tachycardia, and adventitious breath sounds.

Early detection and intervention may prevent occurrence of excessive fluctuation in fluid balance. *Note:* Severely malnourished clients have an increased risk of developing refeeding syndrome, such as life-threatening fluid overload, intracellular electrolyte shifts, and cardiac strain occurring during initial 3 to 5 days of therapy.

Incorporate knowledge of caloric density of enteral formulas into assessment of fluid balance.

Enteric solutions are usually concentrated and do not meet free water needs.

Provide additional water and flush tubing, as indicated.

With higher calorie formula, additional water is needed to prevent dehydration or hyperglycemic complications.

Record intake and output (I&O), calculate fluid balance, and measure urine specific gravity.

Excessive urinary losses may reflect developing HHNC. Specific gravity is an indicator of hydration and renal function.

Weigh daily, or as indicated; evaluate changes.

Rapid weight gain reflecting fluid retention can predispose or potentiate heart failure (HF) or pulmonary edema. Gain of more than 0.5 lb/day indicates fluid retention and not deposition of lean body mass.

ACTIONS/INTERVENTIONS (continued)

RATIONALE (continued)

Collaborative

Monitor laboratory studies, such as the following:
  Serum potassium and phosphorus

Hypokalemia and phosphatemia can occur because of intracellular shifts during initial refeeding and may compromise cardiac function if not corrected.

  Hematocrit (Hct)

Reflects hydration and circulating volume.

  Serum albumin

Hypoalbuminemia and decreased colloidal osmotic pressure leads to third spacing of fluid and edema.

  Serum transferrin

Reacts quickly to changes in protein status.

  Prealbumin

Sensitive to low levels of protein.

Dilute formula or change from hypertonic to isotonic formula, as indicated.

May decrease gastric intolerance, reducing occurrence of diarrhea and associated fluid losses.

NURSING DIAGNOSIS: **Fatigue**

May be related to

Decreased metabolic energy production; increased energy requirements—hypermetabolic states, healing process

Altered body chemistry: medications, chemotherapy

Possibly evidenced by

Overwhelming lack of energy, inability to maintain usual routines or accomplish routine tasks

Lethargy, impaired ability to concentrate

Desired Outcomes/Evaluation Criteria—Client Will

Endurance (NOC)

Report increased sense of well-being and energy level.

Demonstrate measurable increase in physical activity.

ACTIONS/INTERVENTIONS

RATIONALE

Energy Management (NIC)

Independent

Monitor physiological response to activity, including changes in blood pressure (BP) or heart and respiratory rates.

Tolerance varies greatly, depending on the stage of the disease process, nutritional state, and fluid balance.

Establish realistic activity goals with client.

Provides for a sense of control and feelings of accomplishment.

Plan care to allow for rest periods. Schedule activities for periods when client has most energy. Involve client and caregiver in planning schedule.

Frequent rest periods are needed to restore or conserve energy. Planning allows client to be active during times when energy level is higher, which may restore a feeling of well-being and a sense of control.

Encourage client to do self-care when appropriate, such as sitting up in chair and walking. Increase activity level, as indicated.

Increases strength and stamina and enables client to become more active without undue fatigue.

Provide passive and active range-of-motion (ROM) exercises to bedridden clients.

The development of healthy lean muscle mass depends on the provision of both isotonic and isometric exercises. Prevents muscle wasting.

Keep bed in low position and walkways clear of furniture; assist with ambulation.

Protects client from injury during activities.

Assist with self-care needs, as necessary.

Generalized weakness may make activities of daily living (ADLs) almost impossible for client to complete.

Collaborative

Provide supplemental O₂, as indicated.

Presence of anemia or hypoxemia reduces O_2 available for cellular uptake and contributes to fatigue and decreased immune response.

Refer to physical or occupational therapy.

Programmed daily exercises and activities help client maintain or increase strength and muscle tone and enhance sense of well-being.

NURSING DIAGNOSIS: deficient Knowledge [Learning Need] regarding condition, prognosis, treatment, self-care, and discharge needs

May be related to

Lack of exposure and recall, information misinterpretation

Cognitive limitation

Possibly evidenced by

Request for information, questions and statement of misconception

Inaccurate follow-through of instructions or development of preventable complications

Desired Outcomes/Evaluation Criteria—Client Will

Knowledge: Disease Process (NOC)

Verbalize understanding of condition or the disease process and individual nutritional needs.

Knowledge: Treatment Procedure (NOC)

Correctly perform necessary procedures and explain reasons for the actions.

ACTIONS/INTERVENTIONS	RATIONALE
Teaching: Prescribed Diet (NIC)	
Independent	
Assess client's and significant other's (SO's) knowledge of nutritional state.	Determines content matter to be presented.
Review individual situation, signs and symptoms of malnutrition, future expectations, and transitional feeding needs.	Provides information from which client and SO can make informed choices. Knowledge of the interaction between malnutrition and illness is helpful in understanding need for special therapy.
Discuss reasons for use of parenteral or enteral nutrition support.	May experience anxiety regarding inability to eat and may not comprehend the nutritional value of the prescribed TPN or tube feedings.
Provide adequate time for teaching client and SO when client is going home on enteral or parenteral feedings. Document client's and SO's understanding, ability, and competence to deliver safe home therapy.	Generally, 3 to 4 days is sufficient for client and SO to become proficient with tube feedings. Parenteral therapy is more complex, and client and SO may require a week or longer to feel ready for home management; follow-up in the home is required.
Discuss proper handling, storage, and preparation of nutritional solutions or food prepared by a blender; also discuss aseptic or clean techniques for care of insertion sites and use of dressings.	Reduces risk of formula or solution-related problems, metabolic complications, and infection.
Review use and proper care of nutritional support devices.	Client understanding and cooperation are key to the safe insertion and maintenance of nutritional support access devices and prevention of complications.
	Promotes safe self-care and reduces risk of complications.
Review specific precautions, depending on type of feeding, such as checking placement of tube, sitting upright for enteral feeding, maintaining patency of tube, anchoring of tubing, and adequate length of tubing for nighttime feeding.	
Discuss and demonstrate reinsertion of enterostomal feeding tube, if appropriate.	Tube may be changed routinely or inserted only for feedings. Intermittent feedings enhance client mobility and aid in transition to regular feeding pattern.
Identify signs and symptoms requiring medical evaluation— nausea and vomiting, abdominal cramping or bloating, diarrhea, rapid weight changes, erythema, drainage, foul odor at tube insertion site, fever and chills, coughing and choking, or difficulty breathing during enteral feeding.	Early evaluation and treatment of problems such as feeding intolerance, infection, and aspiration may prevent progression to complications that are more serious.
Instruct client and SO in glucose monitoring, if indicated.	Timely recognition of changes in blood glucose levels reduces risk of hyperglycemic or hypoglycemic reactions in client on hyperalimentation.
Discuss signs, symptoms, and treatment of hyperglycemia and hypoglycemia.	Hyperglycemia is more common for clients receiving parenteral feedings and those who have pancreas or liver disease or are taking large doses of corticosteroids. Rebound hypoglycemia can occur when feedings are intentionally or accidentally discontinued.

ACTIONS/INTERVENTIONS (continued)

Encourage use of diary for recording test results, physical feelings and any reactions, activity level, oral intake if any, I&O, and weekly weight.

Recommend daily exercise and activity to tolerance, scheduling of adequate rest periods.

Ascertain that all supplies are in place in the home before discharge; make arrangements as needed with suppliers, such as hospital, pharmacy, medical equipment company, and laboratory.

Refer to nutritional support team, home healthcare agency, and counseling resources. Provide with immediate access phone numbers.

RATIONALE (continued)

Provides resource for review by healthcare providers for optimal management of individual situation.

Enhances gastric motility for enteral transition feedings, promotes feelings of general well-being, and prevents undue fatigue.

Provides for successful, smooth transition from acute care setting to home and competent home therapy.

Client and SO needs readily available support persons to assist with nutrition therapy, equipment problems, and emotional adjustments in long-term or home-based therapy.

POTENTIAL CONSIDERATIONS following acute hospitalization (dependent on client's age, physical condition and presence of complications, personal resources, and life responsibilities)

- *Fatigue*—decreased metabolic energy production, increased energy requirements (hypermetabolic states, healing process), altered body chemistry, such as due to medications, chemotherapy
- *risk for Injury*—catheter-related complications (catheter breaks, dislodgement, occlusion), effects of therapy (such as electrolyte and fluid shifts, diarrhea), drug interactions, aspiration
- *risk for Infection*—invasive tubes, environmental exposure, malnutrition, chronic disease
- *interrupted Family Processes*—situational crises

METABOLIC ACID-BASE IMBALANCES

I. Pathophysiology
  a. The body has the remarkable ability to maintain plasma pH within the narrow range of 7.35 to 7.45; this is accomplished by means of chemical buffering mechanisms involving the kidneys and the lungs.

  b. Although single acid-base (such as metabolic acidosis) imbalances do occur, mixed acid-base imbalances are more common—metabolic acidosis and respiratory acidosis as occurs with cardiac arrest.

METABOLIC ACIDOSIS—PRIMARY BASE BICARBONATE (HCO_3^-) DEFICIENCY

I. Pathophysiology
  a. Reflects a relative excess of acid or hydrogen (H^+) and a deficit of base or bicarbonate (HCO_3^-)
  b. Gain of strong acid may be *endogenous* (for example, ketoacids from lipid metabolism) or *exogenous* (for example, NH_4Cl infusion).
  c. Bicarbonate loss may occur via the bowel or kidneys.

II. Etiology—characterized by normal or high anion gap situations (Priestley, 2007; Thomas & Hamwai, 2007)
  a. *Normal anion gap* (or nonanion gap) acidosis is associated with loss of bicarbonate from the body, gain of chloride, or decreased ammonia production.
    i. Gastrointestinal (GI) losses: vomiting, diarrhea, small-bowel and pancreatic or biliary fistulas, ileal loop bladder
    ii. Early renal failure
    iii. Obstructed ileostomy
    iv. Infusion of ammonium chloride, hyperalimentation; intravenous (IV) sodium chloride in presence of preexisting kidney dysfunction; acidifying drugs

  b. *High anion gap* acidosis reflects accumulation of organic anions.
    i. Diabetic ketoacidosis
    ii. Severe malnutrition or starvation, high-fat, low-carbohydrate diets; parenteral lipid administration
    iii. Alcoholic lactic acidosis
    iv. Renal tubular necrosis
    v. Poisoning: salicylate intoxication (after initial stage), paraldehyde intoxication; drug therapy including acetazolamide (Diamox), isoniazid (INH); or NH_4Cl
  c. Compensatory mechanisms
    i. Hyperventilation to reduce $PaCO_2$
    ii. Decreased renal secretion of H^+, less production of ammonia, and excretion of HCO_3^-
    iii. Treatment of underlying condition

III. Statistics: Morbidity and mortality are primarily related to the underlying disease; therefore, separate statistics are not collected.

Acidemia: Blood disorder characterized by an increased concentration of H^+ ions in the blood.

Acidosis: An increased acidity or increased H^+ ion concentration. If not further qualified, it refers to acidity of the blood plasma. Acidosis is said to occur when arterial pH falls below 7.35.

Base excess/deficit: A calculated number that represents a sum total of the metabolic buffering agents (anions) in the blood; these anions include hemoglobin, proteins, phosphates, and HCO_3^- (the dominant anion); these anions try to compensate for imbalances in the pH caused by diseases or conditions that affect the lungs (respiratory acidosis and alkalosis) or kidneys (metabolic acidosis and alkalosis).

Carbonic acid (H_2CO_3): If too much acid is present, the HCO_3^- ions take up the H^+ ions, creating H_2CO_3, which is then excreted through the lungs in the form of carbon dioxide (CO_2) and water (H_2O). Conversely, if too little acid is present in extracellular fluid, the H_2CO_3 portion of the HCO_3^- buffer system releases H^+ ions. For the pH to remain within normal range (7.35 to 7.45), the ratio of HCO_3^- ions to H_2CO_3 must be 20:1 (Felver, 2005).

CO_2: Respiratory acid—the only acid that can be exhaled via the lungs.

Endogenous: Produced or originating from within the body.

Exogenous: Originating outside the body.

H^+: The ion that is left when the hydrogen atom loses its electron, forming a proton.

HCO_3^-: A measurement of the metabolic component of the acid-base balance. HCO_3^- is excreted and reabsorbed or conserved by the kidneys in response to pH imbalances and is directly related to the pH level; as the amount of HCO_3^- rises, so does the pH.

Kussmaul's respiration: An abnormal respiratory pattern characterized by rapid, deep breathing; often seen in metabolic acidosis.

Partial pressure of carbon dioxide ($PaCO_2$): Reflects the balance between the production of CO_2 and its elimination. Unless the metabolic rate changes, the amount of CO_2 produced is roughly constant and determines the amount of ventilation required and the level of PCO_2. The normal value in arterial blood is 40 mm Hg. In the healthy, awake individual, the end-exhaled value is usually similar.

pH: A measure of the level of H^+ ion, which indicates the acid-base status of blood; the pH decreases (becomes more acidic) with increased amounts of PCO_2 and other acids, and the pH increases (blood becomes more alkaline) with decreased PCO_2 or increased amounts of bases like HCO_3^-.

Care Setting

This condition does not occur in isolation but rather is a complication of a broader problem that may require inpatient care in a medical-surgical or subacute unit.

Related Concerns

Plans of care are specific to predisposing factors.
Fluid and electrolyte imbalances, page 903
Renal dialysis—general considerations, page 560
Respiratory acidosis (primary carbonic acid excess), page 195
Respiratory alkalosis (primary carbonic acid deficit), page 200

Client Assessment Database

Data depend on the underlying cause.

DIAGNOSTIC DIVISION MAY REPORT	MAY EXHIBIT
ACTIVITY/REST • Lethargy, fatigue • Muscle weakness	
CIRCULATION	• Hypotension, wide pulse pressure • Pulse may be weak, irregular • Jaundiced sclera, skin, mucous membranes (liver failure)
ELIMINATION • Diarrhea	• Dark/concentrated urine
FOOD/FLUID • Anorexia • Nausea, vomiting	• Poor skin turgor, dry mucous membranes

Client Assessment Database (continued)

DIAGNOSTIC DIVISION MAY REPORT (continued)	MAY EXHIBIT (continued)
NEUROSENSORY • Drowsiness, changes in thinking ability	• Changes in sensorium—stupor, confusion, lethargy, depression, delirium, coma • Decreased deep-tendon reflexes, muscle weakness
PAIN/DISCOMFORT • Headache • Abdominal pain	
RESPIRATION • Dyspnea on exertion	• Hyperventilation, Kussmaul's respiration
SAFETY • Transfusion of blood and blood products • Exposure to hepatitis virus	• Fever, signs of sepsis
TEACHING/LEARNING • History of diabetes, alcohol abuse, or prolonged starvation • Use of carbonic anhydrase inhibitors or anion-exchange resins—cholestyramine (Questran) • Ingestion of drugs or toxins, such as salicylates, acetazolamide, cyclosporine, ethylene glycol, methanol	
DISCHARGE PLAN CONSIDERATIONS • May require change in therapies for underlying disease process, condition ▶ Refer to section at end of plan for postdischarge considerations.	

Diagnostic Studies

TEST WHY IT IS DONE	WHAT IT TELLS ME
BLOOD TESTS • *Arterial pH:* Adult normal range is 7.35 to 7.45.	Decreased in uncompensated metabolic acidosis (below 7.35) because of excess metabolic acids.
• HCO_3^-: Adult normal range is 22 to 26 mEq/L.	Decreased, less than 22 mEq/L.
• $PaCO_2$: Adult normal range is 36 to 44 mm Hg.	Level is below 35 mm Hg.
• *Base excess:* Adult normal base values are between -2.3 and $+2.3$ $mmol/L^{-1}$.	Value of more than $+3$ $mmol/L^{-1}$ indicates metabolic acidosis.
• *Anion gap:* A calculation of the difference between the sum of cations (sodium, potassium, chloride, and HCO_3^- ions) and anions (sulfates, phosphates, proteinates, organic acids) found in plasma or serum. Adult normal range is 8 to 16 mmol/L.	Level is above 14 mmol/L (high anion gap) or range of 10 to 14 mmol/L (normal anion gap).
• *Serum potassium:* Essential electrolyte needed to regulate water balance, levels of acidity, and blood pressure (BP).	Client may have a low serum potassium level due to excessive body losses of potassium or an elevated serum potassium level secondary to renal insufficiency, tissue breakdown, and shift of potassium from the intracellular space to the extracellular space as a result of acidemia (Priestley, 2006).

(continues on page 486)

TEST WHY IT IS DONE (continued)	WHAT IT TELLS ME (continued)
• *Serum chloride: (Cl⁻):* Negatively charged ion in the fluid outside the body's cells that works with other substances, including sodium, to help control the body's fluid level and acid-base balance.	Level is increased.
• *Serum glucose:* Simple sugar in the blood.	Hypoglycemia associated with a metabolic acidosis can be caused by adrenal insufficiency or liver failure. Hyperglycemia will be present in metabolic acidosis in the presence of diabetic ketoacidosis.
• *Serum ketones:* Acidic substances produced when the body uses fat instead of sugar for energy.	Increased in ketoacidosis, starvation, and alcohol intoxication.
• *Plasma lactic acid:* Acid produced by glucose-burning cells when these cells have an insufficient supply of oxygen.	Elevated in lactic acidosis.
OTHER DIAGNOSTIC STUDIES • *Urinalysis:* Measures pH and renal function in presence of diabetic ketoacidosis.	Urine pH is decreased, less than 4.5, in absence of renal disease. Glucose and ketones may be present.
• *Eletrocardiogram (ECG):* Provides a record of the electrical activity of the heart.	Cardiac dysrhythmias (bradycardia) and pattern changes associated with hyperkalemia, such as with a tall T wave.

Nursing Priorities

1. Achieve homeostasis.
2. Prevent or minimize complications.
3. Provide information about condition, prognosis, and treatment needs, as appropriate.

Discharge Goals

1. Physiological balance restored.
2. Free of complications.
3. Condition, prognosis, and treatment needs understood.
4. Plan in place to meet needs after discharge.

Because no current nursing diagnosis speaks clearly to metabolic imbalances, the following interventions are presented in a general format for inclusion in the primary plan of care.

NURSING DIAGNOSIS:

Desired Outcomes/Evaluation Criteria—Client Will

Electrolyte & Acid/Base Balance (NOC)
Display serum HCO_3^- and electrolytes within normal limits (WNL).
Be free of symptoms of imbalance—absence of neurological impairment and vital signs WNL.

ACTIONS/INTERVENTIONS	RATIONALE
Acid-Base Management: Metabolic Acidosis (NIC) *Independent* Monitor BP.	Arteriolar dilation or decreased cardiac contractility (such as occurs with sepsis), and hypovolemia occur, resulting in systemic shock, evidenced by hypotension and tissue hypoxia.
Assess level of consciousness (LOC) and note progressive changes in neuromuscular status—strength, tone, and movement.	Decreased mental function, confusion, seizures, weakness, and flaccid paralysis can occur because of hypoxia, hyperkalemia, and decreased pH of cerebrospinal and interstitial fluids (Felver, 2005).
Provide seizure and coma precautions—bed in low position, use of padded side rails, and frequent observation.	Protects client from injury resulting from decreased mentation and convulsions.

ACTIONS/INTERVENTIONS (continued)	RATIONALE (continued)
Monitor heart rate and rhythm.	Acidemia may be manifested by changes in ECG configuration and presence of bradydysrhythmias as well as increased ventricular irritability such as fibrillation—signs of hyperkalemia. Life-threatening cardiovascular collapse may also occur because of vasodilation and decreased cardiac contractility. *Note:* Hypokalemia can occur as acidosis is corrected, resulting in premature ventricular contractions (PVCs) or ventricular tachycardia.
Observe for altered respiratory excursion, rate, and depth.	Hyperventilation, or Kussmaul's respiration, may be noted as a compensatory mechanism to eliminate excess acid; however, as potassium shifts out of cells in an attempt to correct acidosis, respiration may become depressed. Transient respiratory depression may be the result of overcorrection of metabolic acidosis with sodium bicarbonate.
Assess skin temperature, color, and capillary refill.	Evaluates circulatory status, tissue perfusion, and effects of hypotension.
Auscultate bowel sounds; measure abdominal girth, as indicated.	In the presence of coexisting hyperkalemia, GI distress, including abdominal distention, diarrhea, and colicky pain, may be present.
Monitor intake and output (I&O) closely and weigh regularly.	Marked dehydration may be present because of GI losses. Therapy needs are based on underlying cause and fluid balance.
Monitor urine pH.	Kidneys attempt to compensate for acidosis by excreting excess hydrogen in the form of weak acids and ammonia. Maximum urine acidity is pH of 4.
Provide oral hygiene with sodium bicarbonate washes and lemon and glycerin swabs.	Neutralizes mouth acids and provides protective lubrication.
Collaborative	
Assist with identification and treatment of underlying cause.	Treatment of disorder is directed at mild correction of acidosis until organ(s) function is improved. Addressing the primary condition, such as diabetic ketoacidosis (DKA), liver or renal failure, drug poisoning, and sepsis, promotes correction of the acid-base disorder.
Monitor and graph serial arterial blood gases (ABGs).	Evaluates therapy needs and effectiveness. Blood bicarbonate and pH should slowly move toward normal levels.
Monitor serum electrolytes, such as potassium.	As acidosis is corrected, serum hypokalemia may occur as potassium shifts back into the cells.
Replace fluids, as indicated, depending on underlying etiology.	Choice of solution varies with cause of acidosis. *Note:* Lactate-containing solutions may be contraindicated in the presence of lactic acidosis.
Administer medications, as indicated, such as:	
Sodium bicarbonate/lactate or saline IV	May be given in life-threatening hypokalemia and severe lactic acidosis, but is used rarely to correct severe acidosis with pH less than 7.2 because sodium bicarbonate can cause rebound metabolic alkalosis.
Potassium	May be required as potassium re-enters the cell, causing a serum deficit.
Phosphate	May be administered to enhance acid excretion in presence of chronic acidosis with hypophosphatemia.
Calcium	May be given to improve neuromuscular conduction and function.
Modify diet as indicated, such as low-protein, high-carbohydrate diet in presence of renal failure, or adjust medical nutritional therapy for the person with diabetes.	Restriction of protein may be necessary to decrease production of acid waste products, whereas addition of complex carbohydrates will correct acid production from the metabolism of fats.
Administer exchange resins and assist with dialysis, as indicated.	May be desired to reduce acidosis by decreasing excess potassium and acid waste products if pH less than 7.1 and other therapies are ineffective or heart failure (HF) develops.

POTENTIAL CONSIDERATIONS:
Refer to Potential Considerations relative to underlying cause of acid-base disorder.

METABOLIC ALKALOSIS—PRIMARY BASE BICARBONATE EXCESS

I. Pathophysiology

a. Increase in base or bicarbonate (HCO_3^-) concentration, generally reflecting a relative loss or shift of hydrogen (H^+) and/or gain in HCO_3^-.

b. Organ systems most often involved are the kidneys and the gastrointestinal (GI) tract.

c. Consequences of the condition on organ systems dependent on degree of alkalemia and underlying pathology.

II. Etiology

a. Chloride-responsive: Urine chloride is less than 20 mEq/L and decreased extracellular fluid (ECF) volume.

  i. GI acid losses: vomiting, nasogastric suction, diarrhea associated with villous adenoma

  ii. Diuretics: Thiazides and loop diuretics interfere with reabsorption of sodium and chloride in the renal tubules, causing loss of chloride.

  iii. HCO_3^- excess: correction of respiratory acidosis, chronic ingestion of large doses of antacids

  iv. Laxative abuse

b. Chloride-resistant: Urine chloride is greater than 20 mEq/L and increased ECF volume.

  i. Renal acid loss: primary or secondary hyperaldosteronism, thiazides or loop diuretics, hypokalemia and hypomagnesemia; genetic deficiency of 11-B-HSD2 or inhibition by licorice, chewing tobacco

  ii. Renal artery stenosis

c. Other causes

  i. Carbohydrate feeding after starvation

  ii. Hypercalcemia

  iii. Multiple blood transfusions

d. Compensatory mechanisms

  i. Rapid excretion of HCO_3^- by the kidneys whenever plasma level exceeds 24 mmol/L—requires normal kidney function, with the ability to filter HCO_3^- and to excrete excess H^+

  ii. Hypoventilation: slow, shallow respirations to increase retention of carbonic acid

III. Statistics

a. Morbidity: Primarily related to the underlying disease; therefore, separate statistics are not collected; most common acid-base imbalance in hospitalized adults (Huang & Priestley, 2007).

b. Mortality: 45% for arterial pH over 7.55; 80% for arterial pH over 7.65 (Yaseen & Thomas, 2007).

GLOSSARY

Base: Chemical opposite of acid.

Base excess/deficit: A calculated number that represents a sum total of the metabolic buffering agents or anions in the blood, including hemoglobin, proteins, phosphates, and HCO_3^- (dominant anion). These anions try to compensate for imbalances in the pH caused by diseases or conditions that affect the lungs (respiratory acidosis/alkalosis) or kidneys (metabolic acidosis/alkalosis).

Chvostek's sign: In tetany, tapping the muscles of the face causes them to go into spasm, reflecting severe hypocalcemia.

Electroneutrality: The principle that in an electrolytic solution, the concentrations of all the ions are such that the solution as a whole is neutral.

Extracellular fluid (ECF): All body fluid located outside of cells, including fluid inside blood vessels and between cells.

HCO_3^-: Measurement of the metabolic component of the acid-base balance. HCO_3^- is excreted and reabsorbed (conserved) by the kidneys in response to pH imbalances and is directly related to the pH level; as the amount of HCO_3^- rises, so does the pH.

H^+: The ion that is left when the hydrogen atom loses its electron, forming a proton.

Intracellular fluid: Fluid located inside the cell.

Kussmaul's respiration: An abnormal respiratory pattern characterized by rapid, deep breathing; often seen in metabolic acidosis.

Partial pressure of carbon dioxide ($PaCO_2$): Reflects the balance between the production of carbon dioxide and its elimination.

pH: Measure of the level of H^+ ion, which indicates the acid-base status of blood. The pH decreases or becomes more acidic with increased amounts of $PaCO_2$ and other acids, and the pH increases or blood becomes more alkaline with decreased $PaCO_2$ or increased amounts of bases such as HCO_3^-.

Tetany: Hyperexcitability of nerves and muscles because of decreased extracellular calcium.

Trousseau's sign: Compression of upper arm causes spasm of the hand, reflecting hidden tetany.

Care Setting

This condition does not occur in isolation but rather is a complication of a broader problem that may require inpatient care in a medical-surgical or subacute unit.

Related Concerns

Plans of care are specific to predisposing factors.
Fluid and electrolyte imbalances, page 903
Renal dialysis—general considerations, page 560
Respiratory acidosis (primary carbonic acid excess), page 195
Respiratory alkalosis (primary carbonic acid deficit), page 200

Client Assessment Database

DIAGNOSTIC DIVISION MAY REPORT	MAY EXHIBIT
CIRCULATION	• Tachycardia, irregularities, or dysrhythmias • Hypotension • Cyanosis
ELIMINATION • Diarrhea—with high chloride content • Use of potassium-losing diuretics (Diuril, Hygroton, Lasix, Edecrin) • Laxative abuse	
FOOD/FLUID • Anorexia, nausea, prolonged vomiting • High salt intake, excessive ingestion of licorice • Recurrent indigestion or heartburn with frequent use of antacids or baking soda	
NEUROSENSORY • Tingling of fingers and toes, circumoral paresthesia • Muscle twitching, weakness • Dizziness	• Hypertonicity of muscles, tetany, tremors, convulsions, loss of reflexes • Confusion, irritability, restlessness, belligerence, apathy, coma • Picking at bedclothes
SAFETY • Recent blood transfusions with citrated blood	
RESPIRATION	• Hypoventilation—increases $PaCO_2$ and conserves carbonic acid; periods of apnea
TEACHING/LEARNING • History of primary aldosteronism, Cushing's syndrome, primary reninism, Bartter's syndrome, milk-alkali syndrome, corticosteroid therapy, pyloric stenosis or ulcers, self-induced vomiting (bulimia), long-term use of diuretics	
DISCHARGE PLAN CONSIDERATIONS • May require change in therapy for underlying disease process, condition ◗ Refer to section at end of plan for postdischarge considerations.	

TEST WHY IT IS DONE	WHAT IT TELLS ME
BLOOD TESTS	
• *Arterial pH:* Adult normal range is 7.35 to 7.45.	Increased, higher than 7.55.
• *HCO₃⁻:* Adult normal range is 22 to 26 mEq/L.	Increased, higher than 26 mEq/L (primary).
• *PaCO₂:* Adult normal range is 36 to 44 mm Hg.	Slightly increased, above 45 mm Hg (compensatory).
• *Base excess:* Adult normal base values are between −2.3 and +2.3 mmol/L⁻¹.	Level is increased.
• *Serum chloride:* Negatively charged ion in the fluid outside the body's cells. It works with other substances, including sodium, to help control the body's fluid level and acid-base balance.	Decreased, less than 98 mEq/L, disproportionately to serum sodium decreases (if alkalosis is hypochloremic).
• *Serum sodium and potassium:* Essential electrolytes needed to regulate water balance, levels of acidity, and blood pressure (BP).	Levels are decreased.
• *Serum calcium:* Important in maintaining acid-base balance.	Usually decreased. Prolonged hypercalcemia (nonparathyroid) may be a predisposing factor.
OTHER DIAGNOSTIC STUDIES	
• *Urinalysis:* Measures level of pH in urine.	Increased pH, higher than 7.0.
• *Urine chloride:* Helpful in determining therapeutic choices.	Levels less than 10 mEq/L suggest chloride-responsive alkalosis, whereas levels above 20 mEq/L suggest chloride resistance.
• *Electrocardiogram (ECG):* A record of the electrical activity of the heart.	May show hypokalemic changes, including peaked P waves, flat T waves, depressed ST segment, low T wave merging to P wave, and elevated U waves.

Nursing Priorities

1. Achieve homeostasis.
2. Prevent or minimize complications.
3. Provide information about condition, prognosis, and treatment needs, as appropriate.

Discharge Goals

1. Physiological balance restored.
2. Free of complications.
3. Condition, prognosis, and treatment needs understood.
4. Plan in place to meet needs after discharge.

Because no current nursing diagnosis speaks clearly to metabolic imbalances, the following interventions are presented in a general format for inclusion in the primary plan of care.

NURSING DIAGNOSIS:

Desired Outcomes/Evaluation Criteria—Client Will

Electrolyte & Acid/Base Balance NOC
Display serum HCO₃⁻ and electrolytes within normal limits (WNL).
Be free of symptoms of imbalance—absence of neurological impairment and irritability.

ACTIONS/INTERVENTIONS	RATIONALE
Metabolic Alkalosis Management NIC *Independent* Monitor respiratory rate, rhythm, and depth.	Hypoventilation is a compensatory mechanism to conserve carbonic acid and represents definite risks to the individual, such as hypoxemia and respiratory failure.

ACTIONS/INTERVENTIONS (continued)	RATIONALE (continued)
Assess level of consciousness and neuromuscular status—strength, tone, and movement; note presence of Chvostek's and Trousseau's signs.	The central nervous system (CNS) may be hyperirritable related to increased pH of CNS fluid, resulting in tingling, numbness, dizziness, restlessness, or apathy and confusion. Hypocalcemia may contribute to tetany, although occurrence is rare.
Monitor heart rate and rhythm.	Atrial or ventricular ectopic beats and tachydysrhythmias may develop.
Record amount and source of output.	Helpful in identifying source of acid loss—potassium and hydrochloric (HCl) acid are lost in vomiting and GI suctioning.
Monitor intake and daily weight.	Useful in monitoring fluid status.
Restrict oral intake and reduce noxious environmental stimuli, use intermittent or low suction during nasogastric (NG) suctioning, and irrigate gastric tube with isotonic solutions rather than water.	Limits gastric losses of HCl, potassium, and calcium.
Provide seizure safety precautions, as indicated—padded side rails, airway protection, bed in low position, and frequent observation.	Changes in mentation and neuromuscular hyperirritability may result in client harm, especially if tetany or convulsions occur.
Encourage intake of foods and fluids high in potassium and possibly calcium, dependent on blood level—canned grapefruit and apple juices, bananas, cauliflower, dried peaches, figs, and wheat germ.	Useful in replacing potassium losses when oral intake permitted.
Review medication regimen for use of diuretics, such as thiazides (Diuril, Hygroton), furosemide (Lasix), and ethacrynic acid (Edecrin).	Discontinuation of these potassium-wasting drugs may prevent recurrence of imbalance.
Instruct client to avoid use of excessive amounts of sodium HCO_3^- antacids, such as Alka-Seltzer or baking soda.	Ulcer clients can cause alkalosis by taking over-the-counter (OTC) products containing sodium HCO_3^-, especially when taken in addition to prescribed alkaline antacids.
Collaborative	
Assist with identification and treatment of underlying disorder.	Addressing the primary condition, such as prolonged vomiting and diarrhea, hyperaldosteronism, and Cushing's syndrome, promotes correction of the acid-base disorder.
Monitor laboratory studies as indicated, such as arterial blood gases (ABGs)/pH, serum electrolytes, especially potassium, and blood urea nitrogen (BUN).	Evaluates therapy needs and effectiveness and monitors renal function.
Administer medications, as indicated, for example:	
Chloride solutions, such as sodium chloride by mouth (PO) or Lactated Ringer's solution intravenously (IV), unless contraindicated	Correcting sodium, water, and chloride defects may be all that is needed to permit kidneys to excrete HCO_3^- and correct alkalosis, but must be used with caution in clients with heart failure (HF) or renal insufficiency.
Potassium chloride	Hypokalemia is frequently present. Chloride is needed so kidneys can absorb sodium with chloride, enhancing excretion of HCO_3^-.
Ammonium chloride or arginine hydrochloride	Although used only in severe cases, ammonium chloride may be given to increase amount of circulating H^+ ions. Monitor administration closely to prevent too rapid a decrease in pH and hemolysis of red blood cells. *Note:* May cause rebound metabolic acidosis and is usually contraindicated in clients with renal or hepatic failure.
Carbonic anhydrase inhibitor, such as acetazolamide (Diamox), or a potassium-sparing diuretic, such as spironolactone (Aldactone)	Blocks HCO_3^- reabsorption in the proximal convoluted renal tubules, promoting renal excretion of HCO_3^-. Effective in treating chloride-resistant alkalosis and its excess fluid volume effects.
Avoid or limit use of sedatives or hypnotics.	If respirations are depressed, may cause hypoxia or respiratory failure.
Encourage fluids IV and PO.	Replaces ECF losses, and adequate hydration facilitates removal of pulmonary secretions to improve ventilation.

(continues on page 492)

Administer supplemental oxygen (O$_2$), as indicated, and respiratory treatments to improve ventilation.

Prepare client for and assist with dialysis, as needed.

Respiratory compensation for metabolic alkalosis is hypoventilation, which may cause decreased PaO$_2$ levels and hypoxemia.

Useful when renal dysfunction prevents clearance of HCO$_3^-$.

POTENTIAL CONSIDERATIONS:
Refer to Potential Considerations relative to underlying cause of acid-base disorder.

CHAPTER 9

Diseases of the Blood/Blood-Forming Organs

ANEMIAS—IRON DEFICIENCY, ANEMIA OF CHRONIC DISEASE, PERNICIOUS, APLASTIC, HEMOLYTIC

I. **Pathophysiology:** decreased number of circulating red blood cells (RBCs), reduction in the amount of hemoglobin (Hgb) in the RBCs, or a combination of both, resulting in diminished oxygen-carrying capacity of the blood

  a. Iron deficiency anemia (ID): inadequate iron stores, which results in insufficient Hgb (key molecule in RBCs), causing cells to appear abnormal, unusually small (microcytic), and pale (hypochromic)

  b. Anemia of chronic disease (ACD): accompanies chronic inflammatory, infectious, or neoplastic disorders

  c. Pernicious anemia (PA): lack of intrinsic factor in the stomach results in inability to absorb vitamin B_{12} causing abnormal RBC formation

  d. Aplastic anemia: failure of bone marrow to produce cells, including RBCs and white blood cells (WBCs) and platelets

  e. Hemolytic anemia: premature destruction of RBCs

II. **Etiology**

  a. Adult anemia is usually defined as a Hgb level lower than 11 g/dL, with severe anemia defined as Hgb lower than 8 g/dL.

  b. Associated with many physiological complications, including dyspnea, fatigue, dizziness, decreased cognition, impaired sleep, sexual dysfunction, and significant debilitation

  c. ID

    i. Lack of iron in the body due to a variety of causes

      1. Blood loss due to disease, such as gastric or duodenal ulcers, diverticula, hemorrhoids, ulcerative colitis; injury or trauma; or certain medications, including aspirin or nonsteroidal anti-inflammatory drugs (NSAIDs)

      2. Inadequate nutrition, such as not eating enough foods that contain iron

      3. Malabsorption syndromes, such as not utilizing iron from food that is eaten

      4. Lead exposure

    ii. Most frequently occurring form of anemia

  d. ACD

    i. Primarily due to slowed production of RBCs as a result of low reticulocyte production

    ii. Develops slowly and is only evident after time

    iii. Symptoms are usually associated with the disease causing the anemia rather than the anemia itself.

    iv. Second most prevalent form of anemia (Hebbar & Gibson, 2006; Krantz, 1994)

  e. PA—an autoimmune disorder

    i. Characterized by the production of autoantibodies to gastric parietal cells and their secretory product—intrinsic factor—which is needed for vitamin B_{12} absorption

    ii. Conditions that interfere with the body's absorption and use of B_{12} include Crohn's and Whipple's diseases, gastrectomy or gastric bypass, and the use of chemotherapeutic medications.

  f. Aplastic anemia—bone marrow failure

    i. May be associated with conditions that affect erythropoietin production and secretion, such as certain cancers and cancer treatments and renal, hepatic, or endocrine disorders

    ii. Other known causes include exposure to chemicals, such as benzene, insecticides, solvents; certain drugs, such as chemotherapy, gold, seizure medications, some antibiotics; viruses, such as HIV, Epstein-Barr; immune conditions, such as systemic lupus erythematosus, rheumatoid arthritis; radiation; and certain inherited disorders, such as Fanconi's anemia.

  g. Hemolytic anemia—marked by an accelerated destruction of RBCs

    i. Several types of hemolytic anemias, including sickle cell anemia (see Sickle Cell Crisis)

    ii. Causes include hereditary factors, such as sickle cell trait or disease; blood transfusion reactions; acute viral or infectious agents; certain drugs, such as quinidine, penicillin, and methyldopa; and toxins, such as chemicals and venoms.

(text continues on page 494)

III. Statistics

a. Morbidity: Approximately 3.5 million Americans have anemia (National Heart, Lung and Blood Institute [NHLBI], 2007); in 1996, an estimated 2.1 million individuals younger than age 45 had anemia (Montoya et al, 2002); in 1999, 174,600 nursing home residents had anemia in the United States (CureResearch, 2003).

b. Morbidity: 4,627 people die from anemia annually in the United States (CureResearch, 2003).

c. Cost: $6.4 billion is spent annually (CureResearch, 2003).

GLOSSARY

Cheilitis: Inflammation of the lips with cracking at the corners of the mouth.

Ecchymosis: Superficial bleeding (bruising) under the skin or mucous membrane.

Erythropoiesis: Red blood cell (RBC) production in the bone marrow.

Glossitis: Inflammation of tongue.

Hematemesis: Bloody vomitus.

Koilonychia: Dystrophy of the nails, resulting in thinning and concave or spoon shape.

Lymphadenopathy: Enlargement of the lymph nodes.

Melena: Black, tarry stools due to digested of blood in the gastrointestinal (GI) tract.

Petechiae: Small, purplish, hemorrhagic spots on the skin.

Pica: Insatiable craving to eat nonfood items, such as starch, clay, crayons, and paper.

Romberg's sign: Inability to maintain body balance when eyes are shut and feet are close together.

Stomatitis: Inflammation, ulceration of mucosal lining of any structures in the mouth.

Care Setting

Clients are treated at the community level except in the presence of severe cardiovascular or immune compromise. Although the medical treatments vary widely due to the many variations in anemia presentation, nursing care for the anemic client has a common theme: managing physical symptoms and maximizing quality-of-life issues.

Related Concerns

Acquired immunodeficiency syndrome (AIDS), page 709

Burns: thermal, chemical, and electrical—acute and convalescent phases, page 667

Cancer, page 846

Cirrhosis of the liver, page 445

Heart failure: chronic, page 48

Psychosocial aspects of care, page 749

Renal failure: acute, page 536

Renal failure: chronic, page 548

Rheumatoid arthritis (RA), page 729

Pulmonary tuberculosis (TB), page 186

Upper gastrointestinal/esophageal bleeding, page 306

Client Assessment Database

DIAGNOSTIC DIVISION MAY REPORT	MAY EXHIBIT
ACTIVITY/REST • Fatigue, weakness, general malaise • Loss of productivity, diminished enthusiasm for work • Low exercise tolerance • Greater need for rest and sleep	• Tachycardia and tachypnea, dyspnea on exertion or at rest (severe or aplastic anemia) • Lethargy, withdrawal, apathy, lassitude, and lack of interest in surroundings • Muscle weakness and decreased strength • Ataxia, unsteady gait • Slumping of shoulders, drooping posture, slow walk, and other cues indicative of fatigue
CIRCULATION • History of chronic blood loss, such as chronic GI bleeding, heavy menses (ID) • Angina (particularly in elderly) • History of chronic infective endocarditis • Palpitations (compensatory tachycardia)	• Tachycardia • Blood pressure (BP)—increased systolic with stable diastolic and a widened pulse pressure, postural hypotension

Client Assessment Database (continued)

| DIAGNOSTIC DIVISION
MAY REPORT (continued) | MAY EXHIBIT (continued) |

• Cold hands and feet
• Brittle nails

• Bounding pulse and throbbing carotid pulsations reflect increased cardiac output as a compensatory mechanism to provide oxygen and nutrients to cells
• Dysrhythmias, electrocardiogram abnormalities—ST-segment depression and flattening or depression of the T wave, tachycardia
• Systolic murmur (ID)
• *Extremities:* color—pallor of the skin, palms, and nailbeds, or grayish cast in black client; waxy, pale skin (aplastic, PA) or bright lemon-yellow (PA)
• Sclera blue or pearl white (ID), jaundice (PA), pale mucous membranes—conjunctiva, mouth, pharynx, lips
• Capillary refill delayed due to diminished blood flow to the periphery, resulting in vasoconstriction
• Nails brittle, spoon-shaped or koilonychia (ID)

EGO INTEGRITY
• Negative feelings about self, ability to handle situation, events

• Depression

ELIMINATION
• History of pyelonephritis, renal failure (ACD)
• Flatulence, malabsorption syndrome (ID)
• Hematemesis, fresh blood in stool, melena
• Diarrhea or constipation
• Diminished urine output

• Abdominal distention

FOOD/FLUID
• Low food intake, low intake of animal protein, high intake of cereal products (ID)
• Mouth or tongue soreness, difficulty swallowing, ulcerations in pharynx (PA)
• Nausea, vomiting, dyspepsia, anorexia
• Recent weight loss
• Pica

• Beefy red, smooth appearance of tongue (PA, folic acid and vitamin B_{12} deficiencies)
• Dry, pale mucous membranes
• Skin turgor poor with dry, shriveled appearance and loss of elasticity (ID)
• Stomatitis and glossitis (deficiency states)
• Cheilitis (ID)

HYGIENE
• Difficulty maintaining activities of daily living (ADLs)

• Unkempt appearance, poor personal hygiene
• Hair dry, brittle, thinning; premature graying (PA)

NEUROSENSORY
• Headaches, fainting, dizziness, vertigo, tinnitus, inability to concentrate
• Insomnia, diminished vision, and spots before eyes
• Weakness, poor balance, wobbly legs, paresthesias of hands or feet (PA)
• Sensation of being cold

• Irritability, restlessness, depression, drowsiness, apathy
• Mentation—notable slowing and dullness in response
• Retinal hemorrhages (aplastic, PA)
• Epistaxis, bleeding from other orifices (aplastic)
• Disturbed coordination, ataxia, decreased vibratory and position sense, positive Romberg's sign, paralysis (PA)

PAIN/DISCOMFORT
• Vague abdominal pains, headache (ID)
• Oral pain

RESPIRATION
• Shortness of breath at rest and with activity

• Tachypnea
• Dyspnea, particularly during and after exercise
• Orthopnea

SAFETY
• History of occupational exposure to chemicals—benzene, lead, insecticides, phenylbutazone, naphthalene (aplastic, hemolytic)

• Low-grade fever
• Generalized lymphadenopathy

(continues on page 496)

DIAGNOSTIC DIVISION MAY REPORT (continued)	MAY EXHIBIT (continued)
• History of exposure to radiation, either as a treatment modality or by accident (aplastic, hemolytic) • History of cancer, cancer therapies (aplastic, hemolytic) • Cold and heat intolerance • Previous blood transfusions • Impaired vision • Poor wound healing, frequent infections • Skin problems, including cracks in side of mouth (PA)	• Petechiae and ecchymosis (aplastic)
SEXUALITY • Changes in menstrual flow—menorrhagia or amenorrhea in women (ID) • Loss of libido—both men and women • Impotence	• Pale cervix and vaginal walls • Impotence
TEACHING/LEARNING • Family tendency for anemia (ID, PA) • Past or present use of anticonvulsants, antibiotics, chemotherapeutic agents (bone marrow failure), aspirin, anti-inflammatory drugs, or anticoagulants • Chronic use of alcohol • Religious or cultural beliefs affecting treatment choices—refusal of blood transfusions • Recent or current episode of active bleeding (ID) • Prior surgeries—splenectomy, tumor excision, prosthetic valve replacement, surgical excision of duodenum or gastric resection, partial or total gastrectomy for weight loss or diseases (ID, PA) • Problems with wound healing or bleeding, chronic infections	
DISCHARGE PLAN CONSIDERATIONS • May require assistance with treatment, such as injections, self-care activities, homemaker and maintenance tasks; changes in dietary plan ▶ Refer to section at end of plan for postdischarge considerations.	

Diagnostic Studies

TEST WHY IT IS DONE	WHAT IT TELLS ME
BLOOD TESTS • *Complete blood count (CBC):* Battery of screening tests, which typically includes Hgb; hematocrit (Hct); RBC count, morphology, indices, and distribution width index; platelet count and size; and WBC count and differential.	Evaluates for known or suspected anemia.
• *Hgb:* The oxygen-carrying pigment and predominant protein in the RBCs. • *Hematocrit (Hct):* The proportion of packed RBCs to serum.	Both are decreased in blood loss and some anemias and bone marrow suppression. Hct is decreased in blood loss and overhydration.
• *Hgb electrophoresis:* Identifies type of Hgb structure.	Aids in determining source of hemolytic anemia or anemias related to deficiencies in dietary intake or malabsorption.

TEST **WHY IT IS DONE** (continued)	**WHAT IT TELLS ME** (continued)
• *RBC (also called erythrocyte) count:* Number of RBCs per unit volume.	Decreased in ID and PA; severely decreased in aplastic anemia.
• *Reticulocyte count:* Immature RBCs. Helps assess bone marrow function.	Decreased in PA and aplastic anemia. Elevated in blood loss and hemolytic and compensated anemias.
• *RBC survival time:* Evaluates age of RBCs.	Useful in the differential diagnosis of anemias because RBCs have shortened life spans in pernicious and hemolytic anemias.
• *Erythrocyte fragility test:* Evaluates susceptibility of RBCs to break down (hemolysis) under certain conditions.	Decreased in ID. Increased fragility confirms hemolytic and autoimmune anemias.
• *WBCs:* Total cell count and specific WBCs, called differential.	May be increased as in hemolytic anemia or decreased in aplastic anemia.
• *Platelet count:* Platelets have essential function in coagulation.	Decreased in blood loss and aplastic anemias. Increased in ID, posthemorrhagic, and hemolytic anemias.
• *Erythrocyte sedimentation rate (ESR):* Measures rate at which RBCs settle.	While not specific to a certain anemia, higher ESR indicates presence of inflammatory reaction, such as increased RBC destruction or malignant disease.
• *Serum iron:* Measures the level of iron in the liquid part of blood.	Iron is needed to help form adequate numbers of normal RBCs. Iron may be decreased or absent (ID) or elevated (hemolytic and aplastic anemias).
• *Total iron-binding capacity (TIBC):* Measures the amount of iron that can be carried through blood by transferrin.	Increased in ID; normal or slightly reduced in PA.
• *Serum ferritin:* Reflects the amount of stored iron in body.	Decreased in ID.
• *Vitamin B$_{12}$ (cobalamin) and folate (folic acid, RBC folate):* Measures the concentration of vitamin B$_{12}$ and folate in the serum. The amount of folate inside RBCs may also be measured; it will normally be at a higher concentration inside the cell than in the serum.	Help diagnose the cause of anemia or neuropathy (nerve damage) or to evaluate nutritional status in some clients.
• *Serum bilirubin:* Product that results from the breakdown of Hgb.	Direct or total bilirubin is elevated in PA and hemolytic anemia.
• *Serum lactate dehydrogenase (LDH):* Serum LDH levels may occasionally be ordered to monitor damage caused by muscle trauma or injury and to help identify hemolytic anemia.	May be elevated in PA and hemolytic anemia.

OTHER DIAGNOSTIC STUDIES

• *Schilling's test:* Evaluates vitamin B$_{12}$ excretion by measuring urinary excretion.	Decreased urinary excretion of vitamin B$_{12}$ in PA. *Note:* Once ordered fairly routinely, it is now ordered only occasionally because it involves the administration of radioactive B$_{12}$.
• *Guaiac:* Tests for hidden or occult blood.	May be positive in urine, stools, and gastric contents, reflecting acute or chronic bleeding (ID).
• *Gastric analysis:* Test specifically determines the presence of gastric acid as well as the amount of gastric acid secreted.	Complete absence of secretion (achlorhydria) may suggest PA.
• *Bone marrow aspiration/biopsy examination:* May be done by needle aspirate or biopsy to identify changes in number, size, and shape of blood cells, helping to differentiate type of anemia.	Megaloblasts increased in PA; fatty marrow, with diminished or absence of blood cells at several sites, found in aplastic anemia.
• *Upper endoscopy—also called esophagogastroduodenoscopy (EGD):* Visualizes esophagus, stomach, and duodenum, using a thin flexible tube that can be looked through or seen on a TV monitor.	Checks for bleeding sites—acute or chronic GI bleeding—causing blood loss anemia.
• *Lower endoscopy—also called colonoscopy:* Visualizes rectum and colon using a thin flexible tube that can be looked through or seen on a TV monitor.	

Nursing Priorities

1. Enhance tissue perfusion.
2. Provide nutritional and fluid needs.
3. Prevent complications.
4. Provide information about disease process, prognosis, and treatment regimen.

Discharge Goals

1. ADLs met by self or with assistance of others.
2. Complications prevented or minimized.
3. Disease process, prognosis, and therapeutic regimen understood.
4. Plan in place to meet needs after discharge.

NURSING DIAGNOSIS: **Activity Intolerance**

May be related to
Imbalance between oxygen supply or delivery and demand

Possibly evidenced by
Weakness and fatigue
Reports of decreased exercise or activity tolerance
Greater need for sleep or rest
Palpitations, tachycardia, increased BP, and increased respiratory response with minor exertion

Desired Outcomes/Evaluation Criteria—Client Will

Endurance (NOC)
Report an increase in activity tolerance, including ADLs.
Demonstrate a decrease in physiological signs of intolerance—pulse, respirations, and BP remain within client's normal range.
Display laboratory values (Hgb/Hct) within acceptable range.

ACTIONS/INTERVENTIONS	RATIONALE
Energy Management (NIC)	
Independent	
Assess client's ability to perform normal tasks and ADLs, noting reports of weakness, fatigue, and difficulty accomplishing tasks.	Influences choice of interventions and needed assistance.
Note changes in balance, gait disturbance, and muscle weakness.	May indicate neurological changes associated with vitamin B_{12} deficiency, affecting client safety and increasing risk of injury.
Monitor BP, pulse, and respirations during and after activity. Note adverse responses to increased levels of activity—increased heart rate and BP, dysrhythmias, dizziness, dyspnea, tachypnea, and cyanosis of mucous membranes and nailbeds.	Cardiopulmonary manifestations result from attempts by the heart and lungs to supply adequate amounts of oxygen to the tissues.
Recommend quiet atmosphere and bedrest, if indicated. Monitor and limit visitors, phone calls, and repeated unplanned interruptions.	Activity may need to be curtailed until severe anemia is at least partially corrected to lower body's oxygen requirements and reduce strain on the heart and lungs.
Elevate head of bed, as tolerated.	Enhances lung expansion to maximize oxygenation for cellular uptake. *Note:* May be contraindicated if hypotension is present.
Suggest client change position slowly; monitor for dizziness.	Postural hypotension or cerebral hypoxia may cause dizziness, fainting, and increased risk of injury.
Assist client to prioritize ADLs and desired activities. Alternate rest periods with activity periods.	Promotes adequate rest, maintains energy level, and alleviates strain on the cardiac and respiratory systems.
Provide or recommend assistance with activities and ambulation as necessary, allowing client to be an active participant as much as possible.	Although help may be necessary, self-esteem is enhanced when client does some things for self.
Plan activity progression with client, including activities that client views as essential. Increase activity levels, as tolerated.	Promotes gradual return to normal activity level and improved muscle tone and stamina without undue fatigue. Increases self-esteem and sense of control.
Identify and implement energy-saving techniques: shower chair and sitting to perform tasks.	Encourages client to do as much as possible, while conserving limited energy and preventing fatigue.
Instruct client to stop activity if palpitations, chest pain, shortness of breath, weakness, or dizziness occur.	Cellular ischemia potentiates risk of infarction, and excessive cardiopulmonary strain and stress may lead to decompensation and failure.
Discuss importance of maintaining environmental temperature and body warmth, as indicated.	Vasoconstriction with shunting of blood to vital organs decreases peripheral circulation, impairing tissue perfusion. Client's comfort and need for warmth must be balanced with need to avoid excessive heat with resultant vasodilation, which reduces organ perfusion.

ACTIONS/INTERVENTIONS (continued)	RATIONALE (continued)
Collaborative	
Monitor laboratory studies, such as Hgb/Hct, RBC count, and arterial blood gases (ABGs).	Identifies deficiencies in RBC components affecting oxygen transport, treatment needs, and response to therapy.
Provide supplemental oxygen as indicated.	Maximizing oxygen transport to tissues improves ability to function.
Administer the following, as indicated:	
Whole blood, packed RBCs (PRCs); blood products as indicated. Monitor closely for transfusion reactions.	Increases number of oxygen-carrying cells; corrects deficiencies to reduce risk of hemorrhage in acutely compromised individuals. *Note:* Transfusions are reserved for severe blood loss anemias with cardiovascular compromise and are used after other therapies have failed to restore homeostasis.
Erythropoiesis-stimulating therapies, such as epoetin-Alpha (Procrit, EPO)	Large-scale clinical studies have shown the effectiveness of EPO in increasing erythrocyte and Hgb levels, relieving clinical and quality-of-life manifestations associated with ACD (National Institute of Diabetes and Digestive and Kidney Diseases [NIDDK], 2005).
Prepare for surgical intervention, if indicated.	Surgery is useful to control bleeding in clients who are anemic because of bleeding, such as in ulcers and uterine bleeding; or to remove spleen as treatment of autoimmune hemolytic anemia. Bone marrow and stem cell transplantation may be done in presence of bone marrow failure—aplastic anemia.

NURSING DIAGNOSIS: imbalanced Nutrition: Less than Body Requirements

May be related to
Failure to ingest or inability to digest food or absorb nutrients necessary for formation of normal RBCs

Possibly evidenced by
Weight loss or weight below normal for age, height, and build
Decreased triceps skinfold measurement
Changes in gums, oral mucous membranes
Decreased tolerance for activity, weakness, and loss of muscle tone

Desired Outcomes/Evaluation Criteria—Client Will

Nutritional Status (NOC)
Demonstrate progressive weight gain or stable weight, with normalization of laboratory values.
Experience no signs of malnutrition.
Demonstrate behaviors or lifestyle changes to regain and maintain appropriate weight.

ACTIONS/INTERVENTIONS	RATIONALE
Nutrition Therapy (NIC)	
Independent	
Review nutritional history, including food preferences.	Identifies deficiencies and suggests possible interventions. *Note:* Daily meal diary over period of time may be necessary to identify anemia related to nutrient deficiencies such as no meat in diet—iron and vitamin B_{12} deficiency, or few leafy vegetables in diet—folic acid deficiency.
Observe and record client's food intake.	Monitors caloric intake or insufficient quality of food consumption.
Weigh periodically as appropriate, such as weekly.	Monitors weight loss and effectiveness of nutritional interventions.
Recommend small, frequent meals and between-meal nourishment.	May reduce fatigue and thus enhance intake while preventing gastric distention. Use of Ensure, Isomil, or similar product provides additional protein and calories.
Suggest bland diet, low in roughage, avoiding hot, spicy, or very acidic foods, as indicated.	When oral lesions are present, pain may restrict type of foods client can tolerate.
Have client record and report occurrence of nausea or vomiting, flatus, and other related symptoms, such as irritability or impaired memory.	May reflect effects of anemias, such as hypoxia or vitamin B_{12} deficiency, on organs.
Encourage or assist with good oral hygiene before and after meals; use soft-bristled toothbrush for gentle brushing. Provide dilute, alcohol-free mouthwash if oral mucosa is ulcerated.	Enhances appetite and oral intake. Diminishes bacterial growth, minimizing possibility of infection. Special mouth-care techniques may be needed if tissue is fragile, ulcerated, or bleeding and pain is severe.

(continues on page 500)

ACTIONS/INTERVENTIONS (continued)

Collaborative

Consult with dietitian.

Monitor laboratory studies, such as Hgb/Hct, blood urea nitrogen (BUN), prealbumin and albumin, protein, transferrin, serum iron, vitamin B_{12}, folic acid, TIBC, and serum electrolytes.

Administer medications, as indicated, for example:

Vitamin and mineral supplements, such as cyanocobalamin (vitamin B_{12}), folic acid (Folvite), and ascorbic acid (vitamin C)

Oral iron supplements, such as ferrous sulfate (Feosol, Mol-Iron, Fer-In-Sol), ferrous gluconate (Fergon), and ferrous fumarate (Ircon, Femiron)

Iron dextran (InFeD) intramuscularly/intravenously (IM/IV)

Antifungal or anesthetic mouthwash, if indicated

RATIONALE (continued)

Aids in establishing dietary plan to meet individual needs.

Evaluates effectiveness of treatment regimen, including dietary sources of needed nutrients.

Replacements needed depend on type of anemia and presence of poor oral intake and identified deficiencies.

May be useful in some types of iron deficiency anemias. Oral preparations are taken between meals to enhance absorption and usually correct anemia and replace iron stores over a period of several months.

Administered until estimated deficit is corrected. Reserved for those who cannot absorb or comply with oral iron therapy or when blood loss is too rapid for oral replacement to be effective.

May be needed in the presence of stomatitis or glossitis to promote oral tissue healing and facilitate intake.

NURSING DIAGNOSIS: **Constipation/Diarrhea**

May be related to

Decreased dietary intake, changes in digestive processes

Drug therapy side effects

Possibly evidenced by

Changes in frequency, characteristics, and amount of stool

Nausea, vomiting, decreased appetite

Reports of abdominal pain, urgency, cramping

Altered bowel sounds

Desired Outcomes/Evaluation Criteria—Client Will

Bowel Elimination (NOC)

Establish return to normal patterns of bowel functioning.

Demonstrate changes in behaviors or lifestyle, as necessitated by causative or contributing factors.

ACTIONS/INTERVENTIONS

Bowel Management (NIC)

Independent

Determine stool color, consistency, frequency, and amount.

Auscultate bowel sounds.

Monitor intake and output (I&O) with specific attention to food and fluid intake.

Encourage fluid intake of 2,500 to 3,000 mL/day within cardiac tolerance.

Recommend avoiding gas-forming foods.

Assess perianal skin condition frequently, noting changes or beginning breakdown. Encourage and assist with perineal care after each bowel movement (BM) if diarrhea is present.

Discuss use of stool softeners, mild stimulants, bulk-forming laxatives, or enemas, as indicated. Monitor effectiveness.

Collaborative

Consult with dietitian to provide well-balanced diet high in fiber and bulk.

Administer antidiarrheal medications, such as diphenoxylate hydrochloride with atropine (Lomotil), and water-absorbing drugs, such as Metamucil.

RATIONALE

Assists in identifying causative or contributing factors and appropriate interventions.

Bowel sounds are generally increased in diarrhea and decreased in constipation.

May identify dehydration and excessive loss of fluids or aid in identifying dietary deficiencies.

Assists in improving stool consistency if constipated. Helps maintain hydration status if diarrhea is present.

Decreases gastric distress and abdominal distention.

Prevents skin excoriation and breakdown.

Facilitates defecation when constipation is present.

Fiber resists enzymatic digestion and absorbs liquids in its passage along the intestinal tract and thereby produces bulk, which acts as a stimulant to defecation.

Decreases intestinal motility when diarrhea is present.

NURSING DIAGNOSIS: risk for Infection

Risk factors may include
Inadequate secondary defenses—decreased Hgb, leukopenia, or decreased granulocytes (suppressed inflammatory response)
Inadequate primary defenses—broken skin, stasis of body fluids, invasive procedures, chronic disease, malnutrition

Possibly evidenced by
(Not applicable; presence of signs and symptoms establishes an *actual* diagnosis)

Desired Outcomes/Evaluation Criteria—Client Will

Risk Control (NOC)
Identify behaviors to prevent and reduce risk of infection.

Immune Status (NOC)
Be free of signs of infection; achieve timely wound healing if present.

ACTIONS/INTERVENTIONS	RATIONALE
Infection Protection (NIC)	
Independent	
Perform and promote meticulous hand washing by caregivers and client.	Prevents cross-contamination or bacterial colonization. *Note:* Client with severe or aplastic anemia may be at risk from normal skin flora.
Maintain strict aseptic techniques with procedures and wound care.	Reduces risk of bacterial colonization and infection.
Provide meticulous skin, oral, and perianal care.	Reduces risk of skin or tissue breakdown and infection.
Encourage frequent position changes and ambulation, coughing, and deep-breathing exercises.	Promotes ventilation of all lung segments and aids in mobilizing secretions to prevent pneumonia.
Promote adequate fluid intake.	Assists in liquefying respiratory secretions to facilitate expectoration and prevent stasis of body fluids in lungs and bladder.
Emphasize need to monitor and limit visitors, as indicated. Provide protective isolation, if appropriate. Restrict live plants and cut flowers.	Limits exposure to infectious agents. Protective isolation may be required in aplastic anemia, when immune response is most compromised.
Monitor temperature. Note presence of chills and tachycardia with or without fever.	Reflective of inflammatory process or infection, requiring evaluation and treatment. *Note:* With bone marrow suppression, leukocytic failure may lead to fulminating infections.
Observe for wound erythema and drainage.	Indicators of local infection. *Note:* Pus formation may be absent if granulocytes are depressed.
Collaborative	
Obtain specimens for culture and sensitivity, as indicated.	Verifies presence of infection, identifies specific pathogen, and influences choice of treatment.
Administer topical antiseptics and systemic antibiotics.	May be used prophylactically to reduce colonization or used to treat specific infectious process.

NURSING DIAGNOSIS: deficient Knowledge [Learning Need] regarding condition, prognosis, treatment, self-care, prevention of crisis, and discharge needs

May be related to
Lack of exposure, recall
Information misinterpretation
Unfamiliarity with information resources

Possibly evidenced by
Questions, request for information, statement of misconception
Inaccurate follow-through of instructions, development of preventable complications

Desired Outcomes/Evaluation Criteria—Client Will

Knowledge: Illness Care (NOC)
Verbalize understanding of the nature of the disease process, diagnostic procedures, and potential complications.
Identify causative factors.
Verbalize understanding of therapeutic needs.
Initiate necessary behaviors or lifestyle changes.

ACTIONS/INTERVENTIONS	RATIONALE

Teaching: Disease Process (NIC)
Independent

Provide information about specific anemia and explain that therapy depends on the type and severity of the anemia.

Provides knowledge base from which client can make informed choices. Allays anxiety and may promote cooperation with therapeutic regimen.

Discuss effects of anemias on preexisting conditions.

Anemias aggravate heart, lung, and cerebrovascular disease.

Review purpose and preparations for diagnostic studies.

Anxiety or fear of the unknown increases stress level, which, in turn, increases the cardiac workload. Knowledge of what to expect can diminish anxiety.

Explain that blood taken for laboratory studies will not worsen anemia.

This is often an unspoken concern that can potentiate client's anxiety.

Review required diet alterations to meet specific dietary needs, as determined by type of anemia and deficiency.

Red meat, liver, seafood, green leafy vegetables, whole wheat bread, and dried fruits are sources of iron. Green vegetables, whole grains, liver, and citrus fruits are sources of folic acid and vitamin C, which enhances absorption of iron.

Discuss foods to avoid, such as coffee, tea, egg yolks, milk, fiber, and soy protein, at the time when client is eating high-iron foods.

These foods block absorption of iron and should be taken at a different meal. For example, red meat and milk taken at the same time can block absorption of the iron from the meat.

Assess resources, including financial, and ability to obtain and prepare food.

Inadequate resources may affect ability to purchase and prepare appropriate food items.

Encourage cessation of smoking.

Smoking decreases available oxygen and causes vasoconstriction.

Provide information about purpose, dosage, schedule, precautions, and potential side effects, interactions, and adverse reactions to all prescribed medications.

Information enhances cooperation with regimen. Recovery from anemias can be slow, requiring lengthy treatment and prevention of secondary complications.

Stress importance of reporting signs of fatigue, weakness, paresthesias, irritability, and impaired memory.

Indicates that anemia is progressing or failing to resolve, necessitating further evaluation and treatment changes.

Instruct and demonstrate self-administration of oral iron preparations:

Iron replacement usually takes 3 to 6 months, whereas vitamin B_{12} injections may be necessary for the rest of client's life.

Discuss importance of taking only prescribed dosages.

Overdose of iron medication can be toxic.

Advise taking with meals or immediately after meals.

Iron is best absorbed on an empty stomach. However, iron salts are gastric irritants and may cause dyspepsia, diarrhea, and abdominal discomfort if taken on an empty stomach.

Dilute liquid preparations, preferably with orange juice, and administer through a straw.

Undiluted liquid iron preparations may stain the teeth. Ascorbic acid promotes iron absorption.

Suggest use of protective devices, such as sheepskin, egg-crate, alternating air pressure, or water mattress; heel and elbow protectors; and pillows, as indicated.

Avoids skin breakdown by preventing or reducing pressure against skin surfaces.

Review good oral hygiene and necessity for regular dental care.

Effects of anemia such as oral lesions and use of iron supplements increase risk of infection and bacteremia.

Instruct to avoid use of aspirin products.

Increases bleeding tendencies.

Refer to appropriate community resources when indicated, such as social services for food stamps and Meals on Wheels.

May need assistance with groceries and meal preparation.

POTENTIAL CONSIDERATIONS following acute hospitalization (dependent on client's age, physical condition and presence of complications, personal resources, and life responsibilities)

- *Activity Intolerance*—imbalance between oxygen supply or delivery and demand
- *imbalanced Nutrition: Less than Body Requirements*—failure to ingest or inability to digest food or absorb nutrients necessary for formation of normal RBCs
- *risk for Infection*—inadequate secondary defenses, such as decreased Hgb, leukopenia, or decreased granulocytes (suppressed inflammatory response); inadequate primary defenses, such as broken skin, stasis of body fluids; invasive procedures; chronic disease; malnutrition
- *ineffective self Health Management*—economic difficulties, perceived benefits

SICKLE CELL CRISIS

I. Pathophysiology

a. Formation of abnormal hemoglobin chains containing hemoglobin S: When red blood cells (RBCs) are exposed to low oxygen saturation states, hemoglobin S causes the beta cells to contract and clump together inside the cell, thus distorting its shape.

b. Hemolysis occurs as the sickled cells clump together and obstruct blood flow, rendering the individual vulnerable to repeated painful crises, which can progressively destroy vital organs.

   i. Vaso-occlusive and thrombocytic crisis
   ii. Hypoplastic and aplastic crisis
   iii. Hyperhemolytic crisis
   iv. Splenic sequestration crisis

c. Plasma clotting factors likely participate in the microthrombi in the prearterioles.

d. After recurrent episodes of sickling, membrane damage occurs, and the cells are no longer capable of resuming their normal shape upon reoxygenation.

II. Etiology

a. Sickle hemoglobinopathies compose a group of genetic diseases, with the most common forms being homozygous hemoglobin SS disease (HbSS) or sickle cell anemia, hemoglobin SC disease, and sickle cell beta-thalassemia or Thal.

b. Primarily affects black populations of African descent as well as people of South and Central American, Caribbean, Mediterranean, Arabian, and East Indian descent (Distenfeld & Woermann, 2007, Taher & Kazzi, 2007)

c. Vaso-occlusive crisis is often triggered by infection, dehydration, fever, or local trauma.

III. Statistics

a. Morbidity: 1 in 500 African Americans has inherited sickle cell hemoglobin from both parents and therefore has the disease; more than 70,000 people in the United States have sickle cell disease (National Heart, Lung and Blood Institute [NHLBI], 2008), accounting for over 83,000 hospital admissions in 2004 (Steiner & Miller, 2006).

b. Mortality: In 2004, there were 699 adult deaths (Steiner & Miller, 2006).

c. Cost: In 2004, approximately $488 million was spent for hospital costs (Steiner & Miller, 2006).

GLOSSARY

Bruit: Abnormal sound heard over an artery or vascular channel, reflecting turbulence of blood flow.

Genetic disease: The ultimate unit of inheritance, carried by the chromosome. Genes determine various characteristics, such as hair texture, skin color, height, shape of nose, lips, and so on, including the kind of hemoglobin in red blood cells (RBCs).

Hemoglobin (Hgb): An iron-containing protein of the RBC, which carries oxygen to the tissues and gives the cell its red color.

Hemolysis: Destruction of RBCs and subsequent release of hemoglobin.

Hyperhemolytic crisis: A rapid, higher-than-normal rate of hemolysis; reticulocytes are increased in peripheral blood, and bone marrow is hyperplastic, leading to anemia and jaundice due to effects of hemolysis. Often associated with vaso-occlusive crisis.

Hypoplastic/aplastic crisis: May be secondary to severe (usually viral) infection or folic acid deficiency, resulting in cessation of production of RBCs and bone marrow.

Icterus (jaundice): Yellowing of the skin and the whites of the eyes caused by an accumulation of bile pigment in the blood.

Kyphosis: Exaggerated outward curvature of the spine.

Lordosis: Curvature of spinal column characterized by an abnormal hollow at the small of the back; also known as swayback.

Priapism: Abnormal, painful, sustained erection of the penis, usually occurring without sexual desire.

Reticulocytes: Immature RBCs, typically composing about 1% of the red cells in the human body. Reticulocytes develop and mature in the red bone marrow and then circulate for about a day in the bloodstream before developing into mature RBCs.

Sickle cell disease: An inherited disorder of the RBCs where the individual inherits two genes for hemoglobin S, or a single S gene is combined with a second variant gene such as C, or Thal. The following are examples of sickle cell disease: SS, SC, SD, Sβ Thal.

Sickle cell trait: The inheritance of one gene for the usual hemoglobin (A) and one gene for sickle hemoglobin (S). A person who has sickle cell trait (AS) is a carrier of the sickle gene but does not have the disease or incur painful episodes and is generally not affected by the sickle hemoglobin.

Splenic sequestration crisis: Occurs when the spleen suddenly traps large numbers of RBCs, causing splenomegaly, a drop in hemogloblin greater than or equal to 20%, hypovolemia, shock, and possible death.

Thalassemia (Thal): An inherited disorder of the gene in the RBCs, which results in the impaired ability to produce hemoglobin.

Vaso-occlusive/thrombocytic crisis: Related to infection, dehydration, fever, hypoxia, and characterized by multiple infarcts of bones, joints, and target organs, with tissue pain and necrosis caused by plugs of sickled cells in the microcirculation.

Care Setting

Sickle cell disease is generally managed at the community level, with many of the interventions included here being appropriate for this focus; however, this plan of care addresses sickle cell crisis, which usually requires hospitalization during the acute phase to address oxygenation and severe pain.

Related Concerns

Cerebrovascular accident (CVA)/stroke, page 238

Cholecystitis with cholelithiasis, page 357

Chronic obstructive pulmonary disease (COPD) and asthma, page 120

Cirrhosis of the liver, page 445

Heart failure: chronic, page 48

Pneumonia, page 131

Psychosocial aspects of care, page 749

Seizure disorders, page 210

Sepsis/septicemia, page 686

Client Assessment Database

Depends on severity of condition and presence of complications.

DIAGNOSTIC DIVISION MAY REPORT	MAY EXHIBIT
ACTIVITY/REST • Lethargy, fatigue, weakness, general malaise • Loss of productivity • Decreased exercise tolerance • Greater need for sleep and rest	• Listlessness, severe weakness, and increasing pallor (aplastic crisis) • Gait disturbances (pain, kyphosis, lordosis), inability to walk (pain) • Poor body posture • Decreased range of motion (ROM) • Joint, bone deformities • Generalized retarded growth, tower-shaped skull with frontal bossing, disproportionately long arms and legs, short trunk, narrowed shoulders and hips, and long, tapered fingers
CIRCULATION • Palpitations or anginal chest pain due to concomitant coronary artery disease (CAD), myocardial ischemia, or acute chest syndrome • Intermittent pain in legs when walking	• Apical pulse—point of maximal impulse (PMI) may be displaced to the left • Tachycardia • Systolic heart murmurs may be heard over entire precordium • Blood pressure (BP)—widened pulse pressure • Generalized symptoms of shock—hypotension; rapid, thready pulse; and shallow respirations during sequestration crisis • Peripheral pulses throbbing on palpation • Bruits—reflects compensatory mechanisms of anemia; may also be auscultated over the spleen because of multiple splenic infarcts • Capillary refill delayed (anemia or hypovolemia) • *Skin color:* Pallor or cyanosis of skin, mucous membranes, and conjunctiva (*Note:* Pallor may appear as yellowish-brown color in brown-skinned clients and as ashen gray in black-skinned clients.) • Scleral icterus, generalized icteric coloring due to excessive RBC hemolysis • Dry skin and mucous membranes
ELIMINATION • Frequent voiding, voiding in large amounts • Nocturia	• Right upper quadrant (RUQ) abdominal tenderness, enlargement due to hepatomegaly or ascites • Left upper quadrant (LUQ) abdominal fullness; spleen may be enlarged and nonfunctional and may eventually become fibrotic and shrunken • Dilute, pale, straw-colored urine, hematuria or smoky appearance from multiple renal infarcts

Client Assessment Database (continued)

DIAGNOSTIC DIVISION
MAY REPORT (continued)

EGO INTEGRITY
- Resentment and frustration with disease, fear of rejection from others
- Negative feelings about self, ability to deal with life or situation
- Concern regarding being a burden to significant others (SOs), financial concerns, possible loss of insurance benefits, lost time at work or school, fear of genetic transmission of disease

FOOD/FLUID
- Thirst
- Anorexia
- Nausea, vomiting

HYGIENE
- Difficulty maintaining activities of daily living (ADLs) (pain or severe anemia)

NEUROSENSORY
- Headaches or dizziness
- Visual disturbances due to retinal vascular changes
- Tingling in the extremities
- Disturbances in pain and position sense

PAIN/DISCOMFORT
- Pain may be acute and severe, throbbing, of varied locations; may be localized, migratory, or generalized in long bones of extremities, abdomen, back, chest
- Recurrent, sharp, transient headaches
- Joint or bone pain may be low-level and chronic or acute and accompanied by warmth, tenderness, erythema, and occasional effusions (vaso-occlusive crisis)
- Gallbladder tenderness and pain

RESPIRATION
- Dyspnea on exertion or at rest
- History of repeated pulmonary infections, infarctions, pulmonary fibrosis, pulmonary hypertension or cor pulmonale

MAY EXHIBIT (continued)

- Anxiety, restlessness, irritability, apprehension, withdrawal, narrowed focus, self-focusing, unresponsiveness to questions, regression, depression, decreased self-concept
- Dependent relationship with whomever can offer security and protection

- Height and weight usually in the lower percentiles
- Poor skin turgor with visible tenting during sequestration crisis, infection, and dehydration
- Dry skin and mucous membranes
- Jugular vein distention (JVD) and general peripheral edema (concomitant heart failure [HF])

- Unkempt appearance, poor personal hygiene

- Mental status usually unaffected except in cases of severe sickling (cerebral infarction and intracranial hemorrhage)
- Weakness of the mouth, tongue, and facial muscles; aphasia (in cerebral infarction of dominant hemisphere)
- Abnormal reflexes, decreased muscle strength and tone, abnormal involuntary movements, hemiplegia or sudden hemiparesis, quadriplegia
- Ataxia, seizures
- Meningeal irritation (intracranial hemorrhage)—decreasing level of consciousness (LOC), nuchal rigidity, focal neurological deficits, vomiting, severe headache

- Sensitivity to palpation over affected areas
- Guarding or holding joints in position of comfort, decreased ROM, resulting from joint pain and swelling
- Maladaptive pain behaviors—guilt for being ill, denial of any aspect of disease, indulgence in precipitating factors such as overwork, strenuous exercise

- Acute respiratory distress—dyspnea, chest pain, and cyanosis (especially in crisis)
- Bronchial or bronchovesicular sounds in lung periphery, diminished breath sounds (pulmonary fibrosis)
- Crackles, rhonchi, wheezes, diminished breath sounds (HF)
- Increased anteroposterior (AP) diameter of the chest (barrel chest)

(continues on page 506)

DIAGNOSTIC DIVISION
MAY REPORT (continued)

SAFETY
- History of repeated, frequent transfusions
- Jaundice with skin itching
- Leg ulcers
- Impaired vision (sickle retinopathy), decreased visual acuity (temporary or permanent blindness)

SEXUALITY
- Loss of libido
- Amenorrhea
- Complications of pregnancy, including placenta previa and abruption; premature birth or fetal death
- Priapism, impotence

TEACHING/LEARNING
- Chronic anemic state
- Pulmonary hypertension or cor pulmonale (multiple pulmonary infections and infarctions)
- Chronic leg ulcers, delayed healing

DISCHARGE PLAN CONSIDERATIONS
- May need assistance with shopping, transportation, self-care, homemaker and maintenance tasks

‣ Refer to section at end of plan for postdischarge considerations.

MAY EXHIBIT (continued)

- Low-grade fever
- Leg ulcers—especially common on the internal and external malleoli and the medial aspect of the tibia

- Delayed sexual maturity
- Pale cervix and vaginal walls (anemia)

Diagnostic Studies

TEST
WHY IT IS DONE

WHAT IT TELLS ME

BLOOD TESTS
- *Complete blood count (CBC):* Battery of screening tests, which typically includes Hgb; hematocrit (Hct); RBC count, morphology, indices, and distribution width index; platelet count and size; and white blood cell (WBC) count and differential.

Hgb and total RBCs are decreased. Young RBCs (reticulocytes) can be low or elevated if anemia is long-standing. Young WBCs (leukocytes) are elevated, especially in vaso-occlusive crisis. Platelets are often increased. *Note:* Anemia is often well tolerated by the client; however, a major drop in Hgb from previously recorded values indicates a hematologic crisis. If the reticulocyte count is normal, splenic sequestration is the probable cause. If the reticulocyte count is low, an aplastic crisis is the probable cause (Taher & Kazzi, 2007).

- *Stained RBC (erythrocyte) examination:* Evaluates changes in morphology of RBCs.

Demonstrates partially or completely sickled, crescent-shaped cells, Howell-Jolly bodies, basophilic stippling, and occasional nucleated RBCs (normoblasts).

- *Hemoglobin electrophoresis:* Determines type of hemoglobin the individual has. When an electric charge is passed through a solution of hemoglobin, distinct hemoglobins move different distances, depending on their composition. This technique differentiates between usual hemoglobin (A), sickle hemoglobin (S), and many other different kinds of hemoglobin.

Identifies any abnormal hemoglobin types and differentiates between sickle cell trait and sickle cell anemia. Results may be inaccurate if client has received a blood transfusion within 3 to 4 months before testing.

Diagnostic Studies (continued)

TEST WHY IT IS DONE (continued)	WHAT IT TELLS ME (continued)
• *Sickle-turbidity tube test (Sickledex):* Detects the presence of hemoglobin S in blood.	Positive if 10% of hemoglobin S is present, but does not differentiate between sickle cell anemia and sickle cell trait.
• *Erythrocyte sedimentation rate (ESR):* Measures how fast RBCs fall to the bottom of a test tube; indicative of inflammatory process.	ESR is elevated.
• *Erythrocyte fragility:* Measures susceptibility of RBCs to hemolysis under certain conditions.	Diagnoses hemolytic anemia.
• *Acid phosphatase (ACP):* Enzyme needed to trigger specific chemical reactions.	Moderately elevated.
• *Alkaline phosphatase (ALP):* Enzyme found primarily in the liver.	Elevated during vaso-occlusive crisis, reflecting bone and liver damage.
• *Lactate dehydrogenase (LDH):* Indicator of the existence and severity of acute or chronic tissue damage.	Elevated because of RBC hemolysis.
• *Serum iron:* Iron balance is not easily achieved in sickle cell disease.	Deficiency is associated with premature destruction of young RBCs. However, the iron stores released by hemolysis may be available for reuse; therefore, serum iron deficiency is not always present. A very high iron level is associated with frequent blood transfusions for sickle cell anemia—a condition more common in children than adults (Iron Disorders Institute, 2006; Mohanty et al, 2008).

OTHER DIAGNOSTIC STUDIES
• *Urine/fecal urobilinogen:* Substance formed in the intestine from the breakdown of bilirubin; some is excreted in feces and some is reabsorbed and excreted in bile or urine.	These sensitive indicators of RBC destruction are increased.
• *Abdominal/pelvic ultrasound:* Performed to evaluate condition of organs.	Documents spleen size and presence of biliary or kidney stones.
• *Bone x-rays:* Evaluate skeletal changes.	May demonstrate bone infarction, osteomyelitis, avascular necrosis of hip, and so forth.

Nursing Priorities

1. Promote adequate cellular oxygenation and perfusion.
2. Alleviate pain.
3. Prevent complications.
4. Provide information about disease process, prognosis, and treatment needs.

Discharge Goals

1. Oxygenation and perfusion are adequate to meet cellular needs.
2. Pain relieved or controlled.
3. Complications prevented or minimized.
4. Disease process, future expectations, potential complications, and therapeutic regimen understood.
5. Plan in place to meet needs after discharge.

NURSING DIAGNOSIS: impaired Gas Exchange

May be related to
Decreased oxygen-carrying capacity of the blood, reduced RBC life span or premature destruction, abnormal RBC structure, sensitivity to low oxygen tension due to strenuous exercise, increase in altitude
Increased blood viscosity—occlusions created by sickled cells packing together within the capillaries
Pulmonary congestion—impairment of surface phagocytosis
Predisposition to bacterial pneumonia, pulmonary infarcts

Possibly evidenced by
Dyspnea, use of accessory muscles
Restlessness, confusion
Tachycardia
Cyanosis (hypoxia)

(continues on page 508)

Desired Outcomes/Evaluation Criteria—Client Will

Respiratory Status: Gas Exchange (NOC)
Demonstrate improved ventilation and oxygenation as evidenced by respiratory rate within normal limits, absence of cyanosis, use of accessory muscles, and clear breath sounds.
Participate in ADLs without weakness and fatigue.
Display improved or normal pulmonary function tests.

ACTIONS/INTERVENTIONS	RATIONALE
Respiratory Monitoring (NIC)	
Independent	
Monitor respiratory rate and depth, use of accessory muscles, and areas of cyanosis.	Indicators of adequacy of respiratory function or degree of compromise and therapy needs and effectiveness.
Auscultate breath sounds, noting presence or absence, and adventitious sounds.	Development of atelectasis and stasis of secretions can impair gas exchange.
Monitor vital signs; note changes in cardiac rhythm.	Changes in vital signs and development of dysrhythmias reflect effects of hypoxia on cardiovascular system.
Investigate reports of chest pain and increasing fatigue. Observe for signs of increased fever, cough, and adventitious breath sounds.	Reflective of developing acute chest syndrome, which increases the workload of the heart and oxygen demand.
Assess LOC and mentation regularly.	Brain tissue is very sensitive to decreases in oxygen, and changes in mentation may be an early indicator of developing hypoxia.
Ventilation Assistance (NIC)	
Assist in turning, coughing, and deep-breathing exercises.	Promotes optimal chest expansion, mobilization of secretions, and aeration of all lung fields; reduces risk of stasis of secretions and pneumonia.
Evaluate activity tolerance; limit activities to those within client's tolerance or place client on bedrest. Assist with ADLs and mobility, as needed.	Reduction of the metabolic requirements of the body reduces the oxygen requirements and degree of hypoxia.
Encourage client to alternate periods of rest and activity. Schedule rest periods, as indicated.	Protects from excessive fatigue and reduces oxygen demands and degree of hypoxia.
Demonstrate and encourage use of relaxation techniques, such as guided imagery and visualization.	Relaxation decreases muscle tension and anxiety and, hence, the metabolic demand for oxygen.
Promote adequate fluid intake, such as 2 to 3 L/day within cardiac tolerance.	Sufficient hydration is necessary to provide for mobilization of secretions and to prevent hyperviscosity of blood with associated capillary occlusion.
Screen health status of visitors and staff.	Protects client from potential sources of respiratory infection.
Collaborative	
Administer supplemental humidified oxygen, as indicated.	Maximizes oxygen transport to tissues, particularly in presence of pulmonary insults or pneumonia. *Note:* Oxygen should be given only in the presence of confirmed hypoxemia because oxygen can suppress erythropoietin levels, further reducing the production of RBCs.
Monitor laboratory studies—CBC, cultures, arterial blood gases (ABGs) or pulse oximetry, chest x-ray, and pulmonary function tests.	Client is particularly prone to pneumonia, which is potentially fatal because of its hypoxemic effect of increasing sickling.
Perform or assist with chest physiotherapy, intermittent positive-pressure breathing (IPPB), and incentive spirometry.	Mobilizes secretions and increases aeration of lung fields.
Administer packed RBCs (PRCs) or exchange transfusions, as indicated.	Simple blood transfusion is indicated in client in aplastic crisis and acute sequestration crisis. Transfusion increases the number of oxygen-carrying cells, dilutes the percentage of hemoglobin S, and improves circulation. PRCs are used because they are less likely to create circulatory overload. Exchange blood transfusions are indicated in cases of stroke and acute chest syndrome. Exchange transfusion consists of replacing the client's RBCs by normal donor RBCs, thereby decreasing hemoglobin S to less than 30% (Taher & Kazzi, 2007). *Note:* Partial transfusions are sometimes used prophylactically in high-risk situations, such as chronic, severe leg ulcers, preparation for general anesthesia, and third trimester of pregnancy.

ACTIONS/INTERVENTIONS (continued)	RATIONALE (continued)
Administer medications, as indicated, for example: Antipyretic, such as acetaminophen (Tylenol)	Maintains normothermia to reduce metabolic oxygen demands without affecting serum pH, which may occur with aspirin.
Antibiotics, such as amoxicillin plus clavulanic acid (Augmentin), cefaclor (Ceclor), among others	Broad-spectrum antibiotics are started immediately pending culture results of suspected infections, then may be changed when the specific pathogen is identified.

NURSING DIAGNOSIS: acute/chronic Pain

May be related to
Intravascular sickling with localized stasis, occlusion, infarction, and necrosis
Activation of pain fibers due to deprivation of oxygen and nutrients, accumulation of noxious metabolites

Possibly evidenced by
Localized, migratory, or more generalized pain, described as throbbing, gnawing, or severe and incapacitating; affecting peripheral extremities, bones, joints, back, abdomen, or head, with headaches recurrent and transient
Decreased ROM, guarding of the affected areas
Facial grimacing, narrowed or self-focus

Desired Outcomes/Evaluation Criteria—Client Will

Pain Level (NOC)
Verbalize relief or control of pain.
Demonstrate relaxed body posture, freedom of movement, and ability to sleep and rest appropriately.

ACTIONS/INTERVENTIONS	RATIONALE
Pain Management (NIC) *Independent*	
Assess reports of pain, including location, duration, and intensity (scale of 0 to 10). Have client help differentiate current pain from typical or usual pain problems.	Vaso-occlusive pain is the most common manifestation of sickle cell crises, where sickling potentiates cellular hypoxia, resulting in severe pain. Typically, pain occurs deep in the bones and muscles of back, ribs, and limbs and lasts 5 to 7 days. However, client may also have acute pain from another cause (ulcers, appendicitis), chronic pain from sickle cell damage (usually bone pain that is present daily), chronic pain from other causes (old injuries, arthritis), and chronic nerve pain caused by damage from sickle cell blockage or other conditions, such as diabetes.
Observe nonverbal pain cues, such as gait disturbances, body positioning, reluctance to move, facial expressions; and physiological manifestations of acute pain—elevated BP, tachycardia, and increased respiratory rate. Explore discrepancies between verbal and nonverbal cues.	Nonverbal cues may aid in evaluation of pain and effectiveness of therapy. Pain is unique to each client; therefore, one may encounter varying descriptions because of individualized perceptions.
Discuss with the client/SO what pain relief measures were effective in the past.	Involves client/SO in care and allows for identification of remedies that have already been found to relieve pain. Helpful in establishing individualized treatment needs.
Explore alternative pain relief measures, such as relaxation techniques, biofeedback, yoga, meditation, and distraction—visual, auditory, tactile, kinesthetic, guided imagery, and breathing techniques.	Cognitive-behavioral interventions may reduce reliance on pharmacological therapy and enhance client's sense of control.
Provide support for and carefully position affected extremities.	Reduces edema, discomfort, and risk of injury, especially if osteomyelitis is present.
Apply local massage gently to affected areas.	Helps reduce muscle tension.
Encourage ROM exercises.	May reduce joint stiffness and possible contracture formation.
Plan activities during peak analgesic effect.	Maximizes movement of joints, enhancing mobility.
Maintain adequate fluid intake.	Dehydration increases sickling vaso-occlusion and corresponding pain.

(continues on page 510)

Collaborative

Apply warm, moist compresses to affected joints or other painful areas. Avoid use of ice or cold compresses.

Administer medications, as indicated, for example: opioids, such as continuous infusion or around-the-clock morphine (Astramorph, Duramorph), hydromorphone (Dilaudid), and nalbuphine (Nubain); long-acting opiate combinations, such as morphine (MS Contin) and oxycodone (Oxycontin); nonopioid analgesics, such as acetaminophen (Tylenol); oral opiate combination analgesics, such as acetaminophen with codeine (Tylenol No. 3) and hydrocodone (Vicodin); and antiseizure medications, such as gabapentin (Neurontin).

Consult with or refer to physical therapy.

Administer and monitor RBC transfusion.

Warmth causes vasodilation and increases circulation to hypoxic areas. Cold causes vasoconstriction and compounds the crisis.

Various types of analgesics are needed to manage different types of pain. Opioids are the mainstay of pain control during crisis and are usually administered via patient-controlled analgesia (PCA). Acetaminophen can be used for control of headache, pain, and fever. Aspirin should be avoided because it alters blood pH and can make cells sickle more easily. *Note:* Meperidine (Demerol) should not be used because its metabolite, normeperidine, can cause central nervous system (CNS) excitation—anxiety, tremors, and seizures.

Determines and provides appropriate therapies, such as massage, heat therapies, and guided exercise.

Although transfusion does not halt the pain in an acute crisis, frequency of painful crises may be reduced by regular partial exchange transfusions to maintain population of normal RBCs.

NURSING DIAGNOSIS: ineffective tissue Perfusion (specify)

May be related to
Vaso-occlusive nature of sickling, inflammatory response
Arteriovenous (AV) shunts in both pulmonary and peripheral circulation
Myocardial damage from small infarcts, iron deposits, and fibrosis

Possibly evidenced by
Changes in vital signs, diminished peripheral pulses and capillary refill, general pallor
Decreased mentation, restlessness
Angina, palpitations
Tingling in extremities, intermittent claudication, bone pain
Transient visual disturbances
Ulcerations of lower extremities, delayed healing

Desired Outcomes/Evaluation Criteria—Client Will

Circulation Status (NOC)
Demonstrate improved tissue perfusion as evidenced by stabilized vital signs, strong and palpable peripheral pulses, adequate urine output, absence of pain; usual mentation; normal capillary refill; skin warm and dry; nailbeds and lips of natural pale, pink color; and absence of paresthesias.

ACTIONS/INTERVENTIONS

RATIONALE

Circulatory Care: Arterial [or] Venous Insufficiency (NIC)
Independent

Monitor vital signs carefully. Assess pulses for rate, rhythm, and volume. Note hypotension; rapid, weak, thready pulse; and tachypnea with shallow respirations.

Assess skin for coolness, pallor, cyanosis, diaphoresis, and delayed capillary refill.

Note changes in LOC; reports of headaches, dizziness; development of sensory or motor deficits, such as hemiparesis or paralysis; and seizure activity.

Maintain adequate fluid intake. (Refer to ND: risk for deficient Fluid Volume, below.) Monitor urine output.

Assess lower extremities for skin texture, edema, and ulcerations, especially of internal and external ankles.

Sludging and sickling in peripheral vessels may lead to complete or partial obliteration of a vessel with diminished perfusion to surrounding tissues. Sudden massive splenic sequestration of cells can lead to shock.

Changes reflect diminished circulation and hypoxia potentiating capillary occlusion. (Refer to ND: impaired Gas Exchange.)

Changes may reflect diminished perfusion to the CNS due to ischemia or infarction (stroke).

Dehydration not only causes hypovolemia but increases sickling and occlusion of capillaries. Decreased renal perfusion and failure may occur because of vascular occlusion.

Reduced peripheral circulation often leads to skin and underlying tissue changes and delayed healing.

ACTIONS/INTERVENTIONS (continued)	RATIONALE (continued)
Investigate reports of change in character of pain, or development of bone pain, angina, tingling of extremities, and eye pain or vision disturbances.	Changes may reflect increased sickling of cells and impaired circulation with further involvement of organs, such as myocardial infarction (MI), pulmonary infarction, or occlusion of vasculature of the eye.
Maintain environmental temperature and body warmth without overheating. Avoid hypothermia.	Prevents vasoconstriction, aids in maintaining circulation and perfusion. Excessive body heat may cause diaphoresis, adding to insensible fluid losses and risk of dehydration. Hypothermia may exacerbate cardiovascular compromise with severe anemia.
Evaluate for developing edema—including genitals in men.	Vaso-occlusion or circulatory stasis may lead to edema of extremities and priapism in men, potentiating risk of tissue ischemia and necrosis.

Collaborative

Monitor laboratory studies, such as the following: Blood gases, liver and kidney function tests	Decreased tissue perfusion may lead to gradual infarction of organ tissues, such as the brain, liver, spleen, kidney, skeletal muscle, and so forth, with consequent release of intracellular enzymes.
Serum electrolytes; provide replacements as indicated	Electrolyte losses, especially sodium, are increased during crisis because of fever, diarrhea, vomiting, and diaphoresis.
Administer intravenous (IV) solutions, such as 0.45 normal saline, via an infusion pump.	Hydration lowers the hemoglobin S concentration, which decreases the sickling tendency and also reduces blood viscosity, which helps to maintain perfusion. Infusion pump may prevent circulatory overload. *Note:* Lactated Ringer's solution or D_5W may cause RBC hemolysis and potentiate thrombus formation.
Administer hydroxyurea (Droxia) or experimental antisickling agents, such as sodium cyanate, carefully and observe for possible lethal side effects.	Hydroxyurea, a cytotoxic agent, dramatically decreases the number of sickle cell episodes, and is given to prevent crises. Antisickling agents currently under investigational use are aimed at prolonging erythrocyte survival and preventing sickling by affecting cell membrane changes.
Administer deferoxamine (Desferal) and vitamin C.	Chelation therapy may be indicated to correct iron overload associated with regular, frequent transfusions. Vitamin C may enhance excretion, especially in clients who are vitamin deficient. *Note:* Phlebotomy and exchange transfusions may be used in conjunction with chelation therapy.
Prepare for and assist with needle aspiration of blood from corpora cavernosa.	Sickling within the penis can cause priapism and edema. Removal of sludged sickled cells can improve circulation, decreasing psychological trauma and risk of necrosis and infection.
Prepare for surgical intervention.	Direct incision and ligation of the dorsal arteries of the penis and saphenous-cavernous shunting may be necessary in severe cases of priapism to prevent tissue necrosis.

NURSING DIAGNOSIS: risk for deficient Fluid Volume

Risk factors may include
Increased fluid needs—hypermetabolic state or fever, inflammatory processes
Renal parenchymal damage or infarctions limiting the kidney's ability to concentrate urine (hyposthenuria)

Possibly evidenced by
(Not applicable; presence of signs and symptoms establishes an *actual* diagnosis)

Desired Outcomes/Evaluation Criteria—Client Will

Hydration (NOC)
Maintain adequate fluid balance as evidenced by individually appropriate urine output with a near-normal specific gravity, stable vital signs, moist mucous membranes, good skin turgor, and prompt capillary refill.

Fluid Monitoring (NIC)
Independent

Maintain accurate intake and output (I&O). Weigh daily.	Client may reduce fluid intake during periods of crisis because of malaise and anorexia. Dehydration from vomiting, diarrhea, and fever may reduce urine output and precipitate a vaso-occlusive crisis.
Note urine characteristics and specific gravity.	The kidney can lose its ability to concentrate urine, resulting in excessive losses of dilute urine and fixation of the specific gravity.
Monitor vital signs, comparing with client's usual or previous readings. Take BP in lying, sitting, and standing positions, if possible.	Reduction of circulating blood volume can occur from increased fluid loss, resulting in hypotension and tachycardia.
Observe for fever, changes in level of consciousness, poor skin turgor, dryness of skin and mucous membranes, and pain.	Symptoms are reflective of dehydration and hemoconcentration with consequent vaso-occlusive state.
Monitor vital signs closely during blood transfusions and note presence of dyspnea, crackles, rhonchi, wheezes, diminished breath sounds, cough, frothy sputum, and cyanosis.	Client's heart may already be weakened and prone to failure because of chronic demands placed on it by the anemic state. Heart may be unable to tolerate the added fluid volume from transfusions or rapid IV fluid administered to treat crisis or shock.

Collaborative

Administer IV fluids, as indicated.	Replaces fluid deficits; may reverse renal concentration of RBCs and reduce potential for kidney failure. Fluids must be given immediately, especially in CNS involvement, to decrease hemoconcentration and prevent further infarction.
Monitor laboratory studies, for example: Hgb/Hct	Elevations may indicate hemoconcentration. Post-transfusion Hgb level of 8 to 9 g/dL is generally recommended to avoid the risk of hyperviscosity that may occur several days after transfusion when RBCs sequestered in the spleen may return to the circulation and increase the Hgb levels.
Serum and urine electrolytes	Kidneys' loss of ability to concentrate urine may result in serum depletions of Na+, K−, and Cl−, necessitating replacement.

NURSING DIAGNOSIS: impaired physical Mobility

May be related to
Multiple, recurrent bone infarctions or infections—weight-bearing bones
Pain and discomfort: kyphosis of upper back and lordosis of lower back, possible joint effusions
Osteoporosis with fragmentation or collapse of femoral head or vertebra, compression deformities
Bacterial infections (osteomyelitis)

Possibly evidenced by
Reports of pain
Limited joint ROM, reluctance to move, inability to walk or perform ADLs, guarding of joints, gait disturbances
Generalized weakness, therapeutic restrictions—bedrest

Desired Outcomes/Evaluation Criteria—Client Will

Mobility (NOC)
Maintain or increase strength and function of affected body parts.
Participate in activities with absence of or improvement in gait disturbances, increased joint ROM, and absence of inflammatory signs.

Refer to CP: Extended Care, ND: impaired physical Mobility for appropriate actions and interventions.

NURSING DIAGNOSIS: risk for impaired Skin Integrity

Risk factors may include
Impaired circulation—venous stasis and vaso-occlusion; altered sensation
Decreased mobility, bedrest

Possibly evidenced by
(Not applicable; presence of signs and symptoms establishes an *actual* diagnosis)

Desired Outcomes/Evaluation Criteria—Client Will

Tissue Integrity: Skin and Mucous Membranes (NOC)
Prevent dermal ischemic injury.
Display improvement in wound or lesion healing if present.

Risk Control (NOC)
Participate in behaviors to reduce risk factors and skin breakdown.

ACTIONS/INTERVENTIONS	RATIONALE
Skin Surveillance (NIC)	
Independent	
Reposition frequently, even when sitting in chair.	Prevents prolonged tissue pressure where circulation is already compromised, reducing risk of tissue trauma and ischemia.
Inspect skin pressure points regularly for redness and provide gentle massage.	Poor circulation may predispose to rapid skin breakdown.
Protect bony prominences with sheepskin, heel and elbow protectors, or pillows, as indicated.	Decreases pressure on tissues, preventing skin breakdown.
Keep skin surfaces dry and clean and linens dry and wrinkle free.	Moist, contaminated areas provide excellent media for growth of pathogenic organisms.
Monitor ischemic areas, leg bruises, cuts, and bumps closely for ulcer formation.	Potential entry sites for pathogenic organisms. In presence of altered immune system, this increases risk of infection and delayed healing.
Elevate lower extremities when sitting.	Enhances venous return, reducing venous stasis and edema formation.
Collaborative	
Provide egg-crate, alternating air pressure, or water mattress.	Reduces tissue pressure and aids in maximizing cellular perfusion to prevent dermal injury.
Provide wound care as indicated, such as cleansing and débriding open wounds and ulcers according to protocol.	Improvement or delayed healing reflects status of tissue perfusion and effectiveness of interventions. *Note:* These clients are at increased risk of serious complications because of lowered resistance to infection and decreased nutrients for healing.
Prepare for and assist with hyperbaric oxygenation of ulcer sites.	Maximizes oxygen delivery to tissues, enhancing healing.

NURSING DIAGNOSIS: risk for Infection [sepsis]

Risk factors may include
Chronic disease process, tissue destruction, such as infarction, fibrosis, loss of spleen (autosplenectomy)
Inadequate primary defenses—broken skin, stasis of body fluids, decreased ciliary action

Possibly evidenced by
(Not applicable; presence of signs and symptoms establishes an *actual* diagnosis)

Desired Outcomes/Evaluation Criteria—Client Will

Knowledge: Infection Control (NOC)
Verbalize understanding of individual causative or risk factors.
Identify interventions to prevent or reduce risk of infection.

Refer to CPs: Pneumonia, Sepsis/Septicemia, Fractures, ND: risk for Infection.

NURSING DIAGNOSIS: deficient Knowledge [Learning Need] regarding condition, prognosis, treatment, self-care, and discharge needs

May be related to
Lack of exposure or recall
Information misinterpretation
Unfamiliarity with resources

Possibly evidenced by
Questions, request for information, statement of misconceptions
Inaccurate follow-through of instructions; development of preventable complications
Verbal or nonverbal cues of anxiety

Desired Outcomes/Evaluation Criteria—Client Will

Knowledge: Disease Process (NOC)
Verbalize understanding of disease process, including symptoms of crisis and potential complications.

Knowledge: Treatment Regimen (NOC)
Verbalize understanding of therapeutic needs.
Initiate necessary behaviors or lifestyle changes to prevent complications.
Participate in continued medical follow-up, genetic counseling, and family planning services.

ACTIONS/INTERVENTIONS	RATIONALE
Teaching: Disease Process (NIC) *Independent* Review disease process and treatment needs.	Provides knowledge base from which client can make informed choices. *Note:* The median age at death is 48 years for women and 42 years for men, with death often being due to organ failure. However, a significant number of individuals are living much longer.
Review precipitating factors, such as the following: Cold environmental temperatures, failure to dress warmly when engaging in winter activities; wearing tight, restrictive clothing; stressful situations	Causes peripheral vasoconstriction, which may result in sludging of the circulation, increased sickling, and may precipitate a vaso-occlusive crisis.
Strenuous physical activity or contact-type sports, and extremely warm temperatures	Increases metabolic demand for oxygen and increases insensible fluid losses (evaporation and perspiration) leading to dehydration, which may increase blood viscosity and tendency to sickle.
Travel to places more than 7,000 ft above sea level or flying in unpressurized aircraft	Decreased oxygen tension present at higher altitudes causes hypoxia and potentiates sickling of cells. *Note:* Even though commercial airline cabins are pressurized, low cabin humidity increases risk of dehydration.
Encourage consumption of at least 3 to 4 L of fluid daily, during a steady state, increasing to 6 to 8 L during a painful crisis or while engaging in activities that might precipitate dehydration.	Prevents dehydration and consequent hyperviscosity that can potentiate sickling and crisis.
Discuss use of antimetabolites, such as hydroxyurea (Hydrea).	May reduce frequency of pain episodes in adults.
Encourage ROM exercise and regular physical activity with a balance between rest and activity.	Prevents bone demineralization and may reduce risk of fractures. Aids in maintaining level of resistance and decreases oxygen needs.
Review client's current diet, reinforcing the importance of diet including liver, green leafy vegetables, citrus fruits, and wheat germ. Provide necessary instruction regarding supplementary vitamins such as folic acid.	Nutritious foods, including vitamins folate and B$_{12}$ in greater quantities than usual, are essential because of increased demands placed on bone marrow. Folic acid supplements are frequently ordered to prevent aplastic crisis.
Emphasize importance of avoiding smoking and alcohol consumption; identify appropriate medical assistance and community support groups for smoking cessation.	Nicotine induces peripheral vasoconstriction and decreases oxygen tension, which may contribute to cellular hypoxia and sickling. Alcohol increases the possibility of dehydration which precipitates sickling. Maintaining these changes in behavior or lifestyle may require prolonged support.
Discuss principles of skin and extremity care, and protection from injury. Encourage prompt treatment of cuts, insect bites, sores, and lesions.	Because of impaired tissue perfusion, especially in the periphery, distal extremities are especially susceptible to altered skin integrity and infection.
Include instructions on care of leg ulcers that might develop.	Fosters independence and maintenance of self-care at home.
Instruct client to avoid persons with infections such as upper respiratory infections (URIs).	Altered immune response places client at risk for infections, especially bacterial bronchitis and pneumonia.

ACTIONS/INTERVENTIONS (continued)	RATIONALE (continued)
Recommend avoiding cold remedies and decongestants containing ephedrine and large amounts of caffeine. Stress the importance of reading labels on over-the-counter (OTC) drugs and consulting healthcare provider before consuming any drugs or herbal supplements.	Those remedies containing vasoconstrictors may decrease peripheral tissue perfusion and cause sludging of sickled cells.
Discuss conditions for which medical attention should be sought, such as the following:	
Urine that appears blood tinged or smoky	Symptoms suggestive of sickling in the renal medulla.
Indigestion, persistent vomiting, diarrhea, high fever, and excessive thirst	Dehydration may trigger a vaso-occlusive crisis.
Severe joint or bone pain	May signify a vaso-occlusive crisis due to sickling in the bones or spleen, leading to ischemia or infarction or onset of osteomyelitis.
Severe chest pain, with or without cough	May reflect acute chest syndrome, with pulmonary infiltrates or pneumonia.
Abdominal pain; gastric distress following meals	Cholelithiasis, primarily with bilirubin stones, is present in more than 50% of adults.
Priapism episode persisting over 4 hours with no resolution	Suggestive of sickling in the penis.
Persistent fever greater than 100°F (38°C); increasing fatigue and pallor; dizziness, drowsiness, and nonhealing leg ulcers	Suggestive of infections that may precipitate a vaso-occlusive crisis if dehydration develops. *Note:* Severe infections are the most frequent cause of aplastic crisis.
Any neurological symptom or sign	Stroke can occur due to cerebral infarction, although it is more common in children than adults. Without long-term transfusion therapy, approximately one-third of clients will experience recurrent strokes.
Review and strengthen coping abilities, such as how to deal appropriately with anxiety, getting adequate information, and using relaxation techniques.	Promotes client's sense of control and may avert a crisis.
Recommend wearing a medical alert bracelet or carrying a wallet card.	May prevent inappropriate treatment in emergency situation.
Discuss genetic implications of the condition. Encourage SO and family members to seek testing to determine presence of hemoglobin S.	Screening may identify other family members with sickle cell trait. Hereditary nature of the disease with the possibility of transmitting the mutation may have a bearing on reproductive decisions.
Explore concerns regarding childbearing and family planning. Refer to community resources and obstetrician knowledgeable about sickle cell disease, as indicated.	Provides opportunity to correct misconceptions and present information necessary to make informed decisions. Pregnancy can precipitate a vaso-occlusive crisis because the placenta's tortuous blood supply and low oxygen tension potentiate sickling, which in turn can lead to fetal hypoxia. Client also has increased risk of maternal infection, pregnancy-induced hypertension, HF, and pulmonary infarction. The fetus is at risk for growth retardation, premature birth, and low birth weight (Beers, 2006).
Encourage client to have routine follow-ups, such as the following:	
Periodic laboratory studies, such as CBC	Monitors changes in blood components; identifies need for changes in treatment regimen. When using hydroxylurea, frequent monitoring of CBC is required because of narrow margin between acceptable degree of bone marrow suppression and toxicity including neutropenia, anemia, and thrombocytopenia.
Biannual dental examination	Sound oral hygiene limits opportunity for bacterial invasion and sepsis.
Annual ophthalmological examination	Detects development of sickle retinopathy with either proliferative or nonproliferative ocular changes predisposing to retinal hemorrhage and increased intraocular pressure.
Determine need for vocational and career guidance.	Sedentary career may be necessary because of decreased oxygen-carrying capacity and diminished exercise tolerance.
Encourage participation in community support groups available to clients and SO, such as the Sickle Cell Disease Association of America, March of Dimes, public health nurse, and visiting nurse.	Helpful in adjustment to long-term situation; reduces feelings of isolation and enhances problem-solving through sharing of common experiences. *Note:* Failure to resolve concerns and deal with situation may require more intensive therapy and psychological support.

ADULT LEUKEMIAS

I. **Pathophysiology**: malignant disorder of the blood and bone marrow characterized by the uncontrolled accumulation of white blood cells (WBCs)
  a. Blood cells originate primarily in the marrow of bones, such as the sternum, iliac crest, and cranium, and begin as immature cells (blasts or stem cells) that differentiate and mature into red blood cells (RBCs), platelets, and various types of WBCs.
  b. Production of normal blood cells markedly decreased, leading to anemia, thrombocytopenia, neutropenia
  c. Rapid growth of immature or ineffective WBCs and delayed cell death lead to their accumulation in bone marrow, blood, spleen, and liver.

II. **Categories**
  a. Dependent on the type of cell involved—myelogenous or lymphocytic—as well as duration: *acute* (acute myelogenous leukemia [AML], acute lymphocytic leukemia [ALL]); or *chronic* (chronic myelogenous leukemia [CML], chronic lymphocytic leukemia [CLL])
    i. Acute
      1. WBCs proliferate so rapidly that they lose the ability to regulate cell division and do not differentiate into mature cells.
      2. Most common form in adults is AML, which affects different types of WBCs, with the exception of lymphocytes.
      3. Progresses rapidly without treatment
    ii. Chronic
      1. Chronic forms have few or no blast cells.
      2. Most common form is CLL, which is characterized by abnormal increase in lymphocytes.
      3. Develops gradually and progresses more slowly than acute forms

III. **Etiology**
  a. Exact cause is unknown.
  b. Risk factors (Seiter, 2006)
    i. Antecedent histological disorders: diseases of the bone marrow, such as myelodysplastic syndrome (MDS)
    ii. Environmental exposures: radiation, smoking, benzene
    iii. Prior chemotherapy
    iv. Genetics or congenital disorders: develop more often in children

IV. **Statistics**
  a. Morbidity: In 2007, an estimated 44,240 new cases of leukemia (all types) were diagnosed in the United States; diagnosed more often in males than females; chronic leukemias account for 7% more cases than acute; most cases occur in older adults, with more than half occurring after age 67 (The Leukemia & Lymphoma Society's SEER Facts 2007–2008); with AML, the median age of onset is 65 years (Seiter, 2006).
  b. Mortality: In 2005, an estimated 9,000 deaths from AML in the United States were reported (Seiter, 2006); majority of those with CLL live 5 to 10 years; however, presence of complications may shorten survival to 2 to 3 years (Perry & Rasool, 2005).
  c. Cost: Projected cost for care was $2.6 billion in 2004 (National Cancer Institute [NCI], 2007).

GLOSSARY

Blast cell: Blood cell that is not fully developed and is still immature.

Lymphocytic or lymphoblastic: A cancerous change takes place in a type of marrow cell that forms lymphocytes.

Lymphopenia: Low number of lymphocytes in the blood.

Myelogenous or myeloid: Cancerous change takes place in a type of marrow cell that normally goes on to form red cells, some types of white cells, and platelets.

Neutropenia: Abnormal decrease in the number of neutrophils (type of white blood cell [WBC] that fights infection) in the blood.

Normocytic, normochromic anemia: Anemia associated with disturbances of red cell formation and related to endocrine deficiencies, chronic inflammation, and condition in which cancer is spread widely throughout the body or, in some cases, to a relatively large region of the body.

GLOSSARY (continued)

Progenitor stem cell transplant: Reestablishment of normal bone marrow function through the infusion of cells committed to forming a specific type of blood cell line—red blood cells (RBCs), WBCs, or platelets. The source of the cells may be from the peripheral blood, bone marrow, or umbilical cord and placenta. The donor may be the client himself or herself (autologous transplant), a genetically compatible relative or individual (allogeneic transplant), or donated cord blood. Syngeneic transplant describes the use of an identical twin as donor.

Thrombocytopenia: Disorder in which there are not enough platelets. This condition is sometimes associated with abnormal bleeding.

Tumor lysis syndrome: Metabolic derangement produced by rapid tumor breakdown as a consequence of therapy. It is characterized by hyperuricemia because of DNA breakdown; hyperkalemia because of cytosol breakdown; hyperphosphatemia because of protein breakdown; and hypocalcemia secondary to hyperphosphatemia. As phosphate level goes up, serum calcium goes down. These derangements can result in acute renal failure, cardiac dysrhythmias, and sudden death from hyperkalemia or hypocalcemia.

Care Setting

Client receives acute inpatient care on medical or oncology unit for initial evaluation and treatment, typically for 4 to 6 weeks, and then at the community level.

Related Concerns

Cancer, page 846

Psychosocial aspects of care, page 749

Transplantation considerations—postoperative and lifelong, page 739

Client Assessment Database

Data depend on degree and duration of the disease and other organ involvement.

DIAGNOSTIC DIVISION MAY REPORT	MAY EXHIBIT
ACTIVITY/REST • Fatigue, malaise • Weakness, inability to engage in usual activities • Flu-like symptoms	• Muscle wasting • Increased need for sleep, somnolence
CIRCULATION • Palpitations	• Tachycardia, heart murmurs • Pallor of skin, mucous membranes • Cranial nerve deficits and signs of cerebral hemorrhage
EGO INTEGRITY • Feelings of helplessness, hopelessness	• Depression, withdrawal, anxiety, fear, anger, irritability • Mood changes, confusion
ELIMINATION • Diarrhea, perianal tenderness, pain • Bright red blood on tissue paper, tarry stools • Blood in urine, decreased urine output	• Perianal abscess, hematuria
FOOD/FLUID • Loss of appetite, anorexia, vomiting • Change in taste • Weight loss • Sore throat, difficulty swallowing	• Abdominal distention, decreased bowel sounds • Splenomegaly, hepatomegaly, jaundice • Stomatitis, oral ulcerations • Gum hypertrophy (gum infiltration may be indicative of AML)
NEUROSENSORY • Lack of or decreased coordination • Mood changes, confusion, disorientation, lack of concentration • Dizziness; numbness, tingling, paresthesias	• Muscle irritability • Seizure activity • Uncoordinated movements

(continues on page 518)

DIAGNOSTIC DIVISION MAY REPORT (continued)	MAY EXHIBIT (continued)
PAIN/DISCOMFORT • Abdominal pain • Headaches • Bone, joint pain—knees, hips, shoulders • Sternal tenderness • Muscle cramping	• Guarding or distraction behaviors, restlessness • Self-focus
RESPIRATION • Shortness of breath with minimal exertion	• Dyspnea, tachypnea • Cough • Crackles, rhonchi • Decreased breath sounds
SAFETY • History of recent or recurrent infections, falls • Visual disturbances or impairment • Nosebleeds or other hemorrhages, spontaneous uncontrollable bleeding with minimal trauma • Swollen gums	• Fever, infections • Bruises, purpura, retinal hemorrhages, gum or nose bleeding • Papilledema and exophthalmos • Leukemic infiltrates in the dermis
SEXUALITY • Changes in libido • Changes in menstrual flow, menorrhagia • Impotence	
TEACHING/LEARNING • History of exposure to chemicals—benzene (commercially used toxic liquid that is also present in lead-free gasoline), excessive levels of ionizing radiation, previous treatment with chemotherapy—especially alkalizing agents • Chromosomal disorder—Down syndrome or Fanconi's aplastic anemia • Exposure to virus—human T-cell leukemia or lymphoma virus-1 (HTLV-1)	
DISCHARGE PLAN CONSIDERATIONS • May need assistance with therapy and treatment needs and supplies, shopping, food preparation, self-care activities, homemaker and maintenance tasks, transportation ▶ Refer to section at end of plan for postdischarge considerations.	

Diagnostic Studies

TEST WHY IT IS DONE	WHAT IT TELLS ME
BLOOD TESTS • *Complete blood count (CBC):* Battery of screening tests, which typically includes hemoglobin (Hgb); hematocrit (Hct); RBC count, morphology, indices, and distribution width index; platelet count and size; and WBC count and differential.	Full blood count is used to establish the number of different blood cell types within the circulation. RBC production can be decreased by the leukemic cells and suppression of normal bone marrow activity. Client may have mild to severe normocytic, normochromic anemia associated with hypersplenism.

Diagnostic Studies (continued)

TEST WHY IT IS DONE (continued)	WHAT IT TELLS ME (continued)
• *Reticulocytes:* Young RBCs.	Count is usually low. "Teardrop" and nucleated RBCs may be seen.
• *WBC count and differential:* Percentage of each of the five types of mature WBCs: neutrophils, lymphocytes (B cells and T cells), monocytes, eosinophils, and basophils within the bloodstream. In particular, the percentage of immature leukemic blast cells is noted.	Persons with ALL or AML often have too many leukocytes—count may be more than 50,000/cm—with increased numbers of immature WBCs ("shift to left"). Leukemic blast cells may be present.
• *Platelet count:* Platelets have essential function in coagulation.	May vary from normal to very low, less than 50,000/mm.
• *Prothrombin time (PT)/activated partial thromboplastin time (aPTT):* Determines bleeding and clotting time.	May be prolonged. Disseminated intravascular coagulation (DIC) may occur with AML, but it is especially common in acute promyelocytic leukemia.
• *Blood chemistries:* Measures the type and amount of enzymes, minerals, and other substances within the blood.	Identifies kidney or liver damage that may be caused by leukemic cell breakdown or by drugs used for chemotherapy.
• *Alkaline phosphatase (ALP):* Aids in differential diagnosis.	Elevated with CML.
• *Lactic dehydrogenase (LDH):* Substance released by tumors and found in blood.	May be elevated.
• *Serum vitamin B$_{12}$:* May aid in differential diagnosis of type of leukemia and other myeloproliferative conditions.	Can be increased with CML and some forms of acute leukemia; normal in CLL and undifferentiated stem cell leukemia.
• *Uric acid:* Waste product resulting from the breakdown of nitrogen-containing compounds (purines).	Commonly elevated in client with ALL or as a result of chemotherapy.

OTHER DIAGNOSTIC STUDIES

• *Computed tomography (CT) scan:* Computer-assisted x-ray that produces cross-sectional images of the body.	CT scans are not usually used in client with leukemia unless metastasis is suspected. In such cases, CT scan may detect changes in the lymph nodes around the heart, trachea, or abdomen. Lymph node enlargement is more common in patients with ALL or CLL with potential for compression of organs or internal structures, such as airway obstruction or obstructive uropathy. Scans of liver and spleen may reveal splenomegaly (Perry & Rasool, 2005).
• *X-rays:* Determine areas of involvement.	May reveal enlarged lymph nodes in the chest, a localized mass in the lungs, or evidence that leukemia has spread to bones or joints.
• *Bone marrow aspiration and biopsy:* May be done by needle aspirate or biopsy for microscopic examination of fluid and tissues within the marrow to determine the number, size, and shape of the various cell types as well as the proportion of mature to immature cells.	Abnormal WBCs usually make up 50% or more of the WBCs in the bone marrow. Often 60% to 90% of the cells are blast cells, with erythroid precursors, mature cells, and megakaryocytes reduced.

DEFINITIVE DIAGNOSTIC STUDIES

• *Cytogenetic analysis:* Cells are studied to see if chromosomal abnormalities are present.	Examination of chromosome abnormalities from samples of peripheral blood, bone marrow, or lymph nodes can indicate prognostic features and direct treatment options.
• *Immunocytochemistry:* Uses antibodies to treat the bone marrow or biopsy samples; specific cells undergo a color change that can be identified under microscope.	Allows pathologist to identify specific types of leukemia.
• *Lumbar puncture:* Determines if cancer has spread to spinal column or brain.	May reveal leukemic cells in cerebrospinal fluid (CSF).
• *Bence Jones protein (urine):* Protein produced by neoplastic cells.	May be increased.

Nursing Priorities

1. Prevent infection during acute phases of disease and treatment.
2. Maintain circulating blood volume.
3. Alleviate pain.
4. Promote optimal physical functioning.
5. Provide psychological support.
6. Provide information about disease process, prognosis, and treatment needs.

Discharge Goals

1. Complications prevented or minimized.
2. Pain relieved or controlled.
3. Activities of daily living (ADLs) met by self or with assistance.
4. Dealing with disease realistically.
5. Disease process, prognosis, and therapeutic regimen understood.
6. Plan in place to meet needs after discharge.

Refer to CP: Cancer, for further discussion and expansion of interventions related to cancer care and for client teaching.

NURSING DIAGNOSIS: **risk for Infection**

Risk factors may include

Inadequate secondary defenses—alterations in mature WBCs with low granulocyte and abnormal lymphocyte count, increased number of immature lymphocytes; immunosuppression, bone marrow suppression (effects of therapy, transplant)
Inadequate primary defenses—stasis of body fluids, traumatized tissue
Invasive procedures
Malnutrition; chronic disease

Possibly evidenced by

(Not applicable; presence of signs and symptoms establishes an *actual* diagnosis)

Desired Outcomes/Evaluation Criteria—Client Will

Knowledge: Infection Control (NOC)
Identify actions to prevent or reduce risk of infection.
Demonstrate techniques or lifestyle changes to promote safe environment and achieve timely healing.

ACTIONS/INTERVENTIONS	RATIONALE
Infection Protection (NIC)	
Independent	
Place in private room. Screen and limit visitors, as indicated. Prohibit use of live plants or cut flowers. Restrict fresh fruits and vegetables or make sure they are washed or peeled.	Protect client from potential sources of pathogens and infection. *Note:* Profound bone marrow suppression, neutropenia, and chemotherapy place client at great risk for infection.
Model and require good hand-washing protocol for all personnel and visitors.	Prevents cross-contamination and reduces risk of infection.
Monitor temperature. Note correlation between temperature elevations and chemotherapy treatments. Observe for fever associated with tachycardia, hypotension, and subtle mental changes.	Although fever may accompany some forms of chemotherapy, progressive hyperthermia occurs in some types of infections, and fever unrelated to drugs or blood products occurs in most leukemia clients. *Note:* Septicemia may occur without fever.
Prevent chilling. Force fluids and administer tepid sponge bath.	Helps reduce fever, which contributes to fluid imbalance, discomfort, and central nervous system (CNS) complications.
Encourage frequent turning and deep breathing.	Prevents stasis of respiratory secretions, reducing risk of atelectasis and pneumonia.
Auscultate breath sounds, noting crackles and rhonchi; inspect secretions for changes in characteristics, such as increased sputum production or change in sputum color. Observe urine for signs of infection: cloudy, foul-smelling, or presence of urgency or burning with voids.	Early intervention is essential to prevent sepsis or septicemia in immunosuppressed person.
Handle client gently. Keep linens dry and wrinkle free.	Prevents sheet burns and skin excoriation.
Inspect skin for tender, erythematous areas and open wounds. Cleanse skin with antibacterial solutions.	May indicate local infection. *Note:* Open wounds may not produce pus because of insufficient number of granulocytes.
Inspect oral mucous membranes. Provide good oral hygiene. Use a soft toothbrush, sponge, or swabs for frequent mouth care.	The oral cavity is an excellent medium for growth of organisms and is susceptible to ulceration and bleeding.
Promote good perianal hygiene. Examine perianal area at least daily during acute illness. Provide sitz baths, using Betadine or Hibiclens, if indicated. Avoid rectal temperatures and use of suppositories.	Promotes cleanliness, reducing risk of perianal abscess; enhances circulation and healing. *Note:* Perianal abscess can contribute to septicemia and death in immunosuppressed clients.

ACTIONS/INTERVENTIONS (continued)

Coordinate procedures and tests to allow for uninterrupted rest periods.

Encourage increased intake of fluids and foods high in protein with adequate fiber.

Avoid or limit invasive procedures, such as venipuncture and injections, as possible.

Collaborative

Monitor laboratory studies, such as the following:
CBC, noting whether WBC count falls or sudden changes occur in neutrophils

Gram's stain cultures and sensitivity

Review serial chest x-rays.

Prepare for and assist with leukemia-specific treatments, such as chemotherapy, radiation, and stem cell transplant.

Administer medications, as indicated, for example:
Anti-infectives, such as ofloxacin (Ocuflox) and rifampin (Rifadin)

Colony-stimulating factors (CSFs), such as sargramostim (Leukine), filgrastim (Neupogen), and pegfilgrastim (Neulasta)
Avoid use of aspirin-containing antipyretics.

Provide nutritious diet, high in protein and calories, avoiding raw fruits, vegetables, or uncooked meats.

RATIONALE (continued)

Conserves energy for healing and cellular regeneration.

Promotes healing and prevents dehydration. *Note:* Constipation potentiates retention of toxins and risk of rectal irritation and tissue injury.
Break in skin could provide an entry for pathogenic and potentially lethal organisms. Use of central venous lines, such as tunneled catheter or implanted port, can effectively reduce need for frequent invasive procedures and risk of infection. *Note:* Myelosuppression may be cumulative in nature, especially when multiple drug therapy, including steroids, is prescribed.

Decreased numbers of normal or mature WBCs can result from the disease process or chemotherapy, compromising the immune response and increasing risk of infection.
Verifies presence of infections; identifies specific organisms and appropriate therapy.
Indicator of development or resolution of respiratory complications.
Leukemia is usually treated with a combination of these agents, each requiring specific safety precautions for client and care providers.

May be given prophylactically or to treat specific infection, especially in client who has prolonged granulocytopenia or too few mature neutrophils (Seiter, 2006).
Restores WBCs destroyed by chemotherapy and reduces risk of severe infection and death in certain types of leukemia.
Aspirin can cause gastric bleeding and further decrease platelet count.
Proper nutrition enhances immune system. Minimizes potential sources of bacterial contamination (Seiter, 2006).

NURSING DIAGNOSIS: **risk for deficient Fluid Volume**

Risk factors may include
Excessive losses—vomiting, hemorrhage, diarrhea
Decreased fluid intake—nausea, anorexia
Increased fluid need—hypermetabolic state, fever, predisposition for kidney stone formation and tumor lysis syndrome

Possibly evidenced by
(Not applicable; presence of signs and symptoms establishes an *actual* diagnosis)

Desired Outcomes/Evaluation Criteria—Client Will

Hydration (NOC)
Demonstrate adequate fluid volume, as evidenced by stable vital signs; palpable pulses; urine output, specific gravity, and pH within normal limits.

Risk Control (NOC)
Identify individual risk factors and appropriate interventions.
Initiate behaviors or lifestyle changes to prevent development of dehydration.

ACTIONS/INTERVENTIONS

Fluid Management (NIC)
Independent
Monitor intake and output (I&O). Calculate insensible losses and fluid balance. Note decreased urine output in presence of adequate intake. Measure urine specific gravity and pH.

RATIONALE

Tumor lysis syndrome occurs when destroyed cancer cells release toxic levels of potassium, phosphorus, and uric acid. Elevated phosphorus and uric acid levels can cause crystal formation in the renal tubules, impairing filtration and leading to renal failure.

(continues on page 522)

Weigh daily.	Measure of adequacy of fluid replacement and kidney function. Continued intake greater than output may indicate renal insult or obstruction.
Monitor blood pressure (BP) and heart rate.	Changes may reflect effects of hypovolemia associated with bleeding or dehydration.
Evaluate skin turgor, capillary refill, and general condition of mucous membranes.	Indirect indicators of fluid status.
Note presence of nausea or fever.	Affects intake, fluid needs, and route of replacement.
Encourage fluids of up to 3 to 4 L/day when oral intake is resumed.	Promotes urine flow, prevents uric acid precipitation, and enhances clearance of antineoplastic drugs.

Bleeding Precautions (NIC)

Inspect skin and mucous membranes for petechiae and ecchymotic areas; note bleeding gums, frank or occult blood in stools and urine, and oozing from invasive line sites.

Suppression of bone marrow and platelet production places client at risk for spontaneous or uncontrolled bleeding.

Implement measures to prevent tissue injury and bleeding: gentle brushing of teeth or gums with soft toothbrush, cotton swab, or sponge-tipped applicator; using electric razor instead of sharp razors when shaving; avoiding forceful nose blowing and needlesticks when possible; and using sustained pressure such as sandbags or pressure dressings on oozing puncture or intravenous (IV) sites.

Fragile tissues and altered clotting mechanisms increase the risk of hemorrhage following even minor trauma.

Limit oral care to mouth rinse, if indicated, such as a mixture of 1/4 tsp baking soda and 1/8 tsp salt in 8 oz water, or may use hydrogen peroxide in water or saline for bleeding or infected oral tissue. Avoid mouthwashes with alcohol.

When bleeding is present, even gentle brushing may cause more tissue damage. Alcohol has a drying effect and may be painful to irritated tissues.

Provide soft diet.

May help reduce gum irritation.

Fluid Management (NIC)
Collaborative

Administer IV fluids as indicated.

Maintains fluid and electrolyte balance in the absence of oral intake. Prevents or minimizes tumor lysis syndrome and reduces risk of renal complications.

Administer medications, as indicated, for example:
Antiemetics: 5-HT$_3$ receptor antagonist drugs, such as ondansetron (Zofran) or granisetron (Kytril)

Relieves nausea and vomiting associated with administration of chemotherapy agents and may enhance oral intake.

Allopurinol (Zyloprim)

Improves renal excretion of toxic by-products from breakdown of leukemia cells. Reduces the chances of nephropathy as a result of uric acid production.

Potassium acetate or citrate and sodium bicarbonate

May be used to alkalinize the urine, preventing or minimizing tumor lysis syndrome and kidney stones.

Bleeding Precautions (NIC)

Monitor laboratory studies: platelets, Hgb/Hct, and clotting.

When the platelet count is less than 20,000/mm because of proliferation of WBCs or bone marrow suppression, client is prone to spontaneous life-threatening bleeding. Decreasing Hgb/Hct is indicative of occult bleeding.

Administer RBCs, platelets, and clotting factors.

Restores or normalizes RBC count and oxygen-carrying capacity to correct anemia. Platelets or fresh frozen plasma (FFP) may be used to prevent or treat hemorrhage (Seiter, 2006).

Maintain external central vascular access device, such as with subclavian or tunneled catheter or implanted port.

Eliminates peripheral venipuncture as source of bleeding.

Administer medications, as indicated, for example:
Stool softeners

Helps reduce straining at stool, which can cause trauma to rectal tissues.

Oral contraceptives

Minimizes blood loss by stopping or slowing menstrual flow.

NURSING DIAGNOSIS: acute Pain

May be related to
Physical agents—enlarged organs and lymph nodes, bone marrow packed with leukemic cells
Chemical agents—antileukemic treatments
Psychological manifestations—anxiety, fear

Possibly evidenced by
Reports of pain—bone, nerve, headaches, and so forth
Guarding or distraction behaviors, facial grimacing, alteration in muscle tone
Autonomic responses

Desired Outcomes/Evaluation Criteria—Client Will

Pain Level (NOC)
Report pain is relieved or controlled.
Appear relaxed and able to sleep and rest appropriately.

Pain Control (NOC)
Demonstrate behaviors to manage pain.

ACTIONS/INTERVENTIONS	RATIONALE
Pain Management (NIC)	
Independent	
Investigate reports of pain. Note changes in degree (use scale of 0 to 10) and site.	Helpful in assessing need for intervention and may indicate developing complications.
Monitor vital signs and note nonverbal cues, such as muscle tension and restlessness.	May be useful in evaluating verbal comments and effectiveness of interventions.
Provide quiet environment and reduce stressful stimuli: noise, lighting, and constant interruptions.	Promotes rest and enhances coping abilities.
Place in position of comfort, and support joints and extremities with pillows and other padding.	May decrease associated bone and joint discomfort.
Reposition periodically and provide or assist with gentle range-of-motion (ROM) exercises.	Improves tissue circulation and joint mobility.
Provide comfort measures, such as massage, cool packs, and psychological support, including encouragement and presence, as appropriate.	Enhances effects of medication.
Review and promote client's own comfort interventions—position and physical activity or nonactivity.	Successful management of pain requires client involvement. Use of effective techniques provides positive reinforcement, promotes sense of control, and prepares client for interventions to be used after discharge.
Evaluate and support client's coping mechanisms.	Using own learned perceptions and behaviors to manage pain can help client cope more effectively.
Encourage use of stress management techniques, such as deep-breathing exercises, guided imagery, visualization, and therapeutic touch.	Facilitates relaxation, augments pharmacological therapy, and enhances coping abilities.
Assist with or provide diversional activities and relaxation techniques.	Helps with pain management by redirecting attention.
Collaborative	
Monitor uric acid level as appropriate.	Rapid turnover and destruction of leukemic cells during chemotherapy can elevate uric acid, causing swollen painful joints in some clients. *Note:* Massive infiltration of WBCs into joints can also result in intense pain.
Administer medications, as indicated, for example: Analgesics, such as acetaminophen (Tylenol)	Given for mild pain not relieved by comfort measures. *Note:* Avoid aspirin-containing products because they may potentiate hemorrhage.
Opioids, such as codeine, morphine, and hydromorphone (Dilaudid)	Routinely scheduled medication administration or patient-controlled analgesia (PCA) is beneficial in preventing peaks and valleys associated with intermittent drug administration and increases client's sense of control.
Anti-anxiety agents, such as diazepam (Valium) and lorazepam (Ativan)	May be given to enhance the action of analgesics and opioids.

NURSING DIAGNOSIS: Activity Intolerance

May be related to
Generalized weakness; reduced energy stores, increased metabolic rate from massive production of leukocytes
Imbalance between oxygen supply and demand (anemia and hypoxia)
Therapeutic restrictions—isolation, bedrest; effect of drug therapy

Possibly evidenced by
Verbal report of fatigue or weakness
Exertional discomfort or dyspnea
Abnormal heart rate or BP response

Desired Outcomes/Evaluation Criteria—Client Will

Endurance (NOC)
Report a measurable increase in activity tolerance.
Participate in ADLs to level of ability.
Demonstrate a decrease in physiological signs of intolerance—pulse, respiration, and BP remain within client's normal range.

ACTIONS/INTERVENTIONS	RATIONALE
Energy Management (NIC)	
Independent	
Evaluate reports of fatigue, noting inability to participate in activities or ADLs.	Effects of leukemia, anemia, and chemotherapy may be cumulative, especially during acute and active treatment phase, necessitating assistance.
Encourage client to keep a diary of daily routines and energy levels, noting activities that increase fatigue.	Helps client prioritize activities and arrange them around fatigue pattern.
Provide quiet environment and uninterrupted rest periods. Encourage rest periods before meals.	Restores energy needed for activity and cellular regeneration and tissue healing.
Implement energy-saving techniques, such as sitting, rather than standing and use of shower chair. Assist with ambulation or other activities, as indicated.	Maximizes available energy for self-care tasks.
Recommend small, nutritious, high-protein meals and snacks throughout the day.	Smaller meals require less energy for digestion than larger meals. Increased intake provides fuel for energy. (Refer to CP: Cancer, ND: imbalanced Nutrition: Less than Body Requirements.)
Collaborative	
Provide supplemental oxygen.	Maximizes oxygen available for cellular uptake, improving tolerance of activity.
Administer blood and blood components, as indicated.	Correcting anemia improves client's stamina and tolerance for activity.

NURSING DIAGNOSIS: deficient Knowledge [Learning Need] regarding disease, prognosis, treatment, self-care, and discharge needs

May be related to
Lack of exposure to resources
Information misinterpretation, lack of recall

Possibly evidenced by
Verbalization of problem, request for information
Statement of misconception

Desired Outcomes/Evaluation Criteria—Client Will

Knowledge: Illness Care (NOC)
Verbalize understanding of condition, disease process, and potential complications.
Verbalize understanding of therapeutic needs.
Initiate necessary lifestyle changes.
Participate in treatment regimen.

ACTIONS/INTERVENTIONS	RATIONALE

Teaching: Disease Process (NIC)
Independent

Review client's specific form of leukemia and various treatment options:

Treatments can include various individual and combinations of therapies.

Chemotherapy, using a combination of drugs, such as daunorubicin (Cerubidine), cytarabine (Ara-C), idarubicin (Idamycin), and imatinib (Gleevec)

Kills leukemic cells.

Monoclonal antibodies and interferon (INF-α)

Biological therapy slows the reproduction of leukemic cells and promotes the immune system's antileukemic activity.

Radiation therapy

Kills cancer cells by exposure to high-energy radiation.

Stem cell transplantation (SCT), including peripheral stem cell transplant or umbilical cord blood transplant

After chemotherapy and/or radiation, the injured bone marrow is replenished by a transplant of stem cells, which can manufacture the necessary new blood cells.

Surgery (rare)

Surgery may be performed to remove an enlarged spleen or to install a venous access device to give medications and withdraw blood samples (Swierzewski, 2007).

Discuss side effects of treatment, as indicated, and possible solutions.

Client may want opportunity to prepare for certain side effects, such as temporary hair loss. Client and significant other (SO) may benefit from knowledge that certain discomforts, such as nausea, vomiting, weakness, mouth sores, bruising, and anorexia, are treatment related, not indications of escalating disease, and will subside.

Inform client and SO of potential sexual side effects of treatment and provide opportunity to consider options. Discuss sperm banking and pregnancy issues, when appropriate, before beginning treatment.

In males, permanent sterility can occur as a result of radiation when combined with certain chemotherapeutic agents. In females, menstruation may cease during the active phase of treatment, with older women subsequently experiencing menopause. Pregnancy should be avoided during treatment and for 2 to 3 years after treatment as that is when recurrence is most common. Vaginal dryness can be a distressing side effect as well (Katz, 2007; Visovsky, 2006).

For additional interventions refer to CP: Cancer, ND: deficient Knowledge.

POTENTIAL CONSIDERATIONS following acute hospitalization (dependent on client's age, physical condition and presence of complications, personal resources, and life responsibilities)

- *risk for Infection*—inadequate secondary defenses: alterations in mature WBCs (low granulocyte and abnormal lymphocyte count), increased number of immature lymphocytes, immunosuppression, bone marrow suppression (effects of therapy/transplant)
- *ineffective Role Performance*—situational crisis, health alterations, change in physical capacity
- *ineffective self Health Management*—complexity of therapeutic regimen, decisional conflicts, economic difficulties, excessive demands made on individual or family, perceived benefits, powerlessness
- *interrupted Family Processes*—situational crisis (illness, disabling and expensive treatments)

LYMPHOMAS

I. Pathophysiology

a. Malignant growth involving reticuloendothelial and lymphoid system, resulting in accumulation of abnormal lymphocytes in lymph tissue forming masses; may travel to distant sites, including the lungs, liver, gastrointestinal (GI) tract, meninges, skin, and bones

b. Major sites of lymphoid tissue are lymph nodes, spleen, thymus gland, adenoids and tonsils, and digestive tract.

II. Classification

a. Defined by clinical, immunological, molecular, genetic, and histological characteristics

b. Based on histological characteristics, lymphomas are divided into two major categories: Hodgkin's disease or Hodgkin lymphoma (HL), with five subtypes, and non-Hodgkin lymphoma (NHL) with 30 subtypes.

i. HL

1. Slow, insidious onset; superficial lymphadenopathy in cervical, supraclavicular, or mediastinal lymph nodes, which are firm, rubbery, and freely movable

2. Spreads in a generally predictable manner to contiguous lymph nodes via lymphatic channels

(text continues on page 526)

ii. NHL

    1. Most fall into two broad categories related to the clinical features: nodular indolent lymphomas and diffuse, aggressive lymphomas.

    2. When normal follicular structure of the nodes remains intact, the lymphoma is called *follicular* or *nodular,* whereas if malignant cells destroy the follicles, the lymphoma is considered *diffuse.*

    3. May be separated into two categories—low-grade lymphomas and aggressive lymphomas, which includes intermediate-grade and high-grade lymphomas

        a. With or without treatment, low-grade lymphomas can transform into more aggressive lymphomas or the tumor replaces blood or lymph tissue leading to multiple systemic dysfunction and death.

        b. Intermediate- and high-grade lymphomas tend to be more responsive to treatment.

        c. Further staging is done to determine treatment options and prognosis.

   iii. Stages I to IV reflect the microscopic appearance of involved lymph nodes and the extent and severity of the disorder.

   iv. May be further classified by letters of the alphabet (A, B, etc.) according to symptoms present at the time of diagnosis

III. Etiology (Hu & Hale, 2005)

  a. Exact causes are unknown.

  b. Several factors have been linked to an increased risk.

    i. Age: Risk of NHL generally increases with advancing age; HL in the elderly population is associated with a poorer prognosis than in younger clients.

    ii. Infection: human immunodeficiency virus (HIV); human T-lymphocytic virus type 1 (HTLV-1); Epstein-Barr virus (EBV), one of the etiological factors in mononucleosis; *Helicobacter pylori*; hepatitis B or C virus

    iii. Medical conditions that compromise the immune system: HIV; autoimmune diseases; conditions requiring immunosuppressive therapy, such as following organ transplant; inherited immunodeficiency diseases; or treatment with phenytoin

    iv. Exposure to toxic chemicals: occupational exposure to pesticides, herbicides, or benzene and other solvents; woodworking

IV. Statistics

  a. Morbidity: In 2007, 71,380 people were diagnosed with lymphoma in the United States (Leukemia & Lymphoma Society, 2006); the 5-year survival rate is 77% to 83% for HL and 42% to 53% for NHL (Dunleavy et al, 2007); incidence of NHL is consistently higher than HL, with NHL the fifth most common cancer in the United States (Leukemia & Lymphoma Society: Facts 2007–2008).

  b. Mortality: In 2001, there were an estimated 26,300 deaths from NHL (Gajra et al, 2007); mortality rate increases with age (Dunleavy et al, 2007).

  c. Cost: In 2004, projected costs for care were $4.6 billion (National Cancer Institute [NCI], 2007).

GLOSSARY

ABVD therapy: Chemotherapy combination of Adriamycin, bleomycin, vinblastine, and decarbazine (DTIC-Dome) commonly used to treat HL.

Aggressive lymphoma: The National Cancer Institute (NCI) designation for high-grade and some intermediate-grade lymphomas. Aggressive lymphomas grow more quickly than indolent lymphomas, but do respond well to chemotherapy.

Bone marrow transplant (BMT): Bone marrow is taken from a compatible donor or the client's own body, prior to high-dose chemotherapy and/or radiation treatment. After treatment, the marrow, which may or may not have been treated with chemotherapy, is reinfused into the patient to restore the immune system.

Hilar lymphadenopathy: Enlargement of the tracheobronchial and pulmonary lymph nodes.

Lymphopenia: Low number of lymphocytes in the blood.

Neuralgia: Pain in the distribution of a nerve or nerve pathway.

Normocytic, normochromic anemia: Anemia associated with disturbances of red blood cell (RBC) formation, which is related to endocrine deficiencies, chronic inflammation, and condition in which cancer is spread widely throughout the body, or, in some cases, to a relatively large region of the body.

Pel-Ebstein fever: Fever pattern common in HL, in which temperature varies during each 24-hour period, but never reaches normal.

Peripheral blood cell transplantation: The most common form of stem cell transplant with the source of stem cells being the circulating blood, rather than the bone marrow. Client with NHL can have either an autologous or an allogeneic peripheral blood cell transplant, depending on whether or not his or her own stem cells are suitable for use and whether a suitable donor can be found.

Progenitor stem cell transplant: Reestablishment of normal bone marrow function through the infusion of cells committed to forming a specific type of blood cell line—RBCs, white blood cells (WBCs), or platelets. The source of the cells may be from the peripheral blood, bone marrow, or umbilical cord and placenta. The donor may be the client himself or herself (autologous transplant), a genetically compatible relative or individual (allogeneic transplant), or donated cord blood. Syngeneic transplant describes the use of an identical twin as donor.

Superior vena cava syndrome: Obstruction of venous drainage from enlarged lymph nodes.

Tumor burden (also called tumor load): Refers to the number of cancer cells, the size of a tumor, or the amount of cancer in the body. Treatment has a better chance of working when a patient's tumor burden is low.

Care Setting

The client receives acute inpatient care on a medical unit for initial evaluation and treatment and then at the community level. This plan of care addresses potential complications that may be encountered in acute care or hospice settings.

Related Concerns

Anemias—iron deficiency, anemia of chronic disease, pernicious, aplastic, hemolytic, page 493

Cancer, page 846

Adult leukemias, page 516

Psychosocial aspects of care, page 749

Sepsis/septicemia, page 686

Spinal cord injury (acute rehabilitative phase), page 271

Transplantation considerations—postoperative and lifelong, page 739

Upper gastrointestinal/esophageal bleeding, page 306

Client Assessment Database

DIAGNOSTIC DIVISION MAY REPORT	MAY EXHIBIT
ACTIVITY/REST • Fatigue • Weakness or general malaise • Loss of productivity and decreased exercise tolerance	• Diminished strength, slumping of the shoulders, slow walk, and other cues indicative of fatigue
CIRCULATION • Palpitations, chest pain	• Tachycardia, dysrhythmias • Painless swelling of the lymph nodes, beginning in the neck and progressing to axillary, inguinal, mediastinal, and mesenteric regions • Cyanosis and edema of the face and neck or arms due to superior vena cava syndrome, a rare occurrence, but more common in lymphomas with large mediastinal mass • Pallor • Diaphoresis, night sweats
EGO INTEGRITY • Increased stress from school, job, family • Fear related to diagnosis and possibility of dying • Concerns about diagnostic testing and treatment modalities—chemotherapy, radiation therapy, surgery • Financial concerns—hospital costs, treatment expenses, fear of losing job-related benefits because of lost time from work • Relationship status—fear and anxiety related to being a burden on family and significant other (SO)	• Varied behaviors—angry, withdrawn, passive
ELIMINATION • Changes in characteristics of urine or stool • History of intestinal obstruction, such as intussusception or malabsorption syndrome (infiltration from retroperitoneal lymph nodes)	• *Abdomen:* Right upper quadrant (RUQ) tenderness and enlargement on palpation (hepatomegaly); left upper quadrant (LUQ) tenderness and enlargement on palpation (splenomegaly) • Decreased output, dark and concentrated urine, anuria • Bowel and bladder dysfunction (spinal cord compression occurs late)
FOOD/FLUID • Anorexia • Dysphagia (pressure on the esophagus) • Recent unexplained weight loss • Night sweats • Severe nausea and vomiting, often treatment related	• Ascites and edema of the lower extremities (inferior vena cava obstruction from intra-abdominal lymph node enlargement associated with NHL)

(continues on page 528)

DIAGNOSTIC DIVISION
MAY REPORT (continued)

NEUROSENSORY
- Nerve pain reflecting compression of nerve roots by enlarged lymph nodes in the brachial, lumbar, and sacral plexuses
- Muscle weakness, paresthesia

PAIN/DISCOMFORT
- Tenderness or pain over involved lymph nodes—in or around the mediastinum (chest)
- Stiff neck; generalized bone pain (bone involvement)
- Abdominal pain

RESPIRATION
- Dyspnea on exertion or at rest, chest pain

SAFETY
- History of frequent or recurrent infections (abnormalities in cellular immunity predispose client to systemic herpes virus infections, tuberculosis [TB], toxoplasmosis, or bacterial infections); history of infectious mononucleosis (higher risk of HL in client with high titers of EBV)
- HIV—risk of NHL is 60 to 100 times higher in these clients compared with the general population
- Administration of immunosuppressive drugs after organ transplantation
- History or presence of ulcers, *H. pylori*
- Waxing and waning pattern of lymph node size
- Cyclical pattern of evening temperature elevations lasting a few days to weeks (Pel-Ebstein fever) followed by alternate afebrile periods; drenching night sweats without chills
- Itchy skin

SEXUALITY
- Concern about sterility, fertility, and pregnancy (although disease does not affect either, treatment does)
- Decreased libido

TEACHING/LEARNING
- Familial risk factors—higher incidence among families of HL than in general population
- Occupational exposure to pesticides and herbicides or other chemicals—benzene, creosote, lead, formaldehyde, paint thinner

DISCHARGE PLAN CONSIDERATIONS
- May need assistance with medical therapies and supplies, self-care activities, and homemaker or home maintenance tasks, transportation, shopping

- ◗ Refer to section at end of plan for postdischarge considerations.

MAY EXHIBIT (continued)

- *Mental status:* lethargy, withdrawal, general lack of interest in surroundings

- Self-focusing; guarding behaviors

- Dyspnea, tachypnea
- Dry, nonproductive cough (hilar lymphadenopathy)
- Hoarseness, laryngeal paralysis (pressure from enlarged nodes on the laryngeal nerve)

- Unexplained, intermittent persistent fever without symptoms of infection
- Tonsillar or other lymph node enlargement
- Generalized pruritus and urticaria (HL)
- Scleral icterus and a generalized jaundice related to liver damage and consequent obstruction of bile ducts by enlarged lymph nodes (may be a late sign)
- Patchy areas of loss of melanin pigmentation (vitiligo)

TEST / WHY IT IS DONE	WHAT IT TELLS ME
BLOOD TESTS Blood studies may vary from completely normal to marked abnormalities.	In stage I, few clients have abnormal blood findings.
• *Complete blood count (CBC):* Battery of screening tests, which typically includes hemoglobin (Hgb); hematocrit (Hct); RBC count, morphology, indices, and distribution width index; platelet count and size; and WBC count and differential.	RBC production may be decreased due to the lymphoma and suppression of bone marrow activity. Client with HL may have mild to severe normocytic, normochromic anemia associated with hypersplenism. WBCs are variable; that is, they may be normal, decreased, or markedly elevated.
• *Differential WBCs:* Percentage of each of the five types of mature WBCs: neutrophils, lymphocytes (B cells and T cells), monocytes, eosinophils, and basophils.	Increased percentage of neutrophils, monocytes, basophils, and eosinophils may be found initially, but these lymphocytes can be profoundly decreased by suppression marrow activity or by lymphoma treatments. A relative or absolute lymphopenia is a late sign.
• *Platelets:* Platelets have essential function in coagulation.	Decreased in bone marrow involvement or as a side effect of therapy.
• *Erythrocyte sedimentation rate (ESR):* Useful to monitor clients in remission and to detect early evidence of recurrence of disease.	Elevated during active stages and indicates inflammatory or malignant disease.
• *Gamma globulin:* Class of proteins in the blood; also called immunoglobulin.	Hypergammaglobulinemia is common; may occur in advanced disease.
• *Serum cryoglobulins:* Abnormal blood protein, which precipitates from the blood serum when chilled.	May be positive with HL.
• *Coombs' test (antiglobulin test):* Looks for antibodies that act against RBCs.	Positive reaction (hemolytic anemia) may occur; however, a negative result usually occurs in advanced disease.
• *C-reactive protein (CRP):* Antibody found in blood in certain acute and chronic conditions, including infections and cancers. It is a nonspecific indicator of inflammation and therefore not diagnostic of any one disease.	May be positive with HL.
• *Serum iron and total iron-binding capacity (TIBC):* Measures the amount of iron in the liquid portion of blood. Iron is necessary for the production of healthy RBCs. Serum iron is almost always measured with the TIBC, from which the transferrin saturation is calculated. The transferrin saturation is a more reliable measure of iron deficiency than measuring iron by itself.	Decreased.
• *Serum cytokines—interleukin-6 (IL-6), IL-10, IL-2 receptors:* Messenger chemicals released by T cells that mobilize other components of the immune system.	Correlates with tumor burden, systemic symptoms, and prognosis.
• *Serum lactate dehydrogenase (LDH):* Substance released by tumors; important prognostic indicator in NHL.	Elevated; may indicate a more aggressive form of NHL.
OTHER DIAGNOSTIC STUDIES	
• *Chest x-ray:* Determines lung involvement, status of airway, and presence of complications.	May reveal mediastinal or hilar adenopathy, nodular infiltrates, or pleural effusions.
• *X-rays or bone scans of thoracic, lumbar vertebrae, proximal extremities, pelvis, or areas of bone tenderness:* Determines areas of involvement and assists in staging.	Bone lesions often associated with acute form of adult T-cell or diffuse large B-cell lymphomas.
• *Whole lung, chest, abdomen, neck computed tomography (CT) scan:* Generally accepted as the primary staging modality for suspected lymphoma and for evaluating therapy response.	Identifies presence of enlarged lymph nodes as well as detects enlargement of liver and spleen.
• *FDG-positron emission tomography (FDG-PET) scan:* Reveals the differences in glucose metabolism between cancer cells and normal cells via radioactive substance (an analogue) of glucose called FDG (2-deoxy-2[18F] fluoro-D-glucose).	The increased FDG uptake in lymphoma cells makes FDG-PET an effective tool for detecting primary lymphoma and recurrent disease (Mullen, 2007).

(continues on page 530)

TEST WHY IT IS DONE (continued)	WHAT IT TELLS ME (continued)
• *Abdominal ultrasound:* Aids in identifying additional sites and assesses organ status.	Evaluates extent of involvement of retroperitoneal lymph nodes and determines size of kidneys and patency of urinary tract in preparation for chemotherapy.
• *Thoracentesis:* May be performed with cytological studies of pleural fluid for differential diagnosis of effusion.	May reveal infectious process, chylous effusion due to lymphatic obstruction, side effects of radiation or chemotherapy, heart failure (HF), or fluid overload.
• *Biopsies:* Aid in diagnosis as well as determining prognosis.	
• *Lymph node:* Establishes the diagnosis of lymphoma and cell type involved.	Presence of Reed-Sternberg cells from blood and lymph cells confirms diagnosis of HL (Visovsky, 2006).
• *Bone marrow:* Sampling may be done by needle aspirate or biopsy to determine bone involvement and staging.	Changes seen in advanced stages. Presence of Reed-Sternberg cells in bone marrow diagnostic for HL (Visovsky, 2006).
• *Fluorescence in situ hybridization (FISH):* Measures the presence of a specific chromosome or gene in cells and helps determine prognosis.	Detects different types of chromosome aberrations and can be used to plan treatment and measure the results of treatment.
• *Cytogenetic analysis:* Cells are studied to see if chromosomal abnormalities are present.	Important in identifying the specific type of lymphoma present, which may help in the choice of drugs for treatment.
• *Flow cytometry:* Method of counting types of cells with fluorescent tags on the surfaces of the cells.	Often used to determine the type of lymphoma cells present. For example, each disease subtype has a specific pattern of markers on its cell surface. Flow cytometry can also detect residual levels of disease after treatment. For some of the more aggressive types of lymphoma, it can sometimes detect residual disease long before it grows large enough to be detected by any other means.
• *Staging laparotomy:* Although rarely performed, may be done to obtain specimens of retroperitoneal nodes and for staging.	May reveal occult lesions in NHL and provides a more complete picture of nodal and splenic involvement.

Nursing Priorities

1. Provide physical and psychological support during extensive diagnostic testing and treatment regimen.
2. Prevent complications.
3. Alleviate pain.
4. Provide information about disease process, prognosis, and treatment needs.

Discharge Goals

1. Complications prevented or minimized.
2. Dealing with individual situation realistically.
3. Pain relieved or controlled.
4. Disease process, prognosis, possible complications, and therapeutic regimen understood.
5. Plan in place to meet needs after discharge.

Refer to CPs: Cancer and Leukemias for shared nursing diagnoses such as Fear/Anxiety, Self-Esteem, Grieving, Pain, and Nutrition to accomplish corresponding nursing priorities and discharge goals. See also other related cancer care plans for nursing interventions related to treatments such as radiation, chemotherapy, and bone marrow transplant.

NURSING DIAGNOSIS: **risk for impaired Gas Exchange**

Risk factors may include
Altered oxygen-carrying capacity of blood
Tracheobronchial obstruction—enlarged mediastinal nodes and airway edema (HL and NHL), superior vena cava syndrome (NHL)

Possibly evidenced by
(Not applicable; presence of signs and symptoms establishes an *actual* diagnosis)

Desired Outcomes/Evaluation Criteria—Client Will

Respiratory Status: Ventilation (NOC)
Maintain a normal, effective respiratory pattern, free of dyspnea, cyanosis, or other signs of respiratory distress, and arterial blood gases (ABGs) within normal limits (WNL).

ACTIONS/INTERVENTIONS	RATIONALE

Ventilation Assistance (NIC)

Independent

Assess and monitor respiratory rate, depth, and rhythm. Note reports of dyspnea or use of accessory muscles, nasal flaring, and altered chest excursion.

Place client in position of comfort, usually with head of bed elevated or sitting upright, leaning forward with weight supported on arms, and feet dangling.

Reposition and assist with turning periodically.

Instruct in and assist with deep-breathing techniques and pursed-lip or abdominal diaphragmatic breathing, if indicated.

Evaluate skin color, noting pallor or development of cyanosis, particularly in nailbeds, ear lobes, and lips.

Assess respiratory response to activity. Note reports of dyspnea and increased fatigue. Schedule rest periods between activities.

Encourage energy-saving techniques, such as rest periods before and after meals, use of shower chair, and sitting for care.

Promote bedrest and provide care as indicated during acute or prolonged exacerbation.

Encourage expression of feelings. Acknowledge reality of situation and normality of feelings.

Provide calm, quiet environment.

Observe for neck vein distention, headache, dizziness, periorbital or facial edema, dyspnea, and stridor.

Provide support to family and SOs. Encourage open expression of feelings.

Changes such as tachypnea, dyspnea, and use of accessory muscles, may indicate progression of respiratory involvement requiring prompt intervention.

Maximizes lung expansion, decreases work of breathing, and reduces risk of aspiration.

Promotes aeration of all lung segments and mobilizes secretions.

Helps promote gas diffusion and expansion of small airways. Provides client with some control over respiration, helping to reduce anxiety.

Proliferation of WBCs and anemia can reduce oxygen-carrying capacity of the blood, leading to hypoxemia.

Decreased cellular oxygenation reduces activity tolerance. Rest reduces oxygen demands and minimizes fatigue and dyspnea.

Aids in reducing fatigue and dyspnea and conserves energy for cellular regeneration and respiratory function.

Worsening respiratory involvement and hypoxia may necessitate cessation of activity to prevent more serious respiratory compromise.

Anxiety increases oxygen demand, and hypoxemia potentiates respiratory distress or cardiac symptoms, which in turn escalates anxiety.

Promotes relaxation, conserving energy and reducing oxygen demand.

NHL client is at risk for superior vena cava syndrome, which may result in tracheal deviation and airway obstruction, representing an oncological emergency.

Development of this complication is very frightening for client and family because it may indicate end-stage of disease process or approaching death, especially in the hospice setting. Keeping family informed may diminish their anxiety and minimize transmission to client.

Collaborative

Assist with treatment of disease process and side effects of therapies.

Provide supplemental oxygen.

Monitor laboratory studies, such as ABGs and pulse oximetry.

Administer analgesics and tranquilizers, as indicated.

Assist with respiratory treatments and adjuncts, such as intermittent positive-pressure breathing (IPPB) and incentive spirometer, if appropriate.

Assist with intubation and mechanical ventilation.

Prepare for other procedures—thrombolysis, emergency radiation, endovascular stenting, or thoracentesis when indicated.

Interventions to correct or manage anemia can improve oxygenation.

Maximizes oxygen available for circulatory uptake, aids in reducing hypoxemia.

Measures adequacy of respiratory function and effectiveness of therapy.

Reducing physiological responses to pain and anxiety decreases oxygen demands and may limit respiratory compromise.

Promotes maximal aeration of all lung segments, preventing atelectasis.

May be necessary to support respiratory function until airway edema is resolved in acutely ill hospitalized client.

Superior vena cava syndrome, rarely presents as an acute emergency, but when it does, life-saving treatments must be immediately carried out. Thoracentesis may also be done if pleural effusion is present.

NURSING DIAGNOSIS: Nausea

May be related to
Chemotherapeutic agents; radiation therapy
Gastric irritation

Possibly evidenced by
Report of nausea, gagging sensation
Aversion toward food

Desired Outcomes/Evaluation Criteria—Client Will

Nausea & Vomiting Severity (NOC)
Be free of nausea.

Nausea & Vomiting Disruptive Effects (NOC)
Manage nausea as evidenced by acceptable level of dietary intake.
Maintain weight, as appropriate.

ACTIONS/INTERVENTIONS	RATIONALE
Nausea Management (NIC) *Independent* Control environmental factors, such as strong or noxious odors or noise. Avoid overly sweet, fatty, or spicy foods.	Can trigger nausea and vomiting response.
Encourage use of relaxation techniques, such as visualization, guided imagery, and moderate exercise before meals.	May prevent onset or reduce severity of nausea, decrease anorexia, and enable client to increase oral intake.
Provide or encourage frequent oral hygiene.	Prevents drying of mucosa, promotes comfort, and reduces sour taste.
Evaluate effectiveness of antiemetic agents.	Individuals respond differently to all medications. First-line antiemetics may not work, requiring alteration in or use of combination drug therapy.
Identify client who experiences anticipatory nausea or vomiting and take appropriate measures.	Psychogenic nausea and vomiting occurring before chemotherapy generally does not respond to antiemetic drugs. Change of treatment environment or client routine on treatment day may be effective.
Obtain client's height and weight. Weigh daily, or as indicated.	Weight loss may indicate client's fat tissues, the chief source of stored energy, are depleted.
Monitor daily food intake and have client keep food diary, as indicated.	Identifies nutritional strengths and deficiencies.
Encourage client to eat high-calorie, nutrient-rich diet, with adequate fluid intake. Encourage use of supplements and frequent, smaller meals spaced throughout the day.	Metabolic tissue needs are increased, as well as fluids, in order to eliminate waste products. Supplements can play an important role in maintaining adequate caloric and protein intake.
Encourage open communication regarding anorexia.	Often a source of emotional distress, especially for SO who wants to feed client frequently. When client refuses, SO may feel rejected or frustrated.
Adjust diet before and immediately after treatment, providing such foods as clear, cool liquids; light or bland foods; candied ginger; dry crackers; toast; and carbonated drinks. Give liquids 1 hour before or 1 hour after meals.	The effectiveness of diet adjustment is very individualized in relief of posttherapy nausea. Clients must experiment to find best solution or combination. Avoiding fluids during meals minimizes becoming "full" too quickly.
Collaborative Administer medications, as indicated, for example:	
5-HT3 receptor antagonists, such as ondansetron (Zofran), granisetron (Kytril), and palonosetron (Aloxi); NK-1 receptor antagonist aprepitant (Emend); phenothiazines, such as prochlorperazine (Compazine) and thiethylperazine (Torecan); and antidopaminergics, such as metoclopramide (Reglan)	Most antiemetics act to interfere with stimulation of true vomiting center, and chemoreceptor trigger zone agents also act peripherally to inhibit reverse peristalsis. These medications are often prescribed routinely before, during, and after chemotherapy to prevent nausea and vomiting.
Antacids and proton pump inhibitors, such as esomeprazole (Nexium), lansoprazole (Prevacid), and pantoprazole (Protonix)	Minimizes gastric irritation, decreases nausea, and reduces risk of mucosal ulceration.
Administer antiemetic on a regular schedule before, during, and after administration of antineoplastic agent, as appropriate.	Nausea and vomiting are frequently the most disabling and psychologically stressful side effects of chemotherapy.

NURSING DIAGNOSIS: Sexual Dysfunction

May be related to
Altered body structure or function related to drugs, surgery, disease process, radiation; loss of sexual desire; disruption of sexual response pattern

Possibly evidenced by
Verbalization of problem
Actual or perceived limitation imposed by disease or therapy
Alteration in relationship with SO

Desired Outcomes/Evaluation Criteria—Client Will

Sexual Functioning (NOC)
Verbalize understanding of individual reasons for sexual problems.
Identify stressors in lifestyle that may contribute to the dysfunction.
Discuss concerns about body image, sex role, and desirability as a sexual partner with partner or SO.

ACTIONS/INTERVENTIONS	RATIONALE
Sexual Counseling (NIC)	
Independent	
Assess knowledge of client and SO regarding sexual function and effects of current situation.	Because lymphomas often affect the relatively young who are in their reproductive years, these clients are affected more by these problems and may be less knowledgeable about the possibilities of change.
Inform client and partner of potential sexual side effects of treatment and provide opportunity to consider options. Discuss sperm banking and pregnancy issues, when appropriate, before beginning treatment.	In males, permanent sterility can occur as a result of radiation when combined with certain chemotherapeutic agents. In females, menstruation may cease during the active phase of treatment, with older women subsequently experiencing menopause. Vaginal dryness can be a distressing side effect as well (Katz, 2007; Visovsky, 2006). Pregnancy should be avoided during treatment and for 2 to 3 years after treatment, as that is when recurrence is most common.
Identify preexisting and current stress factors that may be affecting the relationship.	Client may be concerned about other issues, such as job, financial, and illness-related problems.
Determine specific pathophysiology involved and impact on, or perception of, individual.	Client's perception of the individual effects of this illness is crucial to planning interventions that will be appropriate to those affected.
Assist with treatment of underlying condition.	As illness is treated and client can see improvement, hope is restored and client can begin to look to the future.
Provide factual information.	Promotes trust in caregivers.
Encourage and accept expressions of concern, anger, grief, and fear.	Helps client identify feelings and begin to deal with them.
Encourage client to share thoughts and concerns with partner and to clarify values and impact of condition on relationship.	Helps couple begin to deal with issues that can strengthen or weaken relationship.
Collaborative	
Refer to appropriate community resources or support groups for sexual dysfunction, such as the American Cancer Society.	Provides information about resources that are available to help with individual needs. Meeting with others who are dealing with the effects of devastating illness can help client and family.
Provide written material, informational Web sites such as Fertile Hope, and other resources appropriate to age and situation.	Reinforces information client has received regarding sexual and fertility issues.
Refer to psychiatric clinical nurse specialist or professional sexual therapist, as indicated.	May need additional in-depth assistance to resolve existing problems.

NURSING DIAGNOSIS: **deficient Knowledge [Learning Need] regarding disease process, prognosis, treatment regimen, self-care, and discharge needs**

May be related to
Lack of exposure, recall
Information misinterpretation
Unfamiliarity with information resources
Cognitive limitations

Possibly evidenced by
Request for information, verbalization of problem, statements reflecting misconceptions
Inaccurate follow-through of instruction, development of preventable complications

Desired Outcomes/Evaluation Criteria—Client Will

Knowledge: Illness Care (NOC)
Verbalize understanding of condition, prognosis, and potential complications.
Identify relationship of signs and symptoms to disease process.
Initiate necessary lifestyle changes.

ACTIONS/INTERVENTIONS	RATIONALE
Teaching: Disease Process (NIC) *Independent*	
Review with client and SO their understanding of client's diagnosis and outlook.	Although lymphomas are complex and have intensive treatment regimens, the outlook has improved in recent years. The 5-year survival rate after treatment in both categories of lymphomas has improved significantly, and many people live with lymphoma in remission.
Review potential treatments client may be considering, such as the following:	May assist client and SO in making informed choices. Although medical treatments are fairly standardized, different doctors have different philosophies and practices. In general, the goal of therapy is remission of the lymphoma, and treatments vary according to the disease process and stage.
Radiation therapy	Generally, for stage I and II disease, the treatment of choice is radiation.
Chemotherapy with ABVD	With more extensive disease, radiation may be combined with two to four cycles of chemotherapy.
Interferon-alpha (INF-α) and monoclonal antibodies, such as rituximab (Rituxan) and alemtuzumab (Campath)	Biological therapies may be used to treat HL or NHL.
Bortezomib (Velcade)	Proteasome inhibitor is useful in the treatment of select forms of NHL.
Valproic acid (VPA) and depsipeptide (Romidespin)	Research suggests histone deacetylase (HDAC) inhibitors have potent and specific anticancer capabilities (McIntyre et al, 2007). Some of the newer drugs being investigated are better tolerated than conventional chemotherapy because they can be given orally, have fewer side effects, and do not require frequent blood count monitoring (Mullen, 2007).
Peripheral progenitor (stem) cell transplant	Stem cell transplant from bone marrow is now standard therapy for selected clients with NHL. May be combined with high-dose chemotherapy for clients with HL who have relapsed or who have experienced a failed primary chemotherapy regimen.
Discuss potential complications relative to specific therapeutic regimen.	Receiving radiation or chemotherapy for HL increases the risk of contracting another type of lymphoma, so client will continue to need monitoring after treatment. After 5 disease-free years, however, risk becomes close to normal. Radiation therapy also increases the risk of developing a solid malignancy, such as a breast or lung tumor, or thyroid disease if the radiation field during treatment included these regions (Rogers, 2005).

ACTIONS/INTERVENTIONS (continued)

Emphasize need for ongoing medical follow-up, posttreatment surveillance, and testing.

Identify signs and symptoms requiring further evaluation, such as cough, fever, chills, malaise, dyspnea, weight gain, slow pulse, decreased energy level, intolerance to cold; or moderate fever, chest pain, dry cough, dyspnea, rapid pulse (pericarditis [rare]); or dyspnea, fatigue, chest pain, dizziness, or syncope (cardiomyopathy [rare]).

Recommend regular exercise in moderation, with adequate rest. Discuss energy conservation techniques. Refer for physical therapy or cancer exercise program, as indicated.

Determine financial needs or concerns. Identify community resources and vocational services.

Recommend or refer to appropriate community resources— support groups, social worker, counselor, pastor; home health assistance, medical equipment and supplies; hospice; and Lymphoma Research Foundation and American Cancer Society.

RATIONALE (continued)

After completion of primary therapy, appropriate tests will be repeated to determine efficacy of therapy. Also, certain monitoring tests are continued; for example, thyroid-stimulating hormone (TSH) levels should be monitored yearly starting 8 to 10 years after radiation therapy. Yearly Pap smears are recommended for female clients because Hodgkin's cells may be found on the cervix. Women receiving radiation therapy are at higher risk of developing breast cancer and should receive yearly mammograms starting 8 years after the completion of treatment, or yearly beginning at age 40, depending on age at time of diagnosis (American Cancer Society [ACS], 2007).

Prompt intervention can identify recurrence, or perhaps limit, progression of complications, thereby reducing further debilitating effects.

Promotes general well-being. *Note:* Fatigue is associated with disease process and treatment regimen as well as developing complications. Therefore, balancing activity with rest enhances client's ability to perform activities of daily living (ADLs).

Although survival rates are relatively good, clients often have limitations in physical activities and employment because of dyspnea, chronic fatigue, and difficulties in concentration or memory. Presence of the disease can also impact client's ability to work or qualify for bank loans or obtain insurance.

Client and SO may benefit from many available resources and networks for such help as care assistance, transportation to treatments, sources of financial resources, and long-term support or counseling.

POTENTIAL CONSIDERATIONS following acute hospitalization (dependent on client's age, physical condition and presence of complications, personal resources, and life responsibilities)

• *Fatigue*—decreased metabolic energy production, overwhelming psychological or emotional demands, states of discomfort, altered body chemistry, such as due to chemotherapy

• *interrupted Family Processes*—situational crisis (illness, disabling and expensive treatments)

Refer to CPs: Adult Leukemia and Cancer for additional postdischarge concerns.

CHAPTER 10

Renal and Urinary Tract

RENAL FAILURE: ACUTE

I. Pathophysiology

a. Sudden decrease in kidney function, which may or may not be associated with a decrease in urine output and results in a buildup of toxic wastes, such as urea and creatinine in the blood

b. Three well-defined stages: oliguric or anuric, diuretic, and convalescent (Choka, 2005)

  i. Oliguric

    1. Filtration capability is reduced because of debris and damage to renal tubules.

    2. Output is greatly reduced—may be less than 400 mL/day.

    3. If anuria present, catastrophic injury has likely occurred in both kidneys—as in obstructive uropathy or, less commonly, in bilateral renal artery occlusion, acute cortical necrosis, or rapidly progressive glomerulonephritis (Agraharkar & Gupta, 2007).

  ii. Diuretic

    1. May skip oliguric phase and begin to make large quantities (may be several liters) of urine

    2. Client with oliguria will progress through diuretic phase during recovery.

    3. Urine is dilute because of kidney's inability to concentrate.

  iii. Convalescent

    1. Renal blood flow and filtration improves.

    2. Process of recovery is gradual, often weeks to months; in many cases, some degree of renal insufficiency persists.

II. Classification—dependent on site

a. Prerenal failure (azotemia): decreased renal perfusion manifested by reduced urine output because of decreased glomerular filtration rate (GFR)

b. Renal or intrinsic failure: associated with parenchymal changes with damage to the renal tubules (acute tubular necrosis [ATN]) caused by ischemia or nephrotoxic substances

c. Postrenal failure: results from an obstruction in the urinary tract anywhere from the tubules to the urethral meatus

III. Etiology

a. Multiple causes: ischemia and toxicity (most common), obstructions

  i. Prerenal failure: blood volume depletion due to hemorrhage, "third-space" sequestration of fluid as in edema or ascites in advanced liver disease, or burns; dehydration due to gastrointestinal (GI) losses or overuse of diuretics; septic or anaphylactic shock; heart failure (HF) with renal insufficiency, myocardial infarction (MI), trauma; renal artery obstruction; and use of certain drugs, such as nonsteroidal anti-inflammatory drugs (NSAIDs), cyclooxygenase inhibitors, angiotensin-converting enzyme (ACE) inhibitors

  ii. Intrinsic failure: ischemia and hypoperfusion similar to prerenal hypoperfusion (except that correction of the causative factor may be followed by continued oliguria for up to 30 days) associated with prolonged acute renal failure (ARF), blood transfusion reaction, or renal artery stenosis; and direct damage from nephrotoxic substances, such as radiocontrast media, cyclosporine, heavy metals (e.g., lead, mercury), cytotoxic drugs (e.g., certain chemotherapy agents), certain antibiotics (e.g., carbenicillins, aminoglycosides)

  iii. Postrenal failure: most commonly occurs with stones in the ureters, bladder, or urethra; from trauma or edema associated with infection, prostatic hypertrophy, or cancer; cervical cancer; strictures of renal artery

  iv. If underlying cause is corrected, the nephrons may recover; however, in some cases, damage is permanent and renal failure becomes chronic.

b. Community- or hospital-acquired

  i. Most community-acquired ARF is secondary to volume depletion; as many as 90% of cases are estimated to have a potentially reversible cause (Sinert & Peacock, 2006).

  ii. Hospital-acquired ARF often occurs in the intensive care unit (ICU) setting and is commonly the end result of multiorgan failure.

c. Risk factors: advanced age, chronic infection, diabetes, hypertension, immune disorders such as lupus or scleroderma

IV. Statistics (Agraharkar & Gupta, 2007; Sinert, 2006)

a. Morbidity: Upon hospital admission, approximately 1% of clients have ARF, whereas during hospitalization, the estimated incidence of ARF is 2% to 5%.

b. Mortality: The rate for hospital-acquired ARF is as high as 40% to 80% and is directly correlated to the severity of comorbidities; with the advent of dialysis, the most common causes of death associated with ARF include sepsis, cardiac failure, and pulmonary failure; rates are generally lower for nonoliguric ARF than for oliguric ARF because the former is usually caused by drug-induced nephrotoxicity and interstitial nephritis, which are associated with fewer systemic complications; individuals with ARF who are older than age 80 have mortality rates similar to younger adults.

GLOSSARY

Acute tubular necrosis (ATN): Structural injury or tissue necrosis within the kidney, caused by ischemia or toxic injury. Necrosis is usually patchy, but injury can be widespread.

Anuria: Urine output less than 100 mL/day.

Azotemia: Buildup of nitrogenous waste products, specifically urea, in the blood.

Calculus: Mass of solid material or metabolic substance—kidney or bladder stone.

Catabolic: Destructive metabolism, or breakdown, of proteins for energy, resulting in muscle wasting, loss of lean muscle mass, and negative nitrogen balance.

Glomerular filtration rate (GFR): Rate of fluid filtration through the kidney glomeruli.

Glomerulonephritis: Inflammation of the glomerular capillary walls, causing impaired filtration.

Hydronephrosis: Kidney enlargement caused by urine backing up from the bladder into the kidney or inability of urine to drain from the kidney into bladder; excessive reflux stretches the kidney, causing functional damage to it.

Myoglobin: Form of hemoglobin found in muscle tissue and released into urine when tissue damage occurs.

Nephrotoxins: Chemical substances, including medications, that can cause kidney damage.

Nonoliguric ARF: Urinary output more than 400 mL/day.

Oliguria: Urinary output less than 400 mL/day.

Orthostatic hypotension: Decrease in blood pressure when person rises from seated or lying position; often associated with hypovolemia.

Parenchymal disease: Connective tissue of the kidney is damaged and scarred.

Polyuria: Excretion of large amounts (2 to 6 L/24 hours) of urine, lacking concentration and regulation of waste products; occurs during diuretic phase of ARF.

Porphyrins: Nitrogen-containing chemical components of hemoglobin.

Pyelonephritis: Infection of the kidney's medulla or cortex.

Uremia: Toxic clinical syndrome associated with fluid, electrolyte, and hormone imbalances, and metabolic abnormalities due to deterioration of renal function and the deleterious effects of azotemia on organ systems.

Care Setting

Client will be treated in inpatient acute medical or surgical unit.

Related Concerns

Metabolic acidosis—primary base bicarbonate deficiency, page 483

Fluid and electrolyte imbalances, page 903

Psychosocial aspects of care, page 749

Renal dialysis—general considerations, page 560

Renal failure: chronic, page 548

Sepsis/septicemia, page 686

Total nutritional support: parenteral/enteral feeding, page 469

Upper gastrointestinal/esophageal bleeding, page 306

DIAGNOSTIC DIVISION MAY REPORT	MAY EXHIBIT
ACTIVITY/REST • Fatigue, weakness, malaise	• Muscle weakness, loss of tone
CIRCULATION	• Hypotension or hypertension, including accelerated (malignant) hypertension, eclampsia, or pregnancy-induced hypertension (PIH) • Cardiac dysrhythmias associated with hyperkalemia and hypocalcemia • Weak, thready pulses; orthostatic hypotension (hypovolemia) • Jugular vein distention (JVD), full and bounding pulses (hypervolemia) • Generalized tissue edema, including periorbital area, ankles, sacrum • Pallor (anemia); bleeding tendencies
ELIMINATION • History of benign prostatic hyperplasia (BPH) or kidney or bladder stones • Change in usual urination pattern—increased frequency (early failure and early recovery), or decreased frequency or oliguria (later phase) • Dysuria, hesitancy, urgency, and retention (obstruction or infection) • Abdominal bloating, diarrhea, or constipation	• Change in urinary color; for example, ranges from absence of color to deep yellow, reddish-brown, and cloudy • Oliguria • Polyuria • Anuria
FOOD/FLUID • Weight gain (edema), weight loss (dehydration) • Nausea, anorexia, heartburn • Vomiting • Use of diuretics	• Changes in skin turgor and moisture • Edema—generalized, dependent
NEUROSENSORY • Headache, blurred vision • Muscle cramps or twitching, "restless leg" syndrome, numbness, tingling	• Altered mental state—decreased attention span, inability to concentrate, loss of memory, confusion, decreasing level of consciousness (LOC) (azotemia, electrolyte and acid-base imbalance) • Twitching, muscle fasciculation, seizure activity
PAIN/DISCOMFORT • Flank pain, headache	• Guarding or distraction behaviors, restlessness
RESPIRATION • Shortness of breath	• Tachypnea, dyspnea, increased rate and depth; Kussmaul's respiration can be compensatory mechanism because of metabolic acidosis • Cough productive of pink-tinged sputum (pulmonary edema)
SAFETY • Recent transfusion reaction	• Fever (sepsis, dehydration) • Petechiae, ecchymotic areas on skin • Pruritus, dry skin

Client Assessment Database (continued)

DIAGNOSTIC DIVISION MAY REPORT (continued)	MAY EXHIBIT (continued)
TEACHING/LEARNING • Family history of polycystic disease, hereditary nephritis, urinary calculus, malignancy • History of exposure to toxins, such as drugs (cyclosporine, amphotericin B, cocaine), environmental poisons (e.g., ethyl alcohol, ethylene glycol, mercury vapors, lead, cadmium or other heavy metals), substance abuse • Current or recent use of nephrotoxic drugs, such as aminoglycoside antibiotics, amphotericin B; anesthetics; ACE inhibitors and vasodilators; NSAIDs • Recent diagnostic testing with radiographic contrast media reaction • Concurrent conditions—tumors in the urinary tract, gram-negative sepsis, trauma or crush injuries, hemorrhage, disseminated intravascular coagulation (DIC), burns, electrocution injury, autoimmune disorders (e.g., scleroderma, vasculitis), vascular occlusion or surgery, diabetes mellitus (DM), cardiac or liver failure **DISCHARGE PLAN CONSIDERATIONS** • May require alteration or assistance with medications, treatments, supplies, transportation, and homemaker or maintenance tasks ▶ Refer to section at end of plan for postdischarge considerations.	

Diagnostic Studies

TEST WHY IT IS DONE	WHAT IT TELLS ME
BLOOD TESTS • *Blood urea nitrogen (BUN):* Measures the by-product of protein metabolism in the liver, filtered by the kidneys and excreted in urine. • *Cr:* End product of muscle and protein metabolism, filtered by the kidneys and excreted in urine. • *BUN/Cr ratio:* Ratio helps determine whether factors other than kidney failure are causing changes in the levels. Normal ratio is 10:1. • *Complete blood count (CBC):* Battery of screening tests, which typically includes hemoglobin (Hgb); hematocrit (Hct); red blood cell (RBC) count, morphology, indices, and distribution width index; platelet count and size; and white blood cell (WBC) count and differential. • *Arterial blood gases (ABGs):* Determines the pH and the percentage of oxygen, carbon dioxide, and bicarbonate in arterial blood.	Elevated BUN is highly suggestive of kidney dysfunction, although BUN levels may also be affected by liver disorders, hydration, and other factors. ARF presents clinically as a rapidly rising creatinine (Cr) over several hours or days. No common pathological condition other than renal disease raises Cr. In normal individuals, and in client with intrinsic renal disease, the BUN will be approximately 10 times that of Cr. Therefore, a BUN/Cr ratio considerably greater than 10 suggests a prerenal (decreased renal perfusion) or postrenal (obstruction) cause of renal failure. When the ratio is considerably less than 10, liver disease, low protein intake, or fluid volume excess may be present. Hgb is decreased in presence of anemia, which is the main hematologic effect of ARF. RBCs are often decreased because of increased fragility and decreased survival time. Elevated WBC count (leukocytosis) is common in ARF. Metabolic acidosis (pH less than 7.2) may develop because of decreased renal ability to excrete hydrogen and end products of metabolism. Bicarbonate is decreased.

(continues on page 540)

TEST **WHY IT IS DONE** (continued)	**WHAT IT TELLS ME** (continued)
• *Electrolytes or renalytes:* Electrically charged minerals found in body tissues and blood in the form of dissolved salts. They help move nutrients into and wastes out of the body's cells, maintain water balance, and stabilize the body's pH level.	Sodium—usually increased, but may vary. Potassium—elevated related to retention and cellular shifts (acidosis) or RBC hemolysis. Rapid increase in K^+ is common with ARF. Chloride, phosphorus, and magnesium—usually elevated. Calcium—commonly decreased in ARF and may require replacement.
• *Serum osmolality:* Measures the amount of chemicals dissolved in the serum. Kidneys excrete or reabsorb water to keep osmolality in range of 280 to 300 mOsm/kg. Chemicals that affect serum osmolality include sodium, chloride, bicarbonate, protein, and glucose.	Higher than normal levels can indicate dehydration or renal tubular necrosis. Lower-than-normal levels are associated with fluid volume overload or syndrome of inappropriate antidiuretic hormone secretion (SIADH).

URINE TESTS

• *Volume:* In ARF, volume is variable.	Often less than 400 mL/24 hours (oliguric phase), which occurs within 24 to 48 hours after renal insult. May be less than 100 mL/24 hours (anuric phase), or more than 400 mL/24 hours (nonoliguric) when renal damage is associated with nephrotoxic agents such as contrast media or antibiotics.
• *Color:* Determine presence of RBCs, Hgb, myoglobin, and porphyrins.	Reddish-brown, cola- or tea-colored urine is suggestive of glomerular damage and ATN.
• *Specific gravity:* Measures density of urine compared to water with normal range of 1.005 to 1.030.	Increased in poor renal perfusion. Decreased in kidney disease, such as glomerulonephritis and pyelonephritis with loss of ability to concentrate. Specific gravity that is fixed at 1.010 reflects severe renal damage.
• *pH:* Measures level of acidity.	Alkaline urine (pH greater than 7) can be found in urinary tract infections (UTIs) and renal tubular necrosis.
• *Osmolality or osmolarity:* Measures the ratio of water and solutes, such as electrolytes, acids, and other metabolic wastes, procressed by the kidneys and released in urine. When body fluid is balanced, normal urine osmolarity is in the range of 300 to 900 mOsm/L.	Urine with higher osmolarity is concentrated with less water and a higher solute load, indicating a prerenal cause. Urine with decreased osmolarity is dilute with few solutes, indicating that the cause of renal failure resides in the kidney itself.
• *Cr clearance:* Calculates GFR by measuring the amount of Cr cleared from the blood and filtered into urine in 24 hours.	Best indicator of overall kidney function as reduced Cr clearance correlates with increased circulating creatinine.
• *Sodium:* Determines hydration status and ability to conserve or excrete Na.	Usually increased if ATN is cause of ARF and if kidney is not able to reabsorb sodium, although it is typically decreased in other causes of prerenal azotemia.
• *Fractional sodium (FeNa):* Calculated measure of renal tubule function.	Reveals inability of tubules to reabsorb sodium. Readings of less than 1% indicate prerenal disorders; higher than 1% reflects intrarenal disorders.
• *RBCs:* Presence of RBCs is pathologic.	May be present because of infection, stones, trauma in the renal system, inflammation, tumors, or altered GFR.
• *Protein:* The protein most likely to appear in urine is albumin. The term *albuminuria* is sometimes used when a urine test detects albumin specifically.	High-grade proteinuria (3 to 4+) strongly indicates glomerular damage when RBCs and casts are also present. Low-grade proteinuria (1 to 2+) and WBCs may be indicative of infection or interstitial nephritis. In ATN, proteinuria is usually minimal.
• *Casts:* Tubules in the kidneys secrete proteins. Under some circumstances, these proteins precipitate out to form cylindrical impressions of the tubules called casts.	Usually signal renal disease or infection. Cellular casts with brownish pigments and numerous renal tubular epithelial cells are diagnostic of ATN. Red casts suggest acute glomerular nephritis.

OTHER DIAGNOSTIC STUDIES

• *Kidney/abdominal ultrasound:* Imaging technique that uses high-frequency sound waves and a computer to create images of blood vessels, tissues, and organs.	Evaluates existing renal disease and obstruction of the urinary collecting system. The degree of hydronephrosis does not necessarily correlate with the degree of obstruction.

Diagnostic Studies (continued)

TEST WHY IT IS DONE (continued)	WHAT IT TELLS ME (continued)
• *Voiding cystourethrogram (VCUG):* Specific x-ray that examines the bladder and urethra while the bladder fills and empties.	Shows bladder size and identifies backflow or reflux into ureters or retention caused by postrenal obstruction or failure.
• *Kidney, ureter, bladder (KUB) x-ray:* X-ray of the abdomen, showing the kidneys, ureters, and bladder.	Demonstrates size and structure of kidneys, ureters, and bladder; reveals presence of abnormalities, such as cysts, tumors, or stones.
• *Intravenous pyelogram (IVP) and retrograde pyelogram:* X-ray examination and fluoroscopic visualization of the kidneys, ureters, and bladder using contrast material. Retrograde pyelogram requires cystoscopy and the placement of a small tube into the lower part of the ureter to inject contrast and make opaque the ureter and renal pelvis.	Shows size, shape, and location of urinary structures. Identifies filling defects such as caused by stones or tumors. Retrograde pyelogram may also be done therapeutically during the placement of ureteral stents for renal artery obstruction or during ureteroscopy. May also be performed to delineate renal anatomy in preparation for surgery.
• *Computed tomography (CT) scan, with or without enhancement:* X-ray procedure that uses a computer to produce a detailed picture of a cross-section of the body.	Evaluates kidney size and contour to assess for masses or other obstructions.
• *Radionuclide imaging scan:* Nuclear medicine exam of kidney structure and function.	May reveal structural abnormalities, renal blood flow, kidney stones, tubular dysfunction, and delayed filling or emptying as a cause of ARF.
• *Aortorenal angiography:* Fluoroscopic examination using contrast to examine the renal blood vessels for signs of blockage or abnormalities.	Determines if blood vessel blockage is reducing renal flow.
• *Endourology:* Diagnostic and therapeutic operative procedures performed through instruments—cystoscopic, pelviscopic, or laparoscopic.	Provides direct visualization of urethra, bladder, ureters, and kidneys to diagnose problems or to biopsy or remove small lesions or calculi.
• *Electrocardiogram (ECG):* Record of the electrical activity of the heart.	May be abnormal, reflecting electrolyte (particularly potassium) and acid-base imbalances.

Nursing Priorities

1. Reestablish or maintain fluid and electrolyte balance.
2. Prevent complications.
3. Provide emotional support for client and significant other (SO).
4. Provide information about disease process, prognosis, and treatment needs.

Discharge Goals

1. Homeostasis achieved.
2. Complications prevented or minimized.
3. Dealing realistically with current situation.
4. Disease process, prognosis, and therapeutic regimen understood.
5. Plan in place to meet needs after discharge.

NURSING DIAGNOSIS: excess Fluid Volume

May be related to
Compromised regulatory mechanism (renal failure)

Possibly evidenced by
Intake greater than output, oliguria; changes in urine specific gravity
Venous distention; blood pressure (BP) and central venous pressure (CVP) changes
Generalized tissue edema, weight gain
Changes in mental status, restlessness
Decreased Hgb/Hct, altered electrolytes, pulmonary congestion on x-ray

Desired Outcomes/Evaluation Criteria—Client Will

Fluid Overload Severity (NOC)
Display appropriate urinary output with specific gravity and other laboratory studies near normal; stable weight and vital signs within client's normal range; and absence of edema.

Fluid/Electrolyte Management (NIC)
Independent

Record accurate intake and output (I&O). Include "hidden" fluids, such as intravenous (IV) antibiotic additives, liquid medications, ice chips, and frozen treats. Measure GI losses and estimate insensible losses, such as diaphoresis.

Low urine output less than 400 mL/24 hours may be first indicator of acute failure, especially in a high-risk client. Accurate I&O is necessary for determining fluid replacement needs and reducing risk of fluid overload. *Note:* Hypervolemia occurs in the anuric phase of ARF.

Monitor urine specific gravity.

Measures the kidney's ability to concentrate urine. In intrarenal failure, specific gravity is usually equal to or less than 1.010, indicating loss of ability to concentrate the urine.

Weigh daily at same time of day, on same scale, with same equipment and clothing.

Daily body weight is best monitor of fluid status. A weight gain of more than 0.5 kg/day suggests fluid retention.

Assess skin, face, and dependent areas for edema. Evaluate degree of edema (on scale of +1 to +4).

Edema occurs primarily in dependent tissues of the body, such as hands, feet, and lumbosacral area. Client can gain up to 10 lb (4.5 kg) of fluid before pitting edema is detected. Periorbital edema may be a presenting sign of this fluid shift because these fragile tissues are easily distended by even minimal fluid accumulation.

Monitor heart rate, BP, and CVP.

Tachycardia and hypertension can occur because of (1) failure of the kidneys to excrete urine, (2) excessive fluid resuscitation during efforts to treat hypovolemia or hypotension, and (3) changes in the renin-angiotensin system, which helps regulate long-term blood pressure and blood volume. *Note:* Invasive monitoring may be needed for assessing intravascular volume, especially in clients with poor cardiac function.

Auscultate lung and heart sounds.

Fluid overload may lead to pulmonary edema and HF, as evidenced by development of adventitious breath sounds and extra heart sounds. (Refer to ND: risk for decreased Cardiac Output, below.)

Assess level of consciousness; investigate changes in mentation and presence of restlessness.

May reflect fluid shifts, accumulation of toxins, acidosis, electrolyte imbalances, or developing hypoxia.

Plan oral fluid replacement with client, within multiple restrictions. Intersperse desired beverages throughout 24 hours. Vary offerings, such as hot, cold, and frozen.

Helps avoid periods without fluids, minimizes boredom of limited choices, and reduces sense of deprivation and thirst.

Collaborative

Correct any reversible cause of ARF, such as replacing blood losses, maximizing cardiac output, discontinuing nephrotoxic drug, and removing obstruction via surgery.

Kidneys may be able to return to normal functioning, thus preventing or limiting long-term residual effects.

Insert and maintain indwelling catheter, as indicated.

Catheterization excludes lower tract obstruction and provides means of accurate monitoring of urine output during acute phase; however, indwelling catheterization may be contraindicated because of increased risk of infection.

Monitor laboratory and diagnostic studies, such as the following:
   BUN, Cr

Assesses progression and management of renal dysfunction, failure. *Note:* Dialysis is indicated if ratio is higher than 10:1 or if therapy fails to correct fluid overload or metabolic acidosis.

   Serum sodium

Hyponatremia may result from fluid overload (dilutional) or kidney's inability to conserve sodium. Hypernatremia indicates total body water deficit.

   Serum potassium

Lack of renal excretion or selective retention of potassium by the tubules leads to hyperkalemia, requiring prompt intervention.

   Hgb/Hct

Decreased values may indicate hemodilution associated with hypervolemia; however, during prolonged failure, anemia frequently develops as a result of decreased RBC production. Other possible causes—active or occult hemorrhage—should also be evaluated.

   Serial chest x-rays

Increased cardiac size, prominent pulmonary vascular markings, pleural effusion, and infiltrates indicate acute responses to fluid overload or chronic changes associated with renal failure and HF.

ACTIONS/INTERVENTIONS (continued)	RATIONALE (continued)
Administer and restrict fluids, as indicated.	Fluid management is usually calculated to replace output from all sources as well as estimate insensible losses due to metabolism and diaphoresis. Prerenal failure is treated with volume replacement and vasopressors. The oliguric client with adequate circulating volume or fluid overload who is unresponsive to fluid restriction and diuretics requires dialysis. *Note:* During oliguric phase, "push/pull" therapy or pushing IV fluids and diuresing with diuretics may be tried to stimulate kidney function.
Administer medication, as indicated, for example:	
Diuretics, such as furosemide (Lasix), bumetanide (Bumex), torsemide (Demadex), and mannitol (Osmitrol)	Given early in oliguric phase of ARF in an effort to convert to diuretic phase, flush the tubular lumen of debris, reduce hyperkalemia, and promote adequate urine volume.
Antihypertensives, such as clonidine (Catapres), methyldopa (Aldomet), and prazosin (Minipress)	May be given to treat hypertension by counteracting effects of decreased renal blood flow and/or circulating volume overload.
Vasodilators, such as dopamine (Intropin) and fenoldopam (Corlopam)	Given in small doses, dopamine causes selective dilation of the renal vasculature, enhancing renal perfusion. Fenoldopam maintains or increases renal perfusion while it lowers BP, which may be particularly beneficial in clients with renal sufficiency who present in hypertensive crisis.
Calcium channel blockers, such as nifedipine (Adalat)	Given early in nephrotoxic ATN to reduce influx of calcium into kidney cells, thereby helping to maintain cell integrity and improve GFR.
Prepare for dialysis as indicated, such as hemodialysis, peritoneal dialysis (PD), or continuous renal replacement therapy (CRRT).	Done to reduce volume overload, correct electrolyte and acid-base imbalances, and remove toxins. The type of dialysis chosen for ARF depends on the degree of hemodynamic compromise and client's ability to withstand the procedure. (Refer to CP: Renal Dialysis.)

NURSING DIAGNOSIS: risk for decreased Cardiac Output

Risk factors may include
Fluid overload—kidney dysfunction or failure, overzealous fluid replacement
Fluid shifts, fluid deficit (excessive losses)
Electrolyte imbalance (potassium, calcium), severe acidosis
Uremic effects on cardiac muscle, oxygenation

Possibly evidenced by
(Not applicable; presence of signs and symptoms establishes an *actual* diagnosis)

Desired Outcomes/Evaluation Criteria—Client Will

Circulation Status (NOC)
Maintain cardiac output as evidenced by BP and HR and rhythm within client's normal limits and peripheral pulses strong and equal, with adequate capillary refill time.

ACTIONS/INTERVENTIONS	RATIONALE
Hemodynamic Regulation (NIC)	
Independent	
Monitor BP and heart rate.	Fluid volume excess, combined with hypertension, which often occurs in renal failure, and effects of uremia increase cardiac workload and can lead to cardiac failure. In ARF, cardiac failure is usually reversible.
Observe ECG or telemetry for changes in rhythm.	Changes in electromechanical function may become evident in response to accumulation of toxins and electrolyte imbalance. For example, hyperkalemia is associated with a peaked T wave, wide QRS complex, prolonged PR interval, and flattened or absent P wave. Hypokalemia is associated with flattened T wave, peaked P wave, and appearance of U waves. Prolonged QT interval may reflect calcium deficit.
Auscultate heart sounds.	Development of S_3/S_4 is associated with congestive HF. Pericardial friction rub may be only manifestation of uremic pericarditis, requiring prompt intervention and, possibly, acute dialysis.

(continues on page 544)

Assess color of skin, mucous membranes, and nailbeds. Note capillary refill time.

Pallor may reflect vasoconstriction or anemia—common in ARF, whether associated with actual blood loss or abnormalities in life of RBCs. Cyanosis is a late sign and is related to pulmonary congestion or cardiac failure. A long capillary refill time is associated with hypovolemic states.

Note occurrence of slow pulse, hypotension, flushing, nausea or vomiting, and depressed LOC—central nervous system (CNS) depression.

Magnesium is typically decreased with ARF. If client is also using drugs (e.g., antacids) containing magnesium, the result can be significant hypomagnesemia, potentiating neuromuscular dysfunction and risk of respiratory or cardiac arrest.

Investigate reports of muscle cramps, numbness or tingling of fingers, with muscle twitching and hyperreflexia.

These are symptoms of hypocalcemia. Calcium levels are typically somewhat decreased with ARF. If phosphorus levels are also high, hypocalcemia can become severe, which can also affect cardiac contractility and function.

Maintain bedrest or encourage adequate rest and provide assistance with care and desired activities.

Reduces oxygen consumption and cardiac workload.

Collaborative

Monitor laboratory studies, such as the following:

Potassium

During oliguric phase, hyperkalemia is present, but often shifts to hypokalemia in diuretic or recovery phase. Any potassium value associated with ECG changes requires intervention. *Note:* A serum level of 6.5 mEq or higher constitutes a medical emergency.

Calcium

In addition to its own cardiac effects, calcium deficit enhances the toxic effects of potassium.

Phosphorus

May be abnormal because of reduced renal excretion or excess release of cellular phosphate.

Magnesium

Dialysis or calcium administration may be necessary to combat the CNS-depressive effects of an elevated serum magnesium level.

Administer and restrict fluids as indicated. (Refer to NDs: excess Fluid Volume and risk for deficient Fluid Volume.)

Cardiac output depends on circulating volume—affected by both fluid excess and deficit—and myocardial muscle function.

Provide supplemental oxygen, if indicated.

Maximizes available oxygen for myocardial uptake to reduce cardiac workload and cellular hypoxia.

Administer medications, as indicated, such as:

Inotropic agents

May be used to improve cardiac output by increasing myocardial contractility and stroke volume.

Calcium gluconate

Serum calcium is often low but usually does not require specific treatment in ARF. Calcium gluconate may be given to treat hypocalcemia and to offset the effects of hyperkalemia by modifying or reducing cardiac irritability.

Aluminum hydroxide gels (Amphojel, Basalgel)

Increased phosphate levels may occur as a result of failure of glomerular filtration and require use of phosphate-binding antacids to limit phosphate absorption from the GI tract.

Glucose and insulin solution

Temporary measure to lower serum potassium by driving potassium into cells when cardiac rhythm is endangered.

Sodium bicarbonate or sodium citrate

May be used to correct metabolic acidosis or hyperkalemia by increasing serum pH if client is severely acidotic. Used with caution as it can exacerbate fluid overload and cause tetany by decreasing the ionized calcium concentration. Acidosis that does not respond to medical therapy is an indication for dialysis.

Sodium polystyrene sulfonate (Kayexalate) with or without sorbitol

Exchange resin trades sodium for potassium in the GI tract to lower serum potassium level. Sorbitol may be included to cause osmotic diarrhea to help excrete potassium.

Prepare for and assist with dialysis, as necessary.

May be indicated for persistent dysrhythmias and progressive HF unresponsive to other therapies.

NURSING DIAGNOSIS: **risk for imbalanced Nutrition: Less than Body Requirements**

Risk factors may include

Protein catabolism, dietary restrictions to reduce nitrogenous waste products

Increased metabolic needs

Anorexia, nausea and vomiting, ulcerations of oral mucosa

Possibly evidenced by

(Not applicable; presence of signs and symptoms establishes an *actual* diagnosis)

Desired Outcomes/Evaluation Criteria—Client Will

Nutritional Status (NOC)

Maintain or regain weight as indicated by individual situation; be free of edema.

ACTIONS/INTERVENTIONS	RATIONALE
Nutrition Therapy (NIC)	
Independent	
Assess and document dietary intake.	Aids in identifying deficiencies and dietary needs. Uremic symptoms (such as, nausea, anorexia, altered taste) and multiple dietary restrictions affect food intake.
Provide frequent, small feedings.	Minimizes anorexia and nausea associated with uremic state and diminished peristalsis.
Give client and SO a list of permitted foods and fluids and encourage involvement in menu choices.	Provides client with a measure of control within dietary restrictions. Food from home may enhance appetite.
Offer frequent mouth care and rinse with dilute (0.25%) acetic acid solution; provide gum, hard candy, or breath mints between meals.	Mucous membranes may become dry and cracked. Mouth care soothes, lubricates, and helps freshen mouth taste, which is often unpleasant because of uremia and restricted oral intake. Rinsing with acetic acid helps neutralize ammonia formed by conversion of urea.
Weigh daily, preferably in the morning before breakfast.	The fasting and catabolic client normally loses 0.2 to 0.5 kg/day. Changes in excess of 0.5 kg may reflect shifts in fluid balance.
Collaborative	
Monitor laboratory studies, such as BUN, prealbumin or albumin, transferrin, sodium, and potassium.	Indicators of nutritional needs, restrictions, and necessity for, and effectiveness of, therapy.
Consult with dietitian or nutritional support team.	Determines individual calorie and nutrient needs within the restrictions and identifies most effective route and product—oral supplements, enteral or parenteral nutrition.
Provide high-calorie, low- or moderate-protein diet. Include complex carbohydrates and fat sources to meet caloric needs (avoiding concentrated sugar sources) and to provide essential amino acids.	The amount of needed exogenous protein is less than normal unless client is on dialysis. Carbohydrates meet energy needs and limit tissue catabolism, preventing ketoacid formation from protein and fat oxidation. Carbohydrate intolerance mimicking diabetes mellitus may occur in severe renal failure. Essential amino acids improve nitrogen balance and nutritional status, stimulate repair of tubular epithelial cells, and enhance client's ability to fight systemic complications.
Restrict potassium, sodium, and phosphorus intake, as indicated.	Restriction of these electrolytes may be needed to prevent further renal damage, especially if dialysis is not part of treatment, and during recovery phase of ARF.
Administer medications as indicated, for example:	
Iron preparations	Iron deficiency may occur if protein is restricted, client is anemic, or GI function is impaired.
Calcium carbonate	Restores normal serum levels to improve cardiac and neuromuscular function, blood clotting, and bone metabolism. *Note:* Low serum calcium is often corrected as phosphate absorption is decreased in the GI system. Calcium may be substituted as a phosphate binder.
Vitamin D	Necessary to facilitate absorption of calcium from the GI tract.
B complex and C vitamins and folic acid	Vital as coenzyme in cell growth and actions. Intake is decreased because of protein restrictions.
Antiemetics, such as prochlorperazine (Compazine) and trimethobenzamide (Tigan)	Given to relieve nausea and vomiting, and may enhance oral intake.

NURSING DIAGNOSIS: risk for Infection

Risk factors may include
Depression of immunological defenses (secondary to uremia)
Invasive procedures or devices, such as urinary catheter
Changes in dietary intake, malnutrition

Possibly evidenced by
(Not applicable; presence of signs and symptoms establishes an *actual* diagnosis)

Desired Outcomes/Evaluation Criteria—Client Will

Immune Status (NOC)
Experience no signs or symptoms of infection.

ACTIONS/INTERVENTIONS	RATIONALE
Infection Protection (NIC)	
Independent	
Promote good hand washing by client and staff.	Reduces risk of cross-contamination.
Avoid invasive procedures, instrumentation, and manipulation of indwelling catheters whenever possible. Use aseptic technique when caring for IV and invasive lines. Change site and dressings per protocol. Note edema and purulent drainage.	Limits introduction of bacteria into body. Early detection and treatment of developing infection may prevent sepsis.
Provide routine catheter care and promote meticulous perianal care. Keep urinary drainage system closed and remove indwelling catheter as soon as possible.	Reduces bacterial colonization and risk of ascending UTI.
Encourage deep breathing, coughing, and frequent position changes.	Prevents atelectasis and mobilizes secretions to reduce risk of pulmonary infections.
Assess skin integrity. (Refer to CP: Renal Failure: Chronic; ND: risk for impaired Skin Integrity.)	Excoriations from scratching may become secondarily infected.
Monitor vital signs.	Fever higher than 100.4°F (38.0°C) with increased pulse and respirations is typical of increased metabolic rate resulting from inflammatory process, although sepsis can occur without a febrile response.
Collaborative	
Monitor laboratory studies, such as WBC count with differential.	Although elevated WBCs may indicate generalized infection, leukocytosis is commonly seen in ARF and may reflect inflammation or injury within the kidney. A shifting of the differential to the left is indicative of infection.
Obtain specimen(s) for culture and sensitivity and administer appropriate antibiotics, as indicated.	Verification of infection and identification of specific organism aids in choice of the most effective treatment. *Note:* A number of anti-infective agents require adjustments of dose or time while renal clearance is impaired.

NURSING DIAGNOSIS: risk for deficient Fluid Volume

Risk factors may include
Excessive loss of fluid (diuretic phase of ARF, with rising urinary volume and delayed return of tubular reabsorption capabilities)

Possibly evidenced by
(Not applicable; presence of signs and symptoms establishes an *actual* diagnosis)

Desired Outcomes/Evaluation Criteria—Client Will

Fluid Balance (NOC)
Display I&O near balance, good skin turgor, moist mucous membranes, palpable peripheral pulses, stable weight and vital signs, and electrolytes within normal range.

ACTIONS/INTERVENTIONS	RATIONALE
Fluid Monitoring (NIC)	
Independent	
Measure I&O accurately. Weigh daily. Calculate insensible fluid losses.	Helps estimate fluid replacement needs. Fluid intake should approximate losses through urine, nasogastric (NG) or wound drainage, and insensible losses—diaphoresis and metabolism. *Note:* Some sources believe that fluid replacement should not exceed two-thirds of the previous day's output to prevent prolonging the diuresis.
Encourage fluid intake. Provide allowed fluids throughout 24-hour period.	Diuretic phase of ARF may revert to oliguric phase if fluid intake is not maintained or nocturnal dehydration occurs.
Monitor BP, noting postural changes, and heart rate.	Orthostatic hypotension and tachycardia suggest hypovolemia.
Note signs and symptoms of dehydration, such as dry mucous membranes, thirst, dulled sensorium, and peripheral vasoconstriction.	In diuretic or postobstructive phase of renal failure, urine output can exceed 3 L/day. Extracellular fluid (ECF) volume depletion activates the thirst center, and sodium depletion causes persistent thirst, unrelieved by drinking water. Continued fluid losses and inadequate replacement may lead to hypovolemic state.
Control environmental temperature; limit bed linens, as indicated.	May reduce diaphoresis, which contributes to overall fluid losses.
Collaborative	
Monitor laboratory studies, such as sodium.	In nonoliguric ARF or in diuretic phase of ARF, large urine losses may result in sodium wasting, while elevated urinary sodium acts osmotically to increase fluid losses. Restriction of sodium may be indicated to break the cycle.

NURSING DIAGNOSIS: **deficient Knowledge [Learning Need] regarding condition, prognosis, treatment, self-care, and discharge needs**

May be related to
Lack of exposure or recall
Information misinterpretation
Unfamiliarity with information resources

Possibly evidenced by
Questions, request for information, statement of misconception
Inaccurate follow-through of instructions, development of preventable complications

Desired Outcomes/Evaluation Criteria—Client Will

Knowledge: Disease Process (NOC)
Verbalize understanding of condition, disease process, prognosis, and potential complications.
Identify relationship of signs and symptoms to the disease process and correlate symptoms with causative factors.

Knowledge: Treatment Regimen (NOC)
Verbalize understanding of therapeutic needs.
Initiate necessary lifestyle changes and participate in treatment regimen.

ACTIONS/INTERVENTIONS	RATIONALE
Teaching: Disease Process (NIC)	
Independent	
Review disease process, prognosis, and precipitating factors, if known.	Provides knowledge base from which client can make informed choices.
Explain level of renal function after acute episode is over.	Client may experience residual defects in kidney function, which may or may not be permanent.
Discuss renal dialysis or transplantation if these are likely options for the future.	Although these options would have been previously presented by the physician, client may now be at a point when options need to be considered and decisions made and may desire additional input.
Review dietary plan and restrictions. Include fact sheet listing food and fluid restrictions.	Adequate nutrition is necessary to promote healing and tissue regeneration; adherence to restrictions may prevent complications.

(continues on page 548)

Encourage client to observe characteristics of urine and amount and frequency of output.

Changes may reflect alterations in renal function and need for dialysis.

Establish regular schedule for weighing.

Useful tool for monitoring fluid and dietary status and needs.

Review fluid intake and restriction. Remind client to spread fluids over entire day and to include all fluids (e.g., ice) in daily fluid counts.

Depending on the cause and phase of ARF, client may need to either restrict or increase intake of fluids.

Discuss activity restriction and gradual resumption of desired activity. Encourage use of energy-saving and relaxation techniques and diversional activities.

Client with severe ARF may need to restrict activity and may feel weak for an extended period during lengthy recovery phase, requiring measures to conserve energy and reduce boredom and depression.

Discuss reality of continued presence of fatigue.

Decreased metabolic energy production, presence of anemia, and states of discomfort commonly result in fatigue.

Determine and prioritize activities of daily living (ADLs) and personal responsibilities. Identify available resources and support systems.

Helps client manage lifestyle changes that may be needed to meet personal and family needs.

Recommend scheduling activities with adequate rest periods.

Prevents excessive fatigue and conserves energy for healing and tissue regeneration.

Review medication use. Encourage client to discuss all medications, including over-the-counter (OTC) drugs and herbal supplements, with healthcare provider.

Medications that are concentrated in or excreted by the kidneys can cause toxic cumulative reactions and permanent damage to kidneys. Some supplements may interact with prescribed medications and may contain electrolytes.

Stress necessity of follow-up care and laboratory studies.

Renal function can be slow to return—up to 12 months following ARF—and deficits may persist, requiring frequent monitoring to avoid complications.

Identify symptoms requiring medical intervention, such as decreased urinary output, sudden weight gain, presence of edema, lethargy, bleeding, signs of infection, and altered mental status.

Prompt evaluation and intervention may prevent serious complications and progression to chronic renal failure (CRF).

POTENTIAL CONSIDERATIONS following acute hospitalization (dependent on client's age, physical condition and presence of complications, personal resources, and life responsibilities)
- *deficient Fluid Volume (specify)*—dependent on cause, duration, and stage of recovery
- *Fatigue*—decreased metabolic energy production and dietary restriction, anemia, increased energy requirements, such as fever and inflammation, tissue regeneration
- *risk for Infection*—depression of immunological defenses (secondary to uremia), changes in dietary intake and malnutrition, increased environmental exposure
- *ineffective self Health Management*—complexity of therapeutic regimen, economic difficulties, perceived benefit

---

RENAL FAILURE: CHRONIC

I. Pathophysiology
a. End result of the gradual, progressive destruction of nephrons and decrease in glomerular filtration rate (GFR), resulting in loss of kidney function that produces major changes in all body systems
b. Chronic kidney disease (CKD), although ultimately irreversible, may be slowed by improved standardized blood tests and availability of new drugs to control blood pressure

II. CKD stages correspond to the degree of nephron loss (Choka, 2005; Verrelli, 2006).
a. Decreased renal reserve
  i. GFR may be normal; slightly higher than normal, stage I: greater than or equal to 90 mL/min/1.73 m²; or somewhat less than normal, stage II: 60 to 89 mL/min/1.73 m².
  ii. Kidney dysfunction is present; however, it may be undiagnosed due to lack of symptoms—blood urea nitrogen/creatinine (BUN/Cr) ratio is normal and nephron loss at less than 75%.

b. Renal insufficiency
  i. Nephron loss at 75% to 90%; GFR is moderately (stage III: 30 to 59 mL/min/1.73 m²) to severely (stage IV: 15 to 29 mL/min/1.73 m²) reduced.
  ii. Slight elevation in BUN/Cr
  iii. Polyuria and nocturia present—high output failure
c. End-stage renal disease (ESRD)
  i. Nephron loss at greater than 90% with a GFR of only 10% to 15% (stage V: less than 15 mL/min/1.73 m²)
  ii. Fluid and electrolyte abnormalities
  iii. Azotemia and uremia present
  iv. Dialysis required

III. Etiology (Holcomb, 2005; Verrelli, 2006)
a. Multiple causes
  i. Acute tubular necrosis (ATN) from unresolved acute renal failure (ARF)
  ii. Chronic infections: glomerulonephritis, pyelonephritis, beta-hemolytic *streptococci* infection

iii. Vascular diseases: hypertensive nephrosclerosis, renal artery stenosis, renal vein thrombosis, vasculitis

iv. Obstructive processes: long-standing renal calculi, benign prostatic hyperplasia (BPH)

v. Cystic disorders: polycystic or medullary kidney disease

vi. Collagen diseases: systemic lupus erythematosus (SLE) and collagen vascular disease

vii. Tumors: malignant (multiple myeloma) or benign

viii. Nephrotoxic agents: drugs, such as aminoglycosides, tetracyclines; contrast dyes; heavy metals

ix. Endocrine diseases: diabetes mellitus (DM), hyper-parathyroidism

x. Long-standing systemic hypertension

b. Such comorbidities as diabetes and hypertension are responsible for more than 70% of all cases of ESRD.

c. Highest incidence of ESRD occurs in individuals older than age 65 years (Verrelli, 2006); over the last decade, there has been a 98% increase in incidence in those aged 75 years and older (Alper & Young, 2008).

IV. Statistics

a. Morbidity: In 2005, 485,000 individuals were treated for ESRD in the United States; with 90,000 new cases reported annually, 341,000 receiving dialysis, and more than 140,000 having a functioning kidney transplant (National Kidney Foundation [NFK], 2008); renal transplantation success rates exceed 90% (National Institutes of Health [NIH], 2007).

b. Mortality: In 2005, 81,500 deaths were associated with ESRD in the United States (Morbidity and Mortality Weekly Report [MMWR], 2007) due to (1) cardiovascular disease, (2) sepsis, and (3) cerebrovascular disease (Alper, 2008).

c. Cost: The Medicare program spends approximately $19 billion for care of patients with ESRD, representing 6% of Medicare expenditures (NIH, 2007)

GLOSSARY

Acute tubular necrosis (ATN): Structural injury or tissue necrosis within the kidney, caused by ischemia or toxic injury. Necrosis is usually patchy, but injury can be widespread.

Anuria: Urine output less than 100 mL/24 hours.

Azotemia: Buildup of nitrogenous waste products, specifically urea, in the blood (BUN).

Chronic kidney disease or chronic renal failure: Kidney damage or decreased kidney GFR of less than 60 mL/min/1.73 m² for 3 or more months (Verrelli, 2006).

Ecchymosis: Superficial bleeding under the skin—purple or black-and-blue bruise.

End-stage renal disease (ESRD): GFR less than 15 mL/min, or receiving dialysis.

Glomerular filtration rate (GFR): Rate of fluid filtration through the kidney glomeruli.

Nephrotoxins: Chemical substances, including medications, that can cause kidney damage.

Nocturia: Frequent urination after retiring to bed.

Oliguria: Urinary output less than 400 mL/24 hours.

Osteitis fibrosa: Bones become soft and deformed due to increased metabolism or high bone turnover associated with increased levels of parathyroid hormone. Leads to bone pain, tenderness, and increased risk of fractures.

Polyuria: Excretion of large amounts (2 to 6 L/24 hours) of urine, lacking concentration and regulation of waste products. Occurs during diuretic phase of ARF.

Porphyrins: Nitrogen-containing chemical components of hemoglobin.

Purpura: Hemorrhagic state characterized by patches of purplish discoloration, resulting from extravasation of blood into the skin. Purpura does not blanch with pressure.

Pyelonephritis: Infection of the kidney medulla or cortex.

Renal osteodystrophy: Bone disease that occurs when the kidneys fail to maintain the proper levels of calcium and phosphorus in the blood.

Uremia: Toxic clinical syndrome associated with fluid, electrolyte, and hormone imbalances and metabolic abnormalities due to deterioration of renal function and the deleterious effects of azotemia on organ systems.

Care Setting

Primary focus is at the community level, although inpatient acute hospitalization may be required for life-threatening complications.

Related Concerns

Anemias—iron deficiency, anemia of chronic disease, pernicious, aplastic, hemolytic, page 493

Fluid and electrolyte imbalances, page 903

Heart failure: chronic, page 48

Hypertension: severe, page 37

Metabolic acidosis—primary base bicarbonate deficiency, page 483

Psychosocial aspects of care, page 749

Upper gastrointestinal/esophageal bleeding, page 306

Additional associated nursing diagnoses are found in:

Renal dialysis—general considerations, page 560

Renal failure: acute, page 536

Seizure disorders, page 210

Clients with chronic renal failure may not have any symptoms at all until normal kidney function declines to 20% or less. At that stage, an array of symptoms, such as the following, may appear.

DIAGNOSTIC DIVISION MAY REPORT	MAY EXHIBIT
ACTIVITY/REST • Extreme fatigue, weakness, malaise • Sleep disturbances—insomnia, restlessness, somnolence	• Muscle weakness, loss of tone, decreased range of motion (ROM)
CIRCULATION • History of prolonged or severe hypertension • Palpitations, chest pain (angina)	• Hypertension, jugular vein distention (JVD) • Full or bounding pulses • Generalized tissue and pitting edema of feet, legs, and hands • Cardiac dysrhythmias, distant heart sounds • Pericardial friction rub if uremic pericarditis is present • Enlargement of liver, spleen, and heart • Pallor, bronze-gray, yellow skin • Bleeding tendencies
EGO INTEGRITY • Stress factors—financial, relationship • Feelings of helplessness, hopelessness, powerlessness	• Denial, anxiety, fear, anger, irritability, personality changes
ELIMINATION • Decreased urinary frequency, oliguria, anuria (advanced failure) • Abdominal bloating, diarrhea, or constipation	• Change in urine color—deep yellow, red, brown, cloudy • Oliguria, may become anuric
FOOD/FLUID • Rapid weight gain (edema), weight loss (malnutrition) • Anorexia • Heartburn, nausea, vomiting, unpleasant metallic taste in mouth • Use of diuretics	• Abdominal distention, ascites, liver enlargement (end-stage) • Changes in skin turgor and moisture • Edema—generalized, dependent • Gum ulcerations; bleeding of gums, tongue • Ammonia breath • Muscle wasting, decreased subcutaneous fat, debilitated appearance
HYGIENE • Difficulty performing activities of daily living (ADLs)	• Thin, dry, brittle nails and hair
NEUROSENSORY • Headache, blurred vision • Muscle cramps or twitching, "restless leg" syndrome, burning numbness of soles of feet • Numbness, tingling and weakness, especially of lower extremities (peripheral neuropathy)	• Altered mental state—continuum of symptoms can be present, depending on stage of disease, such as decreased attention span, inability to concentrate, loss of memory, confusion, decreasing level of consciousness, stupor, coma • Gait abnormalities • Twitching, muscle fasciculation, seizure activity
PAIN/DISCOMFORT • Flank pain, headache, muscle cramps or leg pain—worse at night	• Guarding, distraction behaviors, restlessness
RESPIRATION • Shortness of breath, sudden nighttime dyspnea • Cough with or without thick, tenacious sputum	• Tachypnea, dyspnea, increased rate and depth (Kussmaul's respiration may be associated with metabolic acidosis) • Cough productive of pink-tinged sputum (pulmonary edema)
SAFETY • Itching skin, frequent scratching • Recent or recurrent infections • Bleeding tendencies	• Scratch marks, petechiae, ecchymotic areas on skin • Fever (sepsis, dehydration); normothermia may actually represent an elevation in client who has developed a lower than normal body temperature (effect of chronic renal failure [CRF] and depressed immune response) • Bone fractures; calcium phosphate deposits (metastatic calcifications) in skin, soft tissues, joints; limited joint movement

Client Assessment Database (continued)

DIAGNOSTIC DIVISION MAY REPORT (continued)	MAY EXHIBIT (continued)

SEXUALITY
- Decreased libido, amenorrhea, infertility
- Erectile dysfunction

SOCIAL INTERACTION
- Difficulties imposed by condition, such as unable to work, maintain social contacts, or usual role function in family

TEACHING/LEARNING
- Family history of polycystic disease, hereditary nephritis, urinary calculus, malignancy
- History of poorly controlled hypertension or diabetes (high risk for renal failure), exposure to toxins, such as nephrotoxic drugs, drug overdose, environmental poisons
- Current or recent use of nephrotoxic antibiotics, angiotensin-converting enzyme (ACE) inhibitors, chemotherapy agents, heavy metals, nonsteroidal anti-inflammatory drugs (NSAIDs), radiocontrast agents

DISCHARGE PLAN CONSIDERATIONS
- May require alteration or assistance with medications, treatments, supplies; transportation; homemaker or maintenance tasks

▶ Refer to section at end of plan for postdischarge considerations.

Diagnostic Studies

TEST WHY IT IS DONE	WHAT IT TELLS ME

BLOOD TESTS
- *BUN:* Measures the by-product of protein metabolism in the liver, filtered by the kidneys and excreted in urine.
- *Cr:* End product of muscle and protein metabolism, filtered by the kidneys and excreted in urine.
- *BUN/Cr ratio:* Ratio helps determine whether factors other than kidney failure are causing changes in numbers. Normal ratio is 10:1.
- *GFR:* Calculated from serum Cr levels and adjusted for mean normal body surface area. GFR is approximately 90 mL/min in the healthy adult.

- *Complete blood count (CBC):* Battery of screening tests, which typically includes hemoglobin (Hgb); hematocrit (Hct); red blood cell (RBC) count, morphology, indices, and distribution width index; platelet count and size; and white blood cell (WBC) count and differential.

- *Arterial blood gases (ABGs):* Determines the pH and the percentage of oxygen, carbon dioxide, and bicarbonate in arterial blood.

ESRD is present when about 90% of nephrons are lost and is characterized by marked elevation of BUN.

Can be quite elevated before symptoms of CRF are present in unmonitored client. Markedly elevated in late stage

Ratio is less than 10:1, especially in later stages of CRF. Impaired filtration causes reduced BUN reabsorption, thereby lowering BUN/Cr ratio.

GFR is used to stage renal failure. Symptoms are typically absent until GFR falls below 60 (stage II). The client in severe CRF with a GFR between 15 and 29 (stages IV to V) is a candidate for dialysis or transplantation.

Hgb decreased because of anemia, usually less than 7 to 8 g/dL. Anemia develops from decreased renal synthesis of erythropoietin, the hormone responsible for bone marrow stimulation for RBC production. RBC survival is decreased, and bleeding tendency is increased from the uremia-induced platelet dysfunction (Verrelli, 2006).

Decreased pH. Metabolic acidosis (less than 7.2) occurs because of loss of renal ability to excrete hydrogen and ammonia or end products of protein catabolism. Bicarbonate and PCO_2 decreased.

(continues on page 552)

TEST **WHY IT IS DONE** (continued)	**WHAT IT TELLS ME** (continued)

- *Electrolytes (renalytes):* Electrically charged minerals found in body tissues and blood in the form of dissolved salts that help move nutrients into and wastes out of the body's cells, maintain water balance, and stabilize the body's pH level.
- *Sodium:* Helps to evaluate hydration status and progression of renal failure.

May be low if kidney "wastes sodium" or normal, reflecting dilutional state of hypernatremia.

- *Potassium:* Fluctuation in levels can create life-threatening situations, affecting therapeutic choices.

Elevated related to retention, with decline in GFR below 20 to 25 mL/min, cellular shifts (acidosis), or tissue release (RBC hemolysis). In ESRD, electrocardiogram (ECG) changes may not occur until potassium is 6.5 mEq or higher. The resulting hyperkalemia poses a life-threatening emergency, which requires frequent and immediate intervention. Potassium may also be decreased if client is on potassium-wasting diuretics or when client is receiving dialysis treatment.

- *Phosphorus:* Has a direct impact on parathyroid function and bone health.

As GFR declines, less phosphate is filtered and excreted; however, serum levels may remain normal initially because of increased parathyroid hormone (PTH) secretion and the associated increase in renal excretion of phosphorus. As CRF advances to stages IV and V, serum levels rise and bone complications such as osteitis fibrosa may develop.

- *Calcium:* Important in feedback mechanism for inhibiting PTH synthesis and skeletal bone turnover.

Hypocalcemia may become severe as a result of low plasma calcitriol levels impairing intestinal absorption or from calcium binding to elevated serum phosphate levels.

- *Proteins (especially albumin):* Evaluates nutritional status and predicts mortality in clients receiving dialysis.

Decreased serum level may reflect protein loss via urine, fluid shifts, decreased intake, or decreased synthesis because of malnutrition.

- *Serum osmolality:* Measures the amount of chemicals dissolved in the serum. Kidneys excrete or reabsorb water to keep osmolality in range of 285 to 295 mOsm/kg. Chemicals that affect serum osmolality include sodium, chloride, bicarbonate, proteins, and glucose.

Higher than 285 mOsm/kg; often equal to urine.

URINE TESTS

- *Volume:* Reflection of declining renal function, possible development of ARF superimposed on CRF.

Usually less than 400 mL/24 hours (oliguria) or urine is absent (anuria).

- *Color:* Changes in color or clarity indicate developing complications.

Abnormally cloudy urine may be caused by pus, bacteria, fat, colloidal particles, phosphates, or urates. Dirty, brown sediment indicates presence of RBCs, Hgb, myoglobin, and porphyrins.

- *Specific gravity:* Measures density of urine compared to water, with normal range of 1.005 to 1.030.

Less than 1.015 or fixed at 1.010 reflects severe renal damage.

- *Protein (albuminuria):* Dipstick test used as a screening tool to detect glomerular injury (prevalent in persons with diabetes, hypertension, or glomerular disease) that has caused glomeruli to lose selective permeability and leak protein, particularly albumin, which is excreted in the urine.

High-grade persistent proteinuria (3 to 4+) strongly indicates glomerular damage, especially when RBCs and casts are also present. Low-grade proteinuria (1 to 2+) and WBCs may be indicative of infection or interstitial nephritis.

- *Total protein-Cr (albumin-Cr) ratio:* Spot urine collection for total protein-to-creatinine ratio allows reliable approximation (extrapolation) of total 24-hour urinary protein excretion.

A value greater than 3.0 to 3.5 g is within the nephrotic range; less than 2.0 g is characteristic of tubulointerstitial problems.

- *Osmolality:* Measures the ratio of water and solutes, such as electrolytes, acids, and other metabolic wastes, procressed by the kidneys and released in urine. When body fluid is balanced, normal urine osmolarity is in the range of 300 to 900 mOsm/kg.

Less than 350 mOsm/kg is indicative of tubular damage, and urine/serum ratio is often 1:1.

- *Cr clearance:* Calculates GFR by measuring the amount of Cr cleared from the blood and filtered into urine in 24 hours.

Best indicator of overall kidney function, as reduced Cr clearance correlates with increased circulating Cr. May be significantly decreased—less than 80 mL/min in early failure; less than 10 mL/min in ESRD.

Diagnostic Studies (continued)

TEST WHY IT IS DONE (continued)	WHAT IT TELLS ME (continued)
• *Sodium:* Determines hydration status and ability to conserve or excrete Na.	More than 40 mEq/L because kidney is not able to reabsorb sodium.
• *Fractional sodium (FeNa):* Calculated measure of renal tubule function.	Reveals inability of tubules to reabsorb sodium. Readings of less than 1% indicate prerenal problems, whereas higher than 1% reflects intrarenal disorders.
OTHER DIAGNOSTIC STUDIES • *Renal ultrasound:* Imaging technique that uses high-frequency sound waves and a computer to create images of blood vessels, tissues, and organs.	Kidney size can be correlated with certain conditions—large kidney may be present in hyperfiltration, or small, echogenic kidney may be associated with advanced kidney disease. Ultrasound can also document presence of tumors, polycystic disease, or other obstruction in upper urinary system.
• *Computed tomographic (CT) scans:* X-ray procedure that uses a computer to produce a detailed picture of a cross-section of the body.	Demonstrates vessel disorders and kidney mass.
• *Kidney, ureter, bladder (KUB) x-ray:* X-ray of the abdomen, showing the kidneys, ureters, and bladder.	Demonstrates size and structure of kidneys, ureters, and bladder; reveals presence of abnormalities, such as cysts, tumors, or stones.
• *Aortorenal angiography:* Fluoroscopic examination, which uses contrast to examine the renal blood vessels for signs of blockage or abnormality.	Assesses renal circulation and identifies extravascularities and masses. *Note:* Contrast media can precipitate renal failure in damaged kidney.
• *Voiding cystourethrogram (VCUG):* Specific x-ray that examines the bladder and urethra while the bladder fills and empties.	Shows bladder size and identifies backflow (reflux) into ureters or retention caused by postrenal obstruction or failure.
• *Renal biopsy:* Percutaneous renal biopsy currently is performed most often with ultrasound guidance.	Biopsy is generally indicated when renal impairment or proteinuria approaching the nephrotic range is present and diagnosis is still unclear.
• *ECG:* Record of the electrical activity of the heart.	May be abnormal, reflecting electrolyte and acid-base imbalances.
• *X-ray of feet, skull, spinal column, and hands:* Identify presence of associated complications or adverse effects of condition.	May reveal demineralization or calcifications resulting from electrolyte shifts associated with CRF.

Nursing Priorities

1. Maintain homeostasis.
2. Prevent complications.
3. Provide information about disease process, prognosis, and treatment needs.
4. Support adjustment to lifestyle changes.

Discharge Goals

1. Fluid and electrolyte balance stabilized.
2. Complications prevented or minimized.
3. Disease process, prognosis, and therapeutic regimen understood.
4. Dealing realistically with situation and initiating necessary lifestyle changes.
5. Plan in place to meet needs after discharge.

NURSING DIAGNOSIS: **risk for decreased Cardiac Output**

Risk factors may include
Fluid imbalances affecting circulating volume, myocardial workload, and systemic vascular resistance (SVR)
Alterations in rate, rhythm, cardiac conduction (electrolyte imbalances, hypoxia)
Accumulation of toxins (urea), soft tissue calcification (deposition of calcium phosphate)

Possibly evidenced by
(Not applicable; presence of signs and symptoms establishes an *actual* diagnosis)

(continues on page 554)

Desired Outcomes/Evaluation Criteria—Client Will

Circulation Status (NOC)
Maintain cardiac output as evidenced by blood pressure (BP) and heart rate within client's normal range; peripheral pulses strong and equal with prompt capillary refill time.

In addition to interventions here, refer to CP: Renal Failure: Acute; ND: risk for decreased Cardiac Output.

ACTIONS/INTERVENTIONS	RATIONALE
Hemodynamic Regulation (NIC)	
Independent	
Auscultate heart and lung sounds. Evaluate presence of peripheral edema, vascular congestion, and reports of dyspnea.	S_3/S_4 heart sounds with muffled tones, tachycardia, irregular heart rate, tachypnea, dyspnea, crackles, wheezes, and edema or jugular distention suggest heart failure (HF).
Assess presence and degree of hypertension: Monitor BP and note postural changes, such as sitting, lying, and standing.	Significant hypertension can occur because of disturbances in the renin-angiotensin-aldosterone system caused by renal dysfunction. Although hypertension is common, orthostatic hypotension may occur because of intravascular fluid deficit, response to effects of antihypertensive medications, or uremic pericardial tamponade.
Investigate reports of chest pain, noting location, radiation, severity (0 to 10 scale), and whether or not it is intensified by deep inspiration and supine position.	Although hypertension and chronic HF may cause myocardial infarction (MI), approximately half of CRF clients on dialysis develop pericarditis, potentiating risk of pericardial effusion and tamponade.
Evaluate heart sounds for friction rub, BP, peripheral pulses, JVD, capillary refill, and mentation.	Presence of sudden hypotension with paradoxical pulse, narrow pulse pressure, diminished or absent peripheral pulses, marked JVD, pallor, and a rapid mental deterioration indicate tamponade, which is a medical emergency.
Assess activity level and response to activity.	Weakness can be attributed to heart failure and anemia.
Collaborative	
Monitor laboratory and diagnostic studies, such as the following: Electrolytes—potassium, sodium, calcium, magnesium; BUN/Cr	Imbalances can alter electrical conduction and cardiac function.
Chest x-rays	Useful in identifying developing cardiac failure or soft tissue calcification.
Collaborate in treatment of underlying disease or conditions, where possible.	Delaying or halting progression of CRF in early stages can be aided by interventions, such as controlling BP, managing diabetes, treating hyperlipidemia, and avoiding toxins such as NSAIDs, intravenous (IV) contrast dye, aminoglycosides, and so on.
Administer medications, as indicated, for example: Antihypertensive drugs, such as prazosin (Minipress), captopril (Capoten), clonidine (Catapres), and hydralazine (Apresoline)	Aggressive treatment of hypertension is needed to reduce SVR or renin release to decrease myocardial workload and aid in prevention of HF and MI.
ACE inhibitors, such as enalapril (Vasotec), or angiotensin receptor blockers (ARBs), such as irbesartan (Avapro) and losartan (Cozaar)	These drugs may be prescribed not only to lower the patient's BP but more importantly to protect kidneys from further damage, especially in presence of diabetic nephropathy (Polzein, 2007).
Erythropoietin (Epogen, EPO) or erythropoietin-stimulating proteins, such as somatropin (Nutropin) or darbepoetin alpha (Aranesp)	May be given to treat anemia associated with CRF to improve oxygen-carrying capacity of circulating hemoglobin and reduce left ventricular strain.
Administer oxygen, as indicated.	Cardiac function can be improved with use of oxygen if client is severely anemic or metabolic acidosis and electrolyte abnormalities are causing dysrhythmias.
Prepare for renal replacement therapy, such as hemodialysis.	Reduction of uremic toxins and correction of electrolyte imbalances and fluid overload may limit or prevent cardiac manifestations, including hypertension and pericardial effusion.
Assist with pericardiocentesis, as indicated.	Accumulation of fluid within pericardial sac can compromise cardiac filling and myocardial contractility, impairing cardiac output and potentiating risk of cardiac arrest.

NURSING DIAGNOSIS: risk for ineffective Protection

Risk factors may include

Abnormal blood profile—decreased RBC production and survival, altered clotting factors (suppressed erythropoietin production or secretion)

Increased capillary fragility

Possibly evidenced by

(Not applicable; presence of signs and symptoms establishes an *actual* diagnosis)

Desired Outcomes/Evaluation Criteria—Client Will

Coagulation Status (NOC)

Experience no signs and symptoms of bleeding or hemorrhage.

Maintain or demonstrate improvement in laboratory values.

ACTIONS/INTERVENTIONS	RATIONALE
Energy Management (NIC)	
Independent	
Note reports of increasing fatigue and weakness. Observe for tachycardia, pallor of skin and mucous membranes, dyspnea, and chest pain. Plan client activities to avoid fatigue.	May reflect effects of anemia and cardiac response necessary to keep cells oxygenated.
Monitor level of consciousness (LOC) and behavior.	Anemia may cause cerebral hypoxia manifested by changes in mentation, orientation, and behavioral responses.
Evaluate response to activity and ability to perform tasks. Assist as needed and develop schedule for rest.	Anemia decreases tissue oxygenation and increases fatigue, which may require intervention, changes in activity, and rest.
Limit vascular sampling; combine laboratory tests when possible.	Recurrent and excessive blood sampling can worsen anemia.
Bleeding Precautions (NIC)	
Observe for oozing from venipuncture sites, bleeding or ecchymotic areas following slight trauma, petechiae, and joint swelling or mucous membrane involvement—bleeding gums, recurrent epistaxis, hematemesis, melena, and hazy or red urine.	Bleeding can occur easily because of capillary fragility and altered clotting functions and may worsen anemia.
Hematest gastrointestinal (GI) secretions and stool for blood.	Mucosal changes and altered platelet function due to uremia may result in gastric mucosal erosion and GI hemorrhage.
Provide soft toothbrush and electric razor. Use smallest needle possible and apply prolonged pressure following injections or vascular punctures.	Reduces risk of bleeding and hematoma formation.
Collaborative	
Monitor laboratory studies, such as the following:	
RBCs, Hgb/Hct	Uremia decreases production of erythropoietin and depresses RBC production and survival time. In CRF, Hgb and Hct are usually low, but tolerated, such as client may not be symptomatic until Hgb is below 7.
Platelet count, clotting factors	Suppression of platelet formation and inadequate levels of factors III and VIII impair clotting and potentiate risk of bleeding. *Note:* Bleeding may become intractable in ESRD.
Prothrombin time (PT) level	Abnormal prothrombin consumption lowers serum levels and impairs clotting.
Administer fresh blood and packed red cells (PRCs), as indicated.	May be necessary when client is symptomatic with anemia. PRCs are usually given when client is experiencing fluid overload or receiving dialysis treatment. Washed RBCs are used to prevent hyperkalemia associated with stored blood.
Administer medications, as indicated, for example:	
Erythropoietin preparations (Epogen, EPO, Procrit)	Stimulates the production and maintenance of RBCs, thus decreasing the need for transfusion.
Iron preparations, such as folic acid (Folvite) and cyanocobalamin (Rubesol-1000)	Useful in managing symptomatic anemia related to nutritional and dialysis-induced deficits. *Note:* Iron should not be given with phosphate binders because they may decrease iron absorption.

(continues on page 556)

ACTIONS/INTERVENTIONS (continued)

Cimetidine (Tagamet), ranitidine (Zantac), and antacids

Hemostatics or fibrinolysis inhibitors, such as aminocaproic acid (Amicar)
Stool softeners, such as Colace and bulk laxative, such as Metamucil

RATIONALE (continued)

May be given prophylactically to reduce or neutralize gastric acid and thereby reduce the risk of GI hemorrhage.
Inhibits bleeding that does not subside spontaneously or respond to usual treatment.
Straining to pass hard-formed stool increases likelihood of mucosal or rectal bleeding.

NURSING DIAGNOSIS: disturbed Thought Processes

May be related to
Physiological changes—accumulation of toxins, such as urea, ammonia; metabolic acidosis; hypoxia; electrolyte imbalances; calcifications in the brain

Possibly evidenced by
Disorientation to person, place, time, situation
Memory deficit, altered attention span, decreased ability to grasp ideas
Impaired ability to make decisions, problem-solve
Changes in sensorium—somnolence, stupor, coma
Changes in behavior—irritability, withdrawal, depression, psychosis

Desired Outcomes/Evaluation Criteria—Client Will

Cognition (NOC)
Regain or maintain optimal level of mentation.
Identify ways to compensate for cognitive impairment and memory deficits.

ACTIONS/INTERVENTIONS

RATIONALE

Reality Orientation (NIC)
Independent
Assess extent of impairment in thinking ability, memory, and orientation. Note attention span.

Ascertain from significant other (SO) client's usual level of mentation.
Provide SO with information about client's status.

Provide quiet, calm environment and judicious use of TV, radio, and visitation.
Reorient to surroundings, person, and so forth. Provide calendars, clocks, and outside window.
Present reality concisely and briefly, and do not challenge illogical thinking.
Communicate information and instructions in simple, short sentences. Ask direct, yes or no questions. Repeat explanations as necessary.
Establish a regular schedule for expected activities.

Promote adequate rest and undisturbed periods for sleep.

Collaborative
Monitor laboratory studies, such as BUN/Cr, serum electrolytes, glucose level, and ABGs (PO_2, pH).
Provide supplemental oxygen (O_2) as indicated.
Avoid use of barbiturates and opiates.

Prepare for dialysis.

Uremic syndrome's effect can begin with minor confusion or irritability and progress to altered personality, inability to assimilate information or participate in care. Awareness of changes provides opportunity for evaluation and intervention.
Provides comparison to evaluate progression or resolution of impairment.
Some improvement in mentation may be expected with restoration of more normal levels of BUN, electrolytes, and serum pH.
Minimizes environmental stimuli to reduce sensory overload and confusion while preventing sensory deprivation.
Provides clues to aid in recognition of reality.

Confrontation potentiates defensive reactions and may lead to client mistrust and heightened denial of reality.
May aid in reducing confusion and increases possibility that communications will be understood and remembered.
Aids in maintaining reality orientation and may reduce fear and confusion.
Sleep deprivation may further impair cognitive abilities.

Correction of imbalances can have profound effects on cognition.
Correction of hypoxia alone can improve cognition.
Drugs normally detoxified in the kidneys will have increased half-life and cumulative effects, worsening confusion.
Marked deterioration of thought processes may indicate worsening of azotemia and general condition, requiring prompt intervention to regain homeostasis.

NURSING DIAGNOSIS: **risk for impaired Skin Integrity**

Risk factors may include
Altered metabolic state, circulation (anemia with tissue ischemia), and sensation (peripheral neuropathy)
Changes in fluid status; alterations in skin turgor—edema
Reduced activity, immobility
Accumulation of toxins in the skin

Possibly evidenced by
(Not applicable; presence of signs and symptoms establishes an *actual* diagnosis)

Desired Outcomes/Evaluation Criteria—Client Will

Tissue Integrity: Skin and Mucous Membranes (NOC)
Maintain intact skin.

Risk Management (NOC)
Demonstrate behaviors and techniques to prevent skin breakdown or injury.

ACTIONS/INTERVENTIONS	RATIONALE
Skin Surveillance (NIC)	
Independent	
Inspect skin for changes in color, turgor, and vascularity. Note redness and excoriation. Observe for ecchymosis and purpura.	Indicates areas of poor circulation and early breakdown that may lead to decubitus formation and infection.
Monitor fluid intake and hydration of skin and mucous membranes.	Detects presence of dehydration or overhydration that affects circulation and tissue integrity at the cellular level.
Inspect dependent areas for edema. Elevate legs, as indicated.	Edematous tissues are more prone to breakdown. Elevation promotes venous return, limiting venous stasis and edema formation.
Change position frequently, move client carefully, pad bony prominences with sheepskin, and use elbow and heel protectors.	Decreases pressure on edematous, poorly perfused tissues to reduce ischemia.
Provide soothing skin care, restrict use of soaps, and apply ointments or creams such as lanolin or Aquaphor.	Baking soda and cornstarch baths decrease itching and are less drying than soaps. Lotions and ointments may be desired to relieve dry, cracked skin.
Keep linens dry and wrinkle free.	Reduces dermal irritation and risk of skin breakdown.
Investigate reports of itching.	Although dialysis has largely eliminated skin problems associated with uremic frost, itching can occur because the skin is an excretory route for waste products, such as phosphate crystals associated with hyperparathyroidism in ESRD.
Recommend client use cool, moist compresses to apply pressure to, rather than scratch, pruritic areas. Keep fingernails short; encourage use of gloves during sleep, if needed.	Alleviates discomfort and reduces risk of dermal injury.
Suggest wearing loose-fitting cotton garments.	Prevents direct dermal irritation and promotes evaporation of moisture on the skin.
Collaborative	
Provide foam or flotation mattress.	Reduces prolonged pressure on tissues, which can limit cellular perfusion, potentiating ischemia and necrosis.

NURSING DIAGNOSIS: **risk for impaired Oral Mucous Membrane**

Risk factors may include
Lack of or decreased salivation, fluid restrictions
Chemical irritation, conversion of urea in saliva to ammonia

Possibly evidenced by
(Not applicable; presence of signs and symptoms establishes an *actual* diagnosis)

Desired Outcomes/Evaluation Criteria—Client Will

Oral Health (NOC)
Maintain integrity of mucous membranes.
Identify and initiate specific interventions to promote healthy oral mucosa.

ACTIONS/INTERVENTIONS	RATIONALE

Oral Health Maintenance (NIC)
Independent

Inspect oral cavity: note moistness, character of saliva, presence of inflammation, ulcerations, and leukoplakia.

Provide fluids throughout 24-hour period within prescribed limit.

Offer frequent mouth care or rinse with 0.25% acetic acid solution. Provide gum, hard candy, or breath mints between meals.

Encourage good dental hygiene after meals and at bedtime. Recommend avoidance of dental floss.

Recommend client stop smoking and avoid lemon and glycerin products or mouthwash containing alcohol.

Provide artificial saliva as needed, such as Ora-Lube.

Provides opportunity for prompt intervention and prevention of infection.

Prevents excessive oral dryness from prolonged period without oral intake.

Mucous membranes may become dry and cracked. Mouth care soothes, lubricates, and helps freshen mouth taste, which is often unpleasant because of uremia and restricted oral intake. Rinsing with acetic acid helps neutralize ammonia formed by conversion of urea.

Reduces bacterial growth and potential for infection. Dental floss may cut gums, potentiating bleeding.

These substances are irritating to the mucosa and have a drying effect, potentiating discomfort.

Prevents dryness, buffers acids, and promotes comfort.

NURSING DIAGNOSIS: **deficient Knowledge [Learning Need] regarding condition, prognosis, treatment, self-care, and discharge needs**

May be related to
Lack of exposure or recall, information misinterpretation
Cognitive limitation

Possibly evidenced by
Questions, request for information, statement of misconception
Inaccurate follow-through of instructions, development of preventable complications

Desired Outcomes/Evaluation Criteria—Client Will

Knowledge: Disease Process (NOC)
Verbalize understanding of condition, disease process, and potential complications.

Knowledge: Treatment Regimen (NOC)
Verbalize understanding of therapeutic needs.
Correctly perform necessary procedures and explain reasons for the actions.
Demonstrate and initiate necessary lifestyle changes.
Participate in treatment regimen.

In addition to interventions here, refer to interventions outlined in CP: Renal Failure: Acute, ND: deficient Knowledge.

ACTIONS/INTERVENTIONS	RATIONALE

Teaching: Disease Process (NIC)
Independent

Review disease process, prognosis, and future expectations. Educate regarding natural disease progression, different dialysis modalities, renal transplantation, and client's option to refuse or discontinue chronic dialysis.

Address client's and SO's feelings, concerns, and methods of dealing with situation. Offer compassionate listening and honest answers to questions. Refer to appropriate support resources.

Review dietary modifications or restrictions, including the following:

Phosphorus—milk, cheese, carbonated drinks, processed foods, poultry, corn, and peanuts

---

Provides knowledge base from which client can make informed choices. Kidney failure choices depend on stage of disease and include doing no treatment, hemodialysis, peritoneal dialysis, and kidney transplantation. No matter which option is chosen, the client faces many lifestyle changes, including a complicated treatment plan involving several medications, diet and exercise modification, and appointments with numerous healthcare providers. *Note:* Client at stage IV must be evaluated and prepared for renal replacement therapy—dialysis or transplantation.

Common reactions to diagnosis include disbelief, anxiety, anger at self and others, and mild to severe depression (including suicidal ideation). (Refer to CP: Psychosocial Aspects of Care, ND: risk for self-/other-directed Violence.)

Retention of phosphorus stimulates the parathyroid glands to shift calcium from bones (renal osteodystrophy).

ACTIONS/INTERVENTIONS (continued)

Magnesium—whole grain products and legumes

Fluid, potassium, and sodium restrictions, when indicated

Discuss other nutritional concerns such as regulating protein intake according to level of renal function—generally 0.6 to 0.7 g/kg of body weight per day of good quality protein, such as meat, chicken, fish, and eggs.

Encourage adequate calorie intake, especially from carbohydrates in the nondiabetic client.

Discuss drug therapy, including use of vitamin D, calcium supplements, and phosphate binders, such as aluminum hydroxide antacids (Amphojel, Basalgel), and avoidance of magnesium antacids (Mylanta, Maalox, Gelusil).

Emphasize importance of reading all product labels—drugs and foods—and not taking medications without prior approval of healthcare provider.

Instruct in or review BP or glucose monitoring at home and provide information on obtaining monitoring equipment, as indicated.

Emphasize need for smoking cessation, if client smokes. Refer for nicotine medications and support resources.

Review strategies to prevent constipation, including stool softeners, such as Colace, and bulk laxatives, such as Metamucil, but avoiding magnesium products (milk of magnesia).

Review measures to prevent bleeding or hemorrhage, such as use of soft toothbrush, electric razor, avoidance of constipation, forceful blowing of nose, strenuous exercise, or contact sports.

Caution against exposure to external temperature extremes, such as heating pad and snow.

Discuss role of fatigue in client's daily or desired activities. Advise establishing a routine exercise program within limits of individual ability and rest periods with activities. Instruct in energy conservation techniques.

Address sexual concerns.

Identify available resources such as nephrologist, nutritionist, and other specialists, as indicated. Stress necessity of medical and laboratory follow-up.

Discuss quality of life concerns, such as pros and cons of each treatment option, refusing or withdrawing dialysis, medical care advance directives, and durable power of attorney.

RATIONALE (continued)

Accumulation of magnesium can impair neuromuscular function and mentation.

If fluid retention is a problem, client may need to restrict intake of fluid, such as previous day's output plus 500 mL for insensible losses, and restrict dietary potassium and sodium as prescribed. If fluid overload is present, diuretic therapy or dialysis will be part of the regimen. (Refer to CP: Renal Failure, Acute, ND: excess Fluid Volume.)

Metabolites that accumulate in blood derive almost entirely from protein catabolism; as renal function declines, proteins may be restricted proportionately. Too little protein can result in malnutrition. *Note:* Client on dialysis may not need to be as vigilant with protein intake.

Spares protein, prevents wasting, and provides energy. *Note:* Use of special glucose polymer powders can add calories to enhance energy level without extra food or fluid intake.

Prevents serious complications, such as reducing phosphate absorption from the GI tract and supplying calcium to maintain normal serum levels, reducing risk of bone demineralization and fractures and tetany; however, use of aluminum-containing products should be monitored because accumulation in the bones potentiates osteodystrophy. Magnesium products potentiate risk of hypermagnesemia. *Note:* Supplemental vitamin D may be required to facilitate calcium absorption.

It is difficult to maintain electrolyte balance when exogenous intake is not factored into dietary restrictions; for example, hypercalcemia can result from routine supplement use in combination with increased dietary intake of calcium-fortified foods and medications containing calcium.

Because hypertension and poor glycemic control are high risk factors in kidney disease progression, self-monitoring and management are important. Also, hypertension is worsened by CRF, often requiring management with antihypertensive drugs, necessitating close observation of treatment effects, such as vascular response to medication.

Smoking increases renal vasoconstriction and exacerbates hypertension.

Reduced fluid intake, changes in dietary pattern and use of phosphate-binding products often result in constipation that is not responsive to nonmedical interventions. Use of products containing magnesium increases risk of hypermagnesemia.

Reduces risks related to alteration of clotting factors and decreased platelet count.

Peripheral neuropathy may develop, especially in lower extremities, because of effects of uremia and electrolyte/acid-base imbalances impairing peripheral sensation and potentiating risk of tissue injury.

Fatigue due to anemia, sleep disturbances, malnutrition, and failure of kidneys to clear toxins can greatly reduce client's tolerance for activity. At the same time, exercise is needed to maintain muscle tone and joint flexibility; reduces risks associated with immobility including bone demineralization.

Physiological effects of uremia and antihypertensive therapy may impair sexual desire and performance.

Close monitoring of renal function and electrolyte balance is necessary to adjust dietary prescription, treatment, and to make decisions about possible options such as dialysis or transplantation.

When kidney failure is chronic or end-stage, client and SO may want to discuss issues with others, such as family, social worker, religious counselor, and should have the opportunity to receive information to make informed choices.

(continues on page 560)

Identify signs and symptoms requiring immediate medical evaluation, such as the following:

Low-grade fever, chills, changes in characteristics of urine or sputum, tissue swelling or drainage, and oral ulcerations

Numbness or tingling of digits, abdominal and muscle cramps, carpopedal spasms, and pain and tenderness in extremities

Joint swelling or tenderness, decreased ROM, and reduced muscle strength

Headaches, blurred vision, periorbital or sacral edema, and red eyes

Provide client and family information resources, such as books, articles, and informational Web sites; the National Kidney Foundation; and the American Association of Kidney Patients.

Depressed immune system, anemia, and malnutrition all contribute to increased risk of infection.

Uremia and decreased absorption of calcium may lead to peripheral neuropathies. *Note:* Client is also at risk for development of thrombophlebitic complications.

Hyperphosphatemia with corresponding calcium shifts from the bone may result in deposition of the excess calcium phosphate as calcifications in joints and soft tissues. Symptoms of skeletal involvement are often noted before impairment in organ function is evident.

Suggestive of development and poor control of hypertension and changes in eyes caused by calcium.

Offers client and SO opportunity to obtain information, support, and sources of funding.

POTENTIAL CONSIDERATIONS following acute hospitalization (dependent on client's age, physical condition and presence of complications, personal resources, and life responsibilities)

- *excess Fluid Volume*—compromised regulatory mechanism
- *Fatigue*—decreased metabolic energy production and dietary restriction, anemia, increased energy requirements, such as due to fever, inflammation, tissue regeneration
- *ineffective self Health Management*—complexity of therapeutic regimen, decisional conflicts: client value system, health beliefs, cultural influences; powerlessness, economic difficulties, family conflict, lack of or refusal of support systems
- *Hopelessness*—deteriorating physiological condition, long-term stress, prolonged activity limitations

---

RENAL DIALYSIS—GENERAL CONSIDERATIONS

I. Procedure
a. Process that substitutes for kidney function by removing excess fluid and accumulated endogenous or exogenous toxins
b. Type of fluid and solute removal depends on the client's underlying pathophysiology, current hemodynamic status, vascular access, availability of equipment and resources, and healthcare providers' training

II. Indications
a. Treatment for acute renal failure (ARF) or chronic end-stage renal disease (ESRD)
b. Emergency removal of toxins due to drug overdose, acute life-threatening hyperkalemia, severe acidosis, and uremia

III. Types
a. Choice of dialysis is determined by three main factors.
  i. Type of renal failure (acute or chronic)
  ii. Client's particular physical condition
  iii. Access to dialysis resources
b. Two primary types of dialysis
  i. Hemodialysis (HD)
    1. Requires placement of a venous access and a machine removing the blood from the body, running it through a dialyzer, and then returning it to the body

    2. Conventional HD may be done three times a week over 3 to 4 hours, either at a facility or in the home; or, daily dialysis may be done during the day or night hours (nocturnal dialysis).
  ii. Peritoneal dialysis (PD)
    1. Requires a surgically placed abdominal catheter for infusing dialysate fluid into the peritoneal cavity for a predetermined dwell time and then draining it out
    2. Procedure may be carried out at home through gravity or automated pump.

IV. Statistics (National Kidney and Urologic Diseases Information Clearinghouse [NKUDIC], 2005; U.S. Renal Data System [USRDS], 2007)
a. Morbidity: In 2005, 341,319 individuals with ESRD reportedly received dialysis in the United States, with 314,000 receiving HD (most of them in dialysis centers) and approximately 26,000 receiving PD.
b. Mortality: The probability of survival of clients receiving dialysis at 1 year is 78.3%; at 2 years, 63.6%; at 5 years, 32.1%; and at 10 years, 10.3% (NKUDIC, 2008).
c. Costs: In 2002, Medicare payments for outpatient HD and PD were approximately $3.6 billion (USRDS, 2004).

GLOSSARY

Access: Point on the body where a needle or catheter is inserted to gain entry to the bloodstream. Arteriovenous (AV) access is via graft, fistula, or central vein line.

Dialysate: Fluid used in both PD and HD that cleanses the blood and replaces needed electrolytes.

Disequilibrium syndrome: Nausea, vomiting, and hypertension, occasionally with convulsions, which develops within several hours after starting HD for renal failure; it is apparently caused by too rapid removal of urea from the extracellular fluid (ECF) compartment, with movement of water into cells and cerebral edema.

Dry weight: The lowest weight a patient can tolerate without the development of symptoms or hypotension. Because physiological dry weight is that weight resulting from normal renal function, vascular permeability, serum protein concentration, and body volume regulation, dry weight in HD should, theoretically, be lower.

Fistula: Access is made by joining an artery to a vein under the skin to make a bigger blood vessel.

Graft: Soft plastic tube to join an artery and a vein under the skin.

Intradialytic parenteral nutrition (IDPN): Involves infusing hyperalimentation fluids during the time of dialysis—through the vascular shunt or intraperitoneally—to normalize the amounts of albumin, glucose, and other nutrients in the bloodstream and to decrease the associated morbidity and mortality associated with protein-calorie malnutrition.

Ultrafiltration: Blood management method that removes noncellular water and low-molecular-weight solutes from anticoagulated blood through an extracorporeal (external from the body) filter.

Care Setting

Primary focus is at the community level at the dialysis center, although inpatient acute stay may be required during initiation of therapy.

Related Concerns

Anemias—iron deficiency, anemia of chronic disease, pernicious, aplastic, hemolytic, page 493

Heart failure: chronic, page 48

Peritonitis, page 349

Psychosocial aspects of care, page 749

Sepsis/septicemia, page 686

Total nutritional support: parenteral/enteral feeding, page 469

Transplantation considerations—postoperative and lifelong, page 739

Client Assessment Database

Refer to CPs: Renal Failure: Acute and/or Renal Failure: Chronic, for assessment information.

DIAGNOSTIC DIVISION MAY REPORT	MAY EXHIBIT
DISCHARGE PLAN CONSIDERATIONS • May require assistance with treatment regimen, transportation, activities of daily living (ADLs), homemaker and maintenance tasks, end-of life decisions, palliative care ▶ Refer to section at end of plan for postdischarge considerations.	

Diagnostic Studies

Studies and results are variable, depending on reason for dialysis, for example, removal of excess fluid or toxins and drugs, degree of renal involvement, and client considerations, such as distance from treatment center, cognition, available support, and insurance options.

Nursing Priorities

1. Promote homeostasis.
2. Maintain comfort.
3. Prevent complications.
4. Support client independence and self-care.
5. Provide information about disease process, prognosis, and treatment needs.

Discharge Goals

1. Fluid and electrolyte balance maximized.
2. Complications prevented or minimized.
3. Discomfort alleviated.
4. Dealing realistically with current situation; independent within limits of condition.
5. Disease process, prognosis, and therapeutic regimen understood.
6. Plan in place to meet needs after discharge.

This section addresses the general nursing management issues of client receiving some form of dialysis.

NURSING DIAGNOSIS: **imbalanced Nutrition: Less than Body Requirements**

May be related to
Gastrointestinal (GI) disturbances (result of uremia or medication side effects)—anorexia, nausea, vomiting, and stomatitis
Sensation of feeling full—abdominal distention during continuous ambulatory peritoneal dialysis (CAPD)
Dietary restrictions—bland, tasteless food; lack of interest in food
Loss of peptides and amino acids (building blocks for proteins) during dialysis

Possibly evidenced by
Inadequate food intake, aversion to eating, altered taste sensation
Poor muscle tone, weakness
Sore, inflamed buccal cavity; pale conjunctiva and mucous membranes

Desired Outcomes/Evaluation Criteria—Client Will

Nutritional Status (NOC)
Demonstrate stable weight or gain toward goal with normalization of laboratory values and no signs of malnutrition.

ACTIONS/INTERVENTIONS	RATIONALE
Nutrition Therapy (NIC)	
Independent	
Monitor food and fluid ingested and calculate daily caloric intake.	Identifies nutritional deficits and therapy needs, which are extremely variable, depending on client's age, stage of renal disease, other coexisting conditions, and the type of dialysis being planned.
Recommend client/significant other (SO) keep a food diary, including estimation of ingested calories, protein, and electrolytes of individual concern—sodium, potassium, chloride, magnesium, and phosphorus.	Helps client realize "big picture" and allows opportunity to alter dietary choices to meet individual desires within identified restriction.
Note presence of nausea and anorexia.	Symptoms accompany accumulation of endogenous toxins that can alter or reduce intake and require intervention.
Encourage client to participate in menu planning.	May enhance oral intake and promote sense of control.
Recommend small, frequent meals. Schedule meals according to dialysis needs.	Smaller portions may enhance intake. Type of dialysis influences meal patterns; for instance, clients receiving HD might not be fed directly before or during procedure because this can alter fluid removal, and clients undergoing PD may be unable to ingest food while abdomen is distended with dialysate.
Encourage use of herbs and spices such as garlic, onion, pepper, parsley, cilantro, and lemon.	Adds zest to food to help reduce boredom with diet, while reducing potential for ingesting too much potassium and sodium.
Suggest socialization during meals.	Provides diversion and promotes social aspects of eating.
Encourage frequent mouth care.	Reduces discomfort of oral stomatitis and metallic taste in mouth associated with uremia, which can interfere with food intake.
Collaborative	
Refer to nutritionist or dietitian to develop diet appropriate to client's needs.	Necessary to develop complex and highly individual dietary program to meet cultural and lifestyle needs within specific kilocalorie and protein restrictions while controlling phosphorus, sodium, and potassium.

ACTIONS/INTERVENTIONS (continued)	RATIONALE (continued)
Perform complete nutrition assessment—measure muscle mass via triceps skinfold or similar procedure. Determine muscle to fat ratio.	Assesses need and adequacy of nutrient utilization by measuring changes that may suggest presence or absence of tissue catabolism.
Provide a balanced diet, usually of 2,000 to 2,200 calories/day of complex carbohydrates and ordered amount of high-quality protein and essential amino acids.	Provides sufficient nutrients to improve energy and prevent muscle wasting (catabolism); promotes tissue regeneration and healing and electrolyte balance. Although client with kidney disease is often advised to limit protein intake, that changes with the start of dialysis. Protein-rich foods, such as fresh meats, poultry, fish and other seafood, eggs and egg whites, and small servings of dairy products are needed for building muscles, repairing tissue, and fighting infection. However, some protein-rich foods may contain a high level of phosphorus, so a dietitian's input is essential in determining the right amount to eat (Paton, 2007).
Restrict sodium and potassium as indicated; for example, avoid bacon, ham, other processed meats and foods, orange juice, and tomato soup.	These electrolytes can quickly accumulate, causing fluid retention, weakness, and potentially lethal cardiac dysrhythmias. *Note:* PD is not as effective in lowering elevated Na^+ level, necessitating tighter control of Na^+ intake.
Administer multivitamins, including folic acid; vitamins B_6, C, and D; and iron supplements, as indicated.	Replaces vitamin and mineral deficits resulting from malnutrition, anemia, or lost during dialysis.
Administer parenteral supplements, as indicated, or IDPN, as necessary.	Hyperalimentation may be needed to enhance renal tubular regeneration and resolution of underlying disease process and to provide nutrients if oral or enteral feeding is contraindicated. IDPN may be required when parenteral route is also unavailable or contraindicated. Research suggests IDPN may be more efficient at increasing protein synthesis and decreasing proteolysis, resulting in a shift from an essentially catabolic state to a positive nitrogen balance (How & Lau, 2005).
Monitor laboratory studies, for example: Serum protein, prealbumin or albumin levels	Indicators of protein needs. *Note:* PD is associated with significant protein loss. Serum albumin levels below 3.4 g/dL suggest need for IDPN infusions.
Hemoglobin (Hgb), red blood cell (RBC), and iron levels	Anemia is the most pervasive complication affecting energy levels in ESRD.
Administer medications, as appropriate, for example: Antiemetics, such as prochlorperazine (Compazine) Histamine blockers, such as famotidine (Pepcid)	Reduces stimulation of the vomiting center. Gastric distress is common and may be a neuropathy-induced gastric paresis. Hypersecretion can cause persistent gastric distress and digestive dysfunction.
Hormones and supplements as indicated, such as erythropoietin (EPO, Epogen) and iron supplement (Niferex)	Although EPO is given to increase numbers of RBCs, it is not effective without iron supplementation. Niferex is preferred because it can be given once daily and has fewer side effects than many iron preparations.
Insert and maintain nasogastric (NG) or enteral feeding tube, if indicated.	May be necessary when persistent vomiting occurs or when enteral feeding is desired.

NURSING DIAGNOSIS: impaired physical Mobility

May be related to
Restrictive therapies—lengthy dialysis procedure
Fear of or real danger of dislodging dialysis lines or catheter
Decreased strength and endurance; musculoskeletal impairment
Perceptual or cognitive impairment

Possibly evidenced by
Reluctance to attempt movement
Inability to move within physical environment
Decreased muscle mass, tone, and strength
Impaired coordination
Pain, discomfort

Desired Outcomes/Evaluation Criteria—Client Will

Mobility (NOC)
Maintain optimal mobility and function.
Display increased strength and be free of associated complications—contractures and decubitus ulcers.

563

ACTIONS/INTERVENTIONS	RATIONALE

Bed Rest Care (NIC)
Independent

Assess activity limitations, noting presence and degree of restriction or ability.

Encourage frequent change of position when on bedrest or chair rest; support affected body parts and joints with pillows, rolls, sheepskin, and elbow and heel pads, as indicated.

Provide gentle massage. Keep skin clean and dry. Keep linens dry and wrinkle free.

Encourage deep breathing and coughing. Elevate head of bed, as appropriate.

Suggest and provide diversion as appropriate to client's condition—visitors, radio or TV, and books. Take time to interact with client, showing interest in client's life.

Instruct in and assist with active and passive range-of-motion (ROM) exercises.

Influences choice of interventions.

Decreases discomfort, maintains muscle strength and joint mobility, enhances circulation, and prevents skin breakdown.

Stimulates circulation; prevents skin irritation.

Mobilizes secretions, improves lung expansion, and reduces risk of respiratory complications, such as atelectasis or pneumonia.

Decreases boredom; promotes relaxation.

Maintains joint flexibility, prevents contractures, and aids in reducing muscle tension. *Note:* A high level of phosphorus may cause calcium-phosphorus crystals to build up in the joints, muscles, and other body organs, leading to bone and joint pain. To avoid these risks, client may be prescribed a phosphate binder such as Basalgel or Renagel (Leydig, 2005).

Exercise Promotion (NIC)

Institute a planned activity or exercise program as appropriate, with client's input.

Increases client's energy and sense of well-being. Studies have shown that regular exercise programs have benefited clients with ESRD, both physically and emotionally. Stable clients have not been shown to have adverse effects (Goodman & Ballou, 2004).

Bed Rest Care (NIC)
Collaborative

Provide foam, water, or air flotation mattress or soft chair cushion.

Reduces tissue pressure and may enhance circulation, thereby reducing risk of dermal ischemia and breakdown.

NURSING DIAGNOSIS: Self-Care Deficit (specify)

May be related to
Intolerance to activity, decreased strength and endurance, pain or discomfort
Perceptual or cognitive impairment (accumulated toxins)

Possibly evidenced by
Reported inability to carry out ADLs
Disheveled and unkempt appearance, strong body odor

Desired Outcomes/Evaluation Criteria—Client Will

Self-Care: Activities of Daily Living (ADLs) (NOC)
Participate in ADLs within level of own ability and constraints of the illness.

ACTIONS/INTERVENTIONS	RATIONALE

Self-Care Assistance (NIC)
Independent

Determine client's ability to participate in self-care activities (scale of 0 to 4).

Provide assistance with activities as necessary.

Encourage use of energy-saving techniques: sitting, not standing; using shower chair; and doing tasks in small increments.

Recommend scheduling activities to allow client sufficient time to accomplish tasks to fullest extent of ability.

Underlying condition dictates level of deficit, affecting choice of interventions. *Note:* Psychological factors, such as depression, motivation, and degree of support, also have a major impact on the client's abilities.

Meets needs while supporting client participation and independence.

Conserves energy, reduces fatigue, and enhances client's ability to perform tasks.

Unhurried approach reduces frustration and promotes client participation, enhancing self-esteem.

NURSING DIAGNOSIS: risk for Constipation

Risk factors may include
Decreased fluid intake, altered dietary pattern
Reduced intestinal motility, compression of bowel (peritoneal dialysate), electrolyte imbalances, decreased mobility

Possibly evidenced by
(Not applicable; presence of signs and symptoms establishes an *actual* diagnosis)

Desired Outcomes/Evaluation Criteria—Client Will

Bowel Elimination (NOC)
Maintain usual or improved bowel function.

ACTIONS/INTERVENTIONS	RATIONALE
Constipation/Impaction Management (NIC)	
Independent	
Auscultate bowel sounds. Note consistency and frequency of bowel movements (BMs) and presence of abdominal distention.	Decreased bowel sounds; passage of hard-formed or dry stools suggests constipation and requires ongoing intervention to manage.
Review current medication regimen.	Side effects of some drugs, such as iron products and some antacids, may compound problem.
Ascertain usual dietary pattern and food choices.	Although restrictions may be present, thoughtful consideration of menu choices can aid in controlling problem.
Suggest adding fresh fruits, vegetables, and fiber to diet within restrictions, when indicated.	Provides bulk, which improves stool consistency.
Encourage or assist with ambulation, when able.	Activity may stimulate peristalsis, promoting return to normal bowel activity.
Provide privacy at bedside commode and bathroom.	Promotes psychological comfort needed for elimination.
Collaborative	
Administer stool softeners, such as Colace or bulk-forming laxatives, such as Metamucil, as appropriate.	Produces a softer, more easily evacuated stool.
Keep client nothing by mouth (NPO) status; insert NG tube, as indicated.	Decompresses stomach when recurrent episodes of unrelieved vomiting occur. Large gastric output suggests ileus, a common early complication of PD, with accumulation of gas and intestinal fluid that cannot be passed rectally.

NURSING DIAGNOSIS: risk for disturbed Thought Processes

Risk factors may include
Physiological changes—presence of uremic toxins, electrolyte imbalances, hypervolemia or fluid shifts, hyperglycemia (infusion of a dialysate with a high glucose concentration)

Possibly evidenced by
(Not applicable; presence of signs and symptoms establishes an *actual* diagnosis)

Desired Outcomes/Evaluation Criteria—Client Will

Cognition (NOC)
Regain usual or improved level of mentation.
Recognize changes in thinking and behavior and demonstrate behaviors to prevent or minimize changes.

ACTIONS/INTERVENTIONS	RATIONALE
Delirium Management (NIC)	
Independent	
Assess for behavioral changes or change in level of consciousness (LOC)—disorientation, lethargy, decreased concentration, memory loss, and altered sleep patterns.	May indicate level of uremic toxicity, response to or developing complication of dialysis such as "dialysis dementia," and need for further assessment and intervention.
Keep explanations simple and reorient frequently as needed. Provide "normal" day or night lighting patterns, clock, and calendar.	Improves reality orientation.
Provide a safe environment, restrain as indicated, and pad side rails during procedure, as appropriate.	Prevents client trauma and inadvertent removal of dialysis lines or catheter.

(continues on page 566)

ACTIONS/INTERVENTIONS (continued)

Drain peritoneal dialysate promptly at end of specified equilibration period.

Investigate reports of headache, associated with onset of dizziness, nausea and vomiting, confusion or agitation, hypotension, tremors, or seizure activity.

Monitor changes in speech pattern, development of dementia, and myoclonus activity during HD.

Collaborative

Monitor BUN/Cr and serum glucose levels, and determine urea reduction ratio (URR).

Alternate or change dialysate concentrations and add insulin, as indicated.

Administer normal saline intravenously (IV), as appropriate.

Administer medication, as indicated, such as phenytoin (Dilantin), mannitol (Osmitrol), and barbiturates.

Obtain aluminum level, as indicated.

RATIONALE (continued)

Prompt outflow will decrease risk of hyperglycemia or hyperosmolar fluid shifts affecting cerebral function.

May reflect development of disequilibrium syndrome, which can occur near completion of or following HD and is thought to be caused by ultrafiltration or by the too-rapid removal of urea from the bloodstream not accompanied by equivalent removal from brain tissue. The hypertonic cerebrospinal fluid (CSF) causes a fluid shift into the brain, resulting in cerebral edema and increased intracranial pressure.

Occasionally, accumulation of aluminum may cause dialysis dementia, progressing to death if untreated.

Follows progression or resolution of azotemia. Pre- and post-dialysis BUN levels are used to determine efficacy of procedure. URR greater than 65% is desirable (NKUDIC, 2005).

Hyperglycemia may develop secondary to glucose crossing peritoneal membrane and entering circulation. May require initiation of insulin therapy.

Volume restoration may be sufficient to reverse effects of disequilibrium syndrome.

If disequilibrium syndrome occurs during dialysis, medication may be needed to control seizures in addition to a change in dialysis prescription or discontinuation of therapy. After the procedure, an osmotic diuresis may be required to reduce cerebral edema, along with anticonvulsant therapy and barbiturates to slow brain metabolism.

Elevation may warn of impending cerebral involvement or dialysis dementia.

NURSING DIAGNOSIS: **Anxiety [specify level]/Fear**

May be related to
Situational crisis, threat to self-concept, change in health status, role functioning, socioeconomic status
Threat of death, unknown consequences or outcome

Possibly evidenced by
Increased tension, apprehension, uncertainty, fear
Expressed concerns
Sympathetic stimulation, focus on self

Desired Outcomes/Evaluation Criteria—Client Will

Anxiety [or] Fear Self-Control (NOC)
Verbalize awareness of feelings and reduction of anxiety or fear to a manageable level.
Demonstrate problem-solving skills and effective use of resources.
Appear relaxed and able to rest and sleep appropriately.

ACTIONS/INTERVENTIONS

Anxiety Reduction (NIC)
Independent
Assess level of fear of both client and SO. Note signs of denial, depression, or narrowed focus of attention.

Explain procedures and care as delivered. Repeat explanations frequently, as needed. Provide information in multiple formats, including pamphlets and films.

Acknowledge normalcy of feelings in this situation.

Provide opportunities for client and SO to ask questions and verbalize concerns.

RATIONALE

Helps determine the kind of interventions required.

Fear of unknown is lessened by information and knowledge and may enhance acceptance of permanence of ESRD and necessity for dialysis. Alteration in thought processes and high levels of anxiety or fear may reduce comprehension, requiring repetition of important information. *Note:* Uremia can impair short-term memory, requiring repetition or reinforcement of information provided.

Knowing feelings are normal can allay fear that client is losing control.

Creates feeling of openness and cooperation and provides information that will assist in problem identification and solving.

ACTIONS/INTERVENTIONS (continued)	RATIONALE (continued)
Encourage SO to participate in care, as able and desired.	Involvement promotes sense of sharing, strengthens feelings of usefulness, provides opportunity to acknowledge individual capabilities, and may lessen fear of the unknown.
Acknowledge concerns of client and SO.	Prognosis and possibility of need for long-term dialysis and resultant lifestyle changes are major concerns for this client and those who may be involved in future care.
Point out positive indicators of treatment—improvement in laboratory values, stable BP, and lessened fatigue.	Promotes sense of progress in an otherwise chronic process that seems endless while client still is experiencing physical deterioration and depression.
Collaborative	
Arrange for visit to dialysis center and meeting with another dialysis client, as appropriate.	Interaction with others who have encountered similar problems may assist client and SO to work toward acceptance of chronic condition and focus on problem-solving activities.
Address financial considerations. Refer to appropriate resources.	Treatment for kidney failure is expensive, although Medicare and other health insurance programs pay much of the cost.

NURSING DIAGNOSIS: disturbed Body Image/situational low Self-Esteem

May be related to
Situational crisis, chronic illness with changes in usual roles and body image

Possibly evidenced by
Verbalization of changes in lifestyle, focus on past function, negative feelings about body, feelings of helplessness and powerlessness
Continuous physical deterioration, premature aging, disfigurement
Extension of body boundary to incorporate environmental objects (such as dialysis equipment)
Change in social involvement
Overdependence on others for care, not taking responsibility for self-care, lack of follow-through, self-destructive behavior

Desired Outcomes/Evaluation Criteria—Client Will

Self-Esteem (NOC)
Identify feelings and methods for coping with negative perception of self.
Verbalize acceptance of self in situation.
Demonstrate adaptation to changes and events that have occurred, as evidenced by setting realistic goals and active participation in care and life in general.

ACTIONS/INTERVENTIONS	RATIONALE
Body Image [or] Self-Esteem Enhancement (NIC) *Independent*	
Assess level of client's knowledge about condition and treatment and anxiety related to current situation.	Identifies extent of problem or concern and necessary interventions.
Discuss meaning of loss and change to client.	Many clients and their families have difficulty dealing with changes in life and role performance as well as the client's loss of ability to control own body.
Note withdrawn behavior, ineffective use of denial, or behaviors indicative of overconcern with body and its functions. Investigate reports of feelings of depersonalization or the bestowing of humanlike qualities on machinery.	Indicators of developing difficulty handling stress of what is happening. *Note:* Client may feel tied to and controlled by the technology central to his or her survival, even to the point of extending body boundary to incorporate dialysis equipment.
Assess for use of addictive substances, primarily alcohol, other drugs, and self-destructive or suicidal behavior.	May reflect dysfunctional coping and attempt to handle problems in an ineffective manner.
Determine stage of grieving. Note signs of severe or prolonged depression.	Identification of grief stage client is experiencing provides guide to recognizing and dealing appropriately with behavior as client and SO work to come to terms with loss and limitations associated with condition. Prolonged depression may indicate need for further intervention.
Acknowledge normalcy of feelings.	Recognition that feelings are to be expected helps client accept and deal with them more effectively.
Encourage verbalization of personal and work conflicts that may arise. Active-listen concerns.	Helps client identify problems and problem-solve solutions. *Note:* Home dialysis may provide more flexibility and enhance sense of control for clients who are appropriate candidates for this form of therapy.

(continues on page 568)

ACTIONS/INTERVENTIONS (continued)	RATIONALE (continued)
Determine client's role in family constellation and client's perception of expectation of self and others.	Long-term and permanent illness or disability alter client's ability to fulfill usual role(s) in family and work setting. Unrealistic expectations can undermine self-esteem and affect outcome of illness.
Recommend SO treat client normally and not as an invalid.	Conveys expectation that client is able to manage situation and helps maintain sense of self-worth and purpose in life.
Assist client to incorporate disease management into lifestyle.	Necessities of treatment assume a more normal aspect when they are a part of the daily routine.
Identify strengths, past successes, and previous methods client has used to deal with life stressors.	Focusing on these reminders of own ability to deal with problems can help client deal with current situation.
Help client identify areas over which he or she has some measure of control. Provide opportunity to participate in decision-making process.	Provides sense of control over seemingly uncontrollable situation, fostering independence.
Collaborative	
Recommend participation in local support group.	Reduces sense of isolation as client learns that others have been where client is now. Provides role models for dealing with situation, problem-solving, and "getting on with life." Reinforces that therapeutic regimen can be beneficial.
Refer to healthcare and community resources, such as social service, vocational counselor, and psychiatric clinical nurse specialist.	Provides additional assistance for long-term management of chronic illness and change in lifestyle.

NURSING DIAGNOSIS: **deficient Knowledge [Learning Need] regarding condition, prognosis, treatment, self-care, and discharge needs**

May be related to
Lack of exposure or recall
Unfamiliarity with information resources
Cognitive limitations

Possibly evidenced by
Questions, request for information, statement of misconception
Inaccurate follow-through of instruction, development of preventable complications

Desired Outcomes/Evaluation Criteria—Client Will

Knowledge: Disease Process (NOC)
Verbalize understanding of condition and relationship of signs and symptoms of the disease process and potential complications.

Knowledge: Treatment Regimen (NOC)
Verbalize understanding of therapeutic needs.
Correctly perform necessary procedures and explain reasons for actions.

ACTIONS/INTERVENTIONS	RATIONALE
Teaching: Disease Process (NIC)	
Independent	
Note level of anxiety or fear and alteration of thought processes. Time teaching appropriately.	These factors directly affect ability to access and use knowledge. In addition, during the dialysis procedure, client's cognitive function may be impaired, and clients themselves state that they feel "fuzzy." Therefore, learning may not be optimal during this time.
Review particular disease process, prognosis, and potential complications in clear concise terms, periodically repeating and updating information, as necessary.	Providing information at the level of the client's and SO's understanding will reduce anxiety and misconceptions about what client is experiencing. *Note:* Research suggests nocturnal home HD is associated with improved left ventricular function, decreased BP and pulse pressure, and reduced used of antihypertensive medications.
Encourage and provide opportunity for questions.	Enhances learning process, promotes informed decision making, and reduces anxiety associated with the unknown.
Acknowledge that certain feelings and patterns of response are normal during course of therapy.	Client and SO may initially be hopeful and positive about the future, but as treatment continues and progress is less dramatic, they can become discouraged and depressed, and conflicts of dependence versus independence may develop.

ACTIONS/INTERVENTIONS (continued)

Emphasize necessity of reading all product labels—food, beverage, and over-the-counter (OTC) drugs—and not taking medications or herbal supplements without checking with healthcare provider.

Stress importance of establishing and adhering to medication schedule reflecting the specific form of renal disease, timing of dialysis, and properties of the individual medications.

Discuss significance of maintaining nutritious eating habits, preventing wide fluctuation of fluid and electrolyte balance, and avoidance of crowds or people with infectious processes.

Instruct client about epoetin (Epogen) or darbepoetin (Aransep), when indicated. Have client or SO demonstrate ability to administer and state adverse side effects and healthcare practices associated with this therapy.

Identify healthcare and community resources, such as dialysis support group, social services, and mental health clinic.

Teaching: Procedure/Treatment (NIC)

Discuss procedures and purpose of dialysis in terms understandable to client. Repeat explanations as required.

Instruct client and SO in home dialysis, as indicated:

Operation and maintenance of equipment (including vascular shunt), sources of supplies

Aseptic or clean technique

Self-monitoring of effectiveness of procedure

Management of potential complications

Contact persons

Sources for supplies when away from home

RATIONALE (continued)

It is difficult to maintain electrolyte balance when exogenous intake is not factored into dietary restriction; for example, hypercalcemia can result from routine supplement use in combination with increased dietary intake of calcium-fortified foods and medicines.

This is necessary to ensure that therapeutic levels of the drugs are reached and that toxic levels are avoided.

Depressed immune system, presence of anemia, invasive procedures, and malnutrition potentiate risk of infection.

Epogen is used for the management of the anemia associated with chronic renal failure (CRF) and ESRD. The drug is given to increase and maintain RBC production, which allows client to feel better and stronger. Darbepoetin is a non-natural recombinant protein that can stimulate RBC production, but the half-life is about three times longer than erythropoietin, resulting in less frequent dosing. Contraindications may include adverse side effects such as polycythemia, increased clotting, failure to administer correctly or have appropriate follow-up.

Knowledge and use of these resources assist client and SO to manage care more effectively. Interaction with others in similar situation provides opportunity for discussion of options and making informed choices, including stopping dialysis or renal transplantation.

A clear understanding of the purpose, process, and what is expected of client and SO facilitates their cooperation with regimen and may enhance outcomes.

Home dialysis is associated with better outcomes in general and better survival rates as dialysis is usually performed 5 to 7 days/week and is more intensive. This decreases fluctuations in fluid, solute, and electrolyte balance, more closely mimicking renal function. However, specific criteria for client and SO participation and training, home resources, and professional oversight must be met in order to consider this option.

Information diminishes anxiety of the unknown and provides opportunity for client to be knowledgeable about own care.

Prevents contamination and reduces risk of infection.

Provides information necessary to evaluate effects of therapy and need for change.

Reduces concerns regarding personal well-being; supports efforts at self-care.

Readily available support person can answer questions, troubleshoot problems, and facilitate timely medical intervention, when indicated, reducing risk and severity of complications. *Note:* Home dialysis clients usually are monitored by conventional dialysis center or interdisciplinary team.

Home dialysis clients are often capable of travel, even overseas, with proper preplanning and support.

Refer to Renal Dialysis: Peritoneal, below, or Hemodialysis, to complete the plan of care.

POTENTIAL CONSIDERATIONS following acute hospitalization (dependent on client's age, physical condition and presence of complications, personal resources, and life responsibilities)

- *Fatigue*—decreased metabolic energy production, states of discomfort, overwhelming psychological or emotional demands, altered body chemistry
- *excess Fluid Volume*—fluid retention and excessive intake, inadequate therapeutic regimen
- *risk for Infection*—invasive procedures, decreased hemoglobin, chronic disease, malnutrition
- *risk for ineffective self Health Management*—complexity of therapeutic regimen, economic difficulties, excessive demands made on individual and family
- *risk for Caregiver Role Strain*—severity of illness of care receiver, discharge of family member with significant home care needs, caregiver is spouse, presence of situational stressors

PERITONEAL DIALYSIS (PD)

I. Procedure

a. Requires a surgically placed abdominal catheter and uses the peritoneum to filter toxins and excess fluid from the body

b. Fluid removal is controlled by adjusting the dextrose concentration in the dialysate (e.g., 1.5%, 2.5%, 4.25%) to create an osmotic gradient for water with higher dextrose concentrations and more frequent exchanges increasing the rate of fluid removal.

c. May be preferred over hemodialysis because it uses a simpler technique and provides more gradual physiological changes

d. Long-term PD typically calls for four exchanges a day (or night), each with a dwell time of 4 to 6 hours.

e. Manual single-bag method is usually done as an inpatient procedure with short dwell times of only 30 to 40 minutes and is repeated until desired effects achieved.

II. Types

a. Continuous ambulatory peritoneal dialysis (CAPD)

  i. Most commonly used type of long-term PD, allowing client to manually manage the procedure at home with bag and gravity flow

  ii. Some clients experience problems with the long overnight dwell time because, as dextrose in the solution crosses into body, it becomes glucose and starts to draw fluid from the peritoneal cavity back into the body, thereby reducing the efficiency of the exchange and requiring a mini-cycler machine during the night.

b. Automated peritoneal dialysis (APD)

  i. Continuous cycler-assisted peritoneal dialysis (CCPD)

    1. Allows individual to walk around during extended daytime cycle with solution in abdomen

    2. May be method of choice for younger individuals engaged in school or work activities

  ii. Nocturnal intermittent peritoneal dialysis (NIPD)

    1. Usually reserved for individuals with substantial remaining renal function

    2. May improve uremia-associated sleep apnea (Perl & Chan, 2007)

III. Statistics

a. Morbidity: In 2005, more than 25,000 Americans received PD (National Kidney and Urologic Diseases Information Clearinghouse [NKUDIC], 2008).

b. Costs: In 2002, Medicare payments for outpatient PD were approximately $200 million (U.S. Renal Data System [USRDS], 2004).

GLOSSARY

Automated peritoneal dialysis (APD): Uses a machine to control the time of exchanges; warm, infuse, and drain the used solution at preset intervals; and fill the peritoneal cavity with new solution.

Continuous ambulatory peritoneal dialysis (CAPD): Uses three to five cycles daily and one long overnight dwell time, 7 days/week.

Continuous cycler-assisted peritoneal dialysis (CCPD): Mechanically cycles shorter dwell times during the night (three to six cycles) with one 8-hour dwell time during daylight hours, thus increasing the client's independence.

Nocturnal intermittent peritoneal dialysis (NIPD): Similar to CCPD, except the number of overnight exchanges is greater (six to eight) and no exchange is performed during the day.

Peritoneal dialysis (PD): Treatment for both acute renal failure (ARF) and end-stage renal disease (ESRD) using the peritoneum as the semipermeable membrane permitting transfer of nitrogenous waste products, toxins, and fluid from the blood into a dialysate solution.

NURSING DIAGNOSIS: risk for excess Fluid Volume

Risk factors may include
Inadequate osmotic gradient of dialysate
Fluid retention—malpositioned, kinked or clotted catheter; bowel distention, peritonitis, scarring of peritoneum
Excessive oral (PO) or intravenous (IV) intake

Possibly evidenced by
(Not applicable; presence of signs and symptoms establishes an *actual* diagnosis)

Desired Outcomes/Evaluation Criteria—Client Will

Fluid Balance (NOC)
Demonstrate dialysate outflow exceeding or approximating infusion.
Experience no rapid weight gain, edema, or pulmonary congestion.

ACTIONS/INTERVENTIONS	RATIONALE

Peritoneal Dialysis Therapy (NIC)
Independent

Maintain a record of inflow and outflow volumes and cumulative fluid balance.

In most cases, the amount drained should equal or exceed the amount instilled. A positive balance with more fluid in than out indicates need for further evaluation.

Record serial weights, compare with intake and output (I&O) balance. Weigh client when abdomen is empty of dialysate providing a consistent reference point.

Serial body weights are an accurate indicator of fluid volume status. A positive fluid balance with an increase in weight indicates fluid retention.

Assess patency of catheter, noting difficulty in draining. Note presence of fibrin strings or plugs.

Slowing of flow rate or presence of fibrin suggests partial catheter occlusion requiring further evaluation or possible intervention.

Check tubing for kinks; note placement of bags. Anchor catheter so that adequate inflow and outflow is achieved.

Improper functioning of equipment may result in retained fluid in abdomen and insufficient clearance of toxins.

Turn from side to side, elevate the head of the bed, and apply gentle pressure to the abdomen.

May enhance outflow of fluid when catheter is malpositioned or obstructed by the omentum.

Note abdominal distention associated with decreased bowel sounds, changes in stool consistency, and reports of constipation.

Bowel distention or constipation may impede outflow of effluent. (Refer to CP: Renal Dialysis; ND: risk for Constipation.)

Monitor blood pressure (BP) and pulse, noting hypertension, bounding pulses, neck vein distention, and peripheral edema; measure central venous pressure (CVP), if available.

Elevations indicate hypervolemia. Assess heart and breath sounds, noting S_3 and crackles and rhonchi. Fluid overload may potentiate heart failure (HF) or pulmonary edema.

Evaluate development of tachypnea, dyspnea, and increased respiratory effort. Drain dialysate and notify physician.

Abdominal distention or diaphragmatic elevation may cause respiratory distress.

Assess for headache, muscle cramps, mental confusion, and disorientation.

Symptoms suggest hyponatremia or water intoxication.

Collaborative

Alter dialysate regimen, as indicated.

Changes may be needed in the glucose or sodium concentration to facilitate efficient dialysis.

Monitor serum sodium.

Hypernatremia may be present, although serum levels may reflect dilutional effect of fluid volume overload.

Add heparin to initial dialysis runs; assist with irrigation of catheter with heparinized saline.

May be useful in preventing fibrin clot formation, which can obstruct peritoneal catheter.

Maintain fluid restriction, as indicated.

Fluid restrictions may have to be continued to decrease fluid volume overload. Between dialysis treatments, fluids accumulate in the body, particularly in the heart, lungs, and ankles. Therefore, most nephrologists recommend restricting fluid to about 1,500 mL/day (Leydig, 2005).

NURSING DIAGNOSIS: risk for deficient Fluid Volume

Risk factors may include
Use of hypertonic dialysate with excessive removal of fluid from circulating volume

Possibly evidenced by
(Not applicable; presence of signs and symptoms establishes an *actual* diagnosis)

Desired Outcomes/Evaluation Criteria—Client Will

Systemic Toxin Clearance: Dialysis (NOC)
Achieve desired alteration in fluid volume and weight with BP and electrolyte levels within acceptable range.
Experience no symptoms of dehydration.

ACTIONS/INTERVENTIONS	RATIONALE

Peritoneal Dialysis Therapy (NIC)
Independent

Maintain record of inflow and outflow volumes and individual and cumulative fluid balance.

Provides information about the status of client's loss or gain at the end of each exchange.

Adhere to schedule for draining dialysate from abdomen.

Prolonged dwell times, especially when 4.5% glucose solution is used, may cause excessive fluid loss.

Weigh when abdomen is empty, following initial 6 to 10 runs, then as indicated.

Detects rate of fluid removal by comparison with baseline body weight.

(continues on page 572)

ACTIONS/INTERVENTIONS (continued)	RATIONALE (continued)
Monitor BP lying and sitting and pulse. Note level of jugular pulsation.	Decreased BP, postural hypotension, and tachycardia are early signs of hypovolemia.
Note reports of dizziness, nausea, and increasing thirst.	May indicate hypovolemia or hyperosmolar syndrome.
Inspect mucous membranes, evaluate skin turgor, peripheral pulses, and capillary refill.	Dry mucous membranes, poor skin turgor, and diminished pulses and capillary refill are indicators of dehydration and need for increased intake or changes in strength of dialysate.
Collaborative	
Monitor laboratory studies, as indicated, such as:	
Serum sodium and glucose levels	Hypertonic solutions may cause hypernatremia by removing more water than sodium. In addition, dextrose may be absorbed from the dialysate, thereby elevating serum glucose.
Serum potassium levels	Hypokalemia may occur and can cause cardiac dysrhythmias.

NURSING DIAGNOSIS: risk for Trauma

Risk factors may include
Catheter inserted into peritoneal cavity
Site near the bowel and bladder with potential for perforation during insertion or manipulation of the catheter

Possibly evidenced by
(Not applicable; presence of signs and symptoms establishes an *actual* diagnosis)

Desired Outcomes/Evaluation Criteria—Client Will

Risk Control (NOC)
Experience no injury to bowel or bladder.

ACTIONS/INTERVENTIONS	RATIONALE
Peritoneal Dialysis Therapy (NIC)	
Independent	
Have client empty bladder before peritoneal catheter insertion if indwelling catheter not present.	An empty bladder is more distant from insertion site and reduces likelihood of being punctured during catheter insertion.
Anchor catheter and tubing with tape. Stress importance of client avoiding pulling or pushing on catheter. Restrain hands if indicated.	Reduces risk of trauma by manipulation of the catheter.
Note presence of fecal material in dialysate effluent or strong urge to defecate, accompanied by severe, watery diarrhea.	Suggests bowel perforation with mixing of dialysate and bowel contents.
Note reports of intense urge to void or large urine output following initiation of dialysis run. Test urine for sugar, as indicated.	Suggests bladder perforation with dialysate leaking into bladder. Presence of glucose-containing dialysate in the bladder will elevate glucose level of urine.
Stop dialysis if there is evidence of bowel or bladder perforation, leaving peritoneal catheter in place.	Prompt action will prevent further injury. Immediate surgical repair may be required. Leaving catheter in place facilitates diagnosing and locating the perforation.

NURSING DIAGNOSIS: acute Pain

May be related to
Insertion of catheter through abdominal wall, catheter irritation, improper catheter placement
Irritation, infection within the peritoneal cavity
Infusion of cold or acidic dialysate, abdominal distention, rapid infusion of dialysate

Possibly evidenced by
Reports of pain
Self-focusing
Guarding, distraction behaviors, restlessness

Desired Outcomes/Evaluation Criteria—Client Will

Pain Control (NOC)
Verbalize decrease of pain and discomfort.
Demonstrate relaxed posture and facial expression; be able to sleep and rest appropriately.

ACTIONS/INTERVENTIONS	RATIONALE
Pain Management (NIC)	
Independent	
Investigate client's reports of pain; note intensity (0 to 10), location, and precipitating factors.	Assists in identification of source of pain and appropriate interventions.
Explain that initial discomfort usually subsides after the first few exchanges.	Information may reduce anxiety and promote relaxation during procedure.
Monitor for pain that begins during inflow and continues during equilibration phase. Slow infusion rate, as indicated.	Pain will occur if acidic dialysate causes chemical irritation of peritoneal membrane.
Note reports of discomfort that are most pronounced near the end of inflow, and instill no more than 2,000 mL of solution at a single time.	Likely the result of abdominal distention from dialysate. Amount of infusion may have to be decreased initially.
Prevent air from entering peritoneal cavity during infusion. Note report of pain in area of shoulder blade.	Inadvertent introduction of air into the abdomen irritates the diaphragm and results in referred pain to shoulder blade. This type of discomfort may also be reported during initiation of therapy or during infusions and usually is related to stretching or irritation of the diaphragm with abdominal distention. Smaller exchange volumes may be required until client adjusts.
Elevate head of bed at intervals. Turn client from side to side. Provide back care and tissue massage.	Position changes and gentle massage may relieve abdominal and general muscle discomfort.
Warm dialysate to body temperature before infusing.	Warming the solution increases the rate of urea removal by dilating peritoneal vessels. Cold dialysate causes vasoconstriction, which can cause discomfort and excessively lower the core body temperature, precipitating cardiac arrest.
Monitor for severe or continuous abdominal pain and temperature elevation, especially after dialysis has been discontinued.	May indicate developing peritonitis. (Refer to ND: risk for Infection [peritonitis], following.)
Encourage use of relaxation techniques, such as deep-breathing exercises, guided imagery, and visualization. Provide diversional activities.	Redirects attention and promotes sense of control.
Collaborative	
Administer analgesics.	Relieves pain and discomfort.
Add sodium hydroxide to dialysate, if indicated.	Occasionally used to alter pH if client is not tolerating acidic dialysate.

NURSING DIAGNOSIS: risk for Infection [peritonitis]

Risk factors may include
Contamination of the catheter during insertion, periodic changing of tubing and bags
Skin contaminants at catheter insertion site
Sterile peritonitis (response to the composition of dialysate)

Possibly evidenced by
(Not applicable; presence of signs and symptoms establishes an *actual* diagnosis)

Desired Outcomes/Evaluation Criteria—Client Will

Risk Control (NOC)
Identify interventions to prevent or reduce risk of infection.
Experience no signs or symptoms of infection.

ACTIONS/INTERVENTIONS	RATIONALE
Infection Protection (NIC)	
Independent	
Observe meticulous aseptic technique and wear masks during catheter insertion, dressing changes, and whenever the system is opened. Change tubing per protocol.	Prevents the introduction of organisms and airborne contamination that may cause infection, the most common complication of PD.
Change dressings as indicated, being careful not to dislodge the catheter. Note character, color, odor, or drainage from insertion site.	Moist environment promotes bacterial growth. Purulent drainage at insertion site suggests presence of local infection, often involving skin organisms, which can be difficult to treat and sometimes require catheter removal and temporary HD. *Note:* Polyurethane adhesive film (e.g., blister film) dressings have been found to decrease amount of pressure on catheter and exit site as well as incidence of site infections.

(continues on page 574)

ACTIONS/INTERVENTIONS (continued)	RATIONALE (continued)
Observe color and clarity of effluent.	Cloudy effluent is suggestive of peritoneal infection.
Apply povidone-iodine (Betadine) barrier in distal, clamped portion of catheter when intermittent dialysis therapy used.	Reduces risk of bacterial entry through catheter between dialysis treatments when catheter is disconnected from closed system.
Investigate reports of nausea or vomiting, increased or severe abdominal pain, rebound tenderness, or fever.	Signs and symptoms suggesting peritonitis, requiring prompt intervention.
Collaborative	
Monitor white blood cell (WBC) count of effluent.	Presence of WBCs initially may reflect normal response to a foreign substance; however, continued or new elevation of WBCs suggests developing infection.
Obtain specimens of blood, effluent, and drainage from insertion site, as indicated, for culture and sensitivity.	Identifies types of organism(s) present and influences choice of interventions.
Monitor renal blood urea nitrogen (BUN) and creatinine (Cr) clearance.	Choice and dosage of antibiotics are influenced by level of clearance.
Administer antibiotics systemically or in dialysate, as indicated.	Treats infection and prevents sepsis.

NURSING DIAGNOSIS: risk for ineffective Breathing Pattern

Risk factors may include
Abdominal pressure, restricted diaphragmatic excursion, rapid infusion of dialysate, pain
Inflammatory process, such as atelectasis and pneumonia

Possibly evidenced by
(Not applicable; presence of signs and symptoms establishes an *actual* diagnosis)

Desired Outcomes/Evaluation Criteria—Client Will

Respiratory Status: Ventilation (NOC)
Display an effective respiratory pattern with clear breath sounds and arterial blood gases (ABGs) within client's normal range.
Experience no signs of dyspnea or cyanosis.

ACTIONS/INTERVENTIONS	RATIONALE
Respiratory Monitoring (NIC)	
Independent	
Monitor respiratory rate and effort. Reduce infusion rate if dyspnea is present.	Tachypnea, dyspnea, shortness of breath, and shallow breathing during dialysis suggest diaphragmatic pressure from distended peritoneal cavity or may indicate developing complications.
Auscultate lungs, noting decreased, absent, or adventitious breath sounds, such as crackles, wheezes, and rhonchi.	Decreased areas of ventilation suggest presence of atelectasis, whereas adventitious sounds may suggest fluid overload, retained secretions, or infection.
Note character, amount, and color of secretions.	Client is susceptible to pulmonary infections as a result of depressed cough reflex and respiratory effort, increased viscosity of secretions, as well as altered immune response and chronic, debilitating disease.
Elevate head of bed or have client sit up in chair. Promote deep-breathing exercises and coughing.	Facilitates chest expansion and ventilation and mobilization of secretions.
Collaborative	
Review ABGs, pulse oximetry, and serial chest x-rays.	Changes in PaO_2 and $PaCO_2$ and appearance of infiltrates and congestion on chest x-ray suggest developing pulmonary problems.
Administer supplemental oxygen, as indicated.	Maximizes oxygen for vascular uptake, thus preventing or lessening hypoxia.
Administer analgesics, as indicated.	Alleviates pain and promotes comfortable breathing and maximal cough effort.

HEMODIALYSIS (HD)

I. Procedure
a. Removal of urea and other toxic products and correction of fluid and electrolyte imbalances
b. Blood is shunted through an artificial kidney or membrane (dialyzer) for removal of toxins and excess fluid and then returned to the venous circulation.
c. Requires placement of vascular access
   i. Arteriovenous (AV) fistula: usually requires at least 2 to 4 months to heal before it can be used, providing sufficient time so that those involved are prepared and can perform home hemodialysis, if appropriate
   ii. AV graft: may be indicated in presence of small veins, usually ready for use within 2 to 3 weeks
   iii. Temporary access: provides immediate access with insertion of a catheter into a vein in the neck, chest, or groin

II. Types
a. Intermittent HD procedure
   i. Requires permanent AV access, such as primary AV fistula or synthetic graft
   ii. Usually performed three times per week for 3 to 5 hours per procedure, or six to seven times per week for 1.5 to 2 hours
b. Continuous renal replacement therapy (CRRT) (Paton, 2007)
   i. Blood is usually accessed via a central venous catheter.
   ii. Treatment for acute renal failure (ARF) with fluid and toxins removed at a continuous and slower rate than intermittent HD
   iii. May be indicated for clients with ARF and who are too hemodynamically unstable to tolerate conventional hemodialysis
   iv. Commonly used types of CRRT
      1. Slow continuous ultrafiltration (SCUF)
      2. Continuous venovenous hemofiltration via ultrafiltration and convection
      3. Continuous venovenous hemofiltration
      4. Continuous venovenous hemodialysis
      5. Continuous venovenous hemodiafiltration

III. Statistics
a. Morbidity: In 2005, and estimated 312,000 Americans received in-center hemodialysis and 2,000 received home dialysis (National Kidney and Urologic Diseases Information Clearinghouse [NKUDIC], 2008).
b. Cost: Estimates vary from $35,000 to $60,000 annually per client; in 2002, Medicare payments for outpatient hemodialysis were approximately $3.4 billion (U.S. Renal Data System [USRDS], 2004).

GLOSSARY

Arteriovenous (AV) fistula: An artery, usually in the forearm, is surgically connected to a vein.

Arteriovenous (AV) graft: A synthetic tube or graft is surgically implanted in the arm connecting an artery and vein.

Continuous renal replacement therapy (CRRT): Continuous 24-hour dialysis therapy, which provides a more normal physiological response by removing plasma water more slowly, thus compensating for the loss of intravascular volume; particularly useful in intensive care setting.

Continuous venovenous hemodiafiltration: Removes fluid and toxins via ultrafiltration and convection using a dialysate to enhance toxin removal and a replacement fluid to help titrate fluid and electrolyte balance.

Continuous venovenous hemodialysis: Removes fluid and toxins via ultrafiltration and convection. A dialysate is added to enhance the removal of toxins via diffusion.

Continuous venovenous hemofiltration: Removes both fluid and toxins via ultrafiltration and convection with a replacement fluid infused to help titrate fluid removal and maintain electrolyte balance.

Slow continuous ultrafiltration (SCUF): Uses ultrafiltration to remove fluid only.

Thrill: Palpable vibration or buzzing sensation caused by turbulence of high-pressure arterial blood flow entering low-pressure venous system, indicating AV shunt is patent.

Venous access: The point on the body where a needle or catheter is inserted to gain entry to the bloodstream. AV access is via graft, fistula, or central vein line.

This plan of care addresses the typical HD procedure usually performed three times per week and carried out in the hospital, community dialysis center, or at home.

NURSING DIAGNOSIS: **risk for Injury [loss of vascular access]**

Risk factors may include
Clotting, hemorrhage related to accidental disconnection, infection

Possibly evidenced by
(Not applicable; presence of signs and symptoms establishes an *actual* diagnosis)

Desired Outcomes/Evaluation Criteria—Client Will

Hemodialysis Access (NOC)
Maintain patent vascular access.
Be free of infection.

Hemodialysis Therapy (NIC)

Independent

Clotting

Assess client's pulse and tissue color distal to shunt.	Determines general circulatory status of limb.
Monitor internal AV fistula or graft patency at frequent intervals:	Clotting (thrombosis) of the AV access is the most common complication.
Palpate for thrill.	Should be palpable above venous exit site. If the thrill stops, or even feels different, this could indicate clotting. With early intervention, many clots can be dissolved or removed.
Auscultate for a bruit.	Bruit is the sound caused by the turbulence of arterial blood entering the venous system and should be audible by stethoscope, although may be very faint. If the bruit gets higher in pitch, it could mean narrowing of the blood vessels; if it stops, clot may have formed.
Note color of blood and obvious separation of cells and serum.	Change of color from uniform medium red to dark purplish red suggests sluggish blood flow and early clotting. Separation in tubing is indicative of clotting. Very dark reddish-black blood next to clear yellow fluid indicates full clot formation. *Note:* Prior to insertion of an AV fistula or graft, client may have a temporary or permanent central catheter, which is maintained with heparin to inhibit clot formation. Because heparin remains active in the body for 4 to 6 hours, the client is at risk for hemorrhage during and immediately after dialysis (Leydig 2005).
Palpate skin around shunt for warmth.	Diminished blood flow results in "coolness" of shunt.
Notify physician and initiate declotting procedure if there is evidence of loss of shunt patency.	Rapid intervention may save access; however, declotting must be done by experienced personnel.
Evaluate reports of pain, numbness, and tingling; note extremity swelling distal to access.	May indicate inadequate blood supply.
Avoid trauma to shunt; for example, handle tubing gently and maintain cannula alignment. Limit activity of extremity. Avoid taking blood pressure (BP) or drawing blood samples in shunt extremity. Instruct client not to sleep on side with shunt or carry packages, books, or purse on affected extremity.	Decreases risks of clotting and disconnection. It is critical that the catheter be used only for dialysis as it is the client's lifeline (Leydig, 2005).

Hemorrhage

Attach two cannula clamps to shunt dressing. Have tourniquet available. If cannulae separate, clamp the arterial cannula first, then the venous. If tubing comes out of vessel, clamp cannula that is still in place and apply direct pressure to bleeding site. Place tourniquet above site or inflate BP cuff to pressure just above client's systolic BP.	Prevents massive blood loss while awaiting medical assistance if cannula separates or shunt is dislodged.

Infection

Assess skin around vascular access, noting redness, swelling, local warmth, exudate, and tenderness.	Signs of local infection, which can progress to sepsis if untreated.
Avoid contamination of access site. Use aseptic technique and masks when giving shunt care, applying and changing dressings, and when starting and completing dialysis process.	Prevents introduction of organisms that may cause infection.
Monitor temperature. Note presence of fever, chills, and hypotension.	Signs of infection or sepsis requiring prompt medical intervention.

Collaborative

Culture the site and obtain blood samples, as indicated.	Determines presence of pathogens and how best to treat.
Monitor prothrombin time (PT) and activated partial thromboplastin time (aPTT), as appropriate.	Provides information about coagulation status, identifies treatment needs, and evaluates effectiveness.
Administer medications, as indicated, for example:	
Lowdose heparin	Infused on arterial side of filter to prevent clotting in the filter without systemic side effects.
Antibiotics—systemic and topical.	Prompt treatment of infection may save access and prevent sepsis.
Discuss use of acetylsalicylic acid (ASA) or warfarin sodium (Coumadin), as appropriate.	Ongoing low-dose anticoagulation may be useful in maintaining patency of shunt.

NURSING DIAGNOSIS: risk for deficient **Fluid Volume**

Risk factors may include
Ultrafiltration
Fluid restrictions, actual blood loss—systemic heparinization or disconnection of the shunt

Possibly evidenced by
(Not applicable; presence of signs and symptoms establishes an *actual* diagnosis)

Desired Outcomes/Evaluation Criteria—Client Will

Hydration (NOC)
Maintain fluid balance as evidenced by stable vital signs, good skin turgor, moist mucous membranes, absence of bleeding, and appropriate weight.

ACTIONS/INTERVENTIONS	RATIONALE
Fluid Monitoring (NIC)	
Independent	
Measure all sources of intake and output (I&O). Have client keep diary.	Aids in evaluating fluid status, especially when compared with weight. *Note:* Urine output is an inaccurate evaluation of renal function in dialysis clients. Some individuals have water output with little renal clearance of toxins, whereas others have oliguria or anuria.
Weigh daily as well as before and after dialysis run.	Weight loss over precisely measured time is a measure of ultrafiltration and fluid removal. Dry weight determines how much excess fluid has been removed and serves as a guide for subsequent dialysis run time and solution.
Monitor BP, pulse, and hemodynamic pressures, if available, during dialysis.	Hypotension, tachycardia, and falling hemodynamic pressures suggest volume depletion.
Hemodialysis Therapy (NIC)	
Ascertain whether diuretics and antihypertensives are to be withheld.	Dialysis potentiates hypotensive effects if these drugs have been administered.
Verify continuity of shunt or access catheter.	Disconnected shunt or open access permits exsanguination.
Apply external shunt dressing. Permit no puncture of shunt.	Minimizes stress on cannula insertion site to reduce inadvertent dislodgement and bleeding from site.
Place client in a supine or Trendelenburg position, as necessary.	Maximizes venous return if hypotension occurs.
Assess for oozing or frank bleeding at access site, mucous membranes, or incisions and wounds. Hematest stools or any drainage.	Systemic heparinization during dialysis prolongs clotting times and places client at risk for bleeding, especially during the first 4 hours after procedure.
Fluid Monitoring (NIC)	
Collaborative	
Monitor laboratory studies, as indicated, such as the following: Hemoglobin/hematocrit (Hgb/Hct)	May be reduced because of anemia, hemodilution, or actual blood loss.
Serum electrolytes and pH	Imbalances may require changes in the dialysate solution or supplemental replacement to achieve balance.
Clotting times—PT/aPTT and platelet count.	Use of heparin to prevent clotting in blood lines and hemofilter alters coagulation and potentiates active bleeding.
Administer IV solutions during dialysis, as indicated, for example: Normal saline (NS)	Saline or dextrose solutions, electrolytes, and $NaHCO_3$ may be infused in the venous side of continuous arteriovenous hemofilter when high ultrafiltration rates are used for removal of extracellular fluid (ECF) and toxic solutes.
Volume expanders, such as albumin	Volume expanders may be required during or following hemodialysis if sudden or marked hypotension occurs.
Packed red blood cells (RBCs), if needed	Destruction of RBCs (hemolysis) by mechanical dialysis, hemorrhagic losses, or decreased RBC production may result in profound and progressive anemia requiring corrective action.
Reduce rate of ultrafiltration during dialysis, as indicated.	Reduces the amount of water being removed and may correct hypotension or hypovolemia.
Administer protamine sulfate, as appropriate.	May be needed to return clotting times to normal or if heparin rebound occurs within 16 hours after hemodialysis.

Risk factors may include
Rapid and excessive fluid intake—IV, blood, plasma expanders, saline given to support BP during dialysis

Possibly evidenced by
(Not applicable; presence of signs and symptoms establishes an *actual* diagnosis)

Desired Outcomes/Evaluation Criteria—Client Will

Fluid Balance (NOC)
Maintain "dry weight" within client's normal range; be free of edema; **and** have clear breath sounds and serum sodium levels within normal limits.

ACTIONS/INTERVENTIONS	RATIONALE
Fluid Management (NIC)	
Independent	
Measure all sources of I&O. Weigh routinely.	Aids in evaluating fluid status, especially when compared with weight. Weight gain between treatments should not exceed 0.5 kg or approximately 1 lb/day.
Monitor BP and pulse.	Hypertension and tachycardia between hemodialysis runs may result from fluid overload and heart failure (HF).
Note presence of peripheral or sacral edema, respiratory rales, dyspnea, orthopnea, distended neck veins, and electrocardiogram (ECG) changes indicative of ventricular hypertrophy.	Fluid volume excess due to inefficient dialysis or repeated hypervolemia between dialysis treatments may cause or exacerbate HF, as indicated by signs and symptoms of respiratory and systemic venous congestion.
Note changes in mentation. (Refer to CP: Renal Dialysis; ND: risk for disturbed Thought Processes.)	Fluid overload or hypervolemia may potentiate disequilibrium syndrome.
Collaborative	
Monitor serum sodium levels. Restrict sodium intake, as indicated.	High sodium levels are associated with fluid overload, edema, hypertension, and cardiac complications.
Restrict fluid intake as indicated, spacing allowed fluids throughout a 24-hour period.	The intermittent nature of hemodialysis results in fluid retention and volume overload between procedures and may require fluid restriction. Spacing fluids helps reduce thirst.

URINARY DIVERSIONS/UROSTOMY (POSTOPERATIVE CARE)

I. Procedure
  a. Diversion of urine out of the body through an opening in the abdominal wall bypassing the bladder, which requires a pouch to be worn outside the body; or, a continent diversion involving the creation of a pouch or bladder inside the body, usually using part of the digestive tract
  b. Types
    i. Incontinent urinary diversions
      1. Ileal conduit
      2. Colonic conduit
      3. Ureterostomy
    ii. Continent urinary diversions
      1. Catheterizable urinary reservoir: Kock reservoir or Indiana (ileocecal) pouch
      2. Orthotopic continent urinary diversion: neobladder

II. Etiology (Costa & Kreder, 2006)
  a. Bladder cancer, primary or metastatic, requiring cystectomy—fourth most common cancer in the United States
  b. Neurogenic bladder, such as may occur following spinal cord injury
  c. Severe radiation injury to the bladder
  d. Intractable incontinence
  e. Chronic pelvic pain syndromes

III. Statistics
  a. Morbidity: In 2008, an estimated 68,810 new cases of bladder cancer were reported in the United States; male-to-female ratio is 2.6:1; in 2005, median age at diagnosis was age 73 (National Cancer Institute [NCI], 2008).
  b. Mortality: Rate is reportedly 1% to 3% for radical cystectomy, often associated with advanced age and comorbidities (Lohr & Sherk, 2004).

GLOSSARY

Appliance: Pouch and accessories worn over stoma to collect urine.

Clean intermittent catheterization (CIC): Placement of a catheter to remove urine from the body. This is usually done by placing the catheter through the urethra, but may also be done by inserting the catheter through the opening of the reservoir.

Colonic conduit: Similar to an ileal conduit, but uses a segment of colon instead of ileum.

Continent urinary diversions: Ureters carry urine to a pouch or reservoir created inside the body from a section of stomach or small or large intestine. A stoma may or may not be required.

Cystectomy: Surgical removal of the urinary bladder.

Ileal conduit: Ureters are anastomosed to a segment of ileum, usually 15 to 20 cm long, and resected with the blood supply intact. The proximal section is closed, and the distal end is brought through an opening in the skin to form a stoma or a passageway, not a storage reservoir.

Incontinent or noncontinent urinary diversions: Urine flows through ureters directly anastomosed to the abdominal wall (cutaneous ureterostomy), or into a short segment of ileum or colon also attached to the abdominal wall where the urine drains into an external collecting device through a permanent stoma.

Interrupted anastomosis: Loss of the surgical connection of two hollow organs.

Intractable incontinence: Loss of bladder control that becomes impossible to manage, alleviate, or remedy.

Kegel exercises: Pelvic muscle exercises intended to improve pelvic muscle tone and prevent urine leakage for sufferers of stress urinary incontinence.

Kock reservoir or Indiana (ileocecal) pouch: A section of intestine is used to form a pouch inside the client's abdomen, creating a reservoir that the client periodically drains by inserting a catheter through the nipple valve—or a one-way valve integrated into a stoma—thus negating the need for an external collecting device.

Neobladder: Most closely resembles the normal urinary anatomy by using a section of intestine to form a pouch inside the abdomen, creating a reservoir that is then attached to the urethra. The client is able to urinate spontaneously using abdominal muscles to push the urine through the urethra to void; however, intermittent catheterization may be required to manage incomplete emptying of the reservoir.

Peristomal: Skin around and closest to the stoma.

Stoma: An opening which, when used in reference to ostomy care, is the segment of bowel or ureter brought to the surface of the abdomen. It is formed of mucosal tissue and is red and moist in appearance.

Ureterostomy: The ureter(s) is brought directly through the abdominal wall to form its own stoma.

Urostomy: Surgically constructed method of bypassing a dysfunctional or removed bladder in order to discharge urine. Most commonly, a conduit is created from a section of the ileum, and the ureters are connected to it. The open end of the conduit is brought to the abdomen to create a stoma.

Valsalva's maneuver: Performed by holding the breath and bearing down as may be done when straining with bowel movements or to force urine from continent reservoir out through urethra.

Care Setting

Client is treated in acute surgical unit.

Related Concerns

Cancer, page 846
Peritonitis, page 349
Psychosocial aspects of care, page 749
Surgical intervention, page 782

Client Assessment Database

Data depend on underlying problem, duration, and severity, for example, malignant bladder tumor, congenital malformations, trauma, chronic infections, or intractable incontinence due to injury or disease of other body systems, such as with multiple sclerosis. (Refer to appropriate CP.)

DIAGNOSTIC DIVISION MAY REPORT	MAY EXHIBIT
TEACHING/LEARNING	
• *Discharge plan considerations:* May require assistance with management of ostomy and acquisition of supplies	
▸ Refer to section at end of plan for postdischarge considerations.	

TEST WHY IT IS DONE	WHAT IT TELLS ME
URINE TESTS • *Urine cytology:* Urine is examined under a microscope to look for cancerous or precancerous cells.	Detects cancer markers in urine for determining presence and type of tumor.
OTHER DIAGNOSTIC STUDIES • *Intravenous pyelogram (IVP) and retrograde pyelogram:* X-ray examination and fluoroscopic visualization of the kidneys, ureters, and bladder using contrast material. Retrograde pyelogram requires cystoscopy and the placement of a small tube into the lower part of the ureter to inject contrast and opacify the ureter and renal pelvis.	Shows size, shape, and location of urinary structures. Identifies filling defects caused by tumors or other obstructive disorders. Retrograde pyelogram may also be done to delineate urinary tract system anatomy in preparation for surgery.
• *Cystoscopy with biopsy:* Diagnostic procedure that uses a cystoscope (endoscope), which is specially designed to examine the bladder, lower urinary tract, and prostate gland. It can also be used to perform biopsies. Ultraviolet cystoscopy outlines bladder lesions. Bladder washings can also be done during cystoscopy for cytological evaluation.	Initially, may be done to evaluate painless hematuria. If bladder tumor is detected, biopsy will be done to stage the malignancy.
• *Pelvic magnetic resonance imaging (MRI) or computed tomography (CT) scans:* Imaging techniques that use x-rays, or magnetic energy, and computer analysis to provide a complete picture of pelvic body tissues and structures.	Defines size of tumor mass and degree of cancer spread into surrounding tissues.

Nursing Priorities

1. Prevent complications.
2. Assist client and significant other (SO) in physical and psychosocial adjustment.
3. Support independence in self-care.
4. Provide information about procedure, prognosis, treatment needs, potential complications, and resources.

Discharge Goals

1. Complications prevented or minimized.
2. Adjusting to perceived or actual changes.
3. Self-care needs met by self or with assistance, as necessary.
4. Procedure, prognosis, therapeutic regimen, and potential complications understood and sources of support identified.
5. Plan in place to meet needs after discharge.

This plan of care primarily addresses the nursing care of the client with incontinent urinary diversion with a permanent stoma and urine-collecting device.

NURSING DIAGNOSIS: risk for impaired Skin Integrity

Risk factors may include
Absence of sphincter at stoma (actual) with continuous flow of urine
Character and flow of urine from stoma
Reaction to product or chemicals, improper fitting of appliance or removal of adhesive

Possibly evidenced by
(Not applicable; presence of signs and symptoms establishes an *actual* diagnosis)

Desired Outcomes/Evaluation Criteria—Client Will

Tissue Integrity: Skin and Mucous Membranes (NOC)
Maintain skin integrity.

Ostomy Self-Care (NOC)
Identify individual risk factors.
Demonstrate behaviors and techniques to promote healing and prevent skin breakdown.

ACTIONS/INTERVENTIONS	RATIONALE

Ostomy Care (NIC)

Independent

Inspect stoma and peristomal skin. Note irritation, bruises, rashes, and status of sutures.

Stoma should be pink or reddish, similar to mucous membranes. Color changes may be temporary, but persistent changes may require surgical intervention. Early identification of stomal ischemia or fungal infection provides for timely interventions to prevent skin necrosis.

Clean with water and pat dry, or use hair dryer on cool setting.

Maintaining a clean and dry peristomal area helps prevent skin breakdown.

Touch stoma gently to prevent irritation.

Mucosa has good blood supply and bleeds easily with rubbing or trauma.

Measure stoma periodically, for example, each appliance change for first 6 weeks, then monthly times six.

As postoperative edema resolves, size of appliance must be altered to ensure proper fit so that urine is collected as it flows from the stoma and contact with the skin is prevented.

Apply effective sealant barrier, such as Skin Prep or similar product, as recommended by appliance manufacturer.

Protects skin from pouch adhesive, enhances adhesiveness of pouch, and facilitates removal of pouch when necessary. *Note:* Some barriers are designed to be used without skin sealant.

Ensure proper opening for adhesive backing of pouch. Using a stoma-measuring guide or ostomy sizer, find the smallest opening that fits over the stoma and does not allow any skin exposure. Cut the barrier to size with adequate adhesive area left to apply pouch.

Prevents trauma to the stoma tissue and protects the peristomal skin. Adequate adhesive area is important to maintain a seal. *Note:* Too tight a fit may cause stomal edema or stenosis.

Use a transparent, odor-proof drainable pouch. Keep gauze square over stoma while cleansing area, and have client cough or strain before applying skin barrier wafer.

A transparent appliance during first 4 to 6 weeks allows easy observation of stoma and stents when used, without necessity of removing appliance and irritating skin. Covering stoma prevents urine from wetting the peristomal area during pouch changes. Coughing empties distal portion of conduit, followed by a brief pause in drainage to facilitate application of appliance.

Avoid use of karaya-type appliances.

Will not protect skin because urine melts karaya.

Apply waterproof tape around pouch edges, if desired.

Reinforces anchoring to help maintain seal.

Connect collecting pouch to continuous bedside drainage system when necessary.

May be needed during times when rate of urine formation is increased, such as while intravenous (IV) fluids are administered. Weight of the urine can cause pouch to pull loose and leak when pouch becomes more than half full.

Cleanse ostomy pouch on a routine basis, using vinegar solution or commercial solution designed for this purpose.

Frequent pouch changes are irritating to the skin and should be avoided. Emptying and rinsing the pouch with vinegar or commercial solution not only removes bacteria but also deodorizes the pouch.

Change appliance every 3 to 5 days, or as needed for leakage. Remove appliance gently while supporting skin. Use adhesive removers as indicated and wash off completely.

Prevents tissue irritation or damage associated with pulling skin barrier wafer off.

Investigate reports of burning or itching around stoma.

Suggests peristomal irritation or possibly *Candida* infection, both requiring intervention. *Note:* Continuous exposure of skin to urine can cause hyperplasia around stoma, affecting pouch fit and increasing risk of infection.

Evaluate adhesive product and appliance fit on an ongoing basis.

Provides opportunity for problem-solving. Determines need for further intervention.

Monitor for distention of lower abdomen in presence of ileal conduit; assess bowel sounds.

Intestinal distention can cause tension on new suture lines with possibility of rupture.

Collaborative

Consult with ostomy nurse specialist.

Ostomy nurse specialist can help client and caregiver by providing support and education, helping with problem-solving and choosing products appropriate for client's stoma characteristics, evaluating physical and mental status, and seeking financial resources. The client or caregiver should be capable of changing ostomy appliance prior to discharge or receive home care until such time as the client is competent (Colwell et al, 2001).

Apply antifungal spray or powder, as indicated.

Assists in healing if peristomal irritation is caused by fungal infection. *Note:* These products can have potent side effects and should be used sparingly. Creams and ointments are to be avoided because they interfere with adhesion of the appliance.

NURSING DIAGNOSIS: disturbed Body Image

May be related to

Biophysical—presence of stoma, loss of control of urine elimination

Psychosocial—altered body structure

Disease process and associated treatment regimen, such as cancer

Possibly evidenced by

Verbalization of change in body image, fear of rejection and reaction of others, and negative feelings about body

Actual change in structure and function (ostomy)

Not touching or looking at stoma, refusal to participate in care

Desired Outcomes/Evaluation Criteria—Client Will

Body Image NOC

Demonstrate beginning acceptance by viewing and touching stoma and participating in self-care.

Verbalize feelings about stoma and illness; begin to deal constructively with situation.

Verbalize acceptance of self in situation, incorporating change into self-concept without negating self-esteem.

ACTIONS/INTERVENTIONS	RATIONALE
Body Image Enhancement NIC	
Independent	
Review reason for surgery and future expectations.	Client may find it easier to accept and deal with an ostomy done for chronic or long-term disease, such as intractable incontinence or infections, than for traumatic injury or cancer.
Ascertain whether counseling was initiated when the possibility or necessity of urinary diversion was first discussed.	Provides information about client's and SO's levels of knowledge about individual situation and process of acceptance. Client with new ostomy is also often struggling to adjust to cancer or other devastating medical condition requiring the diversion.
Answer all questions concerning urostomy and its function.	Establishes rapport and conveys interest and concern of caregiver. Provides additional information for client to consider.
Encourage client and SO to verbalize feelings. Acknowledge normality of feelings of anger, depression, and grief over loss.	Provides opportunity to deal with issues and misconceptions. Helps client and SO to realize that feelings are not unusual and that feeling guilty for them is not helpful.
Note behaviors of withdrawal, increased dependency, manipulation, or noninvolvement in care.	Suggestive of problems in adjustment that may require further evaluation and more extensive therapy. May reflect grief response to loss of body part and function, worry over acceptance by others, and fear of further disability or loss of life from cancer.
Provide opportunities for client and SO to view and touch stoma, using the moment to point out positive signs of healing, normal appearance, and so forth.	Although integration of stoma into body image can take months or even years, looking at the stoma and hearing comments made in a normal, matter-of-fact manner can help client with this process. Touching stoma reassures client and SO that it is not fragile and that slight movements of stoma actually reflect normal peristalsis.
Provide opportunity for client to deal with ostomy through participation in self-care.	Independence in self-care helps improve self-esteem. In the case of a continent diversion, client needs the energy, ability, and time to intubate the stoma a minimum of four times a day.
Maintain positive approach during care activities, avoiding expressions of disdain or revulsion. Do not take client's angry expressions personally.	Assists client and SO to accept body changes and feel all right about self. Anger is most often directed at the situation and lack of control individual has over what has happened.
Plan stoma care activities with client.	Promotes client's sense of control and gives message that client can handle this situation, enhancing self-esteem.
Discuss contacting ostomy or urostomy visitor and make arrangements for visit if client desires.	Can provide a good support system. Shared experiences can facilitate acceptance of change as client realizes "life does go on" and can be relatively normal.
Discuss sexual functioning and potential physical changes that may occur or medications that effect sexual function, if applicable. (Refer to ND: risk for Sexual Dysfunction.)	Client may experience anticipatory anxiety and fear of failure in relation to sex after surgery, usually because of lack of knowledge. Surgery that removes the bladder and prostate (removed with the bladder) may disrupt parasympathetic nerve fibers that control erection in men, although newer techniques are available that may be used in individual cases to preserve nerve function.

NURSING DIAGNOSIS: acute Pain

May be related to

Physical factors—disruption of skin and tissues (incisions and drains)

Biological factors—activity of disease process (cancer, trauma)

Psychological factors—fear, anxiety

Possibly evidenced by

Reports of pain

Guarding, distraction behaviors, restlessness

Self-focusing

Autonomic responses, such as changes in vital signs

Desired Outcomes/Evaluation Criteria—Client Will

Pain Level (NOC)

Verbalize relief or control of pain.

Appear relaxed and be able to sleep and rest appropriately.

Pain Control (NOC)

Perform general comfort measures.

ACTIONS/INTERVENTIONS	RATIONALE
Pain Management (NIC) *Independent* Assess pain, noting location, characteristics, and intensity (0 to 10 scale).	Helps evaluate degree of discomfort and effectiveness of analgesia or may reveal developing complications. Surgical causes for abdominal pain usually subside gradually as healing begins. Continued or increasing pain may be a sign of infection or intestinal obstruction.
Auscultate bowel sounds; note passage of flatus.	Indicates reestablishment of bowel function. Lack of return of bowel sounds and function within 72 hours may indicate presence of complication, such as peritonitis, hypokalemia, or mechanical obstruction.
Note urine flow and characteristics, and evaluate need for more intensive interventions.	Decreased flow may reflect urinary retention due to edema with increased pressure in upper urinary tract organs or leakage into peritoneal cavity with failure of anastomosis. Cloudy urine may be normal with presence of mucus from intestinal tract or may indicate infectious process.
Encourage client to verbalize concerns. Active-listen these concerns and provide support by acceptance, remaining with client and giving appropriate information.	Reduction of anxiety and fear can promote relaxation and comfort.
Provide comfort measures, such as back rub, repositioning, and ambulating. Assure client that position change will not injure stoma.	Activity, movement, and comfort measures can reduce muscle tension, promote relaxation, and enhance coping abilities.
Encourage use of relaxation techniques, such as guided imagery, visualization, and diversional activities.	Helps client rest more effectively and refocuses attention, which may enhance coping ability, reducing pain and discomfort.
Assist with range-of-motion (ROM) exercises and encourage early ambulation.	Reduces muscle and joint stiffness. Ambulation returns organs to normal position, promotes return of gastrointestinal (GI) peristalsis, and enhances feelings of general well-being.
Investigate and report abdominal muscle rigidity, involuntary guarding, and rebound tenderness.	Suggestive of peritoneal inflammation, requiring prompt medical intervention.
Collaborative Administer medications as indicated, such as opioids, analgesics, and patient-controlled analgesia (PCA).	Relieves pain, enhances comfort, and promotes rest. PCA may be more beneficial than intermittent analgesia, especially following radical resection.
Provide sitz baths, if indicated.	Relieves local discomfort, reduces edema, and promotes healing of perineal wound associated with radical procedure.
Apply and monitor effects of transcutaneous electrical nerve stimulator (TENS) unit.	Cutaneous stimulation may be used to block transmission of pain stimulus.
Maintain patency of nasogastric (NG) tube.	Decompresses stomach and intestines; prevents abdominal distention when intestinal function is impaired.

NURSING DIAGNOSIS: risk for Infection

Risk factors may include
Inadequate primary defenses—break in skin or incision, reflux of urine into urinary tract

Possibly evidenced by
(Not applicable; presence of signs and symptoms establishes an *actual* diagnosis)

Desired Outcomes/Evaluation Criteria—Client Will

Immune Status (NOC)
Achieve timely wound healing, be free of purulent drainage or erythema, and be afebrile.

Knowledge: Infection Control (NOC)
Verbalize understanding of individual causative or risk factors.
Demonstrate techniques or lifestyle changes to reduce risk.

ACTIONS/INTERVENTIONS	RATIONALE
Infection Protection (NIC)	
Independent	
Empty ostomy pouch when it becomes one-third full, once continuous pouch drainage is discontinued.	Reduces risk of urinary reflux and maintains integrity of appliance seal if pouch does not have an antireflux valve.
Document urine characteristics and note whether changes are associated with reports of flank pain.	Cloudy, odorous urine indicates infection, possibly pyelonephritis; however, urine normally contains mucus after a conduit procedure because of normal secretions of the intestine.
Report sudden cessation of urethral drainage.	Constant drainage usually subsides within 10 days; however, abrupt cessation may indicate plugging and lead to abscess formation.
Note red rash around stoma.	Rash is most commonly caused by yeast. Urine leakage or allergy to appliance or products may also cause red, irritated areas.
Inspect incision line around stoma. Observe and document wound drainage, signs of incisional inflammation, and systemic indicators of sepsis.	Provides baseline and comparative reference. Complications may include interrupted anastomosis of intestine or ureteral conduit, with leakage of bowel contents into abdomen or urine into peritoneal cavity.
Change dressings, as indicated, when used.	Moist dressings act as a wick to the wound and provide media for bacterial growth.
Assess skinfold areas in groin, perineum, and under arms and breasts.	Use of antibiotics and trapping of moisture in skinfold areas increases risk of *Candida* infections.
Monitor vital signs.	An elevated temperature suggests incisional infection, urinary tract infection (UTI), or respiratory complications.
Auscultate breath sounds.	Client is at high risk for development of respiratory complications because of length of time under anesthesia. Often this client is older and may already have a compromised immune system. Also, painful abdominal incisions cause client to breathe more shallowly than normal and to limit coughing effort. Accumulation of secretions in respiratory tract predisposes to atelectasis and infections.
Collaborative	
Use pouch with antireflux valve, if available.	Prevents backflow of urine into stoma, reducing risk of infection.
Obtain specimens of exudates, urine, sputum, and blood, as indicated.	Identifies source of infection and most effective treatment. Infected urine may cause pyelonephritis. *Note:* Urine specimen must be obtained from the conduit because the pouch is considered contaminated.
Administer medications, as indicated, for example:	
Cephalosporins, such as cefoxitin (Mefoxin) and cefazolin (Ancef)	Given to treat identified infection or may be given prophylactically, especially with history of recurrent pyelonephritis.
Antifungal powder	Used to treat yeast infections around stoma.

NURSING DIAGNOSIS: impaired Urinary Elimination

May be related to
Surgical diversion, tissue trauma, postoperative edema

Possibly evidenced by
Loss of continence
Changes in amount, character of urine; urinary retention

Desired Outcomes/Evaluation Criteria—Client Will

Urinary Elimination
Display continuous flow of urine, with output adequate for individual situation.

ACTIONS/INTERVENTIONS	RATIONALE
Urinary Elimination Management (NIC)	
Independent	
Evaluate and maintain urinary catheters and drains in the immediate postoperative period.	Most clients have Foley catheter, possibly a suprapubic catheter, and pelvic drains during perioperative phase, especially when neobladder has been constructed. Although pelvic drains and ureteral stents are usually removed within 7 to 10 days, the catheters will stay in place during the healing time (Costa & Kreder, 2006).
Note presence of stents or ureteral catheters. Label "right" and "left" and observe urine flow through each.	Stents and ureteral catheters are placed during surgery to facilitate healing of internal anastomosis by keeping it urine free. It is necessary to verify that both kidneys and ureters are functional.
Record urinary output. Investigate sudden reduction or cessation of urine flow.	Sudden decrease in urine flow may indicate obstruction or dysfunction, such as blockage by edema or mucus, or dehydration. *Note:* Reduced urinary output not related to hypovolemia, associated with abdominal distention, fever, and clear, watery discharge from incision, suggests urinary fistula, also requiring prompt intervention.
Observe and record color of urine. Note hematuria or bleeding from stoma.	Urine may be slightly pink, which should clear up in 2 to 3 days. Rubbing or washing stoma may cause temporary oozing because of vascular nature of mucosal tissues. Continued bleeding, frank blood in the pouch, or oozing around the base of stoma requires medical evaluation and intervention.
Position tubing and drainage pouch so that it allows unimpeded flow of urine. Monitor and protect stents.	Blocked drainage allows pressure to build within urinary tract, risking anastomosis leakage and damage to renal parenchyma. *Note:* Stents inserted to maintain patency of ureters during period of postoperative edema may be inadvertently dislodged, compromising urine flow.
Demonstrate self-catheterization techniques and reservoir irrigations, as appropriate.	After a healing time of several weeks, catheters will be removed, and new voiding techniques initiated. Some clients with neobladders can void spontaneously, whereas others void by sitting down and performing Valsalva's maneuver. Clients should learn CIC in the event they cannot void spontaneously. Periodic irrigations with sterile water or saline are needed in the continent reservoir to remove accumulated mucus.
Encourage increased fluids and maintain accurate intake.	Maintains hydration and good urine flow.
Monitor vital signs. Assess peripheral pulses, skin turgor, capillary refill, and oral mucosa. Weigh daily.	Indicators of fluid balance. Reflects level of hydration and effectiveness of fluid replacement therapy.
Collaborative	
Administer fluids, as indicated.	Assists in maintaining hydration and adequate circulating volume and urinary flow.
Monitor electrolytes and arterial blood gases (ABGs).	Impaired renal function in client with intestinal conduit increases risk of severe electrolyte or acid-base problems, such as hyperchloremic acidosis.
Prepare for diagnostic testing and procedures, as indicated.	Retrograde ileogram may be done to evaluate patency of conduit; nephrostomy tube or stents may be inserted to maintain urine flow until edema or obstruction is resolved.

NURSING DIAGNOSIS: risk for Sexual Dysfunction

Risk factors may include
Altered body structure and function, radical resection, treatment procedures
Vulnerability, psychological concern about response of SO
Disruption of sexual response pattern, such as erection difficulty

Possibly evidenced by
(Not applicable; presence of signs and symptoms establishes an *actual* diagnosis)

Desired Outcomes/Evaluation Criteria—Client Will

Sexual Functioning (NOC)
Verbalize understanding of relationship of physical condition to sexual problems.
Identify satisfying, acceptable sexual practices and explore alternative methods.
Resume sexual relationship, as appropriate.

ACTIONS/INTERVENTIONS	RATIONALE
Sexual Counseling (NIC)	
Independent	
Ascertain client and SO's sexual relationship before surgery, if possible. Identify future expectations and desires.	Mutilation and loss of control of a bodily function can affect client's view of personal sexuality. When coupled with the fear of rejection by a partner, the desired level of intimacy can be greatly impaired. Sexual needs are very basic, and client will be rehabilitated more successfully when a satisfying sexual relationship is continued or developed. *Note:* Even with nerve-sparing procedures, 15% to 50% of men will experience erectile dysfunction, and 30% to 40% of women will experience painful intercourse (Costa & Kreder, 2006).
Review with client and SO anatomy and physiology of sexual functioning in relation to own situation.	Understanding normal physiology helps client and SO understand the mechanisms of nerve damage and need for exploring alternative methods of satisfaction.
Reinforce information given by the physician. Encourage questions. Provide additional information as needed.	Reiteration of previously given information assists client and SO to hear and process the knowledge again, moving toward acceptance of individual limitations or restrictions and prognosis; for example, that it may take months to regain potency after a radical procedure or that a penile prosthesis may be necessary.
Discuss resumption of sexual activities, beginning slowly and progressing, such as cuddling and caressing until both partners are comfortable with body image and function changes. Include alternative methods of stimulation, as appropriate.	Knowing what to expect in progress of recovery helps client avoid performance anxiety and reduce risk of "failure." If the couple is willing to try new ideas, this can assist with adjustment and may help achieve sexual fulfillment.
Encourage dialogue between client and SO. Suggest wearing pouch cover, T-shirt, or short nightgown.	Disguising urostomy appliance may aid in reducing feelings of self-consciousness and embarrassment during sexual activity.
Stress awareness of factors that might be distracting— unpleasant odors and pouch leakage.	Promotes resolution of solvable problems.
Encourage use of sense of humor.	Laughter can help individuals deal more effectively with difficult situation and promote a positive sexual experience.
Problem-solve alternative positions for coitus.	Minimizing awkwardness of appliance and physical discomfort can enhance satisfaction.
Discuss and role-play possible interactions or approaches when dealing with new sexual partners.	Rehearsal helps deal with actual situations when they arise, preventing self-consciousness about "different" body image.
Provide birth control information, as appropriate, and stress that impotence does not mean client is necessarily sterile.	Confusion about impotency and sterility can lead to an unwanted pregnancy.
Collaborative	
Arrange meeting with an ostomy visitor or support group, if appropriate.	Sharing of how these problems have been resolved by others can be helpful and reduce sense of isolation.
Refer for counseling or sex therapy, as indicated.	If problems persist longer than several months after surgery, a trained therapist may be required to facilitate communication between client and partner.

NURSING DIAGNOSIS: **deficient Knowledge [Learning Need] regarding condition, prognosis, treatment, self-care, and discharge needs**

May be related to
Lack of exposure or recall, information misinterpretation
Unfamiliarity with information resources

Possibly evidenced by
Questions, statement of misconception or misinformation
Inaccurate follow-through of instruction or performance of urostomy care
Inappropriate or exaggerated behaviors—hostile, agitated, apathetic, withdrawn

Desired Outcomes/Evaluation Criteria—Client Will

Knowledge: Disease Process (NOC)
Verbalize understanding of condition, disease process, prognosis, and potential complications.

Ostomy Self-Care (NOC)
Verbalize understanding of therapeutic needs.
Correctly perform necessary procedures and explain reasons for the action.
Initiate necessary lifestyle changes.

ACTIONS/INTERVENTIONS	RATIONALE
Teaching: Disease Process (NIC)	
Independent	
Evaluate client's emotional and physical capabilities.	These factors affect client's ability to master tasks and willingness to assume responsibility for ostomy care.
Review anatomy, physiology, and implications of surgical intervention. Discuss future expectations.	Provides knowledge base from which client can make informed choices and an opportunity to clarify misconceptions regarding individual situation.
Include written and picture resources.	Provides references after discharge to support client efforts for independence in self-care.
Instruct client/SO in stomal care, as appropriate. Allow time for return demonstrations and provide positive feedback for efforts.	Promotes positive management and reduces risk of improper ostomy care.
Ensure that stoma and appliance are odorless and nonleaking.	When client feels confident about urostomy, energy and attention can be focused on other tasks.
Demonstrate padding to absorb urethral drainage; ask client to report changes in amount, odor, and character.	Small amount of leakage may continue for several weeks after prostate surgery with bladder left in place—a temporary diversion procedure.
Recommend routine trimming of hair around stoma to edges of pouch adhesive.	Hair can be pulled out when the pouch is changed, causing irritation of hair follicles and increasing risk of local infection.
Encourage clients with Kock pouch to lengthen voiding interval each week unless discomfort noted.	Increases capacity of reservoir to achieve a more normal voiding pattern. Presence of discomfort suggests reservoir is full, necessitating prompt emptying.
Review signs of reservoir overdistention and need for immediate medical intervention.	Client and caregiver will need to recognize signs, such as lower abdominal pain accompanied by feelings of fullness, bloating, or nausea associated with reservoir overdistention. Severe overdistention can result in neobladder rupture, a life-threatening complication (Clark & DuBois, 2005).
Instruct client in a progressive exercise program to include Kegel exercises that stop and start urinary stream.	Improves tone of pelvic muscles and the external sphincter to enhance continence when client voids through urethra.
Encourage optimal nutrition.	Promotes wound healing and increases utilization of energy to facilitate tissue repair. Anorexia may be present for several months postoperatively, requiring conscious effort to meet nutritional needs.
Discuss use of acid-ash diet: cranberries, prunes, plums, cereals, rice, peanuts, noodles, cheese, poultry, and fish; avoidance of salt substitutes, sodium bicarbonate, and antacids; and cautious use of products containing calcium.	May be useful in acidifying urine to decrease risk of infection and crystal or stone formation. Products containing bicarbonate or calcium potentiate risk of crystal and stone formation affecting both urinary flow and tissue integrity. *Note:* Use of sulfa drugs requires alkaline urine for optimal absorption, necessitating acid-ash diet and vitamin C supplements withheld.
Discuss importance of maintaining normal weight.	Changes in weight can affect size of stoma and appliance fit. *Note:* Weight loss of 10 to 20 lb is not uncommon because of intestinal involvement and anorexia.

(continues on page 588)

ACTIONS/INTERVENTIONS (continued)	RATIONALE (continued)
Stress necessity of increased fluid intake of at least 2 to 3 L/day and cranberry juice or ascorbic acid and vitamin C tablets. Explain to client that urine should be pale yellow to almost colorless.	Maintains urinary output and promotes acidic urine to reduce risk of infection and stone formation. *Note:* Oranges and citrus fruits make urine alkaline and are therefore contraindicated. Large doses of vitamin C can inhibit vitamin B_{12} absorption, requiring periodic monitoring of vitamin B_{12} levels.
Discuss resumption of presurgery level of activity and possibility of sleep disturbance, anorexia, and loss of interest in usual activities.	Client should be able to manage same degree of activity as previously enjoyed and in some cases increase activity level, except for contact sports. "Homecoming depression" may occur, lasting for up to 3 months after surgery, requiring patience, support, and ongoing evaluation.
Encourage regular activity and exercise program.	Immobility or inactivity increases urinary stasis and calcium shift out of bones, potentiating risk of stone formation and resultant urinary obstruction or infection.
Emphasize need for smoking cessation, if indicated. Refer for medication and smoking cessation assistance, if client is cooperative.	Smoking cessation is critical to the health of the new bladder, ureters, and kidneys because of the vasoconstrictive, acidic, and carcinogenic effects of smoking (Costa & Kreder, 2006).
Identify signs and symptoms requiring medical evaluation: changes in character, amount, and flow of urine; unusual drainage from wound; fatigue or muscle weakness; anorexia; abdominal distention; and confusion.	Early detection and prompt intervention of developing problems such as UTI, stricture, and intestinal fistula, may prevent more serious complications. Urinary electrolytes, especially chloride, are reabsorbed in the intestinal conduit, which leads to compensatory bicarbonate loss, lowered serum pH or metabolic acidosis, and potassium deficit.
Stress importance of follow-up appointments.	Monitors healing and disease process and provides opportunity for discussion of appliance problems, general health, and adaptation to condition. *Note:* Bowel resection of the distal ileum creating ileal conduit can lead to vitamin B_{12} malabsorption. Therefore, long-term monitoring may be necessary as deficiency can lead to anemia, neurological problems, and anorexia (Clark & DuBois, 2005; Pieper et al, 2006).
Identify community resources, such as the United Ostomy Association, local ostomy support group, enterostomal therapist, visiting nurse, and pharmacy or medical supply house.	Continued support after discharge is essential to facilitate the recovery process and client's independence in care. Enterostomal nurse can be very helpful in solving appliance problems and identifying alternatives to meet individual client needs.

POTENTIAL CONSIDERATIONS following acute hospitalization (dependent on client's age, physical condition and presence of complications, personal resources, and life responsibilities)

In addition to postsurgical concerns:
- *impaired Urinary Elimination*—anatomic diversion
- *situational low Self-Esteem*—loss of or altered control of body function

BENIGN PROSTATIC HYPERPLASIA (BPH)

I. **Pathophysiology**
   a. Overgrowth of normal, nonmalignant cells that cause progressive enlargement of the prostate gland, resulting in bladder outlet obstruction with urinary retention, leakage, and frequency (Shiller, 2007)
   b. Additional complications: bladder wall trabeculation, detrusor muscle enlargement, narrowing of urethra, incontinence, and acute or chronic renal failure (Springhouse, 2005)

II. **Classification** (American Urological Association [AUA], 2003)
   a. International scoring system has been adopted worldwide.

   b. Questions, and subsequent scoring, focus on degree of incomplete emptying, frequency, intermittency, urgency, weak stream, straining, nocturia, as well as impact on quality of life.
      i. Score of 0 to 7: mildly symptomatic
      ii. Score of 8 to 19: moderately symptomatic
      iii. Score of 20 to 35: severely symptomatic

III. **Etiology**
   a. Cause is unknown, although testosterone and other hormones may affect growth.
   b. Microscopically characterized as a hyperplastic process with the number of cells in the gland increasing with age
   c. Most commonly seen in men older than age 50 years

IV. Statistics

a. Morbidity: An estimated 14 million men in the United States have symptoms related to benign enlargement (Leveillee et al, 2006); symptoms present in 50% of males by age 50 and 80% of males by age 80; accounts for 375,000 hospitalizations annually (Gilchrist, 2004).

b. Mortality: Generally related to renal failure, infection, and complications of surgery.

c. Cost: Direct and indirect costs to private sector related to BPH treatment estimated to be $3.9 billion (Saigal & Joyce, 2005).

GLOSSARY

Bladder outlet obstruction (BOO): Blockage at the base of the bladder causing compression of the urethra, thus reducing or preventing urine flow into the urethra.

Bladder wall trabeculation: Characterized by thick wall and hypertrophied muscle bundles; typically seen in instances of long-standing obstruction.

Dysuria: Painful, difficult urination.
Prostatitis: Inflammation of the prostate gland.

Care Settings

Client is treated at the community level, with more acute care provided during outpatient procedures.

Related Concerns

Prostatectomy, page 596
Psychosocial aspects of care, page 749
Renal failure: acute, page 536

Client Assessment Database

DIAGNOSTIC DIVISION MAY REPORT	MAY EXHIBIT
CIRCULATION	• Elevated blood pressure (BP)
ELIMINATION	• Firm mass in lower abdomen (distended bladder), bladder tenderness
• Feeling need to urinate urgently, sensation of imminent loss of urine without control	• Inguinal hernia, hemorrhoids—result of increased abdominal pressure required to empty bladder against resistance
• Hesitancy or straining in initiating voiding, having to stand at or sit on the toilet for some time prior to producing a urinary stream	
• Decreased force or caliber of urinary stream, intermittent flow, dribbling	
• Usually voiding only small amounts of urine with each episode, sensation of incomplete emptying	
• Need to urinate frequently during the day or night (nocturia), resulting in interrupted sleep	
• Dysuria, hematuria	
• Chronic constipation, resulting from protrusion of prostate into rectum	
FOOD/FLUID	
• Anorexia, nausea, vomiting	
• Recent weight loss	
PAIN/DISCOMFORT	
• Suprapubic, flank, or back pain; sharp, intense, with acute prostatitis	
• Low back pain	

(continues on page 590)

DIAGNOSTIC DIVISION MAY REPORT (continued)	MAY EXHIBIT (continued)
SAFETY • Fever **SEXUALITY** • Concerns about effects of condition or therapy on sexual abilities • Fear of incontinence or dribbling during intimacy • Decrease in force of ejaculatory contractions **TEACHING/LEARNING** • Family history of cancer, hypertension, kidney disease • Use of antihypertensive or antidepressant medications, over-the-counter (OTC) cold and allergy medications containing sympathomimetics, urinary antibiotics or antibacterial agents • Use of nutrients or herbal supplements for self-treatment of BPH and urinary flow—saw palmetto, pygeum, pumpkin seed oil, or soy products **DISCHARGE PLAN CONSIDERATIONS** • May need assistance with management of therapy—catheter ⬥ Refer to section at end of plan for postdischarge considerations.	• Enlarged, tender prostate

Diagnostic Studies

TEST WHY IT IS DONE	WHAT IT TELLS ME
BLOOD TESTS • *Prostate-specific antigen (PSA):* Substance manufactured solely by prostate gland cells. An elevated reading indicates an abnormal condition of the prostate gland, either benign or malignant. • *White blood cells (WBCs):* Responsible for fighting infection.	Level is greatly increased in prostatic cancer, but can also be elevated in BPH. May be more than 11,000, which indicates infection if client is not immunosuppressed.
URINE TESTS • *Urinalysis:* Laboratory examination of urine for red blood cells (RBCs) and WBCs or presence of infection or excessive protein. • *Post-void residual (PVR):* Volume of urine remaining in bladder immediately after voiding.	Yellow, dark brown, dark or bright red (bloody) in color; appearance may be cloudy, pH of 7 or greater suggests infection; and bacteria, WBCs, and RBCs may be present microscopically. Determines the severity of bladder decompensation; may be done by catheterization or by transabdominal ultrasound.
OTHER DIAGNOSTIC STUDIES • *Transrectal prostatic ultrasound (TRUS):* Examination where a fingerlike probe is placed in the rectum, and ultrasound pictures are made of the prostate. • *Digital rectal exam (DRE):* Test performed by inserting gloved finger into rectum to detect prostate abnormalities.	Measures size of prostate and amount of residual urine, locates lesions unrelated to BPH. For client with elevated PSA levels, a TRUS-guided biopsy may be indicated. Prostate size and contour can be assessed, nodules evaluated, and areas of suspected malignancy detected; also helps determine pelvic floor tone and fluctuance, such as in prostate abscess, and pain and sensitivity of gland can be assessed.

Diagnostic Studies (continued)

TEST WHY IT IS DONE (continued)	WHAT IT TELLS ME (continued)
• *Uroflowmetry:* Measures urine amount and flow rate via a collection device and scale. The equipment creates a graph that shows changes in flow rate from second to second, measuring peak flow rate and how long it took to get there. • *Intravenous pyelography (IVP):* Series of x-rays of the kidney, ureters, and bladder after injection of a contrast dye into a vein. • *Cystourethrography:* Allows visualization of the bladder and urethra on x-ray, using radiopaque contrast material injected through the urethra. • *Cystourethroscopy:* Direct visualization of the bladder and urethra by means of a flexible fiber-optic scope.	Results of this test will be abnormal if the bladder muscle is weak or urine flow is obstructed. Helps distinguish poor bladder contractibility (detrusor underactivity) from BOO caused by prostate hyperplasia. Shows any blockage in the urinary tract causing delayed emptying of bladder, urinary retention, or presence of prostatic enlargement May be used instead of IVP to visualize bladder and urethra because it uses localized, rather than systemic, radiopaque contrast media. Shows degree of prostatic enlargement and bladder wall changes associated with bladder trabeculation.

Nursing Priorities

1. Relieve acute urinary retention.
2. Promote comfort.
3. Prevent complications.
4. Help client deal with psychosocial concerns.
5. Provide information about disease process, prognosis, and treatment needs.

Discharge Goals

1. Voiding pattern normalized.
2. Pain or discomfort relieved.
3. Complications prevented or minimized.
4. Dealing with situation realistically.
5. Disease process, prognosis, and therapeutic regimen understood.
6. Plan in place to meet needs after discharge.

NURSING DIAGNOSIS: **[acute/chronic] Urinary Retention**

May be related to
Mechanical obstruction, enlarged prostate
Decompensation of detrusor musculature
Inability of bladder to contract adequately

Possibly evidenced by
Frequency, hesitancy, inability to empty bladder completely, incontinence and dribbling
Bladder distention, residual urine

Desired Outcomes/Evaluation Criteria—Client Will

Urinary Elimination (NOC)
Void in sufficient amounts with no palpable bladder distention.
Demonstrate postvoid residuals of less than 50 mL, with absence of dribbling or overflow.

ACTIONS/INTERVENTIONS	RATIONALE
Urinary Retention Care (NIC) *Independent* Encourage client to void every 2 to 4 hours and when urge is noted. Ask client about stress incontinence when moving, sneezing, coughing, laughing, or lifting objects. Observe urinary stream, noting size and force. Have client document time and amount of each voiding. Note diminished urinary output. Measure specific gravity, as indicated.	May minimize urinary retention and overdistention of the bladder. High urethral pressure inhibits bladder emptying or can inhibit voiding until abdominal pressure increases enough for urine to be involuntarily lost. Useful in evaluating degree of obstruction and choice of intervention. Urinary retention increases pressure within the ureters and kidneys, which may cause renal insufficiency. Any deficit in blood flow to the kidney impairs its ability to filter and concentrate substances.

(continues on page 592)

ACTIONS/INTERVENTIONS (continued)

Percuss and palpate suprapubic area.

Encourage oral fluids up to 3,000 mL daily, within cardiac tolerance, if indicated.

Monitor vital signs closely. Observe for hypertension, peripheral or dependent edema, and changes in mentation. Weigh daily. Maintain accurate intake and output (I&O).

Provide and encourage meticulous catheter and perineal care.

Recommend sitz bath, as indicated.

Collaborative

Administer medications, as indicated, for example:

5-α-reductase inhibitors, such as finasteride (Proscar) and dutasteride (Avodart)

Alpha-adrenergic antagonists, such as alfuzosin (UroXatral), terazosin (Hytrin), doxazosin (Cardura), and tamsulosin (Flomax)

Antispasmodics, such as oxybutynin (Ditropan)

Rectal suppositories (B&O)

Antibiotics and antibacterials

Catheterize for residual urine and leave indwelling catheter, as indicated.

Monitor laboratory studies, such as the following:

Blood urea nitrogen (BUN), creatinine (Cr), and electrolytes

Urinalysis and culture

Prepare for and assist with urinary drainage, such as emergency cystostomy.

Prepare for procedures, such as the following:

Heat therapies, such as laser, transurethral microwave thermotherapy (TUMT), Cortherm, Prostatron, and transurethral needle ablation (TUNA)

Other procedures, such as photoselective vaporization, also called laser ablation

RATIONALE (continued)

A distended bladder can be felt in the suprapubic area.

Increased circulating fluid maintains renal perfusion and flushes kidneys, bladder, and ureters of sediment and bacteria. *Note:* Fluids may be restricted to prevent bladder distention if severe obstruction is present or until adequate urinary flow is reestablished.

Loss of kidney function results in decreased fluid elimination and accumulation of toxic wastes; may progress to complete renal shutdown.

Reduces risk of ascending infection.

Promotes muscle relaxation, decreases edema, and may enhance voiding effort.

Medications have long been used as a first-line therapy for clients with mild to moderate symptoms, chosen primarily because of the perceived reduced risk of adverse events and the desire to avoid surgery.

Reduces the size of the prostate and decreases symptoms if taken long-term; however, side effects, such as decreased libido and ejaculatory dysfunction, may influence client's choice for long-term use. Studies indicate combination therapy with doxazosin and finasteride is superior to taking either drug alone for prevention of BPH-related disease progression (National Institute of Diabetes and Digestive and Kidney Diseases [NIDDK], 2003).

These agents block effects of postganglionic synapses that affect smooth muscle and exocrine glands. This action can decrease adverse urinary tract symptoms and increase urinary flow.

Relieves bladder spasms related to irritation by the catheter.

Suppositories are absorbed easily through mucosa into bladder tissue to produce muscle relaxation and to relieve bladder spasms.

Given to combat infection. May be used prophylactically.

Relieves and prevents urinary retention and rules out presence of ureteral stricture. Coudé catheter may be required because the curved tip eases passage of the tube around the enlarged prostate. *Note:* Bladder decompression should be done with caution to observe for signs of adverse reaction, such as hematuria due to rupture of blood vessels in the mucosa of the overdistended bladder and syncope due to excessive autonomic stimulation.

Prostatic enlargement with obstruction eventually causes dilation of upper urinary tract, ureters, and kidneys, potentially impairing kidney function and leading to uremia.

Urinary stasis potentiates bacterial growth, increasing risk of urinary tract infection (UTI).

May be indicated to drain bladder during acute episode with azotemia or when surgery is contraindicated because of client's health status.

Most minimally invasive therapies rely on heat to cause destruction of prostatic tissue. Heat is delivered in a limited and controlled fashion to the central portion of the prostate. Treatment is often completed in a one-time procedure carried out in the physician's office. Long-term outcomes are variable in terms of adequately treating urinary tract symptoms.

Procedure is done to quickly create a wide open prostatic fossa, often resulting in immediate restoration of normal urine flow. The procedure can be performed on an outpatient basis or short-stay settings. *Note:* Open prostate resection procedures, such as TURP, are typically performed on clients with very large prostate glands (Shiller, 2007). (Refer to CP: Prostatectomy, below.)

ACTIONS/INTERVENTIONS (continued)	RATIONALE (continued)
Urethral stent	Placement of urethral stent is simple and immediately effective for restoring patency of the urethral lumen. However, because long-term failure rate is high, this should be used only as a temporary measure until a more definitive procedure can be performed (AUA, 2003).

NURSING DIAGNOSIS: acute Pain

May be related to
Mucosal irritation—bladder distention, renal colic, urinary infection, radiation therapy

Possibly evidenced by
Reports of pain (bladder or rectal spasm)
Narrowed focus, altered muscle tone, grimacing, distraction behaviors, restlessness
Autonomic responses

Desired Outcomes/Evaluation Criteria—Client Will

Pain Level (NOC)
Report pain relieved or controlled.
Appear relaxed.
Be able to sleep and rest appropriately.

ACTIONS/INTERVENTIONS	RATIONALE
Pain Management (NIC)	
Independent	
Assess pain, noting location, intensity (scale of 0 to 10), characteristics, and duration.	Provides information to aid in determining choice and effectiveness of interventions.
Tape drainage tube to thigh and catheter to the abdomen, if traction not required.	Prevents accidental dislodging of catheter with attendant urethral trauma.
Provide comfort measures, such as back rub, helping client assume position of comfort. Suggest use of relaxation and deep-breathing exercises and diversional activities.	Promotes relaxation, refocuses attention, and may enhance coping abilities.
Encourage use of sitz baths and warm soaks to perineum.	Promotes muscle relaxation.
Collaborative	
Insert catheter and attach to straight drainage, as indicated.	Draining bladder reduces bladder tension and irritability.
Administer medications, as indicated, for example:	
Opioids, such as meperidine (Demerol)	Given to relieve severe pain; provide physical and mental relaxation.
Antibacterials, such as methenamine hippurate (Hiprex)	Reduces bacteria present in urinary tract and those introduced by drainage system.
Antispasmodics and bladder sedatives, such as flavoxate (Urispas) and oxybutynin (Ditropan)	Relieves bladder irritability.

NURSING DIAGNOSIS: risk for deficient Fluid Volume

Risk factors may include
Postobstructive diuresis from rapid drainage of a chronically overdistended bladder
Endocrine, electrolyte imbalances, such as in renal dysfunction

Possibly evidenced by
(Not applicable; presence of signs and symptoms establishes an *actual* diagnosis)

Desired Outcomes/Evaluation Criteria—Client Will

Hydration (NOC)
Maintain adequate hydration as evidenced by stable vital signs, palpable peripheral pulses, good capillary refill, and moist mucous membranes.

ACTIONS/INTERVENTIONS	RATIONALE

Fluid Management (NIC)

Independent

Monitor output carefully. Note outputs of 100 to 200 mL/hour.

Encourage increased oral intake based on individual needs.

Monitor BP and pulse. Evaluate capillary refill and oral mucous membranes.

Promote bedrest with head elevated.

Collaborative

Monitor electrolyte levels, especially sodium.

Administer intravenous (IV) fluids—hypertonic saline as needed.

Rapid or sustained diuresis could cause client's total fluid volume to become depleted and limits sodium reabsorption in renal tubules.

Client may have restricted oral intake in an attempt to control urinary symptoms, reducing homeostatic reserves and increasing risk of dehydration and hypovolemia.

Enables early detection of and intervention for systemic hypovolemia.

Decreases cardiac workload, facilitating circulatory homeostasis.

As fluid is pulled from extracellular spaces, sodium may follow the shift, causing hyponatremia.

Replaces fluid and sodium losses to prevent or correct hypovolemia following outpatient procedures.

NURSING DIAGNOSIS: **Fear/Anxiety [specify level]**

May be related to

Change in health status: possibility of surgical procedure or malignancy

Embarrassment; loss of dignity associated with genital exposure before, during, and after treatment; concern about sexual ability

Possibly evidenced by

Increased tension, apprehension, and worries

Expressed concerns regarding perceived changes

Fear of unspecific consequences

Desired Outcomes/Evaluation Criteria—Client Will

Anxiety [or] Fear Self-Control (NOC)

Appear relaxed.

Verbalize accurate knowledge of the situation.

Demonstrate appropriate range of feelings and lessened fear.

Report anxiety is reduced to a manageable level.

ACTIONS/INTERVENTIONS	RATIONALE

Anxiety Reduction (NIC)

Independent

Be available to client. Establish trusting relationship with client and significant other (SO).

Provide information about specific procedures and tests and what to expect afterward, such as catheter, bloody urine, and bladder irritation. Be aware of how much information client wants.

Maintain matter-of-fact attitude in doing procedures and dealing with client. Protect client's privacy.

Encourage client and SO to verbalize concerns and feelings.

Reinforce previous information client has been given.

Demonstrates concern and willingness to help. Encourages discussion of sensitive subjects.

Helps client understand purpose of what is being done and reduces concerns associated with the unknown, including fear of cancer. However, overload of information is not helpful and may increase anxiety.

Communicates acceptance and eases client's embarrassment.

Defines the problem, providing opportunity to answer questions, clarify misconceptions, and problem-solve solutions.

Allows client to deal with reality and strengthens trust in caregivers and information presented.

NURSING DIAGNOSIS: **deficient Knowledge [Learning Need] regarding condition, prognosis, treatment, self-care, and discharge needs**

May be related to

Lack of exposure or recall, information misinterpretation

Unfamiliarity with information resources

Concern about sensitive area

NURSING DIAGNOSIS: deficient Knowledge [Learning Need] regarding condition, prognosis, treatment, self-care, and discharge needs (continued)

Possibly evidenced by

Questions, request for information, verbalization of the problem

Inappropriate behaviors—apathetic, withdrawn

Inaccurate follow-through of instructions, development of preventable complications

Desired Outcomes/Evaluation Criteria—Client Will

Knowledge: Disease Process (NOC)

Verbalize understanding of disease process, prognosis, and potential complications.

Identify relationship of signs and symptoms to the disease process.

Knowledge: Treatment Regimen (NOC)

Verbalize understanding of therapeutic needs.

Initiate necessary lifestyle or behavior changes.

Participate in treatment regimen.

ACTIONS/INTERVENTIONS	RATIONALE
Teaching: Disease Process (NIC)	
Independent	
Review disease process and client expectations.	Provides knowledge base from which client can make informed therapy choices.
Encourage verbalization of fears, feelings, and concerns.	Helping client work through feelings can be vital to rehabilitation.
Give information that the condition is not sexually transmitted.	May be an unspoken fear.
Review drug therapy, use of herbal products, and diet, such as increasing intake of fruits and soybeans.	Some clients may prefer to treat with complementary therapy because of decreased occurrence and lessened severity of side effects, such as impotence. *Note:* Nutrients known to inhibit prostate enlargement include zinc, soy protein, essential fatty acids, flaxseed, and lycopene. Herbal supplements that client may use include saw palmetto, pygeum, stinging nettle, and pumpkin seed oil. *Note:* A recent study found no difference in efficacy or side effects between saw palmetto and a placebo, indicating a need for further research as to benefit versus variability of potency or purity of botanical products (Bent, 2006).
Recommend avoiding spicy foods, coffee, alcohol, long automobile rides, and rapid intake of fluids.	May cause prostatic irritation with resulting congestion. Sudden increase in urinary flow can cause bladder distention and loss of bladder tone, resulting in episodes of acute urinary retention.
Address sexual concerns—during acute episodes of prostatitis, intercourse should be avoided, but may be helpful in treatment of chronic condition.	Sexual activity can increase pain during acute episodes but may serve as massaging agent in presence of chronic disease. *Note:* Medications, such as finasteride (Proscar), are known to interfere with libido and erections. Alternatives include terazosin (Hytrin), doxazosin mesylate (Cardura), and tamsulosin (Flomax), which do not affect testosterone levels.
Provide information about sexual anatomy and function as it relates to prostatic enlargement. Encourage questions and promote a dialogue about concerns.	Having information about anatomy involved helps client understand the implications of proposed treatments because they might affect sexual performance.
Review signs and symptoms requiring medical evaluation—cloudy, odorous urine; diminished urinary output; inability to void; and presence of fever or chills.	Prompt interventions may prevent more serious complications.
Discuss necessity of notifying other healthcare providers of diagnosis.	Reduces risk of inappropriate therapy, such as the use of decongestants, anticholinergics, and antidepressants, which can increase urinary retention and may precipitate an acute episode.
Reinforce importance of medical follow-up for at least 6 months to 1 year, including rectal examination and urinalysis.	Recurrence of hyperplasia and infection caused by same or different organisms is not uncommon and requires changes in therapeutic regimen to prevent serious complications.
Discuss personal safety issues and potential environmental changes.	Recent research reports increased risk of falls in presence of moderate to severe BPH associated with urgency, nocturia, and straining to void, with fall risk increasing with age and symptom severity (Parsons et al, 2008).

595

POTENTIAL CONSIDERATIONS following acute hospitalization (dependent on client's age, physical condition and presence of complications, personal resources, and life responsibilities)
- *[acute/chronic] Urinary Retention*—urethral obstruction, decompensation of detrusor musculature, loss of bladder tone
- *risk for Infection*—urinary stasis, invasive procedure (periodic catheterization)

PROSTATECTOMY

I. Indications

a. Benign prostatic hyperplasia (BPH)-related complications
  i. Urinary retention
  ii. Frequent urinary tract infections
  iii. Bladder stones
  iv. Recurrent gross hematuria
  v. Kidney damage from long-standing blockage
  vi. Failure to respond to medical or minimally invasive treatments

b. Prostate cancer is the second leading cause of cancer death in the United States.

II. Procedures

a. Minimally invasive prostatectomy
  i. Transurethral therapy using microwave
  ii. Transurethral needle ablation (TUNA) using low-level frequency thermal energy
  iii. Laser ablation
  iv. Cryotherapy—freezing of cancerous cells
  v. Electrovaporization
  vi. Transurethral resection of the prostate (TURP)
    1. Most common procedure for the long-term treatment of BPH
    2. Obstructive prostatic tissue of the medial lobe surrounding the urethra is removed by means of a cystoscope introduced through the urethra.

b. Open surgical approaches performed when the prostate is overly enlarged (greater than 75 g), the bladder has been damaged, or when there are complicating factors, such as cancer.
  i. Robot assisted—nerve sparing, uses a laparoscope, and several incisions are made in the abdomen
  ii. Suprapubic prostatectomy
    1. Obstructing prostatic tissue is removed through a low midline incision made through the bladder.
    2. Preferred approach if bladder stones are present
  iii. Retropubic prostatectomy
    1. Hypertrophied prostatic tissue mass located high in the pelvic region is removed through a low abdominal incision without opening the bladder.
  iv. Perineal prostatectomy
    1. Laparoscopy removal of larger tumors or in presence of cancerous lymph nodes or nerve invasion
    2. Large prostatic masses low in the pelvic area are removed through an incision between the scrotum and the rectum.

III. Statistics

a. Morbidity: In 2005, 155,000 prostatectomy procedures were performed in short-stay hospitals in the United States (Centers for Disease Control and Prevention [CDC], 2007); in 2007, 50,000 procedures were robotic assisted.

b. Mortality: Prostatectomy is a relatively low-risk procedure (Guilli et al, n.d.).

c. Cost: In 2004, hospital costs for treatment of prostate cancer totaled $657 million; most commonly performed procedures are prostatectomy and TURP (Milenkovic et al, 2007).

GLOSSARY

Blood dyscrasias: General term used to describe any abnormality in the blood, such as low white blood cell (WBC) count, low red blood cell (RBC) count, or low platelet count.

Continuous bladder irrigation (CBI): Constant flow of normal saline or another bladder irrigant through a three-way urinary catheter to keep the catheter patent.

Hematuria: Blood in the urine.

Kegel exercises: Pelvic muscle exercises intended to improve pelvic muscle tone and prevent urine leakage for sufferers of stress urinary incontinence.

Prostatic fossa: Cavity or depression where the prostate gland lies.

Retropubic: Behind the pubic bone.

Suprapubic: Above the pubic bone.

Transurethral resection of the prostate (TURP) syndrome: Rare complication directly related to this procedure. During the surgery, excess fluid collects in the body, reducing the concentration of sodium in the bloodstream. Common symptoms include nausea, vomiting, and confusion.

Urinary retention: Inability to empty bladder.

Care Setting

Client is treated in inpatient acute surgical unit.

Related Concerns

Benign prostatic hyperplasia (BPH), page 588
Cancer, page 846
Psychosocial aspects of care, page 749
Surgical intervention, page 782

Client Assessment Database

Refer to CP: Benign Prostatic Hyperplasia (BPH), for assessment data.

DIAGNOSTIC DIVISION MAY REPORT	MAY EXHIBIT
DISCHARGE PLAN CONSIDERATIONS • Dependent upon type of procedure, needs may be minimal or client may require assistance with self-care needs, transportation, medical supplies, and home maintenance ▶ Refer to section at end of plan for postdischarge considerations.	

Nursing Priorities

1. Maintain homeostasis and hemodynamic stability.
2. Promote comfort.
3. Prevent complications.
4. Provide information about surgical procedure, prognosis, treatment, and rehabilitation needs.

Discharge Goals

1. Urinary flow restored or enhanced.
2. Pain relieved or controlled.
3. Complications prevented or minimized.
4. Procedure, prognosis, therapeutic regimen, and rehabilitation needs understood.
5. Plan in place to meet needs after discharge.

NURSING DIAGNOSIS: **impaired Urinary Elimination**

May be related to
Mechanical obstruction—blood clots, edema, trauma, surgical procedure
Pressure and irritation of catheter and balloon
Loss of bladder tone due to preoperative overdistention or continued decompression

Possibly evidenced by
Frequency, urgency, hesitancy, dysuria, incontinence, retention
Bladder fullness, suprapubic discomfort

Desired Outcomes/Evaluation Criteria—Client Will

Urinary Elimination (NOC)
Void normal amounts without retention.
Demonstrate behaviors to regain bladder and urinary control.

ACTIONS/INTERVENTIONS	RATIONALE
Urinary Elimination Management (NIC) *Independent* Assess urine output and catheter drainage system, especially during bladder irrigation. Assist client to assume normal position to void; for example, stand and walk to bathroom at frequent intervals after catheter is removed. Record time, amount of voiding, and size of stream after catheter is removed. Note reports of bladder fullness inability to void, and urgency.	Retention can occur because of edema of the surgical area, blood clots, and bladder spasms. Encourages passage of urine and promotes sense of normality. The catheter is usually removed 2 to 5 days after surgery, but voiding may continue to be a problem for some time because of urethral edema and loss of bladder tone.

(continues on page 598)

Encourage client to void when urge is noted but not more than every 2 to 4 hours per protocol.

Voiding with urge prevents urinary retention. Limiting voids to every 4 hours, if tolerated, increases bladder tone and aids in bladder retraining.

Encourage fluid intake to 2,000 to 2,500 mL as tolerated. Limit fluids in the evening once catheter is removed.

Maintains adequate hydration and renal perfusion for urinary flow. "Scheduling" fluid intake reduces need to void during the night.

Instruct client in perineal exercises, such as tightening buttocks and stopping and starting urine stream.

Helps regain bladder sphincter control, minimizing incontinence.

Advise client that "dribbling" is to be expected after catheter is removed and should resolve as recuperation progresses. Provide and instruct in use of continence pads when indicated.

Information helps client deal with the problem. Postoperative incontinence is usually temporary, but stress incontinence—leaking urine when coughing, laughing, and lifting—can persist indefinitely.

Collaborative

Maintain continuous bladder irrigation (CBI), as indicated, in early postoperative period.

Flushes bladder of blood clots and debris to maintain patency of the catheter and urinary flow.

Measure residual volumes via suprapubic catheter, if present, or with Doppler ultrasound.

Monitors effectiveness of bladder emptying. Residuals of more than 50 mL suggest need for continuation of catheter until bladder tone improves.

NURSING DIAGNOSIS: risk for deficient Fluid Volume/Bleeding

Risk factors may include
Vascular nature of surgical area, difficulty controlling bleeding
Restricted intake preoperatively
Postobstructive diuresis

Possibly evidenced by
(Not applicable; presence of signs and symptoms establishes an *actual* diagnosis)

Desired Outcomes/Evaluation Criteria—Client Will

Hydration (NOC)
Maintain adequate hydration as evidenced by stable vital signs, palpable peripheral pulses, good capillary refill, moist mucous membranes, and appropriate urinary output.
Display no active bleeding.

ACTIONS/INTERVENTIONS

RATIONALE

Fluid Management (NIC)
Independent
Monitor intake and output (I&O).

Indicator of fluid balance and replacement needs. With bladder irrigations, monitoring is essential for estimating blood loss and accurately assessing urine output. *Note:* Following release of urinary tract obstruction, marked diuresis may occur during initial recovery period.

Monitor vital signs, noting increased pulse and respiration, decreased blood pressure (BP), diaphoresis, pallor, delayed capillary refill, and dry mucous membranes.

Dehydration and hypovolemia requires prompt intervention to prevent impending shock. *Note:* Hypertension, bradycardia, and nausea or vomiting suggest TURP syndrome, requiring immediate medical intervention.

Investigate restlessness, confusion, and changes in behavior.

May reflect decreased cerebral perfusion (hypovolemia) or indicate cerebral edema from excessive solution absorbed into the venous sinusoids during TUR procedure (TURP syndrome).

Encourage increased fluid intake, preferably water, to 2,000 to 2,500 mL/day unless contraindicated by medical condition.

Flushes bladder of bacteria, blood clots, and debris (Wojcik & Dennison, 2006).

Bleeding Reduction (NIC)
Anchor urethral catheter and avoid excessive manipulation.

After TURP, the client will have special catheter in place that allows traction on the prostatic fossa to minimize bleeding. The catheter also allows irrigation of the bladder. Displacement of the catheter may cause bleeding. With bladder distention, clot formation may cause plugging of the catheter.

ACTIONS/INTERVENTIONS (continued)

Observe urethral and suprapubic catheter drainage, noting excessive or continued bleeding.

Evaluate color, consistency of urine, for example:
Bright red with bright red clots

Dark burgundy with dark clots and increased viscosity

Bleeding with absence of clots

Inspect dressings and wound drains. Weigh dressings, if indicated. Note hematoma formation.

Avoid taking rectal temperatures and use of rectal tubes or enemas.

Collaborative

Monitor laboratory studies, as indicated, such as the following:
Hemoglobin/hematocrit (Hgb/Hct) and RBCs
Coagulation studies and platelet count

Administer intravenous (IV) therapy or blood products, as indicated.

Maintain traction on indwelling catheter; tape catheter to inner thigh.

Release traction within 4 to 5 hours. Document period of application and release of traction, if used.

Administer stool softeners or laxatives, as indicated.

RATIONALE (continued)

Bleeding is not unusual during first 24 hours for all but the perineal approach. Continued or heavy bleeding or recurrence of active bleeding requires medical evaluation and intervention.

Usually indicates arterial bleeding and requires aggressive therapy.

Suggests venous source, which is the most common type of bleeding and usually subsides on its own.

May indicate blood dyscrasias or systemic clotting problems.

Bleeding may be evident or sequestered within tissues of the perineum.

May result in referred irritation to prostatic bed and increased pressure on prostatic capsule with risk of bleeding.

Useful in evaluating blood losses and replacement needs.

May indicate developing complications that can potentiate bleeding or clotting

May need additional fluids, if oral intake inadequate, or blood products, if losses are excessive.

Traction on the 30-mL balloon positioned in the prostatic urethral fossa creates pressure on the arterial supply of the prostatic capsule to help prevent or control bleeding.

Prolonged traction may cause permanent trauma and problems with urinary control.

Prevention of constipation and straining for stool reduces risk of rectal-perineal bleeding.

NURSING DIAGNOSIS: risk for Infection

Risk factors may include
Invasive procedures—instrumentation during surgery, catheter, frequent bladder irrigation
Traumatized tissue, surgical incision, such as perineal

Possibly evidenced by
(Not applicable; presence of signs and symptoms establishes an *actual* diagnosis)

Desired Outcomes/Evaluation Criteria—Client Will

Wound Healing: Primary Intention (NOC)
Experience no signs of infection.
Achieve timely healing.

ACTIONS/INTERVENTIONS

Infection Protection (NIC)
Independent
Maintain sterile catheter system; provide regular catheter and urinary meatus care with soap and water, applying antibiotic ointment around catheter site per protocol.

Ambulate with drainage bag dependent.

Monitor vital signs, noting low-grade fever, chills, rapid pulse and respiration, restlessness, irritability, and disorientation.

Observe drainage from wounds around suprapubic catheter.

Change suprapubic/retropubic and perineal incision dressings frequently, cleaning and drying skin thoroughly each time.

Use ostomy-type skin barriers.

Collaborative
Administer antibiotics, as indicated.

RATIONALE

Prevents introduction of bacteria and resultant infection.

Avoids backward reflux of urine, which may introduce bacteria into the bladder.

Client who has had cystoscopy or TURP is at increased risk for surgical and septic shock related to instrumentation.

Presence of drains and suprapubic incision increases risk of infection, as indicated by erythema or purulent drainage.

Wet dressings cause skin irritation and provide medium for bacterial growth, increasing risk of wound infection.

Provides protection for surrounding skin, preventing excoriation and reducing risk of infection.

May be given prophylactically because of increased risk of infection with prostatectomy.

NURSING DIAGNOSIS: acute Pain

May be related to
Irritation of the bladder mucosa; reflex muscle spasm associated with surgical procedure or pressure from bladder balloon (traction)

Possibly evidenced by
Reports of painful bladder spasms
Facial grimacing, guarding, restlessness
Autonomic responses

Desired Outcomes/Evaluation Criteria—Client Will

Pain Level (NOC)
Report pain is relieved or controlled.
Appear relaxed and sleep and rest appropriately.

Pain Control (NOC)
Demonstrate use of relaxation skills and diversional activities, as indicated, for individual situation.

ACTIONS/INTERVENTIONS	RATIONALE
Pain Management (NIC) *Independent* Assess pain, noting location, intensity (0 to 10 scale), and characteristics.	Changes in pain reports may indicate developing complications requiring further evaluation and intervention. *Note:* Sharp, intermittent pain with urge to void and passage of urine around catheter suggests bladder spasms, which tend to be more severe with suprapubic or TUR approaches and usually decrease within 48 hours.
Maintain patency of catheter and drainage system. Keep tubing free of kinks and clots.	Maintaining a properly functioning catheter and drainage system decreases risk of bladder distention and spasm.
Promote intake of up to 3,000 mL/day, as tolerated.	Decreases irritation by maintaining a constant flow of fluid over the bladder mucosa.
Give client accurate information about catheter, drainage, and bladder spasms.	Allays anxiety and promotes cooperation with necessary procedures.
Provide comfort measures, such as position changes, back rub, Therapeutic Touch, and diversional activities. Encourage use of relaxation techniques, including deep-breathing exercises, visualization, and guided imagery.	Reduces muscle tension, refocuses attention, and may enhance coping abilities.
Collaborative Provide sitz baths or heat lamp, if indicated.	Promotes tissue perfusion and resolution of edema and enhances healing in perineal approach.
Administer antispasmodics, such as the following: Oxybutynin (Ditropan), flavoxate (Urispas), B & O suppositories	Relaxes smooth muscle to provide relief of spasms and associated pain.
Propantheline bromide (Pro-Banthine)	Relieves bladder spasms by anticholinergic action. Usually discontinued 24 to 48 hours before anticipated removal of catheter to promote normal bladder contraction.

NURSING DIAGNOSIS: risk for Sexual Dysfunction

Risk factors may include
Situational crisis—incontinence, leakage of urine after catheter removal, involvement of genital area
Threat to self-concept, change in health status

Possibly evidenced by
(Not applicable; presence of signs and symptoms establishes an *actual* diagnosis)

Desired Outcomes/Evaluation Criteria—Client Will

Sexual Functioning
Report understanding of sexual function and alterations that may occur with surgery in individual situation.
Discuss concerns about possible changes in body image and sexual functioning with partner/significant other (SO) and caregiver.
Demonstrate problem-solving skills regarding solutions to problems that occur.

ACTIONS/INTERVENTIONS

RATIONALE

Sexual Counseling (NIC)
Independent

Provide openings for client and SO to talk about concerns of incontinence and sexual functioning.

Discuss basic anatomy. Be honest in answers to client's questions.

Give accurate information about expectation of return of sexual function.

Discuss retrograde ejaculation if transurethral or suprapubic approach is used.

Instruct in perineal and pelvic floor exercises and interruption of urinary stream exercises.

Collaborative

Refer to sexual counselor as indicated.

May have anxieties about the effects of surgery and may be hesitant about asking necessary questions. Anxiety may have affected ability to access information given previously.

The nerve plexus that controls erection runs posteriorly to the prostate through the capsule. In procedures that do not involve the prostatic capsule, impotence and sterility are usually not consequences. Surgical procedure may not provide a permanent cure, and hypertrophy may recur.

Physiological impotence occurs when the perineal nerves are cut during radical procedures; with other approaches, sexual activity can usually be resumed within weeks. If erectile dysfunction persists after healing is complete, client may want to pursue options to restore function—use of medications such as sildenafil citrate (Viagra).

Seminal fluid goes into the bladder and is excreted with the urine. This does not interfere with sexual functioning, but will decrease fertility and cause urine to be cloudy.

Tightening pelvic floor muscles prior to standing, coughing, and sneezing promotes regaining bladder and, perhaps, erectile function.

Persistent or unresolved problems may require professional intervention.

NURSING DIAGNOSIS: **deficient Knowledge [Learning Need] regarding condition, prognosis, treatment, self-care, and discharge needs**

May be related to
Lack of exposure or recall, information misinterpretation
Unfamiliarity with information resources

Possibly evidenced by
Questions, request for information, statement of misconception
Verbalization of the problem
Inaccurate follow-through of instruction, development of preventable complications

Desired Outcomes/Evaluation Criteria—Client Will

Knowledge: Disease Process (NOC)
Verbalize understanding of surgical procedure and potential complications.

Knowledge: Treatment Regimen (NOC)
Verbalize understanding of therapeutic needs.
Correctly perform necessary procedures and explain reasons for actions.
Initiate necessary lifestyle changes.
Participate in therapeutic regimen.

ACTIONS/INTERVENTIONS

RATIONALE

Teaching: Disease Process (NIC)
Independent

Review implications of procedure and future expectations.

Stress necessity of good nutrition; encourage inclusion of fruits and increased fiber in diet.

Advise client to avoid or limit intake of caffeine, citrus juices, carbonated beverages, and spicy foods for first few weeks after surgery.

Discuss initial activity restrictions, such as avoidance of heavy lifting, strenuous exercise, prolonged sitting, long car trips, and climbing more than two flights of stairs at a time.

Encourage continuation of perineal exercises.

Provides knowledge base from which client can make informed choices.

Promotes healing and prevents constipation, reducing risk of postoperative bleeding.

Acidic substances can lower urine pH, thereby aggravating dysuria (Shiller, 2007).

Increased abdominal pressure and straining places stress on the bladder and prostate, potentiating risk of bleeding.

Facilitates urinary control and alleviation of incontinence.

(continues on page 602)

Instruct in urinary catheter care if present. Identify source for supplies and support.	Promotes independence and competent self-care. Catheter may be in place only on day of surgery when laser procedure is done or for days to weeks with other procedures.
Instruct client to avoid tub baths after discharge.	Decreases the possibility of introduction of bacteria or undue tension on incision.
Review signs and symptoms requiring medical evaluation: erythema, purulent drainage from wound sites; inability to urinate, changes in character or amount of urine, presence of urgency or frequency; and heavy clots or bright red bleeding, fever, or chills.	Prompt intervention may prevent serious complications. *Note:* Urine may appear cloudy for several weeks until postoperative healing occurs and may appear cloudy after intercourse because of retrograde ejaculation.
Provide written information to client and SO regarding recovery expectations and home management, as indicated, regarding pain, incision care, and catheter-related problems and care.	Anxiety related to hospitalization; procedure performed; and associated diagnosis, fatigue, and postoperative pain often makes it difficult for client to absorb necessary self-care information.
Stress importance of follow-up care—evaluation by primary healthcare provider, urologist or oncologist, and laboratory studies.	Monitoring and follow-up can reduce incidence of unaddressed complications. Persistent incontinence and other postoperative issues will require additional evaluation and treatment.
Provide information on available community resources, such as home-health services, medical equipment supply company, housekeeping, and support persons.	Can be helpful in assisting client and SO in coping with challenges they are faced with following prostatectomy, whatever the reason for procedure—BPH, cancer, incontinence, and so forth.

POTENTIAL CONSIDERATIONS following acute hospitalization (dependent on client's age, physical condition, presence of complications, personal resources, and life responsibilities)

In addition to surgical and cancer concerns:
- *impaired Urinary Elimination*—loss of bladder tone, possible discharge with catheter in place
- *Sexual Dysfunction*—leakage of urine, loss of erectile function following radical procedure

---

Sample clinical pathway follows in Table 10.1.

TABLE 10.1 TURP, Hospital. ELOS: 3 Days Urology or Surgical Unit

ND and Categories of Care	Day 1 Day of Surgery _____	Day 2 POD #1_____	Day 3 POD #2_____
Impaired urinary elimination R/T mechanical obstruction, loss of bladder tone, therapeutic intervention	Display urine output individually appropriate, few clots and catheter free-flowing	Verbalize understanding of home care needs, S/S to report to healthcare provider	Void normal amounts w/o retention Demonstrate behaviors to regain bladder/urinary control Plan in place to meet postdischarge needs
Referrals		Home care	
Additional assessments	Characteristics of urinary drainage	→	Voiding frequency, character of urine
	Urinary output q8h	→	Amount per void
	Presence of spontaneous voiding	→	→
Patient education	Foley catheter function, hygiene	Perineal exercises	
		Home care needs, activity/dietary restrictions, sexual concerns	Provide written instructions, schedule for follow-up visits
		S/S to report to healthcare provider → D/C	
Additional nursing actions	Foley catheter to straight drain, irrigate/CBI per protocol	Stand to void q2–4h	→ Per self q4h
	Bedrest if CBI	Ambulate as tolerated	→ Ad lib
	Bed flat × 8 h if epidural anesthesia	Encourage fluids to 3 L/day as indicated	→
Pain R/T increased frequency/force of ureteral contractions, tissue trauma, edema	Report pain relieved/controlled	→	→ Verbalize understanding of pain management post discharge

TABLE 10.1 **TURP, Hospital. ELOS: 3 Days Urology or Surgical Unit** (continued)

ND and Categories of Care	Day 1 Day of Surgery _____	Day 2 POD #1_____	Day 3 POD #2_____
Additional assessments	Pain characteristics/changes, presence of bladder spasms	→	→
	Response to interventions	→	→
		Return of bowel function	→
Medications	Analgesic of choice IM/PO q4h	→ PO analgesic	→
Allergies:	Antispasmotic prn	→ D/C	
		Stool softener/laxative	→
_____			
Patient education	Reporting of pain/effects of intervention		
	Relaxation techniques		
Additional nursing actions	Routine comfort measures	→	→
	Anchor catheter, avoid manipulation		
	Maintain potency of catheter	Sitz bath as indicated	→
Risk for deficient fluid volume, R/T nausea and vomiting, postobstructive diuresis	Maintain adequate hydration with VS stable, palpable pulses, good capillary refill, adequate urinary output	→	→
	Free of active bleeding	→	→
Diagnostic studies		Hb/Hct, RBC	
Additional assessments	Characteristics of catheter drainage	→ Characteristics of urine	→
	VS per postoperative protocol	→ q8h	→
	Peripheral pulses, capillary refill, status of skin q8h	→	→ D/C
	I&O q8h	→	→ D/C
	Mental status/restlessness q4h	→ q8h	→ D/C
	Temperature q8h	→	→
Medications	IV therapy/blood products as indicated	→ D/C	
Patient education	Fluid needs/restrictions		
Additional nursing actions	Maintain catheter traction as indicated, release q4h per protocol	→ D/C	
	Begin PO fluids as tolerated	→ Advance diet/fluids as tolerated	→

Key: ad lib, as desired; CBI, continuous bladder irrigation; D/C, discontinue; Hb/Hct, hemoglobin/hematocrit; IM, intramuscular; I&O, intake & output; PO, by mouth; prn, as needed; q2–4h, every 2 to 4 hours; q4h, every 4 hours; q8h, every 8 hours; RBC, red blood cell; R/T, related to; S/S, signs and symptoms; VS, vital signs.

UROLITHIASIS (RENAL CALCULI)

I. Pathophysiology
 a. Presence of stones anywhere in the urinary tract
   i. Most commonly found in the renal pelvis and calyces
    1. Stones forming in the kidney—nephrolithiasis
    2. Stones formed in the ureters—ureterolithiasis
   ii. May be single or multiple calculi, ranging in size from a grain of salt to the size of a pebble or staghorn calculus
 b. Composition of calculi
   i. Formed of mineral deposits—predominantly calcium oxalate and calcium phosphate
   ii. Uric acid, struvite, and cystine are also calculus formers

II. Etiology
 a. Slow urine flow allows accumulation of crystals—damaging the lining of the urinary tract and decreasing the number of inhibitor substances that would prevent crystal accumulation (Winkleman, 2006).
 b. May remain asymptomatic until passed into a ureter or urine flow is obstructed, at which time the potential for renal damage is acute and the level of pain is at its highest

 c. Causes: dehydration; heredity; excessive intake of vitamins C and D, grapefruit juice, and purines (gout); congenital renal abnormalities; and some medications, such as acetazolamide (Diamox) or indinavir (Crixivan)
 d. Risk factors: men aged 30 to 50, postmenopausal women; gender, male-to-female ratio 3:1; heredity; recurrent urinary tract infections; inflammatory bowel disease; hyperparathyroidism; hypertension; insulin resistance; prolonged bedrest; spinal cord injury; geographic location—southeastern United States; use of antacids or aspirin

III. Statistics (Centers for Disease Control and Prevention [CDC], 2006)
 a. Morbidity: In 2000, there were 2 million doctor visits and outpatient hospital visits by adults with primary diagnosis of "calculus of kidney and ureters"; in 2004, there were 171,000 adult hospital admissions with primary diagnosis of "calculus of kidney and ureters."
 b. Mortality: Rare and related to development of acute renal failure or comorbidities.
 c. Cost: In 2000, $2.07 billion expended for evaluation and treatment of kidney stones.

Calcium oxalate stones: Kidney stones formed by calcium and oxalate crystals, which usually develop in acidic urine.

Calcium phosphate stones: Kidney stones formed by calcium and phosphate crystals, which usually develop in alkaline urine.

Cystine stones: Kidney stones made of cystine crystals.

Extracorporeal shock wave lithotripsy (ESWL): Procedure whereby a shock wave is transmitted through the body to target a stone, thus fragmenting it.

Hematuria: Blood in the urine.

Hypercalciuria: High calcium in the urine—an inherited condition.

Hyperoxaluria: Excretion of excessive amounts of oxalate in the urine.

Polycythemia: Too many red blood cells (RBCs) in the circulation.

Pyuria: Pus in the urine.

Renal calyces: The perimeter of the renal pelvis is interrupted by cuplike projections called calyces. A minor calyx surrounds the renal papillae of each pyramid and collects urine from that pyramid. Several minor calyces converge to form a major calyx. From the major calyces the urine flows into the renal pelvis and from there into the ureter.

Renal colic: Flank (side) pain caused by obstruction to the flow of urine caused by kidney or ureteral stones.

Renal pelvis: The area at the center of the kidney where urine collects and is funneled into the ureter.

Renal tubular acidosis: Condition associated with dehydration, metabolic acidosis, low potassium, and high chloride. Often associated with renal stones due to hypercalciuria (high calcium in urine).

Staghorn calculi: Develops in the center of the kidney or pelvis, filling the entire pelvis and extending out into the calyces.

Stent: Tube inserted into the ureter to bypass a stone or to keep the ureter open so urine flows freely from the kidney to the bladder.

Struvite stone: Also known as magnesium ammonium phosphate—stones that are often present with infection.

Ureterovesical junction: Joining of the ureters and bladder.

Uric acid stones: Kidney stones made of pure uric acid crystals. These stones develop in acidic urine.

Care Setting

Treatment is often handled at the community level or as an outpatient; acute episodes occasionally require inpatient treatment on a medical or surgical unit. On occasion, surgery is necessary to remove the stone(s).

Related Concerns

Fluid and electrolyte imbalances, page 903

Metabolic acidosis—primary base bicarbonate deficiency, page 483

Metabolic alkalosis—primary base bicarbonate excess, page 488

Psychosocial aspects of care, page 749

Renal failure: acute, page 536

Client Assessment Database

Dependent on size, location, and etiology of calculi.

DIAGNOSTIC DIVISION MAY REPORT	MAY EXHIBIT
ACTIVITY/REST • Sedentary occupation or occupation in which client is exposed to high environmental temperatures • Activity restrictions or immobility due to a preexisting condition—debilitating disease, spinal cord injury—causing bones to release more calcium	
CIRCULATION	• Elevated blood pressure (BP) and pulse associated with pain, anxiety, or kidney failure • Warm, flushed skin, pallor
ELIMINATION • History of recent or chronic urinary tract infection (UTI) • Previous kidney stones • Decreased urinary output, bladder fullness • Burning, urgency with urination • Diarrhea	• Oliguria (retention, scant urine), hematuria, pyuria • Alterations in voiding pattern

Client Assessment Database (continued)

DIAGNOSTIC DIVISION MAY REPORT (continued)	MAY EXHIBIT (continued)
FOOD/FLUID • Nausea and vomiting • A high-protein, high-sodium, low-calcium diet, which may increase risk of some types of stones • Insufficient fluid intake, does not drink fluids well	• Abdominal distention, decreased or absent bowel sounds
PAIN/DISCOMFORT • Acute episode of excruciating, colicky pain, with location depending on stone location; in the flank in the region of the costovertebral angle, may radiate to back, abdomen, and down to the groin and genitalia; constant dull pain suggests calculi located in the renal pelvis or calyces • May be described as acute, severe, and not relieved by positioning or any other measures	• Guarding, distraction behaviors, self-focusing • Tenderness in renal areas on palpation
SAFETY • Use of alcohol can contribute to dehydration and to uric acid stone formation • Fever (uncommon)	
TEACHING/LEARNING • Family history of kidney stones, kidney disease, hypertension, gout, chronic UTI, or hereditary disease, such as renal tubular acidosis, cystinuria, hyperoxaluria • History of small-bowel disease, previous abdominal surgery, hyperparathyroidism • Use of antibiotics, antihypertensives, sodium bicarbonate, allopurinol, phosphates, thiazides, excessive intake of calcium or vitamin D • Use of herbal remedies for kidney stones, such as valerian, skullcap, wild yam, khella, marshmallow, slippery elm	
DISCHARGE PLAN CONSIDERATIONS • May require dietary modifications, exercise program, pain management plan ▶ Refer to section at end of plan for postdischarge considerations.	

Diagnostic Studies

TEST WHY IT IS DONE	WHAT IT TELLS ME
BLOOD TESTS • *Serum and urine blood urea nitrogen/creatinine (BUN/Cr):* Helpful in delineating obstructive uropathy due to urolithiasis.	Blockage of urine flow below the kidneys causes postrenal azotemia (ratio greater than 15:1) without intrinsic renal disease. Abnormal levels—high in serum and low in urine—are secondary to high obstructive stones with reduced urine output.
• *Serum chloride and bicarbonate levels:* Used to identify degree of renal involvement and developing complications.	Increased levels of chloride and decreased levels of bicarbonate suggest developing renal tubular acidosis.
• *Complete blood count (CBC):* Battery of screening tests which typically includes hemoglobin (Hb); hematocrit (Hct); RBC count, morphology; and white blood cell (WBC) count and differential.	Hgb/Hct—abnormal if client is severely dehydrated or client is anemic (hemorrhage, kidney dysfunction or failure) RBCs—usually normal WBCs—may be increased, indicating infection

(continues on page 606)

TEST WHY IT IS DONE (continued)	WHAT IT TELLS ME (continued)
• *Blood chemistry:* Measures levels of calcium, phosphate, uric acid, sodium, potassium, chloride, bicarbonate, and albumin. If serum calcium levels are elevated, then testing for hyper-parathyroidism is performed.	These tests are done if complications associated with kidney stones are suspected or present.
URINE TESTS • *Urinalysis:* Simple screening test may suggest type of stone and presence of infection.	Color may be yellow, dark brown, or bloody. Commonly shows RBCs, WBCs, crystals (cystine, uric acid, calcium oxalate), casts, minerals, bacteria, and pus. pH may be less than 5.0, which promotes cystine and uric acid stones, or higher than 7.5, which promotes magnesium, struvite, phosphate, or calcium phosphate stones.
• *Urine (24-hour):* Measures urine volume, pH, and levels of calcium, sodium, uric acid, oxalate, citrate, and creatinine.	Helps identify degree of obstruction and type of stone—especially important for long-term management in client who is prone to stone formation.
• *Urine culture:* Identifies presence of infection and causative agent.	May reveal UTI and identify organism (e.g., *Staphylococcus aureus, Proteus, Klebsiella, Pseudomonas*) as cause for stone development—struvite or infection stone.
OTHER DIAGNOSTIC STUDIES • *Abdominal x-ray of kidneys-ureters-bladder (KUB):* Usually ordered to evaluate hematuria flank pain.	Shows presence of calculi and anatomic changes in the area of the kidneys or along the course of the ureter. May show small stones that can pass unnoticed.
• *Kidney ultrasound and intrarenal Doppler ultrasound:* Determines obstructive changes and location of stone without the risk of kidney failure that can be induced by contrast medium.	Ultrasound is used to show obstruction to the kidney. However, small kidney stones that are not obstructing may be missed. Renal Doppler ultrasound improves the detection of early obstruction by evaluating for elevated resistive index (RI) in kidney with nondilated collecting system.
• *Intravenous urogram (IVU; also known as intravenous pyelogram [IVP]):* Kidney x-ray performed by injecting radiopaque contrast into a vein. Multiple pictures of the kidneys are taken to follow the uptake and excretion of the contrast by the kidneys.	Provides rapid confirmation of urolithiasis as a cause of abdominal or flank pain. Shows abnormalities in anatomical structures, such as distended ureter, and outline of calculi.
• *Renal helical or spiral computerized tomography (CT) scan:* Continuous motion image providing detailed views of the kidneys, ureters, and bladder in a shorter period of time.	Identifies and delineates calculi and other masses, as well as kidney, ureteral, and bladder distention. Contrast is not used because it masks the stones.

Nursing Priorities

1. Alleviate pain.
2. Maintain adequate renal functioning.
3. Prevent complications.
4. Provide information about disease process, prognosis, and treatment needs.

Discharge Goals

1. Pain relieved or controlled.
2. Fluid and electrolyte balance maintained.
3. Complications prevented or minimized.
4. Disease process, prognosis, and therapeutic regimen understood.
5. Plan in place to meet needs after discharge.

NURSING DIAGNOSIS: **acute Pain**

May be related to
Increased frequency and force of ureteral contractions
Tissue trauma, edema formation, cellular ischemia

Possibly evidenced by
Reports of colicky pain
Guarding or distraction behaviors, restlessness, moaning, self-focusing, facial mask of pain, muscle tension
Autonomic responses

NURSING DIAGNOSIS: acute Pain (continued)

Desired Outcomes/Evaluation Criteria—Client Will

Pain Level (NOC)
Report pain is relieved, with spasms controlled.
Appear relaxed and be able to sleep and rest appropriately.

ACTIONS/INTERVENTIONS	RATIONALE
Pain Management (NIC)	
Independent	
Document location, duration, intensity (0 to 10 scale), and radiation. Note nonverbal signs—elevated BP and pulse, restlessness, moaning, and thrashing about.	Helps evaluate site of obstruction and progress of calculi movement. Flank pain suggests that stones are in the kidney area, upper ureter. Flank pain radiates to back, abdomen, groin, and genitalia because of proximity of nerve plexus and blood vessels supplying these areas. Sudden, severe pain may precipitate apprehension, restlessness, and severe anxiety.
Explain cause of pain and importance of notifying caregivers of changes in pain occurrence or characteristics.	Provides opportunity for timely administration of analgesia and alerts caregivers to possibility of passing of stone or developing complications. Sudden cessation of pain usually indicates stone passage.
Provide such comfort measures as back rub and restful environment.	Promotes relaxation, reduces muscle tension, and enhances coping.
Apply warm compresses to back.	Relieves muscle tension and may reduce reflex spasms.
Assist with and encourage use of focused breathing, guided imagery, and diversional activities.	Redirects attention and aids in muscle relaxation.
Encourage and assist with frequent ambulation as indicated; increase fluid intake to at least 3 to 4 L/day within cardiac tolerance.	Renal colic can be worse in the supine position. Vigorous hydration promotes passing of stone, prevents urinary stasis, and aids in prevention of further stone formation.
Note reports of increased or persistent abdominal pain.	Complete obstruction of ureter can cause perforation and extravasation of urine into perirenal space. This represents an acute surgical emergency.
Collaborative	
Administer medications, as indicated, for example:	
Opioids, such as morphine sulfate (Astramorph, Duramorph); oral opioid combination analgesics, such as oxycodone and acetaminophen (Percocet); and nonsteroidal anti-inflammatory drugs (NSAIDs), such as ketorolac (Toradol)	Opioid and NSAID combination is often given intravenously (IV) during acute episode to quickly decrease ureteral colic and promote muscle and mental relaxation.
Antispasmodics, such as flavoxate (Urispas) and oxybutynin (Ditropan); calcium channel blocker, such as nifedipine (Adalat); and alpha-adrenergic blockers, such as tamsulosin (Flomax)	Decreases reflex spasm and relaxes ureteral smooth muscle, which facilitates stone passage. *Note:* Oral analgesics, NSAIDs, and alpha-adrenergic blockers help facilitate stone passage after acute attack
Corticosteroids, such as prednisone (Deltasone)	May be used short-term to reduce tissue edema to facilitate movement of stone.
Maintain patency of catheters when used.	Prevents urinary stasis or retention, reduces risk of increased renal pressure and infection.

NURSING DIAGNOSIS: impaired Urinary Elimination

May be related to
Stimulation of the bladder by calculi, renal or ureteral irritation
Mechanical obstruction, inflammation

Possibly evidenced by
Urgency and frequency, oliguria
Hematuria

Desired Outcomes/Evaluation Criteria—Client Will

Urinary Elimination (NOC)
Void in normal amounts of greater than or equal to 30 mL/hour, and usual pattern.
Experience no signs of obstruction.

ACTIONS/INTERVENTIONS	RATIONALE
Urinary Elimination Enhancement (NIC)	
Independent	
Monitor intake and output (I&O) and characteristics of urine.	Provides information about kidney function and presence of complications—infection and hemorrhage. Bleeding may also indicate increased obstruction or irritation of ureter.
Determine client's normal voiding pattern and note variations.	Calculi may cause urinary tract nerve excitability, which causes sensations of urgent need to void. Frequency and urgency usually increase as calculus nears the ureterovesical junction.
Encourage increased fluid intake, if nausea is not present.	Increased hydration dilutes urine and flushes bacteria, blood, and debris and may facilitate stone passage—especially small stones.
Strain all urine. Document any stones expelled and send to laboratory for analysis.	Retrieval of calculi allows identification of type of stone and influences choice of therapy.
Investigate reports of bladder fullness; palpate for suprapubic distention. Note decreased urine output and presence of periorbital or dependent edema.	Urinary retention may develop, causing bladder, ureteral, and kidney distention, potentiating risk of infection and renal failure.
Observe for changes in mental status, behavior, or level of consciousness (LOC).	Accumulation of uremic wastes and electrolyte imbalances can be toxic to the central nervous system (CNS).
Collaborative	
Maintain patency of indwelling catheters—ureteral, urethral, or nephrostomy—when used.	May be required to facilitate urine flow, preventing retention and corresponding complications. Catheters are positioned above the stone to promote urethral dilation and stone passage. Continuous or intermittent irrigation can be carried out to flush kidneys and ureters and adjust pH of urine to permit dissolution of stone fragments following lithotripsy.
Administer medications, as indicated, for example: Acetazolamide (Diamox) and allopurinol (Zyloprim)	Increases urine pH (alkalinity) to reduce formation of acid stones. Antigout agents such as allopurinol also lower uric acid production and potential of uric acid stone formation.
Hydrochlorothiazide (Esidrix, HydroDiuril) and chlorthalidone (Hygroton)	Diuretics may be used to prevent urinary stasis and decrease calcium stone formation if not caused by underlying disease process such as primary hyperthyroidism or vitamin D abnormalities.
Penicillamine (Cuprimine), tiopronin (Thiola), and potassium citrate (Polycitra-K)	Drugs may be prescribed to make urine more alkaline or bind cystine in the urine, when cystine stones cannot be controlled.
Ammonium chloride and potassium or sodium phosphate	Reduces phosphate stone formation.
Antibiotics	Antibiotics may be needed in presence of UTI or to keep urine bacteria-free to prevent struvite stone formation.
Monitor laboratory studies, for example: Electrolytes, BUN, and Cr	Elevated BUN, Cr, and certain electrolytes indicate presence and degree of kidney dysfunction.
Urine culture and sensitivities	Determines presence of UTI, which may be causing or complicating kidney stone symptoms; determines appropriate antibiotic therapy.
Prepare client for and assist with endoscopic procedures, such as the following: Basket procedure, percutaneous ultrasonic lithotripsy, and stent placement	Calculi in the distal and midureter may be removed by fiber-optic ureteroscope, which shatters the stone with a shock wave and captures it in a basket catheter.
ESWL	ESWL is the most frequently used outpatient procedure for treatment of stones that are not responsive to medical therapy. Kidney stones are pulverized by shock waves delivered from outside the body while client reclines in water bath or on soft cushion. *Note:* ESWL is not ideal for large stones.
Percutaneous or open incision stone removal.	Surgery may be necessary to remove a stone that is (1) too large to pass through ureters, (2) is caught in a difficult place, (3) blocks flow of urine, (4) causes ongoing UTI, (5) causes constant bleeding, or (6) is potentially damaging to kidney tissue. One advantage to the open procedure is that stone fragments are removed at surgery rather than relying on natural passage from the kidneys or urinary tract. Client may have a small drainage tube left in kidney or ureters during the healing process.

NURSING DIAGNOSIS: risk for deficient Fluid Volume

Risk factors may include
Nausea or vomiting—generalized abdominal and pelvic nerve irritation from renal or ureteral colic
Postobstructive diuresis

Possibly evidenced by
(Not applicable; presence of signs or symptoms establishes an *actual* diagnosis)

Desired Outcomes/Evaluation Criteria—Client Will

Hydration (NOC)
Maintain adequate fluid balance as evidenced by vital signs and weight within client's normal range, palpable peripheral pulses,
moist mucous membranes, and good skin turgor.

ACTIONS/INTERVENTIONS	RATIONALE
Fluid/Electrolyte Management (NIC)	
Independent	
Monitor I&O.	Comparing actual and anticipated output may aid in evaluating presence and degree of renal stasis or impairment. *Note:* Impaired kidney functioning and decreased urinary output can result in higher circulating volumes with signs and symptoms of heart failure (HF).
Document incidence and note characteristics and frequency of vomiting and diarrhea, as well as accompanying or precipitating events.	Nausea or vomiting and diarrhea are commonly associated with renal colic because celiac ganglion serves both kidneys and stomach. Documentation may help rule out other abdominal occurrences as a cause for pain or pinpoint calculi.
Increase fluid intake to 3 to 4 L/day within cardiac tolerance.	Maintains fluid balance for homeostasis and "washing" action that may flush the stone(s) out. Reduces problems associated with dehydration and electrolyte imbalance that may occur secondary to vomiting and diarrhea.
Monitor vital signs. Evaluate pulses, capillary refill, skin turgor, and mucous membranes.	Indicators of hydration and circulating volume and need for intervention.
Weigh daily.	Rapid weight changes suggest water loss or retention.
Collaborative	
Monitor Hgb/Hct and electrolytes.	Assesses hydration and effectiveness of, or need for, interventions.
Administer IV fluids.	Maintains circulating volume if oral intake is insufficient, promoting renal function.
Provide appropriate diet, clear liquids, and bland foods, as tolerated.	Easily digested foods decrease gastrointestinal (GI) activity or irritation and help maintain fluid and nutritional balance.
Administer medications, as indicated, for example antiemetics, such as prochlorperazine (Compazine).	Reduces nausea and vomiting.

NURSING DIAGNOSIS: deficient Knowledge [Learning Need] regarding condition, prognosis, treatment, self-care, and discharge needs

May be related to
Lack of exposure or recall; information misinterpretation
Unfamiliarity with information resources

Possibly evidenced by
Questions, request for information, statement of misconception
Inaccurate follow-through of instructions, development of preventable complications

Desired Outcomes/Evaluation Criteria—Client Will

Knowledge: Illness Care (NOC)
Verbalize understanding of disease process and potential complications.
Correlate symptoms with causative factors.
Verbalize understanding of therapeutic needs.
Initiate necessary lifestyle changes and participate in treatment regimen.

ACTIONS/INTERVENTIONS	RATIONALE

Teaching: Disease Process (NIC)

Independent

Review disease process and future expectations.

Provides knowledge base from which client can make informed choices.

Stress importance of increased fluid intake, such as 3 to 4 L/day or as much as 6 to 8 L/day if not contraindicated. Encourage client to notice dry mouth and excessive diuresis or diaphoresis and to increase fluid intake whether or not feeling thirsty.

Flushes renal system, decreasing opportunity for urinary stasis and stone formation. Increased fluid losses or dehydration require additional intake beyond usual daily needs.

Review dietary regimen, as individually appropriate, for example:

Diet depends on the type of stone. Understanding reason for modifications provides opportunity for client to make informed choices, increases cooperation with regimen, and may prevent recurrence.

Low-purine diet, such as limited lean meat, turkey, legumes, whole grains, and alcohol

Decreases oral intake of uric acid precursors.

Low-oxalate diet, such as limited chocolate, caffeine-containing beverages, beets, nuts, rhubarb, strawberries, spinach, and wheat bran

Reduces calcium-oxalate stone formation. *Note:* Research suggests that daily inclusion of coffee, tea, beer, or wine decreases the risk of stone formation, whereas regular intake of apple or grapefruit juice increases the risk (Finkelstein & Goldfarb, 2006).

Limit calcium intake to about 800 mg/day when appropriate. Use calcium citrate when supplements are required.

Although not advocating high-calcium diets, researchers are urging that calcium limitation be reexamined. Research suggests that restricting dietary calcium is not helpful in reducing calcium stone formation and may actually increase oxalate formation. Use of citrate is helpful in binding oxalate and improving calcium absorption.

Shorr regimen: low-calcium and phosphorus diet with aluminum carbonate gel 30 to 40 mL 30 minutes after meals and at bedtime

Prevents phosphoric calculi by forming an insoluble precipitate in the GI tract, reducing the load to the kidney nephrons. Also effective against other forms of calcium calculi. *Note:* May cause constipation.

Encourage foods rich in magnesium and vitamins B and K.

These nutrients reduce stone formation.

Discuss medication and herbal supplement regimen; avoidance of over-the-counter (OTC) drugs, and reading all product and food ingredient labels.

Drugs will be given to acidify or alkalize urine, depending on underlying cause of stone formation. Ingestion of products containing individually contraindicated ingredients, such as calcium and phosphorus, potentiates recurrence of stones. *Note:* Some herbal supplements—valerian, skullcap, wild yam, khella, and marshmallow—are known to have antispasmodic properties or are soothing to irritated urinary tissues.

Encourage client to reveal all medications and herbals to physician or pharmacist.

To reduce risk of dangerous interactions and side effects.

Emphasize need for smoking cessation, when indicated.

Cigarette smoking may contribute to kidney stones because it increases urine levels of cadmium, a heavy metal.

Encourage regular activity and exercise program.

Inactivity contributes to stone formation through calcium shifts and urinary stasis.

Active-listen concerns about therapeutic regimen and lifestyle changes.

Helps client work through feelings and gain a sense of control over what is happening.

Identify signs and symptoms requiring medical evaluation, such as recurrent pain, hematuria, and oliguria.

With increased probability of stone recurrence, prompt interventions may prevent serious complications. *Note:* Rate of recurrence at 1 year is 14%; at 2 years, 35%; and at 10 years, 52% (Craig, 2006).

Demonstrate proper care of incisions or catheters if present.

Promotes competent self-care and independence.

POTENTIAL CONSIDERATIONS following acute hospitalizations (dependent on client's age, physical condition and presence of complications, personal resources, and life responsibilities)

• *impaired Urinary Elimination*—recurrence of calculi

CHAPTER 11

Women's Reproductive

HYSTERECTOMY

I. Indications—surgical removal of the uterus
  a. Malignancies: 11% of hysterectomies
  b. Nonmalignant conditions, such as endometriosis, fibroid tumors; pelvic relaxation with uterine prolapse that leads to disabling levels of pain, discomfort, uterine bleeding, emotional stress
  c. Life-threatening bleeding or hemorrhaging, such as obstetric or traumatic complication; irreparable rupture of the uterus
  d. Treatment of intractable pelvic infection
II. Procedures
  a. Abdominal hysterectomy
    i. Subtotal or partial: removal of body of uterus; cervical stump remains
    ii. Total: removal of the uterus and cervix
    iii. Total with bilateral salpingo-oophorectomy: removal of uterus, cervix, fallopian tubes, and ovaries
    iv. Total pelvic exenteration (TPE): Complex, aggressive surgical procedure involving radical hysterectomy with dissection of pelvic lymph nodes, bilateral salpingo-oophorectomy, total cystectomy, and abdominoperineal resection of the rectum; colostomy and/or urinary conduit are created, and vaginal reconstruction may or may not be performed. (Refer to additional care plans regarding fecal or urinary diversions, as appropriate.)

  b. Vaginal hysterectomy or laparoscopically assisted vaginal hysterectomy (LAVH)
    i. Limited to certain conditions, such as uterine prolapse, cystocele or rectocele, carcinoma in situ, and high-risk obesity
    ii. Requires removal of cervix
    iii. Advantages: less pain, no visible (or much smaller) scars, shorter hospital stay, and shorter recovery period of about 3 to 4 weeks (vaginal) and 2 weeks (LAVH) versus approximately 6 weeks (abdominal)
    iv. Research suggests laparoscopic procedure is associated with a higher rate of complications than abdominal hysterectomy.
  c. Laparoscopic supracervical hysterectomy (LSH)
    i. Can be performed in presence of mild to moderate adhesions or large uterus
    ii. Three or four small abdominal incisions with uterus removed in small pieces through a tube in the umbilical incision
    iii. Removal of cervix not required
    iv. Usually done on outpatient basis, with a recovery period of about 1 week
III. Statistics (Gor et al, 2006; National Uterine Fibroids Foundation, 2004)
  a. Morbidity: 600,000 are performed annually; 37% of all women undergo hysterectomy by age 60 in the United States.
  b. Mortality: Approximately 660 women die annually.
  c. Cost: $5 billion annually in the United States

GLOSSARY

Cervix: Lower end or neck of the uterus, which protrudes into the vagina.
Endometriosis: Ectopic endometrial tissue found outside the uterine cavity, usually in the ovaries, fallopian tubes, and other pelvic structures.
Fibroids: Benign tumors that form in the uterine muscle.

Laparoscopy: Use of a slender, light-transmitting tube to view abdominal organs or perform surgery.
Menopause: Permanent cessation of menstrual activity.
Uterine prolapse: Displacement or sagging of the uterus into the vagina.

Care Setting

Procedure is performed in inpatient acute surgical unit or short-stay unit or outpatient, depending on type performed.

Related Concerns

Cancer, page 846
Psychosocial aspects of care, page 749
Surgical intervention, page 782 (for general considerations and interventions)
Thrombophlebitis: deep vein thrombosis, page 111

Client Assessment Database

Data depend on the underlying disease process and the need for surgical intervention—cancer, prolapse, dysfunctional uterine bleeding, severe endometriosis, or pelvic infections unresponsive to medical management—and associated complications, such as anemia.

TEACHING/LEARNING

DISCHARGE PLAN CONSIDERATIONS
- May need temporary help with transportation and homemaker and maintenance tasks

▶ Refer to section at end of plan for postdischarge considerations.

Diagnostic Studies

TEST / WHY IT IS DONE	WHAT IT TELLS ME
• *Pelvic examination:* Identifies uterine and/or other pelvic organ irregularities.	May reveal masses, tender nodules, visual changes of cervix, requiring further diagnostic evaluation.
• *Pap smear:* Screening test for cervical cancer and certain vaginal or uterine infections.	Cellular dysplasia reflects possibility of or actual presence of cancer, which may affect choice of procedure.
• *Pelvic ultrasound or computed tomography (CT) scan:* Creates an electronic picture of the organs and structures within the pelvis.	Aids in identifying size and location of pelvic mass.
• *Sonohysterogram:* A saline-enhanced sonogram or ultrasound.	Evaluates abnormal growths inside the uterus, lining of the uterus, and deeper tissue layers. Delineates polyps and submucosal fibroids.
• *Hysteroscopy:* Uses fiberoptic viewing scope and a distending medium, such as carbon dioxide, to directly view the uterine cavity and/or biopsy growths.	Viewed by some to be the "gold standard." Determines cause of abnormal bleeding.
• *Laparoscopy:* Visualizes pathology, obtains biopsies, or performs laser treatment for endometriosis.	May reveal source of bleeding, presence of tumors, and superficial peritoneal implants of endometriosis; determines cancer staging and assesses effects of chemotherapy.
• *Endometrial sampling:* Dilation and curettage (D&C) with biopsy of endometrial or cervical tissue for histopathological study of cells.	Determines presence and location of cancer.
• *Schiller's test (staining of cervix with iodine):* Useful in identifying abnormal cells.	Cervix turns dark brown in noncancerous areas and white or yellow in possible cancerous areas.
• *Complete blood count (CBC):* Useful in determining general health status.	Decreased hemoglobin (Hgb) may reflect chronic anemia; decreased hematocrit (Hct) suggests active blood loss; and elevated white blood cell (WBC) count may indicate inflammation and infectious process.
• *Sexually transmitted disease (STD) screen:* Determines presence of infection.	Human papillomavirus (HPV) is present in 80% of clients with cervical cancer.

Nursing Priorities———————

1. Support adaptation to change.
2. Prevent complications.
3. Provide information about procedure, prognosis, and treatment needs.

Discharge Goals———————

1. Dealing realistically with situation.
2. Complications prevented or minimized.
3. Procedure, prognosis, and therapeutic regimen understood.
4. Plan in place to meet needs after discharge.

In addition to the NDs, see nursing actions and interventions listed in CP: Surgical Intervention.

NURSING DIAGNOSIS: situational low Self-Esteem

May be related to
Concerns about changes in femininity, effect on sexual relationship, inability to have children
Religious conflicts

Possibly evidenced by
Expressions of specific concerns and vague comments about result of surgery; fear of rejection or reaction of significant other (SO)
Withdrawal, depression

Desired Outcomes/Evaluation Criteria—Client Will

Self-Esteem (NOC)
Verbalize concerns and indicate healthy ways of dealing with them.
Verbalize acceptance of self in situation and adaptation to change in body and self-image.

ACTIONS/INTERVENTIONS	RATIONALE
Self-Esteem Enhancement (NIC)	
Independent	
Provide time to listen to concerns and fears of client and SO. Discuss client's perceptions of self related to anticipated changes and her specific lifestyle.	Research supports the idea that hysterectomy is physiologically and psychologically stressful for a woman, even when she desires the procedure. Indeed, the prospect of hysterectomy is said to engender more stress than other comparable surgeries (Parker & Parker, 2003). Cultural beliefs may even result in delaying needed surgery, increasing risk of complications and negatively impacting recovery (Augustus, 2002). Although preoperative instruction and interaction are often performed at the community level, the postoperative care providers can convey interest and concern and make opportunities for support, teaching, and correction of misconceptions, such as loss of femininity and sexuality, weight gain, and menopausal body changes.
Provide accurate information, reinforcing information previously given.	Provides opportunity for client to question and assimilate information.
Ascertain individual strengths and identify previous positive coping behaviors.	Helps to build on strengths already available for client to use in coping with current situation.
Provide open environment for client to discuss concerns about sexuality.	Promotes sharing of beliefs or values about sensitive subject and identifies misconceptions or myths that may interfere with adjustment to situation. (Refer to ND: risk for Sexual Dysfunction.)
Collaborative	
Refer to pastoral staff, psychiatric clinical nurse specialist, and other professionals for counseling, as necessary.	May need additional help to resolve feelings about loss.

NURSING DIAGNOSIS: impaired Urinary Elimination/[acute] Urinary Retention

May be related to
Mechanical trauma, surgical manipulation, presence of local tissue edema, hematoma
Sensory and motor impairment—nerve paralysis

(continues on page 614)

NURSING DIAGNOSIS: **impaired Urinary Elimination/[acute] Urinary Retention** (continued)

Possibly evidenced by
Sensation of bladder fullness, urgency
Small, frequent voiding or absence of urinary output
Overflow incontinence
Bladder distention

Desired Outcomes/Evaluation Criteria—Client Will

Urinary Elimination NOC
Empty bladder regularly and completely.

ACTIONS/INTERVENTIONS	RATIONALE
Urinary Elimination Management NIC	
Independent	
Note voiding pattern and monitor urinary output, once surgical catheter is removed.	May indicate urinary retention if voiding frequently in small or insufficient amounts less than 100 mL.
Palpate bladder. Investigate reports of discomfort, fullness, and inability to void.	Perception of bladder fullness and distention of bladder above symphysis pubis indicates urinary retention.
Provide routine voiding measures, such as privacy, normal position, running water in sink, and pouring warm water over perineum.	Promotes relaxation of perineal muscles and may facilitate voiding efforts.
Provide and/or encourage good perineal cleansing and catheter care when present.	Promotes cleanliness, reducing risk of ascending urinary tract infection (UTI).
Assess urine characteristics, noting color, clarity, and odor.	Urinary retention, vaginal drainage, and possible presence of intermittent or indwelling catheter increase risk of infection, especially if client has perineal sutures.
Collaborative	
Catheterize when indicated per protocol if client is unable to void or is uncomfortable.	Edema or interference with nerve supply may cause bladder atony or urinary retention requiring decompression of the bladder. *Note:* Indwelling urethral or suprapubic catheter may be inserted intraoperatively if complications are anticipated.
Maintain patency of indwelling catheter; keep drainage tubing free of kinks.	Promotes free drainage of urine, reducing risk of urinary stasis or retention and infection.
Check residual urine volume after voiding, as indicated.	May not be emptying bladder completely; retention of urine increases possibility for infection and is uncomfortable, even painful.

NURSING DIAGNOSIS: **risk for Constipation/Diarrhea**

Risk factors may include
Physical factors—abdominal surgery, with manipulation of bowel, weakening of abdominal musculature
Pain or discomfort in abdomen or perineal area
Changes in dietary intake

Possibly evidenced by
(Not applicable; presence of signs and symptoms establishes an *actual* diagnosis)

Desired Outcomes/Evaluation Criteria—Client Will

Bowel Elimination NOC
Display active bowel sounds and peristaltic activity.
Maintain usual pattern of elimination.

ACTIONS/INTERVENTIONS	RATIONALE
Bowel Management NIC	
Independent	
Auscultate bowel sounds. Note abdominal distention, and presence of nausea or vomiting.	Indicators of presence or resolution of ileus, affecting choice of interventions.
Assist client with sitting on edge of bed and walking.	Early ambulation helps stimulate intestinal function and return of peristalsis.

ACTIONS/INTERVENTIONS (continued)

Encourage adequate fluid intake, including fruit juices, when oral intake is resumed.

Provide sitz baths.

Collaborative

Restrict oral intake as indicated.

Maintain nasogastric (NG) tube, if present.

Provide clear or full liquids and advance to solid foods as tolerated.

Administer medications, such as stool softeners, mineral oil, and laxatives, as indicated.

RATIONALE (continued)

Promotes softer stool; may aid in stimulating peristalsis.

Promotes muscle relaxation and minimizes discomfort.

Prevents nausea and vomiting until peristalsis returns in 1 to 2 days.

May be inserted in surgery to decompress stomach.

When peristalsis begins, food and fluid intake promote resumption of normal bowel elimination.

Promotes formation and passage of softer stool.

NURSING DIAGNOSIS: risk for ineffective tissue Perfusion (specify)

Risk factors may include

Hypovolemia

Reduction or interruption of blood flow—pelvic congestion, postoperative tissue inflammation, venous stasis

Intraoperative trauma or pressure on pelvic or calf vessels—lithotomy position during vaginal hysterectomy

Possibly evidenced by

(Not applicable; presence of signs and symptoms establishes an *actual* diagnosis)

Desired Outcomes/Evaluation Criteria—Client Will

Tissue Perfusion: (Specify) (NOC)

Demonstrate adequate perfusion, as evidenced by stable vital signs, palpable pulses, good capillary refill, usual mentation, and individually adequate urinary output.

Be free of edema and signs of thrombus formation.

ACTIONS/INTERVENTIONS

Postanesthesia Care (NIC)

Independent

Monitor vital signs, palpate peripheral pulses and note capillary refill, assess urinary output and characteristics, and evaluate changes in mentation.

Inspect dressings and perineal pads, noting color, amount, and odor of drainage. Weigh pads and compare with dry weight if client is bleeding heavily.

Turn client and encourage frequent coughing and deep-breathing exercises.

Assist with and/or encourage use of incentive spirometer.

Embolus Prevention (NIC)

Avoid high Fowler's position and pressure under the knees or crossing of legs.

Assist with and instruct in foot and leg exercises and ambulate as soon as able.

Note erythema, swelling of extremity, or reports of sudden chest pain with dyspnea.

Collaborative

Apply sequential compression devices (SCDs): antiembolism stockings or pneumatic compression stocking and boots.

Postanesthesia Care (NIC)

Administer intravenous (IV) fluids and blood products, as indicated.

RATIONALE

Indicators of adequacy of systemic perfusion, fluid or blood needs, and developing complications.

Proximity of large blood vessels to operative site and/or potential for alteration of clotting mechanism (e.g., cancer) increases risk of postoperative hemorrhage.

Prevents stasis of secretions and respiratory complications.

Promotes lung expansion and minimizes atelectasis.

Creates vascular stasis by increasing pelvic congestion and pooling of blood in the extremities, potentiating risk of thrombus formation.

Movement enhances circulation and prevents stasis complications.

May be indicative of development of thrombophlebitis and pulmonary embolus.

Aids in venous return; reduces stasis and risk of thrombosis.

Replacement of blood losses maintains circulating volume and tissue perfusion.

NURSING DIAGNOSIS: risk for Sexual Dysfunction

Risk factors may include
Altered body structure or function such as shortening of vaginal canal, changes in hormone levels, decreased libido
Possible change in sexual response pattern—absence of rhythmic uterine contractions during orgasm, vaginal discomfort or pain (dyspareunia)

Possibly evidenced by
(Not applicable; presence of signs and symptoms establishes an *actual* diagnosis)

Desired Outcomes/Evaluation Criteria—Client Will

Sexual Functioning (NOC)
Verbalize understanding of changes in sexual anatomy or function.
Discuss concerns about body image, sex role, and desirability as a sexual partner with SO.
Identify satisfying and acceptable sexual practices and some alternative ways of dealing with sexual expression.

ACTIONS/INTERVENTIONS	RATIONALE
Sexual Counseling (NIC)	
Independent	
Listen to comments of client and SO.	Sexual concerns are often disguised as humor and/or offhand remarks.
Assess client's and SO's information regarding sexual anatomy, function, and effects of surgical procedure.	May have misinformation or misconceptions that can affect adjustment. Negative expectations are associated with poor overall outcome. Changes in hormone levels can affect libido and decrease suppleness of the vagina. Although a shortened vagina can eventually stretch, intercourse initially may be uncomfortable or painful.
Identify cultural or value factors and conflicts present.	May affect return to satisfying sexual relationship.
Assist client to be aware of and deal with stage of grieving.	Acknowledging normal process of grieving for actual or perceived changes may enhance coping and facilitate resolution.
Encourage client to share thoughts or concerns with partner.	Open communication can identify areas of agreement and problems and promote discussion and resolution.
Problem-solve solutions to potential problems, such as postponing sexual intercourse when fatigued, substituting alternative means of expression, using positions that avoid pressure on abdominal incision, and using vaginal lubricant or vaginal estrogen product.	Helps client return to desired and satisfying sexual activity.
Discuss expected physical sensations or discomforts and changes in response, as appropriate to the individual.	Vaginal pain may be significant following vaginal procedure, or sensory loss may occur because of surgical trauma. Research data show a trend toward more problems with lubrication, arousal, and altered genital sensation after total hysterectomy as compared to vaginal hysterectomy. Altered hormone levels and loss of sensation of rhythmic contractions of the uterus during orgasm can impair sexual satisfaction for some women (American College of Obstetricians and Gynecologists [ACOG], 2008). *Note:* Many women experience few negative effects because fear of pregnancy is gone, and relief from symptoms often improves sexual pleasure.
Collaborative	
Refer to counselor or sex therapist as needed.	May need additional assistance to promote a satisfactory outcome.

NURSING DIAGNOSIS: risk for Grieving

Risk factors may include
Loss of body part/perceived sexual role or identity

Possibly evidenced by
Making meaning of loss
Experiencing relief

Desired Outcomes/Evaluation Criteria—Client Will

Grief Resolution (NOC)
Verbalize reality of perceived loss.
Report sense of acceptance and hope for future.

ACTIONS/INTERVENTIONS	RATIONALE
Grief Work Facilitation (NIC) *Independent* Provide open environment in which client feels free to discuss realistic feelings and concerns without confrontation.	Therapeutic communication skills, such as active-listening, silence, being available, and acceptance, provide opportunity and encouragement for the client to talk freely and deal with the perceived loss. Provides opportunity for reflection aiding resolution and acceptance.
Determine client's perception and meaning of current and past losses. Note cultural factors and expectations.	Affects client's response and needs to be acknowledged in planning care. Perceptions and way of expressing self may be result of cultural expectations.
Assess emotional stress client is experiencing.	Being aware of what this operation means to client helps avoid inadvertent casualness or oversolicitude by care providers.
Encourage client to vent feelings appropriately, identifying meaning of loss.	Depending on the reason for the surgery (e.g., cancer or long-term, heavy bleeding), the client may be frightened or relieved. She may mourn the loss of ability to fulfill her reproductive role whether or not she has borne children. She may also worry about her wholeness as a woman or have heard stories about problems others have had with the procedure (ACOG, 2008; Mayo Clinic, 2008).
Assist family/SO to cope with client's responses.	Family may not share client's perspective and be intolerant, not recognizing needs of client.
Identify and problem-solve solutions to existing physical responses—eating, sleeping, activity levels, and sexual desire.	May need additional assistance to deal with the physical aspects of the potential for grieving.
Note withdrawn behavior, negative self-talk, and overconcern with actual or perceived changes.	May indicate difficulty in working through the grief process and need for additional interventions or support.
Discuss healthy ways of dealing with difficult situation.	Provides opportunity to look toward the future and incorporate perceived loss into lifestyle.
Collaborative Refer to other resources for counseling, spiritual or pastoral care, and psychotherapy, as indicated.	May need additional help to prevent development of dysfunctional grieving and help client move toward a positive future.

NURSING DIAGNOSIS: **deficient Knowledge [Learning Need] regarding condition, prognosis, treatment, self-care, and discharge needs**

May be related to
Lack of exposure or recall
Information misinterpretation
Unfamiliarity with information resources

Possibly evidenced by
Questions or request for information, statement of misconception
Inaccurate follow-through of instructions, development of preventable complications

Desired Outcomes/Evaluation Criteria—Client Will

Knowledge: Disease Process (NOC)
Verbalize understanding of condition and potential complications.
Identify relationship of signs and symptoms related to surgical procedure and actions to deal with them.

Knowledge: Treatment Regimen (NOC)
Verbalize understanding of therapeutic needs.

ACTIONS/INTERVENTIONS	RATIONALE
Teaching: Disease Process (NIC) *Independent* Review effects of surgical procedure and future expectations; for example, the client needs to know that she will no longer menstruate or bear children, whether surgical menopause will occur, and whether hormonal replacement will be necessary.	Provides knowledge base from which client can make informed choices.

(continues on page 618)

Discuss complexity of problems anticipated during recovery, including emotional lability and expectation of feelings of depression or sadness, excessive fatigue, sleep disturbances, and urinary problems.

Physical, emotional, and social factors can have a cumulative effect, which may delay recovery, especially if hysterectomy was performed because of cancer. Providing an opportunity for problem-solving may facilitate the process. Client and SO may benefit from the knowledge that a period of emotional lability is normal and expected during recovery.

Discuss resumption of activity. Encourage light activities initially, with frequent rest periods, increasing activities and exercise as tolerated. Stress importance of individual response in recuperation.

Client can expect to feel tired when she goes home and needs to plan a gradual resumption of activities, with return to work an individual matter. Prevents excessive fatigue; conserves energy for healing and tissue regeneration. *Note:* Some studies suggest that recovery from hysterectomy, especially when oophorectomy is performed, may take up to four times as long as recovery from other major surgeries—or 12 months versus 3 months.

Identify individual restrictions, such as avoiding heavy lifting and strenuous activities (such as vacuuming, straining at stool) and prolonged sitting or driving. Avoid tub baths and douching until physician authorizes.

Strenuous activity intensifies fatigue and may delay healing. Activities that increase intra-abdominal pressure can strain surgical repairs, and prolonged sitting potentiates risk of thrombus formation. Showers are permitted, but tub baths and douching may cause vaginal or incisional infections and are a safety hazard.

Encourage client to report bowel dysfunction—constipation, loss of urge to defecate, severe straining, incomplete evacuation, and digital evacuation—to healthcare providers if it occurs.

Constipation is a frequent symptom after hysterectomy and may be related to undiagnosed irritable bowel syndrome, which is often present preoperatively and/or associated with the particular procedure performed—vaginal hysterectomy with posterior repair.

Discuss dietary modifications, medicinal bulk agents, and stimulation by suppository, as indicated.

Postsurgical bowel dysfunction may be short-term or long-term and may require simple home management measures, or referral for medical intervention.

Review recommendations of resumption of sexual intercourse. (Refer to ND: risk for Sexual Dysfunction.)

When sexual activity is cleared by the physician, it is best to resume activity easily and gently, expressing sexual feelings in other ways or using alternative coital positions.

Identify dietary needs, such as high-quality protein, complex carbohydrates, and additional iron. Provide information about foods to include and avoid in managing menopausal symptoms.

Facilitates healing and tissue regeneration, helps correct anemia when present. *Note:* Certain vegetables, such as broccoli, cabbage, cauliflower, brussels sprouts, and turnips, may have protective action against excessive estrogen effects. Some foods and substances to avoid or limit include rich dairy products, sugar, fried foods, caffeine, alcohol, and nicotine.

Review hormone replacement therapy (HRT) and route (oral, injection, patch) when used. Clarify distinction between long-term HRT use for preventive therapy and short-term use for symptom relief.

Total hysterectomy with bilateral salpingo-oophorectomy results in surgically induced menopause requiring replacement hormones. Benefits of HRT, particularly estrogen, include protection against osteoporosis and the amelioration of certain postmenopausal discomforts such as sleep disturbance, hot flashes, mood disorders, problems with memory and concentration, reduced libido, and urinary symptoms. However, it is generally recognized that HRT is not cardioprotective, and risks may outweigh benefits (Institute for Clinical Systems Improvement [ICSI], 2006).

Encourage taking prescribed drug(s) routinely, for example with meals or at bedtime. Determine when patch should be changed, wearing time altered.

Establishes routine for taking drug and reduces potential for discontinuing drug because of nausea that is often an early side effect.

Discuss potential side effects, such as weight gain, increased skin pigmentation or acne, breast tenderness, headaches, and photosensitivity.

Development of some side effects is expected but may require problem-solving for the client to continue the hormones, such as change in dosage; change of delivery method; and use of analgesics, sunscreen, and sunglasses.

Recommend cessation of smoking, especially when receiving estrogen therapy.

Some studies suggest an increased risk of thrombophlebitis, myocardial infarction (MI), stroke, and pulmonary emboli associated with smoking and concurrent estrogen therapy (ICSI, 2006).

Inquire if client is taking or planning to take vitamins and/or herbal supplements for menopause, such as vitamin C with bioflavonoids, calcium, magnesium, selenium, evening primrose oil, black cohosh, angelica, and wild yam.

Client may express desire to use "natural hormones" and feel confused over choices. These substances are numerous and available and have been the object of media attention. They should be reviewed in terms of expected action, potential interaction, or adverse effects, depending on client's particular situation and reason for the hysterectomy.

Review incisional care, when appropriate.

Facilitates competent self-care, promoting independence.

ACTIONS/INTERVENTIONS (continued)	**RATIONALE** (continued)
Stress importance of follow-up care.	Provides opportunity to ask questions, clear up misunderstandings, and detect developing complications. *Note:* Client needs to discuss with the physician her particular requirements for follow-up pelvic exams with Pap smear, once surgical healing has occurred. The need and rationale for these exams depends upon the client's reason for hysterectomy—benign fibroids versus cervical neoplasm.
Identify signs and symptoms requiring medical evaluation, such as fever or chills, change in character of vaginal or wound drainage, and bright red bleeding.	Early recognition and treatment of developing complications, such as infection or hemorrhage, may prevent life-threatening situations. *Note:* Hemorrhage may occur as late as 2 weeks postoperatively.
Identify support group and appropriate Web sites, as indicated.	May desire additional information or opportunity to discuss feelings or concerns with women with similar experiences. However, instruct client to exercise caution when choosing Internet resources and sharing personal information online (Bunde et al, 2007).

POTENTIAL CONSIDERATIONS following acute hospitalization (dependent on client's age, physical condition, and presence of complications, personal resources, and life responsibilities)

In addition to surgical and cancer concerns (if appropriate):
- *Sexual Dysfunction*—altered body structure and function, changes in hormone levels, decreased libido, possible change in sexual response pattern, vaginal discomfort or pain (dyspareunia)
- *situational low Self-Esteem*—concerns about changes in femininity, effect on sexual relationship, inability to have children, religious conflicts

---

MASTECTOMY

I. Purpose
  a. Removal of breast tissue due to presence of malignant or cancerous tumor changes
  b. Surgical procedures: dependent on tumor type, size, and location as well as clinical characteristics or staging
   i. Breast-conserving therapy
   ii. Lumpectomy
   iii. Partial or segmental mastectomy
   iv. Lymph node surgery
   v. Mastectomy (Mayo Clinic, 2007)
    1. Simple or total
    2. Modified radical
    3. Radical
    4. Skin-sparing mastectomy

II. Pathology—Tumor growth originates in cells of the breast tissue occurring primarily in women, although men may also be affected.
  a. Types (National Comprehensive Cancer Network [NCCN], 2007)
   i. Ductal
    1. Occurs in the ducts that connect the lobes and the nipple
    2. Represents 80% of all breast cancers (invasive ductal carcinoma)
   ii. Lobular
    1. Occurs in the lobes where milk is produced
    2. Represents 10% to 15% of all cancers
  b. Clinical staging (NCCN, 2007)
   i. Classification: noninvasive, invasive, or infiltrating
   ii. Size and spread of tumor: T stage
   iii. Number of lymph nodes involved: N stage
   iv. Metastasis: M stage
   v. Grade measured from 0–IV, with zero resembling normal breast tissue
   vi. Some stages further divided by letters of the alphabet (A, B, C, etc.)

III. Statistics (National Cancer Institute [NCI], 2008)
  a. Morbidity: As of January 2005, approximately 2,477,847 American women had a history of breast cancer; in 2008, an estimated 182,460 new cases of breast cancer were diagnosed in women and 1,990 in men.
  b. Mortality: In 2007, breast cancer was the second-leading cause of death in women in the United States; an estimated 40,480 women and 450 men died of breast cancer in 2008.
  c. Cost: Projected $8.1 billion spent in United States in 2004, averaging $11,000 per Medicare client in first year following diagnosis (Brown et al, 2002)

Breast-conserving therapy: Treatment of choice for most women with stage I or stage II breast cancer and usually followed with radiation therapy.

Grade: Determined by cellular differentiation; the lower the grade, the more it resembles normal breast tissue and the least likely it is to spread.

Infiltrating: Breast cancer that extends into the surrounding breast tissue and may metastasize.

In situ: Breast cancer that is encapsulated within the breast.

Lumpectomy: Removes only the breast lump and a rim of normal surrounding breast tissue.

Lymph node surgery: Removal of lymph node(s) to determine if breast cancer has spread to the lymph ducts or lymph nodes in the axilla. In tumors 2 cm or smaller in size, a *sentinel* procedure may be performed to remove only the node(s) deemed most likely to contain cancerous cells. In larger tumors, or if sentinel biopsy is positive, a traditional axillary lymph node dissection is performed.

Metastasis: Cancer that has spread to other parts of the body.

Modified radical mastectomy: Removal of entire breast and some axillary (underarm) lymph nodes.

Partial or segmental mastectomy: Removes more breast tissue than a lumpectomy—up to one-quarter of the breast—which is then called a quadrantectomy.

Radical mastectomy: All the muscle under the breast is removed; however, it is rarely used today because it is no more effective than the more limited forms of mastectomy.

Simple or total mastectomy: Entire breast is removed, but no lymph nodes from under the arm or muscle tissue from beneath the breast are removed.

Skin-sparing mastectomy: Removal of the entire breast, nipple, and areola, without removal of the breast skin for immediate or delayed breast reconstruction.

Staging: Method to classify progression of cancer in order to select treatment options and predict a prognosis.

Care Setting

Client is treated at inpatient acute surgical unit.

Related Concerns

Cancer, page 846 (for additional nursing interventions regarding cancer treatments, including chemotherapy and radiation)

Psychosocial aspects of care, page 749

Surgical intervention, page 782

Client Assessment Database

DIAGNOSTIC DIVISION MAY REPORT	MAY EXHIBIT
ACTIVITY/REST • Ineffective activity involving frequent or repetitive arm movements • Altered sleep style such as sleeping in a prone position	
CIRCULATION	• Unilateral engorgement in affected arm as a result of lymph node involvement
EGO INTEGRITY • Constant stressors in work or home life • Stress and fear involving diagnosis, prognosis, and future expectations	
FOOD/FLUID • Loss of appetite, recent weight loss	
PAIN/DISCOMFORT • Pain may be reported in advanced metastatic disease but rarely occurs in early malignancy • Discomfort or "funny feeling" in breast tissue occurs in some clients	

Client Assessment Database (continued)

DIAGNOSTIC DIVISION MAY REPORT (continued)	MAY EXHIBIT (continued)

SAFETY

- Nodular axillary masses
- Edema, erythema of involved skin

SEXUALITY

- Presence of a usually painless breast lump
- Changes in breast symmetry or size, pitting or dimpling of breast skin, color changes such as erythema or temperature, unusual nipple discharge, itching, burning, retracted nipple
- History of early menarche younger than age 12, late menopause after age 50, late first pregnancy such as after age 30
- Concerns about sexuality and intimacy

- Change in breast contour or symmetry
- Retraction of nipple, discharge from nipple

TEACHING/LEARNING

- Family history of genetically transmitted breast cancer. *Note:* BRCA1 and BRCA2 genes that have mutated account for 80%–90% of hereditary cancers and present a lifetime risk factor 10 times that of the population (NCI, 2008); however, most breast cancer clients have no relatives with the disease, with only 5%–10% attributable to hereditary factors
- Previous unilateral breast cancer, endometrial cancer, or ovarian cancer
- History of prolonged hormone replacement therapy, radiation, or multiple breast biopsies or procedures

DISCHARGE PLAN CONSIDERATIONS

- May need assistance with treatments and rehabilitation, decisions, self-care activities, and homemaker or maintenance tasks.

- Refer to section at end of plan for postdischarge considerations.

Diagnostic Studies

TEST WHY IT IS DONE	WHAT IT TELLS ME

BLOOD TESTS

- *Hormone receptor assay:* Test to determine whether a breast cancer's growth is influenced by hormones or if it can be treated with hormones.

Reveals whether cells of excised tumor or biopsy specimens contain hormone receptors (estrogen and progesterone). In malignant cells, the estrogen-plus receptor complex stimulates cell growth and division. About two-thirds of all women with breast cancer are estrogen-receptor positive and tend to respond favorably to the addition of hormone blocking therapy, which extends the disease-free period and increases survival time.

- *Human epidermal growth factor receptor 2 (HER2/neu):* A growth-promoting protein.

Cancer cells with too many copies of this gene tend to grow and spread more aggressively than do other breast cancers. HER2/neu–positive breast cancers can be treated with the drug Herceptin (trastuzumab), which prevents the HER2/neu protein from stimulating breast cancer cell growth.

(continues on page 622)

TEST
WHY IT IS DONE (continued)

- *Breast cancer genes—BRCA-1 and BRCA-2:* Normal genes that are associated with familial breast cancer when inherited in mutated state.

- *Ploidy:* Chromosome test that refers to the amount of DNA that cancer cells contain.

OTHER DIAGNOSTIC STUDIES
- *Mammography:* Visualizes internal structure of the breast; capable of detecting nonpalpable cancers or tumors that are in early stages of development.
  - *Digital mammography:* Creates computer images, rather than images on film, which can be manipulated and transmitted for further review.
  - *Ultrasound:* Uses sound waves to produce images for both screening and diagnostic staging.

- *Magnetic resonance imaging (MRI):* Creates images that capture multiple cross-sectional pictures using a computer to generate detailed two- and three-dimensional images.

- *Biopsy:* Removal of a sample of suspicious tissue for examination by a pathologist.

  - *Fine-needle aspiration biopsy:* A fine, hollow needle is inserted into a lump or lesion and cells are withdrawn for evaluation.

  - *Core-needle biopsy:* A hollow needle is used to take several rice- or grain-sized cores of tissue.

  - *Stereotactic biopsy:* Computer-guided procedure that uses a core needle to obtain a larger tissue sample (than the fine-needle procedure), or, a vacuum-assisted device (VAD) that allows collection of multiple tissue samples during one needle insertion.
  - *Ultrasound-guided core-needle biopsy:* Core-needle biopsy that uses ultrasound to produce precise images of structures within the body.
  - *Surgical biopsy:* All or part of the suspicious tissues may be removed by surgery for cytological examination.
  - *Sentinel node biopsy:* The lymph ducts of the breast usually drain to one lymph node first before draining to the remaining axillary lymph nodes. Lymph node mapping helps to identify that specific lymph node to determine presence of cancerous cells.

WHAT IT TELLS ME (continued)

Associated with a high risk of female breast cancer and ovarian cancer, as well as male breast cancer (BRCA2), and other cancers. The tests may be performed on young women with more than one family member who has developed breast cancer at an early age.

Helps predict how aggressive a cancer is likely to be. If the amount is abnormal, the cells are aneuploid. Aneuploid breast cancers tend to be faster growing and more likely to recur than other forms of breast cancers.

Women with dense breasts may benefit from digital, rather than a film, mammography.

Complements findings of mammograms. Distinguishes fluid-filled cysts from solid tumors. Ongoing studies are evaluating whether whole-breast ultrasound should be used in conjunction with mammography to screen high-risk women with dense breast tissue (Mayo Clinic, 2008).

Performed when more information is needed than a mammogram, ultrasound, or clinical breast exam can provide. Ductal cancer in situ is usually better detected with an MRI than with a mammography.

Biposy may be done if a mammography, surgery, or other screening method reveals a mass or lesion to determine whether it is benign or cancerous.

This is usually performed when a fluid-filled mass is seen on an ultrasound image or a lesion is detected during a clinical breast exam.

With this type of biopsy, tissue structure and cells can be evaluated. When a solid mass has been detected, ultrasound may be used to guide the placement of the needle.

When a suspicious area cannot be palpated or located by ultrasound—but is visible through mammography—the physician uses digital x-rays to guide the needle to the abnormality and perform the biopsy.

May be used in place of fine-needle biopsy or surgical biopsy to verify diagnosis.

Total removal of the tissue is called an excisional biopsy, whereas partial removal is called an incisional biopsy.

If the first node is benign, it is likely that all other nodes are the same, thereby limiting removal of additional nodes, preventing damage to the ducts and the increased potential for lymphedema, and avoiding an axillary node dissection (Mayo Clinic, 2008).

Nursing Priorities

1. Assist client and significant other (SO) in dealing with stress of situation and prognosis.
2. Prevent complications.
3. Establish individualized rehabilitation program.
4. Provide information about disease process, procedure, prognosis, and treatment needs.

Discharge Goals

1. Dealing realistically with situation.
2. Complications prevented or minimized.
3. Exercise regimen implemented.
4. Disease process, surgical procedure, prognosis, and therapeutic regimen understood.
5. Plan in place to meet needs after discharge.

Preoperative

NURSING DIAGNOSIS: Anxiety/death Anxiety

May be related to
Threat to self-concept—change of body image; scarring, loss of body part, sexual attractiveness
Threat of death—extent of disease, impact on others; uncertainty of prognosis; denial of own mortality
Situational crisis

Possibly evidenced by
Increased tension, apprehension, feelings of helplessness, inadequacy
Decreased self-assurance, powerlessness
Self-focus, restlessness, sympathetic stimulation, crying, aggression, withdrawal
Expressed concerns regarding actual or anticipated changes in life

Desired Outcomes/Evaluation Criteria—Client Will

Anxiety Level (NOC)
Demonstrate appropriate range of feelings regarding possibility of death or increasing hope related to prognosis.
Acknowledge acceptance of health status.

Anxiety Self-Control (NOC)
Communicate thoughts and feelings utilizing available support systems such as family, spiritual leaders, and other resources.
Demonstrate coping behaviors that reduce anxiety.

ACTIONS/INTERVENTIONS	RATIONALE
Anxiety Reduction (NIC)	
Independent	
Ascertain what information client has about diagnosis, expected surgical intervention, and future therapies. Note presence of denial or extreme anxiety.	Provides knowledge base for the nurse to enable reinforcement of needed information, helps identify client with high anxiety, or a low capacity for information processing, and need for special attention. *Note:* Denial may be useful as a coping method intially; however, extreme anxiety needs to be dealt with immediately.
Explain purpose and preparation for diagnostic tests or procedures.	Promotes clear understanding of procedures and what is happening, increases feelings of control, and lessens anxiety and fear of the ukown.
Provide an atmosphere of concern and anticipatory guidance and privacy for client and family.	Facilitates therapeutic communication, active-listening, and expression of underlying unresolved issues. Privacy is needed to encourage open discussion related to feelings of anticipated loss and other concerns.
Encourage questions and provide time for expression of fears.	Provides opportunity to identify and clarify misconceptions and offer emotional support.
Offer relaxation techniques such as back massage, guided imagery, and use of touch, if culturally acceptable.	Encourages verbalization of feelings when client is relaxed, thus reducing anxiety and fear.
Explore previously used coping mechanisms as perceived by the client.	Reinforces effective coping mechanisms previously used for coping in a new situation.
Explore spiritual support as a resource.	Provides calmness and peace in times of uncertainty.
Discuss role of rehabilitation after surgery and use of community resources.	Promotes support systems in place in the rehabilitation process as an essential component of therapy intended to meet physical, social, emotional, and vocational needs so that client can achieve the best possible level of physical and emotional functioning.

NURSING DIAGNOSIS: impaired Skin/Tissue Integrity

May be related to
Surgical removal of skin and tissue; altered circulation, presence of edema, drainage; changes in skin elasticity, sensation; tissue destruction (radiation)

Possibly evidenced by
Disruption of skin surface, destruction of skin layers and subcutaneous tissues

Desired Outcomes/Evaluation Criteria—Client Will

Wound Healing: Primary Intention (NOC)
Achieve timely wound healing free of purulent drainage or erythema.

Knowledge: Treatment Procedures (NOC)
Verbalize understanding of treatment plan to promote wound healing.
Demonstrate wound care techniques that facilitate increased tissue granulation at incision site.
Demonstrate behaviors that prevent complications.

ACTIONS/INTERVENTIONS	RATIONALE
Incision Site Care (NIC) *Independent*	
Assess dressings and wound for amount and characteristics of drainage.	Use of dressings depends on the extent of surgery and the type of wound closure. Pressure dressings are usually applied initially and are reinforced, not changed. Drainage occurs because of the trauma of the procedure and manipulation of the numerous blood vessels and lymphatics in the area.
Provide drain care, instructing client/family in the process, as indicated.	The Jackson-Pratt drain is most commonly used for mastectomies to maintain negative pressure in the wound and is easily managed. Simple mastectomies use one drain, whereas more complex procedures, such as those involving removal of lymph nodes, may require several drains. Drains are usually removed around the third day or when drainage ceases, possibly after client is discharged. Teaching facilitates self-care, reducing a major concern of client.
Monitor temperature.	Early recognition of developing infection enables rapid institution of treatment.
Place in semi-Fowler's position on back or unaffected side; avoid letting the affected arm dangle.	Assists with drainage of fluid through use of gravity.
Prevent or minimize edema of involved arm.	Reduces the discomfort and associated complications.
Elevate hand and arm with shoulder positioned at appropriate angles at no more than 65 degrees of flexion, 45–65 degrees of abduction, 45–60 degrees of internal rotation, and forearm resting on wedge or pillow, as indicated.	Elevation of affected arm facilitates drainage and resolution of edema. Lymphedema is present in approximately 24% to 49% postmastectomy depending on surgical procedure performed (Warren et al, 2007). This may develop immediately after surgery or years later.
Avoid measuring blood pressure (BP), injecting medications, or inserting intravenous (IV) lines in affected arm.	Increases potential of constriction, infection, and lymphedema on affected side.
Inspect donor and graft site, if done, for color and blister formation; note drainage from donor site.	Assesses circulation of affected area. Blister formation identifies bacterial growth and infection.
Encourage wearing of loose-fitting, nonconstrictive clothing. Inform the client not to wear wristwatch or other jewelry on affected arm.	Reduces pressure on compromised tissues, which may improve circulation and healing, and minimize lymphedema.
Collaborative	
Administer antibiotics, as indicated.	Provides prophylaxis to treat specific infection and enhance healing.

NURSING DIAGNOSIS: acute Pain

May be related to
Surgical procedure; tissue trauma, interruption of nerves, dissection of muscles

Possibly evidenced by
Reports of stiffness, numbness, or burning in chest area, shoulder and affected arm pain, alteration of muscle tone
Self-focusing, distraction or guarding behaviors

NURSING DIAGNOSIS: acute Pain (continued)

Desired Outcomes/Evaluation Criteria—Client Will

Pain Level (NOC)
Express reduction in pain or discomfort.
Identify factors that aggravate or relieve pain.
Appear relaxed and be able to sleep or rest appropriately.

ACTIONS/INTERVENTIONS	RATIONALE
Pain Management (NIC)	
Independent	
Assess reports of pain and sensory alterations, noting location, duration, and intensity (scale of 0–10). Note reports of stiffness, swelling, and numbness or burning in chest, shoulder, and affected arm. Identify verbal and nonverbal cues.	Examines the degree of discomfort and verifies the need for analgesia and evaluates its effectiveness. The amount of tissue, muscle, and lymphatic system removed can affect the amount of pain experienced. The need to elevate arm, the size of dressings, and the presence of drains all affect client's ability to relax and rest or sleep effectively.
Explain the causes of pain to the client.	Provides understanding of sensory alterations. Destruction of nerves in axillary region causes numbness in upper arm and scapular region, which may be more intolerable than surgical pain. Pain in chest wall can occur from muscle tension, be affected by extremes in heat and cold, and continue for several months.
Acknowledge the presence of phantom breast sensations.	Provides reassurance that sensations are not imaginary and that relief can be obtained.
Provide basic comfort and diversional activities. Encourage early ambulation and use of relaxation techniques, guided imagery, and Therapeutic Touch.	Promotes relaxation, refocuses attention away from the discomfort, and may enhance coping abilities.
Provide opportunities for uninterrupted sleep.	Relieves fatigue, increasing coping ability.
Splint or support chest during coughing and deep-breathing exercises.	Facilitates participation in activity without undue discomfort.
Provide appropriate pain medication on a regular schedule before pain is severe and before activities are scheduled.	Maintains comfort level and permits client to exercise arm and to ambulate without pain hindering efforts.
Provide accurate information related to patient-controlled analgesia (PCA) or opioids to reduce fear of addiction.	Reduces fear, augmenting appropriate pain relief, to enhance mobility and coping abilities.
Describe the adverse effects of unrelieved pain.	Explains complications resulting from poor pain management both physiologically and emotionally (NCI, 2008).
Discuss previous successful methods of coping with pain.	Provides pain-relieving methods to employ based on past experiences.
Collaborative	
Administer PCA, opioids, or nonopioids, as indicated.	Provides relief from discomfort or pain and facilitates rest and participation in postoperative therapy.

NURSING DIAGNOSIS: situational low Self-Esteem

May be related to
Surgical change in structure or body contour
Fear of rejection or reaction by others
Behaviors inconsistent with self-value system

Possibly evidenced by
Reports of current situational challenge to self-worth
Self-negating verbalizations

Desired Outcomes/Evaluation Criteria—Client Will

Self-Esteem (NOC)
Distinguish between self-perceptions and societal stigmas.
Identify strategies to cope with self-acceptance in present situation.
Verbalize progress toward acceptance of self.
Participate in setting realistic goals involving the postoperative therapy program.

ACTIONS/INTERVENTIONS	RATIONALE

Self-Esteem Enhancement (NIC)

Independent

Provide active-listening when surgical dressings are removed.	Provides emotional support and client safety.
Assess for grief, depression, and ineffective coping.	Common reactions that need to be recognized immediately for timely intervention, as indicated. Grief may resurface when subsequent procedures are done, such as fitting for prosthesis or reconstructive procedure if postponed.
Validate client's feelings and address any misinformation that is revealed.	Encourages client to express feelings and provides opportunity to give or reinforce information.
Encourage questions about current situation and future expectations.	Loss of the breast causes many reactions, including feeling disfigured, fear of viewing scar, and fear of partner's reaction to change in body. Loss of body part, disfigurement, and perceived loss of sexual desirability engender grieving process that needs to be dealt with so that client can make plans for the future.
Identify role concerns as woman, wife, mother, career woman, and so forth.	Explores possible alteration in client's self-perception.
Provide positive reinforcement for gains and improvement and participation in self-care and treatment program.	Encourages continuation of healthy behaviors.
Review possibilities for reconstructive surgery and/or prosthetic augmentation.	If feasible, reconstruction provides less disfiguring or "near-normal" cosmetic result. Variations in skin flap may be done for facilitation of reconstructive procedure, which is often performed at the same time as mastectomy. The associated emotional boost may help the client through the more complex surgical recovery process and adjunctive therapies. *Note:* On occasion, reconstruction may not be done for 3 to 6 months. A prolonged delay may result in increased tension in relationships and impair client's incorporation of changes into self-concept.
Identify concerns of client and SO regarding sexual dysfunction in order to provide acceptable practices for self and SO. Encourage communication of needs and fears of both partners.	Negative responses directed at client may actually reflect SO's concern about hurting client, fear of cancer or death, difficulty in dealing with personality, behavior changes in client, or inability to look at operative area.
Discuss and refer to support groups, as appropriate.	Provides a place to exchange concerns and feelings with others who have had a similar experience and identifies ways SO can facilitate client's recovery.

Collaborative

Provide temporary soft prosthesis, if indicated.	Prosthesis of nylon and Dacron fluff may be worn in bra until incision heals if reconstructive surgery is not performed at the time of mastectomy. This may promote social acceptance and allow client to feel more comfortable about body image at the time of discharge.

NURSING DIAGNOSIS: impaired physical Mobility

May be related to
Neuromuscular impairment; pain, discomfort; edema formation

Possibly evidenced by
Reluctance to attempt movement
Limited range of motion (ROM), decreased muscle mass and strength

Desired Outcomes/Evaluation Criteria—Client Will

Motivation (NOC)
Display willingness to participate in therapy.
Demonstrate techniques that enable resumption of activities.

Body Mechanics Performance (NOC)
Demonstrate increased muscle strength of affected body parts.

ACTIONS/INTERVENTIONS	RATIONALE

Exercise Therapy: Muscle Control (NIC)

Independent

Elevate affected arm, as indicated.

Promotes venous return, lessening possibility of lymphedema.

Perform passive ROM, such as flexion and extension of elbow, pronation and supination of wrist, and clenching and extending fingers, as soon as possible.

Early postoperative exercises are usually started in the first 24 hours to prevent joint stiffness that can further limit movement and mobility.

Encourage client to move fingers, noting sensations and color of hand on affected side.

Lack of movement may reflect problems with the intercostal brachial nerve. Discoloration can indicate impaired circulation.

Encourage client to use affected arm for personal hygiene: feeding, combing hair, and washing face.

Increases circulation, minimizes edema, and maintains strength and function of the arm and hand. These activities use the arm without abduction, eliminating stress on the suture line in the early postoperative period.

Assist with self-care activities, as necessary.

Conserves client's energy and prevents undue fatigue.

Assist with ambulation and encourage correct posture.

Client will feel unbalanced and may need assistance until accustomed to change. Keeping back straight prevents shoulder from moving forward, avoiding permanent limitation in movement and posture.

Advance exercise, as indicated, for example, active extension of arm and rotation of shoulder while lying in bed, pendulum swings, rope turning, and elevating arms to touch fingertips behind head.

Prevents joint stiffness, increases circulation, and maintains muscle tone of the shoulders and arm.

Instruct in proper breathing technique of slow, deep breaths during exercise.

Contraction of abdominal muscles helps push fluid out of the cisterna chyli, a lymphatic reservoir, and through the thoracic duct, creating a vacuum effect enhancing drainage.

Progress to hand climbing or walking fingers up wall, clasping hands behind head, and full abduction exercises as soon as client can manage.

Because this group of exercises can cause excessive tension on the incision, they are usually delayed until healing process is well established.

Evaluate degree of exercise-related pain and changes in joint mobility. Measure upper arm and forearm if edema develops.

Monitors progression and resolution of complications. May need to postpone increasing exercises and wait until further healing occurs.

Discuss types of exercises to be done at home to regain strength and enhance circulation in the affected arm.

Exercise program needs to be continued to regain optimal function of the affected side.

Coordinate exercise program into self-care and homemaker activities such as dressing self, washing, dusting, and mopping; and leisure activities, such as swimming.

Client is usually more willing to participate or finds it easier to maintain an exercise program that fits into her lifestyle and accomplishes tasks as well.

Assist client to identify signs/symptoms of shoulder tension, such as an inability to maintain posture or a burning sensation in the postscapular region. Instruct client to avoid sitting or holding arm in dependent position for extended periods.

Altered weight and support put tension on surrounding structures.

Collaborative

Administer medications, as indicated, for example:
  Analgesics

Pain needs to be controlled before exercise or client may not participate optimally and incentive to exercise may be lost.

  Diuretics

May be useful in treating and preventing fluid accumulation or lymphedema.

Maintain integrity of elastic bandages or custom-fitted, pressure-gradient elastic sleeve.

Promotes venous return and decreases risk or effects of edema formation.

Refer to physical and occupational therapist and lymphedema clinic or specialist.

Provides an individualized exercise program. Assesses limitations or restrictions regarding employment requirements.

NURSING DIAGNOSIS: **deficient Knowledge [Learning Need] regarding condition, prognosis, treatment, self-care, and discharge needs**

May be related to
Lack of exposure or recall
Information misinterpretation

Possibly evidenced by
Questions and requests for information, statement of misconception
Inaccurate follow-through of instructions, development of preventable complications

(continues on page 628)

Desired Outcomes/Evaluation Criteria—Client Will

Knowledge: Illness Care (NOC)
Verbalize understanding of disease process and potential complications.
Perform necessary procedures correctly and explain reasons for actions.
Initiate necessary lifestyle changes and participate in treatment regimen.

ACTIONS/INTERVENTIONS	RATIONALE
Teaching: Disease Process (NIC)	
Independent	
Review disease process, surgical procedure, and future expectations.	Provides knowledge base from which client can make informed choices, including participation in radiation and/or chemotherapy programs. (Refer to CP: Cancer.)
Review and have client demonstrate care of drains and wound sites.	Shorter hospital stays may result in discharge with drains in place, requiring more complex care by client and caregivers. Drains may be removed 7 to 10 days after surgery.
Encourage continuation of exercises, increasing program as healing progresses, for at least 1 year.	Good muscle tone enhances development of collateral lymphatic channels, reduces the tightening of scar tissue, and maintains muscle strength and function. Moderation is important because strenuous activity or exercise increases heart rate and body temperature, which can potentially increase edema. Some evidence suggests that exercise lowers the risk of recurrence of breast cancer (Ligibel, 2008).
Discuss necessity for well-balanced, nutritious meals and adequate fluid intake.	Provides optimal nutrition and maintains circulating volume to enhance tissue regeneration and the healing process.
Suggest alternating schedule of frequent rest and activity periods, especially in situations when sitting or standing is prolonged.	Prevents or limits fatigue, promotes healing, and enhances feelings of general well-being. Positions in which arm is dangling or extended intensify stress on stuture lines, creating muscle tension and stiffness, and may interfere with healing.
Instruct client to protect hands and arms, for example:	
Wear long sleeves and gloves when gardening, use thimble when sewing, and do not carry purse or wear jewelry or wristwatch on affected side.	Compromised lymphatic system causes tissues to be more susceptible to infection and/or injury, which may lead to lymphedema.
Use potholders when handling hot items; use plastic gloves when doing dishes.	Sensory alterations place client at risk for burns and infections.
Avoid lifting, moving heavy objects, or prolonged sitting and standing.	Prevents venous stasis.
Demonstrate holding affected arm appropriately, for example, not dangling the arm, swinging arms with elbows bent when walking, and placing arm above heart level when sitting or lying down.	Helps prevent or minimize lymphedema and "frozen shoulder."
Warn against having blood withdrawn or receiving IV fluids and medications or BP measurements on the affected side.	May restrict the criculation and increase risk of infection when the lymphatic system is compromised.
Recommend wearing of a medical identification device.	Prevents unnecessary trauma to affected arm from BP measurements, injections, and so on, in emergency situations.
Demonstrate use of intermittent sequential pumping or low-stretch compression custom-made garments, as appropriate.	Used in managing lymphedema by promoting circulation and venous return.
Suggest gentle massage of healed incision with emollients.	Stimulates circulation, promotes elasticity of skin, and reduces discomfort associated with phantom breast sensations.
Recommend use of sexual positions that avoid pressure on chest wall. Encourage alternative forms of sexual expression such as cuddling or touching during initial healing process and while operative area is still tender.	Promotes feelings of femininity and sense of ability to resume sexual contact.
Encourage regular self-examination of remaining breast. Determine recommended schedule for mammography.	Identifies changes in breast tissue indicative of recurrent or new tumor development.
Stress importance of regular medical follow-up.	Other treatment may be required as adjunctive therapy, such as radiation. Recurrence of malignant breast tumors also can be identified and managed by an oncologist.
Identify signs and symptoms requiring medical evaluation: breast or arm red, warm, and swollen; edema and purulent wound drainage; and fever or chills.	Lymphangitis can occur as a result of infection, causing lymphedema.

ACTIONS/INTERVENTIONS (continued)

Address additional concerns as indicated—ongoing therapies and expected and/or adverse side effects.

RATIONALE (continued)

Some medications, such as tamoxifen (Nolvadex), used as follow-up to surgery or radiation, require ongoing involvement in care. *Note:* Estrogen-blocking treatment may be used in some instances. The female hormone estrogen promotes the growth of breast cancer cells in some women. For these women, several agents, such as tamoxifen or letrozole, are available to block the effect of estrogen or to lower its levels.

POTENTIAL CONSIDERATIONS following acute hospitalization (dependent on client's age, physical condition and presence of complications, personal resources, and life responsibilities)

In addition to surgical and cancer concerns:
- *impaired Skin/Tissue Integrity*—surgical removal of skin/tissue, altered circulation, presence of edema, drainage; changes in skin elasticity, sensation, tissue destruction (radiation)
- *situational low Self-Esteem*—biophysical, disfiguring surgical procedure, concern about sexual attractiveness
- *Self-Care Deficit (specify)*—decreased strength and endurance, pain, muscular impairment

Sample clinical pathway follows in Table 11.1.

TABLE 11.1 Sample CP: Mastectomy—Modified Radical, Hospital. ELOS: 2 Days

ND and Categories of Care	Day of Surgery _____	Postop Day 1 _____	Postop Day 2 _____ (Discharge)
impaired Skin/Tissue Integrity R/T therapeutic interventions	Display wound drainage w/in established limits Maintain usual color, sensation and motion in affected fingers/hand	Participate in self-care activities/beginning exercise program Identify ways to maximize healing/minimize risk of injury to arm	Display minimal erythema, absence of purulent drainage, edema resolving Report plan in place to meet postdischarge needs
Referrals	Physical Therapist Occupational Therapist Home Care		
Additional assessments	Dressing/drainage q4h Presence/degree of edema q8h	→ q8h Wound characteristics → 8d & Measure upper arm/forearm if edema present	→ →
	Donor/graft site if used q4h	→ q8h	→ D/C
	VS q1h × 4 → q4h	→ q8h	→ q12h
	I&O and wound drainage system q8hr	→	→ Discharge with drain in place/remove when less than 30 mL/24 h
	Neurovascular check—UE q1h × 4 → q4h × 2	→ q8h	→
Medications	Diuretic if edema present	→	→ D/C
Client teaching	Protection of affected arm: shaving, use of deodorant/creams, activity limitations, avoidance of heat/cold, proper posture/positioning of arm, sexual positions to prevent pressure on chest wall, wearing loose-fitting clothing	Wound care	Management of wound drain if not removed
	Graduated exercise program incorporating ADLs/homemaking activities	Gentle massage of healed incision	S/S to report to healthcare provider

(continues on page 630)

ND and Categories of Care	Day of Surgery _____	Postop Day 1 _____	Postop Day 2 _____ (Discharge)
		General healthcare needs to promote healing, dietary intake, fluids, rest/pacing self	Use of medical alert device
		Breast self-examination	Provide written instructions, schedule for follow-up visits/additional treatment modalities
Additional nursing actions	Position per protocol; HOB elevated 30° or more	→	→
	BRP/chair w/assist	→ Ambulate/up ad lib	→
	Elevate affected arm	→	→
	Turn, cough, deep breath or incentive spirometry q2hr	→ DB/IS q2h WA	→
	Maintain elastic bandages/custom-fitted, pressure-gradient sleeve if used	→	→
	Reinforce dressing PRN	→ Assist w/dressing chg	→ D/C dressing
	Encourage progressive exercises & ambulate as tolerated	→	→
	Advance diet as tolerated	→	→
Acute Pain R/T tissue trauma, muscle dissection	Report pain reduced to manageable level	→	Verbalize understanding of therapeutic regimen
	Participate in activities to manage pain	→	→
Additional assessments	Pain characteristics/chges	→	→
Medications	Response to interventions	→	→
Allergies:_____	Analgesic of choice	→ PO analgesic	→
	IV/PO		
Client education	Orient to unit/room	S/S of shoulder tension; possibility of phantom breast pain	Medication: dose, time/ frequency, purpose, side effects
	Reporting of pain/effects of interventions	Progression of exercises as tolerated	
	Initial exercises of fingers/wrist of affected arm; ROM exercises of unaffected limbs	Home exercise program	
	Relaxation techniques		
	Splinting of chest w/ coughing, exercise		
	Routine comfort measures	→	→
Additional nursing actions	Passive ROM/exercises per protocol	→ Advance exercises as tolerated	→
	Assist w/self-care	→	→
situational low Self-Esteem, R/T perceived disfigure-ment, psychosocial concerns	Verbalize feelings, verbal/nonverbal com-munication congruent	→	→ Verbalize acceptance of self
		Participate in care/planning for future	→ Plan in place to meet post-discharge needs
		View incision	
Referrals	Social services		
	Reach to Recovery		
Additional assessments	Response to surgical proce-dure by client and SO	Future expectations, role con-cerns, usual coping strate-gies, past coping successes	
	Availability/effectiveness of support systems	Understanding of diagnosis	

TABLE 11.1 **Sample CP: Mastectomy—Modified Radical, Hospital. ELOS: 2 Days** (continued)

Client education	Postoperative routines	Community resources for client and SO	S/S to report to healthcare provider (depression)
	Extent/outcome of surgical procedure		Written information regarding diagnosis/treatment options
	Future treatment needs		
	Use of/sources for temporary prosthesis		
	Possibilities for reconstructive surgery/prosthetic augmentation		
Additional nursing actions	Discuss normalcy of feelings	Role-play ways of handling responses of others	Identify options for managing home/work responsibilities; importance of taking time for self
	Encourage participation in self-care at level of ability	Provide support/answer questions when dressing removed	
	Provide positive reinforcement for participation in therapeutic regimen		

Key: ADLs, activities of daily living; BRP, bathroom privileges; DB/IS, deep breath/insentive spirometry; D/C, discontinue; HOB, head of bed; I&O, intake and output; IV, intravenous; PO, per mouth; PRN, as needed; q1h × 4, every hour 4 times a day; q4h, every 4 hours; q8h, every 8 hours; q12h, every 12 hours; qd, every day; ROM, range of motion; R/T, related to; SO, significant other; S/S, signs and symptoms; UE, upper extremity; VS, vital signs; WA, while awake.

CHAPTER 12

Orthopedic

FRACTURES

I. Pathophysiology
a. Discontinuity or break in a bone
b. May be associated with serious injury to nerves, blood vessels, muscles, and/or organs
c. More than 150 fracture classifications with five major types: incomplete, complete, closed, open, and pathologic

II. Etiology
a. Common causes: trauma, including abuse; overuse injury; osteoporosis; bone tumors; infections
b. Severity of fracture increases with age.

III. Statistics
a. Morbidity: Approximately 6.8 million Americans seek treatment for fractures annually; in the United States, osteoporosis accounts for 70% of fractures in people over age 45; there were more than 2 million cases of fractures in the United States in 2005 (National Osteoporosis Foundation [NOF], n.d.).
b. Mortality: Dependent upon multiple factors including the specific bone affected—humerous versus veterbra—and severity of fracture, associated soft tissue and organ involvement, age of individual, and presence of comorbidities; of the 80,000 males who suffer a hip fracture annually, one-third will die within 1 year (National Institute of Arthritis and Musculoskeletal and Skin Diseases [NIAMS], 2007).
c. Cost: In 2005, osteoporosis-related fractures were responsible for an estimated $19 billion in costs (NOF, n.d.).

GLOSSARY

Closed fracture: Fracture does not extend through the skin.

Closed reduction: Nonsurgical method for reduction and stabilization of fracture through a wide range of interventions, such as simple braces or aluminum splints, plaster or fiberglass casts, metal braces, and/or traction devices.

Comminuted fracture: Bone fragments into three or more pieces.

Compartment syndrome: Excessive swelling in the tissues associated with a fracture or crush injury to a limb, which elevates tissue pressure, resulting in decreased arteriovascular pressure and impaired tissue perfusion.

Complete fracture: Fracture line involves entire cross-section of the bone, and bone fragments are usually displaced.

Compression fracture: Collapsing of bone usually involves vertebra of the thoracic or lumbar spine and is often seen in elderly people as a result of osteoporosis, but may also occur traumatically.

Crepitation: Grating sound heard with movement of ends of fractured bones.

Incomplete or greenstick fracture: Involves only a portion of the cross-section of the bone; one side breaks and the other usually just bends.

Oblique fracture: Break occurs diagonally.

Open fracture: Bone fragments extend through the muscle and skin and are potentially infected.

Open reduction: Surgical method for stabilization of a fracture using pins, screws, and plates.

Pathological fracture: Fracture occurs in diseased bone—such as in cancer and osteoporosis—with no (spontaneous) or only minimal trauma.

Simple fracture: Bone breaks into two pieces.

Spiral fracture: Break follows a helical line along and around the bone; commonly associated with a twisting motion.

Stress fracture: Hairline fracture due to overuse or repeated microtrauma, such as those seen in gymnasts, runners, and tennis or basketball players, as well as those who participate in marching bands or drill teams.

Transverse fracture: Break occurs in a straight line across the bone.

Care Setting

Most fractures are managed at the community level. Although many of the interventions listed here are appropriate for this population, this plan of care addresses more complicated injuries encountered on an inpatient acute medical-surgical unit.

Related Concerns

Craniocerebral trauma—acute rehabilitative phase, page 220
Pneumonia, page 131
Psychosocial aspects of care, page 749
Renal failure: acute, page 536
Spinal cord injury (acute rehabilitative phase), page 271
Surgical intervention, page 782
Thrombophlebitis: deep vein thrombosis, page 111

Client Assessment Database

Symptoms of fracture depend on the site, severity, type, and amount of damage to other structures.

DIAGNOSTIC DIVISION MAY REPORT	MAY EXHIBIT
ACTIVITY/REST • Weakness • Fatigue • Gait and/or mobility problems • Generalized weakness	• Restriction or loss of function of affected part—may be immediate, because of the fracture, or develop secondarily from tissue swelling, pain • Weakness of affected extremity • Range-of-motion (ROM) deficits
CIRCULATION	• Hypertension—occasionally seen as a response to acute pain or anxiety, or hypotension from severe blood loss • Tachycardia—stress response, hypovolemia • Pulse diminished or absent distal to injury in extremity • Delayed capillary refill • Pallor of affected part • Tissue swelling • Bruising or hematoma mass at site of injury
ELIMINATION	• Hematuria • Sediment in urine • Changes in output—acute renal failure (ARF) with major skeletal muscle damage
NEUROSENSORY • Loss of or impaired motion or sensation • Muscle spasms worsening over time • Numbness or tingling (paresthesias)	• Local musculoskeletal deformities—abnormal angulation, posture changes, shortening of limbs, rotation, or crepitation • Muscle spasms • Visible weakness or loss of function • Giving way or collapse, locking of joints, dislocations • Agitation—may be related to pain, anxiety, or other trauma
PAIN/DISCOMFORT • Sudden severe pain at time of injury—may be localized to the area of tissue or skeletal damage and then become more diffuse; however, can diminish on immobilization • Absence of pain—suggests nerve damage • Muscle-aching pain • Muscle spasms or cramping following immobilization	• Guarding or distraction behaviors • Restlessness • Self-focus

(continues on page 634)

DIAGNOSTIC DIVISION **MAY REPORT** (continued)	**MAY EXHIBIT** (continued)
SAFETY • Circumstances of incident may not support type of injury incurred—may be suggestive of abuse • Use of alcohol or other drugs	• Skin lacerations • Tissue avulsion • Bleeding • Color changes of skin • Localized swelling—may increase gradually or suddenly • Presence of risk factors for falling—age, osteoporosis, dementia, arthritis, other chronic conditions; preexisting unrecognized fracture
TEACHING/LEARNING • Use of multiple medications—prescribed and/or over-the-counter (OTC) with interactive effects	
DISCHARGE PLAN CONSIDERATIONS • May require temporary assistance with transportation, self-care activities, and homemaker or maintenance tasks • May require additional therapy or rehabilitation postdischarge • Possible placement in assisted-living or extended-care facility for a period of time ⬧ Refer to section at end of plan for postdischarge considerations.	

Diagnostic Studies

TEST **WHY IT IS DONE**	**WHAT IT TELLS ME**
• *Radiographic examinations:* First-line tool to determine location and extent of fractures/trauma and bone alignment.	May reveal preexisting and yet undiagnosed fracture(s).
• *Bone scans, tomograms, computed tomography (CT), and magnetic resonance imaging (MRI) scans:* Used to visualize changes of structure within the body and bone alignment. May be preferred diagnostic tool because of superior ability to image some types of injuries.	These are used to visualize fractures, bleeding, and soft tissue damage; they differentiate between stress or trauma fractures and bone neoplasms.
• *Arteriograms:* X-rays that use contrast media to evaluate arterial blood flow.	May reveal occult vascular damage.
• *Complete blood count (CBC):* Battery of screening tests, which typically includes hemoglobin (Hgb); hematocrit (Hct); red blood cell (RBC) count, morphology, indices, and distribution width index; platelet count and size; white blood cell (WBC) count and differential.	Hct may be increased, reflecting hemoconcentration or dehydration; or Hct may be decreased, signifying hemorrhage at the fracture site or at distant organs in multiple trauma. Increased WBC count is a normal stress response after trauma.
• *Urine creatinine (Cr) clearance:* Measures filtering ability of the kidneys.	Muscle trauma increases Cr load for renal clearance; decreased renal perfusion or impaired renal function also elevates Cr.
• *Coagulation profile:* Tests that measure blood coagulation. There are many types of coagulation tests, some of which are general and tell only whether a person's blood is clotting normally. Other tests can identify which element within the blood is causing abnormal clotting.	Alterations may occur because of blood loss, multiple transfusions, or liver injury.

Nursing Priorities

1. Prevent further bone/tissue injury.
2. Alleviate pain.
3. Prevent complications.
4. Provide information about condition, prognosis, and treatment needs.

Discharge Goals

1. Fracture stabilized.
2. Pain controlled.
3. Complications prevented or minimized.
4. Condition, prognosis, and therapeutic regimen understood.
5. Plan in place to meet needs after discharge.

NURSING DIAGNOSIS: **risk for [additional] Trauma**

Risk factors may include
Loss of skeletal integrity (fractures); movement of bone fragments

Possibly evidenced by
(Not applicable; presence of signs and symptoms establishes an *actual* diagnosis)

Desired Outcomes/Evaluation Criteria—Client Will

Bone Healing (NOC)
Maintain stabilization and alignment of fracture(s).
Display callus formation/beginning union at fracture site as appropriate.

Risk Control (NOC)
Demonstrate body mechanics that promote stability at fracture site.

ACTIONS/INTERVENTIONS	RATIONALE
Positioning (NIC) *Independent* Maintain bedrest or limb rest as indicated. Provide support of joints above and below fracture site, especially when moving and turning.	Provides stability, reducing possibility of disturbing alignment and aggravating muscle spasms, which enhances healing.
Cast Care: Wet (NIC) Support fracture site with pillows or folded blankets. Maintain neutral position of affected part with sandbags, splints, trochanter roll, or footboard.	Prevents unnecessary movement and disruption of alignment. Proper placement of pillows also can prevent pressure deformities in the drying cast.
Use the palms of the hands, not the fingertips, when touching the wet cast.	Fingertips can dent the cast before it is dry.
Obtain sufficient personnel for turning. Avoid using abduction bar for turning client with spica cast.	Hip, body, or multiple casts can be extremely heavy and cumbersome. Failure to properly support limbs in casts may cause damage to cast or injury to client and staff.
Traction/Immobilization Care (NIC) Evaluate splinted extremity for edema resolution.	Coaptation splint (e.g., Jones-Sugar tong) may be used to provide immobilization of fracture while excessive tissue swelling is present. As edema subsides, readjustment of splint or application of fiberglass or plaster cast may be required for continued alignment of stable fracture.
Maintain position and integrity of traction (e.g., Buck, Dunlop, Pearson, Russell).	Traction permits pull on the long axis of the fractured bone and overcomes muscle tension and shortening to facilitate alignment and union. Skeletal traction using pins, wires, or tongs permits use of greater weight for traction pull than can be applied to skin tissues.
Ascertain that all clamps are functional. Lubricate pulleys and check ropes for fraying. Secure and wrap knots with adhesive tape.	Ensures that traction setup is functioning properly to avoid interruption of fracture approximation.
Keep ropes unobstructed with weights hanging free, avoid lifting and releasing weights.	Optimal amount of traction weight is maintained. *Note:* Ensuring free movement of weights during repositioning of client avoids sudden excess pull on fracture with associated pain and muscle spasm.
Assist with placement of lifts under bed wheels, if indicated.	Helps maintain proper client position and function of traction by providing counterbalance.
Position client so that appropriate pull is maintained on the long axis of the bone.	Promotes bone alignment and reduces risk of complications—delayed healing or nonunion.

(continues on page 636)

ACTIONS/INTERVENTIONS (continued)	RATIONALE (continued)
Review restrictions imposed by therapy, such as not bending at the waist or sitting up with Buck traction, or not turning below the waist with Russell traction.	Maintains integrity of pull of traction.
Assess integrity of external fixation device.	Hoffman external fixator or frame provides stabilization and rigid support for fractured bone without use of ropes, pulleys, or weights, thus allowing for greater client mobility and comfort, and facilitating wound care. Loose or excessively tightened clamps or nuts can alter the compression of the frame, causing misalignment.
Collaborative	
Review follow-up or serial x-rays.	Provides visual evidence of proper alignment or beginning callus formation and healing process to determine level of activity and need for changes in, or additions to, the therapy plan.
Initiate and maintain bone rehabilitation—early ambulation, weight-bearing activities, soft tissue massage, or electrical stimulation if used.	Promotes bone growth and healing.

NURSING DIAGNOSIS: acute Pain

May be related to
Muscle spasms
Movement of bone fragments, edema, and injury to the soft tissue
Traction, immobility device
Stress, anxiety

Possibly evidenced by
Reports of pain
Distraction, self-focusing/narrowed focus, facial mask of pain
Guarding, protective behavior; alteration in muscle tone; autonomic responses

Desired Outcomes/Evaluation Criteria—Client Will

Pain Level (NOC)
Verbalize relief of pain.
Display relaxed manner, able to participate in activities, and sleep and rest appropriately.
Pain Control (NOC)
Demonstrate use of relaxation skills and diversional activities, as indicated for individual situation.

ACTIONS/INTERVENTIONS	RATIONALE
Pain Management (NIC)	
Independent	
Maintain immobilization of affected part by means of bedrest, cast, splint, and traction. (Refer to ND: risk for [additional] Trauma.)	Relieves pain and prevents bone displacement/extension of tissue injury.
Elevate and support injured extremity.	Promotes venous return, decreases edema, and may reduce pain.
Avoid use of plastic sheets/pillows under limbs in cast.	Can increase discomfort by enhancing heat production in the drying cast.
Elevate bed covers and keep linens off toes.	Maintains body warmth without discomfort due to pressure of bedclothes on affected parts.
Evaluate and document reports of pain or discomfort, noting location and characteristics, including intensity (scale of 0–10), relieving, and aggravating factors. Note nonverbal pain cues, such as changes in vital signs and emotions or behavior. Listen to reports of family member/significant other (SO) regarding client's pain.	Influences choice of, and monitors effectiveness of, interventions. Many factors, including level of anxiety, may affect perception of and reaction to pain. *Note:* Absence of pain expression does not necessarily mean lack of pain.
Encourage client to discuss problems related to injury.	Helps alleviate anxiety. Client may feel need to relive the accident experience.
Explain procedures before beginning them.	Allows client to prepare mentally for activity and to participate in controlling level of discomfort.
Medicate before care activities. Let client know it is important to request medication before pain becomes severe.	Promotes muscle relaxation and enhances participation.

ACTIONS/INTERVENTIONS (continued)

Perform and supervise passive or active ROM exercises.

Provide alternative comfort measures, for example, massage, back rub, or position changes.

Provide emotional support and encourage use of stress management techniques—progressive relaxation, deep-breathing exercises, and visualization or guided imagery; provide therapeutic touch.

Identify diversional activities appropriate for client's age, physical abilities, and personal preferences.

Investigate any reports of unusual or sudden pain or deep, progressive, and poorly localized pain unrelieved by analgesics.

Collaborative

Apply cold or ice pack first 24 to 72 hours and as necessary per facility policy or protocol.

Administer medications, as indicated: opioid and nonopioid analgesics, such as morphine, meperidine (Demerol), or hydrocodone (Vicodin); injectable and oral nonsteroidal anti-inflammatory drugs (NSAIDs), such as ketorolac (Toradol) or ibuprofen (Motrin); and/or muscle relaxants, such as cyclobenzaprine (Flexeril) or carisoprodol (Soma).

Maintain continuous intravenous (IV) or patient-controlled analgesia (PCA) using peripheral, epidural, or intrathecal routes of administration. Maintain safe and effective infusions and equipment.

RATIONALE (continued)

Maintains strength and mobility of unaffected muscles and facilitates resolution of inflammation in injured tissues.

Improves general circulation; reduces areas of local pressure and muscle fatigue.

Refocuses attention, promotes sense of control, and may enhance coping abilities in the management of the stress of traumatic injury and pain, which is likely to persist for an extended period.

Prevents boredom, reduces muscle tension, and can increase muscle strength; may also enhance coping abilities.

May signal developing complications, such as infection, tissue ischemia, or compartment syndrome. (Refer to ND: risk for Peripheral Neurovascular Dysfunction, following.)

Reduces edema and hematoma formation, decreases pain sensation. *Note:* Length of application depends on degree of client comfort and whether the skin is carefully protected.

Given to reduce pain and/or muscle spasms. Studies of Toradol have shown it to be effective in alleviating bone pain, with longer action and fewer side effects than opioid agents.

Optimal pain management is essential to permit early mobilization and physical therapy and to maintain adequate blood level of analgesia, preventing fluctuations in pain relief with associated muscle tension or spasms.

NURSING DIAGNOSIS: risk for Peripheral Neurovascular Dysfunction

Risk factors may include
Reduction or interruption of blood flow
Direct vascular injury, tissue trauma, excessive edema, thrombus formation
Hypovolemia

Possibly evidenced by
(Not applicable; presence of signs and symptoms establishes an *actual* diagnosis)

Desired Outcomes/Evaluation Criteria—Client Will

Tissue Perfusion: Peripheral (NOC)
Maintain tissue perfusion as evidenced by palpable pulses; warm, dry skin; normal sensation; usual sensorium; stable vital signs; and adequate urinary output for individual situation.

ACTIONS/INTERVENTIONS

Circulatory Precautions (NIC)
Independent
Remove jewelry from affected limb immediately.

Evaluate presence and quality of peripheral pulse distal to injury via palpation or Doppler. Compare with uninjured limb.

Assess capillary return, skin color, and warmth distal to the fracture.

RATIONALE

May restrict circulation when edema occurs.

Decreased or absent pulse may reflect vascular injury and necessitates immediate medical evaluation of circulatory status. Be aware that occasionally a pulse may be palpated even though circulation is blocked by a soft clot through which pulsations may be felt. In addition, perfusion through larger arteries may continue after increased compartment pressure has collapsed the arteriole and venule circulation in the muscle.

Return of color should be rapid (3–5 seconds). White, cool skin indicates arterial impairment. Cyanosis suggests venous impairment. *Note:* Peripheral pulses, capillary refill, skin color, and sensation may be normal even in the presence of compartment syndrome because superficial circulation is usually not compromised.

(continues on page 638)

ACTIONS/INTERVENTIONS (continued)

Circulatory Care: Arterial [or] Venous Insufficiency (NIC)
Maintain elevation of injured extremity(ies) unless contraindicated by confirmed presence of compartment syndrome.

Assess entire length of injured extremity for swelling and edema formation. Measure injured extremity and compare with uninjured extremity. Note appearance and spread of hematoma.

Note reports of pain extreme for type of injury or increasing pain on passive movement of extremity, development of paresthesia, muscle tension or tenderness with erythema, and change in pulse quality distal to injury. Do not elevate extremity. Report symptoms to physician at once.

Investigate sudden signs of limb ischemia, such as decreased skin temperature, pallor, and increased pain.

Encourage client to routinely exercise digits or joints distal to injury. Ambulate as soon as possible.

Investigate tenderness, swelling, or pain on dorsiflexion of foot (positive Homans' sign).

Monitor vital signs. Note signs of general pallor or cyanosis, cool skin, and changes in mentation.

Test stools and gastric aspirant for occult blood. Note continued bleeding at trauma or injection site(s) and oozing from mucous membranes.

Pressure Management (NIC)
Perform neurovascular assessments, noting changes in motor and sensory function. Ask client to localize pain or discomfort.

Test sensation of peroneal nerve by pinch or pinprick in the dorsal web between the first and second toe, and assess ability to dorsiflex toes, if indicated.

Assess tissues around cast edges for rough places and pressure points. Investigate reports of "burning sensation" under cast.

Monitor position and location of supporting ring of splints or sling.

Circulatory Care: Arterial [or] Venous Insufficiency (NIC)
Collaborative
Apply ice bags around fracture site for short periods of time on an intermittent basis for 24 to 72 hours.

Monitor Hgb/Hct and coagulation studies, such as prothrombin time (PT).

Administer IV fluids and blood products as needed.

Administer medications, as indicated: Low-molecular-weight heparin or heparinoids, such as enoxaparin (Lovenox), dalteparin (Fragmin), or fondaparinux (Arixtra), if indicated.

Apply antiembolic hose, or sequential pressure hose or compression boots, as indicated.

Pressure Management (NIC)
Split or bivalve cast as needed. Be sure to cut through wadding down to the skin.

RATIONALE (continued)

Promotes venous drainage and decreases edema. *Note:* In presence of increased compartment pressure, elevation of the extremity actually impedes arterial flow, decreasing perfusion. Casts or circumferential dressings can also cause arterial venous insufficiency.

Increasing circumference of injured extremity may suggest general tissue swelling or edema but may also reflect hemorrhage. *Note:* A 1-inch increase in an adult thigh can equal approximately 1 unit of sequestered blood.

Continued bleeding or edema formation within a muscle enclosed by tight fascia can result in impaired blood flow and ischemic myositis or compartment syndrome, necessitating emergency interventions to relieve pressure and restore circulation. *Note:* This condition constitutes a medical emergency and requires immediate intervention.

Fracture dislocations of joints, especially the knee, may cause damage to adjacent arteries, with resulting loss of distal blood flow.

Enhances circulation and reduces pooling of blood, especially in the lower extremities.

There is an increased potential for thrombophlebitis and pulmonary emboli in clients who have been immobile for several days. *Note:* The absence of a positive Homans' sign is not a reliable indicator in many people, especially the elderly, because they often have reduced pain sensation.

Inadequate circulating volume compromises systemic tissue perfusion.

Increased incidence of gastric bleeding accompanies fractures and trauma and may be related to stress or occasionally reflects a clotting disorder requiring further evaluation.

Impaired feeling, numbness, tingling, and increased or diffuse pain occur when circulation to nerves is inadequate or nerves are damaged.

Length and position of peroneal nerve increase risk of its injury in the presence of leg fracture, edema, or compartment syndrome, or because of malposition of traction apparatus.

These factors may be the cause of or be indicative of tissue pressure or ischemia, leading to breakdown and necrosis.

Traction apparatus can cause pressure on vessels and nerves, particularly in the axilla and groin, resulting in ischemia and possible permanent nerve damage.

Reduces edema and hematoma formation, which could impair circulation. *Note:* Length of application of cold therapy is usually 20 to 30 minutes at a time.

Assists in calculation of blood loss and needs and effectiveness of replacement therapy. Coagulation deficits may occur secondary to major trauma, in presence of fat emboli, or during anticoagulant therapy

Maintains circulating volume, enhancing tissue perfusion.

Anticoagulants may be given prophylactically to reduce threat of deep venous thrombus.

Decreases venous pooling and may enhance venous return, thereby reducing risk of thrombus formation.

May be done on an emergency basis to relieve restriction and improve impaired circulation resulting from compression and edema formation in injured extremity. The wadding under the cast may also be restrictive.

ACTIONS/INTERVENTIONS (continued)	RATIONALE (continued)
Refer for and monitor intracompartmental pressures as appropriate.	Diagnosis of compartment syndrome requires advanced training and is typically performed by a specialist. It can be measured by means of slit catheter or side-ported catheter. Values that are 10 to 30 mm Hg less than diastolic blood pressure indicate a probable compartment problem, requiring prompt medical attention (Wheeless).
Review electromyography (EMG) and nerve conduction velocity (NCV) studies.	May be performed to evaluate nerve injury or dysfunction and effect on muscle function. *Note:* More likely performed in rehabilitation phase, not typically done in the acute care setting.
Prepare for surgical intervention, such as fasciotomy, as indicated.	Failure to relieve pressure or correct compartment syndrome within 4 to 6 hours of onset can result in severe contractures, loss of function, and disfigurement of extremity distal to injury, possibly necessitating amputation.

NURSING DIAGNOSIS: risk for impaired Gas Exchange

Risk factors may include
Altered blood flow; blood or fat emboli
Alveolar and capillary membrane changes—interstitial, pulmonary edema, congestion

Possibly evidenced by
(Not applicable; presence of signs and symptoms establishes an *actual* diagnosis)

Desired Outcomes/Evaluation Criteria—Client Will

Respiratory Status: Gas Exchange (NOC)
Maintain adequate respiratory function, as evidenced by absence of dyspnea or cyanosis; respiratory rate and arterial blood gases (ABGs) are within client's normal range.

ACTIONS/INTERVENTIONS	RATIONALE
Respiratory Monitoring (NIC) *Independent*	
Monitor respiratory rate and effort. Note stridor, use of accessory muscles, retractions, and development of central cyanosis.	Tachypnea, dyspnea, and changes in mentation are early signs of respiratory insufficiency and may be the only indicator of developing pulmonary emboli in the early stage. Remaining signs and symptoms reflect advanced respiratory distress and impending failure.
Auscultate breath sounds, noting development of unequal, hyperresonant sounds; also note presence of crackles, rhonchi, or wheezes and inspiratory crowing or croupy sounds.	Changes in or presence of adventitious breath sounds reflects developing respiratory complications—atelectasis, pneumonia, emboli, or acute respiratory distress syndrome (ARDS). Inspiratory crowing reflects upper airway edema and is suggestive of fat emboli.
Handle injured tissues and bones gently, especially during first several days.	This may prevent the development of fat emboli associated with fractures, especially of the long bones and pelvis, occasionally seen in the first 12 to 72 hours post injury.
Instruct and assist with deep-breathing and coughing exercises. Reposition frequently.	Promotes alveolar ventilation and perfusion. Repositioning promotes drainage of secretions and decreases congestion in dependent lung areas.
Note increasing restlessness, confusion, lethargy, or stupor.	Impaired gas exchange or presence of pulmonary emboli can cause deterioration in client's level of consciousness as hypoxemia and acidosis develop.
Observe sputum for signs of blood.	Hemoptysis may occur with pulmonary emboli.
Inspect skin for petechiae above nipple line, in axilla, spreading to abdomen or trunk, buccal mucosa and hard palate, and conjunctival sacs and retina.	This is the most characteristic sign of fat emboli, which may appear within 2 to 3 days after injury.
Collaborative	
Instruct in, and encourage regular use of, incentive spirometry.	Maximizes ventilation and minimizes atelectasis.
Administer supplemental oxygen, if indicated.	Increases available O_2 for optimal tissue oxygenation.
Monitor laboratory studies, such as the following: Pulse oximetry or serial ABGs	Identifies situations in which oxygen desaturation is occurring and reveals complications such as impaired gas exchange and developing respiratory failure.

(continues on page 640)

ACTIONS/INTERVENTIONS (continued)

Hgb, calcium, erythrocyte sedimentation rate (ESR), serum lipase, fat screen, and platelets, as appropriate

Administer medications, as indicated, for example:
Low-molecular-weight heparin or heparinoids, such as enoxaparin (Lovenox), dalteparin (Fragmin), or fondaparinux (Arixtra)
Corticosteroids

RATIONALE (continued)

Anemia, hypocalcemia, and elevated ESR and lipase levels; fat globules in blood, urine, or sputum; and decreased platelet count (thrombocytopenia) are often associated with fat emboli.

Used for prevention of thromboembolic phenomena, including deep vein thrombosis and pulmonary emboli.

Steroids have been used with some success to prevent and treat fat embolus.

NURSING DIAGNOSIS: **impaired physical Mobility**

May be related to
Neuromuscular skeletal impairment, pain or discomfort, restrictive therapies—limb immobilization
Psychological immobility

Possibly evidenced by
Inability to move purposefully within the physical environment, imposed restrictions
Reluctance to attempt movement, limited ROM
Decreased muscle strength or control

Desired Outcomes/Evaluation Criteria—Client Will

Mobility (NOC)
Regain and maintain mobility at the highest possible level.
Maintain position of function.
Increase strength and function of affected and compensatory body parts.
Demonstrate techniques that enable resumption of activities, especially activities of daily living (ADLs).

ACTIONS/INTERVENTIONS

Bed Rest Care (NIC)
Independent
Assess degree of immobility produced by injury and/or treatment and note client's perception of immobility.

Encourage participation in diversional or recreational activities. Maintain stimulating environment—radio, TV, newspapers, personal possessions, pictures, clock, calendar, and visits from family and friends.
Instruct client in active, or assist with passive, ROM exercises of affected and unaffected extremities.

Encourage use of isometric exercises, starting with the unaffected limb.

Provide footboard, wrist splints, and trochanter or hand rolls, as appropriate.

Place in supine position periodically if possible when traction is used to stabilize lower limb fractures.
Instruct in, and encourage use of, trapeze and "post position" for lower limb fractures.

Assist with and encourage self-care activities such as bathing, shaving, and oral hygiene.
Assist with mobility by means of wheelchair, walker, crutches, and/or canes as soon as possible. Instruct in safe use of mobility aids.

RATIONALE

Client may be restricted by self-view or self-perception out of proportion with actual physical limitations, requiring information and interventions to promote progress toward wellness.
Provides opportunity for release of energy, refocuses attention, enhances client's sense of self-control and self-worth, and aids in reducing social isolation.

Increases blood flow to muscles and bone to improve muscle tone; maintain joint mobility; and prevent contractures, atrophy, and calcium resorption from disuse.
Isometrics contract muscles without bending joints or moving limbs and help maintain muscle strength and mass. *Note:* These exercises are contraindicated while acute bleeding or edema is present.
Useful in maintaining functional position of extremities, hands or feet, and preventing complications such as contractures or footdrop.
Reduces risk of flexion contracture of hip.

Facilitates movement during hygiene, skin care, and linen changes; reduces discomfort of remaining flat in bed. "Post position" involves placing the uninjured foot flat on the bed with the knee bent while grasping the trapeze and lifting the body off the bed.
Improves muscle strength and circulation, enhances client control in situation, and promotes self-directed wellness.
Early mobility reduces complications of bedrest, such as phlebitis, and promotes healing and normalization of organ function. Learning the correct way to use aids is important to maintain optimal mobility and client safety.

ACTIONS/INTERVENTIONS (continued)	RATIONALE (continued)
Monitor blood pressure (BP) with resumption of activity. Note reports of dizziness.	Postural hypotension is a common problem following prolonged bedrest and may require specific interventions, such as tilt table with gradual elevation to upright position.
Reposition periodically and encourage coughing and deep-breathing exercises.	Prevents or reduces incidence of skin and respiratory complications—decubitus ulcer, atelectasis, or pneumonia.
Auscultate bowel sounds. Monitor elimination habits and provide for regular bowel routine. Place on bedside commode, if feasible, or use fracture pan. Provide privacy.	Bedrest, use of analgesics, and changes in dietary habits can slow peristalsis and produce constipation. Nursing measures that facilitate elimination may prevent or limit complications. Fracture pan limits flexion of hips and lessens pressure on lumbar region and lower extremity cast.
Perform a thorough assessment of client's prior bowel habits.	Provides baseline for comparison with postsurgical concerns. The long-term use of opioids for pain and limited mobility causes constipation in orthopedic clients. Constipation is a major issue and needs immediate and ongoing attention.
Encourage increased fluid intake of 2,000 to 3,000 mL/day within cardiac tolerance, including acid ash juices such as cranberry.	Keeps the body well hydrated, decreasing risk of urinary infection and stone formation, and helps to prevent constipation.
Provide diet high in proteins, carbohydrates, vitamins, and minerals, limiting protein content until after first bowel movement.	In the presence of musculoskeletal injuries, early good feeding is needed as nutrients required for healing are rapidly depleted. This can have a profound effect on muscle mass, tone, and strength. *Note:* Protein foods increase contents in small bowel, resulting in gas formation and constipation. Therefore, gastrointestinal (GI) function should be fully restored before protein foods are increased.
Increase the amount of roughage and fiber in the diet. Limit gas-forming foods.	Adding bulk to stool helps prevent constipation. Gas-forming foods may cause abdominal distention, especially in presence of decreased intestinal motility.
Collaborative	
Consult with physical or occupational therapist and/or rehabilitation specialist.	Useful in creating aggressive individualized activity or exercise program. Client may require long-term assistance with movement, strengthening, and weight-bearing activities as well as use of adjuncts, for example, walkers, crutches, canes; elevated toilet seats; pickup sticks or reachers; special eating utensils; and help for women with actions such as hooking a brassiere.
Refer to dietitian or nutrition team, as indicated.	The client with fractures, especially when associated with trauma, may have special nutritional considerations; for example, he or she may need enteral or parenteral feedings to maximize healing of tissues and bones.
Initiate bowel program—stool softeners, enemas, or laxatives, as indicated.	Important to promote regular bowel evacuation and prevent constipation.
Refer to psychiatric clinical nurse specialist or therapist, as indicated.	Client/SO may require more intensive treatment to deal with reality of current condition, prognosis, prolonged immobility, and perceived loss of control.

NURSING DIAGNOSIS: **[actual/]risk for Impaired Skin/Tissue Integrity**

May be related to
Puncture injury; compound fracture; surgical repair; insertion of traction pins, wires, screws
Altered sensation, circulation; accumulation of excretions or secretions
Physical immobilization

Possibly evidenced by (actual)
Reports of itching, pain, numbness, pressure in affected or surrounding area
Disruption of skin surface; invasion of body structures; destruction of skin layers or tissues

Desired Outcomes/Evaluation Criteria—Client Will

Tissue Integrity: Skin & Mucous Membranes (NOC)
Verbalize relief of discomfort.
Demonstrate behaviors or techniques to prevent skin breakdown and facilitate healing, as indicated.
Achieve timely wound or lesion healing, if present.

ACTIONS/INTERVENTIONS	RATIONALE

Skin Surveillance (NIC)

Independent

Examine the skin for open wounds, foreign bodies, rashes, bleeding, discoloration, duskiness, and/or blanching.

Provides information regarding skin circulation and problems that may be caused by application and/or restriction of cast, splint, or traction apparatus, or edema formation that may require further medical intervention.

Provide specialty beds and Geomatts as indicated.

Used for clients with a high risk of skin breakdown or in whom long-term immobility is expected.

Massage skin and bony prominences. Keep bed linens dry and free of wrinkles. Place water pads or other padding under elbows and heels, as indicated.

Reduces pressure on susceptible areas and risk of abrasions or skin breakdown.

Reposition frequently. Encourage use of trapeze, if possible. If not able to turn independently, a turning schedule must be maintained by the nurse.

Lessens constant pressure on same areas and minimizes risk of skin breakdown. Use of trapeze may reduce risk of abrasions to elbows and heels.

Assess position of traction devices including slings, ropes, as well as the metal bars and wires.

Improper positioning may cause skin injury or breakdown.

Cast Care: Wet (NIC)

Plaster cast application and skin care:

Cleanse skin with soap and water, rubbing gently with alcohol and/or dust with small amount of a zinc or stearate powder.

Provides a dry, clean area for cast application. *Note:* Excess powder may cake when it comes in contact with water or perspiration.

Cut a length of stockinette to cover the area and extend several inches beyond the cast.

Useful for padding bony prominences, finishing cast edges, and protecting the skin.

Use palm of hand to apply, hold, or move cast and support on pillows after application; avoid using fingertips to hold cast.

Prevents indentations or flattening over bony prominences, such as back of heels, and weight-bearing areas, which would cause abrasions or tissue trauma. An improperly shaped or dried cast is irritating to the underlying skin and may lead to circulatory impairment. Fingertips may dent the cast when it is wet.

Trim excess plaster from edges of cast as soon as casting is completed.

Uneven plaster is irritating to the skin and may result in abrasions.

Promote cast drying by removing bed linen, exposing to circulating air.

Prevents skin breakdown caused by prolonged moisture trapped under cast.

Observe for potential pressure areas, especially at the edges of and under the splint/cast.

Pressure can cause ulcerations, necrosis, and/or nerve palsies. These problems may be painless when nerve damage is present.

Pad or petal tape the edges of the cast with waterproof tape or moleskin.

Provides an effective barrier to cast flaking and moisture. Helps prevent breakdown of cast material at edges and reduces skin irritation and excoriation.

Cleanse excess plaster from skin while still wet, if possible.

Dry plaster may flake into completed cast and cause skin damage.

Protect cast and skin in perineal area, providing frequent perineal care.

Prevents tissue breakdown and infection by fecal contamination.

Instruct client/SO to avoid inserting objects inside casts.

"Scratching an itch" may cause tissue injury.

Massage the skin around the cast edges with alcohol.

Has a drying effect, which toughens the skin. Creams and lotions are not recommended because excessive oils can seal cast perimeter, not allowing the cast to "breathe." Powders are not recommended because of potential for excessive accumulation inside the cast.

Turn frequently to include the uninvolved side, back, and prone position, as tolerated, with client's feet over the end of the mattress.

Minimizes pressure on feet and around cast edges.

Traction/Immobilization Care (NIC)

Skin traction application and skin care:

Cleanse the skin with warm, soapy water.

Reduces level of contaminants on skin.

Apply tincture of benzoin.

"Toughens" the skin for application of skin traction.

Apply commercial skin traction tapes lengthwise on opposite sides of the affected limb.

Traction tapes encircling a limb may compromise circulation.

Extend the tapes beyond the length of the limb.

Traction is inserted in line with the free ends of the tape.

Mark the line where the tapes extend beyond the extremity.

Allows for quick assessment of slippage.

Place protective padding under the limb and over bony prominences.

Minimizes pressure on these areas.

Wrap the limb circumference, including tapes and padding, with elastic bandages, being careful to wrap snugly but not too tightly.

Provides for appropriate traction pull without compromising circulation.

ACTIONS/INTERVENTIONS (continued)

Palpate taped tissues daily and document any tenderness or pain.

Remove skin traction every 24 hours or per protocol; inspect and give skin care.

Skeletal traction or fixation application and skin care:

Bend wire ends or cover ends of wires/pins with rubber or cork protectors or needle caps.

Pad slings or frame with sheepskin and foam.

Pressure Management (NIC)
Collaborative

Provide foam mattress, sheepskins, flotation pads, or air mattress, as indicated.

Monovalve, bivalve, or cut a window in the cast, per protocol.

RATIONALE (continued)

If area under tapes is tender, suspect skin irritation, and prepare to remove the bandage system.

Maintains skin integrity. Skin traction is usually short term while stablizing client for surgical clearance.

Prevents injury to other body parts.

Prevents excessive pressure on skin and promotes moisture evaporation that reduces risk of excoriation.

Because of immobilization of body parts, bony prominences other than those affected by the casting may suffer from decreased circulation.

Cutting or hinging the cast allows the release of pressure and provides access for wound and skin care.

NURSING DIAGNOSIS: risk for Infection

Risk factors may include

Inadequate primary defenses—broken skin, traumatized tissues, environmental exposure

Invasive procedures, skeletal traction

Possibly evidenced by

(Not applicable; presence of signs and symptoms establishes an *actual* diagnosis)

Desired Outcomes/Evaluation Criteria—Client Will

Infection Status (NOC)

Achieve timely wound healing, be free of purulent drainage or erythema, and be afebrile.

ACTIONS/INTERVENTIONS

Infection Prevention (NIC)
Independent

Inspect the skin for preexisting irritation or breaks in continuity.

Assess pin sites and skin areas, noting reports of increased pain or burning sensation, or presence of edema, erythema, foul odor, or drainage.

Provide sterile pin and wound care according to protocol, and exercise meticulous hand washing.

Instruct client not to touch the insertion sites.

Line perineal cast edges with plastic wrap.

Observe wounds for formation of bullae, crepitation, bronze discoloration of skin, and frothy or fruity-smelling drainage.

Assess muscle tone, reflexes, and ability to speak.

Monitor vital signs. Note presence of chills, fever, and malaise, and any changes in mentation.

Investigate abrupt onset of pain or limitation of movement with localized edema and erythema in injured extremity.

Institute prescribed isolation procedures.

Collaborative

Monitor laboratory/diagnostic studies, for example:

CBC

ESR

Cultures and sensitivity of wound, serum, and/or bone

Radioisotope scans

RATIONALE

Pins or wires should not be inserted through skin infections, rashes, or abrasions—may lead to bone infection.

May indicate onset of local infection or tissue necrosis, which can lead to osteomyelitis.

May prevent cross-contamination and possibility of infection.

Minimizes risk of contamination.

Damp, soiled casts can promote growth of bacteria.

Signs suggestive of gas gangrene infection.

Muscle rigidity, tonic spasms of jaw muscles, and dysphagia reflect development of tetanus.

Hypotension and confusion may be seen with gas gangrene; tachycardia, chills, and fever reflect developing sepsis.

May indicate development of osteomyelitis.

Presence of purulent drainage requires wound and linen precautions to prevent cross-contamination.

Anemia may be noted with osteomyelitis; leukocytosis is usually present with infective processes.

Elevated in osteomyelitis.

Identifies infective organism and effective antimicrobial agent(s).

Hot spots signify increased areas of vascularity, indicative of osteomyelitis.

(continues on page 644)

ACTIONS/INTERVENTIONS (continued)	RATIONALE (continued)
Administer medications, as indicated, for example: 　IV/topical antibiotics	Wide-spectrum antibiotics may be used prophylactically or may be geared toward a specific microorganism.
Tetanus toxoid	Given prophylactically because the possibility of tetanus exists with any open wound. *Note:* Risk increases when injury or wound(s) occur in "field conditions"—outdoors, rural areas, or the work environment.
Provide wound or bone irrigations, and apply warm, moist soaks, as indicated.	Local debridement and cleansing of wounds reduces microorganisms and incidence of systemic infection. Continuous antimicrobial drip into bone may be necessary to treat osteomyelitis, especially if blood supply to bone is compromised.
Assist with procedures such as incision and drainage, placement of drains, and hyperbaric oxygen therapy.	Numerous procedures may be carried out in treatment of local infections, osteomyelitis, and gas gangrene.
Prepare for surgery, as indicated.	Sequestrectomy, removal of necrotic bone, is necessary to facilitate healing and prevent extension of infectious process.

NURSING DIAGNOSIS: **deficient Knowledge [Learning Need] regarding condition, prognosis, treatment, self-care, and discharge needs**

May be related to
Lack of exposure or recall
Misinterpretation of information or unfamiliarity with information resources

Possibly evidenced by
Questions and requests for information, statement of misconception
Inaccurate follow-through of instructions, development of preventable complications

Desired Outcomes/Evaluation Criteria—Client Will

Knowledge: Treatment Regimen (NOC)
Verbalize understanding of condition, prognosis, and potential complications.
Correctly perform necessary procedures and explain reasons for actions.

ACTIONS/INTERVENTIONS	RATIONALE
Teaching: Disease Process (NIC) *Independent* Review pathology, prognosis, and future expectations.	Provides knowledge base from which client can make informed choices. *Note:* Internal fixation devices can ultimately compromise the bone's strength, and intramedullary nails or rods, and plates may be removed at a future date.
Discuss prophylactic antibiotic use.	When hardware, such as pins, screws, and plates, is implanted, it provides a place for infection to develop. If there are procedures that open the GI tract to the bloodstream, such as dental procedures or a colonoscopy, antibiotics should be given.
Discuss dietary needs.	A low-fat diet adequate in quality protein and rich in calcium promotes healing and general well-being.
Discuss individual drug regimen, as appropriate.	Proper use of pain medication and antiplatelet agents can reduce risk of complications. Long-term use of alendronate (Fosamax) may reduce risk of stress fractures. *Note:* Fosamax should be taken on an empty stomach with plain water because absorption of the drug may be altered by food and some medications, such as antacids and calcium supplements.
Reinforce methods of mobility and ambulation as instructed by physical therapist when indicated.	Most fractures require casts, splints, or braces during the healing process. Further damage and delay in healing could occur secondary to improper use of ambulatory devices.
Suggest use of a backpack.	Provides place to carry necessary articles and leaves hands free to manipulate crutches; may prevent undue muscle fatigue when one arm is casted.
List activities that the client can perform independently and those that require assistance.	Organizes activities around need and who is available to provide help.

ACTIONS/INTERVENTIONS (continued)	RATIONALE (continued)
Identify available community services, such as a rehabilitation team, home nursing care, or homemaker services.	Provides assistance to facilitate self-care and support independence. Promotes optimal self-care and recovery.
Encourage client to continue active exercises for the joints above and below the fracture.	Prevents joint stiffness, contractures, and muscle wasting, promoting earlier return to independence in ADLs.
Discuss importance of clinical and therapy follow-up appointments.	Fracture healing may take as long as a year for completion, and client cooperation with the medical regimen facilitates proper union of bone. Physical therapy and occupational therapy may be indicated for exercises to maintain or strengthen muscles and improve function. Additional modalities such as low-intensity ultrasound may be used to stimulate healing of lower-forearm or lower-leg fractures.
Review proper pin or wound care.	Reduces risk of bone and tissue trauma and infection, which can progress to osteomyelitis.
Recommend cleaning external fixator device regularly.	Keeping device free of dust or contaminants reduces risk of infection.
Identify signs and symptoms requiring medical evaluation, for example, severe pain, fever or chills, or foul odors; changes in sensation, swelling, burning, numbness, tingling, skin discoloration, paralysis, or white/cool toes or fingertips; and warm spots, soft areas, or cracks in the cast.	Prompt intervention may reduce severity of complications such as infection or impaired circulation. *Note:* Some darkening of the skin reflecting vascular congestion may occur normally when walking on the casted extremity or using casted arm; however, this should resolve with rest and elevation.
Discuss care of "green" or wet cast.	Promotes proper curing to prevent cast deformities and associated misalignment or skin irritation. *Note:* Placing a "cooling" cast directly on rubber or plastic pillows traps heat and increases drying time.
Suggest the use of a blow-dryer to dry small areas of dampened cast.	Cautious use can hasten drying.
Demonstrate use of plastic bags to cover plaster cast during wet weather or while bathing. Clean soiled cast with a slightly dampened cloth and some scouring powder.	Protects from moisture, which softens the plaster and weakens the cast. *Note:* Fiberglass casts are being used more frequently. They also need to be thoroughly dried if they get wet to avoid developing mold.
Emphasize the importance of not adjusting clamps or nuts of an external fixator device.	Tampering may alter compression and misalign fracture.
Recommend use of loose-fitting or adaptive clothing.	Facilitates dressing and grooming activities.
Suggest ways to cover toes if appropriate, for example, using stockinette or soft socks.	Helps maintain warmth and protect from injury.
Discuss postcast removal instructions:	
Instruct client to continue exercises as permitted.	Reduces stiffness and improves strength and function of affected extremity.
Inform client that the skin under the cast is commonly mottled and covered with scales or crusts of dead skin.	It will be several weeks before normal appearance returns.
Wash the skin gently with soap and water and lubricate with a protective emollient.	New skin is extremely tender because it has been protected beneath a cast.
Inform client that muscles may appear flabby and atrophied (less muscle mass); recommend supporting the joint above and below the affected part and the use of mobility aids—elastic bandages, splints, braces, crutches, walkers, or canes.	Muscle strength will be reduced and new or different aches and pains may occur for secondary to loss of support.
Elevate the extremity, as needed.	Swelling and edema tend to occur after cast removal.

POTENTIAL CONSIDERATIONS following acute hospitalization (dependent on client's age, physical condition and presence of complications, personal resources, and life responsibilities)

In addition to surgical considerations

• *risk for Trauma*—loss of skeletal integrity, weakness, balancing difficulties, reduced muscle coordination, lack of safety precautions, history of previous trauma
• *impaired physical Mobility*—neuromuscular skeletal impairment, pain/discomfort, restrictive therapies (limb immobilization); psychological immobility
• *Self-Care Deficit*—musculoskeletal impairment, decreased strength/endurance, pain
• *risk for Infection*—inadequate primary defenses: broken skin, traumatized tissues, environmental exposure, invasive procedures, skeletal traction

AMPUTATION

I. **Pathophysiology**—Partial or complete detachment of body part with residual extremity covered with well-vascularized muscle and skin, although reattachment surgery may be possible for fingers, hands, and arms
  a. Primarily two types of amputations
    i. Open or provisional: requires subsequent revisions
    ii. Closed or flap: all surgical revision is performed and the wound closed in one procedure
  b. Five levels currently used in lower-extremity amputation: foot and ankle, below knee (BKA), knee disarticulation and above (thigh), knee-hip disarticulation, and hemipelvectomy and translumbar amputation
  c. Two basic types of prosthetic designs are used: exoskeletal and endoskeletal

II. **Etiology**
  a. Varied causes (Ellis, 2007)
    i. Peripheral vascular disease, often associated with diabetes, usually involves lower extremity; most common in the United States, accounting for 65% of cases
    ii. Trauma: battlefield wounds; upper extremity more common
    iii. Malignant bone tumors
    iv. Infections: osteomyelitis, gangrene
    v. Congenital disorders: approximately 5% of cases
  b. Lower-extremity amputations are performed much more frequently than upper-extremity amputations.
  c. Upper-extremity amputations generally result from trauma caused by industrial accidents.

III. **Statistics**
  a. Morbidity: Approximately 70,000 new major amputations performed annually in the United States (Ellis, 2007); use and early implementation of prosthetic devices are improving long-term outcomes.
  b. Mortality: Dependent on underlying pathology; survival rates decreased in presence of diabetes and end-stage renal disease as well as with above-the-knee amputations (Aulivola et al, 2004).

GLOSSARY

Amputation or traumatic neuromas: Painful proliferation of nerve fibers at the proximal end of a severed nerve.

Complete amputation: Total detachment of appendage or limb from the body.

Endoskeletal prosthetic: Aluminum, titanium, and other tubular materials form the inner structure, providing strength; external shape is removable, usually composed of foam or skin-simulating material.

Exoskeletal prosthetic: Outer plastic laminated skin with wood or urethane foam interiors where the strength is provided by the outer layer.

Partial amputation: Some soft tissue remains attached to the body.

Residual limb: Remaining portion of the amputated limb (once referred to as the stump).

Care Setting

Client is treated in inpatient acute surgical unit and subacute or rehabilitation unit.

Related Concerns

Cancer, page 846
Diabetes mellitus/diabetic ketoacidosis, page 405
Psychosocial aspects of care, page 749
Surgical intervention, page 782

Client Assessment Database

Data depend on underlying reason for surgical procedure, for example severe trauma, peripheral vascular/arterial occlusive disease, diabetic neuropathy, osteomyelitis, and cancer.

DIAGNOSTIC DIVISION MAY REPORT	MAY EXHIBIT
ACTIVITY/REST • Actual or anticipated limitations imposed by condition or amputation	
CIRCULATION	• Presence of edema • Absent or diminished pulses in affected limb or digits

Client Assessment Database (continued)

DIAGNOSTIC DIVISION MAY REPORT (continued)	MAY EXHIBIT (continued)
EGO INTEGRITY • Concern about negative effects or anticipated changes in lifestyle, financial situation, reactions of others • Feelings of helplessness, powerlessness	• Anxiety, apprehension • Irritability • Anger, frustration • Withdrawal, grief • False cheerfulness
NEUROSENSORY • Loss of sensation in affected area • Phantom pain	
SAFETY	• Necrotic or gangrenous area • Nonhealing wound • Local infection
SEXUALITY • Concern about intimate relationships	
SOCIAL INTERACTION • Problems related to illness or condition • Concern about role function • Concern about reaction of others	
TEACHING/LEARNING	
DISCHARGE PLAN CONSIDERATIONS • May require assistance with wound care and supplies, adaptation to prosthesis or other ambulatory devices, transportation, homemaker or maintenance tasks, and possibly self-care activities and vocational retraining ▶ Refer to section at end of plan for postdischarge considerations.	

Diagnostic Studies

Studies depend on the underlying condition necessitating amputation and are used to determine the appropriate level for amputation.

TEST WHY IT IS DONE	WHAT IT TELLS ME
• *X-rays:* Used to visualize pathology and the extent of involvement.	Identify skeletal abnormalities, trauma, or mass or tumor.
• *Computed tomography (CT) scan:* Used to visualize changes of structure within the body and bone alignment.	Identifies soft tissue and bone destruction, neoplastic lesions, osteomyelitis, and hematoma formation.
• *Angiography and blood flow studies:* Evaluates circulation and tissue perfusion.	Helps predict potential for tissue healing after amputation.
• *Doppler ultrasound, laser Doppler flowmetry:* Performed to assess and measure blood flow.	Determines adequacy of skin microcirculation and helps predict tissue or muscle viability and primary wound healing.
• *Transcutaneous oxygen pressure:* Maps out areas of greater and lesser perfusion in the involved extremity.	Helps determine lowest level at which to perform amputation for maximum preservation of limb length and successful healing.
• *Thermography:* Measures temperature differences in an ischemic limb at two sites—the skin and the center of the bone.	The lower that the difference is between the two readings, the greater the chances will be for healing.

(continues on page 648)

TEST WHY IT IS DONE (continued)	WHAT IT TELLS ME (continued)
• *Plethysmography:* Segmental systolic blood pressure (BP) measurements evaluate arterial blood flow.	Helps predict wound healing and need for revision of residual limb.
• *Erythrocyte sedimentation rate (ESR):* Indirect measure of degree of inflammation in body.	Elevation indicates inflammatory response or possible infection.
• *White blood cell (WBC) count/differential:* Assess body's ability to respond to and eliminate infection.	Elevation and "shift to left" suggest infectious process.
• *Wound cultures:* Identify presence of infection.	Reveals causative organism and treatment options.
• *Biopsy:* Determines presence of pathology and treatment needs or options.	Confirms diagnosis of benign or malignant mass.

Nursing Priorities

1. Support psychological and physiological adjustment.
2. Alleviate pain.
3. Prevent complications.
4. Promote mobility and functional abilities.
5. Provide information about surgical procedure, prognosis, and treatment needs.

Discharge Goals

1. Dealing with current situation realistically.
2. Pain relieved or controlled.
3. Complications prevented or minimized.
4. Mobility and function regained or compensated for.
5. Surgical procedure, prognosis, and therapeutic regimen understood.
6. Plan in place to meet needs after discharge.

NURSING DIAGNOSIS: **situational low Self-Esteem**

May be related to
Loss of body part, change in functional abilities

Possibly evidenced by
Anticipated changes in lifestyle, fear of rejection or reaction by others
Negative feelings about body; focus on past strength, function, or appearance
Feelings of helplessness, powerlessness
Preoccupation with missing body part, not looking at or touching residual limb
Perceived change in usual patterns of responsibility or physical capacity to resume role

Desired Outcomes/Evaluation Criteria—Client Will

Grief Resolution (NOC)
Begin to show adaptation and verbalize acceptance of self in situation (amputee).
Recognize and incorporate changes into self-concept in accurate manner without negating self-esteem.
Develop realistic plans for adapting to new role or role modifications.

ACTIONS/INTERVENTIONS	RATIONALE
Grief Work Facilitation (NIC) *Independent* Assess and consider client's preparation for and view of amputation.	Research shows that amputation poses serious threats to client's psychological and psychosocial adjustment. Client who views amputation as life-saving or reconstructive may be able to accept the new self more quickly. Client with sudden traumatic amputation or who considers amputation to be the result of failure in other treatments is at greater risk for disturbances in self-concept.
Encourage expression of fears, negative feelings, and grief over loss of body part.	Venting emotions helps client begin to deal with the fact and reality of life without a limb.

ACTIONS/INTERVENTIONS (continued)

Reinforce preoperative information, including type and location of amputation, type of prosthetic fitting if appropriate (i.e., immediate, delayed), and expected postoperative course, including pain control and rehabilitation.

Assess degree of support available to client.

Discuss client's perceptions of self, related to change, and how client sees self in usual lifestyle and role functioning.

Ascertain individual strengths and identify previous positive coping behaviors.

Self-Esteem Enhancement (NIC)

Encourage participation in activities of daily living (ADLs). Provide opportunities to view and care for residual limb, using the moment to point out positive signs of healing.

Encourage or provide for a visit by another amputee, especially one who is successfully rehabilitating.

Provide open environment for client to discuss concerns about sexuality.

Note withdrawn behavior, negative self-talk, use of denial, or overconcern with actual or perceived changes.

Collaborative

Discuss availability of various resources, for example, psychiatric or sexual counseling, a prosthetist, or an occupational therapist.

RATIONALE (continued)

Provides opportunity for client to question and assimilate information and begin to deal with changes in body image and function, which can facilitate postoperative recovery.

Sufficient support by significant other (SO) and friends can facilitate rehabilitation process.

Aids in defining concerns in relation to previous lifestyle and facilitates problem-solving. For example, client likely fears loss of independence and ability to work or express sexuality and may experience role and/or relationship changes.

Helpful to build on strengths that are already available for client to use in coping with current situation.

Promotes independence and enhances feelings of self-worth. Although integration of residual limb into body image can take months or even years, looking at the residual limb and hearing positive comments made in a normal, matter-of-fact manner can help client with this acceptance.

A peer who has been through a similar experience serves as a role model and can provide validity to comments and hope for recovery and a normal future.

Promotes sharing of beliefs and values about sensitive subject, and identifies misconceptions or myths that may interfere with adjustment to situation.

Identifies stage of grief and need for interventions.

May need assistance for these concerns to facilitate optimal adaptation and rehabilitation.

NURSING DIAGNOSIS: acute Pain

May be related to
Physical injury—tissue and nerve trauma
Psychological impact of loss of body part

Possibly evidenced by
Reports of pain
Narrowed self-focus
Autonomic responses, guarding or protective behavior

Desired Outcomes/Evaluation Criteria—Client Will

Pain Level (NOC)
Report pain is relieved or controlled.
Appear relaxed and able to rest and sleep appropriately.
Verbalize understanding of phantom pain and methods to provide relief.

ACTIONS/INTERVENTIONS

Pain Management (NIC)
Independent

Document location and intensity of pain (scale of 0–10). Investigate changes in pain characteristics—numbness and tingling.

Elevate affected part by raising foot of bed slightly or using a pillow or sling for upper-limb amputation.

Provide or promote general comfort measures (e.g., frequent turning, back rub) and diversional activities. Encourage use of stress management techniques, such as deep-breathing exercises, visualization and guided imagery, and Therapeutic Touch.

RATIONALE

Aids in evaluating need for and effectiveness of interventions. Changes may indicate developing complications, such as necrosis or infection.

Lessens edema formation by enhancing venous return; reduces muscle fatigue and skin or tissue pressure. *Note:* After initial 24 hours and in absence of edema, residual limb may be extended and kept flat.

Refocuses attention, promotes relaxation, may enhance coping abilities, and may decrease occurrence of phantom-limb pain.

(continues on page 650)

Investigate reports of progressive or poorly localized pain unrelieved by analgesics.	May indicate developing compartment syndrome, especially following traumatic injury. (Refer to CP: Fractures; ND: risk for Peripheral Neurovascular Dysfunction.)
Acknowledge reality of residual limb pain and phantom pain and that various modalities will be tried for pain relief.	Residual limb pain is believed to come from injuries to nerves at the amputation site. At the ends of these injured nerve fibers, neuromas send out pain impulses in a random fashion, or when trapped as in excessive compression by other tissues such as muscle, or in the development of the infectious process. In contrast, phantom pain is thought to originate in the part of the brain that controlled the limb before it was amputated. So the client experiences pain and sensation as if the limb were still in place. Phantom pain is often described as crushing, grinding, or burning. It can occur immediately or may not start for several weeks. *Note:* Phantom pain is not well relieved by traditional pain medications.

Collaborative

Administer medications, as indicated, such as the following:	
Opioid analgesics, for example, morphine sulfate (Astramorph, MS Contin), Fentanyl patch; combination agents: oxycodone with acetaminophen (Percocet); and anti-inflammatory agents, for example, acetaminophen (Tylenol) and ibuprofen (Motrin)	Many medications and routes of administration may be used. In acute postamputation pain, opioid analgesics are the mainstay of pain management to reduce pain and muscle spasms.
Antidepressants, for example, amitriptyline (Elavil), nortriptyline (Pamelor), and duloxetine (Cymbalta); antiseizure drugs, for example, carbamazepine (Tegretol), gabapentin (Neurontin), and pregabalin (Lyrica); sedatives/anti-anxiety agents, for example, diazepam (Valium) and alprazolam (Xanax); and local/regional anesthetics, for example, novacaine (Marcaine) and ropivacaine (Naropin)	As surgical pain subsides, other medications will be added to manage more long-term conditions; for example, antidepressants and antiseizure medications appear to help with neuritic pain associated with phantom pain and sensations.
Instruct in, and monitor use of, patient-controlled analgesia (PCA).	PCA provides for continuous and timely drug administration, preventing fluctuations in pain level and muscle tension and spasms associated with surgical procedures.
Refer to interdisciplinary providers as appropriate—pain management specialist, physical therapist, prosthetist, orthopedic surgeon, and neurosurgeon.	A multidisciplinary approach is required, and many therapy modalities may be needed both in the acute and the long-term management of pain.
Discuss and monitor use of transcutaneous electrical nerve stimulation (TENS) of the residual limb.	For some individuals, a TENS unit may help to treat retractable phantom limb pain, especially in combination with medications for neuropathic pain. *Note:* Stimulation of the intact (opposite) limb is often more effective. Indeed, an increase in phantom pain has occasionally been reported when TENS unit has been applied to residual limb.

NURSING DIAGNOSIS: risk for ineffective peripheral tissue Perfusion

Risk factors may include
Reduced arterial or venous blood flow; tissue edema, hematoma formation
Hypovolemia

Possibly evidenced by
(Not applicable; presence of signs and symptoms establishes an *actual* diagnosis)

Desired Outcomes/Evaluation Criteria—Client Will

Tissue Perfusion: Peripheral (NOC)
Maintain adequate tissue perfusion as evidenced by palpable peripheral pulses; warm, dry skin; and timely wound healing.

ACTIONS/INTERVENTIONS	RATIONALE
Circulatory Care: Arterial [or] Venous Insufficiency (NIC)	
Independent	
Monitor vital signs. Palpate peripheral pulses, noting strength and equality.	General indicators of circulatory status and adequacy of perfusion.
Perform periodic neurovascular assessments—sensation, movement, pulse, skin color, and temperature.	Amputation wound healing is a concern because most are performed for compromised circulation; for example, with peripheral vascular disease (PVD) or damaged soft tissue resulting from trauma. Postoperative tissue edema, hematoma formation, or restrictive dressings may impair circulation to residual limb, resulting in tissue necrosis.
Note type of dressing used—soft, soft with pressure wrap, semirigid, or rigid.	Postoperative dressing varies, each with its advantages and disadvantages. For example, a soft dressing does not control edema. Adding a pressure wrap distributes pressure, but requires measures to avoid possible limb strangulation. Semirigid dressings (e.g., plaster splint, Unna bandage) or rigid dressings allow for decreased edema and immediate postoperative prosthesis with early ambulation, but limit access to the wound, and possible excessive pressure may lead to compromised healing.
Inspect dressings and drainage device, noting amount and characteristics of drainage.	Continued blood loss may indicate need for additional fluid replacement and evaluation for coagulation defect or surgical intervention to ligate bleeder.
Apply direct pressure to bleeding site if hemorrhage occurs. Contact physician immediately.	Direct pressure to bleeding site may be followed by application of a bulk dressing secured with an elastic wrap once bleeding is controlled.
Investigate reports of persistent or unusual pain in operative site.	Hematoma can form in muscle pocket under the flap, compromising circulation and intensifying pain.
Evaluate nonoperated lower limb for inflammation and positive Homans' sign.	Increased incidence of thrombus formation in clients with pre-existing peripheral vascular disease or diabetic changes.
Encourage and assist with early ambulation.	Enhances circulation and helps prevent stasis and associated complications. Promotes sense of general well-being.
Collaborative	
Administer intravenous (IV) fluids and blood products as indicated.	Maintains circulating volume to maximize tissue perfusion.
Apply antiembolic or sequential compression hose to nonoperated leg, as appropriate.	Enhances venous return, reducing venous pooling and risk of thrombophlebitis.
Administer low-dose anticoagulant, as indicated.	May be useful in preventing thrombus formation without increasing risk of postoperative bleeding or hematoma formation.
Monitor laboratory studies, for example:	
Hemoglobin/hematocrit (Hgb/Hct)	Indicators of hypovolemia, or dehydration, that can impair tissue perfusion.
Prothrombin time (PT)/activated partial thromboplastin time (aPTT)	Evaluates need for, and effectiveness of, anticoagulant therapy and identifies developing complication such as posttraumatic disseminated intravascular coagulation (DIC).

NURSING DIAGNOSIS: risk for Infection

Risk factors may include
Inadequate primary defenses—broken skin, traumatized tissue
Invasive procedures; environmental exposure
Chronic disease, altered nutritional status

Possibly evidenced by
(Not applicable; presence of signs and symptoms establishes an *actual* diagnosis)

Desired Outcomes/Evaluation Criteria—Client Will

Wound Healing: Primary Intention (NOC)
Achieve timely wound healing, be free of purulent drainage or erythema, and be afebrile.

ACTIONS/INTERVENTIONS	RATIONALE

Wound Care (NIC)

Independent

Maintain aseptic technique when changing dressings and caring for wound.

Minimizes opportunity for introduction of bacteria.

Inspect dressings and wound; note characteristics of drainage.

Early detection of developing infection provides opportunity for timely intervention and prevention of more serious complications such as osteomyelitis.

Maintain patency and routinely empty drainage device.

Hemovac and Jackson-Pratt drains facilitate removal of drainage, promoting wound healing and reducing risk of infection.

Cover dressing with plastic when using the bedpan or if incontinent.

Prevents contamination in lower-limb amputation.

Expose residual limb to air and wash with mild soap and water after dressings are discontinued.

Maintains cleanliness, minimizes skin contaminants, and promotes healing of tender, fragile skin.

Monitor vital signs.

Temperature elevation and tachycardia may reflect developing sepsis.

Collaborative

Obtain wound and drainage cultures and sensitivities, as appropriate.

Identifies presence of infection, specific organisms, and appropriate therapy.

Administer antibiotics, as indicated.

Wide-spectrum antibiotics may be used prophylactically, or antibiotic therapy may be geared toward specific organisms.

NURSING DIAGNOSIS: impaired physical Mobility

May be related to
Loss of a limb (particularly a lower extremity); pain or discomfort; perceptual impairment—altered sense of balance

Possibly evidenced by
Reluctance to attempt movement
Impaired coordination; decreased muscle strength, control, and mass

Desired Outcomes/Evaluation Criteria—Client Will

Risk Control (NOC)
Verbalize understanding of individual situation, treatment regimen, and safety measures.
Maintain position of function as evidenced by absence of contractures.

Mobility (NOC)
Demonstrate techniques and behaviors that enable resumption of activities.
Display willingness to participate in activities.

ACTIONS/INTERVENTIONS	RATIONALE

Amputation Care (NIC)

Independent

Provide residual limb care on a routine basis, for example, inspect the area, clean and dry it thoroughly, and rewrap the residual limb with elastic bandage or air splint. Conversely, apply a "stump shrinker" or heavy stockinette sock for "delayed" prosthesis.

Provides opportunity to evaluate healing and note complications unless covered by immediate prosthesis. Wrapping residual limb controls edema and helps form residual limb into conical shape to facilitate fitting of prosthesis. *Note:* Air splint may be preferred because it permits visual inspection of the wound.

Measure circumference periodically.

Measurement is done to estimate shrinkage to ensure proper fit of sock and prosthesis.

Rewrap residual limb immediately with an elastic bandage, elevate if "immediate or early" cast is accidentally dislodged. Prepare for reapplication of cast.

Edema will occur rapidly, thus delaying rehabilitation.

Assist with specified range-of-motion (ROM) exercises for both the affected and unaffected limbs, beginning early in postoperative stage.

Prevents contracture deformities, which can develop rapidly and could delay prosthesis usage.

Encourage active and isometric exercises for upper torso and unaffected limbs.

Increases muscle strength to facilitate transfers and ambulation and promotes mobility and more normal lifestyle.

Provide trochanter rolls, as indicated.

Prevents external rotation of lower-limb residual limb.

Instruct client to lie in prone position, as tolerated, at least twice a day with pillow under abdomen and lower-extremity residual limb.

Strengthens extensor muscles and prevents flexion contracture of the hip, which can begin to develop within 24 hours of sustained malpositioning.

ACTIONS/INTERVENTIONS (continued)	RATIONALE (continued)
Caution against keeping pillow under lower-extremity residual limb or allowing BKA limb to hang dependently over side of bed or chair.	Use of pillows can cause permanent flexion contracture of hip; a dependent position of residual limb impairs venous return and may increase edema formation.
Demonstrate/assist with transfer techniques and use of mobility aids such as a trapeze, crutches, or a walker.	Facilitates self-care and client's independence. Proper transfer techniques prevent shearing abrasions/dermal injury related to "scooting."
Assist with ambulation based on specific prosthesis used, for example:	
Immediate postoperative fitting	Reduces potential for injury. Ambulation after lower-limb amputation depends on timing of prosthesis placement.
Early postoperative fitting	A rigid plaster of Paris dressing is applied to the residual limb and a pylon and artificial foot are attached. Weight-bearing begins within 24 to 48 hours. Weight-bearing does not occur until 10 to 30 days postoperatively.
Delayed fitting	More common in areas that do not have facilities available for immediate or early application of prosthesis or when the condition of the residual limb and/or client precludes these choices. *Note:* With the advent of new medical techniques at the trauma scene, new surgical techniques, new occupational therapy techniques, and new component and prosthetic technology, such as the C-leg prosthesis that uses computer sensors and hydraulics (enabling client to move around nearly effortlessly), the initial steps for fitting begin when the stitches are removed. Client is fitted with prosthetic 2 weeks after final amputation.
Help client continue preoperative muscle exercises as able or when allowed out of bed; for example, the client should perform abdomen-tightening exercises and knee bends; hop on foot; and stand on toes while holding on to chair for balance.	Contributes to gaining improved sense of balance and strengthens compensatory body parts.
Instruct client in residual limb-conditioning exercises, for example, pushing the residual limb against a pillow initially, then progressing to harder surface.	Hardens the residual limb by toughening the skin and altering feedback of resected nerves to facilitate use of prosthesis.
Collaborative	
Refer to rehabilitation team, for example, physical and occupational therapy and prosthetic specialists.	Provides for creation of exercise and activity program to meet individual needs and strengths and identifies mobility functional aids to promote independence. Early use of a temporary prosthesis promotes activity and enhances general well-being and a positive outlook. *Note:* Vocational counseling and/or retraining also may be indicated.
Provide foam or flotation mattress.	Reduces pressure on skin and tissues that can impair circulation, potentiating risk of tissue ischemia and breakdown.

NURSING DIAGNOSIS: **deficient Knowledge [Learning Need] regarding condition, prognosis, treatment, self-care, and discharge needs**

May be related to
Lack of exposure or recall
Information misinterpretation

Possibly evidenced by
Questions, request for information, verbalization of the problem
Inaccurate follow-through of instructions, development of preventable complications

Desired Outcomes/Evaluation Criteria—Client Will

Knowledge: Disease Process (NOC)
Verbalize understanding of condition, disease process, and potential complications.

Knowledge: Treatment Regimen (NOC)
Verbalize understanding of therapeutic needs.
Correctly perform necessary procedures and explain reasons for the actions.
Initiate necessary lifestyle changes and participate in treatment regimen.

ACTIONS/INTERVENTIONS	RATIONALE

Amputation Care (NIC)

Independent

Review disease process, surgical procedure, and future expectations.

Instruct in dressing and wound care, inspection of residual limb using mirror to visualize all areas, skin massage, and appropriate wrapping of the residual limb.

Discuss general residual limb care, for example:

  Wash daily with mild soap and water; rinse and pat dry. Do this daily, or more often if client sweats a lot, or in treating a rash or infection.

  Massage the residual limb after dressings are discontinued and suture line is healed.

  Avoid the use of alcohol-based lotions, or use of powders.

  Wear only properly fitted, clean, wrinkle-free limb sock.

  Use clean cotton T-shirt under harness for upper-limb prosthesis.

Review common problems and appropriate actions.

Stress importance of well-balanced diet and adequate fluid intake.

Recommend cessation of smoking. Offer referral resources for cessation programs.

Review and demonstrate care of prosthetic device. Stress importance of routine maintenance and periodic refitting.

Encourage continuation of postoperative exercise program.

Identify techniques to manage phantom sensation and phantom pain. (Refer to ND: acute Pain.)

Encourage taking care of whole self: body, mind, and spirit. Emphasize socialization, stress management, relaxation training, or counseling.

Identify signs and symptoms requiring medical evaluation— edema, erythema, increased or odorous drainage from incision, changes in sensation, movement, skin color, and persistent phantom pain.

Identify community and rehabilitation support, such as a certified prosthetist-orthotist, amputee groups, home-care service, and homemaker services, as needed.

Provides knowledge base from which client can make informed choices.

Promotes competent self-care, facilitates healing and fitting of prosthesis, and reduces potential for complications.

Hygiene of residual limb is critical because most of the time it is enclosed in the socket or liner of the prosthesis, rendering it more prone to skin breakdown and infection.

Massage softens the scar and prevents adherence to the bone, decreases tenderness, and stimulates circulation.

Although a small amount of lotion may be indicated if skin is dry, emollients and creams soften skin and may cause maceration when prosthesis is worn. Powder may cake, potentiating skin irritation.

Residual limb may continue to shrink for up to 2 years, and an improperly fitting sock or one that is mended or dirty can cause skin irritation or breakdown.

Absorbs perspiration; prevents skin irritation from harness.

Problems can occur even when client is taking precautions, for example, the development of a red, sore area that does not resolve when prosthesis is off, or a blister caused by pressure between socket liner and skin. These problems need early medical follow-up if home interventions are not effective.

Provides needed nutrients for tissue regeneration and healing, aids in maintaining circulating volume and normal organ function, and aids in maintenance of proper weight. *Note:* Weight changes affect fit of prosthesis.

Smoking potentiates peripheral vasoconstriction, impairing circulation and tissue oxygenation.

Ensures proper fit and alignment, reduces risk of complications, and prolongs life of prosthesis.

Enhances circulation, healing, and function of affected part, facilitating adaptation to prosthetic device.

Persistent and/or recurring pain requires long-term management, with multiple strategies and modalities, including desensitization therapy, intermittent compression, medications, TENS, and nerve blocks. *Note:* Electrical stimulation offers a short-term rerouting or stimulation of different nerve pathways, thus reducing the activity of the usual pain patterns.

Various techniques may be implemented such as relaxation breathing, exercises, visualization, or biofeedback to reduce muscle tension and enhance client's control of situation and coping abilities.

Prompt intervention may prevent serious complications and/or loss of function. *Note:* Chronic phantom-limb pain may indicate neuroma, requiring surgical resection.

Facilitates transfer to home, supports independence, and enhances coping.

POTENTIAL CONSIDERATIONS following acute hospitalization (dependent on client's age, physical condition and presence of complications, personal resources, and life responsibilities)

In addition to considerations in Surgical Intervention plan of care:

- *risk for Trauma*—balancing difficulties/altered gait, muscle weakness, reduced muscle coordination, lack of safety precautions, hazards associated with use of assistive devices
- *disturbed Body Image/situational low Self-Esteem*—loss of body part, change in functional abilities
- *Self-Care Deficit/impaired Home Maintenance* (dependent on location of amputation)—musculoskeletal impairment, decreased strength/endurance, pain, depression

TOTAL JOINT REPLACEMENT

I. Purpose
a. Definitive treatment for advanced, irreversibly damaged joints with loss of function and unremitting pain
b. Commom conditions: degenerative and rheumatoid arthritis (RA); selected fractures, such as with hip and femoral neck; joint instability; congenital hip disorders; avascular necrosis

II. Procedures
a. Performed on any joint except the spine, with hip and knee replacements the most common procedures
b. Prosthesis may be metallic, polyethylene, or ceramic, or a combination
c. Implanted with methylmethacrylate cement or may be a porous, coated implant that encourages bony ingrowth

III. Statistics
a. Morbidity: In 2004, there were more than 1 million primary and revision procedures performed; females accounted for 62% of all procedures, with a mean age (at time of procedure) of 66 to 68 years (U.S. Bone and Joint Decade, 2008).
b. Mortality: Rate is very low, 0.29% in 2004, related to advanced age and comorbidities (Liu et al, 2008).
c. Cost: In 2004, annual hospital cost estimated at over $44 billion (U.S. Bone and Joint Decade, 2008).

GLOSSARY

Arthroplasty: Recontruction or replacement of a diseased or damaged joint.
Primary joint replacement: Initial surgical procedure.

Revision: Second or succeeding procedures to correct loose, unstable hardware or address return of pain in the joint.

Care Setting

Client is treated in inpatient acute surgical unit and subacute or rehabilitation unit.

Related Concerns

Fractures, page 632
Psychosocial aspects of care, page 749
Rheumatoid arthritis (RA), page 729
Sepsis/septicemia, page 686
Surgical intervention, page 782
Thrombophlebitis: deep vein thrombosis, page 111

Client Assessment Database

DIAGNOSTIC DIVISION MAY REPORT	MAY EXHIBIT
ACTIVITY/REST • History of occupation or participation in sports activities that wear on a particular joint • Difficulty walking • Stiffness in joints, which is worse in the morning or after a period of inactivity • Fatigue • Generalized muscle weakness • Inability to participate in occupational and/or recreational activities at desired level • Interruption of sleep, delayed falling asleep or awakened by pain • Does not feel well rested **HYGIENE** • Difficulty performing activities of daily living (ADLs) • Use of special equipment and/or mobility devices • Need for assistance with some or all activities	• Decreased range of motion (ROM) of affected joints • Decreased muscle strength and tone • Gait disturbances—effort to compensate for joint pain

(continues on page 656)

DIAGNOSTIC DIVISION MAY REPORT (continued)	MAY EXHIBIT (continued)
NEUROSENSORY	• Soft tissue swelling, nodules • Muscle spasm, stiffness • Deformity
PAIN/DISCOMFORT • Pain—dull, aching, persistent in affected joint(s) • Pain worsened by movement	
SAFETY • Traumatic injury and/or fractures affecting the joint • Congenital deformities • History of inflammatory, debilitating arthritis—RA or osteoarthritis • Aseptic necrosis of the joint head	• Distorted joints • Joint or tissue swelling • Decreased ROM • Changes in gait
TEACHING/LEARNING • Current medication use—anti-inflammatories, analgesics, opioids, steroids, hormone replacement therapy (HRT), bone resorption inhibitor (e.g., Fosamax), calcium supplements	
DISCHARGE PLAN CONSIDERATIONS • May need assistance with transportation, self-care activities, and homemaker or maintenance tasks • Possible placement in rehabilitation or extended-care facility for continued therapy and assistance ▶ Refer to section at end of plan for postdischarge considerations.	

Diagnostic Studies

TEST WHY IT IS DONE	WHAT IT TELLS ME
• *Radiographs:* Visualize and evaluate skeletal changes or damage, determine treatment options, and guide orthopedic surgery. • *Bone scan, computed tomography (CT) scans, magnetic resonance imaging (MRI):* Assess bone loss and determine presence of comorbidities.	May reveal destruction of articular cartilage, bony demineralization, fractures, soft tissue swelling, narrowing of joint space, joint subluxations, or deformity. Determine extent of degeneration and rule out malignancy or infectious process.

Nursing Priorities

1. Alleviate pain.
2. Prevent complications.
3. Promote optimal mobility.
4. Provide information about diagnosis, prognosis, and treatment needs.

Discharge Goals

1. Mobility increased.
2. Complications prevented or minimized.
3. Pain relieved or controlled.
4. Diagnosis, prognosis, and therapeutic regimen understood.
5. Plan in place to meet needs after discharge.

NURSING DIAGNOSIS: acute Pain

May be related to
Injuring agents—biological, physical, psychological—muscle spasms, surgical procedure, preexisting chronic joint diseases, elderly age, anxiety

Possibly evidenced by
Reports of pain; distraction, guarding behaviors
Narrowed focus, self-focusing
Alteration in muscle tone; autonomic responses

Desired Outcomes/Evaluation Criteria—Client Will

Pain Level (NOC)
Report pain relieved or controlled.
Appear relaxed, able to rest or sleep appropriately.

Pain Control (NOC)
Demonstrate use of relaxation skills and diversional activities, as indicated by individual situation.

ACTIONS/INTERVENTIONS	RATIONALE
Pain Management (NIC)	
Independent	
Perform comprehensive assessment of pain, noting intensity (scale of 0–10), duration, and location. Determine if pain is at operative or different site, associated with ROM or weight-bearing, associated with vascular compromise or fever.	Provides information on which to base and monitor effectiveness of interventions.
Maintain proper position of operated extremity.	Reduces muscle spasm and undue tension on new prosthesis and surrounding tissues.
Provide comfort measures—frequent repositioning, back rub—and diversional activities. Encourage stress management techniques, such as progressive relaxation, guided imagery, visualization, and meditation. Provide Therapeutic Touch, as appropriate.	Reduces muscle tension, refocuses attention, promotes sense of control, and may enhance coping abilities in the management of discomfort or pain, which can persist for an extended period.
Medicate on a regular schedule and before activities or procedures.	Reduces muscle tension, improves comfort, and facilitates participation.
Investigate reports of sudden, severe joint pain with muscle spasms and changes in joint mobility, or sudden, severe chest pain with dyspnea and restlessness.	Early recognition of developing problems, such as dislocation of prosthesis or blood or fat pulmonary emboli, provides opportunity for prompt intervention and prevention of more serious complications.
Collaborative	
Administer medications as indicated, around the clock, such as: Opioids—instruct in and monitor use of patient-controlled analgesia (PCA), epidural administration, and/or pain ball	Relieves surgical pain and reduces muscle tension and spasm, which contribute to overall discomfort. Opioid infusion (including epidural) may be given during the first 24 to 48 hours. The ON-Q PainBuster® ball provides continuous infusion of local anesthetic directly into surgical site for up to 5 days, thus decreasing need for opioids, and allows for earlier ambulation than epidural administration.
Analgesics, such as, oxycodone (Percocet), hycodone and acetaminophen (Vicodin), and muscle relaxants	Oral analgesics are added to pain management program as the client progresses. *Note:* Use of ketorolac (Toradol) or other nonsteroidal anti-inflammatory drug (NSAID) is contraindicated when client is receiving enoxaparin (Lovenox) therapy.
Apply ice packs, as indicated.	Promotes vasoconstriction to reduce bleeding and tissue edema in surgical area and lessens perception of discomfort.
Initiate and maintain extremity mobilization, such as, ambulation, physical therapy, exerciser, or continuous passive motion (CPM) device.	Increases circulation to affected muscles. Minimizes joint stiffness; relieves muscle spasms related to disuse.

ACTIONS/INTERVENTIONS	RATIONALE
Infection Protection (NIC)	
Independent	
Promote good hand washing by staff and client.	Reduces risk of cross-contamination.
Use strict aseptic or clean technique, as indicated, to reinforce or change dressings and when handling drains. Instruct client not to touch or scratch incision.	Prevents contamination and risk of wound infection, which could require removal of prosthesis.
Maintain patency of drainage devices (e.g., Hemovac, Jackson-Pratt) when present. Note characteristics of wound drainage.	Reduces risk of infection by preventing accumulation of blood and secretions in the joint space, which is a medium for bacterial growth. Purulent, nonserous, odorous drainage is indicative of infection, and continuous drainage from incision may reflect developing skin tract, which can potentiate infectious process.
Assess skin and incision color, temperature, and integrity; note presence of erythema, inflammation, and loss of wound approximation.	Provides information about status of healing process and alerts staff to early signs of infection.
Investigate reports of increased incisional pain and changes in characteristics of pain.	Deep, dull, aching pain in operative area may indicate developing infection in joint. *Note:* Infection can be devastating because, once infection sets in, joint may not be salvagable and prosthetic loss may occur.
Monitor temperature. Note presence of chills.	Although temperature elevations are common in early postoperative phase, elevations occurring 5 or more days postoperatively and/or presence of chills usually require intervention to prevent more serious complications, such as sepsis, osteomyelitis, tissue necrosis, and prosthetic failure.
Encourage fluid intake coupled with a high-protein diet with roughage.	Maintains fluid and nutritional balance to support tissue perfusion and provide nutrients necessary for cellular regeneration and tissue healing.
Collaborative	
Maintain reverse or protective isolation, if appropriate.	May be done initially to reduce contact with sources of possible infection, especially in an elderly, immunosuppressed, or diabetic client.
Administer antibiotics, as indicated.	Used prophylactically in the operating room and for the first 24 hours to prevent infection. Late infections may require intravenous (IV) antibiotic treatments for several weeks, in an effort to save the prosthetic joint.

ACTIONS/INTERVENTIONS	RATIONALE
Circulatory Care: Arterial [or] Venous Insufficiency (NIC)	
Independent	
Palpate pulses. Evaluate capillary refill and skin color and temperature. Compare with unoperated limb.	Diminished or absent pulses, delayed capillary refill time, pallor, blanching, cyanosis, and coldness of skin reflect diminished circulation or perfusion. Comparison with unoperated limb provides clues as to whether neurovascular problem is localized or generalized.
Assess motion and sensation of operated extremity.	Increasing pain, numbness or tingling, and/or inability to perform expected movements such as flexing foot suggest nerve injury, compromised circulation, or dislocation of prosthesis, requiring immediate intervention.
Test sensation of peroneal nerve by pinch or pinprick in the dorsal web between first and second toe, and assess ability to dorsiflex toes after hip or knee replacement.	Position and length of peroneal nerve increase risk of direct injury or compression by tissue edema or hematoma.
Monitor vital signs.	Tachycardia and falling blood pressure (BP) may reflect response to hypovolemia or blood loss or suggest anaphylaxis related to absorption of methylmethacrylate into systemic circulation. *Note:* This occurs less often because of the advent of prosthetics having a porous layer that fosters ingrowth of bone instead of total reliance on adhesives to internally fix the device.
Monitor amount and characteristics of drainage on dressings and from suction device. Note swelling in operative area.	May indicate excessive bleeding or hematoma formation, which can potentiate neurovascular compromise. *Note:* Drainage following hip replacement may reach 1,000 mL in early postoperative period, potentially affecting circulating volume.
Ensure that stabilizing devices such as abduction pillow or splint device are in correct position and are not exerting undue pressure on skin and underlying tissue. Avoid use of pillow or bed knee gatch under knees.	Reduces risk of pressure on underlying nerves or compromised circulation to extremities.
Evaluate for calf tenderness, positive Homans' sign, and inflammation.	Although clinical signs are often not reliable in this population, surveillance should be carried out. Early identification of thrombus development and intervention may prevent embolus formation.
Observe for signs of continued bleeding, oozing from puncture sites and mucous membranes, or ecchymosis following minimal trauma.	Depression of clotting mechanisms or sensitivity to anticoagulants may result in bleeding episodes that can affect red blood cell (RBC) level and circulating volume.
Encourage regular "foot pumps" throughout day.	Pushing the foot down, pointing toes, and pulling toes up toward the ceiling causes the calf to tighten and assist venous return to prevent blood pooling and reduce risk of deep vein thrombosis (DVT).
Collaborative	
Administer IV fluids, blood, and plasma expanders, as needed.	Restores circulating volume to maintain perfusion. *Note:* Drainage collected from operative site during first 6 to 10 hours following procedure may be reinfused per protocol, reducing need for transfusion from unknown donor.
Monitor laboratory studies, such as the following: Hematocrit (Hct)	Usually done 24 to 48 hours postoperatively for evaluation of blood loss, which can be quite large because of high vascularity of surgical site in hip replacement.
Coagulation studies	Evaluates presence and degree of alteration in clotting mechanisms and effects of anticoagulant or antiplatelet agents when used.
Administer medications, as indicated, for example, low-molecular-weight heparins, enoxaparin (Lovenox), dalteparin (Fragmin), or tinzaparin (Innohep).	Anticoagulants or antiplatelet agents may be used routinely to reduce risk of thrombophlebitis and pulmonary emboli. *Note:* Incidence of DVT without prophylaxis is around 50% to 80% in client with knee replacement and 47% to 64% in client with hip replacement. Studies have shown significant decrease in these numbers with prophylaxis.
Maintain intermittent compression stocking or compression boots when used.	Promotes venous return and prevents venous stasis, reducing risk of thrombus formation.
Apply cold or heat, as indicated.	Ice packs are used initially to limit edema and hematoma formation. Heat may then be used to enhance circulation, facilitating resolution of tissue edema.
Prepare for surgical procedure, as indicated.	Evacuation of hematoma or revision of prosthesis may be required to correct compromised circulation.

May be related to
Pain and discomfort in surgical site as well as contralateral joint, musculoskeletal impairment
Surgery, restrictive therapies

Possibly evidenced by
Reluctance to attempt movement, difficulty moving purposefully within the physical environment
Reports of pain or discomfort on movement
Limited ROM, decreased muscle strength/control

Desired Outcomes/Evaluation Criteria—Client Will

Mobility (NOC)
Maintain position of function, as evidenced by absence of contracture.
Display increased strength, ROM, and function of affected joint and limb.
Participate in ADLs and rehabilitation program.

ACTIONS/INTERVENTIONS	RATIONALE
Positioning (NIC)	
Independent	
Maintain affected joint in prescribed position and body in alignment when in bed.	Provides for stabilization of prosthesis and reduces risk of injury during recovery from effects of anesthesia.
Medicate around the clock, or significantly before procedures and activities, so that client is able to participate.	Adequate analgesia is a priority to decrease pain, reduce muscle tension and spasm, and facilitate participation in therapy.
Turn on unoperated side using adequate number of personnel and maintaining operated extremity in prescribed alignment. Support position with pillows and wedges.	Prevents dislocation of hip prosthesis and prolonged skin and tissue pressure, reducing risk of tissue ischemia and breakdown.
Demonstrate and assist with transfer techniques and use of mobility aids, such as a trapeze, walker, crutches, or canes.	Facilitates self-care and client's independence. Proper transfer techniques prevent shearing abrasions of skin and falls.
Determine upper body strength and need for equipment to assist with ADLs, as appropriate. Involve in exercise program.	Replacement of lower extremity joint requires increased use of upper extremities for transfer, ADLs, and desired activities as well as use of ambulation devices.
Inspect skin; observe for reddened areas. Keep linens dry and wrinkle-free. Massage skin and bony prominences routinely. Protect operative heel, elevating whole length of leg with pillow and placing heel on water glove if burning sensation reported.	Prevents skin irritation or breakdown.
Exercise Therapy: Joint Mobility (NIC)	
Perform or assist with ROM to unaffected joints.	Client with degenerative joint disease can quickly lose joint function during periods of restricted activity. Contralateral joint may be nearly as painful as the preoperative surgical joint and may require careful and consistent treatment to maximize mobility.
Promote participation in rehabilitative exercise program, such as the following:	
Total hip: Quadriceps and gluteal muscle setting, isometrics, leg lifts, dorsiflexion, and plantar flexion (ankle pumps) of the foot	Strengthens muscle groups, increasing muscle tone and mass; stimulates circulation; and prevents decubitus ulcers.
Total knee: Quadriceps setting, gluteal contraction, flexion and extension exercises, and isometrics	Active use of the joint may be painful but will not injure the joint. CPM exercise may be initiated on the knee joint postoperatively, although its use is dependent on the particular surgeon and on the individual's needs.
Observe appropriate limitations based on specific joint; for example, avoid marked flexion or rotation of hip and flexion or hyperextension of leg; adhere to weight-bearing restrictions; and wear knee immobilizer, as indicated.	Joint stress is to be avoided at all times during stabilization period to prevent dislocation of new prosthesis.
Investigate sudden increase in pain and shortening of limb as well as changes in skin color, temperature, and sensation.	May be indicative of slippage of prosthesis or other complication, requiring medical evaluation and intervention.
Encourage participation in ADLs.	Enhances self-esteem and promotes sense of control and independence.
Provide positive reinforcement for efforts.	Promotes a positive attitude and encourages involvement in therapy.

ACTIONS/INTERVENTIONS (continued)

Collaborative

Consult with physical and occupational therapists and rehabilitation specialist.

Provide foam or flotation mattress.

RATIONALE (continued)

Useful in creating individualized activity and exercise program. Client may require ongoing assistance with movement, strengthening, and weight-bearing activities as well as use of adjuncts, such as walkers, crutches, canes, elevated toilet seat, pickup sticks, and so on.

Reduces skin and tissue pressure; limits feelings of fatigue and general discomfort.

NURSING DIAGNOSIS: **risk for Constipation**

Risk factors may include

Insufficient physical activity; decreased mobility, weakness

Insufficient fiber or fluid intake; dehydration, poor eating habits

Decreased gastrointestinal (GI) motility, effects of medications—anesthesia, opiate analgesics

Environmental changes, inadequate toileting

Possibly evidenced by

(Not applicable; presence of signs and symptoms establishes an *actual* diagnosis)

Desired Outcomes/Evaluation Criteria—Client Will

Bowel Elimination (NOC)

Maintain usual pattern of bowel functioning.

Demonstrate behaviors to prevent problem.

ACTIONS/INTERVENTIONS

Bowel Management (NIC)

Independent

Identify individual risk factors. Determine current situation and possible impact on bowel function—surgery, new and chronic use of medications affecting intestinal functioning, age, or weakness.

Auscultate abdomen for presence, location, and characteristics of bowel sounds.

Determine usual elimination pattern or frequency, characteristics of stool— color, consistency, amount—manner of constipation, and use of laxatives.

Evaluate usual dietary and fluid intake; compare with current intake.

Promote increased fluid intake, including water and high-fiber fruit juices; offer warm stimulating fluids, such as coffee, tea, and hot water.

Encourage activity and exercise within client's limitation of activity. Assist with early mobility.

Provide privacy and routinely scheduled time for defecation based on usual pattern, as appropriate (e.g., bedside commode or toilet with elevated seat, after breakfast).

Collaborative

Consult with dietitian or nutritionist, as indicated.

Implement bowel program: administer routine stool softeners (e.g., docusate [Colace]); stool stimulants (e.g., bisacodyl [Dulcolax]), polyethylene glycol (Miralax); sennosides (e.g., [Senokot, Ex-lax]); bulk-forming agents (e.g., polycarbophil [FiberCon]), psyllium (Metamucil); saline laxatives (e.g., magnesium citrate), and enemas, as indicated.

RATIONALE

Constipation is one of the most frequent complaints following surgery and during rehabilitation. If left untreated, constipation can lead to nausea and vomiting, bowel obstruction, or even sepsis, especially in the elderly.

Reflects activity of GI tract.

Provides baseline for comparison, promotes recognition of changes, and helps to establish a preventative plan.

Client's usual diet and fluid intake may be marginal at best in promoting healthy bowel functioning, especially when combined with current postsurgical status.

Prevents dehydration and decreases reabsorption of water from the bowel, promoting softer stool and facilitating passage of stool.

To stimulate and optimize GI function.

To facilitate return of normalcy in toileting routine.

Helpful in providing a diet with balanced fiber and bulk that client can continue after discharge to improve consistency of stool and facilitate its passage.

Used to prevent or treat constipation.

ACTIONS/INTERVENTIONS	RATIONALE
Teaching: Disease Process (NIC) *Independent* Review disease process, surgical procedure, and future expectations.	Provides knowledge base from which client can make informed choices. The majority of total joint surgeries are elective, and preoperative education is done in some form in the surgeon's office or in the admitting facility. Postsurgical review of process and expectations may be needed, or desired.
Encourage alternating rest periods with activity.	Conserves energy for healing and prevents undue fatigue, which can increase risk of injury or fall.
Stress importance of continuing prescribed exercise and rehabilitation program within client's tolerance—crutch or cane walking, weight-bearing exercises, stationary bicycling, or swimming.	Increases muscle strength and joint mobility. Most clients will be involved in formal outpatient rehabilitation, home-care programs, or be followed in extended-care facilities by physical therapists. *Note:* Muscle aching indicates too much weight-bearing or activity, signaling a need to cut back.
Review activity limitations, depending on joint replaced: for hip or knee—sitting for long periods or in low chair or toilet seat, recliner; jogging, jumping, excessive bending, lifting, twisting, or crossing legs.	Prevents undue stress on implant. Long-term restrictions depend on individual situation and physician protocol.
Discuss need for safe environment in home including removing scatter rugs and unnecessary furniture, and use of assistive devices, such as hand rails in tub and toilet, raised toilet seat, and cane for long walks.	Reduces risk of falls and excessive stress on joints.
Review and have client or caregiver demonstrate incisional or wound care.	Promotes independence in self-care, reducing risk of complications.
Identify signs and symptoms requiring medical evaluation: fever or chills, incisional inflammation, unusual wound drainage, pain in calf or upper thigh, or development of sore throat or dental infections.	Bacterial infections require prompt treatment to prevent progression to osteomyelitis in the operative area and prosthesis failure, which could occur at any time, even years later.
Review procedure for removal of painball catheter if not discontinued before discharge.	Medication may infuse for up to 5 days and if client removes catheter after discharge it is important to check for black marking on tip to ensure tubing is removed intact.
Review drug regimen, for example, anticoagulants or antibiotics for invasive procedures (e.g., tooth extraction).	Prophylactic therapy may be necessary for a prolonged period after discharge to limit risk of thromboemboli and infection. Procedures known to cause bacteremia can lead to osteomyelitis and prosthesis failure.
Identify bleeding precautions—for example, use of soft toothbrush, electric razor, avoidance of trauma, or forceful blowing of nose—and necessity of routine laboratory follow-up.	Reduces risk of therapy-induced bleeding or hemorrhage.
Encourage intake of balanced diet, including roughage and adequate fluids.	Enhances healing and feeling of general well-being. Promotes bowel and bladder function during period of altered activity.
Discuss continuation of supplemental calcium and vitamin D, hormone replacement, bisphosphonates, and the like as indicated.	Promotes bone health in clients with decreased bone density or who are at risk for osteoporosis.

POTENTIAL CONSIDERATIONS following acute hospitalization (dependent on client's age, physical condition and presence of complications, personal resources, and life responsibilities)

In addition to considerations in Surgical Intervention plan of care:
- *risk for Falls*—balancing difficulties/altered gait, weakness, lack of safety precautions, hazards associated with use of assistive devices
- *risk for Constipation*—insufficient physical activity/decreased mobility, weakness, insufficient fiber/fluid intake, poor eating habits
- *Self-Care Deficit/impaired Home Maintenance*—musculoskeletal impairment, decreased strength/endurance, pain in operative site or other joints

Sample clinical pathway follows in Table 12.1.

TABLE 12.1 Sample CP: Total Hip Replacement, Hospital. ELOS: 4 Days Orthopedic or Surgical Unit

ND and Categories of Care	Day of Surgery ____	Day 1 ____	Day 2 ____	Day 3 ____	Day 4 ____ Discharge
risk for Infection R/T broken skin, exposure of joint, long-term steroid use, decreased mobility	Goals: Participate in activities to reduce risk of postoperative infection	→	→	→	→
		Free of purulent drainage	→	→	→
					Display early signs of wound healing, free of erythema or drainage
		Be afrebile	→	→ Verbalize understanding of healthcare needs to enhance healing, promote wellness	→ Plan in place to meet post-discharge needs, self-care
Diagnostics	Hgb/Hct	→	Electrolytes if indicated		
	Pulse oximetry	→ D/C if stable			
Additional assessments	VS/Temp per postoperative protocol	→ q4h	→ q8h	→ bid unless elevated	→
	Breath sounds q8hr	→	→	→ bid	→
	Amount/ characteristic of Hemovac drainage q8hr	→	→ D/C Characteristics of wound/drainage qd and prn	→	→
Medications Allergies: ____ ____	IV antibiotics	→ D/C			
	IV fluids/blood products	→	→ NS lock or D/C	→ D/C lock	
	Tylenol—Temp ≥101°F	→	→	→ D/C	
Client education	Disease process/ surgical procedure		Dietary needs S/S to report of healthcare provider	Wound care Balancing rest/activity	Provide written instructions for home care

(continues on page 664)

ND and Categories of Care	Day of Surgery ___	Day 1 ___	Day 2 ___	Day 3 ___	Day 4 ___ Discharge
	Handwashing technique, avoid touching of dressing/wound		→		
	Respiratory exercises, incentive spirometry				
Additional nursing actions	Aseptic/clean technique	→	→	→	→
	Protective isolation as indicated	→	→ D/C		
	Reinforce dressing	→	→ Change dressing qd and prn	→ D/C if incision dry; Clean incision bid	→; →
	Encourage PO fluids as tolerated	→	→	→	→
	T, C, DB, q2h	→	Per self	→	→
	Incentive spirometry q2h	→ q2h WA	→ q4h WA	→	→
	Supplemental O₂ as indicated	→ D/C if stable	High-calorie/protein diet	→	→
impaired physical Mobility R/T musculoskeletal impairment/ discomfort, therapeutic restrictions	Maintain proper alignment and position of function	→	→	Independent in transfers; →	Independent in ambulation; →
	Participate in rehabilitation/ exercise program	→	→	→; Display increased strength/ function of operated limb	→; Free of DVT/ thromboembolic complications; Establish regular bladder/ bowel elimination
Referrals		PT-assistive devices if not done preop	PT-exercises/ ambulation	OT/rehabilitation specialist; Social Services if placement indicated	Home care
Diagnostic studies		Protime (coumadin use)	→	→	→; CBC w/platelets (if Lovenox used)
Additional assessments	Neurovascular status/ alignment of operated leg per postoperative protocol	→ q4h	→ q8h	→ bid	→
	Skin (especially heels) q8h or per protocol	→	→	→ qd	→
	Voiding/urinary output q8hr	→	→	→ D/C	
	Bowel sounds q8h	→	→ bid	→ qd	→ D/C
	Stool characteristics		→	→	→

TABLE 12.1   Sample CP: Total Hip Replacement, Hospital. ELOS: 4 Days Orthopedic or Surgical Unit (continued)

ND and Categories of Care	Day of Surgery _____	Day 1 _____	Day 2 _____	Day 3 _____	Day 4 _____ Discharge
Medications Allergies: _____ _____	Coumadin (if Lovenox not ordered)	→ Daily order or Lovenox q12h	→	→	→
	Stool softener/ bowel program	→	→	→	→
Client education	Hip precautions	Transfer techniques	Use of mobility aids	Ambulation/weight-bearing exercises	Provide written instructions
	Use of trapeze		S/S to report to healthcare provider	Activity level/ restrictions post discharge	Home exercise program
	Initial exercises— ankle pumps, quad/gluteal sets			Self-administer Lovenox	Coumadin dose, time, purpose, side effects, precautions, monitoring (if used)
					Sexual concerns
Additional nurs-ing actions	Bedrest/HOB elevated 30°	→ Chair/commode elevate operated leg	→ Chair × 3 ambulate with assistance	→ Ambulate × 3 with assistance as needed prn	→
	Pillow between knees	→	→	→	→
	Turn per protocol q2h	→	→	→	→
	ROM to nonoper-ated side q2h	→	→ Per self	→	→
	Initial exercises q1h WA		→	→	→
		CPM to tolerance		Knee exercise × 5 q1h WA	→ Leg strength-ening
		→ While in bed	→	→	→
		→ Assist w/care	→	→ D/C if protime 1.3 or above	
	SCDs to calves	Elevated toilet seat	→ Self-care	→	→ Shower as indicated
	Total care	→ Insert Foley on #3 if no void	→	→	→
	Fracture pan	→	→ D/C Foley-male	→ D/C Foley-female	→ Send home
	Straight catheter if no void q8h × 2		→	→	
	Foam/special mattress				
acute Pain R/T therapeutic interventions, preexisting chronic joint disease	Verbalize pain within man-ageable level	→	→ Participate in action to decrease pain	→ →	→ →
					Verbalize under-standing of medications/ modalities for pain management
					Demonstrate proper use of adjunct comfort measures

(continues on page 666)

ND and Categories of Care	Day of Surgery _____	Day 1 _____	Day 2 _____	Day 3 _____	Day 4 _____ Discharge
Additional assessments	Pain characteristics/ changes	→	→	→	→
	Response to interventions	→	→	→	→
Medications Allergies: _____ _____	PCA—narcotic of choice	→ D/C, begin PO if tolerated	→		
	Painball	→	→ Acetaminophen prn	→	→
	Antiemetic prn	→ D/C	→ for break-through pain		
	Muscle relaxant				
Client education	Orient to unit/room	Relaxation techniques, guided imagery, breathing exercises		Medications: dose, time, route, purpose, side effects	Written instructions for home-care needs, equipment resources, removal of pain ball if still in place
	Proper use of PCA				
	Reporting of pain/effects of interventions				
Additional nursing actions	Maintain position/ alignment of leg per protocol	→	→	→	→
	Ice pack to operated site	→ prn	→ D/C		
	Routine comfort measures prn	→	→	→	→

Key: bid, twice a day; C, cough; CBC, complete blood count; CPM, continuous passive motion; DB, deep breath; D/C, discontinue; DVT, deep vein thrombosis; Hct, hematocrit; Hgb, hemoglobin; HOB, head of bed; IV, intravenous; NS, normal saline; OT, occupational therapist; PCA, patient-controlled analgesia; PO, by mouth; prn, as needed; PT, physical therapist; q1h, every 1 hour; q2h, every 2 hours; q4h, every 4 hours; q8h, every 8 hours; q12h, every 12 hours; qd, every day; ROM, range of motion; R/T, related to; SCD, sequential compression device; S/S, signs and symptoms; T, temp; VS, vital signs; WA, while awake.

Integumentary

BURNS: THERMAL, CHEMICAL, AND ELECTRICAL—ACUTE AND CONVALESCENT PHASES

I. Pathophysiology—Local and systemic response affecting skin and/or other tissues depending on cause of burn injury and physiological response (Hettiaratchy, 2004)

a. Local responses

   i. Coagulation: Occurs at the point of maximum damage, causing irreversible tissue loss due to coagulation of the constituent proteins.

   ii. Stasis: Area characterized by decreased tissue perfusion that is potentially salvageable unless additional insults, such as prolonged hypotension, infection, or edema, occur, converting this zone into an area of complete tissue loss.

   iii. Hyperemia: Outermost area has increased tissue perfusion, and tissue will recover unless severe sepsis or prolonged hypoperfusion occurs.

b. Systemic response—Cytokines and other inflammatory mediators are released at the site of burn injuries with total body surface area (TBSA) of 30% or greater.

   i. Cardiovascular: Increased capillary permeability leads to shift of intravascular proteins and fluids into the interstitial space, followed by vasoconstriction and decreased myocardial contractility; combined with fluid loss from the burn wound, systemic hypotension and organ hypoperfusion occur.

   ii. Respiratory: Bronchoconstriction occurs in response to inflammatory mediators, which, in severe burns, can cause acute respiratory distress syndrome (ARDS).

   iii. Metabolic—Rate increases up to three times the baseline rate, resulting in breakdown of muscle tissue.

   iv. Immunological—Immune suppression response occurs.

II. Classification by burn wound and depth

a. Superficial partial-thickness (first-degree) burns: affect only the epidermis, skin is often warm and dry, and wounds appear bright pink to red with minimal edema and fine blisters, if present

b. Moderate partial-thickness (second-degree) burns: include the epidermis and dermis; wounds appear red to pink with moderate edema and blisters that may be intact or draining

c. Deep partial-thickness (second-degree) burns: extend in to the deep dermis; wounds are dryer than moderate partial-thickness burns and appear pale-pink to pale-ivory, with moderate edema and blisters

d. Full-thickness (third-degree) burns: include all layers of skin and subcutaneous fat and may involve the muscle, nerves, and blood supply; wounds have a dry, leathery texture and appearance varies from white to cherry-red to brown or black, with blistering uncommon; absence of pain in the center, but the edges of the burn wound may have heightened sensation

e. Full-thickness, subdermal (fourth-degree) burns: involve all skin layers as well as muscle, organ tissue, and bone, with charring

III. Etiology

a. Thermal burns: flame, hot fluids or gases, friction, or exposure to extremely cold objects (e.g., snow, nitrogen, dry ice); flame burns are often associated with smoke/inhalation injury

b. Chemical burns: contact with a caustic substance (acid or alkaline); degree of injury dependent on type and content as well as concentration and temperature of injuring agent

c. Electral burns: current travels through the body along the pathway of least resistance (i.e., nerves offer the least resistance and bones the greatest resistance), generating heat in proportion to resistance offered; degree of injury dependent on type/voltage of current with underlying injury more severe than visible injury

d. Radiation burns: exposure to ionizing radiation, most commonly protracted and overexposure to ultraviolet rays—UVA and UVG (e.g., the sun, sunlamps, tanning booths), or high exposure to x-rays including radiotherapy (e.g., cancer therapy)

e. Risk factors: substance abuse, careless smoking, cultural practices, socioeconomic status (e.g., overcrowded living conditions, insufficient parental supervision of children, lack of safety precautions), and violence, including child abuse and neglect, such as with those aged 4 years and under or those aged 65 years and older

IV. Statistics (American Burn Association, 2007)

a. Morbidity: 500,000 burn injuries require medical attention in the United States annually, with approximately 40,000 requiring hospitalization; approximately 25,000 are classified as major burns, involving at least 30% of TBSA.

b. Mortality: There are approximately 4,000 deaths annually.

c. Cost: $7.5 billion is spent annually for fire and burn injuries (Centers for Disease Control and Prevention [CDC], 2007).

Catabolism: Breaking down of muscle tissue.

Dermis: Inner layer of skin, which contains blood and lymph vessels, hair follicles, and glands.

Epidermis: Outermost layer of skin, made up of flat, scale-like cells called squamous cells.

Total body surface area (TBSA): The "rule of nines" estimates the extent of TBSA involved in a burn injury to guide treatment. Major anatomic areas of the body are divided into percentages: in adults, 9% for the head and neck, 9% for each upper extremity, 18% to each of the anterior and posterior portions of the trunk, 18% to each lower extremity, and 1% to the perineum and genitalia. The client's palm area represents approximately 1% of TBSA and can be helpful in calculating scattered areas of involvement.

Care Setting

The following adult clients are admitted for acute care and, during the rehabilitation phase, may be cared for in a subacute or rehabilitation unit: those with partial-thickness burns more than 15% to 25% of TBSA or whose age is considered high risk (older than 50 years and younger than 10 years); full-thickness burns more than 2% to 10% of TBSA; and those clients with second- and third-degree burns of face, both hands, perineum, or both feet; or inhalation and all electrical burns, including lightning injury (Edlich et al, 2006).

Related Concerns

Disaster considerations, page 876

Fluid and electrolyte imbalances, page 903

Metabolic acidosis—primary base bicarbonate deficiency, page 483

Psychosocial aspects of care, page 749

Respiratory acidosis (primary carbonic acid excess), page 195

Sepsis/septicemia, page 686

Surgical intervention, page 782

Total nutritional support: parenteral and enteral feeding, page 469

Upper gastrointestinal/esophageal bleeding, page 306

Client Assessment Database

Data depend on type, severity, and body surface area involved.

DIAGNOSTIC DIVISION MAY REPORT	MAY EXHIBIT
ACTIVITY/REST	• Decreased strength, endurance • Limited range of motion (ROM) of involved areas • Altered muscle mass and tone
CIRCULATION (with burn injury of more than 20% TBSA)	• Hypotension (shock) • Peripheral pulses diminished distal to extremity injury; generalized peripheral vasoconstriction with loss of pulses, mottling of skin, and coolness (electrical shock) • Tachycardia (shock, anxiety, pain) • Dysrhythmias (electrical shock) • Tissue edema formation (all burns)
EGO INTEGRITY • Feeling scared, self-conscious, conspicuous, angry, embarrassed, different • Concerns about family, job, finances, disfigurement	• Anxiety, irritability • Denial, withdrawal • Crying, depression • Hostility, aggressive behavior

DIAGNOSTIC DIVISION MAY REPORT (continued)	MAY EXHIBIT (continued)
ELIMINATION	• Urinary output decreased or absent during emergent phase; color may be pink from damaged red blood cells (RBCs); or reddish-black if myoglobin present, indicating deep-muscle damage • Diuresis—after capillary leak sealed and fluids mobilized back into circulation • Bowel sounds decreased or absent, especially in cutaneous burns of more than 20% TBSA, because stress reduces gastric motility, peristalsis
FOOD/FLUID	• Generalized tissue edema—swelling is rapid and may be extreme in early hours after injury • Weight loss • Anorexia, nausea, vomiting
NEUROSENSORY • Mixed areas of numbness, tingling, burning pain • Changes in vision, decreased visual acuity (electrical shock)	• Changes in orientation, affect, behavior • Decreased deep tendon reflexes (DTRs), reflexes and sensation in injured extremities • Seizure activity (electrical shock) • Corneal lacerations, retinal damage (electrical shock) • Rupture of tympanic membrane (electrical shock) • Paralysis (electrical injury to nerve pathways)
PAIN/DISCOMFORT • Pain varies—first-degree burns are extremely sensitive to touch, pressure, air movement, and temperature changes • Second-degree moderate-thickness burns are very painful, whereas pain response in second-degree deep-thickness burns is dependent on intactness of nerve endings • Third-degree burns are painless, except along the edges of the burn wound	• Guarding behavior, protective positioning • Expressive behavior, such as restlessness, moaning, crying • Self-focusing; facial mask • Changes in blood pressure (BP), pulse, respiratory rate
RESPIRATION • Confinement in a closed space, prolonged exposure (possibility of inhalation injury)	• Hoarseness, wheezy cough, carbonaceous particles on face or in sputum, drooling or inability to swallow oral secretions, and cyanosis (indicative of inhalation injury) • Thoracic excursion may be limited in presence of circumferential chest burns • Upper airway stridor, wheezes (obstruction due to laryngospasm, laryngeal edema) • Breath sounds—crackles (pulmonary edema), stridor (laryngeal edema), profuse airway secretions, wheezing (rhonchi)
SAFETY • Engaging in risky behavior—substance abuse, sporting activities during thunderstorm, working near high power lines • Lack of safety practices; for example, no smoke detector, smoking in bed, wearing loose-fitting clothing around open flame, improper use or storage of caustic chemicals • Sensory impairments limiting detection of heat or cold • Episodes of violence or abuse • History of previous burns or other injuries	**SKIN** • *General:* Exact depth of tissue destruction may not be evident for 3 to 5 days because of the process of microvascular thrombosis in some wounds; unburned skin areas may be cool, clammy and pale, with slow capillary refill in the presence of decreased cardiac output as a result of fluid loss or shock state • *Flame injury:* There may be areas of mixed depth of injury because of varied intensity of heat produced by burning clothing; singed nasal hairs; dry, red mucosa of nose and mouth; blisters on posterior pharynx, circumoral and/or circumnasal edema

(continues on page 670)

DIAGNOSTIC DIVISION
MAY REPORT (continued)

TEACHING/LEARNING
• Use of sedatives, alcohol, tobacco, and street drugs
• Cultural beliefs and practices

DISCHARGE PLAN CONSIDERATIONS
• May require assistance with treatments, wound care and supplies, self-care activities, homemaker and maintenance tasks, transportation, finances, and vocational counseling
• Changes in physical layout of home or living facility other than home during prolonged rehabilitation

▸ Refer to section at end of plan for postdischarge considerations.

MAY EXHIBIT (continued)

• *Chemical injury:* Wound appearance varies according to causative agent; skin may be yellowish-brown with soft leather-like texture; blisters, ulcers, necrosis, or thick eschar. *Note:* Injuries are generally deeper than they appear cutaneously, and tissue destruction can continue for up to 72 hours after injury.
• *Electrical injury:* The external cutaneous injury is usually much less than the underlying necrosis; appearance of wounds varies and may include entry and exit (explosive) wounds of current, arc burns from current moving in close proximity to body, and thermal burns due to ignition of clothing
• *Other:* Presence of fractures, dislocations (concurrent falls, motor vehicle accident; tetanic muscle contractions due to electrical shock)

Diagnostic Studies

TEST
WHY IT IS DONE

WHAT IT TELLS ME

BLOOD TESTS
• *Complete blood count (CBC):* Battery of screening tests, which typically includes hemoglobin (Hgb); hematocrit (Hct); red blood cell (RBC) count morphology, indices, and distribution width index; platelet count and size; white blood cell (WBC) count and differential.

Initial increased Hct suggests hemoconcentration due to fluid shift or loss. Later, Hct and RBCs may be decreased because of heat damage to vascular endothelium. WBCs may be elevated due to inflammatory response to injury.

• *Arterial blood gases (ABGs):* Describe the assessment of arterial blood levels of oxygen (PaO_2) and carbon dioxide ($PaCO_2$). Typically, blood pH (acidity) is measured simultaneously with ABGs.

Baseline is especially important with suspicion of inhalation injury. Reduced Pao_2 and increased $Paco_2$ may be seen with carbon monoxide poisoning. Acidosis may occur because of reduced renal function and loss of compensatory respiratory mechanisms.

• *Carboxyhemoglobin (COHgb):* Compound that is formed when inhaled carbon monoxide combines with Hgb, binding more tightly than oxygen and rendering the Hgb incapable of transporting oxygen.

Elevated percentage reflects the extent to which normal transport of oxygen has been negatively affected. Elevation of more than 10% indicates inhalation injury in a nonsmoker. Toxic exposure with levels greater than 30% indicate carbon monoxide poisoning and can result in loss of consciousness, seizures, coma, and death (Van Leeuwen et al, 2006).

Diagnostic Studies (continued)

TEST WHY IT IS DONE (continued)	WHAT IT TELLS ME (continued)
• *Serum electrolytes:* Substance that will dissociate into ions in solution and acquire the capacity to conduct electricity. Electrolytes include sodium, potassium, chloride, calcium, and phosphate.	Potassium level may be initially elevated because of injured tissues, RBC destruction, and decreased renal function; hypokalemia can occur when diuresis starts; and magnesium level may be decreased. Sodium level may initially be decreased with body water losses; hypernatremia can occur later as renal conservation occurs.
• *Serum glucose:* Simple sugar that is a major energy source for all cellular and bodily functions.	Elevation reflects stress response.
• *Albumin, globulin, and albumin/globulin ratio:* Albumin and globulin make up most of the protein within the body and are measured in the total protein of the blood and other body fluids. Albumin proteins are normally higher than globulin and are expressed in ratio.	Albumin/globulin ratio may be reversed because of loss of protein in edema fluid.
• *Blood urea nitrogen (BUN) and creatinine (Cr):* BUN and Cr are waste products in the blood from the breakdown of protein and are filtered by the kidneys.	Elevation reflects decreased renal perfusion or function; however, the level of Cr can become elevated because of tissue injury.
URINE TESTS • *Urinalysis:* Screening test to evaluate renal function and detect substances or cellular material reflecting injury.	Presence of albumin, Hgb, and myoglobin indicates deep-tissue damage and protein loss—especially seen with serious electrical burns. Reddish-black color of urine indicates presence of myoglobin.
OTHER DIAGNOSTIC STUDIES • *Photographs of burns:* Documents burn wound at time of admission.	Provides baseline to evaluate healing process.
• *Laser Doppler:* Measures microvascular blood flow in dermis.	Laser Doppler flow measurements performed early after burn injury are useful in predicting the depth of burn wounds and the potential for healing. Laser Doppler flowmetry helps with selection of clients for early excision and grafting of burn wounds (Edlich et al, 2006).
• *Magnetic resonance imaging (MRI) scan:* Scan that uses magnetic fields to produce two- or three-dimensional images of organs inside the body.	Detects tissue edema—a manifestation of cell membrane damage that begins to accumulate minutes after electrical injury from increased vascular permeability and extravasation of intracellular contents.
• *Wound cultures:* Drainage or material from burn area is grown in the laboratory on nutrient-enriched media to identify presence of microorganisms such as bacteria or fungi.	May be obtained for baseline data and repeated periodically to evaluate for wound infection and/or effectiveness of antimicrobial therapies.
• *Chest x-ray:* Evaluates organs and structures within the chest for symptoms of disease.	May appear normal in early postburn period even with inhalation injury; however, a true inhalation injury presents as infiltrates, often progressing to whiteout on x-ray (ARDS).
• *Upper airway endoscopy and fiberoptic bronchoscopy—also known as direct or indirect laryngoscopy:* Direct visualization of upper airways by means of either a rigid or a flexible bronchoscope.	Useful in diagnosing extent of inhalation injury in the high-risk client; findings can include edema, hemorrhage, and/or ulceration of upper respiratory tract.
• *Pulmonary function studies—forced expiratory volume (FEV₁) and peak flow volume loop:* Evaluate respiratory status.	Provides noninvasive assessment of effects and extent of inhalation injury. Airway obstruction causes a decrease in FEV_1 and peak flow.
• *Ventilation-perfusion lung scan:* Uses inhaled and injected radioisotopes to measure breathing and circulation in all areas of the lungs.	May be done to determine extent of inhalation injury
• *Electrocardiogram (ECG):* Record of the electrical activity of the heart, providing important information concerning the spread of electricity to the different parts of the heart.	Signs of myocardial ischemia and dysrhythmias may occur with electrical burns.

(continues on page 672)

TEST WHY IT IS DONE (continued)	WHAT IT TELLS ME (continued)
• *Cardiac enzymes (e.g., creatinine phosphokinase [CPK] isoenzyme [MB]):* A group of enzymes normally found in heart tissue and released into the bloodstream in increased concentration when the heart muscle is damaged.	Myocardial infarction (MI) can be a complication of electrical injury or postinjury resuscitation causing elevation of cardiac enzymes. However, recent studies show that skeletal muscle cells contain up to 20% to 25% of CPK-MB fraction, suggesting that electrical damage to skeletal muscle, rather than cardiac muscle, may account for an elevated CPK-MB in electrical injury (Serebrisky & Nazarian, 2006).

Nursing Priorities

1. Maintain patent airway and respiratory function.
2. Restore hemodynamic stability and circulating volume.
3. Alleviate pain.
4. Prevent complications.
5. Provide emotional support for client and significant other (SO).
6. Provide information about condition, prognosis, and treatment.

Discharge Goals

1. Homeostasis achieved.
2. Pain controlled or reduced.
3. Complications prevented or minimized.
4. Current situation dealt with realistically.
5. Condition, prognosis, and therapeutic regimen understood.
6. Plan in place to meet needs after discharge.

NURSING DIAGNOSIS: risk for ineffective Airway Clearance

Risk factors may include
Tracheobronchial obstruction—mucosal edema and loss of ciliary action (smoke inhalation); circumferential full-thickness burns of the neck, thorax, and chest, with compression of the airway or limited chest excursion
Trauma—direct upper-airway injury by flame, steam, hot air, and chemicals or gases
Fluid shifts, pulmonary edema, decreased lung compliance

Possibly evidenced by
(Not applicable; presence of signs and symptoms establishes an *actual* diagnosis)

Desired Outcomes/Evaluation Criteria—Client Will

Respiratory Status: Airway Patency (NOC)
Demonstrate clear breath sounds, respiratory rate will be within normal range and be free of dyspnea and cyanosis.

ACTIONS/INTERVENTIONS	RATIONALE
Respiratory Monitoring (NIC) *Independent*	
Obtain history of injury. Note presence of preexisting respiratory conditions and any history of smoking.	Causative burning agent, duration of exposure, and occurrence in closed or open space predict probability of inhalation injury. Type of material burned, such as wood, plastic, or wool, suggests type of toxic gas exposure. Preexisting conditions increase the risk of respiratory complications.
Assess gag and swallow reflexes; note upper airway burns, drooling, inability to swallow, hoarseness, and wheezy cough.	Suggestive of inhalation injury, which may develop over several days.
Monitor respiratory rate, rhythm, and depth; note presence of pallor or cyanosis and carbonaceous or pink-tinged sputum.	Tachypnea, use of accessory muscles, presence of cyanosis, and changes in sputum suggest developing respiratory distress or pulmonary edema and need for medical intervention.
Auscultate lungs, noting stridor, wheezing, crackles, diminished breath sounds, and brassy cough.	Airway obstruction and respiratory distress can occur very quickly or may be delayed, for example, up to 3 days after burn.
Note presence of pallor or cherry-red color of unburned skin.	Suggests presence of hypoxemia or carbon monoxide.
Investigate changes in behavior and mentation, such as restlessness, agitation, and confusion.	Although often related to pain, changes in consciousness may reflect developing, worsening hypoxia or effects of inhaled toxins, especially carbon monoxide.

ACTIONS/INTERVENTIONS (continued)	RATIONALE (continued)
Monitor 24-hour fluid balance, noting variations or changes.	Fluid shifts or excess fluid replacement increases risk of pulmonary edema. *Note:* Inhalation injury increases fluid demands as much as 35% or more because of edema and fluid shifts.
Airway Management (NIC)	
Elevate head of bed. Avoid use of pillow under head, as indicated.	Promotes optimal lung expansion and respiratory function. When head and neck burns are present, a pillow can inhibit respiration, cause necrosis of burned ear cartilage, and promote neck contractures.
Encourage coughing, deep-breathing exercises, and frequent position changes.	Promotes lung expansion, mobilization, and drainage of secretions.
Suction, if necessary, with extreme care, maintaining sterile technique.	Helps maintain clear airway, but should be done cautiously because of mucosal edema and inflammation. Sterile technique reduces risk of infection.
Promote voice rest, but assess ability to speak and/or swallow oral secretions periodically.	Increasing hoarseness or decreased ability to swallow suggests increasing tracheal edema and may indicate need for prompt intubation.
Collaborative	
Administer humidified oxygen via appropriate mode, for example, a face mask.	Oxygen corrects hypoxemia and acidosis. Humidity decreases drying of respiratory tract and reduces viscosity of sputum.
Monitor continuous pulse oximetry and serial ABGs.	Baseline is essential for further assessment of respiratory status and as a guide to treatment. PaO_2 less than 50, $PaCO_2$ greater than 50, and decreasing pH reflect smoke inhalation and developing pneumonia or ARDS.
Monitor COHgb levels, if indicated.	Client with inhalation injury may be monitored for elevated carbon monoxide levels. If pH is below 7.4 along with elevated COHgb, hyperbaric oxygenation may be considered.
Review serial chest x-rays.	Changes reflecting atelectasis or pulmonary edema may not occur for 2 to 3 days after burn.
Provide or assist with chest physiotherapy and incentive spirometry.	Chest physiotherapy drains dependent areas of the lung, and incentive spirometry may be done to improve lung expansion, thereby promoting respiratory function and reducing atelectasis. *Note:* Bronchoscopy may be done to remove endotracheal debris.
Prepare for, or assist with, intubation or tracheostomy and mechanical ventilation, as indicated.	Intubation and mechanical support is required when airway edema or circumferential burn injury interferes with respiratory function and oxygenation. If client develops signs of respiratory failure or ARDS, mechanical ventilation and intensive respiratory care is required. (Refer to CP: Ventilatory Assistance [Mechanical].)

NURSING DIAGNOSIS: risk for deficient Fluid Volume

Risk factors may include
Loss of fluid through abnormal routes—burn wounds
Increased need—hypermetabolic state, insufficient intake
Hemorrhagic losses

Possibly evidenced by
(Not applicable; presence of signs and symptoms establishes an *actual* diagnosis)

Desired Outcomes/Evaluation Criteria—Client Will

Hydration (NOC)
Demonstrate improved fluid balance as evidenced by individually adequate urinary output with normal specific gravity, stable vital signs, and moist mucous membranes.

ACTIONS/INTERVENTIONS	RATIONALE

Shock Prevention (NIC)

Independent

Monitor vital signs and central venous pressure (CVP). Note capillary refill and strength of peripheral pulses.

Serves as a guide to fluid replacement needs and assesses cardiovascular response. *Note:* Invasive monitoring is indicated for clients with major burns, smoke inhalation, or preexisting cardiac disease, although there is an associated increased risk of infection, necessitating careful monitoring and care of insertion site.

Monitor urinary output and specific gravity. Observe urine color and Hematest, as indicated.

Generally, fluid replacement should be titrated to ensure average urinary output of 30 to 50 mL/hr in the adult. Urine can appear red to black in association with massive muscle destruction because of presence of blood and release of myoglobin. If gross myoglobinuria is present, minimum urinary output should be 75 to 100 mL/hr to reduce risk of tubular damage and renal failure.

Estimate wound drainage and insensible losses.

Increased capillary permeability, protein shifts, inflammatory process, and evaporative losses greatly affect circulating volume and urinary output, especially during initial 24 to 72 hours after burn injury.

Maintain cumulative record of amount and types of fluid intake.

Massive or rapid replacement with different types of fluids and fluctuations in rate of administration require close tabulation to prevent constituent imbalances or fluid overload.

Weigh daily.

Fluid replacement formulas partly depend on admission weight and subsequent changes. A 15% to 20% weight gain can be anticipated in the first 72 hours during fluid replacement, with return to preburn weight approximately 10 days after burn.

Measure circumference of burned extremities, as indicated.

May be helpful in estimating extent of edema and fluid shifts affecting circulating volume and urinary output.

Investigate changes in mentation.

Deterioration in the level of consciousness may indicate inadequate circulating volume and reduced cerebral perfusion.

Observe for gastric distention, hematemesis, and tarry stools. Hematest nasogastric (NG) drainage and stools periodically.

Stress (Curling's) ulcer occurs in up to half of all severely burned clients and can occur as early as the first week. Clients with burns more than 20% of TBSA are at risk for mucosal bleeding in the gastrointestinal (GI) tract during the acute phase because of decreased splanchnic blood flow and reflex paralytic ileus.

Collaborative

Insert and maintain indwelling urinary catheter.

Allows for close observation of renal function and prevents urinary retention. Retention of urine with its by-products of tissue-cell destruction can lead to renal dysfunction and infection.

Insert/maintain large-bore intravenous (IV) catheter(s).

Accommodates rapid infusion of fluids.

Administer calculated IV replacement of fluids, electrolytes, plasma, and albumin.

Fluid resuscitation replaces lost fluids and electrolytes and helps prevent complications, such as shock and acute tubular necrosis (ATN). Replacement formulas vary, such as Brooke, Evans, or Parkland, but are based on extent of injury, amount of urinary output, and weight. *Note:* Once initial fluid resuscitation has been accomplished, a steady rate of fluid administration is preferred to boluses, which may increase interstitial fluid shifts and cardiopulmonary congestion.

Monitor laboratory studies, such as Hgb/Hct, electrolytes, and urine sodium.

Identifies blood loss, RBC destruction, and fluid and electrolyte replacement needs. Urine sodium less than 10 mEq/L suggests inadequate fluid resuscitation. *Note:* During first 24 hours after burn, hemoconcentration is common because of fluid shifts into the interstitial space.

Administer medications, as indicated, such as the following:
Diuretics, for example, mannitol (Osmitrol)

May be indicated to enhance urinary output and clear tubules of debris to prevent necrosis if acute renal failure (ARF) is present.

Potassium

Although hyperkalemia often occurs during first 24 to 48 hours due to tissue destruction, subsequent replacement may be necessary because of large urinary losses.

ACTIONS/INTERVENTIONS (continued)

Antacids, for example, calcium carbonate (Titralac) and magaldrate (Riopan) and histamine inhibitors, for example, cimetidine (Tagamet) and ranitidine (Zantac)

Add electrolytes to water used for wound débridement, as indicated.

RATIONALE (continued)

Antacids may reduce gastric acidity; histamine inhibitors decrease production of hydrochloric acid to reduce risk of gastric irritation or bleeding.

Washing solution that approximates tissue fluids may minimize osmotic fluid shifts.

NURSING DIAGNOSIS: acute Pain

May be related to
Destruction of skin and tissues, edema formation
Manipulation of injured tissues—wound débridement

Possibly evidenced by
Reports of pain
Narrowed focus, facial mask of pain
Alteration in muscle tone; autonomic responses
Distraction, guarding behaviors; anxiety, fear; restlessness, crying

Desired Outcomes/Evaluation Criteria—Client Will

Pain Level (NOC)
Report pain reduced or controlled.
Display relaxed facial expressions and body posture.

Pain Control (NOC)
Participate in activities and sleep and rest appropriately.

ACTIONS/INTERVENTIONS

Pain Management (NIC)
Independent
Cover wounds as soon as possible unless open-air exposure burn care method required.
Elevate burned extremities periodically.

Provide bed cradle, as indicated.
Wrap digits and extremities in position of function, avoiding flexed position of affected joints, using splints and footboards as necessary.

Change position frequently and assist with active and passive range-of-motion (ROM) exercises, as indicated.

Maintain comfortable environmental temperature; provide heat lamps and heat-retaining body coverings.
Assess reports of pain, noting location/character and intensity (scale of 0–10).

Provide medication and/or place in hydrotherapy as appropriate before performing dressing changes and débridement.
Encourage expression of feelings about pain.

Involve client in determining schedule for activities, treatments, and drug administration.
Explain procedures and provide frequent information as appropriate, especially during wound débridement.

Provide basic comfort measures—massage of uninjured areas and frequent position changes.

RATIONALE

Temperature changes and air movement can cause great pain to exposed nerve endings.
Elevation may be required initially to reduce edema formation; thereafter, changes in position and elevation reduce discomfort and risk of joint contractures.
Elevation of linens off wounds may help reduce pain.
Position of function reduces deformities and contractures, and promotes comfort. Although flexed position of injured joints may feel more comfortable, it can lead to flexion contractures.
Movement and exercise reduce joint stiffness and muscle fatigue, but type of exercise depends on location and extent of injury.
Temperature regulation may be lost with major burns. External heat sources may be necessary to prevent chilling.
Pain is nearly always present to some degree because of varying severity of tissue involvement/destruction but is usually most severe during dressing changes and débridement. Changes in location, character, and intensity of pain may indicate developing complications (e.g., limb ischemia) or herald improvement and return of nerve function and sensation.
Reduces severe physical and emotional distress associated with painful procedures.
Verbalization allows outlet for emotions and may enhance coping mechanisms.
Enhances client's sense of control and strengthens coping mechanisms.
Showing empathy and support can help alleviate pain and promote relaxation. Knowing what to expect provides opportunity for client to prepare self and enhances sense of control.
Promotes relaxation and reduces muscle tension and general fatigue.

(continues on page 676)

Encourage use of stress management techniques, such as progressive relaxation, deep breathing, guided imagery, and visualization.

Refocuses attention, promotes relaxation, and enhances sense of control, which may reduce pharmacological dependency.

Provide diversional activities appropriate for age and condition.

Helps lessen concentration on pain experience and refocus attention.

Promote uninterrupted sleep periods.

Sleep deprivation can increase perception of pain and reduce coping abilities.

Collaborative

Administer analgesics (opioid and nonopioid) as indicated, such as morphine, fentanyl (Sublimaze, Ultiva), hydrocodone (Vicodin, Hycodan), or oxycodone (OxyContin, Percocet).

The burned client may require around-the-clock medication and dose titration. IV method is often used initially to maximize drug effect. Concerns of client addiction or doubts regarding degree of pain experienced are not valid during emergent and acute phases of care, but opioids should be decreased as soon as feasible and alternative methods for pain relief initiated.

Provide and instruct in use of patient-controlled analgesia (PCA).

PCA provides for timely drug administration, preventing fluctuations in intensity of pain, often at lower total dosage than would be given by conventional methods.

NURSING DIAGNOSIS: risk for Infection

Risk factors may include
Inadequate primary defenses—destruction of skin barrier, traumatized tissues
Inadequate secondary defenses—decreased Hgb, suppressed inflammatory response
Environmental exposure, invasive procedures

Possibly evidenced by
(Not applicable; presence of signs and symptoms establishes an *actual* diagnosis)

Desired Outcomes/Evaluation Criteria—Client Will

Burn Healing (NOC)
Achieve timely wound healing free of purulent exudate and be afebrile.

ACTIONS/INTERVENTIONS

RATIONALE

Infection Protection (NIC)
Independent
Implement appropriate isolation techniques, as indicated.

Dependent on type and extent of wounds, and the choice of wound treatment (e.g., open versus closed); isolation may range from simple wound and skin to complete or reverse to reduce risk of cross-contamination and exposure to multiple bacterial flora.

Emphasize and model good hand-washing technique for all individuals coming in contact with client.

Prevents cross-contamination and reduces risk of acquired infection.

Use gowns, gloves, masks, and strict aseptic technique during direct wound care and provide sterile or freshly laundered bed linens and gowns.

Prevents exposure to infectious organisms.

Monitor and limit visitors, if necessary. Explain isolation procedure to visitors, if used. Supervise visitor adherence to protocol as indicated.

Prevents cross-contamination from visitors. Concern for risk of infection should be balanced against client's need for family support and socialization.

Wound Care (NIC)
Shave/clip all hair from around burned areas to include a 1-inch border (excluding eyebrows). Shave facial hair (men) and shampoo head daily.

Hair is a good medium for bacterial growth; however, eyebrows act as a protective barrier for the eyes. Regular shampooing decreases bacterial fallout into burned areas.

Examine unburned areas such as groin, neck creases, and mucous membranes; and vaginal discharge routinely.

Opportunistic infections (e.g., yeast) frequently occur because of depression of the immune system and/or proliferation of normal body flora during systemic antibiotic therapy.

Provide special care for eyes, for example, use eye covers and tear formulas as appropriate.

Eyes may be swollen shut and/or become infected by drainage from surrounding burns. If lids are burned, eye covers may be needed to prevent corneal damage.

Prevent skin-to-skin surface contact—wrap each burned finger or toe separately; do not allow burned ear to touch scalp.

Prevents adherence to the surface that it may be touching and encourages proper healing. *Note:* Ear cartilage has limited circulation and is prone to pressure necrosis.

ACTIONS/INTERVENTIONS (continued)

Examine wounds daily; note and document changes in appearance, odor, or quantity of drainage.

Monitor vital signs for fever and increased respiratory rate and depth in association with changes in sensorium, presence of diarrhea, decreased platelet count, and hyperglycemia with glycosuria.

Collaborative

Remove dressings and cleanse burned areas in a hydrotherapy or whirlpool tub, or in a shower stall with handheld shower-head. Maintain temperature of water at 100°F (37.8°C). Wash areas with a mild cleansing agent or surgical soap.

Excise and cover burn wounds quickly.

Débride necrotic and loose tissue, including ruptured blisters, with scissors and forceps. Do not disturb intact blisters if they are smaller than 1 to 2 cm, do not interfere with joint function, and do not appear infected.

Photograph wound initially and at periodic intervals.

Infection Protection (NIC)

Administer topical antimicrobial agents, as indicated, for example:

Silver sulfadiazine (Silvadene)

Mafenide acetate (Sulfamylon) solution or mafenide HCl cream

Acticoat

Aqueous silver nitrate

Poloxamer 188 containing bacitracin and polymixin B

Hydrogels, such as Transorb and Burnfree

Administer other medications, as appropriate, for example:
Subeschar clysis/systemic antibiotics

Tetanus toxoid or clostridial antitoxin, as appropriate

RATIONALE (continued)

Identifies presence of granulation tissue indicating healing and provides for early detection of burn-wound infection. Infection in a partial-thickness burn may cause conversion of burn to full-thickness injury. *Note:* A strong, sweet, musty smell at a graft site is indicative of *Pseudomonas.*

Indicators of sepsis—often occurring with full-thickness burn—requiring prompt evaluation and intervention. *Note:* Changes in sensorium, bowel habits, and respiratory rate usually precede fever and alteration of laboratory studies.

Water softens and aids in removal of dressings, slough layer of dead skin or tissue, and dry scabs or eschar. Sources vary as to whether bath or shower is best. Bath has advantage of water providing support for exercising extremities but may promote cross-contamination of wounds. Showering enhances wound inspection and prevents contamination from floating debris.

Early excision is known to reduce scarring and risk of infection, thereby facilitating healing.

Promotes healing and prevents autocontamination. Small, intact blisters help protect skin and increase rate of re-epithelialization unless the burn injury is the result of chemicals in which case fluid contained in blisters may continue to cause tissue destruction.

Provides baseline and documentation of healing process.

The following agents help control bacterial growth and pre-vent drying of wound, which can cause further tissue destruction.

Still the most common topical antibiotic used in burn care, Silvadene is a broad-spectrum antimicrobial that may allow the wound to heal without need for skin grafting and is relatively painless but has intermediate, somewhat delayed eschar penetration. May cause rash or depression of WBCs.

Antibiotic of choice with confirmed invasive burn wound infection that does not respond to Silvadene. Useful against gram-negative and gram-positive organisms and some fun-gal species. The solution is painless; however, the cream causes burning or pain on application and for 30 minutes thereafter. Can cause rash and is contraindicated in metabolic acidosis.

Acticoat is a nonadherent antimicrobial dressing that stays on the wound for up to 7 days, delivering a low concentration of nanocrystalline silver.

Effective against *Staphylococcus aureus, Escherichia coli,* and *Pseudomonas aeruginosa,* but has poor eschar penetration, is painful, and may cause electrolyte imbalance. Dressings must be constantly saturated. Product stains skin and other surfaces black.

This gel is effective against gram-positive organisms, does not interfere with re-ephithelializaton, and is generally used for tar and asphalt-based residues, other imbedded materials, and for superficial and facial burns.

Useful for partial- and full-thickness burns, in rehydrating dry wound beds, and promoting autolytic debridement. May be used when infection is present.

Systemic antibiotics are given to control general infections identified by culture and sensitivity. Subeschar clysis has been found effective against pathogens in granulated tissues at the line of demarcation between viable and nonviable tissue, reducing risk of sepsis.

Tissue destruction and altered defense mechanisms increase risk of developing tetanus or gas gangrene, especially in deep burns such as those caused by electricity.

(continues on page 678)

ACTIONS/INTERVENTIONS (continued)

Place IV and invasive lines in nonburned area.

Obtain routine cultures and sensitivities of wounds and drainage.
Assist with excisional biopsies when infection is suspected.

RATIONALE (continued)

Decreased risk of infection at insertion site with possibility of progression to septicemia.
Allows early recognition and specific treatment of wound infection.
Bacteria can colonize the wound surface without invading the underlying tissue; therefore, biopsies may be obtained for diagnosing infection.

NURSING DIAGNOSIS: **ineffective peripheral tissue Perfusion/risk for Peripheral Neurovascular Dysfunction**

Risk factors may include
Reduction or interruption of arterial or venous blood flow—circumferential burns of extremities with resultant edema
Hypovolemia

Possibly evidenced by
(Not applicable; presence of signs and symptoms establishes an *actual* diagnosis)

Desired Outcomes/Evaluation Criteria—Client Will

Tissue Perfusion: Peripheral (NOC)
Maintain palpable peripheral pulses of equal quality and strength; good capillary refill and skin color normal in uninjured areas.

ACTIONS/INTERVENTIONS

Circulatory Care: Venous [or] Arterial (NIC)
Independent
Assess color, sensation, movement, capillary refill, and peripheral pulses via Doppler on extremities with circumferential burns. Compare with findings of unaffected limb.

Elevate affected extremities, as appropriate. Remove jewelry or arm band. Avoid taping around a burned extremity or digit.

Obtain BP in unburned extremity when possible. Remove BP cuff after each reading, as indicated.

Investigate reports of deep, throbbing ache and numbness.

Encourage active ROM exercises of unaffected body parts.
Investigate irregular pulses.

Collaborative
Maintain fluid replacement per protocol. (Refer to ND: risk for deficient Fluid Volume.)
Monitor electrolytes, especially sodium, potassium, and calcium. Administer replacement therapy, as indicated.

Avoid use of intramuscular (IM) and subcutaneous (SC) injections.

Measure intracompartmental pressures as indicated. (Refer to CP: Fractures; ND: risk for Peripheral Neurovascular Dysfunction.)
Assist with or prepare for escharotomy or fasciotomy, as indicated.

RATIONALE

Edema formation can readily compress blood vessels, thereby impeding circulation and increasing venous stasis and edema. Comparisons with unaffected limbs aid in differentiating localized versus systemic problems such as hypovolemia and decreased cardiac output.
Promotes systemic circulation and venous return, and may reduce edema or other deleterious effects of constriction of edematous tissues. *Note:* Prolonged elevation can impair arterial perfusion if BP falls or tissue pressures rise excessively.
If BP readings must be obtained on an injured extremity, leaving the cuff in place may increase edema formation, reduce perfusion, and convert partial-thickness burn to a more serious injury.
Indicators of decreased perfusion and/or increased pressure within enclosed space, such as may occur with a circumferential burn of an extremity (compartmental syndrome).
Promotes local and systemic circulation.
Cardiac dysrhythmias can occur as a result of electrolyte shifts, electrical injury, or release of myocardial depressant factor, compromising cardiac output and tissue perfusion.

Maximizes circulating volume and tissue perfusion.

Losses or shifts of these electrolytes affect cellular membrane potential and excitability, thereby altering myocardial conductivity, potentiating risk of dysrhythmias, and reducing cardiac output and tissue perfusion.
Altered tissue perfusion and edema formation impair drug absorption. Injections into potential donor sites may render them unusable because of hematoma formation.
Ischemic myositis may develop because of decreased perfusion.

Enhances circulation by relieving constriction caused by rigid, nonviable tissue (eschar) or edema formation.

NURSING DIAGNOSIS: imbalanced Nutrition: Less than Body Requirements

May be related to

Hypermetabolic state (can be as much as 50% to 60% higher than normal proportional to the severity of injury)

Protein catabolism

Anorexia, restricted oral intake

Possibly evidenced by

Decrease in total body weight, loss of muscle mass/subcutaneous fat, and development of negative nitrogen balance

Desired Outcomes/Evaluation Criteria—Client Will

Nutritional Status (NOC)

Demonstrate nutritional intake adequate to meet metabolic needs as evidenced by stable weight and muscle-mass measurements, positive nitrogen balance, and tissue regeneration.

ACTIONS/INTERVENTIONS	RATIONALE
Nutrition Therapy (NIC)	
Independent	
Auscultate bowel sounds, noting hypoactive or absent sounds.	Ileus is often associated with postburn period but usually subsides within 36 to 48 hours, at which time oral or intragastic feedings can be initiated.
Maintain strict calorie count. Weigh daily. Reassess percentage of open body surface area and wounds weekly.	Appropriate guides to proper caloric intake include 25 kcal/kg body weight, plus 40 kcal per percentage of TBSA burn in the adult. As burn wound heals, energy needs are reevaluated to calculate prescribed dietary formulas, and appropriate adjustments are made.
Monitor muscle mass and subcutaneous fat, as indicated.	Indirect calorimetry, if available, may be useful in more accurately estimating body reserves and losses, and effectiveness of therapy.
Provide small, frequent meals and snacks.	Helps prevent gastric distention or discomfort, and may enhance intake.
Encourage client to view diet as a treatment and to make food and beverage choices high in calories and protein.	Calories and proteins are needed to meet metabolic needs, and promote wound healing.
Ascertain food likes and dislikes. Encourage SO to bring food from home, as appropriate.	Provides client/SO sense of control; enhances participation in care and may improve intake.
Encourage client to sit up for meals and visit with others.	Sitting helps prevent aspiration and aids in proper digestion of food. Socialization promotes relaxation and may enhance intake.
Provide oral hygiene before meals.	Clean mouth and clear palate enhances taste and helps promote a good appetite.
Perform fingerstick glucose and urine testing, as indicated.	Monitors for development of hyperglycemia related to hormonal changes and demands or use of hyperalimentation to meet caloric needs.
Collaborative	
Refer to dietitian or nutritional support team.	Useful in establishing individual nutritional needs based on weight and body surface area of injury, and identifying appropriate routes.
Provide diet high in calories and protein with trace elements and vitamin supplements.	Calories approximating 25 kcal/kg/day, protein up to 2 g/kg/day, and vitamins are needed to meet increased metabolic needs, maintain weight, and encourage tissue regeneration. Zero fat or minimal fat is preferred during early acute phase to minimize the susceptibility to infection.
Insert and maintain small feeding tube for enteral feedings and supplements, if needed.	Provides continuous or supplemental feedings when client is unable to consume total daily calorie requirements orally. *Note:* Research supports use of early intragastric feedings as soon after admission as possible because delayed enteral feeding longer than 18 hours postinjury results in a high rate of gastroparesis and need for IV nutrition. Continuous tube feeding during the night increases calorie intake without decreasing appetite and oral intake during the day.
Administer parenteral nutritional solutions containing vitamins and minerals, as indicated.	Total parenteral nutrition (TPN) maintains nutritional intake and meets metabolic needs in presence of severe complications or sustained esophageal or gastric injuries that do not permit enteral feedings. (Refer to CP: Total Nutritional Support: Parenteral/Enteral Feeding.)

(continues on page 680)

ACTIONS/INTERVENTIONS (continued)

Monitor laboratory studies, such as serum albumin or prealbumin, glucose, electrolytes, magnesium, BUN/Cr, calcium, inorganic phosphorus, transaminase, and triglycerides.

Administer insulin, as indicated.

RATIONALE (continued)

Indicators of nutritional needs, and adequacy of diet and therapy.

Elevated serum glucose levels may develop because of stress response to injury, high caloric intake, and pancreatic fatigue.

NURSING DIAGNOSIS: impaired physical **Mobility**

May be related to
Neuromuscular impairment; pain, discomfort; decreased strength and endurance
Restrictive therapies, limb immobilization; contractures

Possibly evidenced by
Reluctance to move, inability to purposefully move
Limited ROM, decreased muscle strength control and/or mass

Desired Outcomes/Evaluation Criteria—Client Will

Mobility (NOC)
Maintain position of function as evidenced by absence of contractures.
Maintain or increase strength and function of affected and/or compensatory body part.

Self-Care: Activities of Daily Living (ADLs) (NOC)
Verbalize and demonstrate willingness to participate in activities.
Demonstrate techniques and behaviors that enable resumption of activities.

ACTIONS/INTERVENTIONS

Bed Rest Care (NIC)
Independent
Maintain proper body alignment with supports or splints, especially for burns over joints.
Note circulation, motion, and sensation of digits frequently.

Initiate the rehabilitative phase on admission.

Perform ROM exercises consistently, initially passive, then active.

Medicate for pain before activity or exercises.

Schedule treatments and care activities to provide periods of uninterrupted rest.
Encourage family/SO support and assistance with ROM exercises.

Self-Care Assistance (NIC)
Incorporate ADLs with physical therapy, hydrotherapy, and nursing care.
Encourage client participation in all activities as individually able.
Instruct and assist with mobility aids, such as a cane, walker, or crutches, as appropriate.

Bed Rest Care (NIC)
Collaborative
Provide foam or flotation mattress or kinetic therapy bed, as indicated.
Maintain pressure garment when used.

Consult with rehabilitation, physical, and occupational therapists.

RATIONALE

Promotes functional positioning of extremities and prevents contractures, which are more likely over joints.
Edema may compromise circulation to extremities, potentiating tissue necrosis and development of contractures.
It is easier to enlist participation when client is aware of the possibilities that exist for recovery.
Prevents progressively tightening scar tissue and contractures, enhances maintenance of muscle and joint functioning, and reduces loss of calcium from the bone.
Reduces muscle and tissue stiffness and tension, enabling client to be more active and facilitating participation.
Increases client's strength and tolerance for activity.

Enables family/SO to be active in client care and provides more constant and consistent therapy.

Combining activities produces improved results by enhancing effects of each.
Promotes independence, enhances self-esteem, and facilitates recovery process.
Promotes safe ambulation.

Prevents prolonged pressure on tissues, reducing potential for tissue ischemia, necrosis, and decubitus ulcer formation.
Hypertrophic scarring can develop around grafted areas or at the site of deep partial-thickness wounds. Pressure dressings minimize scar tissue by keeping it flat, soft, and pliable, enhancing movement.
Normally members of the burn team, these specialists provide integrated activity and exercise programs and specific assistive devices based on individual needs. Consultation facilitates intensive long-term management of potential deficits.

NURSING DIAGNOSIS: impaired Skin Integrity, [grafts]

May be related to
Disruption of skin surface with destruction of skin layers (partial-/full-thickness burn) requiring grafting

Possibly evidenced by
Absence of viable tissue

Desired Outcomes/Evaluation Criteria—Client Will

Wound Healing: Secondary Intention (NOC)
Demonstrate tissue regeneration.
Achieve timely healing of burned areas.

ACTIONS/INTERVENTIONS	RATIONALE
Wound Care (NIC)	
Independent	
Preoperative	
Assess and document size, color, depth of wound, noting necrotic tissue and condition of surrounding skin.	Provides baseline information about need for skin grafting and possible clues about circulation in area to support graft.
Provide appropriate burn care and infection control measures. (Refer to ND: risk for Infection.)	Prepares tissues for grafting and reduces risk of infection and graft failure.
Collaborative	
Administer topical wound débridement ointment, as indicated, for example enzymatic products—collangenase ointment (Santyl) and papain (Accuzyme).	Early débridement of burn eschar is beneficial to wound healing and some treatment centers suggest use of these products to promote healing. However, despite theoretical advantage, enzymatic débridement results have been highly variable.
Independent	
Postoperative	
Elevate grafted area, if possible and appropriate.	Reduces swelling and limits risk of graft separation.
Maintain desired position and immobility of area when indicated.	Movement of tissue under graft can dislodge it, interfering with optimal healing.
Maintain dressings (mesh, petroleum, nonadhesive) over newly grafted area and/or donor site, as indicated.	Areas may be covered by translucent, nonreactive surface material between graft and outer dressing to eliminate shearing of new epithelium to protect healing tissue. The donor site is usually covered for 4 to 24 hours, then bulky dressings are removed and fine mesh gauze is left in place.
Keep skin free from pressure.	Promotes circulation and prevents ischemia, necrosis, and graft failure.
Evaluate color of grafted and donor site(s); note signs of healing.	Evaluates effectiveness of circulation and identifies developing complications.
Collaborative	
Maintain wound covering as indicated, for example: Biosynthetic dressing (Biobrane)	Biobrane membrane contains collagenous porcine peptides that adhere to wound surface until removed or sloughed off by spontaneous skin re-epithelialization. Useful for eschar-free partial-thickness burns awaiting autografts because it can remain in place for longer periods of time and is permeable to topical antimicrobial agents.
Human fibroblast-derived temporary skin substitute (TransCyte)	Bioengineered skin substitute used on middermal burns after débridement; in prospective trials, shows faster healing with less pain.
Nonbiologic synthetic dressings, such as contact layer dressing (Mepitel) and hydrocolloid dressing (DuoDerm)	These dressings adhere to the skin to cover small partial-thickness burns and interact with wound exudate to form a soft gel that facilitates débridement.
Opsite, Acu-Derm	Thin, transparent, elastic, waterproof, and occlusive dressing is permeable to moisture and air and is used to cover clean partial-thickness wounds and clean donor sites.
Wash sites with mild soap, rinse, and lubricate with cream (e.g., Nivea) several times daily after dressings are removed and healing is accomplished.	Newly grafted skin and healed donor sites require special care to maintain flexibility.
Aspirate blebs under sheet grafts with sterile needle or roll with sterile swab.	Fluid-filled blebs prevent graft adherence to underlying tissue, increasing risk of graft failure.

(continues on page 682)

Prepare for/assist with surgical grafting or biological dressings, such as the following:	
Homograft (allograft)	Skin grafts obtained from living persons or cadavers are used as a temporary covering for extensive burns until individual's own skin is ready for grafting (test graft) to cover excised wounds immediately after escharotomy or to protect granulation tissue.
Heterograft (xenograft, porcine)	Skin grafts may be carried out with animal skin for the same purposes as homografts or to cover meshed autografts.
Cultured epithelial autograft (CEA)	Skin graft obtained from uninjured part of client's own skin and prepared in a laboratory; may be full-thickness or partial-thickness. *Note:* This process takes 20 to 30 days from harvest to application. The new CEA sheets are one to six cell layers thick and thus are very fragile.
Artificial skin (Integra, Dermagraft-TC)	Wound coverings for full-thickness and deep partial-thickness burns provide a permanent, immediate covering that reproduces the skin's normal functions and stimulates the regeneration of dermal tissue.

NURSING DIAGNOSIS: **Fear/Anxiety**

May be related to
Situational crises—hospitalization/isolation procedures, interpersonal transmission and contagion, memory of the trauma experience, threat of death and/or disfigurement

Possibly evidenced by
Expressed concern regarding changes in life, fear of unspecific consequences
Apprehension, increased tension
Feelings of helplessness, uncertainty, decreased self-assurance
Sympathetic stimulation, extraneous movements, restlessness, insomnia

Desired Outcomes/Evaluation Criteria—Client Will

Fear [or] Anxiety Self-Control (NOC)
Verbalize awareness of feelings and healthy ways to deal with them.
Report anxiety and fear are reduced to a manageable level.
Demonstrate problem-solving skills and effective use of resources.

ACTIONS/INTERVENTIONS

RATIONALE

Anxiety Reduction (NIC)
Independent

Provide frequent explanations and information about care procedures. Repeat information as needed or desired.	Knowing what to expect usually reduces fear and anxiety, clarifies misconceptions, and promotes cooperation. *Note:* Because of the shock of the initial trauma, many people do not recall information provided during that time.
Demonstrate willingness to listen and talk to client when free of painful procedures.	Helps client and SO know that support is available and that healthcare provider is interested in the person, not just care of the burn.
Involve client and SO in decision-making process whenever possible. Provide time for questioning and repetition of proposed treatments.	Promotes sense of control and cooperation, decreasing feelings of helplessness or hopelessness.
Assess mental status, including mood and affect, comprehension of events, and content of thoughts, such as illusions or manifestations of terror or panic.	Initially, client may use denial and repression to reduce and filter information that might be overwhelming. Some clients display calm manner and alert mental status, representing dissociation from reality, which is also a protective mechanism.
Investigate changes in mentation and presence of hypervigilance, hallucinations, sleep disturbances (e.g., nightmares), agitation or apathy, disorientation, and labile affect, all of which may vary from moment to moment.	Indicators of extreme anxiety or delirium state in which client is literally fighting for life. Although cause can be psychologically based, pathological life-threatening causes, such as shock, sepsis, or hypoxia, must be ruled out.
Provide constant and consistent orientation.	Helps client stay in touch with surroundings and reality.

ACTIONS/INTERVENTIONS (continued) | **RATIONALE** (continued)

Encourage client to talk about the burn circumstances when ready.

Client may need to tell the story of what happened over and over to make some sense out of a terrifying situation. Adjustment to the impact of the trauma and grief over losses and disfigurement can easily lead to clinical depression, psychosis, and posttraumatic stress disorder (PTSD).

Explain to client what happened. Provide opportunity for questions and give open and honest answers.

Compassionate statements reflecting the reality of the situation can help client and SO acknowledge the reality and begin to deal with what has happened.

Identify previous methods of coping with and handling stressful situations.

Past successful behavior can be used to assist in dealing with the present situation.

Create a restful environment; use guided imagery and relaxation exercises.

Clients experience severe anxiety associated with burn trauma and treatment. These interventions are soothing and helpful for positive outcomes.

Assist the family to express their feelings of grief and guilt.

The family may initially be most concerned about client's dying and/or feel guilty, believing that in some way they could have prevented the incident.

Be empathetic and nonjudgmental in dealing with client and family.

Family relationships are disrupted; financial, lifestyle, and role changes make this a difficult time for those involved with client, and they may react in many different ways.

Encourage family/SO to visit and discuss family happenings. Remind client of past and future events.

Maintains contact with a familiar reality, creating a sense of attachment and continuity of life.

Collaborative

Involve entire burn team in care from admission to discharge, including social worker and psychiatric resources.

Provides a wider support system and promotes continuity of care and coordination of activities.

Administer mild sedation, as indicated, for example, lorazepam (Ativan), alprazolam (Xanax), and midazolam (Versed).

Antianxiety medications may be necessary for a brief period until client is more physically stable and internal locus of control is regained.

NURSING DIAGNOSIS: disturbed Body Image/ineffective Role Performance

May be related to
Situational crisis—traumatic event, dependent client role; disfigurement, pain

Possibly evidenced by
Negative feelings about body and self, fear of rejection or reaction by others
Focus on past appearance, abilities; preoccupation with change/loss
Change in physical capacity to resume role, change in social involvement

Desired Outcomes/Evaluation Criteria—Client Will

Body Image (NOC)
Incorporate changes into self-concept without negating self-esteem.
Verbalize acceptance of self in situation.

Role Performance (NOC)
Talk with family/SO about situation and changes that have occurred.
Develop realistic goals and plans for the future.

ACTIONS/INTERVENTIONS | **RATIONALE**

Body Image [or] Role Enhancement (NIC)
Independent

Assess meaning of loss or change to client and SO, including future expectations and impact of cultural and religious beliefs.

Traumatic episode results in sudden, unanticipated changes, creating feelings of grief over actual or perceived losses. This necessitates support to work through to optimal resolution.

Acknowledge and accept expression of feelings of frustration, dependency, anger, grief, and hostility. Note withdrawn behavior and use of denial.

Acceptance of these feelings as a normal response to what has occurred facilitates resolution. It is not helpful or possible to push client before he or she is ready to deal with the situation. Denial may be prolonged and be an adaptive mechanism because client is not ready to cope with personal problems.

(continues on page 684)

ACTIONS/INTERVENTIONS (continued)

Set limits on maladaptive behavior (e.g., manipulative or aggressive). Maintain nonjudgmental attitude while giving care, and help client identify positive behaviors that will aid in recovery.

Be realistic and positive during treatments, in health teaching, and in setting goals within limitations.

Encourage client and SO to view wounds and assist with care, as appropriate.

Provide hope within parameters of individual situation; do not give false reassurance.

Assist client to identify extent of actual change in appearance/ body function.

Give positive reinforcement of progress and encourage endeavors toward attainment of rehabilitation goals.

Show slides or pictures of burn care or other client outcomes, being selective in what is shown as appropriate to the individual situation. Encourage discussion of feelings about what client has seen.

Encourage family interaction with one another and with rehabilitation team.

Provide support group for SO. Give information about how SO can be helpful to client.

Role-play social situations of concern to client.

Collaborative

Refer to physical or occupational therapy, vocational counselor, and psychiatric counseling, for example, a psychiatric clinical nurse specialist, social services, or a psychologist, as needed.

RATIONALE (continued)

Client and SO tend to deal with this crisis in the same way in which they have dealt with problems in the past. Staff may find it difficult and frustrating to handle behavior that is disrupting and not helpful to recuperation but should realize that the behavior is usually directed toward the situation and not the care provider.

Enhances trust and rapport between client and nurse.

Promotes acceptance of reality of injury and of change in body and image of self as different.

Promotes positive attitude and provides opportunity to set goals and plan for future based on reality.

Helps begin process of looking to the future and how life will be different.

Words of encouragement can support development of positive coping behaviors.

Allows client and SO to be realistic in expectations. Also assists in demonstration of importance of, and necessity for, certain devices and procedures.

Maintains or opens lines of communication and provides ongoing support for client and family.

Promotes ventilation of feelings and allows for more helpful responses to client.

Prepares client and SO for reactions of others and anticipates ways to deal with them.

Helpful in identifying ways and devices to regain and maintain independence. Client may need further assistance to resolve persistent emotional problems—especially posttrauma response.

NURSING DIAGNOSIS: deficient Knowledge [Learning Need] regarding condition, prognosis, treatment, self-care, and discharge needs

May be related to
Lack of exposure or recall
Misinterpretation of information, unfamiliarity with resources

Possibly evidenced by
Questions and request for information, statement of misconception
Inaccurate follow-through of instructions, development of preventable complications

Desired Outcomes/Evaluation Criteria—Client Will

Knowledge: Disease Process (NOC)
Verbalize understanding of condition, prognosis, and potential complications.

Knowledge: Treatment Regimen (NOC)
Verbalize understanding of therapeutic needs.
Correctly perform necessary procedures and explain reasons for actions.
Initiate necessary lifestyle changes and participate in treatment regimen.

ACTIONS/INTERVENTIONS

Teaching: Disease Process (NIC)
Independent
Review condition, prognosis, and future expectations.

Discuss client's expectations of returning home, to work, and to normal activities.

RATIONALE

Provides knowledge base from which client can make informed choices.

Client frequently has a difficult and prolonged adjustment after discharge. Problems, such as sleep disturbances, nightmares, reliving the accident, difficulty with resumption of social interactions or intimacy and sexual activity, and emotional lability, often occur and can interfere with successful adjustment to resuming normal life.

ACTIONS/INTERVENTIONS (continued)	RATIONALE (continued)
Review and have client and SO demonstrate proper burn, skin graft, and wound care techniques. Identify appropriate sources for outpatient care and supplies.	Promotes competent self-care after discharge, enhancing independence.
Discuss skin care, such as scar massage and use of perfume-free moisturizers (e.g., Vaseline Intensive Care, Eucerin), sunscreens, and anti-itching medications (e.g., diphenhydramine [Benadryl], hydroxyzine [Atarax]).	Itching, blistering, and sensitivity of healing wounds and graft sites can be expected for an extended time, and injury can occur because of the lack of natural lubrication and fragility of the new tissue. *Note:* Sun block may be required for life because of potential for hyperpigmentation.
Explain scarring process and necessity for and proper use of silicone gel sheeting, static splint, or pressure garments when used.	Helps minimize and treat hypertrophic scarring and contracture formation. Consistent use of the pressure garment over a long period can reduce the need for reconstructive surgery to release contractures and remove scars. *Note:* Studies show that client compliance is not easily attained and that client may wear garment inappropriately, with resultant failure to demonstrate a difference in scarring with pressure garment therapy.
Encourage continuation of prescribed exercise program and scheduled rest periods.	Maintains mobility, reduces complications, and prevents fatigue, facilitating recovery process.
Identify specific limitations of activity as individually appropriate.	Imposed restrictions depend on the severity and location of the injury and the stage of healing.
Emphasize importance of sustained intake of high-protein and high-calorie meals and snacks.	Optimal nutrition enhances tissue regeneration and general feeling of well-being. *Note:* Client often needs to increase caloric intake to meet calorie and protein needs for healing.
Review medications, including purpose, dosage, route, and expected or reportable side effects.	Reiteration allows opportunity for client to ask questions and be sure understanding is accurate.
Advise client and SO of potential for exhaustion, boredom, emotional lability, and adjustment problems. Provide information about possibility of discussion as well as interaction with appropriate professional counselors.	Provides perspective to some of the problems that client/SO may encounter, and aids awareness that assistance is available when necessary.
Identify signs and symptoms requiring medical evaluation—inflammation, increase or changes in wound drainage, fever, chills, changes in pain characteristics, or loss of mobility or function.	Early detection of developing complications (e.g., infection, delayed healing) may prevent progression to more serious or life-threatening situations.
Stress necessity and importance of follow-up care and rehabilitation program.	Long-term support with continual reevaluation and changes in therapy is required to achieve optimal recovery.
Provide phone number for contact person.	Provides easy access to treatment team to reinforce teaching, clarify misconceptions, and reduce potential for complications.
Identify community resources, such as skin and wound care professionals and crisis centers; recovery groups; and mental health, Red Cross, visiting nurse, Ambli-Cab, and homemaker service.	Facilitates transition to home, provides assistance with meeting individual needs, and supports independence.

POTENTIAL CONSIDERATIONS following acute hospitalization (dependent on client's age, physical condition and presence of complications, personal resources, and life responsibilities)

• *ineffective Coping*—situational crisis, vulnerability
• *risk for Disuse Syndrome*—severe pain, prescribed immobilization or restrictive therapies
• *situational low Self-Esteem*—change in health status/independent functioning, perceived loss of control in some aspect of life
• *ineffective self Health Management*—complexity of medical regimen, added demands made on individual/family, social support deficits
• *Post-Trauma Syndrome*—catastrophic accident/injury to self and possibly others

CHAPTER 14

Systemic Infections and Immunological Disorders

SEPSIS/SEPTICEMIA

I. Pathophysiology (Cunha, 2008; Kleinpell, 2006; Sharma & Mink, 2007; Wood & Lavieri, 2007)

a. Presence of a systemic inflammatory response to documented or presumed infection, which may progress along a continuum

i. Systemic inflammatory response syndrome (SIRS)

1. Infection with release of endo- or exotoxins activating the inflammatory cascade—local release of cytokines into the circulation in attempt to restore homeostasis

2. Failure of mechanism leads to destructive response with loss of circulatory integrity

3. Criteria (two or more)—fever greater than 100.4°F/38°C or less than 96°F/36°C; heart rate greater than 90 beats per minute; respiration greater than 20/min or $PaCO_2$ less than 32 mm Hg; white blood cell (WBC) count greater than 12,000/μL, less than 4,000/μL, or greater than than 10% of bands or immature cells

ii. Severe sepsis—presence of known or suspected infection and two or more SIRS criteria; associated with organ dysfunction, hypoperfusion, hypotension with alteration of mental status, hypoxemia, lactic acidosis, and/or oliguria

iii. Septic shock—characterized by hemodynamic changes and persistent hypotension, development of perfusion abnormalities, and impaired cellular function that fails to respond to adequate fluid resuscitation

iv. Multiple organ dysfunction syndrome (MODS)—organ dysfunction leading to organ failure with inability to maintain homeostasis

II. Etiology

a. Multiple microorganisms associated with sepsis

i. Bacteria, fungi, viruses, or rickettsiae

ii. Common pathogens: *Streptococcus pneumoniae* or *Staphyloccocus aureus, Candida, Salmonella, Escherichia coli, Legionella, Klebsiella, Pseudomonas*

b. Common origin of infections

i. Abdomen: appendicitis, bowel problems (perforated diverticuli), infection of the abdominal cavity, and gallbladder or liver infections

ii. Central nervous system: infections of the brain or the spinal cord, such as encephalitis, meningitis

iii. Lungs: pneumonia

iv. Skin: wounds or cellulitis; punctures, such as from intravenous (IV) lines, intravascular devices, or catheters inserted into the body to administer or drain fluids

v. Urinary tract: kidneys or bladder (glomerulonephritis, pyelonephritis, cystitis), prostatic obstruction

c. Risk factors: unsanitary and/or crowded living conditions, pollution, poor nutrition, immunosuppression, chronic health conditions, improper use of antibiotics

III. Statistics (Angus et al, 2001)

a. Morbidity: A reported 751,000 cases of severe sepsis occur annually in the United States.

b. Mortality: Dependent on progression of condition and degree of organ failure, presence of comorbidities, and age; in 2001, the rate was 28.6%.

c. Cost: Averages $22,100 per case, with approximately $16.7 billion spent annually.

GLOSSARY

Anaerobic infection: An infection caused by bacteria, called anaerobes, which cannot grow in the presence of oxygen.

Bacteremia: The presence of live bacteria in the blood-stream. Bacteremia is similar in some respects to viremia (the presence of a virus in the blood); parasitemia (the presence of a parasite in the blood); or fungemia (presence of a fungus in the blood).

Body substance isolation (BSI): Practice of isolating all body substances—blood, urine, feces, sputum, tears, and so on.

Cytokines: Protein chemical messengers involved in the inflammatory process, usually from white blood cells (WBCs).

Disseminated intravascular coagulation (DIC): Hyperstimulation of coagulation pathways results in diffuse activation and consumption of coagulation factors leading to generalized bleeding.

GLOSSARY (continued)

Endotoxins: Potentially toxic, natural compounds found inside pathogens such as bacteria.

Hyperbaric oxygen therapy: Treatment in which client is placed in a chamber and breathes oxygen at higher-than-atmospheric pressure. This high-pressure oxygen stops bacteria from growing and, at high enough pressure, destroys them.

Infection: Inflammatory response to invasion or host tissue by microorganisms.

Multiple organ dysfunction syndrome (MODS): Organ function is altered in an acutely ill individual, such that homeostasis cannot be achieved without intervention and support.

Oliguria: Urine output less than 30 mL/hr.

Purpura: Hemorrhagic area in the skin, which does not blanch when touched. The area of bleeding within the skin is greater than 3 mm in diameter.

Sepsis: Systemic inflammatory response secondary to infection—symptomatic bacteremia. Sepsis is termed severe if associated with organ dysfunction, hypoperfusion, and hypotension.

Septicemia: Presence of rapidly multiplying microorganisms in the bloodstream, which can result in profound physiological changes.

Septic shock: State that produces an inability to maintain adequate tissue perfusion and oxygenation, ultimately causing cellular, and then organ system, dysfunction.

Systemic inflammatory response syndrome (SIRS): Condition in which there is inflammation throughout the body. Bacteremia may be a factor; other causes include trauma or ischemia.

Third spacing of fluid: Loss of albumin or protein from circulating blood leads to decreased oncotic pressure. Fluid can then leak from the intravascular space into the interstitial space and stay there, causing edema.

Care Setting

Although severely ill individuals will likely receive care in the intensive care unit (ICU), this plan addresses care on an inpatient acute medical-surgical unit.

Related Concerns

Acquired immunodeficiency syndrome (AIDS), page 709

Chronic obstructive pulmonary disease (COPD) and asthma, page 120

Disaster considerations, page 876

Fluid and electrolyte imbalances, page 903

Metabolic acidosis—primary base bicarbonate deficiency, page 483

Peritonitis, page 349

Pneumonia, page 131

Psychosocial aspects of care, page 749

Pulmonary tuberculosis (TB), page 186

Renal failure: acute, page 536

Surgical intervention, page 782

Total nutritional support: parenteral/enteral feeding, page 469

Ventilatory assistance (mechanical), page 173

Client Assessment Database

Data depend on the type, location, and duration of the infective process and organ involvement.

DIAGNOSTIC DIVISION MAY REPORT	MAY EXHIBIT
ACTIVITY/REST • Fatigue • Malaise	• Mental status changes—withdrawn, lethargy • Respiration and heart rate increased with activity, or at rest
CIRCULATION	• Blood pressure (BP) may be normal, slightly low to normal range—as long as cardiac output remains elevated • Profound hypotension (late-stage sign) • Peripheral pulses bounding, rapid (hyperdynamic phase), weak, thready, or easily obliterated • Heart rate elevated (greater than 90); extreme tachycardia may be present, unless blunted by beta blockers or other medications (in septic shock) • Heart sounds may include development of S_3

(continues on page 688)

DIAGNOSTIC DIVISION
MAY REPORT (continued)

MAY EXHIBIT (continued)

- Dysrhythmias suggest myocardial dysfunction and effects of acidosis and electrolyte imbalance
- Skin warm, dry, flushed (vasodilation) or pale, cold, clammy, mottled (vasoconstriction)

ELIMINATION
- Urinary frequency, urgency
- Diarrhea

- Oliguria, anuria

FOOD/FLUID
- Loss of appetite, nausea, vomiting

- Weight loss
- Diminished or absent bowel sounds
- Extremity and generalized edema

NEUROSENSORY
- Headache
- Dizziness, fainting

- Restlessness, apprehension, confusion
- Disorientation, delirium, or coma

PAIN/DISCOMFORT
- Abdominal tenderness, localized pain or discomfort
- Headache, sinus pain
- Pelvic or flank pain
- Localized limb pain or tenderness

RESPIRATION

- Tachypnea (respiratory alkalosis) with decreased respiratory depth
- Dyspnea, rapid labored respirations
- Cough—may be productive if pneumonia is source

SAFETY
- History of recent or current infection, viral illness, cancer therapies, use of corticosteroids, or other immunosuppressant medications
- Presence of invasive lines or catheters

- Temperature usually elevated (greater than 100.4°F [38°C]) but may be normal in elderly or compromised client; may occasionally be lower than normal (less than 96.8°F [36°C])
- Shaking chills
- Poor or delayed wound healing, purulent drainage, or localized erythema
- Petechiae
- Oozing or bleeding from invasive line sites, wounds, and mucous membranes (late sign)

SEXUALITY
- Recent childbirth or abortion
- Vaginal or urethral discharge

- Maceration of vulva or purulent vaginal drainage

TEACHING/LEARNING
- Chronic, debilitating health problems—liver, renal, cardiac disease; cancer, diabetes mellitus (DM), alcoholism
- History of splenectomy
- Recent surgery or invasive procedures, traumatic wounds
- Antibiotic use—recent or long-term

DISCHARGE PLAN CONSIDERATIONS
- May require assistance with wound care and supplies, treatments, self-care, and homemaker tasks

▶ Refer to section at end of plan for postdischarge considerations.

Diagnostic Studies

TEST / WHY IT IS DONE	WHAT IT TELLS ME
BLOOD TESTS	
• *Complete blood count (CBC):* Battery of screening tests, which typically includes hemoglobin (Hgb); hematocrit (Hct); red blood cell (RBC) count, morphology, indices, and distribution width index; platelet count and size; WBC count and differential, which includes neutrophils, lymphocytes, monocytes, eosinophils, and basophils.	Hct may be elevated in hypovolemic states because of hemoconcentration. Leukopenia, decreased WBCs, occurs early and may be followed by a rebound leukocytosis reflecting rapid production of immature WBCs. Neutrophils may be elevated or depressed. Platelets may be elevated initially as an acute-phase reactant, but are decreased in later stages.
• *Serum electrolytes:* Substances that will dissociate into ions in solution and acquire the capacity to conduct electricity. Common electrolytes include sodium, potassium, chloride, calcium, and phosphate.	Various imbalances may occur because of acidosis, fluid shifts, and altered renal function.
• *Acute-phase reactants:*	
• *C-reactive protein (CRP):* Indicator of inflammation, but is not sensitive in distinguishing between causes of SIRS.	CRP is released by the liver in response to pro-inflammatory cytokines and is thought to recruit monocytes in early infection. Elevated levels may have a role in monitoring response to treatment (Burdette & Parilo, 2007).
• *Procalcitonin (PCT):* Peptide precursor to calcitonin.	PCT rises with severity of illness and increases more rapidly than CRP in sepsis. PCT is able to differentiate between infectious and noninfectious SIRS (Burdette & Parilo, 2007).
• *Clotting studies:*	
• *Platelets:* Platelets play an important role in blood coagulation and hemostasis that is often altered by sepsis.	Decreased platelet levels (thrombocytopenia) can occur because of platelet aggregation.
• *Prothrombin time (PT)/activated partial thromboplastin time (aPTT):* Measurement of coagulation times to identify abnormalities common to sepsis and which can lead to life-threatening complications.	Both PT and aPTT may be prolonged, indicating coagulopathy associated with liver ischemia, circulating toxins, or shock state.
• *Fibrin degradation products:* End-product of clot breakdown associated with abnormal coagulation process.	Often elevated and associated with tendency to bleed.
• *Serum lactate:* Product of anaerobic cellular metabolism, thus reflecting tissue hypoperfusion.	Elevated in metabolic acidosis, liver dysfunction, and shock.
• *Serum glucose:* Glucose is a primary energy source and necessary for cellular function.	Hyperglycemia occurs in response to insulin resistance and cellular starvation. The liver mobilizes alternative sources of glucose through gluconeogenesis and glycogenolysis. Hypoglycemia is a predictor of poor prognosis.
• *Blood urea nitrogen (BUN)/Creatinine (Cr):* Measurement of organ involvement and indicator of early stage of endotoxin shock.	Increased levels of BUN and Cr are associated with dehydration, renal impairment or failure, and liver dysfunction or failure.
• *Arterial blood gases (ABGs):* Measures pH level and oxygen and carbon dioxide concentrations in arterial blood.	Early respiratory alkalosis and hypoxemia may occur. In later states, hypoxemia, respiratory acidosis, and lactic and metabolic acidosis occur because of failure of compensatory mechanisms.
OTHER DIAGNOSTIC STUDIES	
• *Culture and sensitivity—wound, sputum, urine, blood, spinal fluid, or invasive lines:* Determine presence of infection and microorganism(s) susceptibility or resistance to specific antimicrobials.	Identifies causative organism(s) and appropriate treatment options. However, clients can deteriorate to full-blown septic shock without an identifiable microbial agent.
• *Urinalysis:* Screening test for common source of infectious process.	Presence of blood cells, protein, and bacteria in the urine suggests infection.
• *Imaging studies:*	
• *Chest and abdominal x-rays:* Screening procedure to help determine source of infection.	Chest x-ray may reveal pneumonia, a common source of infection. Free air in the abdomen may suggest organ perforation caused by infection.
• *Abdominal ultrasound:* Imaging technique that uses high-frequency sound waves to create an image of organs.	Modality of choice when biliary tract source is suspected.
• *Computed tomography (CT) scan or CAT scan:* X-ray procedure that uses a computer to produce a detailed picture of a cross-section of the body.	Modality of choice when intra-abdominal abscess or other gastrointestinal (GI) tract disorders are suspected.

Nursing Priorities

1. Eliminate infection.
2. Support tissue perfusion or circulatory volume.
3. Prevent complications.
4. Provide information about disease process, prognosis, and treatment needs.

Discharge Goals

1. Infection eliminated or controlled.
2. Homeostasis maintained.
3. Complications prevented or minimized.
4. Disease process, prognosis, and therapeutic regimen understood.
5. Plan in place to meet needs after discharge.

NURSING DIAGNOSIS: **risk for Infection [progression of sepsis to septic shock, development of opportunistic infections]**

Risk factors may include
Compromised immune system
Failure to recognize or treat infection and/or exercise proper preventive measures
Invasive procedures, environmental exposure (nosocomial)

Possibly evidenced by
(Not applicable; presence of signs and symptoms establishes an *actual* diagnosis)

Desired Outcomes/Evaluation Criteria—Client Will

Infection Severity (NOC)
Achieve timely healing; be free of purulent secretions, drainage, or erythema; and be afebrile.

ACTIONS/INTERVENTIONS	RATIONALE
Infection Control (NIC)	
Independent	
Examine client for possible source of infection, such as sore throat, sinus pain, burning with urination, localized abdominal pain, burns, open wounds or cellulitis, presence of invasive catheters, or lines.	Respiratory tract and urinary tract infection are the most frequent causes of sepsis, followed by abdominal and soft tissue infections. The use of intravascular devices is also a well-known cause of hospital-acquired sepsis.
Wash hands with antibacterial soap before and after each care activity, even when gloves are used.	Hand washing and hand hygiene reduce the risk of cross-contamination. *Note:* Methicillin-resistant *Staphylococcus aureus* (MRSA) is most commonly transmitted via direct contact with healthcare workers who fail to wash hands between client contacts.
Provide isolation and monitor visitors, as indicated.	BSI should be used for all infectious clients. Wound and linen isolation and hand washing may be all that is required for draining wounds. Clients with diseases transmitted through air may also need airborne and droplet precautions. Reverse isolation and restriction of visitors may be needed to protect the immunosuppressed client.
Encourage or provide frequent position changes, deep-breathing, and coughing exercises.	Good pulmonary toilet may reduce respiratory compromise.
Encourage client to cover mouth and nose with tissue when coughing or sneezing. Place in private room if indicated. Wear mask when providing direct care as appropriate.	Appropriate behaviors, personal protective equipment, and isolation prevent spread of infection via airborne droplets.
Limit use of invasive devices and procedures when possible. Remove lines and devices when infection is present and replace if necessary.	Reduces number of possible entry sites for opportunistic organisms.
Inspect wounds and sites of invasive devices daily, paying particular attention to parenteral nutrition lines. Document signs of local inflammation and infection and changes in character of wound drainage, sputum, or urine.	Catheter-related bloodstream infections (CR-BSIs) are increasing where central venous catheters are used in both acute and chronic care settings. Clinical signs, such as local inflammation or phlebitis, may provide a clue to portal of entry, type of primary infecting organism(s), as well as early identification of secondary infections.
Investigate reports of pain out of proportion to visible signs.	Pressurelike pain over area of cellulitis may indicate development of necrotizing fasciitis due to group A beta hemolytic streptococci (GABS), necessitating prompt intervention.
Maintain sterile technique when changing dressings, suctioning, and providing site care, such as an invasive line or a urinary catheter.	Medical asepsis prevents or limits introduction of bacteria and reduces the risk of nosocomial infection.

ACTIONS/INTERVENTIONS (continued)	RATIONALE (continued)
Wear gloves and gowns when caring for open wounds or anticipating direct contact with secretions or excretions.	Prevents spread of infection and cross-contamination.
Dispose of soiled dressings and other materials in double bag.	Appropriate disposal of contaminated materials reduces contamination and spread of organisms.
Note temperature trends and observe for shaking chills and profuse diaphoresis.	Fever (101°F–105°F [38.5°C–40°C]) is the result of endotoxin effect on the hypothalamus and pyrogen-released endorphins. Hypothermia lower than 96°F (36°C) is a grave sign reflecting advancing shock state, decreased tissue perfusion, and/or failure of the body's ability to mount a febrile response. Chills often precede temperature spikes in presence of generalized infection.
Monitor for signs of deterioration of condition or failure to improve with therapy.	Deterioration of clinical condition or failure to improve with therapy may reflect inappropriate or inadequate antibiotic therapy or overgrowth of resistant or opportunistic organisms.
Inspect oral cavity for white plaques. Investigate reports of vaginal and perineal itching or burning.	Depression of immune system and use of antibiotics increase the risk of secondary infections, particularly yeast—thrush.

Collaborative

Obtain specimens of urine, blood, sputum, wound, and invasive lines or tubes for culture, and sensitivity, as indicated.	Identification of portal of entry and organism causing the septicemia is crucial to effective treatment based on susceptibility to specific medications.
Monitor laboratory studies, such as WBC count with neutrophils and band counts.	The normal ratio of neutrophils to total WBCs is at least 50%; however, when WBC count is markedly decreased, calculating the absolute neutrophil count is more pertinent to evaluating immune status. Likewise, an initial elevation of band cells reflects the body's attempt to mount a response to the infection, whereas a decline indicates decompensation.
Administer medications, as indicated, for example: Anti-infective agents: broad-spectrum antibiotics, such as imipenem and cilastatin (Primaxin), meropenem (Merrem), ticarcillin and clavulanate (Timentin), piperacillin and tazobactam (Zosyn), clindamycin (Cleocin), vancomycin (Vancocin); aminoglycosides, such as tobramycin (Nebcin), gentamicin (Garamycin); cephalosporins, such as cefepime (Maxipime); fluoroquinolones, such as levofloxacin (Levaquin), ciprofloxin (Cipro); antifungals, such as fluconazole (Diflucan), caspofungin acetate (Cancidas)	Specific antibiotics are determined by culture and sensitivity tests, but therapy is usually initiated before obtaining results, using broad-spectrum antibiotics and/or based on most likely infecting organisms. Antifungal therapy may be considered in client who has already been treated with antibiotics, who is neutropenic, receiving total parenteral nutrition (TPN), or who has central venous access in place.
Recombininant human activated protein C (rhAPC) or drotrecogin alpha (Xigris)	Administration of recombinant activated protein C inhibits thrombosis and inflammation, promotes fibrinolysis, and modulates coagulation and inflammation, and may reduce mortality in adult clients with severe sepsis. Drotrecogin alpha is the only widely accepted drug specific to the therapy of sepsis (Sharma & Mink, 2007).
Assist with or prepare for procedures, such as removal of infected devices, incision and drainage of abscess, or débridement of infected wounds, as indicated.	Removal of infection sources promotes healing.
Prepare for hyperbaric therapy, as appropriate.	Exposing wounds to high ambient oxygen tension therapy may be done to combat anaerobic infections.

NURSING DIAGNOSIS: **Hyperthermia**

May be related to
Increased metabolic rate, illness
Dehydration
Direct effect of circulating endotoxins on the hypothalamus, altering temperature regulation

Possibly evidenced by
Increase in body temperature higher than normal range
Flushed skin, warm to touch
Increased respiratory rate, tachycardia

Desired Outcomes/Evaluation Criteria—Client Will

Thermoregulation (NOC)
Demonstrate temperature within normal range and be free of chills.
Experience no associated complications.

ACTIONS/INTERVENTIONS	RATIONALE

Fever Treatment (NIC)
Independent

Monitor client temperature—degree and pattern. Note shaking chills or profuse diaphoresis.

Temperature of 102°F to106°F (38.9°C–41.1°C) suggests acute infectious disease process. Fever pattern may aid in diagnosis: sustained or continuous fever curves lasting more than 24 hours suggest pneumococcal pneumonia, scarlet or typhoid fever; remittent fever varying only a few degrees in either direction reflects pulmonary infections; and intermittent curves or fever that returns to normal once in 24-hour period suggests septic episode, septic endocarditis, or tuberculosis (TB). Chills often precede temperature spikes. *Note:* Use of antipyretics alters fever patterns and may be restricted until diagnosis is made or if fever remains higher than 102°F (38.9°C).

Monitor environmental temperature. Limit or add bed linens, as indicated.

Room temperature and linens should be altered to maintain near-normal body temperature.

Provide tepid sponge baths. Avoid use of alcohol.

Tepid sponge baths may help reduce fever. *Note:* Use of ice water or alcohol may cause chills, actually elevating temperature. Alcohol can also cause skin dehydration.

Collaborative

Administer antipyretics, such as acetylsalicylic acid (ASA) (aspirin) or acetaminophen (Tylenol).

Antipyretics reduce fever by its central action on the hypothalamus; fever should be controlled in clients who are neutropenic or asplenic. However, fever may be beneficial in limiting growth of organisms and enhancing autodestruction of infected cells.

Provide cooling blanket, or hypothermia therapy, as indicated.

Used to reduce fever, especially when higher than 104°F to 105°F (39.5°C–40°C), and when seizures or brain damage are likely to occur.

NURSING DIAGNOSIS: risk for Shock

Risk factors may include
Relative or actual hypovolemia
Reduction of arterial/venous blood flow: selective vasoconstriction, vascular occlusion—intimal damage, microemboli

Possibly evidenced by
(Not applicable; presence of signs and symptoms establishes an *actual* diagnosis)

Desired Outcomes/Evaluation Criteria—Client Will

Circulation Status (NOC)
Display adequate perfusion as evidenced by stable vital signs, palpable peripheral pulses, skin warm and dry, usual level of mentation, individually appropriate urinary output, and active bowel sounds.

ACTIONS/INTERVENTIONS	RATIONALE

Shock Prevention (NIC)
Independent

Maintain bedrest and assist with care activities.

Preventing overexertion decreases myocardial workload and oxygen consumption, thus maximizing effectiveness of tissue perfusion.

Monitor trends in blood pressure (BP), especially noting progressive hypotension and widening pulse pressure.

Hypotension develops as circulating microorganisms stimulate release and activation of chemical and hormonal substances. These endotoxins initially cause peripheral vasodilation, decreased systemic vascular resistance (SVR), and relative hypovolemia. As shock progresses, cardiac output becomes severely depressed due to major alterations in contractility, preload, and/or afterload, thus producing profound hypotension.

Monitor heart rate and rhythm. Note dysrhythmias.

Tachycardia occurs because of sympathetic nervous system stimulation secondary to stress response and to compensate for the relative hypovolemia and hypotension. Cardiac dysrhythmias can occur because of hypoxia, acid-base and electrolyte imbalance, and/or low-flow perfusion state.

ACTIONS/INTERVENTIONS (continued)	RATIONALE (continued)
Note quality and strength of peripheral pulses.	Initially, the pulse is strong and bounding because of increased cardiac output. Pulse may become weak and thready because of sustained hypotension, decreased cardiac output, and peripheral vasoconstriction if the shock state progresses.
Assess respiratory rate, depth, and quality. Note onset of severe dyspnea.	Increased respirations occur in response to direct effects of endotoxins on the respiratory center in the brain, as well as developing hypoxia, stress, and fever. Respirations become shallow as respiratory insufficiency develops, creating risk of acute respiratory failure. (Refer to ND: risk for impaired Gas Exchange.)
Investigate changes in sensorium—mental cloudiness, agitation, restlessness, personality changes, delirium, stupor, and coma.	Changes in mentation reflect alterations in cerebral perfusion, hypoxemia, and/or acidosis.
Assess skin for changes in color, temperature, and moisture.	Vasodilation results in the warm, dry, pink skin characteristic of hyperperfusion in hyperdynamic phase of early septic shock. If shock state progresses, compensatory vasoconstriction occurs, shunting blood to vital organs, reducing peripheral blood flow, and creating cool, clammy, pale and dusky skin.
Record hourly urinary output and specific gravity.	Decreasing urinary output with high specific gravity indicates diminished renal perfusion related to fluid shifts and selective vasoconstriction. There may be transient polyuria during hyperdynamic phase, while cardiac output is elevated, but this may progress to oliguria.
Auscultate bowel sounds.	Reduced blood flow to the mesentery (splanchnic vasoconstriction) decreases peristalsis and may lead to paralytic ileus or possibly trigger MODS.
Hematest gastric secretions and stools for occult blood.	Stress of illness and use of steroids increase risk of gastric mucosal erosion and bleeding.
Evaluate lower extremities for local tissue swelling, erythema, and positive Homan's sign.	Venous stasis, changes in the coagulation processes, and infection may result in the development of thrombosis.
Maintain sequential compression devices (SCDs), as indicated.	These are preventive measures for bedfast client to reduce lower extremity stasis complications.
Monitor for signs of bleeding: oozing from puncture sites or suture lines, petechiae, ecchymoses, hematuria, epistaxis, hemoptysis, and hematemesis.	Coagulopathies such as DIC may occur, related to accelerated clotting in the microcirculation reflecting activation of chemical mediators, vascular insufficiency, and cell destruction creating a life-threatening hemorrhagic situation and multiple emboli.
Note drug effects, and monitor for signs of toxicity.	Massive doses of antibiotics have potentially toxic effects in clients with compromised renal and/or hepatic function.
Collaborative	
Administer parenteral fluids. (Refer to ND: risk for deficient Fluid Volume, following.)	Parenteral fluid therapy helps maintain tissue perfusion and expand circulating volume.
Administer drugs, as indicated, for example: Corticosteroids	Although steroid therapy remains controversial, low-dose steroids may be given for the potential advantages of decreasing capillary permeability, increasing renal perfusion, and inhibiting microemboli formation. *Note:* Adrenal insufficiency occurs in many clients with septic shock. Appropriate dosing of steroids provides support to dysfunctional adrenal glands and enhances vasomotor tone.
Inotropic agents and vasopressors, such as norepinephrine (Levophed), dopamine (Intropin), and vasopressin (Pitressin)	Inotropic agents and vasopressors may be needed to improve organ perfusion and to maintain blood pressure during and after fluid treatment. *Note:* Client needing this level of support is critically ill and will be treated in the ICU.
Low-molecular-weight heparin, such as enoxaparin (Lovenox), dalteparin (Fragmin), and tinzaparin (Innohep); and unfractionated heparin	Low-molecular-weight heparin prevents or treats deep vein thrombosis (DVT).
Histamine 2–receptor blockers, such as cimetidine (Tagamet), famotidine (Pepcid AC), nizatidine (Asid), and rantidine (Zantac)	Histamine receptor blockers prevent or treat stress ulcers.

(continues on page 694)

693

ACTIONS/INTERVENTIONS (continued)	RATIONALE (continued)
Monitor laboratory studies, such as ABGs and lactate levels.	Circulatory collapse reduces tissue perfusion. Inadequate renal perfusion alters filtration, reabsorption, and secretion of various substances resulting in fluid and electrolyte imbalances. ABGs and serum lactate levels indicate acid-base balance and anaerobic metabolism. Respiratory or metabolic acidosis indicates weakened compensatory mechanisms. Lactic acid accumulation is due to inadequate oxygenation and thus accumulation of anaerobic by-products or lactate.
Provide supplemental oxygen.	Supplemental oxygen improves cellular oxygenation.
Maintain stable body temperature, using adjunctive aids as necessary. (Refer to ND: Hyperthermia.)	Temperature elevations increase metabolic and oxygen demands beyond cellular resources, hastening tissue ischemia and cellular destruction.
Prepare for and transfer to critical care setting, as indicated.	Progressive deterioration requires more aggressive therapy including hemodynamic monitoring and vasoactive drug infusions.

NURSING DIAGNOSIS: risk for deficient Fluid Volume

Risk factors may include
Marked increase in vascular compartment, massive vasodilation
Capillary permeability with fluid leaks into the interstitial space (third spacing)

Possibly evidenced by
(Not applicable; presence of signs and symptoms establishes an *actual* diagnosis)

Desired Outcomes/Evaluation Criteria—Client Will

Hydration (NOC)
Maintain adequate circulatory volume as evidenced by vital signs within client's normal range, palpable peripheral pulses of good quality, and individually appropriate urinary output.

ACTIONS/INTERVENTIONS	RATIONALE
Shock Prevention (NIC) *Independent*	
Measure and record urinary output and specific gravity. Note cumulative intake and output (I&O) imbalances (including insensible losses), and correlate with daily weight. Encourage oral fluids, as tolerated.	Decreasing urinary output with a high specific gravity suggests relative hypovolemia associated with vasodilation. Continued positive fluid balance with corresponding weight gain may indicate third spacing and tissue edema, suggesting need to alter fluid therapy or replacement components. *Note:* Excessive diarrhea may lead to a negative fluid balance.
Monitor BP and heart rate. Measure central venous pressure (CVP) if used.	Reduction in the circulating fluid volume reduces BP and CVP, initiating compensatory mechanisms of tachycardia to improve cardiac output and increase systemic blood pressure.
Palpate peripheral pulses.	Weak, easily obliterated pulses suggest hypovolemia.
Assess for dry mucous membranes, poor skin turgor, and thirst.	Hypovolemia and third spacing of fluid give rise to signs of dehydration.
Observe for dependent or peripheral edema in sacrum, scrotum, back, and legs.	Fluid losses from the vascular compartment into the interstitial space create tissue edema.
Collaborative	
Administer IV fluids, such as isotonic crystalloids (D$_5$W, normal saline [NS], lactated Ringer's [LR]) and colloids (albumin, fresh frozen plasma), as indicated.	Fluid therapy is most effective early in the course of severe sepsis because as the condition worsens, there is greater dysfunction at the cellular level. Large volumes of fluid may be required to overcome relative hypovolemia or peripheral vasodilation, and replace losses from increased capillary permeability (e.g., sequestration of fluid in the peritoneal cavity) and increased insensible sources such as fever and diaphoresis.
Monitor laboratory values, such as the following: Hct/RBC count	Evaluates changes in hydration/blood viscosity.
BUN/Cr	The BUN/Cr ratio could indicate dehydration or renal dysfunction and failure.
Monitor cardiac output, as indicated.	Cardiac output, and other functional parameters such as cardiac index, preload, afterload, contractility, and cardiac work, can be measured noninvasively using thoracic electrical bioimpedance (TEB) technique. Cardiac output determination is useful in determining therapeutic needs and effectiveness.

NURSING DIAGNOSIS: risk for impaired Gas Exchange

Risk factors may include

Altered O₂ supply—effects of endotoxins on the respiratory center in the medulla (resulting in hyperventilation and respiratory alkalosis); hypoventilation

Altered blood flow (changes in vascular resistance), alveolar-capillary membrane changes—increased capillary permeability leading to pulmonary congestion

Interference with oxygen delivery and utilization in the tissues (endotoxin-induced damage to the cells and capillaries)

Possibly evidenced by

(Not applicable; presence of signs and symptoms establishes an *actual* diagnosis)

Desired Outcomes/Evaluation Criteria—Client Will

Respiratory Status: Gas Exchange (NOC)

Display ABGs and respiratory rate within client's normal range, with breath sounds clear and chest x-ray clear or improving. Experience no dyspnea or cyanosis.

ACTIONS/INTERVENTIONS	RATIONALE
Respiratory Monitoring (NIC)	
Independent	
Maintain client airway. Place client in position of comfort with head of bed elevated 30 to 45 degrees.	Elevating the head of bed enhances lung expansion and reduces respiratory effort.
Monitor respiratory rate and depth. Note use of accessory muscles or work of breathing.	Rapid, shallow respirations occur because of hypoxemia, stress, and circulating endotoxins. Hypoventilation and dyspnea reflect ineffective compensatory mechanisms and are indications that ventilatory support is needed.
Auscultate breath sounds. Note crackles, wheezes, and areas of decreased or absent ventilation.	Respiratory distress and the presence of adventitious sounds are indicators of pulmonary congestion, interstitial edema, and atelectasis. *Note:* Respiratory complications, including pneumonia and acute respiratory distress syndrome (ARDS), are prime causes of death.
Note presence of circumoral cyanosis.	Circumoral cyanosis indicates inadequate central oxygenation and hypoxemia.
Investigate alterations in sensorium: agitation, confusion, personality changes, delirium, stupor, and coma.	Cerebral function is very sensitive to decreases in oxygenation such as hypoxemia, or reduced perfusion.
Note cough and purulent sputum production.	Pneumonia is a common nosocomial infection that can occur by aspiration of oropharyngeal organisms or spread from other sites.
Reposition frequently. Encourage coughing and deep-breathing exercises. Suction, as indicated.	Good pulmonary toilet is necessary for reducing ventilation/perfusion imbalance and for mobilizing and facilitating removal of secretions to maximize gas exchange.
Collaborative	
Monitor ABGs and pulse oximetry.	Hypoxemia is related to decreased ventilation and pulmonary changes (e.g., interstitial edema, atelectasis, and pulmonary shunting) and increased oxygen demands caused by fever or infection. Respiratory acidosis (pH below 7.35 and PaCO₂ higher than 40 mm Hg) occurs because of hypoventilation and ventilation-perfusion imbalance. As septic condition worsens, metabolic acidosis (pH below 7.35 and HCO₃ less than 22–24 mEq/L) develops as a result of buildup of lactic acid from anaerobic metabolism.
Administer supplemental oxygen via appropriate route: nasal cannula, mask, or high-flow rebreathing mask.	Supplemental oxygen is necessary for correction of hypoxemia with failing respiratory effort or progressing acidosis. *Note:* Intubation and mechanical ventilation may be required if respiratory failure develops.
Administer red blood cells (RBCs), as indicated.	May be required to improve available oxygen to treat sepsis-induced hypoperfusion, or when Hct is less than 30% (Kleinpell, 2006).
Review serial chest x-rays.	Changes on x-ray reflect progression or resolution of pulmonary complications, such as infiltrates and edema.

NURSING DIAGNOSIS: **deficient Knowledge [Learning Need] regarding illness, prognosis, treatment, self-care, and discharge needs**

May be related to
Lack of exposure or recall, information misinterpretation
Cognitive limitation

Possibly evidenced by
Questions, request for information, statement of misconception
Inaccurate follow-through of instructions, development of preventable complications

Desired Outcomes/Evaluation Criteria—Client Will

Knowledge: Infection Control (NOC)
Verbalize understanding of disease process, prognosis, and potential complications.
Correctly perform necessary procedures and explain reasons for the actions.
Initiate necessary lifestyle changes.
Verbalize understanding of therapeutic needs.
Participate in treatment regimen.

ACTIONS/INTERVENTIONS	RATIONALE
Teaching: Disease Process (NIC) *Independent* Review disease process and future expectations.	Open discussion regarding the disease and clinical expectations provides knowledge base from which client can make informed choices.
Review individual risk factors, mode of transmission, and portal of entry of infections.	Awareness of means of infection transmission provides opportunity to plan for and institute protective measures.
Provide information about drug therapy, interactions, side effects, and importance of adherence to regimen.	Adequate and appropriate information promotes understanding and enhances compliance with treatment or prophylaxis, and reduces risk of recurrence and complications.
Discuss need for good nutritional intake or balanced diet.	Good nutrition is necessary for optimal healing, immune system enhancement, and general well-being.
Encourage adequate rest periods with scheduled activities.	Rest prevents fatigue, conserves energy, and facilitates recovery.
Review necessity of personal hygiene and environmental cleanliness, proper cooking techniques, and food storage.	Personal hygiene and environmental cleanliness reduce exposure to pathogens.
Discuss proper use or avoidance of tampons with menstruating women, as indicated.	Superabsorbent tampons or infrequent tampon changing potentiates risk of *Staphylococcus aureus* infection and toxic shock syndrome.
Identify signs and symptoms requiring medical evaluation: persistent temperature elevation(s), tachycardia, syncope, rashes of unknown origin, unexplained fatigue, anorexia, increased thirst, and changes in bladder function.	Early recognition of developing or recurring infection allows for timely intervention and reduces risk for progression to life-threatening situation.
Stress importance of prophylactic immunizations and antibiotic therapy, as needed.	Prophylactic vaccines and antibiotics prevent infection, especially in high-risk groups such as those of advanced age or with chronic illness and/or a past history of infective heart disease and immunosuppression.

POTENTIAL CONSIDERATIONS following acute hospitalization (dependent on client's age, physical condition and presence of complications, personal resources, and life responsibilities)
• *risk for recurrence/opportunistic Infection*—stasis of body fluids, decreased hemoglobin, leukopenia, suppressed inflammatory response, use of anti-infective agents, increased environmental exposure, malnutrition
• *imbalanced Nutrition: Less than Body Requirements*—increased energy needs (hypermetabolic state), anorexia, continuing GI dysfunction, side effects of medication
• *Self-Care Deficit/impaired Home Maintenance*—decreased strength/endurance, pain/discomfort, inadequate support systems, unfamiliarity with neighborhood resources

THE HIV-POSITIVE CLIENT

I. Pathophysiology

a. Infection by a subgroup of retroviruses with a high affinity for CD4 T-lymphocytes and monocytes, with viral DNA incorporating itself into host DNA (Dubin, 2008)

b. Following successful transmission of HIV, the course of subsequent infection is variable and dependent on a number of factors.

c. Main consequence of infection is damage to the immune system.

II. Stages: continuum with progression individually variable (Health24, 2004; Highleyman, 2005)

a. *Infection or initial incubation period* lasts 2 to 4 weeks.
   i. Individual asymptomatic
   ii. HIV test negative but individual is infectious.

b. *Primary infection or acute seroconversion stage* usually occurs 4 to 8 weeks after infection.
   i. Individual may be asymptomatic or develop flu-like symptoms—low-grade fever, sore throat, swollen lymph nodes, rash, joint and muscle pain lasting 1 to 2 weeks
   ii. HIV positive but immune system usually functional.

c. *Latency or asymptomatic stage* can last anywhere from 2 weeks to years.
   i. Virus remains active.
   ii. Individual may be unaware of HIV status.

d. *Mild to moderate stage* usually occurs between 5 to 7 years after infection.
   i. Immune system is compromised.
   ii. Individual symptomatic—skin rashes; fatigue; night sweats; weight loss; mouth ulcers; fungal skin and nail infections, which progress to chronic oral or vaginal thrush; recurrent herpes blisters on mouth or genitals; ongoing fevers; persistent diarrhea

e. *Severe or late stage HIV disease* median occurrence is 11 years postinfection.
   i. Viral load is very high; CD4 count is very low, thus indicating full-blown AIDS.
   ii. Severe immune system damage and development of opportunistic infections (Refer to CP: AIDS for information.)

III. Etiology

a. Infection results from one of two similar retroviruses—HIV-1 and HIV-2—that destroy CD4 lymphocytes and impair cell-mediated immunity, thereby increasing the risk of certain infections and cancers.

b. Mode of transmission
   i. Sexual contact—deposition of HIV on mucosal surfaces, especially the genital mucosa and intestinal epithelium (most common mode)
   ii. Direct inoculation into the blood through intravenous (IV) needle sharing or use of contaminated blood products (rare in United States)
   iii. Mother-to-baby perinatal transmission

c. Worldwide, high-risk populations—sex workers, men who have sex with men, injection drug users, and prisoners (United Nations Programme on HIV/AIDS [UNAIDS] & World Health Organization [WHO], 2006)

d. Risk and severity of opportunistic infections, AIDS, and AIDS-related cancers are determined by the CD4 lymphocyte count and the client's exposure to potentially opportunistic pathogens.

e. Ability of virus to mutate has made disease management challenging, which has hindered efforts at development of a vaccine.

IV. Statistics

a. Morbidity: In 2005, there were an estimated 38.6 million people worldwide with HIV (UNAIDS & WHO, 2006); in 2003, there were approximately 1 million with HIV/AIDS in the United States (Glynn & Rhodes, 2005); annually, 40,000 Americans are newly infected (Armington, 2007); new infections are still increasing in some age ranges (e.g., 40–44), among males (white, black, and Hispanic), and among female adolescent and adult injection drug users (Centers for Disease Control and Prevention [CDC], 2007).

b. Mortality: Associated with progression to AIDS; life expectancy 2 to 3 years in untreated HIV progressing to AIDS (Dubin, 2008); in 2002, AIDS-related deaths were at a rate of 2.2%, with marked increase for non-HIV/AIDS-related causes, such as diabetes, chronic hepatitis, and cardiovascular disease (Highleyman, 2005).

c. Cost: In 2002, $36.4 billion estimated lifetime costs for individuals newly diagnosed in the United States, with $6.7 billion in direct medical costs and almost $30 billion in productivity loss (Hutchinson et al, 2006).

GLOSSARY

Acquired immunodeficiency syndrome (AIDS): Outcome of infection with a retrovirus (HIV).

Acute retroviral syndrome (ACR): Describes a group of symptoms that can resemble mononucleosis—fever, fatigue, muscle aches, loss of appetite, upset stomach, and weight loss.

CD4: Type of protein molecule in the blood that is present on the surface of immune cells. The HIV virus infects cells that have CD4 surface proteins and, as a result, depletes the number of T cells, B cells, natural killer cells, and monocytes in the blood. Most of the damage to the immune system is through destruction of CD4 lymphocytes.

Electrophoresis: Method of separating large molecules, such as DNA fragments or proteins, from a mixture of similar molecules.

Herpes simplex virus (HSV-2): Virus that has deleterious effects with coinfection of HIV.

Human immunodeficiency virus (HIV): Virus that causes a progressive disease leading to AIDS.

(text continues on page 698)

Seroconversion: Development of an antibody response to infection that is measurable in the serum. The HIV seropositive individual is one who is asymptomatic and who does not meet the Centers for Disease Control and Prevention (CDC, 1987) definition for AIDS.

Sexually transmitted diseases (STDs): Group of diseases that includes chlamydia, syphilis, herpes, and gonorrhea, among others.

T cells: Lymphocytes that originate in the thymus gland and regulate the immune system's response to infections, including HIV; CD4 lymphocytes are a subset of T lymphocytes.

Thrush: Fungal infection of the mucous membranes appearing as a patchy, raised white rash or spots.

Viral load tests: Detects viral RNA levels as low as 50 copies.

Care Setting

Client is treated in a community setting, although development of opportunistic infections may require occasional inpatient acute medical care.

Related Factors

Acquired immunodeficiency syndrome (AIDS), page 709
Extended care, page 801
Fluid and electrolyte imbalances, page 903
Pneumonia, page 131
Psychosocial aspects of care, page 749
Sepsis/septicemia, page 686

Client Assessment Database

Although client may be asymptomatic, refer to CP: AIDS for potential signs and symptoms. Refer to section at end of plan for ongoing considerations.

Diagnostic Studies

TEST WHY IT IS DONE	WHAT IT TELLS ME
BLOOD TESTS	
• *HIV antibody test:* Detects HIV antibodies in the blood.	Antibodies to HIV are produced by the body and can be detected in the blood about 2 to 4 weeks after exposure to the virus.
• *Rapid HIV tests—OraQuick ADVANCE Rapid HIV-1/2 Antibody Test, MultiSpot HIV-1/HIV-2 Rapid Test, Clearview COMPLETE HIV-1/2:* Antibody tests that are now available in the United States, with two that are approved for use at point-of-care sites outside a traditional laboratory.	Positive results should be followed up with additional tests (Greenwald et al, 2006).
• *Enzyme-linked immunosorbent assay (ELISA):* Sensitive immunoassay that uses an enzyme linked to an antibody or antigen as a marker for the detection of a specific protein.	Determines exposure to a particular infectious agent, such as the HIV virus, by identifying antibodies present in a blood sample; however, it is not diagnostic because seroconversion can occur between 4 weeks and 6 months after exposure.
• *Rapid plasma reagin test:* Detects antibodies in the blood. Can be used as a rapid screening test with positive results requiring confirmation by Western blot test.	During initial stage, assay test to diagnose acute HIV antibodies will be negative; however, rapid plasma reagin test may identify acute HIV infection before antibodies have developed (Armington, 2007).
• *Western blot test:* Technique for identifying specific antibodies or proteins in which proteins are separated by electrophoresis.	Confirms diagnosis of HIV-1 in individuals with positive ELISA screening.
• *Viral load tests:*	
• *Reverse transcriptase–polymerase chain reaction (RT-PCR):* Highly sensitive technique for detecting and quantifying viral load.	Detects viral RNA levels as low as 50 copies/mL of plasma.
• *Branched DNA (bDNA) 3.0 assay:* Has a wider range—50 to 500,000 copies/mL. (The RI-PCR range is 50–75,000/mL.)	Currently the leading indicator of effectiveness of therapy. Therapy can be initiated, or changes made in treatment approaches, based on rise of viral load or maintenance of a low viral load.

Diagnostic Studies (continued)

TEST WHY IT IS DONE (continued)	WHAT IT TELLS ME (continued)
• *CD8+ CTL (cytopathic suppressor cells):* Current quantitative assays allow for rapid evaluation of levels.	CD8+ (CTL) have been strongly implicated in the control of HIV-1 replications. At late stage of infection, CD8+ (CTL) numbers are reduced.
• *CD4 lymphocyte count (previously T4 helper cells):* CD4 cells are a target for HIV infection and destruction.	Used to diagnose HIV infection and progression and to monitor effects of drug therapy. Clients with counts below 500 benefit from antiretroviral therapy; counts equal to or below 200 define progression to AIDS. Levels are measured immediately before and again 4 to 8 weeks after initiation of antiretroviral therapy.
• *Serum glucose:* Monitor for development of diabetes mellitus (DM) or side effect of protease inhibitors (PIs).	Glucose levels elevated because of insulin resistance. Increased risk for developing DM in presence of HIV infection.
• *Albumin/prealbumin and transferrin levels:* • *Lipids:* Evaluates nutritional status.	Progressively decrease secondary to malabsorption or malnutrition. Lipids rise as HIV infection progresses.
• *Complete blood count (CBC):* Battery of screening tests, which typically includes hemoglobin (Hgb); hematocrit (Hct); red blood cell (RBC) count, morphology, indices, and distribution width index; platelet count and size; white blood cell (WBC) count and differential.	Hgb and RBC counts are decreased. Abnormalities in iron metabolism can result in anemia, which occurs in some asymptomatic clients with HIV and a high percentage of clients with advanced disease.
OTHER DIAGNOSTIC STUDIES • *Pap smear:* Detects precursor lesions that can precede the diagnosis of invasive carcinoma.	Higher incidence of abnormal cells occurs in HIV-infected women.
• *Pelvic/genital examination:* Direct visualization of structures and mucosal membranes.	Identifies presence of lesions from STDs.
• *Chest x-ray:* Procedure used to evaluate organs and structures within the chest for symptoms of disease.	Abnormalities suggest presence of TB, which is common with HIV infection, or other opportunistic infections.

Nursing Priorities

1. Promote acceptance of reality of diagnosis and condition.
2. Support incorporation of behavioral and lifestyle changes to enhance well-being.
3. Provide information about disease process, prognosis, and treatment needs.
4. Assist in developing plan and strategies to meet long-term medical, behavioral, and financial needs and enhancing quality of life.

Goals of Care

1. Dealing with current situation realistically.
2. Participating in and appropriately managing therapeutic regimen.
3. Diagnosis, prognosis, and therapeutic regimen understood.
4. Plan in place to meet medical, behavioral change, and financial needs.

NURSING DIAGNOSIS: risk-prone health Behavior

May be related to
Life-threatening, stigmatized disease, incomplete or ongoing grieving
Assault to self-esteem, altered locus of control
Denial, negative attitudes toward health behavior and/or lifestyle changes
Inadequate support systems
Complex medication regimen and side effects—fatigue and depression

Possibly evidenced by
Verbalization of nonacceptance or denial of diagnosis
Extended period of shock, disbelief, or anger regarding change in health status
Failure to take action to prevent further health problems
Inability to effectively manage medication regimen
Failure to achieve optimal sense of control

(continues on page 700)

Desired Outcomes/Evaluation Criteria—Client Will

Acceptance: Health Status (NOC)
Verbalize reality and acceptance of condition.
Demonstrate increased trust and participation in development of plan of action.
Initiate lifestyle changes that will permit adaptation to present life situations.

ACTIONS/INTERVENTIONS	RATIONALE
Crisis Intervention (NIC)	
Independent	
Evaluate client's ability to understand events and realistically appraise situation.	Provides base to develop plan of action.
Identify real barriers to adjustment.	Promotes opportunity to deal appropriately with real problems in client's individual situation.
Encourage expression of feelings, denial, shock, and fears. Listen without judgment, accepting client's expressions. Focus on positive outcomes.	It is important to convey belief in client's fears and feelings. By focusing on positive outcomes, client is encouraged to take charge of those areas in which changes can be made, such as managing medical regimen and behavior.
Challenge morbid thoughts and reframe into positive statements: "You know why the virus is going to kill me. I deserve to die for what I've done." Response: "The virus may or may not kill you. It's not smart enough to decide when you may die. The virus is 'just there.' It does not have a mind to know what you have or have not done."	Interrupts morbid thoughts and challenges client's self-deprecating ideas. As with any potentially terminal disease, this population is likely to experience depression and is at increased risk for suicide, necessitating ongoing evaluation.
Determine available resources and programs.	Identifies client needs and what comprehensive services might be available and immediately accessible. Services may include education concerning sexual myths, HIV transmission prevention, safer sex practices, and alternate methods of expressing sexuality. Interventions and education may be needed for addictive behaviors, such as the ability of injection drug user to obtain clean "works."
Assess social system as well as presence of support, perception of losses, and stressors.	Partners, friends, and families will have individual responses depending on the individual's lifestyle, knowledge of HIV transmission, and belief systems. *Note:* Belief systems can include values or myths, which affect how the individual approaches the disease and the outcome.
Encourage client to participate in support groups.	Long-term support is critical to dealing with and effectively coping with the reality of being HIV positive and with frequent healthcare evaluations, medical treatments, and ongoing lifestyle changes.
Educate client about drug interactions, HIV, and emotions.	Fatigue and depression can be side effects of some medications and of the infection itself. Knowledge that these effects are usually of short duration can support informed choices and cooperation and promote hope.
Encourage continued or renewed use of familiar effective coping strategies.	Client is supported and given encouragement for past effective behaviors. Positive reinforcement enhances self-esteem.
Explore use and practice of new and different coping strategies.	Using new strategies is uncomfortable in the beginning, but practice fosters self-confidence.
Help client use humor to combat stigmatization of the disease.	Humor defuses the sense of secretiveness people may place on diagnosis of, and dealing with, HIV.
Reinforce structure in daily life. Include exercise as part of routine.	Routines help the client focus. Exercise improves sense of wellness and enhances immune response.
Discuss meaning of high-risk behavior, such as unprotected sexual activity, injection drug use with shared needles, and failure to take medications; and address barriers to change.	Fear of disclosure, need to change usual behaviors, and the difficulty of doing so may prevent the individual from making the changes necessary to prevent transmission of disease and to manage lifestyle.
Assist client to set limits on sexually risky behaviors and explore ways client can achieve change.	Needs for love, comfort, and companionship that are met through sexual expression must be met safely through means that carry a reduced risk of HIV transmission.
Assist client to channel anger to healthy activities.	The increased energy of anger can be used to accomplish other tasks and enhance feelings of self-esteem.
Inform client about new medical advances and treatments.	Promotes hope and helps client make informed decisions.

ACTIONS/INTERVENTIONS (continued)	RATIONALE (continued)
Discuss issues of voluntary disclosure, personal responsibility, needs of others, and federal, state, and local reporting requirements.	Understanding responsibilities and consequences of disclosure is necessary for client to make informed decisions.
Collaborative	
Refer client to nurse practitioner or clinical nurse specialist, psychologist, or social worker knowledgeable about HIV as well as specific HIV programs and resources or appropriate research programs.	May need additional help adjusting to difficult situation.

NURSING DIAGNOSIS: Fatigue

May be related to
Decreased metabolic energy production, increased energy requirements (hypermetabolic state)
Overwhelming psychological and emotional demands
Altered body chemistry—side effects of medications, insulin resistance

Possibly evidenced by
Verbalization of unremitting, overwhelming lack of energy
Inability to maintain usual routines, decreased performance, impaired ability to concentrate

Desired Outcomes/Evaluation Criteria—Client Will

Endurance (NOC)
Report improved sense of energy.
Participate in desired activities at level of ability.

Energy Conservation (NOC)
Identify individual areas of control and engage in energy conservation techniques.

ACTIONS/INTERVENTIONS	RATIONALE
Energy Management (NIC)	
Independent	
Assess sleep patterns and other factors that may be aggravating fatigue.	Multiple factors can cause and aggravate fatigue, including sleep deprivation, emotional distress, side effects of drugs, and developing central nervous system (CNS) disease.
Encourage timely evaluation of fatigue if new medications have been added to regimen.	Fatigue is present in variable degrees as part of HIV infection process, but is often aggravated by nutritional deficiencies and side effects of certain medications. For example, when PIs are added or changed, fatigue may worsen.
Discuss reality of client's feelings of exhaustion and identify limitations imposed by fatigue state. Note daily energy patterns—peaks and valleys.	Helpful in planning activities within tolerance levels. Clients often expect too much of themselves, believing that they should be able to do more.
Assist client to set realistic activity goals, determining individual priorities and responsibilities.	Client may need to alter priorities and delegate some responsibilities to manage fatigue and optimize performance.
Discuss energy conservation techniques, such as sitting instead of standing for activities, as appropriate.	Enables client to become aware of ways in which energy expenditure can be maximized to complete necessary tasks.
Review importance of meeting individual nutritional needs.	Adequate nutrition is needed for optimizing energy production. (Refer to ND: imbalanced Nutrition: risk for less than body requirements, following.)
Encourage adequate rest periods during the day, routine schedule for bedtime and arising, and scheduling activities during time of best energy.	Helps client recoup energy to manage desired activities.
Instruct in stress management techniques, such as breathing exercises, visualization, and music and light therapy.	Reduction of stress factors in client's life can minimize energy output.
Identify available resources and support systems.	May require outside assistance with homemaking and maintenance activities and child care.

Risk factors may include
Inadequate food intake less than recommended daily allowance
Lack of interest in food, anorexia, depression
Lack of information, misinformation, misconceptions
Limited resources (including finances)
Reported altered sensation of taste and smell, nausea, and other side effects of medications
Sore, inflamed buccal cavity (thrush)

Possibly evidenced by
(Not applicable; presence of signs and symptoms establishes an *actual* diagnosis)

Desired Outcomes/Evaluation Criteria—Client Will

Nutritional Status (NOC)
Maintain adequate muscle mass.
Maintain stable weight.
Demonstrate laboratory values within normal limits.
Report improved energy level.

ACTIONS/INTERVENTIONS	RATIONALE
Nutritional Counseling (NIC)	
Independent	
Determine usual weight before client was diagnosed with HIV.	Early wasting is not readily determined by normal weight-to-height charts; therefore, determining current weight in relation to prediagnosis weight is more useful. Recent unexplained or involuntary weight loss may be a factor in seeking initial medical evaluation.
Weigh regularly and establish current anthropometric measurements. Measure resting energy expenditure (REE) using indirect calorimetry.	Helps assess and monitor wasting and determine nutritional needs—40% of HIV-positive clients show substantial weight loss. Indirect calorimetry is more accurate for calculating REE than the Harris-Benedict equation, which underestimates the energy needs of these clients.
Determine client's current dietary pattern and intake and knowledge of nutrition. Use an in-depth dietary assessment tool.	Identification of these factors helps plan for individual needs. Clients with HIV infection have documented vitamin (e.g., vitamin B_{12}, folate) and trace mineral (e.g., zinc, magnesium, selenium) deficits. Alcohol and drug abuse can interfere with adequate intake.
Assess presence and degree of nausea and vomiting.	The causes of nausea and vomiting are numerous and are associated with medications, functional changes in gastrointestinal (GI) system, and endocrine dysfunction. Protracted nausea and vomiting can debilitate a client, leading to loss of lean body mass, electrolyte imbalances, and further deterioration of immune function.
Ascertain current financial status and recent and/or anticipated changes in economic status. Explore related costs of a variety of foods.	Helps in planning for meeting nutritional needs, such as purchasing low-cost foods that are nutritionally rich. Client may need referral to financial aid to help with food stamps or obtaining meals.
Discuss and document nutritional side effects of medications.	Commonly used medications cause anorexia, altered taste, nausea and/or vomiting; some interfere with bone marrow production of RBCs, causing anemia. Protease inhibitors (PIs) increase the risk of developing diabetes. GI symptoms are common with over-the-counter (OTC) drugs, such as nonsteroidal anti-inflammatory drugs (NSAIDs), which may also contribute to anorexia.
Help client plan ways to maintain/improve intake. Identify lactose-free supplements, as appropriate. Provide information about nutritionally dense high-calorie, high-protein, high-vitamin, and high-mineral foods.	Having this information helps client understand importance of a well-balanced diet. Some clients may try macrobiotic and other diets, believing the diarrhea is caused by lactose intolerance. Eliminating dairy products can have detrimental effects when these nutrient components are not replaced from other sources.
Stress importance of maintaining balanced, adequate nutritional intake and fluids rich with electrolytes, such as Gatorade or Pedialyte.	Client may be depressed and discouraged by changed health and social status and find it difficult to eat for many reasons. Knowing how important nutritionally balanced intake is to supporting the immune system and remaining healthy can motivate client to eat.

ACTIONS/INTERVENTIONS (continued)	RATIONALE (continued)
Assist client to formulate dietary plan, taking into consideration increased metabolic demands and energy needs, and hyperlipidemia.	Provides guidance and feedback while promoting sense of control, enhancing self-esteem, and possibly improving intake. HIV infection is continuously stimulating the immune system, increasing metabolic rate and nutritional needs. *Note:* Use of PIs is known to elevate levels of glucose and lipids—especially triglycerides and cholesterol.
Recommend eating frequent small meals, avoiding cooking odors if bothersome, keeping room well ventilated, and removing noxious stimuli. Suggest use of spices, marinating red meat before cooking, and/or substituting other protein sources for red meat.	Reduces possible adverse stimuli or enhances palatability of food and may improve nutritional intake, which is needed to help client restore and maintain nutritional defenses.
Recommend environment conducive to eating. Emphasize importance of sharing mealtime with others. Identify someone who can join client for meals.	A quiet, relaxed, calm, unrushed setting and socialization can enhance appetite/food intake, especially when depression, neglect of self-care, and diminished appetite are present.
Explore complementary therapies and nonpharmacological interventions, such as acupressure, progressive relaxation, and guided imagery, to manage anorexia.	The goal of these interventions is to manage distressing symptoms that interfere with optimal nutritional intake.
Discuss use of *Lactobacillus acidophilus* replacement, such as LactAid dairy products and/or tablets/capsules.	HIV infection changes the structure of the gut wall, resulting in a decreased lactose level. Intolerance causes abdominal cramping, malabsorption, a bloated feeling, and diarrhea. Also, antibiotics taken for prevention of opportunistic infections cause changes in normal bowel flora, contributing to diarrhea.
Collaborative	
Consult with dietitian and nutritional support team.	Provides assistance in planning nutritionally sound diet and identifying nutritional supplements to meet individual needs. Liquid supplements (e.g., Advera) have been specifically formulated for the GI manifestations common to the HIV-positive population.
Monitor laboratory values, such as Hgb, RBCs, albumin or pre-albumin, total iron-binding capacity (TIBC), potassium, and sodium.	These laboratory tests are important in monitoring the client's nutritional immune status and in identifying nutritional therapy needs. For example, anemia may require additional interventions, such as use of epoetin (Epogen or Procrit), to stimulate RBC production.
Provide medications, as indicated, for example:	
Dronabinol (Marinol), megestrol (Megace), and cyproheptadine (Periactin)	Antiemetics or appetite stimulants can improve intake to prevent and correct dietary deficiencies. *Note:* A side effect of Megace may include impotence, necessitating change of drug as desired.
Antidiarrheal medications, such as diphenoxylate/atropine (Lomotil) and octreotide (Sandostatin)	Diarrhea may be present because of altered GI flora and side effects of anti-infective agents. Treatment can correct malabsorption and enhance oral intake.
Acidophilus OTC products	Can be useful in restoration of normal bowel flora.

NURSING DIAGNOSIS: **deficient Knowledge [Learning Need] regarding disease, prognosis, treatment, self-care, and discharge needs**

May be related to
Lack of exposure or recall
Information misinterpretation
Unfamiliarity with information resources
Cognitive limitation

Possibly evidenced by
Statement of misconception, request for information
Inaccurate follow-through of instructions, development of preventable complications
Inappropriate or exaggerated behaviors—hostile, agitated, hysterical, apathetic

Desired Outcomes/Evaluation Criteria—Client Will

Knowledge: Disease Process (NOC)
Verbalize understanding of condition, disease process, and potential complications.
Identify relationship of signs and symptoms to the disease process and correlate symptoms with causative factors.

Knowledge: Treatment Regimen (NOC)
Verbalize understanding of goals of treatment.
Initiate necessary lifestyle changes.
Participate in treatment regimen.

ACTIONS/INTERVENTIONS	RATIONALE

Teaching: Learning Facilitation (NIC)
Independent

Assess emotional ability to assimilate information and understand instructions. Respect client's need to use denial and coping techniques initially.

Initial shock and anxiety can block intake of information. Self-esteem, lifestyle, guilt, and denial of own responsibility in acquiring or transmitting disease become issues that must be dealt with. *Note:* Some initial denial may serve as a protective mechanism promoting more effective self-care.

Provide realistic, optimistic information during each contact with client.

Necessary to provide realistic hope because most clients have been exposed to some inaccurate information about AIDS or may have friends or lovers who have died of the disease.

Plan frequent short sessions for teaching. Include written information—a few pieces at each visit.

Client will likely feel overwhelmed and need time and repeated contacts to absorb information, the scope of, and the requirements for treating the infection. Written materials allow for later review and reinforcement of information presented.

Include significant other (SO) and family in discussions and conferences, as appropriate.

Provides opportunity to learn information first hand, ask questions, and provide support for client.

Teaching: Disease Process (NIC)

Determine current understanding and perception of diagnosis. Discuss difference between HIV positive status and AIDS.

Provides opportunity to clarify misconceptions and myths and make informed choices. People often believe that if they are positive for the virus, they have AIDS; having accurate information about the difference can alleviate fears and allow for development of an individualized plan of care.

Identify and problem-solve potential or actual barriers to accessing healthcare services.

Transportation, distance, child care, work schedule, homelessness, poverty, and lack of insurance or finances are some of the issues that typically interfere with accessing needed primary care and prophylactic interventions.

Provide information about normal immune system response and how HIV affects it, transmission of the virus, behaviors, and factors believed to increase probability of progression. Encourage questions.

Client needs to be aware of own personal risk and risk to others to make immediate and long-range decisions and establish a basis for goal setting. Also, establishes rapport and provides opportunity to identify concerns and assimilate information.

Review signs and symptoms that could be a consequence of HIV infection—mild fever, anorexia, weight loss, fatigue, night sweats, diarrhea, dry cough, rashes, headaches, and sleep disturbances.

Client may experience an acute illness 2 to 6 weeks after becoming infected; however, it is common for infection to be subclinical, with the individual simply feeling unwell.

Discuss management strategies for persistent signs and symptoms.

Client involvement in care increases cooperation and satisfaction with care.

Identify signs and symptoms that require medical evaluation—persistent fever, increasing cough, swollen lymph glands, profound fatigue unrelieved by rest, weight loss of 10 lb or more in less than 2 months, severe or persistent diarrhea, blurred vision, skin discoloration or rash that persists or spreads, open sores anywhere, and symptoms occurring with medication regimen.

Early recognition of progression of disease and development of opportunistic infections provides for timely intervention and may prevent situations that are more serious. *Note:* Most HIV-positive clients are now on medication regimens (usually at least three drugs) and must adhere to the dosages and schedules, which may be difficult and/or cause side effects that tempt client to alter or discontinue them without notifying the physician.

Stress necessity of regular follow-up care and evaluations, including routine CD4 and HIV-RNA viral load counts, and any change in medication regimen including time, frequency, and side effects.

Even though client may be asymptomatic, periodic evaluation may prevent development of complications, slow the progression of the disease, and assist with treatment decisions. *Note:* Clients who change medication dosage and/or frequency in response to side effects can create problems for medication adjustment later with increased viral load and drug resistance.

Discuss need for regular gynecological examinations.

HIV-positive women experience a high prevalence of Pap smear, vaginal, and cervical abnormalities.

Discuss family planning issues and careful selection of oral contraceptives.

Various antiretroviral drugs have differing effects on ethinyl estradiol (EE), either enhancing or decreasing protective effectiveness.

Provide preconception counseling, giving information about risk of vertical transmission and ways to reduce the possibility of perinatal transmission.

The risk of viral rebound with adverse consequences to the fetus increases in women currently receiving treatment at the time of conception. Research shows that when antiretroviral treatment is initiated early in pregnancy, the neonatal transmission rate has dropped to less than 8% of live births. However, there is a lack of research regarding safety of antiretroviral therapy in pregnancy and its effect on the

ACTIONS/INTERVENTIONS (continued)

RATIONALE (continued)

fetus. The majority of drugs are category C—meaning no clinical trial information for therapy. For newly pregnant women, consider withholding medication until after the first trimester. A few studies have evaluated HSV-2 and viral load in serum and cervicovaginal fluids. HSV-2 positive women who take acyclovir during pregnancy have lower HIV levels.

Refer to Antiretroviral Pregnancy Registry, as appropriate.

Collection of information regarding women and pregnancy will increase data on teratogenic effects of medications and antiretrovirals.

Teaching: Prescribed Medication (NIC)

Review drug therapies, including correct dosing and scheduling, side effects, monitoring tests and techniques, and adverse reactions as appropriate:

These drugs interfere with the HIV replication process, and early treatment may be considered when CD4 count is near 500, even if individual is asymptomatic. *Note:* Medication management of HIV is now more individualized, targeting specific HIV isolates, identifying susceptibility, and so forth.

Nucleoside reverse transcriptase inhibitors (NRTIs): zidovudine/ ZDV (Retrovir, AZT), abacovir (Ziagen), emtricitabine (Emtriva), tenofovir (Viread), and lamivudine/3TC (Epivir)

In the past, zidovudine was given alone and as a first-line treatment. Now the drug is usually given in a three-drug treatment regimen, along with another NRTI and a PI. Zidovudine is, however, safe in preventing perinatal HIV infection, so it is an option for the pregnant client.

PIs, such as tipranavir (Aptivus), indinavir (Crixivan), nelfinevir (Viracept), ritonavir/RTV (Norvir), saquinavir(Invirase), and amprenavir/APV (Agenerase)

When combined with NRTIs, PIs control the HIV-RNA viral load by blocking viral replication at two different target sites in the replication process. Immune function is maintained with early intervention, or improved when initiated later.

Non-nucleoside reverse transcriptase inhibitors (NNRTIs), such as delavirdine (Rescriptor), etravirine (Intelence), nevirapine (Viramune), and efavirenz (Sustiva)

These drugs inhibit viral replication by a different mechanism than NRTIs or PIs. They also are used in combination because using them alone seems to encourage drug resistance.

Entry inhibitors, including fusion inhibitors, such as enfuvirtide (Fuzeon), and maraviroc (Selzentry)

These work by preventing HIV from entering healthy CD4 cells (T cells) in the body.

Anti-infectives, such as trimethoprim-sulfamethoxazole/ TMP/SMX (Bactrim, Septra), azithromycin (Zithromax), clarithromycin (Biaxin), foscarnet (Foscavir), rifabutin (Mycobutin), isoniazid (INH), and pyridoxine (Doxine)

These focus on prevention of commonly occurring opportunistic infections, such as *Pneumocystis carinii* pneumonia (PCP), cytomegalovirus (CMV), *Mycobacterium avium* complex (MAC), or TB, and may prolong general wellness. Primary prophylactic therapy aims to prevent or delay onset of symptoms of reactivated or newly acquired infection. The goal of secondary prophylaxis is to prevent or delay recurrent episodes of particular infection.

Provide information about clinical trials available, as individually appropriate.

Scientific research requires HIV-positive test subjects. Participation may provide individual with a sense of contributing to the body of knowledge or search for a cure in addition to no-cost monitoring and medications for those with limited financial resources.

Provide information about pharmaceutical company assistance programs.

Some medications are provided free or at reduced cost, based on income.

Risk Identification (NIC)

Assess potential for inappropriate or high-risk behavior, such as continued injection drug abuse or unsafe sexual practices. Stress need to avoid use of illicit injected drugs or, if unwilling to abstain, to avoid sharing needles and to clean works with bleach solution, rinsing carefully with water.

High levels of denial, anger, or drug addiction may cause client to continue behaviors that are high risk for spread of the virus. Even moderate changes in lifestyle may reduce exposure to other infective agents that can cause additional stress to the immune system. *Note:* Client may intensify substance abuse as a means of denial. A sense of "not me" can contribute to continuation of risky behaviors.

Recommend exploring drug treatment resources—methadone clinics or substance abuse recovery groups or programs.

May help reduce risk of HIV transmission by reducing injection drug use when client substitutes methadone, recovers from drug use, or learns safer injection and needle use techniques. *Note:* Some women may decrease drug use or be amenable to rehabilitation in an attempt to improve relationships with children or family.

Stress necessity of, and methods for, practicing safer sex at all times.

Limits spread of virus and exposure to other STDs. A person's sexual expression and identity are threatened by the discovery of the diagnosis. Therefore, many individuals with HIV will not reveal status to potential sexual partners, contributing to ongoing transmission. Women may not follow guidelines because partner refuses to use condoms.

(continues on page 706)

ACTIONS/INTERVENTIONS (continued)

Discuss active changes in sexual behaviors that client can make that may satisfy sexual needs.

Provide information about other necessary lifestyle changes and health maintenance factors:

Avoid people with infections.

Exercise within ability, alternate rest periods with activity, and get adequate sleep.

Eat regularly, even if appetite is reduced; try small, frequent meals and snacks high in nutritional value; and discuss ways to control nausea and vomiting and improve appetite.

Practice daily oral hygiene, use a soft toothbrush; examine mouth regularly for sores, white film, or changes in color; and have regular dental checkups every 6 months.

Examine skin for rashes, bruises, and breaks in skin integrity.

Identify additional resources—support groups, peer counselors, mental health professionals, and case managers.

RATIONALE (continued)

Learning alternative forms of expression promotes a sense of responsibility and control. May reduce sexual tensions, promote normalcy in sexual relationships, and reduce fear or guilt related to potential transmission of HIV. *Note:* Clients, particularly women, may fear partner will leave, resulting in loss of love and emotional and financial support.

Evidence suggests that specific dietary and lifestyle factors may slow the progression of HIV infection because they support a healthier immune system.

When the immune system is depressed, the person's ability to fight exposure to common communicable diseases is limited.

Helps manage fatigue; maintains strength and sense of well-being. Exercise has also been shown to stimulate the immune system.

Physical and psychological stressors increase metabolic needs; in addition, side effects of medication, presence of nausea or vomiting, and anorexia often limit oral intake. The result is nutritional deficits that can further impair the immune system.

Poor oral hygiene and dental care can affect oral intake adversely and increase the risk of opportunistic and systemic infections.

May indicate developing complications and increase risk of infection.

Client will experience a variety of emotional and psychological responses to the diagnosis and its consequences and may need additional assistance and periodic reinforcement to promote optimal adjustment. *Note:* In early stages of HIV infection, focus may be on social services (e.g., help with housing, employment, legal issues, and finances). Later, as disease progresses, the emphasis switches to medical and related community services.

NURSING DIAGNOSIS: risk for Social Isolation

Risk factors may include
Altered state of wellness, changes in physical appearance
Perceptions of unacceptable social or sexual behavior, values
Inadequate resources and/or fear of losing personal resources

Possibly evidenced by
(Not applicable; presence of signs and symptoms establishes an *actual* diagnosis)

Desired Outcomes/Evaluation Criteria—Client Will

Social Support (NOC)
Identify stable support system and supportive individual(s).
Use resources for assistance, as appropriate.
Express increased sense of self-esteem.

ACTIONS/INTERVENTIONS

Support System Enhancement (NIC)
Independent
Determine client's response to condition, feelings about self, concerns or fears about response of others, sense of ability to control situation, and sense of hope.

Assess coping mechanisms and previous methods of dealing with life problems.

Discuss concerns regarding employment and leisure involvement. Note potential problems involving finances, insurance, and housing.

Identify availability and stability of support systems including SO, immediate and extended family, and community.

RATIONALE

How the individual accepts and deals with the situation will help decide the plan of care and interventions.

May reveal successful techniques that can be used in current situation.

Clients with this potentially terminal illness, which carries a stigma, face major problems with possible loss of employment, medical insurance, housing, and care sources if they become unable to independently care for themselves.

This information is crucial to help client plan future care.

ACTIONS/INTERVENTIONS (continued)	RATIONALE (continued)
Encourage honesty in relationships, as appropriate.	As a rule, acquaintances do not need to be informed of client's health status. However, information should be shared with close relationships such as SO, family, and sexual partners. Honesty can help identify stable support persons.
Encourage contact with SO, family, and friends.	Many clients fear telling SO, family, and friends for fear of rejection, and some clients withdraw because of tumultuous feelings. Contact promotes sense of support, concern, involvement, and understanding. Supporting loved ones as they learn of the diagnosis is beneficial and can provide optimism for the long term.
Assist client to problem-solve solutions to short-term and/or imposed isolations, such as communicable disease measures or severely compromised immune system.	Anticipatory planning can defuse sense of isolation and loneliness that can accompany these situations.
Help client differentiate between isolation and loneliness or aloneness, which may be by choice.	Provides an opportunity for client to realize the control he or she has to make decisions about the choice to take care of self about these issues.
Be alert to verbal and nonverbal cues, such as withdrawal, statements of despair, and sense of aloneness. Determine presence and level of risk of suicidal thoughts.	Indicators of despair and suicidal ideation may be present. When these cues are acknowledged, client is usually willing to divulge thoughts and sense of isolation and hopelessness.

Collaborative

Identify community resources, self-help groups, and rehabilitation or drug cessation programs, as indicated.	Provides opportunities for resolving problems that may contribute to sense of loneliness and isolation, transmission risks, and sense of guilt.
Refer to psychiatric clinical nurse specialist or psychiatrist, as needed.	May require more in-depth support to deal with feelings and manage difficult situations.

NURSING DIAGNOSIS: **ineffective self Health Management/family Therapeutic Regimen Management**

May be related to
Complexity of healthcare system and access to care, economic difficulties
Complexity of therapeutic regimen—confusing or difficult dosing schedule, duration of regimen
Mistrust of regimen and/or healthcare personnel—client and provider interactions
Health beliefs or cultural influences
Perceived seriousness, susceptibility, or benefits of therapy
Decisional conflicts, powerlessness
Family conflict or crises

Possibly evidenced by
Expressed desire to manage situation more appropriately
Verbalized difficulty with regulation or integration of one or more prescribed regimens for treatment of illness and its effects
Failure to take actions to reduce risk factors for progression of illness and sequelae
Evidence of acceleration of illness symptoms, development of complications

Desired Outcomes/Evaluation Criteria—Client/Family Will

Treatment Behavior: Illness or Injury (NOC)
Identify individual factors affecting management of regimen.
Accept personal responsibility for own actions and participate in problem-solving activities.
Develop contract for care with mutually agreeable goals for treatment and mechanisms for changing or terminating elements of plan.

ACTIONS/INTERVENTIONS	RATIONALE
Patient Contracting (NIC)	
Independent	
Make time to listen to client concerns.	Promotes feelings of value and may identify additional factors that affect outcome of therapy. Timing of teaching needs to consider the stage of acceptance.
Note client's stage of acceptance of the diagnosis: Precontemplation stage	Client has just learned of the diagnosis, and may not be able to participate in any discussions.

(continues on page 708)

Contemplation stage

Client can participate in, and may initiate, discussions of therapy. Encourages individual's responsibility to be involved with planning. Promotes increased sense of control and self-esteem.

Action or maintenance stage

Client is actively involved in understanding and managing own care.

Determine client's and SO's perception or understanding of regimen.

Identifies areas of confusion or conflict or lack of accurate information that may impede cooperation with regimen.

Assess perceived and actual barriers to accessing healthcare services and reasons for deviations from prescribed plan.

Provides opportunity to clarify actual problems and develop alternative plan acceptable to healthcare provider.

Instruct client carefully in all aspects of medication regimen, times, interaction with food, and side effects:

Thorough understanding may enhance cooperation with regimen and help in identifying potential for compromise.

Provide written schedule.

Helpful for keeping track of multiple drugs and changes that occur.

Suggest placing doses of medications in various locations.

When client's routine is stable, and he or she engages in activities away from home, it is helpful to keep a supply of medications in more than one location such as work or home of family and friends.

Recommend various methods to alert client to medication time, such as portable pill container or alarms.

Will assist busy or forgetful client to take medications at appropriate intervals.

Reduce dose frequency and number of pills when possible.

Increases ability to manage treatment regimen with little interference.

Stress importance of keeping healthcare provider informed of concerns and ability to continue prescribed medication regimen.

Drug levels quickly fall below therapeutic levels if one dose is missed. Reduces potential for drug resistance or increased viral load. Poor adherence or factors leading to discontinuation of an antiretroviral medication can impede future attempts to reduce viral load. Suboptimal drug exposure increases the potential for drug resistance.

Negotiate a therapy plan client can commit to. Include routines of awakening, meals, work schedule, and medication side effects.

The more individualized the plan is, the greater probability of adherence. *Note:* New dosing regimens are addressing the issues of pill load or number of pills in each dose, dosing frequency, dietary restrictions, and adverse events, resulting in greater individualization of the medication regimen.

Assist client to develop realistic health goals and incorporate wellness activities and practices—exercise, smoking cessation, nutrition, vitamin supplements—into daily routine.

Multiple responsibilities and demands on the client's time, especially with women, make it appear difficult to include any additional activities of self-care.

Review stress management skills.

Client must balance self-care needs and needs of other family members, which may be conflicting.

Provide anticipatory guidance and possible occurrences and choices, if any, to prevent or delay complications.

Reduces crisis events. Provides time for client to prepare for known, usual, or expected changes. Permits earlier initiation of therapies and decreases disruption of schedule.

Identify adaptive interventions valid for progressive long-term care needs.

Builds on coping strategies already effective for this individual.

Monitor adherence to prescribed medical regimen. Alter plan of care as needed.

Regimen is likely to be complicated and time consuming. Thoughtful changes in plan may help enhance cooperation.

Evaluate short-term side effects and their interference with adherence to the medical regimen.

In the past, symptoms were considered part of having the disease and were accepted. Perception is that the side effect symptoms are the "main" effect. Improved options for better client care include the role of new HIV-1 PIs.

Support System Enhancement (NIC)

Identify potential or actual support person(s). Include in teaching and problem-solving activities, as appropriate.

Helpful in planning for future and current needs of client and family.

Help client develop strategies that can gain supportive persons.

The more support persons there are available, the lower the risk of support burnout.

Collaborative

Identify appropriate women's groups and services, social worker, financial resources, respite care, and other community programs.

Often female clients are single parents and caretakers for family. Groups can provide support and tangible help in dealing with issues of child care, parenting, and what to do when client is too ill to parent.

Refer to counselor, therapist, or spiritual advisor, as appropriate.

Opportunity to discuss concerns and fears may aid in problem-solving solutions and living with required changes.

ACQUIRED IMMUNODEFICIENCY SYNDROME (AIDS)

I. Pathophysiology

a. End result of infection with a retrovirus—the human immunodeficiency virus (HIV)

b. Progression from HIV infection to AIDS is highly variable: It may take weeks to years, with median rate of 9 to 11 years after infection in the absence of antiretroviral therapy (United Nations Programme on HIV/AIDS [UNAIDS] & World Health Organization [WHO], 2007).

c. Defined by the Centers for Disease Control and Prevention (CDC) as presence of HIV infection with at least one other criteria.

   i. CD4 T-cell count below 200 cells/μl

   ii. CD4 T-cell percentage of total lymphocytes at less than 14%

   iii. Presence of opportunistic infection (OIs) or AIDS-defining illness

II. Etiology

a. Primary HIV infection: unprotected sex, anal intercourse, contaminated blood products, occupational exposure

b. OIs are major contributors to morbidity and mortality in the HIV-infected client (Powderly, 1999)—undiagnosed HIV, CD4 T-cell count below 200 cells/μl, not taking antiretrovirals, drug resistance or failure of antiretroviral therapy

   i. Infecting microbes: candidiasis, coccidioidomycosis, cryptococcosis, cryptosporidiosis, cytomegalovirus (CMV), herpes simplex, histoplasmosis, isosporiasis, mycobacterium, *Pneumocystis jiroveci* (*Pneumocystis carinii* pneumonia [PCP]), polyomavirus JC (causes progressive multifocal leukoencephalopathy), salmonella, toxoplasmosis

   ii. Other AIDS-defining illnesses: HIV-related encephalopathy, Kaposi's sarcoma (KS), invasive cervical cancer, Burkitt's lymphoma, wasting syndrome due to HIV

III. Statistics (CDC, 2007)

a. Morbidity: As of 2005, an estimated 984,155 individuals had been diagnosed with AIDS, with 433,760 living with AIDS in the United States.

b. Mortality: In 2005, 17,011 deaths resulted from AIDS in the United States, and there have been more than 550,394 deaths since it was first diagnosed.

c. Cost: Yearly healthcare costs average $34,000 per individual with an AIDS diagnosis, with approximately $24,000 going toward antiretroviral therapy (Saag, 2002).

GLOSSARY

AIDS-defining illnesses: Group of over 20 conditions that, when coupled with a diagnosis of HIV, indicates the individual has progressed to AIDS.

AIDS dementia complex (ADC): Progressive mental disorder with different nervous system and mental symptoms—memory loss, speech problems, inabilty to concentrate, or poor judgment. There may be behavior changes, mood changes, and motor difficulties. ADC is considered an AIDS-defining condition in people with HIV. Also known as HIV-associated dementia.

Antigen: Substance that can stimulate the body to produce antibodies against it. Antigens include bacteria, viruses, pollen, and other foreign materials.

Antiretroviral (ARV): Medication that interferes with the ability of a retrovirus (such as HIV) to make more copies of itself.

Co-infection: Infection with more than one virus, bacterium, or other micro-organism at a given time. For example, an HIV-infected individual may be co-infected with hepatitis C virus (HCV) or tuberculosis (TB).

Combination therapy: Two or more drugs used together to achieve optimal results in controlling HIV infection.

Highly active antiretroviral therapy (HAART): Aggressive anti-HIV treatment, using several antiretroviral drugs at one time. Also known as ART, ARV, and HART.

(text continues on page 710)

Immunomodulators: Drugs that strengthen the immune system and help the body to fight off infections or other diseases that attack people living with HIV/AIDS.

Immunosuppression: Inability of the immune system to function normally. May be caused by drugs, such as

chemotherapy, or result from certain diseases, such as HIV infection.

Retrovirus: Type of virus that stores its genetic information in a single-stranded RNA molecule, then constructs a double-stranded DNA version of its genes using a special enzyme called reverse transcriptase. The DNA copy is then integrated into the host cell's own genetic material.

Care Setting

The interventions listed here are appropriate for community care as well as an inpatient or hospice setting. Most of the signs and symptoms and psychosocial issues happen long before inpatient care, which currently, is usually of very short duration.

Related Factors

End-of-life care/hospice, page 866
Extended care, page 801
Fluid and electrolyte imbalances, page 903
The HIV-positive client, page 697
Psychosocial aspects of care, page 749
Sepsis/septicemia, page 686
Total nutritional support: parenteral/enteral feeding, page 469
Upper gastrointestinal/esophageal bleeding, page 306
Ventilatory assistance (mechanical), page 173

Client Assessment Database

Data depend on the organs and body tissues involved, the current viral load, and the specific OI or cancer.

DIAGNOSTIC DIVISION MAY REPORT	MAY EXHIBIT
ACTIVITY/REST • Reduced tolerance for usual activities, progressing to profound fatigue and malaise • Weakness • Altered sleep patterns	• Muscle weakness, wasting of muscle mass • Physiological response to activity— changes in blood pressure (BP), heart rate, and respirations
CIRCULATION • Slow healing (if anemic) • Bruising or bleeding with minor injury	• Tachycardia, postural BP changes • Decreased peripheral pulse volume • Pallor or cyanosis • Delayed capillary refill
EGO INTEGRITY • Stress factors related to lifestyle changes—specifically health-care planning and regimen of multiple medications—losses, including family support, relationships, independence, financial; spiritual concerns, and change in self-concept (loss of control) • Concern about appearance—hair loss, disfiguring lesions, weight loss, altered distribution of body fat associated with protease-inhibiting drug therapy, and wrinkling of skin • Denial of diagnosis • Feelings of hopelessness, helplessness, worthlessness, guilt, depression, and powerlessness	• Denial, anxiety, depression, fear, and withdrawal • Angry behaviors, dejected body posture, crying, and poor eye contact • Failure to keep appointments or multiple appointments for similar symptoms
ELIMINATION • Difficult and painful elimination • Rectal pain, itching • Intermittent, persistent, frequent diarrhea with or without abdominal cramping • Flank pain, burning on urination	• Loose-formed to watery stools with or without mucus or blood; frequent, copious diarrhea • Abdominal tenderness • Rectal, perianal lesions or abscesses • Changes in urinary output, color, or character • Urinary or bowel incontinence

Client Assessment Database (continued)

DIAGNOSTIC DIVISION MAY REPORT (continued)	MAY EXHIBIT (continued)

FOOD/FLUID
- Anorexia, changes in taste of foods; food intolerance
- Nausea or vomiting
- Rapid, progressive weight loss
- Difficulty chewing and swallowing, retrosternal pain with swallowing
- Food intolerance—diarrhea after ingestions of dairy products, nausea, early satiation, or bloating

- Hyperactive bowel sounds
- Abdominal distention
- Thin frame, decreased subcutaneous fat or muscle mass
- Poor skin turgor
- Lesions of the oral cavity, white patches, discoloration
- Poor dental and gum health, loss of teeth
- Edema—generalized, dependent

HYGIENE
- Inability to complete activities of daily living (ADLs) independently

- Deficits in many or all personal care, self-care activities

NEUROSENSORY
- Fainting spells and dizziness
- Headache; stiff neck
- Changes in ability to solve problems, forgetfulness, poor concentration
- Impaired sensation or sense of position
- Muscle weakness, tremors
- Numbness, tingling in extremities
- Changes in vision—light flashes or floaters, photophobia; blurred vision

- Mental status changes ranging from confusion to dementia, delirium with sudden onset
- Forgetfulness, poor concentration, decreased alertness, apathy, psychomotor retardation or slowed responses
- Paranoid ideation, free-floating anxiety, unrealistic expectations
- Abnormal reflexes, decreased muscle strength, ataxic gait
- Fine and/or gross motor tremors, focal motor deficits, hemiparesis
- Seizures
- Retinal hemorrhages and exudates (CMV retinitis); blindness

PAIN/DISCOMFORT
- Generalized or localized pain
- Headache
- Pleuritic chest pain

- Swelling of joints, painful nodules, tenderness
- Decreased range of motion (ROM)
- Gait changes, limp
- Muscle guarding

RESPIRATION
- Frequent, persistent upper respiratory infections (URIs)
- Progressive shortness of breath
- Cough ranging from mild to severe, nonproductive or productive of sputum; spasmodic cough on deep breathing (may be earliest sign of PCP)
- Congestion or tightness in chest
- History of exposure to or prior episode of active TB

- Tachypnea, respiratory distress
- Changes in breath sounds, presence of adventitious breath sounds

SAFETY
- Exposure to infectious diseases, such as TB or sexually transmitted diseases (STDs)
- History of other immune deficiency diseases, such as rheumatoid arthritis, cancer
- History of frequent or multiple blood or blood product transfusions; hemophilia, major vascular surgery, traumatic incident
- History of falls, burns, episodes of fainting, slow-healing wounds
- Easy bruising, prolonged bleeding, and hemorrhage (thrombocytopenia)
- Suicidal or homicidal ideation with or without a plan
- Experiencing anger, disgust, rejection and/or violence from others

- Recurrent fevers, low-grade, intermittent temperature elevations or spikes, night sweats
- Changes in skin integrity—cuts, ulcerations, rashes (eczema), exanthemas, psoriasis; discolorations; changes in size or color of moles; unexplained, easy bruising; multiple injection scars
- Rectal, perianal lesions or abscesses
- Nodules, enlarged lymph nodes in two or more areas of the body—neck, axillae, and groin, for example
- Decline in general strength, muscle tone
- Changes in gait

(continues on page 712)

DIAGNOSTIC DIVISION MAY REPORT (continued)	MAY EXHIBIT (continued)
SEXUALITY • History of high-risk behavior, such as having sex with a partner who is HIV positive, multiple sexual partners, unprotected sexual activity, and anal sex; substance use or abuse, injection drug user • Loss of libido, too sick for sex, afraid to engage in any sexual activities • Inconsistent use of condoms	• Pregnancy or risk for pregnancy (sexually active), pregnancy resulting in HIV-positive infant • Genitalia—herpes, warts, discharge
SOCIAL INTERACTION • Problems related to diagnosis and treatment—loss of family/significant other (SO), friends, support; fear of telling others, fear of rejection; loss of income • Isolation, loneliness, close friends or sexual partners who have died of, or are sick with, AIDS • Questioning of ability to remain independent, unable to plan for needs	• Changes in family or SO interaction pattern • Disorganized activities, difficulty with goal setting
TEACHING/LEARNING • Unaware of HIV infection • Failure to comply with treatment • Continued high-risk behavior (e.g., unchanged sexual behavior or injection drug use) • Injection drug use or abuse, current smoking, alcohol abuse	
DISCHARGE PLAN CONSIDERATIONS • Usually requires assistance with finances, medications and treatments, skin or wound care, equipment, supplies, transportation, food shopping and preparation, self-care, technical nursing procedures, homemaker and maintenance tasks, child care, and changes in living arrangements ❯ Refer to section at end of plan for postdischarge considerations.	

Diagnostic Studies

TEST WHY IT IS DONE	WHAT IT TELLS ME
BLOOD TESTS • *HIV antibody test:* Detects HIV antibodies in the blood. • *Enzyme-linked immunosorbent assay (ELISA):* Sensitive immunoassay that uses an enzyme linked to an antibody or antigen as a marker for the detection of a specific protein. • *Western blot test:* Technique for identifying specific antibodies or proteins in which proteins are separated by electrophoresis.	Antibodies to HIV are produced by the body and can be detected in the blood about 2 to 4 weeks after exposure to the virus. Determines exposure to a particular infectious agent, such as the HIV virus, by identifying antibodies present in a blood sample; however, it is not diagnostic. Confirms presence of HIV in individuals with positive ELISA screening. Based on genetic similarities, the numerous virus strains may be classified into types, groups, and subtypes. *Note:* There are two types of HIV: HIV-1 and HIV-2. Both types are transmitted through sexual contact, through blood, and from mother to child, and they appear to cause clinically indistinguishable AIDS. However, it seems that HIV-2 is less easily transmitted, and the period between initial infection and illness is longer than with HIV-1. Worldwide, the predominant virus is HIV-1 (Noble, 2008).

Diagnostic Studies (continued)

TEST WHY IT IS DONE (continued)	WHAT IT TELLS ME (continued)

VIRAL LOAD TESTS

- *Radioimmunoprecipitation–polymerase chain reaction (RI-PCR):* Detects viral RNA levels as low as 50 copies/mL of plasma.
- *Branched DNA (bDNA):* Currently, the leading indicator of effectiveness of therapy.
- *CD8 CTL (cytopathic suppressor cells):* CD8 CTL have been strongly implicated in the control of HIV-1 replications.
- *CD4 lymphocyte count (previously T4 helper cells):* Used to diagnose HIV infection and progression and to monitor effects of drug therapy.
- *Complete blood count (CBC):* Battery of screening tests, which typically includes hemoglobin (Hgb); hematocrit (Hct); red blood cell (RBC) count, morphology, indices, and distribution width index; platelet count and size; white blood cell (WBC) count and differential.
- *TB skin test/purified protein derivative (PPD):* Antigen used to aid in the diagnosis of TB infection.

- *Sexually transmitted disease (STD) screening tests:* Lifestyle behaviors may increase risk of, or exposure to, infection by STDs.

OTHER DIAGNOSTIC STUDIES

- *Cultures:* Specific cultures (e.g., urine, blood, stool, spinal fluid, lesions, sputum, and secretions) may be done to identify causative organism(s). Sensitivity determines microorganism susceptibility or resistance to specific antimicrobials.
- *Neurological studies—electroencephalogram (EEG), magnetic resonance imaging (MRI), computed tomography (CT) scans of the brain, electromyography (EMG)/nerve conduction studies:* Indicated for persistent headache, changes in mentation, fever of undetermined origin, and/or changes in sensory or motor function.
- *Chest x-rays:* Determines effects of disease process.

- *Pulmonary function tests:* Group of tests (e.g., spirometry, lung volumes, etc.) that measure how well the lungs take in and release air and how well they move oxygen into the blood.
- *Barium swallow, endoscopy, colonoscopy:* Tests for gastrointestinal (GI) function either by direct visualization or imaging studies.
- *Biopsies:* Determines presence of pathology and treatment options.

Determines progression of HIV to AIDS or onset of drug resistance.

Therapy can be initiated, or changes made in treatment approaches, based on rise of viral load or maintenance of a low viral load.
At late stage of infection, CD8 CTL numbers are reduced.

Client with counts below 200 defines progression to AIDS. Levels are measured immediately before and again 4 to 8 weeks after initiation of antiretroviral therapy.
Anemia from blood loss or bone marrow infection (e.g., mycobacterium) and idiopathic thrombocytopenia (anemia occurs in up to 85% of clients with AIDS and may be profound). WBC count is low (leukopenia), and lymphocyte percentage is low (lymphopenia). Neutropenia may be drug induced.
Determines exposure to, or active TB disease. Outside the United States, TB is the leading cause of death among people who are HIV positive (WHO, 2007). *Note:* PPD may be negative because of anergy.
Hepatitis B (HBV) envelope and core antibodies, hepatitis C (HVC), syphilis, and other common STDs (e.g., *Chlamydia,* gonococcus) may be positive.

Done to identify the causative organism causing the OI and to determine best therapies.

Determines effects of HIV infection and/or OIs.

May initially be normal or may reveal progressive interstitial infiltrates secondary to advancing PCP which is the most common opportunistic disease, or other pulmonary complications or disease processes such as TB, spontaneous pneumothorax, and hilar adenopathy.
Useful in early detection of interstitial pneumonias.

May be done to identify OI (e.g., *Candida,* CMV) or to stage KS in the GI system.

May be done for differential diagnosis of KS or other neoplastic lesions.

Nursing Priorities

1. Prevent or minimize development of new infections.
2. Maintain homeostasis.
3. Promote comfort.
4. Support psychosocial adjustment.
5. Provide information about disease process, prognosis, and treatment needs.

Discharge Goals/Goals of Care

1 Infection prevented or resolved.
2. Complications prevented or minimized.
3. Pain and discomfort alleviated or controlled.
4. Dealing with current situation realistically.
5. Diagnosis, prognosis, and therapeutic regimen understood.
6. Plan in place to meet ongoing needs.

NURSING DIAGNOSIS: **risk for Infection [progression to sepsis/onset of new opportunistic infection]**

Risk factors may include
Inadequate primary defenses—broken skin, traumatized tissue, stasis of body fluids
Depression of the immune system, chronic disease, malnutrition, use of antimicrobial agents
Environmental exposure, invasive techniques

Possibly evidenced by
(Not applicable; presence of signs and symptoms establishes an *actual* diagnosis)

Desired Outcomes/Evaluation Criteria—Client Will

Infection Severity (NOC)
Achieve timely healing of wounds or lesions.
Be afebrile and free of purulent drainage or secretions, and other signs of infectious conditions.

Risk Control (NOC)
Identify and participate in behaviors to reduce risk of infection.

ACTIONS/INTERVENTIONS	RATIONALE
Infection Control (NIC)	
Independent	
Assess client knowledge and ability to maintain OI prophylactic regimen.	Multiple medication regimen is difficult to maintain over a long period of time. Clients may adjust medication regimen based on side effects experienced, contributing to inadequate prophylaxis, active disease, and resistance. However, new medication regimens may increase adherence because they require less frequent dosing, fewer pills at each dose, and fewer side effects, thus maximizing quality of life and improving adherence to treatment.
Wash hands before and after all care contacts. Instruct client and SO to wash hands, as indicated.	Reduces risk of cross-contamination.
Provide a clean, well-ventilated environment. Screen visitors and staff for signs of infection and maintain isolation precautions as indicated.	Reduces number of pathogens presented to the immune system and reduces possibility of client contracting a nosocomial infection.
Discuss extent and rationale for isolation precautions and maintenance of personal hygiene.	Promotes cooperation with regimen and may lessen feelings of isolation.
Monitor vital signs, including temperature.	Provides information for baseline and data to track changes. Frequent temperature elevations or onset of new fever indicates that the body is responding to a new infectious process or that medications are not effectively controlling noncurable infections.
Assess respiratory rate and depth; note dry spasmodic cough on deep inspiration, changes in characteristics of sputum, and presence of wheezes or rhonchi. Initiate respiratory isolation when etiology of productive cough is unknown.	Respiratory congestion and distress may indicate developing PCP—the most common opportunistic disease in clients with CD4 count below 200. However, TB is on the rise and other fungal, viral, and bacterial infections may occur that compromise the respiratory system. *Note:* CMV and PCP can reside together in the lungs and, if treatment is not effective for PCP, the addition of CMV therapy may be effective.

ACTIONS/INTERVENTIONS (continued)

Investigate reports of headache, stiff neck, and altered vision. Note changes in mentation and behavior. Monitor for nuchal rigidity or seizure activity.

Examine skin and oral mucous membranes for white patches or lesions. (Refer to ND: actual and/or risk for impaired Skin Integrity; impaired Oral Mucous Membrane.)

Clean client's nails frequently. File, rather than cut, and avoid trimming cuticles.

Monitor reports of heartburn, dysphagia, retrosternal pain on swallowing, increased abdominal cramping, and profuse diarrhea.

Inspect wounds and site of invasive devices, noting signs of local inflammation.

Wear gloves and gowns during direct contact with secretions or excretions, or any time there is a break in skin of caregiver's hands. Wear mask and protective eyewear to protect nose, mouth, and eyes from secretions during procedures (e.g., suctioning) or when splattering of blood may occur.

Dispose of needles and sharps in rigid, puncture-resistant containers.

Label blood bags, body fluid containers, soiled dressings or linens, and package appropriately for disposal per isolation protocol.

Clean up spills of body fluids or blood with bleach solution (1:10); add bleach to laundry.

Collaborative

Administer medications, as indicated, for example:

Nucleoside reverse transcriptase inhibitors (NRTIs): abacavir, lamivudine, zidovudine (Trizivir), zidovudine/ZDV (Retrovir, AZT), abacovir (Ziagen), emtricitabine (Emtriva), and tenofovir (Viread)

PIs, such as lopinavir and ritonavir (Kaletra), tapranavir (Aptivus), indinavir (Crixivan), ritonavir/RTV (Norvir), saquinavir (Invirase), and amprenavir (Agenerase)

Non-nucleoside reverse transcriptase inhibitors (NNRTIs), such as etravirine (Intelence), nevirapine (Viramune), and efavirenz (Sustiva)

Entry inhibitors, including fusion inhibitors, such as enfuvirtide (Fuzeon), maraviroc (Selzentry), and raltegravir (Isentress)

Anti-infectives, such as trimethoprim-sulfamethoxazole (Bactrim), pentamidine (Pentacarinat), flucytosine (Ancobon), and clotrimazole (Femizole)

Refer to and encourage cooperation with local epidemiology agency or public health department.

RATIONALE (continued)

Neurological abnormalities are common and may be related to HIV or secondary infections. Symptoms may vary from subtle changes in mood or sensorium (personality changes or depression) to hallucinations, memory loss, severe dementias, seizures, and loss of vision. Central nervous system (CNS) infections (encephalitis is the most common) may be caused by protozoal and helminthic organisms or fungus.

Oral candidiasis, KS, herpes, CMV, and cryptococcosis are common opportunistic diseases affecting the cutaneous membranes.

Reduces risk of transmission of pathogens through breaks in skin. *Note:* Fungal infections along the nail plate are common.

Esophagitis may occur secondary to oral candidiasis, CMV, or herpes. Cryptosporidiosis is a parasitic infection responsible for watery diarrhea, often more than 15 L/day.

Early identification and treatment of secondary infection may prevent sepsis.

Use of masks, gowns, and gloves is required by the Occupational Safety and Health Administration (OSHA, 1992) for direct contact with body fluids, such as sputum, blood or blood products, semen, or vaginal secretions.

Prevents accidental inoculation of caregivers. Use of needle cutters and recapping is not to be practiced. *Note:* Accidental needle sticks should be reported immediately, with follow-up evaluations done per protocol.

Prevents cross-contamination and alerts appropriate personnel to exercise specific hazardous materials procedures.

Kills HIV and controls other microorganisms on surfaces.

The goal of pharmacotherapy is to inhibit viral replication and to reduce morbidity and development of OIs.

In the past, zidovudine was given alone and as a first-line treatment. Presently the drug is usually given in a three-drug treatment regimen, along with another NRTI and a protease inhibitor (PI) with the combination referred to as HAART.

When combined with NRTIs, PIs control the HIV-RNA viral load by blocking viral replication at two different target sites in the replication process. Immune function is maintained with early intervention, or improved when initiated later.

These drugs inhibit viral replication by a different mechanism than NRTIs or PIs. They also are used in combination to reduce possibility of drug resistance.

These drugs work by preventing HIV from entering healthy CD4 cells, or by blocking enzyme needed for replication.

Early identification and treatment of secondary infection may prevent sepsis.

This is a legal requirement. Accurate information facilitates tracking, disease spread, and groups affected.

NURSING DIAGNOSIS: **risk for deficient Fluid Volume**

Risk factors may include
Excessive losses—copious diarrhea, profuse sweating, vomiting
Hypermetabolic state, fever
Restricted intake—nausea, anorexia, lethargy

Possibly evidenced by
(Not applicable; presence of signs and symptoms establishes an *actual* diagnosis)

(continues on page 716)

Desired Outcomes/Evaluation Criteria—Client Will

Hydration (NOC)
Maintain hydration as evidenced by moist mucous membranes, good skin tugor, stable vital signs, and individually adequate urinary output.

ACTIONS/INTERVENTIONS	RATIONALE
Fluid Management (NIC)	
Independent	
Monitor vital signs, including central venous pressure (CVP) if available. Note hypotension, including postural changes.	Indicators of circulating fluid volume.
Note temperature elevation and duration of febrile episode. Administer tepid sponge baths, as indicated. Keep clothing and linens dry. Maintain comfortable environmental temperature.	Fever is one of the most frequent symptoms experienced by clients with HIV infection. Increased metabolic demands and associated excessive diaphoresis result in increased insensible fluid losses and dehydration.
Assess skin turgor, mucous membranes, and thirst.	Indirect indicators of fluid status.
Measure urinary output and specific gravity. Measure or estimate amount of diarrheal loss. Note insensible losses.	Increased specific gravity and decreasing urinary output reflects altered renal perfusion or circulating volume. *Note:* Monitoring fluid balance is difficult in the presence of excessive GI and insensible losses.
Weigh, as indicated.	Although weight loss may reflect muscle wasting, sudden fluctuations reflect state of hydration. Fluid losses associated with diarrhea can quickly create a crisis and become life threatening.
Monitor oral intake and encourage fluids of at least 2,500 mL/day.	Maintains fluid balance, reduces thirst, and keeps mucous membranes moist.
Make fluids easily accessible to client. Encourage use of fluids that are tolerable to client and that replace needed electrolytes, such as Gatorade or broth.	Enhances intake. Certain fluids such as acidic fruit juices or iced beverages may be too painful to consume because of mouth lesions.
Eliminate foods potentiating diarrhea, such as spicy or high-fat foods, nuts, cabbage, and milk products. Provide lactose-free products, such as Resource or Advera. Adjust rate or concentration of enteral feedings, if indicated.	May help reduce diarrhea. Use of lactose-free products helps control diarrhea in the lactose-intolerant client.
Encourage use of live culture yogurt or an over-the-counter (OTC) product such as *Lactobacillus acidophilus* (Lactaid).	Antibiotic therapies disrupt normal bowel flora balance, leading to diarrhea. *Note:* Must be taken 2 hours before or after antibiotic to prevent inactivation of live culture.
Collaborative	
Administer fluids and electrolytes via feeding tube or intravenously (IV), as appropriate.	May be necessary to support or augment circulating volume, especially if oral intake is inadequate, or nausea or vomiting persists.
Monitor laboratory studies, as indicated, for example: Serum and urine electrolytes	Alerts to possible electrolyte disturbances and determines replacement needs.
Blood urea nitrogen/creatinine (BUN/Cr)	Evaluates renal perfusion and function.
Stool specimen collection	Bowel flora changes can occur with multiple or single antibiotic therapy.
Administer medications, as indicated, for example: Antiemetics, such as prochlorperazine maleate (Compazine)	Reduces incidence of vomiting to reduce further loss of fluids and electrolytes.
Antidiarrheals, such as diphenoxylate (Lomotil), loperamide (Imodium), or paregoric; or antispasmodics, such as mepenzolate bromide (Cantil)	Decreases the amount and fluidity of stool; may reduce intestinal spasm and peristalsis. *Note:* Antibiotics may also be used to treat diarrhea if caused by infection.
Antipyretics, such as acetaminophen (Tylenol)	Helps reduce fever and hypermetabolic response, decreasing insensible losses. *Note:* Studies caution that Tylenol toxicity can occur more frequently in the client with AIDS, so it needs to be used with caution.
Maintain hypothermia blanket if used.	May be necessary when other measures fail to reduce excessive fever and insensible fluid losses.

NURSING DIAGNOSIS: ineffective Breathing Pattern/risk for impaired Gas Exchange

Risk factors may include

Muscular impairment—wasting of respiratory musculature, decreased energy, fatigue, decreased lung expansion

Retained secretions—tracheobronchial obstruction; infectious or inflammatory process; pain

Ventilation perfusion imbalance (PCP, other pneumonias, anemia)

Possibly evidenced by

(Not applicable; presence of signs and symptoms establishes an *actual* diagnosis)

Desired Outcomes/Evaluation Criteria—Client Will

Respiratory Status: Ventilation (NOC)

Maintain effective respiratory pattern.

Experience no dyspnea or cyanosis, with breath sounds and chest x-ray clear or improving and arterial blood gases (ABGs) within client's normal range.

ACTIONS/INTERVENTIONS	RATIONALE
Respiratory Monitoring (NIC)	
Independent	
Auscultate breath sounds, noting areas of decreased or absent ventilation and presence of adventitious sounds—crackles, wheezes, and rhonchi.	Suggests developing pulmonary complications or infections, such as atelectasis or pneumonia. *Note:* PCP is often advanced before changes in breath sounds occur.
Note rate and depth of respiration, use of accessory muscles, increased work of breathing, and presence of dyspnea, anxiety, and cyanosis.	Tachypnea, cyanosis, restlessness, and increased work of breathing reflect respiratory distress and need for increased surveillance or medical intervention.
Assess changes in level of consciousness.	Hypoxemia can result in changes ranging from anxiety and confusion to unresponsiveness.
Investigate reports of chest pain.	Pleuritic chest pain may reflect nonspecific pneumonitis or pleural effusions associated with malignancies.
Ventilation Assistance (NIC)	
Elevate head of bed. Have client turn, cough, and deep breathe as indicated.	Promotes optimal pulmonary function and reduces incidence of aspiration or infection due to atelectasis.
Suction airways as indicated, using sterile technique and observing safety precautions—mask, protective eyewear.	Assists in clearing the ventilatory passages, thereby facilitating gas exchange and preventing respiratory complications.
Allow adequate rest periods between care activities. Maintain a quiet environment.	Reduces oxygen consumption.
Collaborative	
Monitor and graph serial ABGs or pulse oximetry.	Indicators of respiratory status and treatment needs and effectiveness.
Review serial chest x-rays.	Presence of diffuse infiltrates may suggest pneumonia, whereas areas of congestion or consolidation may reflect other pulmonary complications, such as atelectasis or KS lesions.
Assist with and instruct in use of incentive spirometer. Provide chest physiotherapy—percussion, vibration, and postural drainage.	Encourages proper breathing technique and improves lung expansion. Loosens secretions and dislodges mucous plugs to promote airway clearance. *Note:* In the event of multiple skin lesions, chest physiotherapy may be discontinued.
Provide humidified supplemental oxygen via appropriate means—cannula, mask, or intubation with mechanical ventilation.	Maintains effective ventilation and oxygenation to prevent or correct respiratory crisis.
Administer medications, as indicated, for example:	Choice of therapy depends on individual situation and infecting organism(s).
Bronchodilators, expectorants, and cough suppressants	May be needed to improve or maintain airway patency or help clear secretions.
Antimicrobials, such as clarithromycin (Bixian), azithromycin (Zithromaz), or ethambutol (Myambutol)	Bixian or Zithromax may be used prophylactically for prevention of *Mycobacterium avium* complex (MAC) or one drug may be used in combination with Myambutol as treatment of choice for MAC.
Prepare for and assist with procedures as indicated, such as bronchoscopy, lavage, and biopsy.	May be required to clear mucous plugs or obtain specimens for diagnosis.

NURSING DIAGNOSIS: risk for Bleeding

Risk factors may include
Abnormal blood profile—decreased vitamin K absorption, alteration in hepatic function, presence of autoimmune antiplatelet antibodies, malignancies (KS), and/or circulating endotoxins (sepsis)

Possibly evidenced by
(Not applicable; presence of signs and symptoms establishes an *actual* diagnosis)

Desired Outcomes/Evaluation Criteria—Client Will

Risk Control (NOC)
Display homeostasis as evidenced by absence of bleeding.

ACTIONS/INTERVENTIONS	RATIONALE
Bleeding Precautions (NIC)	
Independent	
Avoid injections and rectal temperatures and rectal tubes; administer rectal suppositories with caution.	Protects client from procedure-related causes of bleeding; for example, insertion of thermometers or rectal tubes can damage or tear rectal mucosa. *Note:* Some medications may need to be given via suppository in spite of risk.
Maintain a safe environment—keep all necessary objects and call bell within client's reach and keep bed in low position.	Reduces accidental injury, which could result in bleeding.
Maintain bedrest or chair rest when platelets are low, or as individually appropriate. Assess medication regimen.	Reduces possibility of injury, although activity needs to be maintained. May need to discontinue or reduce dosage of a drug. *Note:* Client can have a surprisingly low platelet count without bleeding.
Hematest body fluids—urine, stool, and vomitus—for occult blood.	Prompt detection of bleeding and initiation of therapy may prevent critical loss of blood.
Observe for and report epistaxis, hemoptysis, hematuria, non-menstrual vaginal bleeding, or oozing from lesions, body orifices, or IV insertion sites.	Spontaneous bleeding may indicate development of disseminated intravascular coagulation (DIC) or immune thrombocytopenia, necessitating further evaluation and prompt intervention.
Monitor for changes in vital signs and skin color, such as BP, pulse, respirations, and skin pallor or discoloration.	Presence of bleeding or hemorrhage may lead to circulatory failure and shock.
Evaluate change in level of consciousness.	May reflect cerebral bleeding.
Collaborative	
Review laboratory studies, such as Prothrombin time (PT), activated partial thromboplastin time (aPTT), clotting time, platelets, and Hgb and Hct.	Detects alterations in clotting capability; identifies therapy needs. *Note:* Many individuals display platelet counts below 50,000 and may be asymptomatic, necessitating regular monitoring.
Administer blood products, as indicated.	Transfusions may be required in the event of persistent or massive spontaneous bleeding.
Avoid use of aspirin products and nonsteroidal anitinflammatory drugs (NSAIDs), especially in presence of gastric lesions.	These medications reduce platelet aggregation, prolonging the coagulation process, and may cause further gastric irritation, increasing risk of bleeding. *Note:* Aspirin is contraindicated even in the short term because of its nonreversible effect on platelets.

NURSING DIAGNOSIS: imbalanced Nutrition: Less than Body Requirements

May be related to
Inability or altered ability to ingest, digest, and/or metabolize nutrients—nausea, vomiting, hyperactive gag reflex, intestinal disturbances, GI tract infections, fatigue
Increased metabolic rate and nutritional needs (fever, infection)

Possibly evidenced by
Weight loss, decreased subcutaneous fat and muscle mass (wasting)
Lack of interest in food, aversion to eating, altered taste sensation
Abdominal cramping, hyperactive bowel sounds, diarrhea
Sore, inflamed buccal cavity
Abnormal laboratory results—vitamin, mineral, and protein deficiencies, electrolyte imbalances

Desired Outcomes/Evaluation Criteria—Client Will

Nutritional Status (NOC)
Maintain weight or display weight gain toward desired goal.
Demonstrate positive nitrogen balance, be free of signs of malnutrition, and display improved energy level.

ACTIONS/INTERVENTIONS	RATIONALE

Nutritional Monitoring (NIC)

Independent

Assess ability to chew, taste, and swallow.

Lesions of the mouth, throat, and esophagus are often caused by candidiasis, herpes simplex, hairy leukoplakia, or KS and other cancers; and metallic or other taste changes caused by medications may cause dysphagia, limiting client's ability to ingest food and reducing desire to eat.

Auscultate bowel sounds.

Hypermotility of intestinal tract is common and is associated with vomiting and diarrhea, which may affect choice of diet or route. *Note:* Lactose intolerance and malabsorption, such as associated with CMV, MAC, or cryptosporidiosis, contribute to diarrhea and may necessitate change in diet or supplemental formula, such as Advera or Resource.

Weigh, as indicated. Evaluate weight in terms of premorbid weight. Compare serial weights and anthropometric measurements.

Indicator of nutritional needs and adequacy of intake. *Note:* Because of immune suppression, some blood tests normally used for testing nutritional status are not useful.

Note drug side effects.

Prophylactic and therapeutic medications can have side effects affecting nutrition, such as altered taste, nausea, and vomiting associated with ZDV; anorexia, glucose intolerance, or glossitis associated with Bactrim; altered taste and smell, nausea, vomiting, and glucose intolerance associated with Pentam; or elevated lipids and blood sugar secondary to insulin resistance associated with PIs.

Nutritional Therapy (NIC)

Plan diet with client and SO, incorporating foods client likes or food from home. Encourage small, frequent meals and snacks of nutritionally dense foods and nonacidic foods and beverages, with choice of foods palatable to client. Encourage high-calorie, nutritious foods, some of which may be considered appetite stimulants. Note time of day when appetite is best, and try to serve a larger meal at that time.

Including client in planning gives a sense of control of environment and may enhance intake. Fulfilling cravings for desired food may also improve intake. *Note:* In this population, foods with a higher fat content may be recommended as tolerated to enhance taste and oral intake.

Limit food(s) that induce nausea or vomiting or are poorly tolerated by client with mouth sores or dysphagia. Avoid serving very hot liquids and foods. Serve foods that are easy to swallow such as eggs, ice cream, or cooked vegetables.

Pain in the mouth or fear of irritating oral lesions may cause client to be reluctant to eat. These measures may be helpful in increasing food intake.

Schedule medications between meals if tolerated and limit fluid intake with meals, unless fluid has nutritional value.

Gastric fullness diminishes appetite and food intake.

Encourage as much physical activity as possible.

May improve appetite and general feelings of well-being.

Provide frequent mouth care, observing secretion precautions. Avoid alcohol-containing mouthwashes.

Reduces discomfort associated with nausea or vomiting, oral lesions, mucosal dryness, and halitosis. A clean mouth may enhance appetite.

Provide rest period before meals. Avoid stressful procedures close to mealtime.

Minimizes fatigue; increases energy available for work of eating.

Remove existing noxious environmental stimuli or conditions that aggravate gag reflex.

Reduces stimulus of the vomiting center in the medulla.

Encourage client to sit up for meals.

Facilitates swallowing and reduces risk of aspiration.

Record ongoing caloric intake.

Identifies need for supplements or alternative feeding methods.

Collaborative

Review laboratory studies, such as BUN, glucose, liver function studies, electrolytes, protein, and albumin or prealbumin.

Indicates nutritional status and organ function and identifies replacement needs. *Note:* Nutritional tests can be altered because of disease processes and response to some medications or therapies. *Note:* Multiple medications are metabolized by the liver and have potential for synergistic damage.

Maintain nothing by mouth (NPO) status when appropriate.

May be needed to reduce nausea or vomiting.

Insert and maintain nasogastric (NG) tube, as indicated.

May be required to reduce vomiting or to administer tube feedings. *Note:* Esophageal irritation from existing infection, such as *Candida,* herpes, or KS, may provide site for secondary infections or trauma; therefore, NG tube should be used with caution.

Consult with dietitian or nutritional support team.

Provides for diet based on nutritional needs and appropriate route.

(continues on page 720)

ACTIONS/INTERVENTIONS (continued)	RATIONALE (continued)
Administer enteral or parenteral feedings, as indicated.	Enteral feedings are preferred because they cost less and carry less risk of exacerbating endocrine dysfunction than total parenteral nutrition (TPN). However, TPN may be required when oral or enteral feedings are not tolerated. TPN is reserved for those whose gut cannot absorb even an elemental formula, such as Vivonex, or those with severe refractory diarrhea.
Administer medications, as indicated, for example: Antiemetics, such as prochlorperazine (Compazine)	Reduces incidence of nausea and vomiting, possibly enhancing oral intake.
Sucralfate (Carafate) suspension, which is a mixture of Maalox, diphenhydramine (Benadryl), and lidocaine (Xylocaine)	Given with meals—swish and hold in mouth—to relieve mouth pain and enhance intake. Mixture may be swallowed in presence of pharyngeal or esophageal lesions.
Vitamin supplements	Corrects vitamin deficiencies resulting from decreased food intake and/or disorders of digestion and absorption in the GI system. *Note:* Avoid megadoses; suggested supplemental level is two times the recommended daily allowance (RDA).
Appetite stimulants, such as dronabinol (Marinol), megestrol (Megace), or oxandrolone (Oxandrin)	Marinol, an antiemetic, and Megace, an antineoplastic, act as appetite stimulants in the presence of AIDS. Oxandrin is currently being studied in clinical trials to boost appetite and improve muscle mass and strength.
Antidiarrheals, such as diphenoxylate (Lomotil), loperamide (Imodium), or octreotide (Sandostatin)	These drugs inhibit GI motility subsequently decreasing diarrhea. Imodium or Sandostatin is an effective treatment for secretory diarrhea with secretion of water and electrolytes by intestinal epithelium.
Antibiotic therapy, such as ketoconazole (Nizoral) or fluconazole (Diflucan)	These may be given to treat or prevent infections involving the GI tract.

NURSING DIAGNOSIS: **acute/chronic Pain**

May be related to
Tissue inflammation or destruction—infections, internal or external cutaneous lesions, rectal excoriation, malignancies, necrosis
Peripheral neuropathies, myalgias, and arthralgias
Abdominal cramping

Possibly evidenced by
Reports of pain
Self-focusing, narrowed focus, guarding behaviors
Alteration in muscle tone, muscle cramping, ataxia, muscle weakness, paresthesias, paralysis
Autonomic responses, restlessness

Desired Outcomes/Evaluation Criteria—Client Will

Pain Level (NOC)
Report pain relieved or controlled.
Demonstrate relaxed posture and facial expression.
Be able to sleep or rest appropriately.

ACTIONS/INTERVENTIONS	RATIONALE
Pain Management (NIC) *Independent*	
Assess pain reports, noting location, intensity (scale of 0–10), frequency, and time of onset. Note nonverbal cues, such as restlessness, tachycardia, or grimacing.	Indicates need for, and effectiveness of, interventions and may signal development or resolution of complications. *Note:* Chronic pain does not produce autonomic changes; however, acute and chronic pain can coexist.
Encourage client to report pain as it develops rather then waiting until level is severe.	Efficacy of comfort measures and medications is improved with timely intervention.
Encourage verbalization of feelings.	Can reduce anxiety and fear and thereby reduce perception of intensity of pain.
Provide diversional activities, such as reading, visiting, music, and television.	Refocuses attention; may enhance coping abilities.
Perform palliative measures—repositioning, massage, or ROM exercises of affected joints.	Promotes relaxation and decreases muscle tension.

ACTIONS/INTERVENTIONS (continued)	RATIONALE (continued)
Instruct client in, and encourage use of, visualization, guided imagery, progressive relaxation, deep-breathing techniques, meditation, and mindfulness.	Promotes relaxation and feeling of well-being. May decrease the need for opioid analgesics (CNS depressants) when a neurological or motor degenerative process is already involved. May not be successful in presence of dementia, even when dementia is minor. *Note:* Mindfulness is the skill of staying in the here and now.
Provide oral care. (Refer to ND: impaired Oral Mucous Membrane.)	Oral ulcerations or lesions may cause severe discomfort.
Apply warm moist packs to pentamidine injection or IV sites for 20 minutes after administration.	These injections are known to cause pain and sterile abscesses.
Collaborative	
Administer analgesics, antipyretics, or opioid analgesics. Use patient-controlled analgesia (PCA) or provide around-the-clock analgesia with rescue doses, as needed.	Provides relief of pain and discomfort; reduces fever. PCA or around-the-clock medication keeps the blood level of analgesia stable, preventing cyclic undermedication or overmedication.

NURSING DIAGNOSIS: [actual/] risk for impaired Skin Integrity

Risk factors may include
Decreased level of activity or immobility, altered sensation, skeletal prominence, changes in skin turgor
Malnutrition, altered metabolic state

May be related to (actual)
Immunological deficit—AIDS-related dermatitis; viral, bacterial, and fungal infections (e.g., herpes, *Pseudomonas, Candida*); opportunistic disease processes (e.g., KS)
Excretions or secretions

Possibly evidenced by
Skin lesions, ulcerations, decubitus ulcer formation

Desired Outcomes/Evaluation Criteria—Client Will

Risk Control (NOC)
Be free of or display improvement in wound or lesion healing.

Tissue Integrity: Skin and Mucous Membranes (NOC)
Demonstrate behaviors or techniques to prevent skin breakdown and promote healing.

ACTIONS/INTERVENTIONS	RATIONALE
Skin Surveillance (NIC)	
Independent	
Assess skin daily. Note color, turgor, circulation, and sensation. Describe and measure lesions and observe changes.	Establishes comparative baseline providing opportunity for timely intervention.
Provide and instruct in good skin hygiene—wash thoroughly, pat dry carefully, and gently massage with lotion or appropriate cream.	Maintaining clean, dry skin provides a barrier to infection. Patting skin dry instead of rubbing reduces risk of dermal trauma to dry, fragile skin. Massaging increases circulation to the skin and promotes comfort. *Note:* Isolation precautions are required when extensive or open cutaneous lesions are present.
Reposition frequently. Use turn sheet as needed. Encourage periodic weight shifts. Protect bony prominences with pillows, heel and elbow pads, or sheepskin.	Reduces stress on pressure points, improves blood flow to tissues, and promotes healing.
Maintain clean, dry, wrinkle-free linen, preferably soft cotton fabric.	Skin friction caused by movement over wet, wrinkled, or rough sheets leads to irritation of fragile skin and increases risk of infection.
Encourage ambulation as tolerated.	Decreases pressure on skin from prolonged bedrest.
Cleanse perianal area by removing stool with water and mineral oil or commercial product. Avoid use of toilet paper if vesicles are present. Apply protective creams—zinc oxide or A & D ointment.	Prevents maceration caused by diarrhea and keeps perianal lesions dry. *Note:* Use of toilet paper may abrade lesions.
File nails regularly.	Long or rough nails increase risk of dermal damage.
Cover open pressure ulcers with sterile dressings or protective barrier, such as Tegaderm or DuoDerm, as indicated.	May reduce bacterial contamination and promote healing.

(continues on page 722)

Collaborative

Provide foam, flotation, or alternate pressure mattress or bed.

Obtain cultures of open skin lesions.

Apply topical or administer systemic drugs, as indicated.

Reduces pressure on skin, tissue, and lesions, decreasing tissue ischemia.

Identifies pathogens and appropriate treatment choices.

Used in treatment of skin lesions. Use of agents, such as Prederm spray, can stimulate circulation, enhancing healing process. *Note:* When multidose ointments are used, care must be taken to avoid cross-contamination.

Provide wound care, as indicated:
Cover ulcerated KS lesions with wet-to-wet dressings or antibiotic ointment and nonstick dressing such as Telfa.
Use Tegasorb Thin or other absorbing product, as indicated.

Protects ulcerated areas from contamination and promotes healing.

If the wound or ulcer is moist with exudate, these products keep the wound slightly moist with no maceration of periwound tissue.

Refer to physical therapy for regular exercise program.

Promotes improved muscle tone and skin health.

NURSING DIAGNOSIS: impaired Oral Mucous Membrane

May be related to
Immunological deficit, presence of lesion-causing pathogens, such as *Candida,* herpes, KS
Dehydration, malnutrition
Ineffective oral hygiene
Side effects of drugs, chemotherapy

Possibly evidenced by
Open ulcerated lesions, vesicles
Oral pain or discomfort
Stomatitis; leukoplakia, gingivitis, carious teeth

Desired Outcomes/Evaluation Criteria—Client Will

Oral Hygiene (NOC)
Display intact mucous membranes, which are pink, moist, and free of inflammation or ulcerations.

Risk Control (NOC)
Demonstrate techniques to restore or maintain integrity of oral mucosa.

ACTIONS/INTERVENTIONS   **RATIONALE**

Oral Health Restoration (NIC)
Independent

Assess mucous membranes and document all oral lesions. Note reports of pain, swelling, and difficulty with chewing or swallowing.

Provide oral care daily and after food intake, using soft toothbrush, nonabrasive toothpaste, nonalcohol mouthwash, floss, and lip moisturizer.

Rinse oral mucosal lesions with saline or dilute hydrogen peroxide or baking soda solutions.

Suggest use of sugarless gum or candy, or commercial salivary substitute.

Plan diet to avoid salty, spicy, abrasive, and acidic foods or beverages. Check for temperature tolerance of foods. Offer cool or cold smooth foods.

Encourage oral intake of at least 2,500 mL/day.

Encourage client to refrain from smoking.

Edema, open lesions, and crusting on oral mucous membranes and throat may cause pain and difficulty with chewing or swallowing.

Alleviates discomfort, prevents acid formation associated with retained food particles, and promotes feeling of well-being.

Reduces spread of lesions and encrustations from candidiasis and promotes comfort.

Stimulates flow of saliva to neutralize acids and protect mucous membranes. Sorbitol in some artificially sweetened products can increase risk for loose stools.

Abrasive foods may open healing lesions. Open lesions are painful and aggravated by salt, spices, and acidic foods and beverages. Extreme cold or heat can cause pain to sensitive mucous membranes.

Maintains hydration; prevents drying of oral mucous membranes.

Smoke is drying and irritating to mucous membranes.

Collaborative

Obtain culture specimens of lesions.

Administer medications, as indicated, such as nystatin (Mycostatin) or ketoconazole (Nizoral).

Apply mixture of Maalox, diphenhydramine (Benadryl), and lidocaine (Xylocaine) to oral lesions.

Refer for dental consultation, if appropriate.

Reveals causative agents and identifies appropriate therapies.

Specific drug choice depends on particular infecting organism(s) such as *Candida.*

Reduces local pain of *Candida* and other oral lesions.

May require additional therapy to prevent dental losses.

NURSING DIAGNOSIS: Fatigue

May be related to
Decreased metabolic energy production, increased energy requirements (hypermetabolic state)
Overwhelming psychological or emotional demands
Altered body chemistry—side effects of medication, chemotherapy, insulin resistance
Sleep deprivation

Possibly evidenced by
Unremitting, overwhelming lack of energy; inability to maintain usual routines, tiredness
Decreased performance, impaired ability to concentrate, lethargy, listlessness
Disinterest in surroundings

Desired Outcomes/Evaluation Criteria—Client Will

Endurance (NOC)
Report improved sense of energy.
Perform ADLs, with assistance as necessary.
Participate in desired activities at level of ability.

In addition to interventions in CP: HIV-Positive Client, ND: Fatigue.

ACTIONS/INTERVENTIONS	RATIONALE
Energy Management (NIC) *Independent* Recommend scheduling activities for periods when client has most energy. Plan care to allow for rest periods. Involve client and SO in schedule planning.	Planning allows client to be active during times when energy level is higher, which may restore a feeling of well-being and a sense of control. Frequent rest periods are needed to restore or conserve energy.
Encourage client to do whatever possible, such as perform self-care, sit in chair, or take short walks. Provide assistance, as needed. Increase activity level, as indicated.	Prevents severe deconditioning, and may conserve strength, increase stamina, and enable client to become more active. *Note:* Weakness may make ADLs almost impossible for client to complete.
Monitor physiological response to activity, such as changes in BP, respiratory rate, or heart rate.	Tolerance varies greatly, depending on the stage of the disease process, nutrition state, fluid balance, and number and type of opportunistic diseases.
Collaborative Refer to physical and/or occupational therapy.	Programmed daily exercises and activities help client maintain or increase strength and muscle tone and enhance sense of well-being.
Refer to community resources, such as grocery delivery, Meals on Wheels, house cleaning or home maintenance services, or home-care agency.	Provides assistance in areas of individual need as ability to care for self becomes more difficult.
Provide supplemental oxygen, as indicated.	Presence of anemia and hypoxemia reduces oxygen available for cellular uptake and contributes to fatigue.

NURSING DIAGNOSIS: disturbed Thought Processes

May be related to
Hypoxemia, CNS infection by HIV, brain malignancies, and/or disseminated systemic OI, stroke, vasculitis
Alteration of drug metabolism or excretion, accumulation of toxic elements, renal failure, severe electrolyte imbalance, hepatic insufficiency

Possibly evidenced by
Altered attention span; distractibility
Memory deficit
Disorientation; cognitive dissonance; delusional thinking
Sleep disturbances
Impaired ability to make decisions or problem-solve; inability to follow complex commands and mental tasks, loss of impulse control

Desired Outcomes/Evaluation Criteria—Client Will

Cognition (NOC)
Maintain usual reality orientation and optimal cognitive functioning.

ACTIONS/INTERVENTIONS	RATIONALE

Cognitive Stimulation (NIC)

Independent

Assess mental and neurological status using appropriate tools.

Establishes functional level at time of admission and provides baseline for future comparison.

Consider effects of emotional distress, such as anxiety, grief, and anger.

May contribute to reduced alertness, confusion, withdrawal, and hypoactivity, requiring further evaluation and intervention.

Monitor medication regimen and usage.

Actions and interactions of various medications, prolonged drug half-life, and altered excretion rates result in cumulative effects, potentiating risk of toxic reactions. Some drugs may have adverse side effects, such as haloperidol (Haldol), which can seriously impair motor function in clients with AIDS dementia complex.

Investigate changes in personality, response to stimuli, orientation, and level of consciousness; or development of headache, nuchal rigidity, vomiting, fever, or seizure activity.

Changes may occur for numerous reasons, including development or exacerbation of opportunistic diseases or CNS infection. *Note:* Early detection and treatment of CNS infection may limit permanent impairment of cognition.

Maintain a pleasant environment with appropriate auditory, visual, and cognitive stimuli.

Providing normal environmental stimuli can help in maintaining some sense of reality orientation.

Provide cues for reorientation such as radio, television, calendars, clocks, or a room with an outside view. Use client's name; identify yourself. Maintain consistent personnel and structured schedules, as appropriate.

Frequent reorientation to place and time may be necessary, especially during fever or acute CNS involvement. Sense of continuity may reduce associated anxiety.

Discuss use of datebooks, lists, and other devices to keep track of activities.

These techniques help client manage problems of forgetfulness.

Encourage family/SO to socialize and provide reorientation with current news and family events.

Familiar contacts are often helpful in maintaining reality orientation, especially if client is hallucinating.

Encourage client to do as much as possible such as dressing and grooming and visiting with friends.

Can help maintain mental abilities for longer period.

Provide support for SO. Encourage discussion of concerns and fears.

Bizarre behavior or deterioration of abilities may be very frightening for SO and makes management of care and dealing with situation difficult. SO may feel a loss of control as stress, anxiety, burnout, and anticipatory grieving impair coping abilities.

Provide information about care on an ongoing basis. Answer questions simply and honestly. Repeat explanations as needed.

Can reduce anxiety and fear of unknown; can enhance client's understanding, involvement, and cooperation in treatment when possible.

Cognitive Restructuring (NIC)

Reduce provocative or noxious stimuli. Maintain bedrest in quiet, darkened room, if indicated.

If client is prone to agitation, violent behavior, or seizures, reducing external stimuli may be helpful.

Decrease noise, especially at night.

Promotes sleep, reducing cognitive symptoms and effects of sleep deprivation.

Set limits on maladaptive or abusive behavior; avoid open-ended choices.

Provides sense of security and stability in an otherwise confusing situation.

Maintain safe environment, such as excess furniture out of the way, call bell within client's reach, bed in low position, rails up; restriction of smoking unless monitored by caregiver and SO; seizure precautions; and soft restraints, if indicated.

Decreases the possibility of client injury.

Discuss future expectations and treatment if dementia is diagnosed. Use concrete terms.

Obtaining information that some medications have been shown to improve cognition can provide hope.

Collaborative

Assist with diagnostic studies, such as MRI, CT scan, and spinal tap, and monitor laboratory studies (BUN/Cr, electrolytes, ABGs), as indicated.

Choice of tests or studies depends on clinical manifestations and index of suspicion, because changes in mental status may reflect a wide variety of causative factors, such as CMV meningitis or encephalitis, drug toxicity, electrolyte imbalances, and altered organ function.

Administer medications, as indicated, for example:

Amphotericin B (Fungizone)

Antifungal useful in treatment of cryptococcosis meningitis.

ZDV (Retrovir) and other antiretrovirals alone or in combination

Shown to improve neurological and mental functioning for undetermined period of time.

Antipsychotics, such as haloperidol (Haldol), and/or anti-anxiety agents, such as lorazepam (Ativan)

Cautious use may help with problems of sleeplessness, emotional lability, hallucinations, suspiciousness, and agitation.

Provide controlled environment and behavioral management.

Team approach may be required to protect client when mental impairment, especially delusions, threatens client safety.

Refer to counseling, as indicated.

May help client gain control in presence of thought disturbances or psychotic symptoms.

NURSING DIAGNOSIS: death Anxiety

May be related to
Confronting reality of potentially terminal disease
Anticipating pain, suffering
Concern about impact of death on others; life after death; or encounter with a higher power

Possibly evidenced by
Negative thoughts related to death and dying
Feeling powerless over dying
Fear of pain or suffering related to dying, or prolonged dying
Deep sadness

Desired Outcomes/Evaluation Criteria—Client Will

Acceptance: Health Status (NOC)
Verbalize acceptance of reality of situation.
Express hopefulness and sense of control.
Appear calm and peaceful.
Participate in decisions about care and death.

ACTIONS/INTERVENTIONS	RATIONALE
Dying Care (NIC)	
Independent	
Assure client of confidentiality within limits of situation.	Provides reassurance and opportunity for client to problem-solve solutions to anticipated situations.
Maintain frequent contact with client. Talk with and touch client. Limit use of isolation clothing and masks.	Provides assurance that client is not alone or rejected; conveys respect for and acceptance of the person, fostering trust.
Provide accurate, consistent information regarding prognosis. Avoid arguing about client's perceptions of the situation.	Can reduce anxiety and enable client to make decisions or choices based on realities.
Be alert to signs of denial or depression including withdrawal, or angry, inappropriate remarks. Determine presence of suicidal ideation and assess potential on a scale of 1 to 10.	Client may use defense mechanism of denial and continue to hope that diagnosis is inaccurate. Feelings of guilt and spiritual distress may cause client to become withdrawn and believe that suicide is a viable alternative. Although client may be too "sick" to have enough energy to implement thoughts, ideation must be taken seriously and appropriate intervention initiated.
Provide open environment in which client feels safe to discuss feelings or to refrain from talking.	Helps client feel accepted in present condition without feeling judged and promotes sense of dignity and control.
Permit expressions of anger, fear, and despair without confrontation. Give information that feelings are normal and are to be appropriately expressed.	Acceptance of feelings allows client to begin to deal with situation.
Recognize and support the stage client and family are at in the grieving process. (Refer to CP: Cancer, ND: Grieving.)	Choice of interventions is dictated by stage of grief and coping behaviors, such as anger, withdrawal, and denial.
Explain procedures, providing opportunity for questions and honest answers. Arrange for someone to stay with client during anxiety-producing procedures and consultations.	Accurate information allows client to deal more effectively with the reality of the situation, thereby reducing anxiety and fear of the unknown.
Identify and encourage client interaction with support systems. Encourage verbalization and interaction with family and SO.	Reduces feelings of isolation. If family support systems are not available, outside sources such as local AIDS task force may be needed.
Provide reliable and consistent information and support for SO.	Allows for better interpersonal interaction and reduction of anxiety and fear.
Include SO as indicated when major decisions are to be made.	Ensures a support system for client, and allows SO the chance to participate in client's life. *Note:* If client, family, and SO are in conflict, separate care consultations and visiting times may be needed.
Discuss advance directives and end-of-life desires and needs. Review specific wishes and explain various options clearly.	May assist client and SO to plan realistically for terminal stages and death. *Note:* Many individuals do not understand medical terminology or options such as percutaneous enodoscopic gastrostomy (PEG) tube for short- or long-term feeding and pain management techniques.
Collaborative	
Refer to counseling—psychiatric clinical nurse specialist, psychiatrist, or social worker.	May require further assistance in dealing with diagnosis/prognosis, especially when suicidal thoughts are present.
Provide contact with other resources, as indicated:	
Spiritual advisor	Provides opportunity for addressing spiritual concerns.
Hospice staff	May help relieve anxiety regarding end-of-life care and support for client and SO.

725

NURSING DIAGNOSIS: Social Isolation

May be related to
Altered state of wellness, changes in physical appearance, alterations in mental status
Perceptions of unacceptable social or sexual behavior or values
Inadequate personal resources or support systems
Physical isolation

Possibly evidenced by
Expressed feeling of aloneness imposed by others, feelings of rejection
Absence of supportive SO—partners, family, acquaintances or friends

Desired Outcomes/Evaluation Criteria—Client Will

Social Support (NOC)
Identify supportive individual(s).
Use resources for assistance.

Social Involvement (NOC)
Participate in activities and programs at level of ability and desire.

ACTIONS/INTERVENTIONS	RATIONALE
Support System Enhancement (NIC)	
Independent	
Ascertain client's perception of situation.	Isolation may be partly self-imposed because client fears rejection or reaction of others. Client may experience physical isolation as a result of current medical status and some degree of social isolation secondary to diagnosis of AIDS.
Spend time talking with client during and between care activities. Be supportive, allowing for verbalization. Treat with dignity and regard for client's feelings.	Reduces client's sense of physical isolation and provides positive social contact, which may enhance self-esteem and decrease negative behaviors.
Limit or avoid use of mask, gown, and gloves when possible, such as when talking to client.	When client has assistance from SO, feelings of loneliness and rejection are diminished. However, for some homosexual clients this may be the first time that the family has been made aware that client lives an alternative lifestyle. *Note:* Client may not receive needed support for coping with life-threatening illness and associated grief because of discrimination, fear, and lack of understanding—AIDS hysteria.
Identify support systems available to client, including presence of, relationship with, immediate and extended family.	
Explain isolation precautions and procedures to client and SO.	Gloves, gowns, and mask are not routinely required with a diagnosis of AIDS, except when contact with secretions or excretions is expected. Misuse of these barriers enhances feelings of emotional and physical isolation. When precautions are necessary, explanations help client understand reasons for procedure and provide feeling of inclusion in what is happening.
Encourage open visitation, as appropriate, telephone contacts, and social activities within level of tolerance.	Participation with others can foster a feeling of belonging.
Encourage active role of contact with SO.	Helps reestablish a feeling of participation in a social relationship. May lessen likelihood of suicide attempts.
Develop a plan of action with client that looks at available resources and supports healthy behaviors. Help client problem-solve solution to short-term or imposed isolation.	Having a plan promotes a sense of control over own life and gives client something to look forward to and actions to accomplish.
Be alert to verbal and nonverbal cues including withdrawal, statements of despair, and sense of aloneness. Ask client if thoughts of suicide are being entertained.	Indicators of despair and suicidal ideation are often present. When these cues are acknowledged by the caregiver, client is usually willing to talk about thoughts of suicide and sense of isolation and hopelessness.
Collaborative	
Refer to resources, such as social services counselors and local and national AIDS organizations.	Establishes support systems; may reduce feelings of isolation.
Provide for placement in sheltered community when necessary.	May need more specific care when unable to be maintained at home or when SO cannot manage care.

NURSING DIAGNOSIS: Powerlessness

May be related to
Confirmed diagnosis of a potentially terminal disease, incomplete grieving process
Social ramifications of AIDS; alteration in body image, desired lifestyle; advancing CNS involvement

Possibly evidenced by
Feelings of loss of control over own life
Depression over physical deterioration that occurs despite client compliance with regimen
Anger, apathy, withdrawal, and passivity
Dependence on others for care and/or decision making, resulting in resentment, anger, guilt

Desired Outcomes/Evaluation Criteria—Client Will

Health Beliefs: Perceived Control (NOC)
Acknowledge feelings and healthy ways to deal with them.
Verbalize some sense of control over present situation.
Make choices related to care and be involved in self-care.

ACTIONS/INTERVENTIONS	RATIONALE
Self-Responsibility Facilitation (NIC)	
Independent	
Identify factors that contribute to client's feelings of powerlessness—diagnosis of a terminal illness, lack of support systems, and lack of knowledge about present situation.	Powerlessness is most prevalent in a client newly diagnosed with HIV and when dying with AIDS. Fear of AIDS (by the general population and the client's family/SO) is the most profound cause of client's isolation. Multiple medications and inconvenient dosing regimens can also reduce a person's sense of control, independence, and general quality of life.
Assess degree of feelings of helplessness noting verbal and nonverbal expressions indicating lack of control ("It won't make any difference"), flat affect, or lack of communication.	Determines the status of the individual client and allows for appropriate intervention when client is immobilized by depressed feelings.
Encourage active role in planning activities, establishing realistic and attainable goals. Encourage client control and responsibility as much as possible. Assist client to identify things that client can and cannot control.	May enhance feelings of control and self-worth and sense of personal responsibility.
Encourage advance directives or living will and durable medical power of attorney documents, with specific and precise instructions regarding acceptable and unacceptable procedures to prolong life.	Many factors associated with the treatments used in this debilitating and often fatal disease process place client at the mercy of medical personnel and other unknown people who may be making decisions for and about client without regard for client's wishes, increasing loss of independence.
Discuss desires and assist with planning for funeral, as appropriate.	The individual can gain a sense of completion and value to his or her life when he or she decides to be involved in planning this final ceremony. This provides an opportunity to include things that are of importance to the client.

NURSING DIAGNOSIS: deficient Knowledge [Learning Need] regarding disease, prognosis, current therapies, and self-care needs

May be related to
Lack of exposure or recall, information misinterpretation
Cognitive limitation
Unfamiliarity with information resources

Possibly evidenced by
Questions or request for information, statement of misconception
Inaccurate follow-through of instructions, development of preventable complications

Desired Outcomes/Evaluation Criteria—Client Will

Knowledge: Disease Process (NOC)
Verbalize understanding of condition, disease process, and potential complications.
Identify relationship of signs and symptoms to the disease process and correlate symptoms with causative factors.

Knowledge: Treatment Regimen (NOC)
Verbalize understanding of therapeutic needs.
Correctly perform necessary procedures and explain reasons for actions.
Initiate necessary lifestyle changes and participate in treatment regimen.

ACTIONS/INTERVENTIONS	RATIONALE

Teaching: Disease Process (NIC)
Independent

Review disease process and future expectations.

Provides knowledge base from which client can make informed choices. *Note:* Clients with AIDS are usually aware of the current literature and prognosis unless newly diagnosed.

Determine level of dependence and physical condition. Note extent of care and support available from family and SO and need for supplemental caregivers.

Helps plan amount of care and symptom management required and need for additional resources.

Review modes of transmission of disease, especially if newly diagnosed.

Corrects myths and misconceptions; promotes safety for client and others. Accurate epidemiological data are important in targeting prevention interventions.

Instruct client and caregivers concerning infection control:
Using good hand-washing techniques for everyone including client, family, and caregivers
Using gloves when handling bedpans, dressings, and soiled linens
Wearing mask if client has productive cough
Placing soiled or wet linens in plastic bag and separating them from family laundry; washing with detergent and hot water
Cleaning surfaces with bleach and water solution of 1:10 ratio, disinfecting toilet bowl or bedpan with full-strength bleach
Preparing client's food in clean area; washing dishes and utensils in hot, soapy water—can be washed with the family dishes

Reduces risk of transmission of diseases; promotes wellness in presence of reduced ability of immune system to control level of flora.

Stress necessity of daily skin care, including inspecting skin-folds, pressure points, and perineum, and of providing adequate cleansing and protective measures such as ointments and padding.

Healthy skin provides barrier to infection. Measures to prevent skin disruption and associated complications are critical.

Ascertain that client/SO can perform necessary oral and dental care. Review procedures, as indicated. Encourage regular dental care.

The oral mucosa can quickly exhibit severe, progressive complications. Studies indicate that 65% of AIDS clients have some oral symptoms. Therefore, prevention and early intervention are critical.

Review high-protein and high-calorie dietary needs and ways to improve intake when anorexia, diarrhea, weakness, or depression interfere with intake.

Promotes adequate nutrition necessary for healing and support of immune system and enhances feeling of well-being.

Discuss medication regimen, interactions, and side effects.

Enhances cooperation and increases probability of success with therapeutic regimen.

Provide information about and assist in developing a plan for symptom management that complements medical regimen; for example, client experiencing intermittent diarrhea should take diphenoxylate (Lomotil) before going to a social event.

Quality of life is an important issue in the management of symptoms of severe HIV infection, such as anemia, pain, fatigue, weakness, sleep disorders, or GI symptoms, and/or the side effects of medications. Having a plan provides client with increased sense of control, reduces risk of embarrassment, and promotes comfort.

Stress importance of adequate rest.

Helps manage fatigue; enhances coping abilities and energy level.

Encourage activity and exercise at level that client can tolerate.

Stimulates release of endorphins in the brain, enhancing sense of well-being.

Stress necessity of continued healthcare and follow-up.

Provides opportunity for altering regimen to meet individual changing needs.

Recommend cessation of smoking.

Smoking increases risk of respiratory infections and can further impair immune system.

Identify signs and symptoms requiring medical evaluation: persistent fever or night sweats, swollen glands, continued weight loss, diarrhea, skin blotches or lesions, headache, and chest pain or dyspnea.

Early recognition of developing complications and timely interventions may prevent progression to life-threatening situation.

Identify community resources such as hospice or residential care centers, visiting nurse, home-care services, Meals on Wheels, and peer group support.

Facilitates transfer from acute care setting for recovery and independence, or end-of-life care.

POTENTIAL CONSIDERATIONS in addition to the nursing diagnoses listed in the plan of care.
- *Grieving*—loss of physiological/psychological well-being, social and lifestyle changes, loss of SO and family, probability of premature death
- *ineffective Protection*—abnormal blood profile—anemia, thrombocytopenia, coagulation; inadequate nutrition, drug therapies (e.g., antineoplastic, immune), chronic disease
- *Caregiver Role Strain*—illness severity of care receiver, significant home-care needs, caregiver health impairment, marginal family adaptation or dysfunction, presence of situational stressors, lack of respite for caregiver, caregiver's competing role commitments

RHEUMATOID ARTHRITIS (RA)

I. Pathophysiology

a. Systemic inflammatory process originating in the synovium or synovial fluid involving connective tissue and characterized by destruction and proliferation of the synovial membrane

b. Phagocytosis produces enzymes within the joint, causing inflammation

c. Collagen is destroyed over time and pannus formations occur, narrowing the joint space

d. May result in joint destruction, ankylosis, and deformity, with loss of articulation and joint motion

e. Inflammatory process can also affect the spine, blood vessels, the pleural membrane of the lungs, or the pericardial sac.

f. Condition may be short lived and limited or progressive and severe.

g. Spontaneous remissions and unpredictable exacerbations can occur.

II. Classification (*New York Times*, 2007)

a. Type 1: benign, less common, milder form lasting a few months at most and leaving no permanent disability

b. Type 2: aggressive, more severe, progressive form lasting for years, often for life

III. Etiology (King & Worthington, 2006)

a. Specific cause unknown

b. Associated factors: infectious triggers, genetic predisposition, autoimmune response

c. Other possible factors: more common in females, with ratio to males approximately 3:1; hormone interaction; psychological stress; heavy, long-term smoking; history of blood transfusions

IV. Statistics

a. Morbidity: Prevalence in United States is approximately 1% or 2.1 million adults (King & Worthington, 2006; NIAMS, 2004); peak incidence occurs at ages 40 to 60 years (Gupta & Bhagia, 2006).

b. Mortality: Dependent on overall deterioration in health and secondary organ dysfunction (King & Worthington, 2006); shortens lifespan by 3 to 10 years.

c. Cost: Annual medical costs are approximately $14 billion (Arthritis Foundation and National Pharmaceutical Council, 2002).

GLOSSARY

Pannus: Inflamed synovial granulation tissue reflecting chronic RA.

Phagocytosis: Cellular process involved in the acquisition of nutrients for certain cells; major mechanism used to remove pathogens and cell debris

Raynaud's phenomenon: Condition in which cold temperatures or strong emotions cause blood vessel spasms that block blood flow to the fingers, toes, ears, and nose. This causes intermittent pallor, cyanosis, and then redness before color returns to normal.

Sjögren's syndrome: Chronic disorder that causes insufficient moisture production in certain glands of the body. This leads to impaired secretion of saliva and tears and results in the sicca complex: dry mouth (xerostomia) and dry eyes (keratoconjunctivitis sicca). Secondary Sjögren's syndrome is often associated with other autoimmune disorders, including RA.

Synovial fluid: A thick, straw-colored substance found in small amounts in joints, bursae, and tendon sheaths.

Synovial membrane: Tissue that lines a joint.

Synovitis: Inflammation of the lining of a joint.

Care Settings

Client is treated at community level unless surgical procedure is required.

Related Concerns

Psychosocial aspects of care, page 749
Total joint replacement, page 655

Data depend on severity and involvement of other organs (e.g., eyes, heart, lungs, kidneys), stage (i.e., acute exacerbation or remission), and coexistence of other forms of arthritis and autoimmune diseases.

DIAGNOSTIC DIVISION MAY REPORT	MAY EXHIBIT
ACTIVITY/REST	
• Joint pain and tenderness, usually symmetrical, worsened by movement	• Malaise
• Morning stiffness often lasting 1 hour or more, and that does not improve with movement	• Impaired ROM of joints, particularly hands—fingers and wrist; hips, knees, ankles, elbows, and shoulders
• Generalized weakness (possible effect of anemia)	• Altered gait and posture
• Fatigue; sleep disturbances	• Muscle weakness, contractures and atrophy
• Functional limitations affecting desired lifestyle, leisure time, and occupation	• Joint deformities
CARDIOVASCULAR	
• Changes in color of fingers, toes	• Raynaud's phenomenon
EGO INTEGRITY	
• Acute and/or chronic stress factors, including financial, employment, disability, and relationship	• Dependence on others
• Hopelessness and powerless over incapacitating situation	
• Threat to self-concept, body image, and personal identity	
FOOD/FLUID	
• Inability to consume adequate food and fluids (temporomandibular joint [TMJ] involvement)	• Weight loss
• Anorexia, nausea	• Dryness of oral mucous membranes, decreased oral secretions, and dental caries
HYGIENE	
• Varying difficulty performing self-care activities	
• Dependence on others	
NEUROSENSORY	
• Numbness, tingling of hands and feet	• Symmetrical joint swelling
• Loss of sensation or burning in fingers	
PAIN/DISCOMFORT	
• Acute episodes of pain that may or may not be accompanied by soft tissue swelling in joints	• Red, swollen, hot joints (during acute exacerbations)
• Symmetrical pattern of pain involving joints on both sides of the body	• Pain limiting ability to perform tasks, such as lifting, using hands, or walking
• Chronic aching pain and stiffness with mornings most difficult	
SAFETY	
• Persistent low-grade fever	• Pale, shiny, taut skin
• Dryness of eyes and mucous membranes	• May have skin problems, especially under nails; or skin rash, ulcers, blisters (reflects a more serious case of RA in general)
• Difficulty managing homemaker or maintenance tasks	• Subcutaneous rounded, nontender nodules on pressure points of elbows, feet, knees
	• Decreased muscle strength, altered gait, reduced ROM
	• Palpation of joint reveals spongy tissue
	• Lymph node enlargement
SEXUALITY	
• Difficulty engaging in sexual activity as desired; abstinence	
• Risk for pregnancy complications	

Client Assessment Database (continued)

DIAGNOSTIC DIVISION MAY REPORT (continued)	MAY EXHIBIT (continued)

SOCIAL INTERACTION
- Impaired interactions with family and others
- Change in roles, responsibilities
- Isolation

TEACHING/LEARNING
- Familial history of RA (in juvenile onset)
- Higher risk of heart and lung disorders, including pericarditis, valvular lesions, pulmonary fibrosis, pleuritis
- Use of health foods, vitamins, untested arthritis "cures"

DISCHARGE PLAN CONSIDERATIONS
- May require assistance with transportation, self-care activities, homemaker, maintenance tasks, and changes in physical layout of home

◗ Refer to section at end of plan for postdischarge considerations.

Diagnostic Studies

TEST WHY IT IS DONE	WHAT IT TELLS ME

BLOOD TESTS

- **Inflammatory markers: Cyclic citrullinated peptide antibody test (also called anti-CCP):** Useful in early detection of RA.
- **Rheumatoid factor (RF):** Macroglobulin type of antibody found in blood of individuals with RA. RF antibodies are usually immunoglobulin (Ig) M, but may also be IgG or IgA (Van Leeuwen et al, 2006).

If both anti-CCP and rheumatoid factor (RF) are positive, it is likely the client has a more severe form of the disease.
Positive in 70% to 80% of cases (Matsumoto et al, n.d.), but may become positive later in disease process than anti-CCP.

- **Erythrocyte sedimentation rate (ESR):** Measures the speed at which red blood cells (RBCs) fall to the bottom of a test tube.

A high ESR indicates inflammation, and the higher it is, the more severe the RA. *Note:* Only about 60% of people with RA have an elevated ESR (Arthritis Foundation, 2007).

- **Antinuclear antibody (ANA) titer:** Presence of ANA indicates presence of collagen vascular and immune complex disorders such as RA.
- **C-reactive protein (CRP):** Glycoprotein produced by the body in response to inflammation.
- **Complement C_3 and C_4:** Act as enzymes that aid in the immunologic and inflammatory response and are used to detect autoimmune disease.

Elevated in 30% to 40% of clients with RA (Arthritis Foundation, 2007). Follow-up tests are needed to pinpoint/diagnose the specific rheumatic disorder.
May be elevated with RA, but is not specific to RA.

C_3 and C_4 are increased in acute onset RA. Normal C_4 and decreased C_3 may be present in chronic RA (Van Leeuwen et al, 2006). Immune disorder or exhaustion results in depressed total complement levels.

- **Complete blood count (CBC):** Battery of screening tests, which typically includes hemoglobin (Hgb); hematocrit (Hct); RBC count and morphology, indices, and distribution width index; platelet count and size; white blood cell (WBC) count and differential.

Hgb may be decreased, revealing anemia, which is a common problem in clients with RA. Platelet count may be elevated when inflammation is present or low because of certain medications. WBCs are elevated when infectious processes are present.

OTHER DIAGNOSTIC STUDIES

- **X-rays/radiographs:** Identify early indicators of RA and changes over time.

Reveals soft tissue swelling, erosion of joints, and osteoporosis of adjacent bone as well as progression to bone cyst formation, narrowing of joint space, and subluxation. Concurrent osteoarthritic changes may also be noted.

(continues on page 732)

TEST **WHY IT IS DONE** (continued)	**WHAT IT TELLS ME** (continued)
• *Joint ultrasound; power Doppler ultrasonography (PDUS); quantitative ultrasound (QUS):* Uses high-energy sound waves bounced off internal tissues to detect arthritis by identifying the presence of fluid in the joints.	Can reveal joint inflammation before x-rays show damage and document early evidence of RA. PDUS may be reliable for monitoring inflammatory activity in the joint. QUS, which is used for osteoporosis, can detect bone loss in fingers, which may prove to be a good indicator of early RA.
• *Computed tomography (CT) scan:* X-ray procedure that produces cross-sectional images of the body layer by layer.	Provides preoperative assessment as to the main indications for surgical intervention, namely, neurological deficit and severe pain.
• *Magnetic resonance imaging (MRI):* Diagnostic technique that provides cross-sectional images of structures within the body without x-ray or other forms of radiation.	MRI can detect early inflammation in the hands before it is even visible on x-ray and is particularly accurate at pinpointing synovitis.
• *Direct arthroscopy:* Surgical technique where a tubelike instrument is inserted into a joint to inspect, diagnose, and repair tissues.	Visualization of area reveals bone irregularities and degeneration of joint.
• *Synovial fluid aspirate:* Needle aspiration of joint fluid to note volume, clarity, and presence of cells (red and white cells), crystals, and bacteria to aid in diagnosing joint-related problems and determining treatment options.	May reveal volume greater than normal; may be opaque, cloudy, or yellow due to inflammatory response, bleeding, or degenerative waste products. WBCs and leukocytes are increased, whereas viscosity and complement (C_3 and C_4) are decreased.

Nursing Priorities

1. Alleviate pain.
2. Increase mobility.
3. Promote positive self-concept.
4. Support independence.
5. Provide information about disease process, prognosis, and treatment needs.

Discharge Goals

1. Pain relieved or controlled.
2. Dealing realistically with current situation.
3. Managing activities of daily living (ADLs) by self or with assistance, as appropriate.
4. Disease process, prognosis, and therapeutic regimen understood.
5. Plan in place to meet needs after discharge.

NURSING DIAGNOSIS: **acute/chronic Pain**

May be related to
Injuring agents—distention of tissues by accumulation of fluid/inflammatory process, destruction of joint

Possibly evidenced by
Reports of pain, discomfort; fatigue
Self-narrowed focus
Distraction behaviors; autonomic responses
Guarding, protective behavior

Desired Outcomes/Evaluation Criteria—Client Will

Pain Level (NOC)
Report pain is relieved or controlled.
Appear relaxed and able to sleep, rest, and participate in activities appropriately.

Pain Control (NOC)
Follow prescribed pharmacological regimen.
Incorporate relaxation skills and diversional activities into pain control program.

ACTIONS/INTERVENTIONS	RATIONALE

Pain Management (NIC)

Independent

Investigate reports of pain, noting location, and intensity using a scale of 0 to 10 or similar. Note precipitating factors and nonverbal pain cues.

Recommend or provide firm mattress or bedboard and small pillow. Elevate linens with bed cradle as needed.

Suggest client assume position of comfort while in bed or sitting in chair. Promote bedrest when indicated, but resume movement as soon as possible.

Place and monitor use of pillows, sandbags, trochanter rolls, and splints.

Encourage frequent changes of position. Assist client to move in bed, supporting affected joints above and below, avoiding jerky movements.

Recommend that client take warm bath or shower on arising and/or at bedtime. Apply warm, moist compresses to affected joints several times a day. Monitor water temperature of compresses, baths, and so on.

Provide gentle massage.

Encourage use of stress management techniques, such as progressive relaxation, biofeedback, visualization, guided imagery, self-hypnosis, and controlled breathing. Provide Therapeutic Touch.

Involve client in diversional activities appropriate for individual situation.

Medicate before planned activities and exercises, as indicated.

Monitor for development of skin rash in clients using cyclo-oxgenase-2 (COX-2) inhibitors, especially those allergic to sulfur.

RATIONALE

Self-report should be the primary source of pain assessment in determining pain management needs and effectiveness of program.

Soft or sagging mattress and large pillows prevent maintenance of proper body alignment, placing stress on affected joints. Elevation of bed linens reduces pressure on inflamed, painful joints.

In severe disease or acute exacerbation, total bedrest may be necessary until objective and subjective improvements are noted to limit pain and injury to joint. *Note:* Immobility is known to worsen arthritis pain and stiffness.

Rests painful joints and maintains neutral position. *Note:* Use of splints can decrease pain and may reduce damage to joint; however, prolonged inactivity can result in loss of joint mobility and function.

Prevents general fatigue and joint stiffness. Stabilizes joint, decreasing joint movement and associated pain.

Heat promotes muscle relaxation and mobility, decreases pain, and relieves morning stiffness. Sensitivity to heat may be diminished and dermal injury may occur.

Promotes relaxation and reduces muscle tension.

Promotes relaxation, provides sense of control, and may enhance coping abilities.

Refocuses attention, provides stimulation, and enhances self-esteem and feelings of general well-being.

Promotes relaxation, reduces muscle tension and spasms, facilitating participation in therapy.

Severe, life-threatening skin reactions, such as toxic epidermal necrolysis, Stevens-Johnson syndrome, and erythema multiforme, may develop within the first 2 weeks of treatment or later on, indicating need for prompt discontinuation of medication.

Collaborative

Administer medications, as indicated, for example:

Analgesics: nonsteroidal anti-inflamtory drugs (NSAIDS), such as aspirin and acetaminophen (Tylenol Arthritis, Panadol); ibuprofen (Advil, Motrin); naproxen (Alleve); meloxicam (Mobic), etodolac (Lodine), and nabumetone (Relafen); indomethicin (Indocin) and Ketoprofen (Orudis)

COX-2 inhibitors, such as celecoxib (Celebrex)

Disease-modifying anti-rheumatic drugs (DMARDS), such as:

Methotrexate (Rheumatrex, Trexall), sulfasalazine (Azulfidine), leflunomide (Arava), hydroxychloroquine (Plaquenil), and anakinra (Kineret)

Gold compounds, such as oral gold—auranofin (Ridaura); injectable gold—sodium thiomalate (Myochrysine) or aurothioglucose(Solganal)

Because irreversible joint damage occurs within the first 2 years, early diagnosis and intervention are necessary. Medications are the mainstay of treatment with a goal of (1) managing pain, (2) slowing joint destruction, and (3) preserving joint function.

These drugs control mild to moderate pain and inflammation by inhibition of prostaglandin synthesis and allow for improvement in mobility and function.

The NSAID class of COX-2 inhibitors are also effective in controlling inflammation. However, Celebrex is the only one currently available in the United States due to Food and Drug Administration (FDA) findings of potential for adverse side effects with other COX-2 drugs, including Viox and Bextra (Flynn & Johnson, 2008).

Although both NSAIDs and DMARDs improve symptoms of active RA, only DMARDs have been shown to alter the disease course and improve radiographic outcomes.

Methotrexate is now considered the first-line DMARD agent for most patients with RA and is usually given in combination with two or three other drugs.

Although gold compounds are effective in the treatment of RA, they have been largely replaced by other DMARDs (Matsumoto et al, n.d.) due to their numerous side effects and monitoring requirements, their limited efficacy, and very slow onset of action.

(continues on page 734)

Corticosteroids, such as prednisone (Deltasone) and methylprednisolone (Medrol)	These drugs have both anti-inflammatory and immunoregulatory activity and are useful in early disease as temporary adjunctive therapy. Corticosteroids may also be used as chronic adjunctive therapy in clients with severe disease not well controlled by NSAIDs and DMARDs. These drugs selectively block parts of the immune system.
Biological response modifiers, such as tumor necrosis factor (TNF) inhibitors—etanercept (Enbrel), infliximab (Remicade), and adalimumab (Humira)	TNF is one of the critical cytokines that mediate joint damage and destruction due to its activities on many cells in the joint as well as effects on other organs and body systems. These drugs are similar in their efficacy at decreasing signs and symptoms of RA, slowing or halting radiographic damage, and improving function and quality of life.
T-cell costimulatory blocker, such as Abatacept (Orencia)	This first-in-class agent works by interfering with the interactions between antigen-presenting cells and T lymphocytes and is specifically indicated for use in the client that has not responded well to TNF inhibitors and methotrexate.
B-cell reducer, such as Rituximab (Rituxan)	The depletion of specific B cells has been shown to limit the immune system's attack, effectively reducing pain and symptoms of RA and slowing radiographic progression.
Immunomodulatory and cytotoxic agents, such as Azathioprine (Imuran) and cyclosporine (Neoral)	Immune suppressants may be used for treatment of severe cases of RA when other medications have failed.
Assist with physical therapies, such as paraffin gloves or whirlpool baths.	Provides sustained heat to reduce pain and improve ROM of affected joints.
Apply ice or cold packs when indicated.	Cold may relieve pain and swelling during acute episodes.
Instruct in use and monitor effect of transcutaneous electrical nerve stimulator (TENS) unit, if used.	Constant low-level electrical stimulus blocks transmission of pain sensations.
Assist with other modalities, as indicated, such as blood filtration.	Prosorba Column is a device similar to a kidney dialysis machine that removes substances from blood plasma that contribute to joint swelling and pain. The plasma is then returned to the client's bloodstream. The offending antibodies are gone, decreasing the immune response.
Prepare for surgical interventions, such as synovectomy, total joint replacement, joint fusion; tunnel release procedures; and tendon repair.	Corrective surgical procedures may be indicated to reduce pain and/or improve joint function and mobility.

NURSING DIAGNOSIS: **impaired physical Mobility/impaired Walking**

May be related to
Skeletal deformity
Pain, discomfort
Intolerance to activity, decreased muscle strength

Possibly evidenced by
Reluctance to attempt movement and inability to purposefully move within the physical environment
Limited ROM; impaired coordination; decreased muscle strength, control and mass (late stages)

Desired Outcomes/Evaluation Criteria—Client Will

Mobility (NOC)
Maintain position of function with absence or limitation of contractures.
Maintain or increase strength and function of affected and/or compensatory body part.
Demonstrate techniques and behaviors that enable resumption or continuation of activities.

ACTIONS/INTERVENTIONS

RATIONALE

Exercise Therapy: Joint Mobility (NIC)
Independent

Evaluate and then continuously monitor degree of joint inflammation and pain.	Level of activity and exercise depends on progression or resolution of inflammatory process.
Maintain bedrest or chair rest when indicated. Schedule activities providing frequent rest periods and uninterrupted nighttime sleep.	Person with RA needs a good balance between rest and exercise, with more rest when disease is active and more exercise when it is not. Systemic rest is mandatory during acute exacerbations and important throughout all phases of disease to reduce fatigue and improve strength.

ACTIONS/INTERVENTIONS (continued)	RATIONALE (continued)
Assist with active, or perform passive, ROM and resistive exercises and isometrics when able.	Maintains and may improve joint function, muscle strength, and general stamina. *Note:* Inadequate exercise leads to joint stiffening, whereas excessive activity can damage joints.
Encourage client to maintain upright and erect posture when sitting, standing, and walking.	Maximizes joint function and maintains mobility.
Discuss and provide safety needs, such as raised chairs and toilet seat, use of handrails in tub or shower and toilet, proper use of mobility aids or wheelchair safety.	Helps prevent accidental injuries and falls.

Positioning (NIC)

Reposition frequently using adequate personnel. Demonstrate and assist with transfer techniques and use of mobility aids, such as walker, cane, or trapeze.	Relieves pressure on tissues and promotes circulation. Facilitates self-care and client's independence. Proper transfer techniques prevent shearing abrasions of skin.
Position with pillows, sandbags, or trochanter roll. Provide joint support with splints.	Promotes joint stability, reducing risk of injury, and maintains proper joint position and body alignment, minimizing contractures.
Suggest using small or thin pillow under neck.	Prevents flexion of neck.

Collaborative

Provide foam or alternating pressure mattress.	Decreases pressure on fragile tissues to reduce risks of immobility and development of decubitus ulcers.

Exercise Therapy: Joint Mobility (NIC)

Consult with physical and occupational therapists and vocational specialist.	Helps with formulating exercise and activity program based on individual needs in identifying and reducing impairments in ROM, flexibility, strength and endurance, and to instruct in joint protection strategies and mobility devices and adjuncts.

Self-Care Assistance: Instrumental Activities of Daily Living (IADLs) (NIC)

Determine appropriateness of, and ability to use, scooter or special enhancements to automobile such as hand controls and wide mirrors.	Facilitates movement within the environment, decreases fatigue, and promotes independence.

NURSING DIAGNOSIS: disturbed Body Image/ineffective Role Performance

May be related to
Changes in ability to perform usual tasks
Increased energy expenditure, impaired mobility

Possibly evidenced by
Change in structure or function of affected parts
Negative self-talk, focus on past strength and function, appearance
Change in lifestyle, physical ability to resume roles; loss of employment, dependence on significant other (SO) for assistance
Change in social involvement; sense of isolation
Feelings of helplessness, hopelessness

Desired Outcomes/Evaluation Criteria—Client Will

Psychosocial Adjustment: Life Change (NOC)
Verbalize increased confidence in ability to deal with illness, changes in lifestyle, and possible limitations.
Formulate realistic goals and plans for future.

ACTIONS/INTERVENTIONS	RATIONALE

Body Image [or] Role Enhancement (NIC)
Independent

Encourage verbalization about concerns of disease process and future expectations.	Provides opportunity to identify fears or misconceptions and deal with them directly.
Discuss meaning of loss or change to client and SO. Ascertain how client views self in usual lifestyle functioning, including sexual aspects.	Identifying how illness affects perception of self and interactions with others will determine need for further intervention or counseling.
Discuss client's perception of how SO perceives limitations.	Verbal and nonverbal cues from SO may have a major impact on how client views self.

(continues on page 736)

ACTIONS/INTERVENTIONS (continued)

Acknowledge and accept feelings of grief, hostility, and dependency.

Note withdrawn behavior, use of denial, or overconcern with body and changes.

Set limits on maladaptive behavior. Assist client to identify positive behaviors that will aid in coping.
Involve client in planning care and scheduling activities.

Assist with grooming needs, as necessary.
Give positive reinforcement for accomplishments.

Collaborative
Refer to psychiatric counseling, such as psychiatric clinical nurse specialist, psychiatrist/psychologist, and social worker.
Administer medications as indicated, such as anti-anxiety and mood-elevating drugs.

RATIONALE (continued)

Constant pain is wearing, and feelings of anger and hostility are common. Acceptance provides feedback that feelings are normal.
May suggest emotional exhaustion or maladaptive coping methods, requiring more in-depth intervention and psychological support.
Helps client maintain self-control, enhancing self-esteem.

Enhances feelings of competency and self-worth and encourages independence and participation in therapy.
Maintaining appearance enhances self-image.
Allows client to feel good about self. Reinforces positive behavior. Enhances confidence.

Client/SO may require ongoing support to deal with long-term debilitating process.
May be needed in presence of severe depression until client develops more effective coping skills.

NURSING DIAGNOSIS: **Self-Care Deficit (specify)**

May be related to
Musculoskeletal impairment, decreased strength and endurance, pain on movement
Depression

Possibly evidenced by
Inability to manage ADLs—feeding, bathing, dressing, and/or toileting

Desired Outcomes/Evaluation Criteria—Client Will

Self-Care: Activities of Daily Living (ADLs) (NOC)
Perform self-care activities at a level consistent with individual capabilities.

Self-Care: Instrumental Activities of Daily Living (IADLs) (NOC)
Demonstrate techniques and lifestyle changes to meet self-care needs.
Identify personal and community resources that can provide needed assistance.

ACTIONS/INTERVENTIONS

Self-Care Assistance (NIC)
Independent
Determine usual level of functioning using Functional Level Classification 0–4 for status before onset or exacerbation of illness and potential changes now anticipated.
Maintain mobility, pain control, and exercise program.
Assess barriers to participation in self-care. Identify and plan for environmental modifications.
Allow client sufficient time to complete tasks to fullest extent of ability. Capitalize on individual strengths.

Collaborative
Consult with rehabilitation specialists, such as occupational therapist.

Arrange home-health evaluation before discharge, with follow-up afterward.

Arrange for consult with other agencies, such as Meals on Wheels, home-care service, or nutritionist.

RATIONALE

May be able to continue usual activities with necessary adaptations to current limitations.

Supports physical and emotional independence.
Prepares for increased independence, which enhances self-esteem.
May need more time to complete tasks by self but provides an opportunity for greater sense of self-confidence and self-worth.

Helpful in determining assistive devices to meet individual needs, such as buttonhooks, long-handled shoehorn, reacher, and handheld showerhead.
Identifies problems that may be encountered because of current level of disability. Provides for more successful team efforts with others who are involved in care, such as occupational therapy team.
May need additional kinds of assistance to continue in home setting.

NURSING DIAGNOSIS: **risk for impaired Home Maintenance**

Risk factors may include
Long-term degenerative disease process
Inadequate support systems

Possibly evidenced by
(Not applicable; presence of signs and symptoms establishes an *actual* diagnosis)

Desired Outcomes/Evaluation Criteria—Client Will

Self-Care: Instrumental Activities of Daily Living (IADLs) (NOC)
Maintain safe, growth-promoting environment.
Demonstrate appropriate, effective use of resources.

ACTIONS/INTERVENTIONS	RATIONALE
Home Maintenance Assistance (NIC)	
Independent	
Determine level of physical functioning using Functional Level Classification 0–4.	Identifies degree of assistance and support required. For example, the level 0 client is completely able to perform usual ADLs including self-care, vocational, and avocational, whereas the level 4 client is limited in all these areas and does not participate in activity.
Evaluate environment to assess ability to care for self.	Determines feasibility of remaining in and changing home layout to meet individual needs.
Determine financial resources to meet needs of individual situation. Identify support systems available to client, such as extended family, friends, and neighbors.	Availability of personal resources and community supports will affect ability to problem-solve and choice of solutions.
Develop plan for maintaining a clean, healthful environment, such as sharing of household repairs and other tasks among family members or by contract services.	Ensures that needs will be met on an ongoing basis.
Identify sources for necessary equipment such as lifts, elevated toilet seat, wheelchair, or scooter.	Provides opportunity to acquire equipment before discharge.
Collaborative	
Coordinate home evaluation by occupational therapist and rehabilitation team.	Useful for identifying adaptive equipment and ways to modify tasks to maintain independence.
Identify and meet with community resources, such as visiting nurse, homemaker service, social services, and senior citizens' groups.	Can facilitate transfer to, and support continuation in, home setting.

NURSING DIAGNOSIS: **deficient Knowledge [Learning Need] regarding disease, prognosis, treatment, self-care, and discharge needs**

May be related to
Lack of exposure or recall
Information misinterpretation

Possibly evidenced by
Questions, request for information, statement of misconception
Inaccurate follow-through of instructions, development of preventable complications

Desired Outcomes/Evaluation Criteria—Client Will

Knowledge: Disease Process (NOC)
Verbalize understanding of condition, prognosis, and potential complications.

Knowledge: Treatment Regimen (NOC)
Verbalize understanding of therapeutic needs.
Develop a plan for self-care, including lifestyle modifications consistent with mobility and/or activity restrictions.

ACTIONS/INTERVENTIONS	RATIONALE

Teaching: Disease Process (NIC)

Independent

Review disease process, prognosis, and future expectations.

Provides knowledge base from which client can make informed choices.

Discuss client's role in management of disease process through nutrition, medication, and balanced program of exercise and rest.

Goal of disease control is to suppress inflammation in joints and other tissues to maintain joint function and prevent deformities.

Assist in planning a realistic and integrated schedule of activity, rest, personal care, drug administration, physical therapy, and stress management.

Provides structure and defuses anxiety when managing a complex chronic disease process.

Identify individually appropriate exercise program components, such as swimming, stationary bike, or nonimpact aerobics.

Can increase client's energy level and mental alertness and minimize functional limitations. Program needs to be customized based on joints involved and client's general condition to maximize effect and reduce risk of injury.

Stress importance of continued pharmacotherapeutic management.

Benefits of drug therapy depend on correct dosage, for example, aspirin must be taken regularly to sustain therapeutic blood levels of 18 to 25 mg/dL.

Recommend use of enteric-coated or buffered aspirin or nonacetylated salicylates, such as choline salicylate (Arthropan) or choline magnesium trisalicylate (Trilisate).

These preparations, ingested with food, minimize gastric irritation, reducing risk of gastric bleeding. *Note:* Nonacetylated products have a longer half-life, requiring less frequent administration in addition to producing less gastric irritation.

Suggest taking medications, such as NSAIDs, with meals, milk products, or antacids and at bedtime.

Limits gastric irritation. Reduction of pain at bedtime enhances sleep and increased blood level decreases early-morning stiffness.

Identify adverse drug effects, such as tinnitus, gastric intolerance, gastrointestinal (GI) bleeding, or purpuric rash.

Prolonged, maximal doses of aspirin may result in overdose. Tinnitus usually indicates high therapeutic blood levels. If tinnitus occurs, the dosage is usually decreased by one tablet every 2 to 3 days until it stops.

Stress importance of reading product labels and refraining from over-the-counter (OTC) drug usage without prior medical approval.

Many products, such as cold remedies or antidiarrheals, contain hidden salicylates that increase risk of drug overdose and harmful side effects.

Review importance of balanced diet with foods high in vitamins, protein, and iron.

Promotes general well-being and tissue repair or regeneration.

Encourage obese client to lose weight and supply with weight reduction information, as appropriate.

Weight loss reduces stress on joints, especially hips, knees, ankles, and feet.

Provide information about and resources for assistive devices, such as wheeled dolly or wagon for moving items, pickup sticks, lightweight dishes and pans, raised toilet seat, and safety handlebars.

Reduces force exerted on joints and enables individual to participate more comfortably in needed or desired activities.

Discuss energy-saving techniques, such as sitting instead of standing to prepare meals, shower, shave, or apply make-up.

Prevents fatigue; facilitates self-care and independence.

Encourage maintenance of correct body position and posture both at rest and during activity—keeping joints extended, not flexed, wearing splints for prescribed periods, avoiding remaining in a single position for extended periods, positioning hands near center of body during use, and sliding rather than lifting objects when possible.

Good body mechanics must become a part of client's lifestyle to lessen joint stress and pain.

Review safety issues related to mobility devices, especially electric scooters. Suggest use of a pennant when traveling on open streets.

Ability to travel over uneven surfaces, gravel or soft ground is dependent upon specific scooter model. In addition, speed and safe maneuvering are equally important for the driver and other individuals in the vicinity. A pennant can be seen by other motorists.

Review necessity of frequent inspection of skin and meticulous skin care under splints, casts, and supporting devices. Demonstrate proper padding.

Reduces risk of skin irritation and breakdown.

Discuss necessity of medical follow-up and laboratory studies.

Drug therapy requires frequent assessment and refinement to ensure optimal effect and to prevent overdose or dangerous side effects.

Provide for sexual and childbirth counseling, as necessary.

Information about different positions and techniques and/or other options for sexual fulfillment may enhance personal relationships and feelings of self-worth and self-esteem. *Note:* A large number of clients with RA are in childbearing years and need counseling, support, and medical interventions.

Identify community resources, such as chapters of the National Institute of Arthritis and Muscular and Skin Diseases (NIAMS) and the Arthritis Foundation.

Assistance and support from others promote maximal recovery.

TRANSPLANTATION CONSIDERATIONS— POSTOPERATIVE AND LIFELONG

I. Procedure

a. Transfer of whole or partial organs—including heart, lung, kidney, liver, pancreas, and intestines—and tissues or cells from one location to another

b. Long considered experimental, heart and other transplant procedures are successfully moving to domain of conventional therapy; however, others, such as hand and limb transplants, are still at the experimental stage

c. Bone, bone marrow, heart valve, cartilage, vein, pancreatic islet, cornea, and stem cell transplantations are also performed on a daily basis (Sharma & Unruh, 2006).

  i. Stem cell use is being investigated for treating a wide range of diseases, tissue damage, or both.

  ii. Two types of stem cells: human embryonic stem cells (hES) and adult somatic stem cells (ASSC), which is the source currently being used (Sullivan & Schoonover-Shoffner, 2007)

d. Major concerns (Workman, 2006)

  i. Immunological response of the client to donor tissues and the ability of the immune system to distinguish self from nonself leading to rejection of the transplant

  ii. Special considerations necessitate meticulous measures to prevent infection and identify early signs of rejection.

II. Types—characterized according to the genetic relationship between the donor and recipient or the anatomical site of the implantation

a. Genetic relationship characterized into four classes (Sharma & Unruh, 2006)

  i. Autograft

  ii. Isograft or syngeneic graft

  iii. Allograft or homograft

  iv. Xenograft or heterograft

b. Site of implantation (Sharma & Unruh, 2006)

  i. Orthotropic: tissue implanted in the anatomically correct position

  ii. Heterotopic: relocation of the implant at a site different from the normal anatomy

III. Statistics (U.S. Organ and Procurement Network [OPTN], 2006)

a. Morbidity: In 2006, 28,291 transplants were performed in all categories—heart, lung, kidney, pancreas, liver, intestine, and multi-organ—in the United States; kidney transplant is the most common (greater than 16,000), followed by liver (greater than 6,000) and heart (greater than 2,100).

b. Mortality: Dependent on type of transplant, level of match and human leukocyte antigen (HLA) status, recipient's age at transplant, preoperative condition, presence of comorbidities (Parimon et al, 2005); in 2005, the 90-day mortality for a live donor kidney was 0.7%; intestinal transplant, 8.6% (U.S. Department of Health and Human Services [USDHHS], 2007).

c. Cost: Varies according to procedure; estimated average first-year medical charges per transplant episode for kidney, $246,400; heart, $658,800; intestine, $908,600 (Hauboldt, 2007).

GLOSSARY

Acute rejection: Usually occurs within 3 to 6 months and is diagnosed through laboratory testing and biopsy of the donated organ. Drug management of the host immune responses may limit damage to the organ so that it can be retained.

Allograft or homograft: Organ or tissue donor and recipient are genetically unrelated but belong to the same species.

Antibody: Protein molecule produced by the immune system in response to a foreign body, such as a transplanted organ.

Anti-rejection drugs: Drugs that are used to prevent and/or treat rejection of a transplanted organ; also called immunosuppressive therapies.

Autograft: Donor and recipient are the same individual.

Chronic rejection: May occur months or years after transplant and is similar to chronic inflammation and scarring where functional tissue of the donated organ is replaced by fibrotic tissue, thus hindering organ function. The process is gradual and can be delayed with drug management of host immune responses. However, if fibrosis causes the donated organ to fail, the only cure is reimplantation.

(text continues on page 740)

Donor: Someone from whom at least one organ or tissue is recovered for the purpose of transplantation. A deceased donor is a person who has been declared dead using either brain death or cardiac death criteria, from whom at least one vascularized solid organ is recovered for the purpose of organ transplantation. A living donor is one who donates an organ or segment of an organ for the intent of transplantation.

Graft: Transplanted organ or tissue.

Heterotopic transplantation: Relocation of the implant in the recipient at a site different from the normal anatomy, such as positioning the donor heart so that the chambers and blood vessels of both hearts are joined.

Human leukocyte antigens (HLAs): Genetic markers found on all cells of the body that determine white blood cell (WBC) types. HLA tissue types are used to match donated organs or bone marrow with transplant recipients.

Hyperactive or hyperacute rejection: Process where an antibody-remediated reaction occurs within minutes to hours and causes widespread clotting in the new organ. It occurs most frequently in transplanted kideys and requires removal of the rejected organ.

Immune response: Body's natural defense against foreign objects or organisms, such as bacteria, viruses, or transplanted organs or tissue.

Isograft or syngeneic graft: Donor and recipient are genetically identical.

Match: Compatibility between the donor and the recipient. The more appropriate the match is, the greater the chance of a successful transplant.

Orthotopic transplantation: Donor tissue is implanted in the anatomically correct position in the recipient.

Retransplantation: Due to rejection or failure of a transplanted organ, some patients receive another transplant.

Stem cell: An unspecialized cell that is capable of replicating or self-renewing itself and developing into specialized cells of a variety of cell types.

Xenograft or heterograft: Organ or tissue procured from a different species for transplantation into a human—use of pig heart valve in humans.

Care Setting

Post-intensive care unit (ICU) plan of care addresses early recovery and long-term postdischarge community or clinic follow-up phases.

Related Concerns

Refer to (1) specific surgical plans of care for general considerations (e.g., cardiac surgery) and (2) organ-specific plans (e.g., heart failure, renal failure, cirrhosis, hepatitis) relative to issues of target organ problems following transplantation.

Peritonitis, page 349
Psychosocial aspects of care, page 749
Sepsis/septicemia, page 686
Surgical intervention, page 782
Thrombophlebitis: deep vein thrombosis, page 111

Client Assessment Database

Refer to specific plans of care for data reflecting specific organ failure necessitating transplantation.

DIAGNOSTIC DIVISION MAY REPORT	MAY EXHIBIT
EGO INTEGRITY • Feelings of anxiety, fearfulness • Multiple stressors—impact of condition on personal relationships, ability to perform expected or needed roles, loss of control, required lifestyle changes, financial concerns, cost of procedure and future treatment needs, uncertainty of outcomes, personal mortality, spiritual conflicts, waiting period for suitable donation • Concerns about changes in appearance—bloating, jaundice, major scars, esthetic side effects of immunosuppressant medications • Spiritual questioning, such as "Why me?" or "Why should I benefit from someone else's death?"	• Anxiety, delirium, depression • Cognitive and emotional behavioral changes

Client Assessment Database (continued)

DIAGNOSTIC DIVISION MAY REPORT (continued)	MAY EXHIBIT (continued)

SEXUALITY
- Loss of libido
- Concerns regarding sexual activity

SOCIAL INTERACTIONS
- Reactions of family members
- Conflicts regarding family member(s) ability and willingness to participate—financial, organ or bone marrow donation, postprocedure support
- Concern about benefiting from other person's death
- Concern for family member who must take on new responsibilities as roles shift

TEACHING/LEARNING
- Previous illnesses, hospitalizations, surgeries
- Lack of improvement or deterioration in condition
- Beliefs about transplantation; previous noncompliance with medical treatment
- History of abuse or current dependency on alcohol or other drug(s) resulting in organ failure

DISCHARGE PLAN CONSIDERATIONS
- May need assistance with activities of daily living (ADLs); shopping, transportation, ambulation; managing medication regimen

▶ Refer to section at end of plan for postdischarge considerations.

Diagnostic Studies (dependent on specific organ involvement)

General preoperative screening studies include the following.

TEST WHY IT IS DONE	WHAT IT TELLS ME
BLOOD TESTS • Blood tests to determine blood type, clotting ability, and biochemical status of blood and to gauge renal and liver function. • *Serology screening tests:* Tests for potentially transmissible infections. • *Complete blood count (CBC):* Battery of screening tests, which typically includes hemoglobin (Hgb); hematocrit (Hct); red blood cell (RBC) count, morphology, indices, and distribution width index; platelet count and size; and WBC count and differential.	Help to predict success of procedure and to identify treatment needs. Detect presence and type of hepatitis; HIV, or viruses (e.g., cytomegalovirus [CMV], herpes). Determines adequacy of RBCs, including oxygen-binding capacity that may affect recovery. WBCs, specifically leukocytes (made up of granulocytes, lymphocytes, and monocytes), are crucial to immune defense.
OTHER DIAGNOSTIC STUDIES • *Donor-recipient matching:* Studies include three distinct areas: (1) blood type, (2) tissue type matching, and (3) cross-matching. • *Blood typing:* Initial screening for compatibility, which is repeated just prior to surgery to varify that recipient has not developed new antibodies that would cause rejection of transplant.	There are four major blood types—A, B, AB, and O. Example of a match is type O for both parties; or, recipient with type AB is a positive match for donor with AB, A, B, or O blood type. Another factor, the Rh factor, adds a plus or a minus following the above blood type letter, such as A+ or B−, and so on.

(continues on page 742)

TEST WHY IT IS DONE (continued)	WHAT IT TELLS ME (continued)
• *Tissue matching:* Complex testing relates to genetic matching between donors and recipients. Prior to a graft or transplant, tissue types of the donor and recipient are examined for compatibility by testing antigens, such as HLAs.	A six-antigen match is not always necessary because rejection can be overcome through the use of immunosuppressive drugs. However, if the recipient has already been exposed to one or more of the donor's HLAs, as might occur due to a previous blood transfusion, there may be antibodies already present that would increase the chances of rejection (Twynman, 2003).
• *Cross-matching:* Involves a mixing of cells and serum.	Positive result indicates donor and recipient are incompatible resulting in immediate loss of transplant.
• *Computed tomography (CT)/magnetic resonance imaging (MRI) scans:* Uses x-ray or magnetic energy to generate images of organs.	Reveals status of body systems and organs, including size, shape, and general function of major blood vessels; organ size for best match with donor organ; and potential sources of postoperative complications. Rules out presence of cancer, which would contraindicate transplantation.
• *Total-body bone scan:* Evaluates status of skeletal system.	Determines presence or absence of bone cancer.
• *Electrocardiogram (ECG):* Measures the electrical activity of the heart.	Screens for cardiac dysrhythmias, infarcts, and hypertrophy.
• *Pulmonary function studies (PFTs):* Battery of studies or maneuvers, including spirometry, lung volume measurement, diffusing capacity for carbon monoxide, and arterial blood gases (ABGs).	Determines lung function and ability to exchange oxygen and carbon dioxide.
• *Renal function studies (e.g., intravenous [IV] pyelogram, creatinine clearance):* Determines functional status of kidneys.	Presence of preexisting renal problems may alter options or medication choices as research suggests an increased risk for developing chronic renal failure following nonkidney transplants and progressing to end-stage renal disease even in individuals with normal renal function preoperatively (Ojo, 2003).
• *Dental evaluation:* Rules out oral infection or abscessed teeth.	Dental work may be required prior to transplantation procedures.

Nursing Priorities

1. Prevent infection.
2. Maximize organ function.
3. Promote independent functioning.
4. Support family involvement and coping.

Discharge Goals

1. Free of signs of infection.
2. Signs of rejection absent or controlled.
3. New organ function adequate.
4. Usual activities resumed.
5. Client and family education plan established.
6. Plan in place to meet individual needs following discharge.

NURSING DIAGNOSIS: risk for Infection

Risk factors may include
Medically induced immunosuppression, suppressed inflammatory response
Antibiotic therapy
Invasive procedures, broken skin, traumatized tissue
Effects of chronic and debilitating disease

Possibly evidenced by
(Not applicable; presence of signs and symptoms establishes an *actual* diagnosis)

Desired Outcomes/Evaluation Criteria—Client Will

Infection Severity (NOC)
Be free of signs of infection.
Achieve timely wound healing.

Client/Caregiver Will

Risk Control (NOC)
Demonstrate techniques and lifestyle changes to promote safe environment.

ACTIONS/INTERVENTIONS

Infection Protection (NIC)
Independent

Screen visitors and staff for signs of infection; make sure nurse caring for client with new transplant is not caring for another client with infection. Maintain protective isolation, as indicated.

Demonstrate and emphasize importance of proper hand-washing techniques by client and caregivers.

Inspect all incisions and puncture sites. Evaluate healing progress.

Provide meticulous care of invasive lines, incisions, and wounds. Remove invasive devices as soon as possible.

Encourage deep breathing and coughing.

Provide or assist with frequent oral hygiene.

Obtain culture specimens of wound drainage, as appropriate.

Collaborative

Monitor laboratory tests, such as WBC count and blood glucose.

Administer antimicrobials, as indicated, such as levofloxacin (Levaquin), cefazolin (Ancef), cefepime (Maxipime), vancomycin (Lyphocin), or ciprofloxacin (Cipro).

RATIONALE

Isolation precautions reduce possibility of client's contracting a nosocomial infection. *Note:* Total isolation is usually restricted to clients with lung transplants or individuals with neutropenia.

Hand washing is the first-line of defense against infection and cross-contamination.

Frequent assessment of incisions and puncture sites promotes early identification of onset of infection and prompt intervention.

Minimizes potential for bacteria to reduce exposure and risk of infection.

Mobilizes respiratory secretions and reduces risk of respiratory problems.

Meticulous oral hygiene reduces the risk for opportunistic infections in clients who are on antibiotic therapy or who are immunocompromised.

Identifying organism allows for appropriate treatment.

Elevated WBC count signals inflammation or infection. However, reduced WBC levels may result from severe immunosuppression and viral infection. *Note:* Use of some medications such as corticosteroids increases risk of insulin resistance. Tight glucose control is required to reduce risk of deep wound infections during the postoperative period.

Antibiotics may be used to treat infections; however, they must be closely monitored for side effects and drug interaction with cyclosporine and other immunosuppressants.

NURSING DIAGNOSIS: **Anxiety [specify level]/Fear**

May be related to
Unconscious conflict about essential values and beliefs
Situational crises, interpersonal transmission or contagion
Perceived or actual threat to self-concept, organ rejection, threat of death
Side effects of steroids and/or cyclosporine

Possibly evidenced by
Increased tension, apprehension, uncertainty
Expressed concerns
Somatic complaints
Sympathetic stimulation

Desired Outcomes/Evaluation Criteria—Client Will

Anxiety [or] Fear Self-Control (NOC)
Appear relaxed and report anxiety is reduced to a manageable level.
Verbalize awareness of feelings.
Identify healthy ways to deal with anxiety.
Use resources and support systems effectively.

ACTIONS/INTERVENTIONS

Anxiety Reduction (NIC)
Independent

Discuss client's posttransplant expectations and fears, including physical appearance, lifestyle changes, and concern about recurrence of disease or condition that precipitated the need for the transplant.

RATIONALE

Depending on past experience and exposure to others with transplants, client may have unrealistic ideas and real concerns about what may happen, for example, rejection of received organ, effects of required medications, or limitations associated with immunosuppression. Even with effective preoperative teaching, client will continue to have new concerns or suppressed thoughts and beliefs, which can surface during recovery. For example, client may fear recurrence of disease, such as hepatitis C, in the transplanted organ or chronic rejection.

(continues on page 744)

Encourage client to discuss feelings and concerns about situation and to express fears.	Open discussion helps identify issues and can lead to problem-solving. Client may experience anxiety about many things such as physical limitations, cognitive changes, or role changes in the family. These anxieties change frequently; some are persistent, and new ones arise. Serious anxiety, delirium, and depression are the most commonly reported postoperative psychiatric problems.
Discuss beliefs and concerns that are commonly held regarding source of organ.	Cultural or spiritual beliefs may lead client to question whether organ from someone of another race or particular group may change own sense of self-identity or sexuality. *Note:* Some clients may use denial to deal with concerns about the organ donor. A lack of interest or curiosity about the donor may indicate donor denial.
Answer client's questions about donor honestly, but refrain from providing unrequested information.	Excess information may add to survivor guilt that could distract the client from focusing on business of recovery.
Identify and encourage use of previously successful coping behaviors.	Prolonged nature of stressors can erode coping abilities. Discussion regarding previous successes may promote repetition of more effective behaviors.
Help client focus on one problem at a time.	Dealing with one issue at a time seems to make it more manageable. Provides sense of success and opportunity to build on each success.
Discuss possibility and normalcy of mood swings.	Feelings of euphoria and depression are not uncommon, especially in the early postoperative period, and can be managed to a large extent by presence, quiet environment, and rest. Medication may be required to promote client safety and comfort.
Encourage open communication between significant other (SO)/family and client within safe environment.	Free expression of feelings and beliefs can lead to clarification and problem-solving of different views. When concerns or beliefs are hidden from one another, additional stress and adverse effects may result.
Provide opportunity for client and SO/family to meet with other(s) who have experienced a similar and successful transplant.	Sharing experiences and hearing about successes and universal problems can lessen client's and SO's anxieties, promote hope, and provide a role model.
Identify possible actions to limit physical effects or manifestations of long-term steroid or cyclosporine use.	Learning about clothing styles, makeup techniques, and the use of bleach or mild depilatory to reduce facial hair can enhance client's appearance and reduce anxiety about social rejection.

Collaborative

Refer to spiritual advisor, as indicated.	Facing one's mortality may provoke feelings of anxiety and questions about one's spiritual beliefs and practices.
Refer to social worker and other professionals, as indicated.	Provides assistance with readjustment to life following major life event.

NURSING DIAGNOSIS: risk for ineffective Coping/compromised [or] disabled family Coping

Risk factors may include
Situational crises, family disorganization and role changes
Prolonged disease exhausting supportive capacity of SO and family

Possibly evidenced by
(Not applicable; presence of signs and symptoms establishes an *actual* diagnosis)

Desired Outcomes/Evaluation Criteria—Client/Family Will

Coping [or] Family Coping (NOC)
Assess current situation accurately.
Verbalize awareness of own coping abilities.
Meet psychological needs as evidenced by appropriate expression of feelings, identifying options and resources.

ACTIONS/INTERVENTIONS	RATIONALE
Coping Enhancement [or] Family Integrity Promotion (NIC)	
Independent	
Encourage and support client and family in evaluating lifestyle. Discuss implications for the future.	Transplant clients sometimes cannot evaluate the seriousness of their condition or do not comprehend the risks or benefits involved in transplantation. Acceptance into a transplant program is often a major stressful event as it signals a "last treatment option." Additionally, there may be denial about the impact of long-term post-transplantation treatment requirements—use of immunosuppressant drugs, biopsies, blood tests, and clinic visits.
Assess client's and family's current functional status and note how transplant is affecting ability to cope.	Provides a starting point to identify needs and plan care. The client's SO/family have been dealing with client's chronic disease, experiencing the uncertainty of organ waiting period, and protracted postoperative recovery course. They are the family members who also face a complicated medical regimen after the client's discharge, factors that place demands on their life routines, time, energy, finances, and relationships.
Determine additional outside stressors—family, social, work environment, or healthcare management.	Illness and treatment demands may affect all areas of life, and problems need to be addressed to enable client and SO to manage current situation optimally.
Provide ongoing information about expected progression of recuperation and potential course of recovery.	Knowing what to expect helps individuals cope more effectively and encourages planning for future needs and lifestyle changes. *Note:* These clients normally require a longer postoperative recovery period because of effects of medication regimen, opportunistic infections, or episodes of acute organ rejection.
Discuss normalcy of, and monitor progression through, states of acceptance of transplanted organ:	
Foreign body stage—organ feels strange, separate from own body	Sense that organ is "outside" body can be very frightening, while fixation on organ can be irritating to others. Understanding normalcy of feelings is reassuring. *Note:* Movement through stages is variable and regression is common, especially during early posttransplant period.
Partial internalization stage—protective of organ, restricts movement or activity, excessive concern regarding organ function or fragility	
Complete internalization—acceptance of organ into self-concept, discusses organ only in response to direct questioning	
Have client and SO list previous methods of dealing with life problems and outcomes of actions.	Identifying previously successful life strategies promotes problem-solving in current situation, and allows client to build on past successes.
Active-listen and identify individual's perceptions of what is happening and how transplant has affected view of self and family member.	Helps those involved to recognize own feelings and concerns regarding use of an organ from someone who died.
Encourage discussion between client and family regarding future expectations.	Period of dependence during illness and concerns over possible acute or chronic organ rejection and other life-threatening complications may lead to conflicts regarding client's return to an independent role.
Collaborative	
Involve in individual and family support groups.	Support groups serve as resources for practical advice and emotional sharing.
Refer to spiritual resource and/or psychiatric clinical nurse specialist, psychiatrist, or social worker, as indicated.	Spiritual and psychological guidance may be helpful in resolving lingering or difficult concerns. *Note:* During waiting period for transplant, relationships may be strained due to various stressors.

NURSING DIAGNOSIS: **deficient Knowledge [Learning Need] regarding prognosis, therapeutic regimen, self-care, and discharge needs**

May be related to
Lack of exposure or recall
Information misinterpretation
Unfamiliarity with information resources
Cognitive limitation

(continues on page 746)

deficient Knowledge [Learning Need] regarding prognosis, therapeutic regimen, self-care, and discharge needs (continued)

Possibly evidenced by
Request for information; statement of misconception
Development of preventable complications

Desired Outcomes/Evaluation Criteria—Client Will

Knowledge: Health Behaviors [or] Health Resources (NOC)
Describe measures to reduce individual risk factors to recovery and general well-being.
Initiate necessary lifestyle changes and participate in treatment regimen.
Identify community resources.
Develop plan to meet follow-up care needs.
Assume responsibility for own learning and begin to look for information and ask questions.

For routine postoperative instructions, refer to CP: Surgical Intervention.

ACTIONS/INTERVENTIONS	RATIONALE
Teaching: Disease Process (NIC)	
Independent	
Include SO and family in teaching.	Successful recovery and long-term wellness require a coordinated effort by client and those regularly involved with client.
Provide information via multiple media, including written format, depending on level of comprehension. Include presentations by various members of the transplant team, as appropriate.	Multiple forms of information enhance learning experience and provides references for postdischarge review and recall. Use of team members, such as dietitian and physical and occupational therapists, provides for personalization of teaching plan to meet individual needs.
Review general signs and symptoms of rejection and infection such as general malaise, fatigue, dyspnea, sudden weight gain, fever, chills, sore throat, delayed healing of wound, nausea, vomiting, and syncope. Review indicators specific to transplanted organ (e.g., liver rejection: pain in liver or back, lighter-colored stools, jaundice, dark-colored urine).	Prompt recognition and timely intervention may limit severity of complication. Acute rejection usually develops within days of transplant or may be delayed for a number of months. If detected early, rejection process can be minimized or reversed with changes in drug regimen. *Note:* Chronic rejection developing after months or years is generally irreversible.
Emphasize necessity for, and verify client's ability to adhere to, medical regimen and appropriate follow-up, including periodic laboratory tests such as drug levels, lipid panels, and organ function studies. Routine examinations, including dental and gynecologic, or specialty examinations, such as ophthalmologic or gastroenterologic, may also be required. Anticipate problems and participate in problem-solving with client and SO.	Because the incidence of medication noncompliance is a major cause of posttransplant complications and mortality, the client and SO need to understand that adherence to regimen is imperative—dosing, timing, length of time after transplant, and addition of this medication regimen to others client requires; and physical and cognitive demands of routine. Routine follow-up care by healthcare providers is necessary to maximize general well-being and to monitor effects of long-term medication regimen on other organ systems such as nephrotoxic effects. Specialty examinations aid in monitoring new organ function and effect on other systems. Additionally, steroid use may cause changes in visual acuity or development of cataracts or glaucoma.
Recommend that results of laboratory tests and diagnostic studies done locally be faxed to transplant center.	Long-term care is very complex and requires coordination and cooperation among all healthcare providers.
Discuss need to seek prompt medical attention.	Generally a "wait-and-see" attitude can be detrimental because a delay in treatment could result in organ damage or rejection.
Discuss managing immunosuppressant therapy, including "do's and don'ts" of specific medications, anticipated and adverse effects, interaction with other drugs, appropriate use of over-the-counter (OTC) products; adjustment of prescribed medication dosage during periods of stress, or with gradual decrease in immunosuppression over months or years, as appropriate.	Multiple medications such as a triple therapy regimen of cyclosporine (Sandimmune), tacrolimus (Prograf), and sirolimus (Rapamune) are typically required on an ongoing, lifelong basis to prevent or manage organ rejection. Additional drugs may be needed to manage side and adverse effects of immunosuppressant therapy such as infection, weight gain, nausea, diarrhea, osteoporosis, peptic ulcers, and hypertension.
Encourage client and SO to maintain a working relationship with transplant team. Include family members and caregivers in education sessions and discharge planning, as appropriate.	Good working relationships among the client, SO, family, and transplant team promote understanding, cooperation, goal setting, and achievement of outcomes.

ACTIONS/INTERVENTIONS (continued)	RATIONALE (continued)
Recommend wearing an ID tag, bracelet, or necklace.	In emergencies, ID tag provides immediate information to care providers relative to surgical and transplant history and medication regimen.
Identify community resources, including transplant club or other support groups.	Community resources provide opportunity for client and SO to share experiences with others who are going through the same process. Providing anticipatory guidance may enhance problem-solving.
Discuss self-monitoring routine and record keeping, such as chart temperature per protocol (twice a day before meals, and when not feeling well), weigh daily before breakfast in like clothing using same scale; record blood pressure and pulse, changes in medication dosage, and changes in health status and functional ability.	Self-monitoring helps identify individual needs and onset of preventable complications.
Recommend frequent oral and dental care and periodic visual inspection of oral mucosa and gums.	Immunosuppression increases susceptibility to common opportunistic infections affecting the mouth (e.g., *Candida*, herpes simplex). Ongoing drug regimen can cause hypertrophy of gums (cyclosporine) or ulcerations of the oral mucosa (rampamune).
Review dietary needs. Determine optimal weight and discuss expected changes associated with medication regimen.	Requirements of normal healing, as well as effects of current stress, medications, and preoperative debilitation, can exacerbate nutritional deficiencies, and cause excessive weight loss; however, undesired weight gain can also occur because food tastes better, dietary restrictions are eliminated, and prednisone stimulates appetite.
Identify risk factors and safety concerns relative to infections, such as avoid changing cat litter box or use of live virus vaccines, use gloves when gardening, and take proper care of wounds and tissue trauma.	Awareness of possible risks including unusual sources enables client and family/SO to plan for avoidance. Cat litter can transmit infectious agents such as *Listeria*. Steroid-induced skin fragility increases risk of injury from minor trauma as a result of thinning of the skin and immunosuppression.
Discuss necessity of handling skin carefully, avoiding strong sunlight and using sunblock with sun protection factor (SPF) of 15 or higher.	Steroid therapy results in skin fragility, sun sensitivity, and risk of developing skin cancers.
Review common postoperative care needs, such as routine wound care and need for adequate rest; avoidance of heavy lifting, physical labor or exercise including contact sports, and activities that stretch or put pressure on incision; when and how to resume driving and sexual activity; and dietary and fluid needs or restrictions.	Reduces likelihood of complications, aids client and SO in determining appropriateness of activities, and enhances client's sense of control and personal responsibility for altering activity level.
Provide information about potential sexual dysfunction and encourage open communication for future discussion and support, as needed.	Decreased libido, erectile dysfunction, and impaired orgasmic ability often occur because of medication regimen, low hormone levels, impaired blood flow, fear of harm to transplanted organ, or emotional disturbances. Initially, client may be too focused on survival to address sexual issues or concerns.
Encourage continuation of pre-illness daily routines and activities, as appropriate.	Continuation of pre-illness activities enhances general well-being, promotes focus on returning to "normal life," and reduces the sense of "everything is different now."
Discuss participation in planned endurance and strength training exercise programs and inform about Transplant Olympics, as appropriate and desired.	Endurance and strength training restores strength, promotes sense of well-being and self-esteem, reduces risk of osteoporosis and inappropriate weight gain, and decreases hypertension.
Identify employment concerns and risks specific to particular transplanted organ, job responsibilities, and workplace environment.	Provides opportunity to problem-solve, plan for modifications, or seek alternative options.
Discuss travel needs, including notifying team contact person in advance regarding plans, hand carrying medications when traveling by airplane, and locating transplant center nearest to travel destination before leaving home.	Transplant clients must carefully integrate their health needs when traveling.
Stress importance of notifying future care providers of medication regimen.	Status of immune system functioning may require prophylactic therapy for procedures (such as antibiotics with dental care).

POTENTIAL CONSIDERATIONS following acute hospitalization (depending on client's age, physical condition and presence of complications, personal resources, and life responsibilities)

- *ineffective self Health Management*—postdischarge concern, complexity of therapeutic regimen, side effects of medications, economic difficulties, prolonged nature of treatment
- *risk for Infection*—immunosuppression, antibiotic therapy
- *ineffective Protection*—drug therapies (corticosteroid, immune)
- *deficient Knowledge [Learning Need]*—participation in support groups, ongoing care in collaboration with transplant team, gradual decrease of immunosuppression over months and years

CHAPTER 15

General

PSYCHOSOCIAL ASPECTS OF CARE

I. Mind-Body-Spirit Connection

a. When a physiological response occurs, there is a corresponding psychological response (Anandarajah & Hight, 2001).

   i. Emotional instability associated with steroid therapy or Cushing's syndrome

   ii. Irritability of hypoglycemia

   iii. Anxiety associated with impaired oxygenation

b. Emotional response during illness is of extreme importance.

   i. The stress of illness is well recognized; however, the effect on the individual is unpredictable.

   ii. The client's perception of, and response to, the event may result in unmet psychological needs that drain energy resources needed for healing.

   iii. Values brought to the interactions between clients, families, and healthcare providers affect the care that a client expects and receives.

II. Psychoneuroimmunology (PNI) provides new information about how interactions between the mind and the neuroendocrine and immune systems influence health and healing.

a. Negative emotions or stressful experiences can intensify health threats, contribute to prolonged infection, and result in delayed healing (Kiecolt-Glaser et al, 1984; Kiecolt-Glaser et al, 2002).

   i. Chronic stress: decreased T and B cells, decreased natural killer (NK) cells, increased blood levels of Epstein-Barr virus

   ii. Depression: decreased T cells, decreased number and function of lymphocytes, decreased NK cells

   iii. Grieving: decreased lymphocyte proliferation

b. Positive emotions can enhance immune response, facilitate healing, and slow disease progression.

   i. Personal sharing of traumatic experience: increased lymphocyte response

   ii. Support group intervention: increased NK cells and activity, increased lymphocyte count

   iii. Humor and laughter: increased immunoglobulin A, increased lymphocyte count and activity

GLOSSARY

Active-listening: Reflecting the underlying feelings in the message that is heard.

Eye movement desensitization and reprocessing (EMDR): Information processing psychotherapy technique that integrates elements of psychodynamic, cognitive behavioral, interpersonal, experiential, and body-centered therapies to assist individuals to deal with anxious feelings and stress associated with traumatic memories.

Guided imagery: Method of helping an individual relax by means of guiding them in a vision of tranquil places.

I-messages: Expression of feelings stated as "I feel . . ." in a nonblameful way.

Implosive therapy (flooding): The individual is "flooded" with a continuous presentation of the phobic stimulus until it no longer elicits anxiety.

Labile affect: Excessive emotional reactivity associated with frequent changes or swings in emotions and mood.

Locus of control: Site of control in an individual, which may be internal or external.

Mindfulness: Method of staying in the moment.

Natural killer (NK) cells: Cytotoxic lymphocytes play a major role in suppressing cancer cells and killing cells infected by viruses.

Psychoneuroimmunology (PNI): Field of study that focuses on relationship between psychosocial processes and nervous, endocrine, and immune system functioning.

Psychosocial: Theory of development proposed by Eric Erickson (1963).

Religiosity: Excessive demonstration of/or obsession with religious ideas and behavior.

Therapeutic Touch: Method of healing by use of the hands moving through the energy field.

Care Setting

Any setting in which nursing contact occurs and care is provided.

Related Concerns

This is an aspect of all care and plans of care.

Assessment Factors to Be Considered

SUBJECTIVE	OBJECTIVE
INDIVIDUAL • Level of knowledge and education, how the individual accesses and incorporates information—auditory, visual, kinesthetic • Religious affiliation—church attendance, importance of religion in client's life, belief in life after death • Perception of body and its functions in health, illness, current situation • Past experience with illness, hospitalization, and healthcare systems • Emotional reactions in feeling (sensory) terms, for example, client states, "I feel scared"	• Age and gender • Client's dominant language, literacy, knowledge and use of other languages, style of speech • Patterns of communication with significant others (SOs), with healthcare givers • How is client experiencing illness versus what illness actually is • Emotional response to current treatment or hospitalization • Behavior when anxious, afraid, impatient, withdrawn, or angry
SIGNIFICANT OTHERS (SOs) • Marital status, SOs, nuclear and extended family, recurring or patterned relationships • Client's role in family tasks and functions • How are SOs affected by the illness and prognosis? • Lifestyle preferences to be considered: dietary, spiritual, sexual preference, other community—religious order, commune, retirement center	• Family development cycle—just married; young, adolescent children, leaving or returning home; retired • Interaction processes within the family may not be supportive.
SOCIOECONOMIC • Employment; finances • Environmental factors—residence, work, and recreation; out of usual environment such as on vacation, visiting	• Social class, value system • Social acceptability of disease or condition—sexually transmitted diseases (STDs), HIV, obesity, substance abuse
CULTURAL • Ethnic background, heritage and residence or locale • Beliefs regarding caring and curing • Values related to health and treatment • Cultural factors related to illness in general and to pain response	• Health-seeking behaviors, illness referral system
DISEASE (ILLNESS) • Kind and cause of illness; how has it been treated and how should it be treated? • Anticipated response to treatment; client's and SO's expectations • If terminal illness, what do the client and SO know and anticipate?	• Is this an acute or chronic condition, is it inherited, what is the threat to self or others? • Is the condition "appropriate" to the afflicted individual, for example, multiple sclerosis, diabetes mellitus (DM), cancer (*Note:* Some theories suggest certain personalities are more prone to certain illnesses.) • Illness related to personality factors, such as type A (may be myth or valid relative to management of stressors); high-risk behaviors
NURSE RELATED • Basic knowledge of human responses and how the current situation is related to response of the individual • Basic knowledge of biological, psychological, social, cultural, and religious issues • Knowledge of own value and belief systems, including prejudices and biases	• Knowledge and use of therapeutic communication skills • Willingness to look at own behavior in relation to interaction with others and make changes as necessary • Respect of client's privacy, confidentiality, human needs

Nursing Priorities

1. Encourage effective coping skills of client and SO.
2. Reduce anxiety or fear.
3. Facilitate integration of self-concept and body-image changes.
4. Support grieving process.
5. Promote safe environment and client well-being.

Discharge Goals

1. Client and family dealing realistically with current situation.
2. Anxiety or fear manageable.
3. Progressing through stages of grieving.
4. Safe environment maintained.
5. Plan in place to meet needs after discharge.

NURSING DIAGNOSIS: **ineffective Coping/decisional Conflict (specify)**

May be related to
Situational crises; high degree of threat; severe pain
Age and developmental stage; lack of experience or interference with decision making; inadequate resources or support system available
Inadequate level of confidence in ability to cope, perception of control
Unclear personal values or beliefs; perceived threat to value system
Lack of relevant information; multiple or divergent sources of information
Impairment of nervous system, memory loss, impaired adaptive behaviors or problem-solving skills

Possibly evidenced by
Verbalization of inability to cope or ask for help; feelings of distress while attempting a decision; questioning personal values or beliefs; chronic worry
Vacillation between alternative actions, delayed decision making
Muscular tension, frequent headaches or neckaches, fatigue, insomnia, anxiety, depression; poor concentration
High illness or accident rate; destructive behavior toward self or others; risk taking; overeating, excessive smoking and/or drinking
Alteration in social participation, change in usual communication patterns
Inappropriate use of defense mechanisms; inability to meet role expectations, problem solve

Desired Outcomes/Evaluation Criteria—Client Will

Coping (NOC)
Identify ineffective coping behaviors and consequences.
Verbalize awareness of own coping and problem-solving abilities.
Meet psychological needs as evidenced by appropriate expression of feelings, identification of options, and use of resources.

Decision Making (NOC)
Make decisions and express satisfaction with choices.

ACTIONS/INTERVENTIONS	RATIONALE

Coping Enhancement (NIC)
Independent

Review pathophysiology affecting the client and extent of feelings of hopelessness, helplessness, and loss of control over life; level of anxiety, and perception of situation.

Indicators of degree of disequilibrium and need for intervention to prevent or resolve the crisis. Studies suggest that 20% to 40% of physically ill individuals are depressed (Robinson & Krishnan, 2002). Impairment of normal functioning for more than 2 weeks, especially in presence of chronic condition, may reflect depression, requiring further evaluation. *Note:* In contrast, depression is believed to contribute to the development and progression of some physical illnesses, such as heart or vascular disease or certain viral infections (Thomas, 2005).

Establish therapeutic nurse-client relationship.

Client may feel less inhibited in the context of this relationship to verbalize feelings of helplessness and powerlessness and feel more freedom to discuss changes that may be necessary in the client's life to improve situation.

Note expressions of indecision, dependence on others, and inability to manage own activities of daily living (ADLs).

May indicate need to lean on others for a time. Early recognition and intervention can help client regain equilibrium.

Assess presence of positive coping skills and inner strengths, such as use of relaxation techniques, willingness to express feelings, and use of support systems.

When the individual has coping skills that have been successful in the past, they may be used in the current situation to relieve tension and preserve the individual's sense of control. However, limitations of condition may impact choices available to client; for example, playing a musical instrument to relieve stress may not be possible for individual with tremors or hemiparesis, but listening to tapes or CDs may provide some degree of comfort.

(continues on page 752)

Encourage client to talk about what is happening at this time and what has occurred to precipitate feelings of helplessness and anxiety.

Evaluate ability to understand events. Correct misperceptions and provide factual information.

Provide quiet, nonstimulating environment. Determine what client needs, and provide, if possible. Give simple, factual information about what client can expect and repeat as necessary.

Allow client to be dependent in the beginning, with gradual resumption of independence in ADLs, self-care, and other activities. Make opportunities for client to make simple decisions about care and other activities when possible, accepting choice not to do so.

Accept verbal expressions of anger, setting limits on maladaptive behavior.

Discuss feelings of self-blame or projection of blame on others.

Note expressions of inability to find meaning in life or reason for living and feelings of futility or alienation from God.

Promote safe and hopeful environment, as needed. Identify positive aspects of this experience and assist client to view it as a learning opportunity.

Provide support for client to problem-solve solutions for current situation. Provide information and reinforce reality as client begins to ask questions and look at what is happening.

Provide for gradual implementation and continuation of necessary behaviors or lifestyle changes. Reinforce positive adaptation and new coping behaviors.

Collaborative

Refer to other resources as necessary such as clergy, psychiatric clinical nurse specialist, psychiatrist, family or marital therapist, and addiction support groups.

Provides clues to assist client to develop coping and regain equilibrium.

Assists in identification and correction of perception of reality and enables problem-solving to begin.

Decreases anxiety and provides control for the client during crisis situation.

Promotes feelings of security—client knows nurse will provide safety. As control is regained, client has the opportunity to develop adaptive coping and problem-solving skills.

Verbalizing angry feelings is an important process for resolution of grief and loss. However, preventing destructive actions, such as striking out at others, preserves client's self-esteem.

Although these mechanisms may be protective at the moment of crisis, they eventually are counterproductive and intensify feelings of helplessness and hopelessness.

Crisis situation may evoke questioning of spiritual beliefs, affecting ability to cope with current situation and plan for the future.

May be helpful while client regains inner control. The ability to learn from the current situation can provide skills for moving forward.

Helping client and SO to brainstorm possible solutions and giving consideration to the pros and cons of each promotes feelings of self-control and strengthens self-esteem.

Reduces anxiety of sudden change and allows for developing new and creative solutions.

Additional assistance may be needed to help client resolve problems or make decisions. *Note:* If untreated, depression may complicate recovery from physical illness (Robinson & Krishnan, 2002).

NURSING DIAGNOSIS: risk for compromised family Coping

May be related to

Inadequate or incorrect information or understanding by a primary person, unrealistic expectations

Temporary family disorganization and role changes, feeling that caregiving interferes with other important roles in their lives

Prolonged disease or disability progression that exhausts the supportive capacity of family members

Possibly evidenced by

(Not applicable; presence of signs and symptoms establishes an *actual* diagnosis)

Desired Outcomes/Evaluation Criteria—Family Will

Family Coping (NOC)

Identify resources within themselves to deal with situation.

Visit regularly and participate positively in care of client, within limits of abilities.

Express more realistic understanding and expectations of the client.

Provide opportunity for client to deal with situation in own way.

ACTIONS/INTERVENTIONS

RATIONALE

Family Involvement Promotion (NIC)
Independent

Establish rapport and acknowledge difficulty of the situation for the family.

Determine current knowledge and perception of the situation.

May assist family to accept what is happening and be willing to share problems with caregivers.

Lack of information or unrealistic perceptions can interfere with family members' and client's response to illness situation.

ACTIONS/INTERVENTIONS (continued)	RATIONALE (continued)
Assess level of anxiety present in family and SO.	Anxiety level needs to be dealt with before problem-solving can begin. Individuals may be so preoccupied with own reactions to situation that they are unable to respond to another's needs.
Evaluate pre-illness and current behaviors that are interfering with care or recovery of the client.	Information about family problems, such as divorce or separation, financial limitations, and substance use, will be helpful in determining options and developing an appropriate plan of care.
Discuss underlying reasons for client behaviors with family.	When family members know why client is behaving in different ways, it helps them understand and accept or deal with situation.
Assist family/client to understand "who owns the problem" and who is responsible for resolution. Avoid placing blame or guilt.	When these boundaries are defined, each individual can begin to take care of own self and stop taking care of others in inappropriate ways.
Reframe negative expressions into positives whenever possible.	Promotes more hopeful attitude and helps family and client look toward the future.
Involve SO in information giving, problem-solving, and care of client as feasible. Identify other ways of demonstrating support while maintaining client's independence.	Information can reduce feelings of helplessness. Involvement in care enhances feelings of control and self-worth.

Collaborative

Refer to appropriate resources for assistance, as indicated, such as counseling, psychotherapy, and financial and spiritual support.	May need additional assistance in resolving family issues.

NURSING DIAGNOSIS: **readiness for enhanced family Coping**

May be related to
Basic needs sufficiently gratified and adaptive tasks effectively addressed to enable goals of self-actualization to surface
Willingness to deal with one's own needs and to begin to problem-solve with the client

Possibly evidenced by
Family member attempting to describe growth impact of crisis on his/her own values, priorities, goals, or relationships
Family member moving in direction of health-promoting and enriching lifestyle and generally choosing experiences that optimize wellness

Desired Outcomes/Evaluation Criteria—Family Will

Family Functioning (NOC)
Express willingness to look at own role in family's growth.
Undertake tasks leading to change.
Verbalize feelings of self-confidence and satisfaction with progress being made.

ACTIONS/INTERVENTIONS	RATIONALE
Family Support (NIC)	
Independent	
Provide opportunities for family to talk with client and/or caregiver(s).	Reduces anxiety and allows expression of what has been learned and how they are managing as well as opportunity to make plans for the future and share support.
Listen to family's expressions of hope, planning, effect on relationships and life, and change of values.	Provides clues to avenues to explore for assistance with growth.
Provide opportunities for, and instruction in, how SOs can care for client. Discuss ways in which they can support client in meeting own needs.	Enhances feelings of control and involvement in situation in which SOs cannot do many things. Also provides opportunity to learn how to be most helpful when client is discharged from care.
Provide a role model with which family may identify.	Having a positive example can help with adoption of new behaviors to promote growth.
Discuss importance of open communication. Role play effective communication skills of active-listening, "I-messages," and problem-solving.	Helps individuals to express needs and wants in ways that will develop family cohesiveness. Promotes solutions in which everyone wins.
Encourage family to learn new and effective ways of dealing with feelings.	Effective recognition and expression of feelings clarify situation for involved individuals.

(continues on page 754)

Encourage seeking support appropriately. Give information about available persons and agencies.

Permission to seek help as needed allows them to choose to take advantage of available assistance and resources.

Collaborative

Refer to specific support group(s) as indicated.

Provides opportunities for sharing experiences, provides mutual support and practical problem-solving, and can aid in decreasing alienation and helplessness.

NURSING DIAGNOSIS: **Anxiety [specify level]/Fear**

May be related to

Unconscious conflict about essential goals and values of life; unmet needs

Situational or maturational crises, stress

Interpersonal transmission and contagion of anxious feelings

Threat of death—perceived or actual

Threat to, or change in, health status—exposure to toxins, substance abuse, progressive or debilitating disease, terminal illness

Separation from support system

Sensory impairment

Possibly evidenced by

Behavioral: Expressed concerns due to change in life events, diminished productivity, restlessness, extraneous movement, insomnia

Affective: Irritability, jittery, rattled, regretful, distressed, apprehensive, worried, feelings of inadequacy, uncertainty, feelings of helplessness

Physiological: Reports of increased tension, quivering voice, trembling

Sympathetic and parasympathetic: Palpitations, urinary frequency, nausea

Cognitive: Blocking of thought, impaired attention, confusion, forgetfulness, rumination, difficulty concentrating, focus on self, fight or flight behavior, dread of an identifiable problem recognized by client, fear of unspecific consequences

Desired Outcomes/Evaluation Criteria—Client Will

Anxiety [or] Fear Self-Control (NOC)

Acknowledge and discuss fears and concerns.

Appear relaxed and report anxiety is reduced to a manageable level.

Verbalize awareness of feelings of anxiety and healthy ways to deal with them.

Demonstrate problem-solving and use resources effectively.

ACTIONS/INTERVENTIONS

RATIONALE

Anxiety Reduction (NIC)

Independent

Note palpitations and elevated pulse or respiratory rate.

Changes in vital signs may suggest the degree of anxiety the client is experiencing or reflect the impact of physiological factors such as pain or endocrine imbalances.

Acknowledge fear and anxieties. Validate observations with client, for example, "You seem to be afraid."

Feelings are real, and it is helpful to bring them out in the open so they can be discussed and dealt with.

Assess degree and reality of threat to client and level of anxiety—mild, moderate, severe—by observing behavior, such as clenched hands, wide eyes, startle response, furrowed brow, clinging to family and staff, or physical and verbal lashing out.

Individual responses can vary according to cultural beliefs and traditions and culturally learned patterns. Distorted perceptions of the situation may magnify feelings.

Note narrowed focus of attention and client concentrating on one thing at a time.

Narrowed focus usually reflects extreme fear or panic.

Observe speech content, vocabulary, and communication patterns, such as rapid or slow, pressured speech; words commonly used, repetition, use of humor or laughter, and swearing.

Provides clues about such factors as the level of anxiety, ability to comprehend what is currently happening, cognition difficulties, and possible language differences.

Assess severity of pain when present. Delay gathering of information if pain is severe.

Severe pain and anxiety leave little energy for critical thinking and other activities.

Determine client's and SO's perception(s) of the situation.

Regardless of the reality of the situation, perception affects how each individual deals with the illness and stress.

Acknowledge reality of the situation as the client sees it, without challenging the belief.

Client may need to deny reality until ready to deal with it. It is not helpful to force the client to face facts.

ACTIONS/INTERVENTIONS (continued)

Evaluate coping and defense mechanisms being used to deal with the perceived or real threat.

Review coping mechanisms used in the past, such as problem-solving skills and recognizing and asking for help.

Assist client to use the energy of anxiety for coping with the situation when possible.

Maintain frequent contact with the client and SO. Be available for listening and talking, as needed.

Acknowledge feelings, as expressed, using active-listening or reflection. If actions are unacceptable, take necessary steps to control or deal with behavior. (Refer to ND: risk for Violence.)

Identify ways in which client can get help when needed, including telephone numbers of contact persons.

Stay with or arrange to have someone stay with client, as indicated.

Provide accurate information as appropriate and when requested by the client and SO. Answer questions freely and honestly and in language that is understandable by all. Repeat information as necessary; correct misconceptions.

Avoid empty reassurances, with statements of "everything will be all right." Instead, provide specific information, such as "Your heart rate is regular, your pain is being easily controlled, and that is what we want," or "Your CD4 count has been stable for the last three visits."

Note expressions of concern or anger about treatment or staff.

Ask client and SO to identify what he or she can or cannot do about what is happening.

Provide as much order and predictability as possible in scheduling care, activities, and visitors.

Instruct in ways to use positive self-talk: "I can manage this pain for now," or "My cancer is shrinking."

Encourage client to develop regular exercise and activity program.

Encourage and instruct in guided imagery or other relaxation methods, such as imagining a pleasant place, use of music, deep breathing, meditation, and mindfulness.

Provide touch, Therapeutic Touch, massage, and other adjunctive therapies as indicated.

Collaborative

Administer medications, as needed, for example:

Anti-anxiety agents, such as diazepam (Valium), clorazepate (Tranxene), or chlordiazepoxide (Librium)

Benzodiazepines, such as palprazolam (Xanax), oxazepam (Serax), lorazepam (Ativan), or temazepam (Restoril)

Selective serotonin reuptake inhibitors (SSRIs), such as fluoxetine (Prozac), sertraline (Zoloft), fluvoxamine (Luvox), citalopram HAABr (Celexa), or paroxetine HCL (Paxil)

Other drugs, such as buspirone (BuSpar) or doxepin (Adapin, Sinequan)

RATIONALE (continued)

May be dealing well with the situation at the moment; for example, denial and regression may be helpful coping mechanisms for a time. However, use of such mechanisms diverts energy the client needs for healing, and problems need to be dealt with at some point in time.

Provides opportunity to build on resources the client and SO may have used successfully.

Moderate anxiety heightens awareness and can help motivate the client to focus on dealing with problems.

Establishes rapport, promotes expression of feelings, and helps client and SO look at realities of the illness and treatment without confronting issues they are not ready to deal with.

Often acknowledging feelings enables client to deal more appropriately with situation. May need chemical or physical control for brief periods.

Provides assurance that staff and resources are available for assistance/support.

Continuous support may help client regain internal locus of control and reduce anxiety and fear to a manageable level.

Complex and/or anxiety-provoking information can be given in manageable amounts over an extended period. As opportunities arise and facts are given, individuals will accept what they are ready for. *Note:* Words and phrases may have different meanings for each individual; therefore, clarification is necessary to ensure understanding.

It is not possible for the nurse to know how the specific situation will be resolved, and false reassurances may be interpreted as lack of understanding or honesty, further isolating the client. Sharing observations used in assessing condition and prognosis provides opportunity for client and SO to feel reassured.

Anxiety about self and outcome may be masked by comments or angry outbursts directed at therapy or caregivers.

Assists in identifying areas in which control can be exercised and those in which control is not possible.

Helps client anticipate and prepare for difficult treatments or movements, as well as look forward to pleasant occurrences.

Internal dialogue is often negative. When this is shared out loud, the client becomes aware and can be directed in the use of positive self-talk, which can help reduce anxiety.

Has been shown to raise endorphin levels to enhance sense of well-being and help reduce level of anxiety.

Promotes release of endorphins and aids in developing internal locus of control, reducing anxiety. May enhance coping skills, allowing body to go about its work of healing.

Aids in meeting basic human need, decreasing sense of isolation, and assisting client to feel less anxious. *Note:* Therapeutic Touch requires the nurse to have specific knowledge and experience to use the hands to correct energy field disturbances by redirecting human energies to help or heal.

Anti-anxiety agents and/or antidepressants may be useful for brief periods to assist the client and SO to reduce anxiety to manageable levels, providing opportunity for initiation of client's own coping skills. *Note:* Use of SSRIs, such as Prozac or Zoloft, have been associated with sexual function complaints. Alternatives may need to be considered. Also, ethnic variations affecting psychotropic drugs require close monitoring to determine therapeutic dosage. For example, East Asians and blacks may be more sensitive or react faster, have higher plasma drug levels, and have increased risk of side effects, necessitating lower dosage than whites in general (Munoz & Hilgenberg, 2005).

May be related to

Loss—health status, body part, independent functioning, sense of control

Maturational transitions; developmental changes (specify)

Behavior inconsistent with values

Unrealistic self-expectations

Possibly evidenced by

Reports current situational challenge to self-worth; evaluates self as unable to deal with situation or event; expressions of helplessness, uselessness

Self-negating verbalizations

Indecisive behavior

Desired Outcomes/Evaluation Criteria—Client Will

Self-Esteem (NOC)

Verbalize realistic view and acceptance of self in situation.

Identify existing strengths and view self as capable person.

Recognize and incorporate change into self-concept in accurate manner without negating self-worth.

Demonstrate adaptation to changes or events that have occurred as evidenced by setting of realistic goals and active participation in work, play, and personal relationships.

ACTIONS/INTERVENTIONS	RATIONALE
Self-Esteem Enhancement (NIC)	
Independent	
Ask how the client would like to be addressed.	Shows courtesy and respect and acknowledges person.
Identify SO from whom the client derives comfort and who should be notified in case of emergency.	Allows provisions to be made for specific person(s) to visit or remain close and provides needed support for client. *Note:* May or may not be legal next of kin.
Identify basic sense of self-esteem and image client has of existential, physical, psychological self. Identify locus of control.	May provide insight into whether this is a single episode or recurrent or chronic situation and can help determine needs and treatment plan. Determining whether the individual's locus of control is internal or external facilitates choosing most effective interventions.
Determine client's perception of threat to self.	Client's perception is more important than what is really happening and needs to be dealt with before reality can be addressed.
Active-listen client concerns and fears.	Conveys sense of caring and can be helpful in identifying the client's needs, problems, and coping strategies and how effective they are. Provides opportunity to develop and begin a problem-solving process.
Encourage verbalization of feelings, accepting what is said.	Helps client and SO begin to adapt to change and reduces anxiety about altered function or lifestyle.
Discuss stages of grief and the importance of grief work. (Refer to ND: Grieving [specify].)	Grieving is a necessary step for integration of change or loss into self-concept.
Provide nonthreatening environment; listen and accept client as presented.	Promotes feelings of safety, encouraging verbalization.
Observe nonverbal communication including body posture and movements, eye contact, gestures, and use of touch.	Nonverbal language is a large portion of communication and therefore is extremely important. How the person uses touch provides information about how it is accepted and how comfortable the individual is with being touched.
Reflect back to the client what has been said, for example, "You were upset when he told you that."	Clarification and verification of what has been heard promotes understanding and allows client to validate information; otherwise, assumptions may be inaccurate.
Observe and describe behavior in objective terms.	All behavior has meaning, some of which is obvious and some of which needs to be identified. This is a process of educated guesswork and requires validation by the client.
Identify age and developmental level.	Age is an indicator of the stage of life client is experiencing, whether it be adolescence or middle age. However, developmental level may be more important than chronological age in anticipating and identifying some of the client's needs. Some degree of regression occurs during illness, depending on many factors, such as the normal coping skills of the individual, the severity of the illness, and family and cultural expectations.

ACTIONS/INTERVENTIONS (continued)	RATIONALE (continued)
Discuss client's view of body image and how illness or condition might affect it.	The client's perception of a change in body image may occur suddenly or over time such as actual loss of a body part through injury or surgery, or a perceived loss, such as a heart attack; or be a continuous subtle process such as chronic illness, eating disorders, or aging. Awareness can alert the nurse to the need for appropriate interventions tailored to the individual need.
Encourage discussion of physical changes in a simple, direct, and factual manner. Give realistic feedback and discuss future options such as rehabilitation services.	Provides opportunity to begin incorporating actual changes in an accepting and hopeful atmosphere.
Acknowledge efforts at problem-solving, resolution of current situation, and future planning.	Provides encouragement and reinforces continuation of desired behaviors.
Recognize client's pace for adaptation to demands of current situation.	Failure to acknowledge client's need to take time and/or pressuring client to "get on with it" conveys a lack of acceptance of the person as an individual and may result in feelings of lowered self-esteem.
Introduce tasks at client's level of functioning, progressing to more complex activities as tolerated.	Provides opportunity for client to experience successes, reaffirming capabilities and enhancing self-worth.
Ascertain how the client sees own role within the family system: breadwinner, homemaker, or husband or wife.	Illness may create a temporary or permanent problem in role expectations. Sexual role and how the client views self in relation to the current illness also play important parts in recovery.
Assist client and SO with clarifying expected roles and those that may need to be relinquished or altered.	Provides opportunity to identify misconceptions and begin to look at options; promotes reality orientation.
Determine client awareness of own responsibility for dealing with situation and personal growth.	Conveys confidence in client's ability to cope. When client acknowledges own part in planning and carrying out treatment plan, he or she has more investment in following through on decisions that have been made.
Assess impact of condition, surgery, or medication regimen on sexuality.	Sexuality encompasses the whole person in the total environment. Many times problems of illness are superimposed on already existing problems of sexuality and can affect client's sense of self-worth. Some problems are more obvious than others, such as illness involving the reproductive parts of the body. Others are less obvious, such as sexual values and role in family: mother, wage earner, or single parent.
Be alert to comments and innuendos, which may mean the client has a concern in the area of sexuality.	People are often reluctant and/or embarrassed to ask direct questions about sexual or sexuality concerns.
Be aware of caregiver's feelings about dealing with the subject of sexuality.	Nurses and caregivers are often as reluctant and embarrassed in dealing with sexuality issues as most clients. (Refer to CP: Extended Care, ND: Sexual Dysfunction.)
Collaborative	
Provide information and referral to hospital and community resources.	Enables client and SO to be in contact with interested groups with access to assistive and supportive devices, services, and counseling.
Support participation in group or community activities, such as assertiveness classes, volunteer work, and support groups.	Promotes skills of coping and sense of self-worth. Provides role models and facilitates problem-solving.
Refer to psychiatric support or therapy group and social services, as indicated.	May be needed to assist client and SO to achieve optimal recovery.
Refer to appropriate resources for sex therapy as need indicates.	May be someone with comfort level and knowledge who is available, or may be necessary to refer to professional resources for additional guidance and support.

NURSING DIAGNOSIS: Grieving [specify]

May be related to
Anticipatory or actual loss—parts or processes of body, independent functioning, status, job; SO

Possibly evidenced by
Verbal expression of distress, unresolved issues
Difficulty in expressing loss; denial of loss
Altered eating habits, sleep or dream patterns, activity levels, and libido
Psychological distress; disorganization; detachment
Alterations in immune or neuroendocrine function

(continues on page 758)

Desired Outcomes/Evaluation Criteria—Client Will

Grief Resolution (NOC)
Identify and express feelings freely and effectively.
Verbalize a sense of progress toward resolution of the grief and hope for the future.
Function at an acceptable level and participate in work and ADLs, as appropriate.

ACTIONS/INTERVENTIONS	RATIONALE
Grief Work Facilitation (NIC)	
Independent	
Provide open environment in which client feels free to realistically discuss feelings and concerns.	Therapeutic communication skills, such as active-listening, silence, being available, and acceptance, provide opportunity and encourage the client to talk freely and deal with the perceived or actual loss.
Determine client perception and meaning of loss—current and past. Note cultural or religious factors and expectations.	Affects client's responses and needs to be acknowledged in planning care.
Identify stage of grieving and effect on functioning:	Awareness allows for appropriate choice of interventions because individuals handle grief in many different ways.
Denial: Be aware of avoidance behaviors, such as anger, withdrawal, and so forth; allow client to talk about what he or she chooses, and do not try to force client to "face the facts."	Denying the reality of diagnosis and/or prognosis is an important phase in which the client protects self from the pain and reality of the threat of loss. Each person does this in an individual manner based on previous experiences with loss and cultural or religious factors.
Anger: Note behaviors of withdrawal, lack of cooperation, and direct expression of anger; be alert to body language and check meaning with client, noting congruency with verbalizations; encourage, and provide opportunity for, verbalization of anger; and acknowledge feelings and set limits regarding destructive behavior.	Denial gives way to feelings of anger, rage, guilt, and resentment. Client may find it difficult to express anger directly and may feel guilty about normal feelings of anger. Although staff may have difficulty dealing with angry behaviors, acceptance allows client to work through the anger and move on to more effective coping behaviors.
Bargaining: Be aware of statements such as ". . . if God will just . . . I will do . . ."; allow verbalization without confrontation about realities.	Bargaining with care providers or God often occurs and may be helpful in beginning resolution and acceptance. Client may be working through feelings of guilt about things done or undone.
Depression: Give client permission to be where he or she is; provide hope within parameters of individual situation without giving false reassurance; and provide comfort and availability as well as caring for physical needs.	When client can no longer deny the reality of the loss, feelings of helplessness and hopelessness replace feelings of anger. The client needs information that this is a normal progression of feelings.
Acceptance: Respect client's needs and wishes for quiet, privacy, and/or talking.	Having worked through the denial, anger, and depression stages, client often prefers to be alone and may not want to talk much at this point. Client may still cling to hope, which can be sustaining through whatever is currently happening.
Active-listen client's concerns and be available for support, as necessary.	The process of grieving does not proceed in an orderly fashion, but fluctuates with various aspects of all stages present at one time or another. If process is dysfunctional or prolonged, more aggressive interventions may be required to facilitate the process.
Determine quality of interactions with others, including family members.	Although periods of withdrawal and loneliness usually accompany grieving, persistent isolation may indicate deepening depression, necessitating further evaluation and intervention. *Note:* Family/SO may not be dysfunctional but may be intolerant of client's behaviors.
Identify and problem-solve solutions to existing physical responses, such as eating, sleeping, activity levels, and sexual desire.	May need additional assistance to deal with the physical aspects of grieving.
Assess needs of SO and assist, as indicated.	Identification of problems indicating dysfunctional grieving allows for individual interventions.
Include family/SO, as appropriate, when determining future needs.	Depending on client's desires and legal requirements, choices regarding future plans (e.g., living situation, continuation of care, end-of-life decisions, funeral arrangements) can provide guidance and peace of mind.
Discuss healthy ways of dealing with difficult situation.	Provides opportunity to look toward the future and plan for family's/SO's needs (e.g., for life after loss).
Collaborative	
Refer to other resources, such as support groups, counseling, spiritual or pastoral care, and psychotherapy, as indicated.	May need additional help to resolve grief, make plans, and look toward the future.

NURSING DIAGNOSIS: risk for impaired Religiosity

Risk factors may include
Physical: Illness, hospitalization, pain
Psychological factors: Ineffective support or coping with condition, personal crisis, anxiety, fear of death, depression
Sociocultural: Lack of social interaction
Spiritual: Spiritual crises, suffering
Developmental and situational: Life transitons, aging; end-stage life crises

Possibly evidenced by
(Not applicable; presence of signs and symptoms establishes an *actual* diagnosis)

Desired Outcomes/Evaluation Criteria—Client Will

Spiritual Health (NOC)
Express ability to once again participate in beliefs and rituals of desired religion.
Discuss beliefs and values about spiritual or religious issues.
Attend religious or worship services of choice as desired.
Verbalize concerns about end-of-life issues and fear of death.

ACTIONS/INTERVENTIONS

Spiritual Suppot (NIC)
Independent
Listen to client's and SO's reports and expressions of anger and concern or alienation from God. Note sense of guilt or retribution.

Discuss differences between grief and guilt and help client to identify and deal with each. Point out consequences of actions based on guilt.

Use therapeutic communication skills of reflection and active-listening.
Encourage expression of feelings about illness/condition and death.
Determine sense of futility, feelings of hopelessness, and lack of motivation to help self.
Assess extent of depression client may be experiencing.

Note recent changes in behavior, such as withdrawal from others and religious activities and dependence on alcohol or medications.

Suggest use of journaling and/or reminiscence.

Encourage client to identify SO(s) and others such as spiritual advisor or parish nurse who can provide needed support.

Religious Ritual Enhancement (NIC)
Identify client's religious affiliation, associated rituals, and beliefs.
Make time for nonjudgmental discussion of philosophical issues related to religious belief patterns and customs.

Discuss desire to continue or reconnect with previous belief patterns and customs.
Involve client in refining healthcare goals and therapeutic regimen, as appropriate.

Provide privacy for meditation, prayer, or performance of rituals, as appropriate.
Explore alternatives to, or modifications for, ritual based on setting and individual needs or limitations.

RATIONALE

May be suffering from severe or terminal illness or accident straining resources and affecting client's ability to cope. Perception of guilt may cause spiritual crisis or suffering resulting in rejection of religious activities and symbols.
As client recognizes consequences of actions, they can be discussed, and desire to change may enhance new coping skills, avoid acting out of false guilt, and enable client to resume desired religious activities.
Communicates acceptance and enables client to find own solutions to concerns.
Allows client to identify how feelings are impacting situation and deal with them appropriately.
Indicators that client may see no, or only limited, options or personal choices available and lack energy to deal with situation.
Some studies suggest that a focus on religion may protect against depression.
Helpful in determining severity and duration of situation and possible need for additional referrals such as substance withdrawal. Lack of connectedness with self or others impairs ability to trust others or feel worthy of trust from others or God.
Promotes life review. Can assist in clarifying values and ideas, recognizing and resolving feelings and situation, and identifying reasons for resuming desired religious activities.
Ongoing support is required to enhance sense of connectedness and strengthen religious ties as desired.

Helps determine individual's needs and possible resources, if desired.
Open communication can assist client to check reality of perceptions and identify personal options and willingness to resume desired activities.
Enables client to identify barriers to participating in desired activities and take appropriate actions to resume them.
Identifies role illness is playing in current concerns about ability to or appropriateness of participating in desired religious activities.
Allows client to engage in spiritual activites in own way without fear of interruption or judgment of others.
Assists client to develop new ways of expressing religious beliefs and satisfying these needs.

(continues on page 760)

759

ACTIONS/INTERVENTIONS (continued)

Collaborative

Refer to spiritual resources, such as spiritual advisor—who has qualifications and experience in dealing with specific problems individual is concerned about—or to facility's chaplain or visiting clergy and parish nurse.

RATIONALE (continued)

Provides answers to spiritual questions, assists in the journey of self-discovery, helps client learn to accept, forgive self, and engage in desired rituals.

NURSING DIAGNOSIS: **risk for ineffective self Health Management**

Risk factors may include

Complexity of therapeutic regimen, knowledge deficits

Decisional conflicts—client and family value system, health beliefs, spiritual values, cultural influences, ethical concerns, perceived seriousness

Perceived barriers, economic difficulties, side effects of therapy, mistrust of regimen and/or healthcare personnel, complexity of healthcare system

Family patterns of healthcare, family conflict, powerlessness

Possibly evidenced by

(Not applicable; presence of signs and symptoms establishes an *actual* diagnosis)

Desired Outcomes/Evaluation Criteria—Client Will

Treatment Behavior: Illness or Injury (NOC)

Participate in the development of goals and treatment plan.

Verbalize accurate knowledge of disease and understanding of treatment regimen.

Demonstrate behaviors or changes in lifestyle necessary to incorporate or maintain therapeutic regimen in daily life.

Identify and use available resources.

ACTIONS/INTERVENTIONS

Values Clarification (NIC)

Independent

Review client's and SO's knowledge and understanding of the need for treatment or medication as well as consequences of actions and choices. Note ability to comprehend information, including literacy, level of education, and primary language.

Be aware of developmental and chronological age.

Determine cultural, spiritual, and health beliefs and ethical concerns.

Self-Modification Assistance (NIC)

Review treatment plan with client and SO.

Contract with client for participation in care.

Establish graduated goals or modified regimen as necessary; work out alternate solutions.

Assess availability and use of support systems. Identify additional resources, as appropriate.

Determine problems that may, or do, interfere with treatment including lack of financial or personal resources, or lack of availability of providers. Assess level of anxiety, locus of control, and sense of powerlessness.

Note length of illness and prognosis.

RATIONALE

Provides opportunities to clarify viewpoints or misconceptions. Verifies that client and SO have accurate and factual information with which to make informed choices.

Impacts ability to understand own needs and incorporate into treatment regimen.

Provides insight into thoughts and factors related to individual situation. Beliefs will affect client's perception of situation and participation in treatment regimen. Treatment may be incongruent with client's social and cultural lifestyle and perceived role/responsibilities.

Provides opportunities to exchange accurate information and to clarify viewpoints or misconceptions.

Client who agrees to own responsibility is more apt to adhere to treatment plan.

Promotes client involvement and independence; provides opportunity for compromise and may enhance cooperation with regimen. When client participates in setting goals, there is a sense of investment that encourages cooperation and willingness to follow through with the program.

Access to and proper use of helpful resources can assist client in meeting treatment goals and provide purpose for living. Presence of caring, empathic family/SO(s) can help client in process of recovery.

Many factors may be involved in behavior that is disruptive to the treatment regimen such as fear of hospitalization or treatment; denial of situation consequences; suspicion about healthcare system; and physical factors such as pain, hypoxemia, and chemical imbalance.

Clients tend to become passive and dependent in long-term, debilitating illness.

ACTIONS/INTERVENTIONS (continued)

Listen to, and active-listen, client's reports and comments.

Develop a system for self-monitoring. Share data pertinent to client's condition such as laboratory results or blood pressure (BP) readings.
Have same personnel care for client as much as possible.

Accept client's choice or point of view even if it appears to be self-destructive, such as a decision to continue smoking.

Be aware of own and caregiver's response to client's treatment choices such as refusal of blood or chemotherapy and living will or advance directive choices.

RATIONALE (continued)

Conveys message of concern and belief in individual's capabilities to resolve situation in positive manner.
Provides a sense of control; enables client to follow own progress and make informed choices.

Enables relationship to develop in which the client can begin to trust and participate in care.
Client has the right to make own decisions, and acceptance may give a sense of control, which can help client look more clearly at consequences. Confrontation is not beneficial and may actually be detrimental to future cooperation and goal achievement.
Negative feelings regarding these choices may create power struggles and be expressed in judgmental behaviors that block or interfere with client's wishes, comfort, and/or care. *Note:* If resolution cannot be found, providers have the right to terminate their services with appropriate notice.

NURSING DIAGNOSIS: risk for self-directed/other-directed Violence

Risk factors may include
Neurological impairment: head trauma, seizure disorders
Cognitive impairment: decreased intellectual functioning, learning disabilities
  Hormonal imbalance; toxic reactions to medication; physical health—chronic or terminal illness
Mental health issues: severe depression, substance abuse or withdrawal; delusions, hallucinations
Emotional responses: hopelessness, despair, increased anxiety, anger, hostility
  Conflictual interpersonal relationships; lack of personal or social resources; employment problems
  Impulsivity; self-destructive behavior; suicidal ideation or behavior
Verbal clues: talking about death, "better off without me," asking questions about lethal dosages of drugs
Behavioral clues: writing forlorn notes, giving away personal items, threatening letters

Possibly evidenced by
(Not applicable; presence of signs and symptoms establishes an *actual* diagnosis)

Desired Outcomes/Evaluation Criteria—Client Will

Impulse Self-Control (NOC)
Acknowledge realities of the situation.
Verbalize understanding of reason(s) for behavior/precipitating factors.
Express increased self-concept.
Demonstrate self-control, as evidenced by relaxed posture and nonviolent behavior.

ACTIONS/INTERVENTIONS

Mood Management (NIC)
Independent
Observe for early signs of distress and investigate possible causes.

Maintain straightforward communication and assist client to learn assertive rather than manipulative, nonassertive, or aggressive behavior.
Help client identify more adequate solutions and behaviors such as motor activities or exercise. Redirect and provide directions for actions client can take.

Give as much autonomy as is possible in the situation.

Monitor for suicidal or homicidal ideation, for example, morbid or anxious feelings while with the client; thoughts expressed by, or warning from, the client, "It doesn't matter, I'd be better off dead"; and mood swings, putting affairs in order, and previous suicide attempt.

RATIONALE

Irritability, pacing, shouting or cursing, lack of cooperation, and demanding behavior may all be signs of increasing anxiety or indicate change in health status of confused client that requires further evaluation.
Avoids reinforcing manipulative behavior and enhances positive interactions with others, accomplishing the goal of getting needs met in acceptable ways.
Promotes release of energies in acceptable ways. Redirecting confused client can minimize escalation of agitation. (Refer to CP: Dementia of the Alzheimer's Type/Vascular Dementia.)
Enhances feelings of power and control in a situation in which many things are not within individual's control.
Indicators of need for further assessment and intervention or psychiatric care.

(continues on page 762)

ACTIONS/INTERVENTIONS (continued)	RATIONALE (continued)
Assess suicidal intent (scale of 1 to 10) by asking directly if client is thinking of killing self, has plan, means, and so on.	Provides guidelines for necessity and urgency of interventions. Direct questioning is most helpful when done in a caring, concerned manner.
Acknowledge reality of suicide or homicide as an option. Discuss consequences of actions if client were to follow through on intent. Ask how it will help client resolve problems.	Client may focus on suicide, or possibly homicide, as the "only" option and this response provides an opening to look at and discuss other options. *Note:* Be aware of own responsibility under Tarasoff's rule to warn possible victim(s) when client is expressing homicidal ideation. (Under Tarasoff's rule, the counselor/care provider has a legal responsibility to notify a third party of a credible threat made by the client.)
Accept client's anger without reacting on an emotional basis.	Responding with anger is not helpful in resolving the situation and may result in escalating client's behavior. Anger is usually not directed at the nurse, but at the situation and feelings of powerlessness.
Remain calm and state limits on behavior in a firm manner. Be truthful and nonjudgmental.	Understanding that helplessness and fear underlie this behavior aids in choosing appropriate response.
Assume that the client has control and is responsible for own behavior.	Often enables the individual to exercise control. *Note:* When violent behavior is the result of drug use, client may not be able to respond appropriately.
Identify conditions that may interfere with ability to control own behavior.	Acute or chronic brain syndrome or drug-induced or postsurgical confusion may precipitate violent behavior that is difficult to control.

Environmental Management: Violence Prevention (NIC)

Provide protection within the environment such as constant observation and removal of objects that might be used to harm self and others.	May need more structure to maintain control until own internal locus of control is regained.
Tell client to stop.	May be sufficient to help client control own actions if exhibiting hostile actions. *Note:* Client is often afraid of own actions and wants staff to set limits.
Use an organized team approach when necessary to subdue client with force. Tell client clearly and concisely what is happening.	Knowing and practicing these actions before they are needed helps prevent untoward problems. Keeping client informed can help client to regain internal control.
Hold client; place in restraints or seclusion if necessary. Do so in a calm, positive, nonstimulating, and nonpunitive manner.	As a last resort, physical restraint may be necessary while the client regains control. *Note:* These measures are meant to protect client, not punish the behavior.
Apply and adjust restraint devices properly.	It is important to maintain body alignment and client safety and comfort.
Document precise reason for restraints, actions taken, and doctor's order. Check restraints frequently per facility protocol, each time documenting the condition and how long the restraints are used.	Restraints are to be used for very specific reasons, which need to be clearly documented to avoid overuse or misuse, and to ensure client safety.

Collaborative

Refer to psychiatric resource(s): —psychiatric clinical nurse specialist, psychiatrist, psychologist, social worker, and classes such as anger management.	More in-depth assistance may be needed to deal with client and defuse situation. Learning new ways to deal with feelings can provide opportunity for individual to manage life in a more optimal way.
Administer medications, such as anti-anxiety or antipsychotic agents, sedatives, and narcotics.	May be indicated to quiet or control behavior. *Note:* May need to be withheld if they are suspected to be the cause of, or contribute to, the behavior.

NURSING DIAGNOSIS: **risk for Post-Trauma Syndrome**

Risk factors may include
Serious injury or threat to self; criminal victimization
Tragic occurance involving violent and/or multiple deaths; disasters; epidemics
Perception of event; survivor's role in event; duration of event

Possibly evidenced by
(Not applicable; presence of signs and symptoms establishes an *actual* diagnosis)

NURSING DIAGNOSIS: risk for Post-Trauma Syndrome (continued)

Desired Outcomes/Evaluation Criteria—Client Will

Coping (NOC)
Verbalize reduced stress.
Demonstrate ability to deal with emotional reactions in an individually appropriate manner.
Express own feelings and reactions avoiding projection.
Demonstrate appropriate changes in lifestyle, getting support from SO and friends as needed.
Participate in plans for follow-up care and counseling.

ACTIONS/INTERVENTIONS	RATIONALE
Crisis Intervention (NIC)	
Independent	
Determine when traumatic event(s) occurred: present or past.	Manifestations of acute and chronic posttrauma responses may require different interventions. *Note:* Event may encompass many forms of trauma, including the diagnosis of life-threatening illness.
Assess physical trauma, if present, and individual reaction to occurrence, for example, physical symptoms such as numbness, headache, and tightness in chest; and psychological responses of anger, shock, acute anxiety, confusion, and denial.	Provides information with which to develop plan of care and make informed choices.
Evaluate behavior (e.g., calm or agitated, excited, hysterical, inappropriate laughter, crying) and expressions of disbelief and/or self-blame.	Indicators of extent of individual response to traumatic incident and degree of disorganization.
Note ethnic background, cultural and religious perceptions, and beliefs about the event.	May influence client's response to what has happened, for example, client may believe it is retribution from God.
Assess signs or stage of grieving.	Client may be suffering from sense of loss of self and/or others.
Tell client that painful emotional reactions are normal. Phrase this information in neutral terms: "You may or may not experience . . ."	Understanding that experiencing these uncomfortable feelings is not unusual after traumatic event may reduce client's anxiety or fear of "going crazy" and enhance coping ability.
Discuss things client can do to feel better such as physical exercise alternated with relaxation, keeping busy with normal activities, talking to others, acknowledging that it is all right to feel upset, writing about the experience in a journal, and being kind to self.	Enhances sense of control and helps client achieve resolution of uncomfortable feelings. Often when the client begins these activities within the first 24 hours of the event, further therapy may not be required.
Assist with learning stress management techniques.	Promotes sense of control and ability to handle existing problems.
Identify supportive persons for client.	Having positive support systems and role models can help client reach optimal recovery.
None signs of severe or prolonged depression, frequency of flashbacks and nightmares, and presence of chronic pain and somatic complaints.	If client did not deal with trauma when it occurred, behavioral manifestations may reveal extent of problem in the present.
Help client identify factors that may have created a vulnerable situation or increased likelihood for event.	Even though individual may not be responsible for what has happened, he or she may have placed self at risk or engaged in activies potentiating negative outcome. Changes in behaviors or lifestyle may decrease potential for recurrence.
Collaborative	
Refer to support groups, counselor, or therapist for further therapy such as psychotherapy in conjunction with medications, implosive therapy, flooding, hypnosis, EMDR, rolfing, memory work, or cognitive restructuring, as indicated.	Client may need more in-depth assistance from sensitive, trained individuals who are skilled in dealing with these problems to prevent progression to, or treat development of, posttrauma syndrome. *Note:* EMDR is recommended for the treatment of trauma, having a direct effect on the way that the brain processes information, so that a person no longer relives the images, sounds, and feelings when the painful event is brought to mind (EMDR Institute, Inc., 2004).

POTENTIAL CONSIDERATIONS
Refer to primary diagnosis for postdischarge concerns.

DEMENTIA OF THE ALZHEIMER'S TYPE/VASCULAR DEMENTIA

I. Pathophysiology

a. Cognitive disorder characterized by impaired memory, language, thinking, and perception

b. Dementia of the Alzheimer's type (DAT) (Hausman, 2006; Nelson-Marsh, 2005)

  i. Characterized by structural and chemical changes in the brain, causing a steady and global decline in function

  ii. Degenerative process occurring primarily in the cells located at the base of the forebrain that sends information to the cerebral cortex and hippocampus

  iii. Decrease in acetylcholine production reduces the amount of neurotransmitter released to cells in the cortex, hippocampus, and nucleus basalis, resulting in a disruption of memory processes.

  iv. Enzyme required to produce acetylcholine is dramatically reduced, especially in the area of the brain where neuritic plaques and neurofibrillary tangles occur in the greatest numbers.

  v. Formation of plaques composed of beta-amyloid and tangles appears to be related to the cholesterol-transporting protein, apolipoprotein-E (ApoE).

c. Vascular dementia

  i. Referred to as multi-infarct, post-stroke dementia, or vascular cognitive impairment, resulting in decreased blood flow to parts of the brain

  ii. Multiple infarcts to various areas of the brain result in a pattern of intermittent deterioration determined by the area of the brain that is affected.

II. Classification

a. Alzheimer's and vascular dementia are irreversible and share common symptomology and therapeutic intervention.

  i. Alzheimer's disease accounts for 70% of dementia diagnoses.

  ii. Vascular dementia accounts for 17% of cases.

b. Criteria for dementia diagnosis (Alzheimer's Association, 2008)

  i. Decline in memory and at least one of the following cognitive abilities

    1. Coherent speech, understand spoken or written language

    2. Recognize or identify objects, assuming intact sensory function

    3. Execute motor activities, assuming intact motor abilities, sensory function, and comprehension of the required task

    4. Abstract thinking, make sound judgments, plan, and carry out complex tasks

  ii. Decline in cognitive abilities must be severe enough to interfere with daily life.

III. Etiology

a. DAT: Exact cause unknown; most likely due to multiple factors rather than a single cause (Alzheimer's Association, 2008).

  i. Lifelong process—incidence increases with longevity, and changes in the brain may develop decades before the onset of dementia

  ii. Genetics—familial pattern four times greater than general population (Nelson-Marsh, 2005)

    1. Familial or early-onset Alzheimer's is linked to defects on genes on chromosome 1, 14, or 21 with some families exhibiting a pattern of inheritance suggesting possible autosomal dominant gene transmission (Kuljis, 2007).

    2. Down syndrome: presents with an extra chromosome 21; may have a relationship to Alzheimer's disease

      a. At autopsy, both disorders have many of the same pathophysiological changes.

      b. High percentage of individuals with Down syndrome who survive to adulthood develop Alzheimer's lesions by age 50 (Alvarez, 2008).

    3. Studies suggest that autoantibodies are produced in the brain, reflecting a possible alteration in the body's immune system.

  iii. Proposed risk factors: Studies to date have not supported causal relationship; however, various factors that have been suggested include head trauma, low educational level, cigarette smoking, cholesterol-reducing drugs (statins), and ingestion of aluminum.

b. Vascular dementia

  i. Predisposing factors: various diseases and conditions that interfere with blood circulation, including cerebral and systemic vascular disease, hypertension, cerebral hypoxia, hypoglycemia, cerebral embolism, and severe head injury

IV. Statistics (Alzheimer's Association, 2008; Centers for Disease Control and Prevention [CDC], 2008)

a. Morbidity: In 2008, an estimated 5.2 million people in the United States were living with Alzheimer's disease; it is projected that 10 million baby boomers will develop Alzheimer's in their lifetime.

b. Mortality: DAT is the sixth-leading cause of death—72,914 Americans died in 2006.

c. Cost: In 2005, $112 billion was spent in direct medical costs to Medicare and Medicaid for Alzheimer's and other dementias and $36.5 billion in indirect costs to businesses; it is estimated that 9.8 million family, friends, and neighbors provided 8.4 billion hours of unpaid care, a contribution valued at $89 billion.

GLOSSARY

apolipoprotein-E (ApoE): Lipoprotein with three isoforms with the ApoE$_4$ variant associated with an earlier-than-average age of onset for the common form of Alzheimer's disease.

Amyloid plaque: Buildup of amyloid protein and a primary hallmark of Alzheimer's disease.

Atrophy: Wasting or a decrease in the size of an organ or tissue.

GLOSSARY (continued)

Beta amyloid: Insoluble protein that is an abnormal breakdown product of the cell membrane constituent, amyloid precursor protein (APP), and is a component of the neurofibrillary tangles and plaques characteristic of Alzheimer's disease.

Catastrophic reactions: Extreme outbursts of emotion, most often anger or agitation.

Emotional lability: Excessive emotional reactivity associated with frequent changes or swings in emotions or mood.

Hippocampus: Part of the limbic system of the brain and one of several structures involved with emotion, memory, and learning.

Hypermetamorphosis: Compulsive exploration of environment, including touching.

Hyperorality: Consists of unexplained movements of the mouth and tongue and the act of placing nonfood items in the mouth.

Neuritic plaques: Extracellular abnormalities composed of beta-amyloid in the gray matter of the brain.

Neurofibrillary tangles: Masses of fine fibrous elements found in cytoplasm signaling an abnormality of the hippocampus and neurons of the cerebral cortex that occurs especially in Alzheimer's disease. Classic finding at autopsy in the brain of client with DAT.

Proprioception: Awareness of posture; movement; changes in equilibrium; and the knowledge of position, weight, and resistance of objects in relation to the body.

Sundowner's syndrome (also called sundowning syndrome): Increased restlessness, wandering, aggression, or exacerbation of behavioral symptoms of Alzheimer's disease in the afternoon and evening.

Tau: Protein that channels chemical messages inside nerve cells.

Care Setting

Client is cared for primarily in the home or assisted living/extended care; however, inpatient care may be required for treatment of other health problems.

Related Concerns

End-of-life/hospice care, page 866

Extended care, page 801

Pneumonia, page 131

Psychosocial aspects of care, page 749

Sepsis/septicemia, page 686

Total nutritional support: parenteral/enteral feeding, page 469

Client Assessment Database

DIAGNOSTIC DIVISION MAY REPORT	MAY EXHIBIT
ACTIVITY/REST • Feeling tired • Decreased interest in usual activities, hobbies; inability to recall what is read or follow plot of television program • Forced to retire from work	• Day-night reversal • Wakefulness disturbance of sleep rhythms • Lethargy • Impaired motor skills • Inability to carry out familiar, purposeful movements • Content sitting and watching others • Repetitive motions, such as folding, unfolding, refolding linen • Wandering
CIRCULATION • History of systemic vascular disease, cerebral vascular disease, hypertension, embolic episodes (may be predisposing factors)	
EGO INTEGRITY • Anxiety, depression—usually during early stages related to the knowledge that cognitive abilities are deteriorating • Multiple losses, such as changes in body image and self-esteem	• Inconsistent behavior • Verbal and nonverbal communication and behavior may be incongruent • Suspicious or fearful of imaginary people and situations • May cling to significant others SO(s) • Misperception of environment, misidentification of objects and people

(continues on page 766)

DIAGNOSTIC DIVISION MAY REPORT (continued)	MAY EXHIBIT (continued)
	• Hoarding objects • Belief that misplaced objects are stolen • Emotional lability—may cry easily or laugh inappropriately • Variable mood changes, such as apathy, lethargy, restlessness, short attention span, or irritability • Catastrophic reactions • May deny significance of early changes and symptoms, especially cognitive changes • May conceal limitations, such as make excuses for not being able to perform tasks, redirect conversation, or avoid direct answers to questions • Feelings of helplessness, strong, depressive overlay, delusions, or paranoia
ELIMINATION	• Incontinence • Diarrhea—related to impaction
FOOD/FLUID • Changes in taste, appetite • Denial of hunger, refusal to eat—may be trying to conceal lost skills	• Hypoglycemic episodes—predisposing factor • Lack of interest in or forgetting mealtimes • Dependence on others for food cooking and preparation at table, feeding, or using utensils • Loss of ability to chew—silent aspiration concerns • Weight loss • Decreased muscle mass; emaciation in advanced stage
HYGIENE • Dependence on others to meet basic hygiene needs	• Disheveled, unkempt appearance • Body odor • Poor personal habits • Inappropriate clothing for situation or weather conditions • Misinterpretation of, or ignoring, internal cues • Forgetting steps involved in toileting self, or inability to find the bathroom
NEUROSENSORY • Family members may report a gradual decrease in cognitive abilities, impaired judgment, or inappropriate decisions; impaired recent memory but good remote memory; behavioral changes and altered or exaggerated individual personality traits	• Concealing inabilities, may make excuses not to perform task or may thumb through a book without actually reading • Loss of proprioception • Primitive reflexes such as positive snout, suck, and palmar reflexes may be present • Facial signs or symptoms dependent on degree of vascular insults • Seizure activity secondary to associated brain damage • Disorientation to time initially then place; usually oriented to person until late in disease process • Impaired recent memory, progressive loss of remote memory • May change answers during the interview • Difficulty in comprehension, abstract thinking • Unable to do simple calculations or repeat the names of three objects; short attention span • Hallucinations, delusions, severe depression, or mania may occur in advanced stage • May have impaired communication—difficulty finding correct words, especially nouns; conversation repetitive or scattered with substituted meaningless words; speech may become inaudible; gradually loses ability to write or read

Client Assessment Database (continued)

DIAGNOSTIC DIVISION MAY REPORT (continued)	MAY EXHIBIT (continued)
SAFETY • Predisposing or factors that may accelerate the condition, such as a history of recent viral illness or serious head trauma, drug toxicity, stress, or nutritional deficits • Incidental trauma such as falls or burns	• Forgets how to negotiate places when away from home • Ignores safety issues • Presence of bruises, lacerations, or other evidence of falling • Disturbance of gait • Striking out or violence directed toward others
SOCIAL INTERACTIONS • Difficulty in relating to others	• Fragmented speech, aphasia, and dysphasia • Demonstrates inappropriate behavior and ignores rules of social conduct • Behavioral pattern alterations related to prior psychosocial factors and individuality and personality • Family roles possibly altered/reversed as individual becomes more dependent
TEACHING/LEARNING • Family history of DAT • May present a total healthy picture, with exception of memory or behavioral changes • Use or misuse of medications, over-the-counter (OTC) drugs, including alcohol • Difficulty managing medications	
DISCHARGE PLAN CONSIDERATIONS • May require support and legal services, financial assistance, caregiver support groups, respite and home healthcare ◗ Following inpatient acute care, refer to underlying condition requiring admission for postdischarge considerations.	

Diagnostic Studies

Although no diagnostic studies are specific for Alzheimer's disease, these studies are used to rule out reversible problems that may be confused with these types of dementia.

TEST WHY IT IS DONE	WHAT IT TELLS ME
BLOOD TESTS • *Antibodies:* Tests for marker for amyloid-â peptide and receptor for advanced glycation end products (Medical College of Georgia, 2004). • *ApoE₄:* Tests for a variant form of ApoE₄, a low penetrance mutation believed to be associated with an increased likelihood of Alzheimer's disease.	Abnormally high levels may be found, leading to a theory of an immunological defect. Investigation of the neuritic plaques gives rise to the possibility that the body has turned against itself. Screens for the presence of a genetic defect associated with the common form of DAT. In rare families, an autosomal dominant inheritance of early onset Alzheimer's disease occurs due to high penetrance mutations. Genetic testing may be helpful in such families.
OTHER DIAGNOSTIC STUDIES • *Neurological mental status examination:* The client is asked to perform maneuvers or answer questions that are designed to elicit information about the condition of specific parts of the brain or peripheral nerves. Testing assesses mental status and alertness, muscle strength, reflexes, sensory-perception, language skills, and coordination.	Many tests may be administered to evaluate client's brain functioning, each measuring a different aspect. One such test, the 7-minute screen (7MS), appears to be highly sensitive to Alzheimer's disease by differentiating between cognitive changes related to the normal aging process and those related to Alzheimer's disease (Solomon et al, 1999).

(continues on page 768)

TEST **WHY IT IS DONE** (continued)	**WHAT IT TELLS ME** (continued)
• *Electroencephalogram (EEG):* Measures electrical activity of the brain.	May reveal slow-wave delta activity indicative of later stages of Alzheimer's disease. May also reveal focal vascular lesions associated with vascular dementia.
• *Skull x-rays:* Determine presence of structural injury.	Usually normal but may reveal signs of head trauma.
• *Positron-emission tomography (PET) scan:* Three-dimensional, computer enhanced, full-color image of the brain.	Traces a positron-emitting chemical that binds effectively to abnormal protein plaques and tangles, thus detecting these Alzheimer markers.
• *Computed tomography (CT) or CAT scan:* X-ray procedure that uses a computer to produce a detailed picture of a cross section of the brain.	May show widening of ventricles or cerebral atrophy. These studies are also used to rule out other central nervous system (CNS) disease.
• *Cerebrospinal fluid (CSF):* Fluid produced within the brain, which surrounds the brain and spinal cord. Samples are obtained by means of lumbar pucture and evaluated for abnormal proteins.	Evidence supports the notion that some cases of mild cognitive impairment may be an early form of Alzheimer's disease. Individuals likely to progress can be identified by measuring tau protein and beta-amyloid-42 proteins in the CSF (Barklay, 2002).

Nursing Priorities

1. Provide safe environment and prevent injury.
2. Promote socially acceptable responses and limit inappropriate behavior.
3. Maintain reality orientation and prevent sensory deprivation or overload.
4. Encourage participation in self-care within individual abilities.
5. Promote coping mechanisms of client/SO(s).
6. Support client and family in grieving process.
7. Provide information about disease process, prognosis, and resources available for assistance.

Discharge Goals

Not indicated in home or community setting. Following inpatient care, based on underlying condition requiring admission.

NURSING DIAGNOSIS: **risk for Injury/Trauma**

Risk factors may include
Inability to recognize or identify danger in environment, impaired judgment
Disorientation, confusion, agitation, irritability, excitability
Weakness, muscular incoordination, balancing difficulties, disturbed perception (e.g., missing chairs, steps)
Seizure activity

Possibly evidenced by:
(Not applicable; presence of signs and symptoms establishes an *actual* diagnosis)

Desired Outcomes/Evaluation Criteria—Family/Caregiver(s) Will

Safe Home Environment (NOC)
Recognize potential risks in the environment.
Identify and implement steps to correct or compensate for individual factors.

Client Will

Physical Injury Severity (NOC)
Be free of injury.

ACTIONS/INTERVENTIONS	RATIONALE
Environmental Management: Safety (NIC) *Independent*	
Assess degree of impairment in ability and competence and presence of impulsive behavior.	Identifies potential risks in the environment and heightens awareness of risks so caregivers are more alert to dangers. Clients demonstrating impulsive behavior are at increased risk of injury because they are less able to control their own behavior/actions.
Assist caregiver to identify any risks or potential hazards and visual-perceptual deficits that may be present.	Visual-perceptual deficits increase the risk of falls.
Eliminate or minimize identified hazards in the environment.	A person with cognitive impairment and perceptual disturbances is prone to accidental injury because of the inability to take responsibility for basic safety needs or to evaluate the unforeseen consequences, such as lighting a stove or cigarette and forgetting about it, mistaking plastic fruit for the real thing and eating it, or misjudging distance involving chairs and stairs. Preventive measures can contain client without constant supervision. Activities promote involvement and keep client occupied.
Lock outside doors as appropriate, especially in evening and night. Do not allow access to stairwell or exit. Provide supervision and activities for client who is regularly awake during the night. Recommend use of "child-proof locks"; secure such items as medications, cleaning products, poisonous substances, tools, and sharp objects. Remove stove knobs and burners.	As the disease worsens, the client may compulsively handle or fidget with objects, including locks, or put small items in mouth, which potentiates possibility of accidental injury and death.
Dementia Management (NIC)	
Monitor behavior routinely, note timing of behavioral changes, increasing confusion, and hyperactivity. Initiate least restrictive interventions before behavior escalates.	Early identification of negative behaviors with appropriate action can prevent need for more stringent measures. *Note:* Sundowner's syndrome develops in late afternoon or early evening, requiring programmed interventions and closer monitoring at this time to redirect and protect client.
Distract or redirect client's attention when behavior is agitated or dangerous, for example climbing out of bed. Place bed in low position and mattress on floor, as indicated.	Maintains safety while avoiding a confrontation that could escalate behavior or increase risk of injury.
Obtain and have client wear identification jewelry, such as bracelet or necklace showing name, phone number, and diagnosis.	Facilitates safe return of client if lost. Because of poor verbal ability and confusion, these persons may be unable to state name, address, and phone number. Client may wander, exhibit poor judgment, and be detained by police, appearing confused, irritable, or having violent outbursts.
Dress according to physical environment and individual need.	The general slowing of metabolic processes results in lowered body heat. The hypothalamic gland may be affected by the disease process or by aging, causing client to feel cold. Client may have seasonal disorientation and may wander out in the cold. *Note:* Leading causes of death in these clients include pneumonia and accidents.
Be attentive to nonverbal physiological symptoms.	Because of sensory loss and language dysfunction, client may express needs nonverbally such as thirst by panting and pain by sweating or doubling over. *Note:* Wandering may be a coping mechanism as client seeks a change in environment if too hot or cold, bored, or overstimulated; or searches for food, or relief from discomfort.
Be alert to underlying meaning of verbal statements.	May direct a question to another, such as, "Are you cold or tired?" meaning client is cold or tired.
Monitor for medication side effects and signs of overmedication—extrapyramidal signs, orthostatic hypotension, visual disturbances, and gastrointestinal (GI) upsets.	Client may not be able to report signs or symptoms, and drugs can easily build up to toxic levels in the elderly. Dosages or drug choice may need to be altered.
Provide quiet room and reduced activity.	Overstimulation increases irritability and agitation, which can escalate to violent outbursts.
Avoid use of restraints. Have SO or others stay with client during periods of acute agitation.	Endangers the individual who succeeds in partial removal of restraints. May increase agitation and potentiate fall risk and fractures in the elderly.

(continues on page 770)

Collaborative

Administer medications as appropriate, such as risperidone (Risperdal), olanzapine (Zyprexa), quetiapine (Seroquel), or ziprasidone (Geodon).

Some antipsychotics are favored to control agitation, aggression, halluncinations, thought disturbances, and wandering because of their lessened propensity to cause anticholinergic and extrapyramidal side effects. May help moderate "sundowning" behaviors. *Note:* Condition may be related to deterioration of the suprachiasmatic nucleus of the hypothalamus which controls the sleep–wake cycle.

NURSING DIAGNOSIS: chronic Confusion

May be related to
Irreversible neuronal degeneration

Possibly evidenced by
Disturbed interpretation or response to stimuli
Progressive, long-standing cognitive impairment; impaired short-term memory
Disturbed personality; impaired socialization
Clinical evidence of organic impairment

Desired Outcomes/Evaluation Criteria— Client Will

Personal Well-Being (NOC)
Experience a decrease in level of frustration, especially when participating in daily activities.

Family/Caregiver Will

Caregiver Performance: Direct Care (NOC)
Verbalize understanding of disease process and client's needs.
Identify and participate in interventions to deal effectively with situation.
Provide for maximal independence while meeting safety need of client.
Initiate behaviors or lifestyle changes to maximize client's cognitive functioning.

ACTIONS/INTERVENTIONS   RATIONALE

Dementia Management (NIC)
Independent

Assess degree of cognitive impairment including changes in orientation to person, place, and time and attention span and thinking ability. Talk with SO and caregiver about changes from usual behavior and length of time problem has existed.

Provides baseline for future evaluation and comparison and influences choice of interventions. *Note:* Repeated evaluation of orientation may actually heighten negative responses and client's level of frustration.

Maintain a pleasant, quiet environment.

Reduces distorted input, whereas crowds, clutter, and noise generate sensory overload that stresses the impaired neurons.

Approach in a slow, calm manner.

This nonverbal gesture lessens the chance of misinterpretation and potential agitation. Hurried approaches can startle and threaten the confused client who misinterprets or feels threatened by imaginary people and/or situations.

Face the individual when conversing.

Maintains reality, expresses interest, and arouses attention, particularly in persons with perceptual disturbances.

Address client by name.

Names form our self-identity and establish reality and individual recognition. Client may respond to own name long after failing to recognize family or caregiver.

Use lower voice register and speak slowly to client.

Increases the chance for comprehension. High-pitched, loud tones convey stress and anger, which may trigger memory of previous confrontations and provoke an angry response.

Give simple directions, one at a time, or step-by-step instructions, using short words and simple sentences.

As the disease progresses, the communication centers in the brain become impaired, hindering the individual's ability to process and comprehend complex messages. Simplicity is the key to communicating, both verbally and nonverbally, with the cognitively impaired person.

Pause between phrases or questions.

Invites a verbal response and may increase comprehension.

Give hints and use open-ended phrases when possible.

Hints stimulate communication and give the person a chance for a positive experience.

Listen with regard despite content of client's speech.

Conveys interest and worth to the individual.

ACTIONS/INTERVENTIONS (continued)

Interpret statements, meanings, and words. If possible, supply the correct word.

Reduce provocative stimuli, such as negative criticism, arguments, and confrontations.

Use distraction. Talk about real people and real events when client begins ruminating about false ideas, unless talking realistically increases anxiety or agitation.

Refrain from forcing activities and communications.

Change activity if client loses interest in present activity.

Use humor with interactions.

Focus on appropriate behavior. Give verbal feedback and positive reinforcement such as a pat on the back or applause. Use touch judiciously and respect individual's personal space and response.

Respect individuality and evaluate individual needs.

Allow personal belongings.

Permit hoarding of safe objects.

Create simple, noncompetitive activities paced to the individual's abilities. Provide entertaining, memory-stimulating music, videos, and TV programs. Engage in old hobbies and preferred activities, such as arts and crafts, music, supervised cooking, gardening, and spiritual programs.

Make useful activities or jobs out of hoarding and repetitive motions, such as collecting junk mail, creating scrapbook, folding and unfolding linen, bouncing balls, dusting, or sweeping floors.

Provide several drawers or baskets that are acceptable to rummage through. Fill with safe items that would be of interest to client, such as yarn balls, quilt blocks, fabrics with different textures and colors; baby clothes, pictures, costume jewelry (without pins), small tools, or sports magazines.

Help client find misplaced items; label drawers and belongings. Do not challenge client.

Monitor phone use closely. Post significant phone numbers in prominent place and secure long-distance numbers.

Evaluate sleep and rest pattern and adequacy. Note lethargy, increasing irritability or confusion, frequent yawning, and dark circles under eyes.

Monitor for medication side effects and signs of overmedication.

Collaborative

Administer medications, as individually indicated, for example:
Acetylcholinesterase (AChE) inhibitors, such as donepezil (Aricept), rivastigmine (Exelon), or galantamine (Razadyne)

RATIONALE (continued)

Assisting the client with word processing aids in decreasing frustration.

Any provocation decreases self-esteem and may be interpreted as a threat, which may trigger agitation or increase inappropriate behavior.

Rumination promotes disorientation. Reality orientation increases client's sense of reality, self-worth, and personal dignity.

Force decreases cooperation and may increase suspiciousness and delusions.

Changing activity maintains interest and reduces restlessness and possibility of confrontation.

Laughter can assist in communication.

Reinforces correctness and appropriate behavior. A focus on inappropriate behavior can encourage repetition. Although touch frequently transcends verbal interchange, and conveys warmth and acceptance, the individual may misinterpret the meaning of touch. Intrusion into personal space may be interpreted as threatening because of the client's distorted perceptions.

Persons experiencing a cognitive decline deserve respect, dignity, and recognition of worth as an individual. Client's past and background are important in maintaining self-concept, planning activities, and communication.

Familiarity enhances security, sense of self, and decreases feelings of loss and deprivation.

This activity may preserve security and counterbalances irrevocable losses.

Motivates client in ways that will reinforce usefulness and self-worth and stimulate reality.

May decrease restlessness and provide option for pleasurable activity. Having a "job" helps client feel useful.

Availability of this kind of assortment provides stimulation that enhances the sense and promotes memories of past life experiences.

May decrease defensiveness when client believes he or she is being accused of stealing a misplaced, hoarded, or hidden item. To refute the accusation will not change the belief and may invite anger.

Can be used as reality orientation. However, client may forget time of day when making calls or may try to call dead relative. Impaired judgment does not allow for distinguishing long-distance numbers and makes client easy prey for phone sales pitches.

Lack of sleep can impair cognitive function and coping abilities. Fatigue may increase severity of symptoms, especially as evening approaches. (Refer to ND: disturbed Sleep Pattern.)

Drugs can easily build up to toxic levels in the elderly, aggravating confusion. Dosages or drug choice may need to be altered.

Cholinesterase inhibitors prevent the breakdown of acetylcholine, a chemical messenger important for learning and memory. These medications are being used for the treatment of mild to moderate cognitive impairment by delaying progression of symptoms in Alzheimer's disease.

(continues on page 772)

N-methyl-D-aspartate (NMDA) inhibitors, such as memantine (Namenda, Axura)

This class of drugs works by regulating the activity of glutamate, a different messenger chemical involved in learning and memory. This medication was approved by the Food and Drug Administration (FDA) in 2003 for treatment of moderate to severe Alzheimer's disease. It slows the progression of the disease and has been shown to improve cognitive and physical abilities in the later stages of the disease.

Antipsychotic agents, such as aripiprazole (Abilify), clozapine (Clozaril), haloperidol (Haldol), quetiapine (Seroquel), or ziprasidone (Geodon)

Psychotic symptoms, such as hallucinations, delusions, aggression, agitation, and hostility may respond to neuroleptic management in most clients with dementia.

Anxiolytic agents, such as buspirone (BuSpar), lorazepam (Ativan), or oxazepam (Serax)

These drugs may be useful for management of anxiety, restlessness, verbally disruptive behavior, and resistance.

Investigational drugs approved for other uses, for example, nonsteroidal anti-inflammatory drugs (NSAIDs), such as ibuprofen (Motrin); estrogen; *Ginkgo biloba;* vitamin E; selegiline (Eldepryl); and prednisone

These drugs are being studied for possible benefit of treatment or for delaying the onset and progression of DAT (NIA, 2008).

NURSING DIAGNOSIS: disturbed Sensory Perception (specify)

May be related to
Altered sensory reception, transmission, and/or integration—neurological disease or deficit
Socially restricted environment—homebound or institutionalized
Sleep deprivation

Possibly evidenced by
Changes in usual response to stimuli—spatial disorientation, confusion, rapid mood swings
Change in problem-solving abilities, altered abstraction and conceptualization
Exaggerated emotional responses—anxiety, paranoia, hallucinations
Inability to tell position of body parts
Diminished or altered sense of taste

Desired Outcomes/Evaluation Criteria—Client Will

Sensory Function Status (NOC)
Demonstrate improved or appropriate response to stimuli.

Caregivers Will

Risk Control (NOC)
Identify and control external factors that contribute to alterations in sensory and/or perceptual abilities.

Reality Orientation (NIC)
Independent

Assess degree of impairment and how it affects the individual, including hearing or visual deficits.

Although brain involvement is usually global, a small percentage of clients may exhibit asymmetrical involvement, which may cause unilateral neglect. Client may not be able to locate internal cues, recognize hunger or thirst, perceive external pain, or locate body within the environment.

Encourage use of corrective lenses and hearing aids, as appropriate.

May enhance sensory input and limit or reduce misinterpretation of stimuli.

Maintain a reality-oriented relationship and environment.

Reduces confusion and promotes coping with the frustrating struggles of misperception and being disoriented or confused.

Provide clues for 24-hour reality orientation with calendars, clocks, notes, cards, signs, music, seasonal hues, and scenic pictures; color-code rooms.

Dysfunction in visual-spatial perception interferes with the ability to recognize directions and patterns, and the client may become lost even in familiar surroundings. Clues are tangible reminders that aid recognition and may permeate memory gaps, increasing independence.

Provide quiet, nondistracting environment when indicated, including soft music, or room with plain but colorful wallpaper or paint.

Helps to avoid visual or auditory overload, by emphasizing qualities of calmness and consistency. *Note:* Patterned wallpaper may be disturbing to the client.

Provide touch in a caring way.

May enhance perception to self and body boundaries.

ACTIONS/INTERVENTIONS (continued)	RATIONALE (continued)
Engage client in individually meaningful activities, supporting remaining abilities and minimizing failures. Examples include meal preparation, setup and cleaning activities, making bed, and gardening or watering plants.	Supports client's dignity, familiarizes individual with home and community events, and enables him or her to experience satisfaction and pleasure.
Use sensory games to stimulate reality, such as smelling mentholated ointment may prompt client to tell of the time mother used it on client; use of spring or fall nature boxes may stimulate reality.	Communicates reality through multiple channels.
Indulge in periodic reminiscence, such as listening to old music; recalling historical events; and looking at photos, mementoes, or videos.	Stimulates recollections, awakens memories, aids in the preservation of self and individuality via past accomplishments, and increases feelings of security. Helpful in easing adaptation to a changed environment.
Provide intellectual activities, such as word games, review of current events, storytime, or travel discussions.	Stimulates remaining cognitive abilities and provides a sense of normalcy.
Include in Bible study group, church activities, and TV services for shut-ins; or arrange for visitation by clergy or spiritual advisor, as appropriate.	Provides opportunity to meet spiritual needs and to maintain connection with religious beliefs; may help reduce sense of isolation from humanity.
Encourage simple outings and short walks. Monitor activity.	Outings refresh reality and provide pleasurable sensory stimuli, which may reduce suspiciousness or hallucinations caused by feelings of imprisonment. Motor functioning may be decreased, because nerve degeneration results in weakness, decreasing stamina.
Promote balanced physiological functions tossing colorful foam or beach balls or beanbags, marching, dancing, or arm dancing with music.	Preserves mobility by reducing the potential for bone loss and muscle atrophy; provides diversional activity and opportunity for interaction with others.
Involve in activities with others as dictated by individual situation—one-to-one visitors; animal visitation; socialization groups at an Alzheimer center; or occupational therapy including crafts, painting or finger paints, and modeling clay.	Provides opportunity for the stimulation of participation with others and may maintain some level of social interaction.

NURSING DIAGNOSIS: Fear

May be related to
Decreases in functional abilities
Public disclosure of disabilities
Further mental and/or physical deterioration

Possibly evidenced by
Social isolation
Apprehension, irritability, defensiveness, suspiciousness
Aggressive behavior

Desired Outcomes/Evaluation Criteria—Client Will

Fear Level (NOC)
Demonstrate more appropriate range of feelings and lessened fear.

ACTIONS/INTERVENTIONS	RATIONALE
Anxiety Reduction (NIC) *Independent* Note change of behavior, suspiciousness, irritability, and defensiveness.	Change in moods may be one of the first signs of cognitive decline, and the client, fearing helplessness, tries to hide the increasing inability to remember and engage in normal activities.
Identify strengths the individual had previously.	Facilitates assistance with communication and management of current deficits.
Deal with aggressive behavior by imposing calm, firm limits.	Acceptance can reduce fear and lessen progression of aggressive behavior.
Provide clear, honest information about actions and events.	Assists in maintaining trust and orientation as long as possible. When the client knows the truth about what is happening, coping is often enhanced, and guilt over what is imagined is decreased.
Discuss feelings of SO and caregivers. Acknowledge normalcy of feelings and concerns and provide information as needed.	Client senses but may not understand reaction of others. This may heighten client's sense of anxiety and fear.

773

NURSING DIAGNOSIS: Grieving

May be related to
Client awareness of something "being wrong" with changes in memory/family reaction, physiopsychosocial well-being
Family perception of potential loss of loved one

Possibly evidenced by
Expressions of distress, anger at potential loss
Choked feelings, crying
Alteration in activity level, communication patterns, eating habits, and sleep patterns

Desired Outcomes/Evaluation Criteria—Client/Family Will

Psychosocial Adjustment: Life Change (NOC)
Express concerns openly.
Discuss loss and participate in planning for the future.

ACTIONS/INTERVENTIONS	RATIONALE
Grief Work Facilitation (NIC)	
Independent	
Assess degree of deterioration or level of coping.	Information is helpful to understand how much the client is capable of doing to maintain highest level of independence and to provide encouragement to help individuals deal with losses.
Provide open environment for discussion. Use therapeutic communication skills of active-listening and acknowledgment.	Encourages client and caregivers to discuss feelings and concerns realistically.
Note statements of despair, hopelessness, "nothing to live for," and expressions of anger.	May be indicative of suicidal ideation. Angry behavior may be client's way of dealing with feelings of despair.
Respect desire not to talk.	May not be ready to deal with or share grief.
Be honest; do not give false reassurances or dire predictions about the future.	Honesty promotes a trusting relationship. Expressions of gloom, such as, "You'll spend the rest of your life in a nursing home," are not helpful because no one knows what the future holds.
Discuss with client and SOs ways they can plan together for the future.	Having a part in problem-solving and planning can provide a sense of control over anticipated events.
Assist client and SO to identify positive aspects of the situation.	Ongoing research, possibility of slow progression may offer some hope for the future.
Identify strengths client and SO see in self and situation and support systems available.	Recognizing these resources provides opportunity to work through feelings of grief.
Collaborative	
Refer to other resources, such as support groups, counseling, and spiritual advisor.	May need additional support or assistance to resolve feelings.

NURSING DIAGNOSIS: Sleep Deprivation

May be related to
Dementia, sundowner's syndrome
Aging-related sleep stage shifts
Inadequate daytime activity

Possibly evidenced by
Changes in behavior and performance, irritability, agitation
Fatigue, daytime drowsiness

Desired Outcomes/Evaluation Criteria—Client Will

Sleep (NOC)
Establish adequate sleep pattern, with wandering reduced.
Report or appear rested.

ACTIONS/INTERVENTIONS	RATIONALE

Sleep Enhancement (NIC)
Independent
Provide for adequate rest. Restrict daytime sleep as appropriate; increase interaction time between client and family and staff during the day, then reduce mental activity late in the day.
Avoid use of continuous restraints.

Although prolonged physical and mental activity results in fatigue, which can increase confusion, programmed activity without overstimulation promotes sleep.
Restraints may potentiate sensory deprivation, agitation, and restrict rest. *Note:* The Health Care Financing Administration's (HCFA) guidelines (1999) require that clients be free from chemical or mechanical restraint unless warranted by a medical diagnosis and that the least restrictive means of control be used.

Evaluate level of stress and orientation as day progresses.

Increasing confusion, disorientation, and uncooperative behaviors may interfere with attaining restful sleep pattern.

Adhere to regular bedtime schedule and rituals. Tell client that it is time to sleep.

Reinforces that it is bedtime and maintains stability of environment. *Note:* Later-than-normal bedtime may be indicated to allow client to dissipate excess energy and facilitate falling asleep.

Provide evening snack, warm milk, bath, or back rub or general massage with lotion.
Reduce fluid intake in the evening. Toilet before retiring.

Promotes relaxation and drowsiness and helps to address skin-care needs.
Decreases need to get up to go to the bathroom/incontinence during the night.

Provide soft music or "white noise."

Reduces sensory stimulation by blocking out other environmental sounds that could interfere with restful sleep.

Allow to sleep in shoes or clothing, if client demands.

Provided no harm is done, altering the "normal" lessens the rebellion and allows rest.

Collaborative
Administer medications, as indicated for sleep, for example:
  Antidepressants, such as trazadone (Desyrel) or quetiapine (Seroquel)
  Sedative-hypnotics, such as zolpidem (Ambien) or zaleplon (Sonata)

May be effective in treating pseudodementia or depression, thus improving ability to sleep.
Used sparingly, low-dose, short-acting, rapid-onset hypnotics may be effective in treating insomnia or sundowner's syndrome.

  Avoid use of diphenhydramine (Benadryl).

Once used for sleep, this drug is now contraindicated because it interferes with the production of acetylcholine, which is already inhibited in the brains of clients with DAT.

NURSING DIAGNOSIS: Self-Care Deficit (specify type/level)

May be related to
Cognitive decline, physical limitations
Frustration over loss of independence, depression

Possibly evidenced by
Impaired ability to perform activities of daily living (ADLs)—frustration; forgetfulness; misuse or misidentification of objects; inability to bring food from receptacle to mouth; inability to wash body part(s), regulate water temperature; impaired ability to put on/take off clothing; difficulty completing toileting tasks

Desired Outcomes/Evaluation Criteria—Client Will

Self-Care Status (NOC)
Perform self-care activities within level of own ability.

Caregiver Will

Caregiver Home Care Readiness (NIC)
Identify and use personal and community resources that can provide assistance; support client's independence.

ACTIONS/INTERVENTIONS	RATIONALE

Self-Care Assistance: [specify] (NIC)
Independent
Identify reason for difficulty in self-care related to physical limitations in motion, depression, cognitive decline, or environment.

Underlying cause affects choice of interventions and strategies. Clients reported to be unable to perform specific ADLs are often able to do so given the right circumstances, such as adequate and knowledgeable caregiver support.

(continues on page 776)

Determine hygienic needs and provide assistance as needed with activities, including care of hair, nails, and skin; brushing teeth, and cleaning glasses.	As the disease progresses, basic hygienic needs may be forgotten. Infection, gum disease, disheveled appearance, or harm may occur when client or caregivers become frustrated, irritated, or intimidated by degree of care required.
Inspect skin regularly.	Presence of such lesions as ecchymoses, lacerations, or rashes may require treatment as well as signal the need for closer monitoring and protective interventions.
Incorporate usual routine into activity schedule as possible. Wait or change the time to initiate dressing and hygiene if a problem arises.	Maintaining routine may prevent worsening of confusion and enhance cooperation. Because anger is quickly forgotten, another time or approach may be successful.
Be attentive to nonverbal physiological symptoms.	Sensory loss and language dysfunction may cause client to express self-care needs in nonverbal manner, such as thirst by panting, need to void by holding self or fidgeting, and pain by facial grimacing.
Be alert to underlying meaning of verbal statements.	May direct a question to another, such as, "Are you cold?" meaning "I am cold and need additional clothing."
Supervise but allow as much autonomy as possible.	Eases the frustration over lost independence.
Allot plenty of time to perform tasks.	Tasks that were once easy, such as dressing or bathing, are now complicated by decreased motor skills or cognitive and physical changes. Time and patience can reduce chaos resulting from trying to hasten this process.
Assist with neat dressing and provide colorful clothes.	Enhances esteem; may diminish sense of sensory loss and convey aliveness.
Offer one item of clothing at a time in sequential order. Talk client through each step of the task. Allow the wearing of extra clothing if client demands.	Simplicity reduces frustration and the potential for rage and despair. Guidance reduces confusion and allows autonomy. Altering the "normal" may lessen rebellion.
Provide reminders for elimination needs. Involve in bowel and bladder program, as appropriate.	Loss of control and independence in this self-care activity can have a great impact on self-esteem and may limit socialization. (Refer to ND: Constipation.)
Assist with and provide reminders for pericare after toileting or incontinence.	Good hygiene promotes cleanliness and reduces risks of skin irritation and infection.

NURSING DIAGNOSIS: **risk for imbalanced Nutrition: Less/More than Body Requirements**

Risk factors may include
Sensory changes
Impaired judgment and coordination
Agitation, forgetfulness, regressed habits, concealment

Possibly evidenced by
(Not applicable; presence of signs and symptoms establishes an *actual* diagnosis)

Desired Outcomes/Evaluation Criteria—Client Will

Nutritional Status (NOC)
Ingest nutritionally balanced diet.
Maintain or regain appropriate weight.

ACTIONS/INTERVENTIONS

RATIONALE

Nutrition Management (NIC)
Independent

Assess caregiver's and client's knowledge of nutritional needs.	Identifies needs to assist in formulating individual teaching plan. Role-reversals may occur: a child now cooks for a parent, or a husband taking over "duties" of his wife, increasing the need for information.
Perform Edinburgh Feeding Evaluation in Dementia (EdFED) scale, as appropriate, if client demonstrates weight loss or decline in mealtime function. Schedule regular repeat reviews at same time of day and in same environment.	Helps establish baseline and monitors behaviors in moderate-to-severe dementia and to determine level of assistance required (Stockdell & Amella, 2008).
Determine amount of exercise or pacing client does.	Nutritional intake may need to be adjusted to meet needs related to individual energy expenditure.

ACTIONS/INTERVENTIONS (continued)

Offer or provide assistance in menu selection.

Provide privacy when eating habits become an insoluble problem. Accept eating with hands, spills, and whimsical mixtures such as salad dressing in milk or salt and pepper on ice cream. Avoid solo dining or separating client from other people too early in the disease process.

Offer small meals and/or snacks of one or two foods around the clock, as indicated.

Simplify steps of eating and serve food in courses.

Anticipate needs, cut foods, and provide soft or finger foods.

Provide ample time for eating.

Place food items in pita bread or paper sack for the client who paces.
Avoid baby food and excessively hot foods.

Observe swallowing ability; monitor oral cavity.

Stimulate oral-suck reflex by gentle stroking of the cheeks or stimulating the mouth with a spoon.

Collaborative
Refer to dietitian or nutritionist, as indicated.

RATIONALE (continued)

Poor judgment may lead to poor choices; client may be indecisive or overwhelmed by choices and/or unaware of the need to maintain elemental nutrition. *Note:* In general, metabolic rate decreases with age, requiring caloric adjustment that must be balanced with activity.

Socially unacceptable and embarrassing eating habits develop as the disease progresses. Acceptance preserves esteem and decreases irritability or refusal to eat as a result of anger or frustration. Early separation can result in client feeling upset and rejected and can actually result in decreased food intake.

Large feedings may overwhelm the client, resulting either in complete abstinence or gorging. Small feedings may enhance appropriate intake. Limiting number of foods offered at a single time reduces confusion regarding which food to choose.

Promotes autonomy and independence; decreases potential frustration or anger over lost abilities.

Coordination decreases as the disease progresses, which impairs the client's ability to chew and handle utensils.

A leisurely approach aids digestion and decreases the chance of anger precipitated by rushing.

Carrying food may encourage client to eat.

Baby foods lack adequate nutritional content, fiber, and taste for adults and can add to client's humiliation. Hot foods may result in mouth burns and/or refusal to eat.

Diminished abilities may result in client or caregiver repeatedly placing food in client's mouth, which is not swallowed, increasing risk of aspiration.

As the disease progresses, the client may clench teeth and refuse to eat. Stimulating the reflex may increase cooperation and intake.

Assistance may be needed to develop nutritionally balanced diet individualized to meet client needs or food preferences.

NURSING DIAGNOSIS: ## Constipation (specify)/Bowel Incontinence/impaired Urinary Elimination

May be related to
Disorientation, inability to locate the bathroom or recognize need
Lost neurological functioning and muscle tone
Changes in dietary and fluid intake

Possibly evidenced by
Urgency, inappropriate toileting behaviors
Incontinence, constipation

Desired Outcomes/Evaluation Criteria—Client Will

Bowel [or] Urinary Elimination (NOC)
Establish adequate or appropriate pattern of elimination.

ACTIONS/INTERVENTIONS

Urinary Elimination [or] Bowel Management (NIC)
Independent
Assess prior pattern and compare with current situation.

Establish bowel and bladder training program. Promote client participation to level of ability.

RATIONALE

Provides information about changes that may require further assessment and intervention.

Stimulates awareness, enhances regulation of body function, and helps to avoid accidents.

(continues on page 778)

Monitor appearance and color of urine. Note amount and consistency of stool.

Detection of changes provides opportunity to alter interventions to prevent complications or acquire treatment, as indicated. *Note:* Although it is difficult, the caregiver must try to monitor frequency of bowel movements during the stage of the illness when the client is still toileting self. It is not enough to ask client, "Did you have a bowel movement today?" Client cannot remember. Monitoring is essential to prevent constipation and potential for impaction.

Encourage adequate fluid intake during the day, with diet high in fiber and fruit juices. Limit intake during the late evening and at bedtime.

Essential for bodily functions and prevents potential dehydration and constipation. Restricting intake in evening may reduce frequency and incontinence during the night.

Self-Care Assistance: Toileting (NIC)

Locate bed near a bathroom when possible; make signs or color code door. Place a picture of a commode on the door. Provide adequate lighting, particularly at night.

Promotes orientation and increases success in finding bathroom. Incontinence may be attributed to inability to find a toilet.

Take client to the toilet at regular intervals. Dictate each step one at a time and use positive reinforcement.

Adherence to a daily and regular schedule may prevent accidents. Frequently, the problem is forgetting how to toilet, such as pushing pants down or positioning.

Avoid a sense of hurrying or being rushed.

Hurrying may be perceived as intrusion, which leads to anger and lack of cooperation with activity.

Be alert to nonverbal cues, such as restlessness, holding self, or picking at clothes.

May signal urgency or inattention to cues and/or inability to locate bathroom.

Be discreet and respect client's privacy.

Although the client is confused, a sense of modesty is often retained.

Convey acceptance when incontinence occurs. Change promptly; provide good skin care.

Acceptance is important to decrease the embarrassment and feelings of helplessness that may occur during the changing process. Prompt changing reduces risk of skin irritation and breakdown.

Collaborative

Administer stool softeners, bulk expanders (e.g., Metamucil), or glycerin suppository, as indicated.

May be necessary to facilitate or stimulate regular bowel movement.

NURSING DIAGNOSIS: risk for Sexual Dysfunction

Risk factors may include
Altered body function, progression of disease—decrease in habit or control of behavior, confusion, forgetfulness, and disorientation to place or person
Lack of intimacy, sexual rejection by SO
Lack of privacy

Possibly evidenced by
(Not applicable; presence of signs and symptoms establishes an *actual* diagnosis)

Desired Outcomes/Evaluation Criteria—Client Will

Sexual Functioning (NOC)
Meet sexuality needs in an acceptable manner.
Experience fewer or no episodes of inappropriate behavior.

ACTIONS/INTERVENTIONS

RATIONALE

Sexual Counseling (NIC)
Independent

Assess individual needs, desires, and abilities of client and partner.

Alternative methods need to be designed for the individual situation to fulfill the need for intimacy and closeness.

Encourage partner to show affection and acceptance.

The cognitively impaired person retains the basic needs for affection, love, acceptance, and sexual expression.

Ensure privacy or encourage home visitation for residential client, as appropriate.

Sexual expression or behaviors may differ. The individual may masturbate or expose self. Privacy allows sexual expression without embarrassment and the objections of others.

Use distraction, as indicated. Remind client that, when in a public area, sexual behavior is unacceptable.

This tool is useful when there is inappropriate or objectionable behavior, such as self-exposure.

Provide time to listen to and discuss concerns of partner.

Partner may need information and/or counseling about alternatives for sexual activity and ways to deal with problems, such as impotence or sexual aggression.

NURSING DIAGNOSIS: compromised/disabled family Coping

May be related to
Disruptive behavior of client
Family grief about their helplessness watching loved one deteriorate
Prolonged disease or disability progression that exhausts the supportive capacity of SO
Highly ambivalent family relationships

Possibly evidenced by
Family becoming embarrassed and socially immobilized
Home maintenance becoming extremely difficult, leading to difficult decisions with legal and financial considerations

Desired Outcomes/Evaluation Criteria—Family Will

Family Coping (NOC)
Identify resources within themselves to deal with the situation.
Acknowledge client's condition and demonstrate positive coping behaviors in dealing with situation.
Use outside support systems effectively.

ACTIONS/INTERVENTIONS	RATIONALE
Family Support (NIC)	
Independent	
Include family in teaching and planning for home care.	Can ease the burden of home management and increase adaptation. A comfortable and familiar lifestyle at home helps preserve the client's need for belonging.
Review past life experiences, role changes, and coping skills.	Identifies skills that may help individuals cope with grief of current situation more effectively.
Focus on specific problems as they occur, the "here and now."	Disease progression follows no set pattern. A premature focus on the possibility of long-term care or possible incontinence, for example, impairs the ability to cope with present issues.
Establish priorities.	Helps to create a sense of order and facilitates problem-solving.
Be realistic and honest in all matters.	Decreases stress that surrounds false hopes, such as that client may regain past level of functioning from advertised or unproven medication.
Reassess family's ability to care for client at home on an ongoing basis.	Behaviors like hoarding, clinging, unjust accusations, and angry outbursts, can precipitate family burnout and interfere with ability to provide effective care.
Provide time to listen with regard to concerns and anxieties.	SO and caregiver require constant support with the multifaceted problems that arise during the course of this illness to ease the process of adaptation and grieving.
Help caregiver/family understand the importance of maintaining psychosocial functioning.	Embarrassing behavior and the demands of care may cause withdrawal from social contact.
Discuss possibility of isolation. Reinforce need for support systems.	The belief that a single individual can meet all the needs of the client increases the potential for physical or mental illness due to caregiver role strain. *Note:* Mortality rate for primary caregivers is actually higher than for the client with DAT.
Provide positive feedback for efforts.	Reassures individuals that they are doing their best and provides reinforcement to continue efforts.
Acknowledge concerns generated by consideration or decision to place client in long-term care facility. Answer questions honestly and explore options, as appropriate.	Constant care requirements may be more than can be managed by the caregiver and support systems. Support is needed for this difficult guilt-producing decision, which may create a financial burden as well as family disruption and dissension.
Encourage visitation by extended family and friends as tolerated by client.	Familiarity forms a base of reality and can provide a reassuring freedom from loneliness. Recurrent contact helps family members realize and accept situation. *Note:* Family members may require ongoing support in dealing with visitation and issues of client's deterioration and their own personal needs.
Collaborative	
Involve SO and family members in planning care and problem-solving. Verify presence of advance directives and durable medical power of attorney.	Consensus may be more readily achieved when family participates in decision making. It is important, however, to keep client's wishes in mind when making choices and to be aware of who actually has the power to make decisions for the cognitively impaired client.

(continues on page 780)

ACTIONS/INTERVENTIONS (continued)

Refer to local resources such as adult day care, respite care, homemaker services, or a local chapter of Alzheimer's Disease Education and Referral (ADEAR) and the National Family Caregivers Association (NFCA).

Refer for family counseling or to appropriate ethical committee, as indicated.

RATIONALE (continued)

Coping with these clients is a full-time, frustrating task. Respite and day care may lighten the burden, reduce potential social isolation, and prevent family burnout and caregiver role strain. ADEAR provides group support and family teaching and promotes research. Local groups provide a social outlet for sharing grief and promote problem-solving with such matters as financial or legal advice and home care. NFCA also provides programs for educating caregivers and health-care providers, and a quarterly publication.

Differing opinions regarding client care and placement can result in conflict requiring professional mediation.

NURSING DIAGNOSIS: **impaired Home Maintenance/ineffective Health Maintenance**

May be related to
Progressively impaired cognitive functioning
Complete or partial lack of gross and/or fine motor skills
Significant alteration in communication skills
Ineffective individual or family coping
Insufficient family organization or planning
Unfamiliarity with resources, inadequate support systems

Possibly evidenced by
Overtaxed family members—exhausted, anxious
Household members express difficulty and request help in maintaining home safely and comfortably
Home surroundings appear disorderly, unsafe
Reported or observed inability to take responsibility for meeting basic health practices
Reported or observed lack of equipment, financial, or other resources, impairment of personal support system

Desired Outcomes/Evaluation Criteria—Family/Caregiver(s) Will

Family Resiliency (NOC)
Verbalize ability to cope adequately with existing situation.
Identify factors related to difficulty in maintaining a safe environment for the client.
Assume responsibility for and initiate changes supporting client safety and healthcare goals.
Demonstrate appropriate, effective use of resources such as respite or day care, homemakers, and support groups.

ACTIONS/INTERVENTIONS

Home Maintenance Assistance (NIC)
Independent
Evaluate level of cognitive, emotional, and physical functioning, including level of independence.

Assess environment, noting unsafe factors and ability of client to care for self.
Identify senior services and community resources for homemaking and cleaning or handyman tasks.

Health System Guidance (NIC)
Assist client to develop plan for keeping track of and dealing with health needs.
Identify support systems available to client and SO, including other family members and friends.

Evaluate coping abilities, effectiveness, and commitment of caregiver(s) and support persons.

RATIONALE

Identifies strengths, areas of need, and how much responsibility the client may be expected to assume. (Refer to ND: Self-Care Deficit.)
Determines what changes need to be made to accommodate disabilities. (Refer to ND: risk for Injury/Trauma.)
As client's condition worsens, caregiver will require additional support to maintain client in home, especially if family support is limited or not available.

Schedule can be helpful to maintain system for managing routine healthcare services.
Planning and constant care is necessary to maintain this client at home. If family system is unavailable or unaware, client health needs, such as nutrition, dental care, or eye exams, can be neglected. Primary caregiver can benefit from sharing responsibilities and constant care with others. (Refer to ND: risk for Caregiver Role Strain, following.)
Progressive debilitation taxes caregiver(s) and may alter ability to meet client's and own needs. (Refer to ND: compromised/disabled family Coping.)

ACTIONS/INTERVENTIONS (continued)

Collaborative

Refer to supportive services, as needed.

Identify in-home healthcare options including medical, dental, and diagnostic services.

RATIONALE (continued)

Medical and social services consultant may be needed to develop ongoing plan or identify resources as needs change.

Delivery of healthcare needs "on site" may prevent exacerbation of confusion, increase cooperation, and provide more accurate picture of client's status.

NURSING DIAGNOSIS: risk for Caregiver Role Strain

Risk factors may include

Illness severity of the care receiver, duration of caregiving required, complexity or amount of caregiving tasks

Caregiver is female, spouse

Care receiver exhibits deviant, bizarre behavior

Family/caregiver isolation, lack of respite and recreation

Possibly evidenced by

(Not applicable; presence of signs and symptoms establishes an *actual* diagnosis)

Desired Outcomes/Evaluation Criteria—Caregiver Will

Caregiver Performance: Direct Care (NOC)

Identify individual risk factors and appropriate interventions.

Demonstrate or initiate behaviors or lifestyle changes to prevent development of impaired function.

Caregiver Performance: Indirect Care (NOC)

Use available resources appropriately.

Report satisfaction with plan and support available.

ACTIONS/INTERVENTIONS

RATIONALE

Caregiver Support (NIC)

Independent

Determine family/caregiver's understanding of condition and expectations for the future.

Identifies teaching needs. Provides opportunity to update information and clarify misconceptions. During the prolonged caregiving experience, 7 of 10 clients with Alzheimer's continue to live at home, where family and friends provide almost 75% of their care. As the individual descends into the disease, he or she cannot translate a thought into a motor action, thus full-time supervision and care is required. For some family members and care partners, this supervision becomes overwhelming and exhausting (Rentz, 2008).

Provide bibliotherapy.

Materials that can be reviewed as time permits or questions arise can be very helpful in expanding knowledge and providing on-going support.

Identify strengths of caregiver and care receiver.

Helps to use positive aspects of each individual to the best of abilities in daily activities.

Facilitate family conference to share responsibilities as indicated and to stress importance of self-nurturing for caregiver, including such factors as pursuing self-development interests, personal needs, hobbies, and social activities.

Helps family to focus on needs of caregiver as well as care receiver. When others are involved in care, the risk of one person becoming overwhelmed is lessened.

Determine available supports and resources currently used.

Organizations including Azheimer's Foundation of America, Alzheimer's Association, NFCA, or local support groups can provide information regarding adequacy of supports, identify needs, and suggest possible options.

Identify alternate-care sources such as sitter or day-care facility; senior care services such as Meals on Wheels and respite care; and Alzheimer's programs or a home-care agency.

As client's condition worsens, caregiver may need additional help from several sources to maintain client at home, even on a part-time basis.

Refer to CP: Multiple Sclerosis, ND: risk for Caregiver Role Strain for additional interventions.

risk for Relocation Stress Syndrome

Risk factors may include
Little or no preparation for transfer to hospital or extended care setting
Changes in daily routine
Sensory impairment, physical deterioration
Separation from support systems

Possibly evidenced by:
(Not applicable; presence of signs and symptoms establishes an *actual* diagnosis)

Desired Outcomes/Evaluation Criteria—Client Will

Stress Level (NOC)
Experience minimal disruption of usual activities.
Display limited increase in agitation.

Family/Caregiver Will

Family Participation in Professional Care (NOC)
Be aware of potential impact of changes on client.
Plan for and coordinate move as situation permits.
Recognize need to provide stability for client during adaptation period.

ACTIONS/INTERVENTIONS	RATIONALE
Relocation Stress Reduction (NIC)	
Independent	
Discuss ramifications of move to new surroundings.	Discussing pros and cons of this decision helps those involved to reach an informed decision and feel better about and plan for the future.
Encourage visitation to facility prior to planned move.	Familiarizes family and client with new options to enable them to make informed decision.
Provide clear, honest information about actions and events.	Decreases "surprises." Assists in maintaining trust and orientation. When the client knows the truth about what is happening, coping may be enhanced.

Refer to CP: Extended Care, ND: risk for Relocation Stress Syndrome for additional interventions.

POTENTIAL CONSIDERATIONS following acute hospitalization (dependent on underlying cause for admission and comorbidities) refer to appropriate care plan.

SURGICAL INTERVENTION

I. Procedure—Therapeutic manipulation or use of instruments to diagnose or remedy physical disorders or defects
  a. Indications
    i. Diagnose or cure a specific disease process
    ii. Correct a structural deformity
    iii. Restore a functional process
    iv. Reduce the level of dysfunction or pain

  b. Classification
    i. Generally elective or preplanned
      1. Inpatient procedure
      2. Ambulatory or outpatient
    ii. Potentially life-threatening conditions can arise requiring emergent intervention.
II. Pathophysiology—Dependent upon the type of injury or disease process that the client has experienced

G L O S S A R Y

Ambulatory surgery: Refers to surgical procedures performed on an outpatient basis in a hospital or freestanding ambulatory surgery center's general or main operating rooms, satellite operating rooms, cystoscopy rooms, endoscopy rooms, cardiac catheterization labs, or laser procedure rooms.

Atelectasis: Collapsed or airless condition of the lung or lung segment.
Bronchospasm: Abnormal narrowing with partial obstruction of the lumen of the bronchi due to spasm of the peribronchial smooth muscle.

GLOSSARY (continued)

Cephalad diffusion: Movement toward the head, in context of spinal anesthesia, indicates advancement of drug effect generally beyond desired level.

Cubital: Refers to the ulna or the forearm.

Dehiscence: Bursting open or separation of surgical incision or wound.

Electrocautery: Cauterization using a variety of electrical modalities to create thermal energy, including a directly heated metallic applicator or bipolar or monopolar electrodes.

Fasciculation: Involuntary contraction or twitching of muscle fibers, which are visible under the skin.

Hemostasis: Arrest or cessation of bleeding from an injured vessel.

Hypercoagulation: Increased ability of blood, for example, to coagulate.

Hypoxia: An oxygen deficiency in body tissues.

Intraoperatively: Occurring during surgery.

Laryngospasm: Spasm of the laryngeal muscles that may be life threatening.

Perioperative: Period of time that constitutes the surgical experience; includes the preoperative, intraoperative, and postoperative phases of nursing care.

Postoperative: Period of time that begins with admission to the postanesthesia care unit (PACU) and ends after a follow-up evaluation in the clinical setting or home.

Preoperative: Period of time from when the decision for surgical intervention is made to when the individual is transferred to the operating room table.

Prophylactically: Any agent or regimen that contributes to the prevention of infection or disease.

Time-out protocol: Procedure for ensuring final verification of the correct client, procedure, site, and, if applicable, implants. Includes active communication among all members of the surgical team; procedure is not started until this has occurred.

Care Setting

Client may be inpatient on a surgical unit or outpatient or have a short stay in an ambulatory surgical setting.

Related Concerns

Alcohol: acute withdrawal, page 819

Cancer, page 846

Diabetes mellitus/diabetic ketoacidosis, page 405

Fluid and electrolyte imbalances, page 903

Pneumothorax/hemothorax, page 154

Metabolic acidosis—primary base bicarbonate deficiency, page 483

Metabolic alkalosis—primary base bicarbonate excess, page 488

Peritonitis, page 349

Pneumonia, page 131

Psychosocial aspects of care, page 749

Respiratory acidosis (primary carbonic acid excess), page 195

Respiratory alkalosis (primary carbonic acid deficit), page 200

Sepsis/septicemia, page 686

Thrombophlebitis: deep vein thrombosis, page 111

Total nutritional support: parenteral/enteral feeding, page 469

Also refer to plan of care for specific surgical procedure performed.

Client Assessment Database

Data depend on the duration and severity of underlying problem and involvement of other body systems. Refer to specific plans of care for data and diagnostic studies relevant to the procedure and additional nursing diagnoses.

DIAGNOSTIC DIVISION MAY REPORT	MAY EXHIBIT
CIRCULATION • History of cardiac problems, heart failure (HF), pulmonary edema, peripheral vascular disease, or vascular stasis, which increase risk of thrombus formation	• Changes in heart rate due to sympathetic stimulation
EGO INTEGRITY • Feelings of anxiety, fear, anger, apathy • Multiple stress factors related to financial, relationship, lifestyle issues	• Restlessness, increased tension or irritability • Sympathetic stimulation—changes in heart or respiratory rate

(continues on page 784)

DIAGNOSTIC DIVISION
MAY REPORT (continued)

ELIMINATION
- History of kidney or bladder conditions
- Use of diuretics and/or laxatives
- Change in bowel habits

FOOD/FLUID
- History of pancreatic insufficiency or diabetes mellitus (DM), which may predispose client to hypoglycemia or ketoacidosis
- Use of diuretics

PAIN/DISCOMFORT
- History of painful body area—often the reason for surgical procedure—due to disease, inflammation, infection, or trauma

RESPIRATION
- History or presence of respiratory infections
- Chronic lung conditions
- Past and/or current smoking

SAFETY
- Differences in personal identifiers, procedure type, and/or site when compared to verification tools, such as the consent form, history and physical examination, surgery schedule
- Allergies or sensitivities to medications, iodine, food, tape, latex, and solution(s)
- Immune deficiencies—increase risk of systemic infections and delayed healing
- Presence of cancer or recent cancer therapy
- Family history of malignant hyperthermia or reaction to anesthesia, autoimmune diseases
- History of hepatic disease which might affect drug detoxification and may alter coagulation
- History of blood transfusion(s) or transfusion reaction

TEACHING/LEARNING
- Use of medications, such as anticoagulants, steroids, non-steroidal anti-inflammatory drugs (NSAIDs), antibiotics, antihypertensives, cardiotonic glycosides, antidysrhythmics, bronchodilators, diuretics, decongestants, analgesics, anti-inflammatory drugs, anticonvulsants, or antipsychotics and anti-anxiety agents as well as over-the-counter (OTC) medications, herbal supplements (e.g., garlic, ginseng, ginkgo biloba, ginger, and feverfew present risk of excessive postoperative bleeding), or alcohol or other drugs of abuse, with risk of liver damage affecting coagulation and choice of anesthesia as well as potential for postoperative withdrawal

DISCHARGE PLAN CONSIDERATIONS
- May require temporary assistance with transportation, dressing(s), supplies, self-care, and homemaker or maintenance tasks
- Possible placement in rehabilitation or extended care facility

▶ Refer to section at end of plan for postdischarge considerations.

MAY EXHIBIT (continued)

- Abdominal tenderness, distention
- Absence of bowel elimination
- Decreased or absent urinary elimination

- Malnutrition, including obesity
- Dry mucous membranes due to limited intake, or nothing-by-mouth (NPO) status preoperatively

- Guarding behavior, facial mask, sleep disturbance, restlessness, moaning

- Changes in respiratory rate (respiratory pathology, pain, or sympathetic stimulation)

- Presence of existing infectious process
- Fever
- Advanced age

Diagnostic Studies

Studies depend on type of operative procedure, underlying medical conditions, current medications, age, and weight. Deviations from normal should be corrected, if possible, for safe administration of anesthetic agents.

TEST WHY IT IS DONE	WHAT IT TELLS ME
BLOOD TESTS • *Complete blood count (CBC):* Battery of screening tests, which typically includes hemoglobin (Hgb); hematocrit (Hct); red blood cell (RBC) count, morphology, indices, and distribution width index; platelet count and size; and white blood cell (WBC) count and differential.	An elevated WBC count is indicative of inflammatory process. It may be diagnostic, as in appendicitis. A decreased WBC count suggests viral processes, requiring further evaluation because immune system may be dysfunctional. Low Hgb suggests anemia or blood loss, which impairs tissue oxygenation and decreases the amount of Hgb available to bind with inhalation anesthetics. It may suggest need for crossmatch for possible blood transfusion. An elevated Hct may indicate dehydration, whereas decreased Hct suggests fluid overload.
• *Electrolytes:* Substances that dissociate into ions in solution and acquire the capacity to conduct electricity. Common electrolytes include sodium, potassium, chloride, calcium, and phosphate.	Imbalances impair organ function; for example, decreased potassium affects cardiac muscle contractility, leading to decreased cardiac output.
• *Arterial blood gases (ABGs):* Measurement of the pH level and the oxygen and carbon dioxide concentrations in arterial blood.	Evaluates current respiratory status, which may be especially important in smokers or clients with chronic lung diseases.
• *Bleeding or coagulation studies—prothrombin time (PT) and activated partial thromboplastin time (aPTT):* Screening for coagulation problems indicated with history of abnormal bleeding, liver or kidney disease, use of anticoagluants, or when medical history is not available as well as for high-risk procedures, such as peripheral vascular surgery, cardiopulmonary bypass, or prostatectomy.	May be prolonged, interfering with intraoperative and/or postoperative hemostasis. Hypercoagulation increases risk of thrombosis formation, especially in conjunction with dehydration and decreased mobility associated with surgery.
OTHER DIAGNOSTIC STUDIES • *Chest x-ray:* Procedure used to evaluate organs and structures within the chest for symptoms of disease.	Should be free of infiltrates or pneumonia. Used for identification of masses and chronic obstructive pulmonary disease (COPD).
• *Electrocardiogram (ECG):* Record of the electrical activity of the heart.	Abnormal findings require attention before administering anesthetics.
• *Urinalysis:* Examination of urine for various cells and chemicals such as RBCs, WBCs, infection, or excessive protein.	Presence of WBCs or bacteria indicates infection. Elevated specific gravity may reflect dehydration.
• *Pregnancy test:* Recommended in presence of recently absent or irregular menses, unreliable use of contraception, or for gynecological procedures to limit fetal exposure to teratogenic agents.	Positive results affect timing of procedure and choice of pharmacological agents.

Nursing Priorities

1. Assure correct client, procedure, and site.
2. Reduce anxiety and emotional trauma.
3. Provide for physical safety.
4. Prevent complications.
5. Alleviate pain.
6. Facilitate recovery process.
7. Provide information about disease process, surgical procedure, prognosis, and treatment needs.

Discharge Goals

1. Client dealing realistically with current situation.
2. Injury prevented.
3. Complications prevented or minimized.
4. Pain relieved or controlled.
5. Wound healing and organ function progressing toward normal.
6. Disease process, surgical procedure, prognosis, and therapeutic regimen understood.
7. Plan in place to meet needs after discharge.

NURSING DIAGNOSIS: deficient Knowledge [Learning Need] regarding condition, prognosis, treatment, self-care, and discharge needs

May be related to
Lack of exposure or recall, information misinterpretation
Unfamiliarity with information resources

Possibly evidenced by
Statement of the problem or concerns, misconceptions
Request for information
Inappropriate, exaggerated behaviors—agitated, apathetic, hostile
Inaccurate follow-through of instructions, development of preventable complications

Desired Outcomes/Evaluation Criteria—Client Will

Knowledge: Treatment Procedure(s) (NOC)
Verbalize understanding of disease process, perioperative process, and postoperative expectations.
Correctly perform necessary procedures and explain reasons for the actions.
Initiate necessary lifestyle changes and participate in treatment regimen.

ACTIONS/INTERVENTIONS	RATIONALE
Teaching: Preoperative (NIC)	
Independent	
Assess client's level of understanding.	Facilitates planning of preoperative teaching program and identifies content needs.
Review specific pathology and anticipated surgical procedure. Verify correct client, procedure, and marked site and that appropriate consent has been signed.	Provides knowledge base from which client can make informed therapy choices and consent appropriate for correct procedure and site. Presents opportunity to clarify misconceptions.
Use institution's Universal Protocol for Preventing Wrong Site, Wrong Procedure, and Wrong Person Surgery and resource teaching materials and audiovisuals, as available.	Institution's Universal Protocol and completion of specific checklists will minimize risk of error. Specifically designed materials can facilitate the client's learning.
Implement individualized preoperative teaching program:	
Preoperative and postoperative procedures and expectations, urinary and bowel changes, dietary considerations, activity levels, transfers, respiratory and cardiovascular exercises; anticipated intravenous (IV) lines and tubes such as nasogastric (NG) tubes, drains, and catheters	Enhances client's understanding and control and can relieve stress related to the unknown or unexpected. *Note:* Absence or limitation of preoperative preparation and teaching increases the need for postoperative support in addition to managing underlying medical conditions.
Preoperative instructions including bowel prep, NPO time, shower and other skin preparation, which routine medications to take or hold—prophylactic antibiotics or anticoagulants; anesthesia premedication	Helps reduce the possibility of postoperative complications and promotes a rapid return to normal body function. *Note:* In some instances, liquids and medications are allowed up to 2 hours before scheduled procedure.
Intraoperative client safety—positional needs due to arthritis, previous injury, or current mobility; not crossing legs during procedures performed under local or light anesthesia	Reduced risk of complications or untoward outcomes, such as muscular, nerve (e.g., injury to the peroneal and tibial nerves with postoperative pain in the calves and feet), or joint soreness.
Expected or transient reactions such as low backache, localized numbness, and reddening or skin indentations	Minor effects of immobilization or positioning should resolve in 24 hours. If they persist, medical evaluation is required.
Inform client and SO about timely arrival on surgical day, itinerary, and physician-SO communications.	Logistical information about preoperative preparation time, operating room (OR) schedule and locations (e.g., recovery room, postoperative room assignment), as well as where and when the surgeon will communicate with SO relieves stress and miscommunications, preventing confusion and doubt over client's well-being.
Discuss and develop individual postoperative pain management plan. Identify misconceptions client may have and provide appropriate information. Review use of 0 to 10 or similar pain assessment scale.	Increases likelihood of successful pain management. Some clients may expect to be pain free or fear becoming addicted to opioid agents.
Provide opportunity to practice coughing, deep-breathing exercises, possible use of incentive spirometry, and muscular exercises.	Enhances learning and continuation of activity postoperatively.

NURSING DIAGNOSIS: Fear/Anxiety [specify level]

May be related to
Situational crisis including wrong client, procedure or site error; unfamiliarity with environment
Change in health status, threat of death
Separation from usual support systems

Possibly evidenced by
Increased tension, apprehension, decreased self-assurance, behavior regression
Expressed concern regarding changes, fear of consequences
Facial tension, restlessness, focus on self
Sympathetic stimulation

Desired Outcomes/Evaluation Criteria—Client Will

Anxiety [or] Fear Self-Control (NOC)
Acknowledge feelings and identify healthy ways to deal with them.
Appear relaxed and be able to rest or sleep appropriately.
Report decreased fear and anxiety reduced to a manageable level.
Demonstrate ability to carry out procedure requirements.

ACTIONS/INTERVENTIONS	RATIONALE
Preoperative Coordination (NIC)	
Independent	
Provide preoperative education, including intentional repetitive verification of client identifiers, procedure, marked site steps, and surgical "time out" process. Visit with OR personnel before surgery when possible. Discuss or demonstrate routine procedures and processes that may frighten or concern client, such as masks, lights, IVs, blood pressure (BP) cuff, electrodes, bovie pad, feel of oxygen cannula or mask on nose or face, autoclave and suction noises, or child crying.	Can provide reassurance that client safety precautions are constantly ongoing, alleviate client's anxiety, as well as provide information for formulating intraoperative care. Acknowledges that foreign environment may be frightening and alleviates associated fears. Decreased anxiety level reduces elevation of glucocorticosteroid levels, which can interfere with healing.
Inform client and SO of nurse's intraoperative advocate role.	Develops trust and rapport, decreasing fear of loss of control in a foreign environment. Provides client and SO with contact person.
Assure client anticipating conscious sedation or spinal anesthesia that drowsiness or sleep occurs, that more sedation may be requested and will be given if needed, and that surgical drapes will block view of the operative field.	Reduces concerns that client may "see" the procedure.
Surgical Preparation (NIC)	
Identify fear levels that may necessitate postponement of surgical procedure.	Overwhelming or persistent fears result in excessive stress reaction and increasing glucocorticosteroid levels, potentiating risk of adverse reaction to procedure and anesthetic agents and impairing healing.
Validate source of fear. Provide accurate factual information. Active-listen concerns.	Identification of specific fear helps client deal realistically with fears, such as misidentification or wrong operation, dismemberment, disfigurement, loss of dignity and control, or being awake or aware with local anesthesia. Client may have misinterpreted preoperative information or have misinformation regarding surgery or disease process. Fears regarding previous experiences of self, family, or acquaintances may be unresolved.
Note expressions of distress or feelings of helplessness, preoccupation with anticipated change or loss, and choked feelings.	Client may already be grieving for the loss represented by the anticipated surgical procedure, diagnosis, or prognosis of illness.
Introduce client to staff at time of transfer to operating suite.	Establishes rapport and psychological comfort with operative team.
Verbalize and document client identifiers to surgery schedule, client identification band, chart, marked site, and signed operative consent for surgical procedure according to facility's protocol and checklist.	Provides for positive identification, reducing fear that wrong procedure may be done as well as minimizing risk for wrong procedure and site.
Prevent unnecessary body exposure during transfer to and in OR suite.	Preserves client's modesty, reduces fear of loss of dignity and inability to exercise control, and reinforces nurse advocacy role.

(continues on page 788)

ACTIONS/INTERVENTIONS (continued)

Give simple, concise directions and explanations to sedated client. Review environmental concerns, as needed.
Control external stimuli.

Collaborative

Refer to surgeon, anesthesiologist, clinical manager, pastoral spiritual care, psychiatric clinical nurse specialist, or psychiatric counseling, if indicated.

Discuss postponement or cancellation of surgery with physician, anesthesiologist, client, and family, as appropriate.
Refer wrong client, procedure, site, or implant discrepancies to surgeon, anesthesiologist, and appropriate persons.
Administer medications, as indicated, for example:
  Sedatives and hypnotics

  IV anti-anxiety agents

  Antacids and H₂ blocker, preoperatively as indicated

RATIONALE (continued)

Impairment of thought processes makes it difficult for client to understand lengthy instructions.
Extraneous noises and commotion may accelerate anxiety.

Further evaluation or counseling may be desired or required for client to deal with fear, especially concerning life-threatening conditions and serious and/or high-risk procedures.
May be necessary if overwhelming fears are not reduced or resolved.
Discrepancies must be corrected and verified by surgeon, client, and SO prior to OR entry.

Used to promote sleep the evening before surgery; may enhance coping abilities.
May be provided in the outpatient admitting or preoperative holding area to reduce nervousness and provide comfort. *Note:* Respiratory depression or bradycardia may occur, necessitating prompt intervention.
Neutralizes gastric acidity and may reduce risk of aspiration or severity of pneumonia should aspiration occur, especially in obese or pregnant clients in whom there is an 85% risk of mortality with aspiration. *Note:* Ranitidine (Zantac) has been found to reduce postoperative infections in acute colorectal surgery.

Intraoperative

NURSING DIAGNOSIS: risk for perioperative positioning Injury

Risk factors may include
Disorientation, sensory and perceptual disturbances due to anesthesia
Immobilization, musculoskeletal impairments
Obesity, emaciation, edema

Possibly evidenced by
(Not applicable; presence of signs and symptoms establishes an *actual* diagnosis)

Desired Outcomes/Evaluation Criteria—Client Will

Physical Injury Severity (NOC)
Be free of injury related to perioperative disorientation.
Be free of untoward skin or tissue injury, or changes lasting beyond 24 to 48 hours following procedure.
Report resolution of localized numbness, tingling, or changes in sensation related to positioning within 24 to 48 hours, as appropriate.

ACTIONS/INTERVENTIONS

Positioning Intraoperative (NIC)
Independent
Note anticipated length of procedure and customary position. Provide for potential complications.

Review client's history, noting age, weight, height, nutritional status, and physical limitation or preexisting conditions that may affect choice of position and skin and tissue integrity during surgery.

Stabilize both client cart and OR table when transferring client to and from OR table, using an adequate number of personnel for transfer and support of extremities.

RATIONALE

Supine position may cause low back pain and skin pressure at heels, elbows, and sacrum; lateral chest position can cause shoulder and neck pain as well as eye and ear injury on the client's downside.
Many conditions, such as lack of subcutaneous padding in elderly person, arthritis, thoracic outlet or cubital tunnel syndrome, diabetes, obesity, presence of abdominal stoma, peripheral vascular disease, level of hydration, and temperature of extremities, can make individual prone to injury.
Unstabilized cart or table can separate, causing client to fall. Both side rails must be in the down position for caregiver(s) to assist client transfer and prevent loss of balance.

ACTIONS/INTERVENTIONS (continued)

Anticipate movement of extraneous lines and tubes during the transfer and secure or guide them into position.

Secure client on OR table with safety belt and arm protection as appropriate, explaining necessity for safety precautions.

Protect body from contact with metal parts of the operating table.

Prepare equipment and padding for required position, according to operative procedure and client's specific needs. Pay special attention to pressure points of bony prominences on arms and ankles, and neurovascular pressure points and soft tissues such as breasts and knees.

Position extremities so they may be periodically checked for safety, circulation, nerve pressure, and alignment. Monitor peripheral pulses and skin color and temperature.

Place legs in stirrups simultaneously when lithotomy position used, adjusting stirrup height to client's legs, maintaining symmetrical position. Pad popliteal space and heels and feet, as indicated.

Provide foot board, elevate drapes off toes, and decrease blanket weight on extremities. Avoid or monitor equipment and instrumentation placement on trunk or extremities during procedure.

Reposition slowly at transfer from table and to bed.

Determine specific postoperative positioning guidelines, such as elevation of head of bed following spinal anesthesia or nose and throat surgery, or turning to unoperated side following pneumonectomy.

Collaborative

Recommend position changes to anesthesiologist and/or surgeon, as appropriate.

RATIONALE (continued)

Prevents undue tension and dislocation of IV lines, NG tubes, catheters, and chest tubes; maintains gravity drainage when appropriate.

OR tables and arm boards are narrow, placing client at risk for injury, especially during fasciculation. Client may become resistive or combative when sedated or emerging from anesthesia, furthering potential for injury.

Reduces risk of electrical injury.

Depending on individual client's size, weight, and preexisting conditions, extra padding materials may be required to protect bony prominences, prevent circulatory compromise or nerve pressure, or to allow for optimal chest expansion for ventilation.

Prevents accidental trauma to hands, fingers, and toes which could inadvertently be scraped, pinched, or amputated by moving table attachments. Reduces risk of positional pressure on brachial plexus, peroneal, and ulnar nerves, which can cause serious neurovascular impairment in extremities; or prolonged plantar flexion which may result in footdrop.

Prevents muscle strain and reduces risk of hip dislocation in elderly clients. Padding helps prevent peroneal and tibial nerve damage. *Note:* Prolonged positioning in stirrups may lead to compartment syndrome in calf muscles.

Pressure may cause neural, circulatory, and skin integrity disruption.

Myocardial depressant effect of various agents increases risk of hypotension and/or bradycardia. Controlling movement enhances volume accommodation.

Reduces risk of postoperative complications, such as headache associated with migration of spinal anesthesia, or loss of maximal respiratory effort.

Close attention to proper positioning can prevent muscle strain, nerve damage, circulatory compromise, and undue pressure on skin and bony prominences. Although the anesthesiologist is responsible for positioning, the nurse may be able to see or have more time to note client needs and provide assistance.

NURSING DIAGNOSIS: risk for Injury

Risk factors may include
Wrong client, procedure, site, implants, equipment, or materials
Interactive conditions between individual and environment
External environment—physical design, structure of environment, exposure to equipment, instrumentation, positioning, use of pharmaceutical agents
Internal environment—tissue hypoxia, abnormal blood profile or altered clotting factors, broken skin

Possibly evidenced by
(Not applicable; presence of signs and symptoms establishes an *actual* diagnosis)

Desired Outcomes/Evaluation Criteria—Caregiver Will

Risk Control (NOC)
Implement surgical Universal "Time Out" Protocol.
Identify individual risk factors.
Modify environment, as indicated, to enhance safety and use resources appropriately.

ACTIONS/INTERVENTIONS	RATIONALE

Surgical Precautions (NIC)

Independent

Remove dentures, partial plates, or bridges, preoperatively per protocol. Inform anesthesiologist of problems with natural teeth such as loose teeth.

Foreign bodies may be aspirated during endotracheal intubation and extubation.

Remove prosthetics or other devices preoperatively or after induction, depending on sensory or perceptual alterations and mobility impairment.

Contact lenses may cause corneal abrasions while under anesthesia; eyeglasses and hearing aids are obstructive and may break; however, clients may feel more in control of environment if hearing and visual aids are left on as long as possible. Artificial limbs may be damaged and skin integrity impaired if left on.

Remove jewelry preoperatively. Tape over, or isolate from skin according to institution protocol. Remove piercing hardware.

Metals conduct electrical current and provide an electrocautery hazard. Piercings may be "snagged," resulting in soft-tissue injury. In addition, loss or damage to client's personal property can easily occur in the foreign environment. *Note:* In some cases (e.g., arthritic knuckles), it may not be possible to remove rings without cutting them off. In this situation, applying tape over the ring may prevent client from "catching" ring and prevent loss of stone or damage to finger and decrease psychological loss because of damage to personal property.

Verify client identity and scheduled operative procedure by comparing client chart, arm band, and surgical schedule. Verbally ascertain correct name, procedure, operative site, and physician.

Ensures correct client, procedure, and appropriate extremity or side.

Document allergies, including risk for adverse reaction to latex, tape, and prep solutions.

Reduces risk for allergic responses that may impair skin integrity or lead to life-threatening systemic reactions.

Give simple and concise directions to the sedated client.

Impairment of thought process makes it difficult for client to understand lengthy directions.

Prevent pooling of prep solutions under and around client.

Antiseptic solutions may chemically burn skin as well as conduct electricity.

Assist with induction as needed, for example, standing by to apply cricoid pressure during intubation or stabilizing position during lumbar puncture for spinal block.

Facilitates safe administration of anesthesia.

Verify electrical safety of equipment used in surgical procedure, which includes intact cords, grounds, and medical engineering verification labels.

Malfunction of equipment can occur during the operative procedure, causing not only delays and unnecessary anesthesia, but also injury or death. Short circuits, faulty grounds, laser malfunctions, or laser misalignment could occur. Periodic electrical safety checks are imperative for all OR equipment.

Place dispersive electrode or electrocautery pad over largest available muscle mass closest to surgical site, ensuring its contact.

Provides for shortest distance and maximum conductivity to ground to prevent electrical burns.

Confirm and document correct sponge, instrument, needle, and blade counts.

Foreign bodies remaining in body cavities at closure may result in inflammation, infection, perforation, abscess formation, and disastrous complications that can lead to death.

Laser Precautions (NIC)

Verify credentials of laser operators for specific wavelength laser required for particular procedure.

Because of the potential hazards of lasers, physician and equipment operators must be certified in the use and safety requirements of specific wavelength laser and procedure including open, endoscopic, abdominal, laryngeal, and intrauterine procedures.

Confirm presence of fire extinguishers and wet fire smothering materials when lasers are used intraoperatively.

Laser beam may inadvertently contact and ignite combustibles outside of surgical site such as drapes and sponges.

Apply client and personnel eye protection before laser activation.

Eye protection for specific laser wavelength must be used to prevent injury.

Protect surrounding skin and anatomy appropriately utilizing wet towels, sponges, dams, and cottonoids.

Prevents inadvertent skin integrity disruption, hair ignition, and adjacent anatomy injury in area of laser beam use.

Specimen Management (NIC)

Handle, label, and document specimens appropriately, ensuring proper medium and transport for tests required.

The OR nurse advocate must properly identify specimens to client, site, and test to ensure validity and maximum client outcome. Loss or mislabeling of specimens renders the surgical procedure fruitless and grossly compromises further treatment and client outcome. Frozen sections, preserved or fresh examination, and cultures all have different medium and transfer requirements.

ACTIONS/INTERVENTIONS (continued)

Fluid Management (NIC)
Observe intake and output (I&O) during procedure. Anticipate need for volume replacement or rapid infusion via infusion pumps and set up appropriately. Ascertain that pumps are functioning accurately.

Collaborative
Administer IV fluids, blood or blood components, and medications such as aprotinin (Trasylol) or desmopressin (DDAVP), as indicated.

Collect autologous blood intraoperatively, as appropriate.

Surgical Precautions (NIC)
Validate surgical field medications and dosages with surgeon and anesthesiologist, including local anesthetics with or without epinephrine in regional blocks.

RATIONALE (continued)

Potential for fluid volume deficit or excess exists, affecting safety of anesthesia, tissue perfusion, organ function, and client well-being.

Maintains homeostasis and adequate level of sedation and muscle relaxation to produce optimal surgical outcome. *Note:* Trasylol or DDAVP may be given before or during procedure to reduce blood loss and promote clotting.
Blood lost intraoperatively may be collected, filtered, and reinfused either intraoperatively or postoperatively. A continuous, closed circuit must be maintained for the procedure to be acceptable for use by Jehovah's Witnesses. *Note:* Alternatively, red blood cell (RBC) production may be increased by the administration of epoetin (Epogen, Procrit) for up to 3 weeks preoperatively, reducing the need for blood transfusion whether autologous or donated.

Prevents administration of contraindicated medications or inappropriate dosages. *Note:* Excessive doses of local anesthetic agents may potentiate cardiovascular compromise.

NURSING DIAGNOSIS: risk for Infection

Risk factors may include
Broken skin, traumatized tissues, stasis of body fluids
Presence of pathogens or contaminants, environmental exposure, invasive procedures

Possibly evidenced by
(Not applicable; presence of signs and symptoms establishes an *actual* diagnosis)

Desired Outcomes/Evaluation Criteria—Caregiver Will

Knowledge: Infection Control (NOC)
Identify individual risk factors and interventions to reduce potential for infection.
Maintain safe aseptic environment.

ACTIONS/INTERVENTIONS

RATIONALE

Infection Control: Intraoperative (NIC)
Independent
Adhere to facility infection control, sterilization, and aseptic policies and procedures.
Verify sterility of all items used in procedure as event related.

Review laboratory studies for systemic infections and scrutinize operative area for possibility of localized infections.

Verify that preoperative skin, vaginal, and bowel cleansing procedures have been done, as needed, depending on specific surgical procedure.
Prepare operative site according to specific procedures.

Established mechanisms designed to prevent infection.

Prepackaged items may appear to be sterile; however, each item must be scrutinized for manufacturer's sterility statement or central sterile processing indicators, package integrity, environmental effect on package, and delivery techniques. *Note:* Package sterilization and expiration dates and lot and serial numbers must be documented on implant items for further follow-up if necessary.
Increased WBC count may indicate ongoing infection, which the operative procedure will alleviate such as appendicitis, abscess, and inflammation from trauma. Presence of local or systemic infection such as an upper respiratory infection (URI), urinary tract infection (UTI), skin lesions, or unknown infections may contraindicate or adversely affect the surgical procedure and/or anesthesia.
Cleansing reduces bacterial counts on the skin, vaginal mucosa, and alimentary tract.

Minimizes bacterial counts at operative site.

(continues on page 792)

Examine skin for breaks or irritation and signs of infection.	Disruptions of skin integrity at or near the operative site are sources of contamination to the incision. Careful shaving or clipping as close as possible to incision time will prevent skin abrasions, which potentiate skin infection.
Maintain dependent gravity drainage of indwelling catheters, tubes, and/or positive pressure of parenteral or irrigation lines.	Prevents stasis and reflux of body fluids.
Identify breaks in aseptic technique and resolve immediately upon occurrence.	Contamination by environmental or personnel contact renders the sterile field unsterile, thereby increasing the risk of infection.
Utilize Universal Precautions, contain contaminated fluids or materials to specific site in operating room suite, and dispose of according to facility protocol.	Containment of blood and body fluids, tissue, and materials in contact with an infected wound or client will prevent spread of infection to environment and other clients or personnel.
Apply sterile dressing.	Prevents environmental contamination of fresh wound.
Monitor blood glucose levels of diabetic clients, and maintain tight glycemic control, as indicated.	Depending on length of procedure and type of IV fluids infused, intervention may be required to maintain preferred glucose levels.

Collaborative

Provide and document copious wound irrigation with saline, water, antibiotic, or antiseptic solution.	May be used intraoperatively to reduce bacterial counts at surgical site and cleanse the wound of bone, ischemic tissue, bowel contaminants, toxins, or other debris.
Obtain specimens for cultures and Gram stain.	Immediate identification of infective organism type by Gram stain allows prompt treatment, whereas more specific identification by cultures can be obtained in hours or days.
Administer antibiotics, as indicated.	May be given prophylactically for suspected infection or contamination.

NURSING DIAGNOSIS: **risk for imbalanced Body Temperature**

Risk factors may include
Exposure to cool environment
Use of medications, anesthetic agents
Extremes of age, weight; dehydration

Possibly evidenced by
(Not applicable; presence of signs and symptoms establishes an *actual* diagnosis)

Desired Outcomes/Evaluation Criteria—Client Will

Thermoregulation (NOC)
Maintain body temperature within normal range.

| ACTIONS/INTERVENTIONS | RATIONALE |

Temperature Regulation: Intraoperative (NIC)
Independent

Note preoperative temperature related to age and disease process.	Used as baseline for monitoring intraoperative temperature. Preoperative temperature elevations may be indicative of disease process, such as appendicitis, abscess, or systemic disease requiring perioperative treatment. *Note:* Effects of aging on hypothalamus may decrease fever response to infection.
Assess environmental temperature and modify, as needed, by providing warming blankets or increasing room temperature.	Manipulating ambient air around client will prevent heat loss.
Cover skin areas outside of operative field.	Heat losses will occur as skin on head, arms, and legs are exposed to cool environmental temperatures.
Provide cooling measures for client with preoperative or intraoperative temperature elevations.	Cool irrigations, exposure of skin surfaces to air, or cooling blanket may be required to decrease temperature.
Increase ambient room temperature (e.g., to 78°F or 80°F [25.6°C to 26.7°C]) at conclusion of procedure.	Minimizes client heat loss when drapes are removed and client is prepared for transfer.
Apply warming blankets at emergence from anesthesia.	Inhalation anesthetics depress the hypothalamus, resulting in poor body temperature regulation.

ACTIONS/INTERVENTIONS (continued)

Collaborative

Monitor temperature throughout intraoperative phase.

Malignant Hyperthermia Precautions (NIC)

Respond promptly to symptoms of malignant hyperthermia (MH)—rapid temperature elevation and persistent high fever:

Provide iced saline to all body surfaces and orifices.

Obtain dantrolene (Dantrium) for IV administration per protocol.

RATIONALE (continued)

Continuous warm or cool humidified inhalation anesthestics are used to maintain humidity and temperature balance within the tracheobronchial tree. Temperature fluctuations may indicate adverse response to anesthesia. *Note:* Use of atropine or scopolamine may further increase temperature.

Prompt recognition and immediate action to control temperature is necessary to prevent serious complications or death.

Iced solution lavage of body surfaces and cavities will reduce body temperature.
Immediate action to control temperature is necessary to prevent intense catabolic process associated with MH.

Postoperative

NURSING DIAGNOSIS: ineffective Breathing Pattern

May be related to
Neuromuscular, perceptual, or cognitive impairment
Decreased lung expansion, energy
Tracheobronchial obstruction

Possibly evidenced by
Changes in respiratory rate and depth
Reduced vital capacity, apnea, cyanosis, noisy respirations

Desired Outcomes/Evaluation Criteria—Client Will

Respiratory Status: Ventilation (NOC)
Establish an effective respiratory pattern free of cyanosis or other signs of hypoxia.

ACTIONS/INTERVENTIONS

Postanesthesia Care (NIC)
Independent
Maintain client airway by head tilt, jaw hyperextension, or oral pharyngeal airway.
Auscultate breath sounds. Listen for gurgling, wheezing, crowing, and/or silence after extubation.

Observe respiratory rate and depth, chest expansion, use of accessory muscles, retraction or flaring of nostrils, and skin color; note airflow.
Monitor vital signs continuously.

Position client appropriately, depending on respiratory effort and type of surgery.

Observe for return of muscle function, especially respiratory.

Initiate "stir-up" regimen—turn, cough, deep breathe—as soon as client is reactive and continue in the postoperative period.

RATIONALE

Prevents airway obstruction.

Lack of breath sounds is indicative of obstruction by mucus or tongue and may be corrected by positioning and/or suctioning. Diminished breath sounds suggest atelectasis. Wheezing indicates bronchospasm, whereas crowing or silence reflects partial to total laryngospasm.
Ascertains effectiveness of respirations immediately so that corrective measures can be initiated.

Increased respirations, tachycardia, and/or bradycardia suggests hypoxia.
Head elevation and left lateral Sims' position prevents aspiration of secretions or vomitus, enhances ventilation to lower lobes, and relieves pressure on diaphragm.
After administration of intraoperative muscle relaxants, return of muscle function occurs first to the diaphragm, intercostals, and larynx; followed by large muscle groups, neck, shoulders, and abdominal muscles; then by midsize muscles, tongue, pharynx, extensors, and flexors; and finally, by eyes, mouth, face, and fingers.
Active deep ventilation inflates alveoli, breaks up secretions, increases O_2 transfer, and removes anesthetic gases; coughing enhances removal of secretions from the pulmonary system. *Note:* Respiratory muscles weaken and atrophy with age, possibly hampering elderly client's ability to cough or deep-breathe effectively.

(continues on page 794)

ACTIONS/INTERVENTIONS (continued)

Observe for excessive somnolence.

Elevate head of bed as appropriate to surgical procedure. Get out of bed as soon as possible.
Suction, as necessary.

Collaborative
Administer supplemental O$_2$, as indicated.

Administer IV medications, such as naloxone (Narcan), doxapram (Dopram), or neostigmine (Prostigmin).

Provide and maintain ventilator assistance, as indicated.

Assist with use of respiratory aids such as incentive spirometer.

RATIONALE (continued)

Opioid-induced respiratory depression or presence of muscle relaxants in the body may be cyclical in recurrence, creating sine-wave pattern of depression and reemergence from anesthesia. In addition, thiopental sodium (Pentothal) is absorbed in the fatty tissues, and, as circulation improves, it may be redistributed throughout the bloodstream.
Promotes maximal expansion of lungs, decreasing risk of pulmonary complications.
Airway obstruction can occur as a result of blood or mucus in throat or trachea.

Maximizes oxygen for uptake to bind with Hgb in place of anesthetic gases to enhance removal of inhalation agents.
Narcan reverses opioid-induced central nervous system (CNS) depression; Dopram stimulates respiratory muscles. The effects of both drugs are cyclic in nature and respiratory depression may return. Prostigmin reverses nonpolarizing muscle blockers.
Depending on cause of respiratory depression or type of surgery (e.g., pulmonary, extensive abdominal, cardiac), endotracheal tube (ET) may be left in place and mechanical ventilation continued for a time.
Maximal respiratory efforts reduce potential for atelectasis and pulmonary infection. Client may need to be reminded and coached to reach specific goal.

NURSING DIAGNOSIS: **disturbed Sensory Perception, (specify)/disturbed Thought Processes**

May be related to
Chemical alteration—use of pharmaceutical agents, hypoxia
Therapeutically restricted environments; excessive sensory stimuli
Physiological stress

Possibly evidenced by
Disorientation to person, place, time; change in usual response to stimuli; impaired ability to concentrate, reason, make decisions
Motor incoordination

Desired Outcomes/Evaluation Criteria—Client Will
Cognition (NOC)
Regain usual level of consciousness and mentation.
Recognize limitations and seek assistance as necessary.

ACTIONS/INTERVENTIONS

Postanesthesia Care (NIC)
Independent
Reorient client continuously when emerging from anesthesia; confirm that surgery is completed.
Speak in normal, clear voice without shouting, being aware of what you are saying. Minimize discussion of negatives about the client or personal or work-related problems within client's hearing. Explain procedures and environmental events even if client does not seem aware.
Evaluate sensation and movement of extremities and trunk, as appropriate.

Use bed rail padding, medical protective devices as necessary.

Secure parenteral lines, ET tube, and catheters, if present, and check for patency.

RATIONALE

As client regains consciousness, support and assurance of current physical status will help alleviate anxiety.
The nurse cannot tell when client is aware, but it is thought that the sense of hearing returns before client appears fully awake, so it is important not to say things that may be misinterpreted. Providing factual information helps client preserve dignity and prepare for next recuperative activity.
Return of function following local or spinal nerve blocks depends on type and amount of agent used and duration of procedure.
Provides for client safety and protection from environment during emergence state. Prevents injury to head and extremities if client becomes combative while disoriented.
Disoriented client may pull on lines and drainage systems, disconnecting or kinking them.

ACTIONS/INTERVENTIONS (continued)

Maintain quiet, calm environment.

Investigate changes in sensorium.

Observe for hallucinations, delusions, depression, or an excited state.

Reassess sensory, motor, and cognitive function thoroughly before discharge.

Collaborative
Evaluate need for extended stay in postoperative recovery area or need for additional nursing care before discharge, as appropriate.
Contact or refer to case manager for alternate care options.

RATIONALE (continued)

External stimuli, such as noise, lights, and touch, may cause psychic aberrations when dissociative anesthetics (e.g., ketamine, tiletamine [Telazol]) have been administered.
Continued confusion, specific to pediatric and geriatric age groups, may reflect drug interactions, hypoxia, anxiety, pain, electrolyte imbalances, or fear.
May develop following trauma and indicate delirium or may reflect sundowner's syndrome in elderly client. In client who has used alcohol or other drugs to excess, may suggest impending delirium tremens.
Phase II recovery or ambulatory surgical client must be able to care for self with the help of SO, if available, to prevent personal injury after discharge.

Disorientation may persist, and SO may not be able to protect the client at home.

May not be ready or able to care for self, especially if no SO and family member is available to provide necessary assistance.

NURSING DIAGNOSIS: risk for deficient Fluid Volume

Risk factors may include
Restriction of oral intake—disease process, medical procedure, presence of nausea
Loss of fluid through abnormal routes—indwelling tubes, drains; through normal routes—vomiting
Loss of vascular integrity, changes in clotting ability
Extremes of age and weight

Possibly evidenced by
(Not applicable; presence of signs and symptoms establishes an *actual* diagnosis)

Desired Outcomes/Evaluation Criteria—Client Will

Hydration (NOC)
Demonstrate adequate fluid balance, as evidenced by stable vital signs, palpable pulses of good quality, normal skin turgor, moist mucous membranes, and individually appropriate urinary output.

ACTIONS/INTERVENTIONS

Fluid Management (NIC)
Independent
Measure and record I&O including tubes and drains. Calculate urine specific gravity, as appropriate. Review intraoperative record for potential causes of imbalance.

Assess urinary output specifically for type of operative procedure done.

Provide voiding assistance measures as needed such as privacy, sitting position, running water in sink, and pouring warm water over perineum, as needed.
Monitor vital signs, noting changes in BP, heart rate and rhythm, and respirations. Calculate pulse pressure.

Note presence of nausea or vomiting.

RATIONALE

Accurate documentation helps identify fluid losses and replacement needs and influences choice of interventions. *Note:* Ability to concentrate urine declines with age, increasing renal losses despite general fluid deficit.
May be decreased or absent after procedures on the genitourinary system and/or adjacent structures, such as ureteroplasty, ureterolithotomy, and abdominal or vaginal hysterectomy, indicating malfunction or obstruction of the urinary system.
Promotes relaxation of perineal muscles and may facilitate voiding efforts.

Hypotension, tachycardia, and increased respirations may indicate fluid deficit—dehydration or hypovolemia. Although a drop in BP is generally a late sign of fluid deficit or hemorrhagic loss, widening of the pulse pressure may occur early, followed by narrowing as bleeding continues and systolic BP begins to fall.
Women, obese individuals, and those prone to motion sickness have a higher risk of postoperative nausea and vomiting. In addition, the longer the duration of anesthesia, the greater the risk for nausea. *Note:* Nausea occurring during first 12 to 24 hours postoperatively is frequently related to anesthesia (including regional anesthesia). Nausea persisting more than 3 days postoperatively may be related to the choice of opioid for pain control or other drug therapy.

(continues on page 796)

Inspect dressings and drainage devices at regular intervals. Assess wound for swelling.	Excessive bleeding can lead to hypovolemia and circulatory collapse. Local swelling may indicate hematoma formation or hemorrhage. *Note:* Bleeding into a cavity (e.g., retroperitoneal) may be hidden and diagnosed only via vital sign depression or client reports of pressure sensation in affected area.
Monitor skin temperature; palpate peripheral pulses.	Cool or clammy skin and/or weak pulses indicate decreased peripheral circulation and need for additional fluid replacement.

Collaborative

Administer parenteral fluids, blood products including autologous collection, and/or plasma expanders, as indicated. Increase IV rate, if needed.	Replaces documented fluid loss. Timely replacement of circulating volume decreases potential for complications of deficit including electrolyte imbalance, dehydration, and cardiovascular collapse. *Note:* Increased volume may be required initially to support circulating volume and prevent hypotension because of decreased vasomotor tone following halothane (Fluothane) administration.
Insert and maintain urinary catheter with or without urimeter, as necessary.	Provides mechanism for accurate monitoring of urinary output.
Resume oral intake gradually, or begin enteral feeding, as indicated.	Following surgical procedures not involving the gastrointestinal (GI) tract, the small bowel may be capable of absorbing nutrients regardless of absence of bowel sounds reflecting GI motility. If there is no evidence of abdominal distention, mechanical obstruction, or GI bleeding, early enteral feeding can hasten resolution of postoperative ileus and reduce risk of infection. As ileus resolves, oral fluids can be started.
Administer medications, as appropriate, for example: Antiemetics	Relieves nausea and vomiting, which may impair intake and add to fluid deficit. *Note:* Naloxone (Narcan) may relieve nausea related to use of anesthetic agents, such as morphine (Duramorph) or fentanyl citrate (Sublimaze).
Epoetin alfa, vitamins B$_{12}$ C, and folic acid	Medications used to stimulate production of RBCs are begun preoperatively and may be administered postoperatively as well.
Monitor laboratory studies, such as Hgb and Hct or electrolytes. Compare preoperative and postoperative blood studies.	Indicators of hydration and circulating volume. Preoperative anemia and/or low Hct combined with unreplaced fluid losses intraoperatively will further potentiate deficit.

NURSING DIAGNOSIS: acute Pain

May be related to
Disruption of skin, tissue, and muscle integrity; musculoskeletal or bone trauma
Presence of tubes and drains

Possibly evidenced by
Reports of pain
Alteration in muscle tone, facial mask of pain
Distraction, guarding, or protective behaviors
Self-focusing, narrowed focus
Autonomic responses

Desired Outcomes/Evaluation Criteria—Client Will

Pain Level (NOC)
Report pain relieved or controlled.
Appear relaxed, able to rest or sleep and participate in activities appropriately.

ACTIONS/INTERVENTIONS   RATIONALE

Pain Management (NIC)
Independent

Note client's age, weight, coexisting medical or psychological conditions, idiosyncratic sensitivity to analgesics, and intraoperative course, including size and location of incision, drain placement, and anesthetic agents used.	Approach to postoperative pain management is based on multiple variable factors. *Note:* Administration of the anticonvulsant lamotrigine (Lamictal) before spinal anesthesia reduces analgesic use and lowers pain scale ratings in the postoperative client.

ACTIONS/INTERVENTIONS (continued)

Review intraoperative and recovery room record for type of anesthesia and medications previously administered.

Evaluate pain frequently in immediate postoperative phase and regularly (e.g., hourly per protocol) following transfer, noting characteristics, location, and intensity (0–10 scale). Emphasize client's responsibility for reporting pain and relief of pain completely.

Note presence of anxiety or fear, and relate with nature of and preparation for procedure.

Assess vital signs, noting tachycardia, hypertension, and increased respiration, even if client denies pain.

Assess causes of possible discomfort other than operative procedure.

Provide information about transitory nature of discomfort, as appropriate.

Reposition as indicated, such as semi-Fowler's or lateral Sims'.

Provide additional comfort measures such as backrub and heat or cold applications.

Encourage use of relaxation techniques such as deep-breathing exercises, guided imagery, visualization, or music.

Provide regular oral care, occasional ice chips or sips of fluids as tolerated.

Document effectiveness and side or adverse effects of analgesia.

Collaborative

Administer medications, as indicated, for example:

IV analgesics after reviewing anesthesia record for contraindications and/or presence of agents that may potentiate analgesia

Around-the-clock analgesia via patient-controlled analgesia (PCA) or epidural analgesia (PCEA) with intermittent rescue doses, as needed

RATIONALE (continued)

Presence of opioids and droperidol in system potentiates opioid analgesia, whereas inhalation anesthetics have no analgesic effects. In addition, intraoperative local and regional blocks have varying duration based on drug choice and dose.

Provides information about need for, and effectiveness of, interventions. *Note:* It may not always be possible to eliminate pain; however, analgesics should reduce pain to a tolerable level. A frontal and/or occipital headache may develop 24 to 72 hours following spinal anesthesia, necessitating recumbent position, increased fluid intake, and notification of the anesthesiologist for alternative pain relief plan.

Concern about the unknown, such as outcome of a biopsy and/or inadequate preparation due to emergent procedure, can heighten client's perception of pain.

Changes in these vital signs often indicate acute pain and discomfort. *Note:* Some clients may have a slightly lowered BP, which returns to normal range after pain relief is achieved.

Discomfort can be caused or aggravated by presence of non-patent indwelling catheters causing bladder pain, NG tube resulting in gastric fluid and gas accumulation, or parenteral lines that have infiltrated IV fluids or medications.

Understanding the cause of the transitory discomfort, such as sore muscles from administration of succinylcholine, which may persist up to 48 hours postoperatively; sinus headache, which may be associated with nitrous oxide; or sore throat, which may be due to intubation, provides emotional reassurance. *Note:* Paresthesia of body parts suggests nerve injury. Symptoms may last hours or months and require additional evaluation.

May relieve pain and enhance circulation. Semi-Fowler's position relieves abdominal muscle tension and arthritic back muscle tension, whereas lateral Sims' will relieve dorsal pressures.

Improves circulation, reduces muscle tension and anxiety associated with pain. Enhances sense of well-being.

Relieves muscle and emotional tension; enhances sense of control and may improve coping abilities.

Reduces discomfort associated with dry mucous membranes due to anesthetic agents and oral restrictions.

Respirations may decrease on administration of opioid, or synergistic effects with anesthetic agents may occur. *Note:* Migration of epidural analgesia toward head may cause respiratory depression or excessive sedation.

Analgesics given IV reach the pain centers immediately, providing more effective relief with smaller doses of medication. *Note:* Initial opioid dosage should be reduced by one-fourth to one-third after use of fentanyl (Innovar) or droperidol (Inapsine) to prevent respiratory depressant effects (Deglin & Valler, 2005).

Research supports need to administer analgesics around the clock initially to prevent rather than merely treat pain. Use of PCA necessitates detailed client instruction. PCA is considered very effective in managing acute postoperative pain with smaller amounts of opioid and increased client satisfaction. *Note:* Continuous epidural infusions may be used for 1 to 5 days following procedures that are known to cause severe pain such as certain types of thoracic or abdominal procedures.

(continues on page 798)

ACTIONS/INTERVENTIONS (continued)

Local anesthetics, such as epidural block or infusion

NSAIDs, such as ketorolate (Toradol), diflunisal (Dolobid), or naproxen (Anaprox)

Monitor use and effectiveness of transcutaneous electrical nerve stimulation (TENS) unit when used.

RATIONALE (continued)

Analgesics may be injected into the operative site, or nerves to the site may be kept blocked in the immediate postoperative phase to prevent severe pain. *Note:* Continuous epidural infusions may be used for 1 to 5 days following procedures that are known to cause severe pain such as certain types of thoracic or abdominal surgeries.

Useful for mild to moderate pain or as adjuncts to opioid therapy in moderate to severe pain. Allows for a lower dosage of opioids, reducing potential for side effects. Use alternating schedule with NSAIDs administered between opioid doses so peak effect occurs at a different time.

TENS may be useful in reducing pain and amount of medication required postoperatively.

NURSING DIAGNOSIS: impaired **Skin/Tissue Integrity**

May be related to
Mechanical interruption of skin and tissues
Altered circulation, effects of medication, accumulation of drainage, altered metabolic state

Possibly evidenced by
Disruption of skin surface/layers and tissues

Desired Outcomes/Evaluation Criteria—Client Will

Wound Healing: Primary Intention (NOC)
Achieve timely wound healing.

Knowledge: Treatment Regimen (NOC)
Demonstrate behaviors or techniques to promote healing and prevent complications.

ACTIONS/INTERVENTIONS

RATIONALE

Incision Site Care (NIC)
Independent

Reinforce initial dressing or change, as indicated. Use strict aseptic techniques.

Gently remove tape in direction of hair growth and dressings when changing.

Apply skin sealants or barriers before tape, if needed. Use hypoallergenic tape, Montgomery straps, or elastic netting for dressings requiring frequent changing.

Check tension of dressings. Apply tape at center of incision to outer margin of dressing. Avoid wrapping tape around extremity.

Inspect incision regularly, noting characteristics and integrity. Note clients at risk for delayed healing such as presence of COPD, anemia, obesity, malnutrition, DM, hematoma formation, vomiting, ETOH (ethyl alcohol) withdrawal; use of steroid therapy; and advanced age.

Assess amounts and characteristics of drainage.

Maintain patency of drainage tubes; apply collection bag over drains or incisions in presence of copious or caustic drainage.

Elevate operative area, as appropriate.

Splint abdominal and chest incisions or area with pillow or pad during coughing and movement.

Protects wound from mechanical injury and contamination. Prevents accumulation of fluids that may cause excoriation. *Note:* Studies suggest clean techniques may be sufficient, but additional research is required before protocols are revised.

Reduces risk of skin trauma and disruption of wound.

Reduces potential for skin trauma or abrasions and provides additional protection for delicate skin and tissues.

Prevents tape skin abrasions. Wrapping tape can impair or occlude circulation to wound and to distal portion of extremity.

Early recognition of delayed healing or developing complications may prevent a more serious situation. Incisions may heal more slowly in clients with comorbidity, or the elderly in whom reduced cardiac output decreases capillary blood flow.

Decreasing drainage suggests evolution of healing process, whereas continued drainage or presence of bloody or odoriferous exudate suggests complications, which may include hemorrhage, infection, and fistula formation.

Facilitates approximation of wound edges; reduces risk of infection and chemical injury to skin and tissues.

Promotes venous return and limits edema formation. *Note:* Elevation in presence of venous insufficiency may be detrimental.

Equalizes pressure on the wound, minimizing risk of dehiscence—especially important during stage I healing during the first 3 to 4 days—and for incisions closed with adhesives.

ACTIONS/INTERVENTIONS (continued)	RATIONALE (continued)
Caution client not to touch incision.	Prevents contamination of area.
Cleanse skin surface, if needed, with diluted hydrogen peroxide solution, or running water and mild soap after incision is sealed.	Reduces skin contaminants; aids in removal of drainage or exudate.
Monitor blood glucose levels of diabetic clients, as indicated.	These clients are at higher risk for nosocomial infections and delayed healing, and the risk increases if glucose level exceeds 220 mg/dL on the first postoperative day.

Collaborative

Apply ice, if appropriate.	Reduces edema formation that may cause undue pressure on incision during initial postoperative period.
Use abdominal binder, if indicated.	Provides additional support for high-risk incisions, especially in obese clients.

Wound Care (NIC)

Irrigate wound; assist with débridement as needed.	Removes infectious exudate and necrotic tissue to promote healing.
Monitor and maintain dressings, whether hydrogel, vacuum dressing, or other types.	May be used to hasten healing in large, draining wound or fistula, to increase client comfort, and to reduce frequency of dressing changes. Also allows drainage to be measured more accurately and analyzed for pH and electrolyte content, as appropriate.

NURSING DIAGNOSIS: risk for ineffective tissue Perfusion

Risk factors may include
Interruption of flow—arterial, venous
Hypovolemia

Possibly evidenced by
(Not applicable; presence of signs and symptoms establishes an *actual* diagnosis)

Desired Outcomes/Evaluation Criteria—Client Will

Circulation Status (NOC)
Demonstrate adequate perfusion evidenced by stable vital signs, peripheral pulses present and strong, warm and dry skin, usual mentation, and individually appropriate urinary output.

ACTIONS/INTERVENTIONS	RATIONALE
Hypovolemia Management (NIC)	
Independent	
Change position slowly initially.	Vasoconstrictor mechanisms are depressed, and quick movement may lead to orthostatic hypotension, especially in the early postoperative period.
Monitor vital signs; palpate peripheral pulses; and note skin temperature, color, and capillary refill. Evaluate urinary output and time of voiding. Document dysrhythmias.	Indicators of adequacy of circulating volume and tissue perfusion or organ function. Effects of medications and electrolyte imbalances may create dysrhythmias, impairing cardiac output and tissue perfusion.
Investigate changes in mentation or failure to achieve usual mental state.	May reflect a number of problems, such as inadequate clearance of anesthetic agent, oversedation with pain medication, hypoventilation, hypovolemia, or intraoperative complications such as emboli.
Embolus Precautions (NIC)	
Assist with range-of-motion (ROM) exercises, including active ankle and leg exercises.	Stimulates peripheral circulation; aids in preventing venous stasis to reduce risk of thrombus formation.
Encourage and assist with early ambulation.	Enhances circulation and return of normal organ function.
Avoid use of knee gatch or pillow under knees. Caution client against crossing legs or sitting with legs dependent for prolonged period.	Prevents stasis of venous circulation and reduces risk of thrombophlebitis.
Assess lower extremities for erythema, edema, and calf tenderness.	Circulation may be restricted by some positions used during surgery, whereas anesthetics and decreased activity alter vasomotor tone, potentiating vascular pooling and increasing risks of thrombus formation.

(continues on page 800)

Collaborative

Apply antiembolic hose or sequential compression device (SCDs), as indicated.

Promotes venous return and prevents venous stasis of legs to reduce risk of thrombosis.

Hypovolemia Management (NIC)

Administer IV fluids and/or blood products, as needed.

Maintains circulating volume and supports perfusion.

NURSING DIAGNOSIS: deficient Knowledge [Learning Need] regarding condition/situation, prognosis, treatment, self-care, and discharge needs

May be related to

Lack of exposure or recall, information misinterpretation
Unfamiliarity with information resources
Cognitive limitation

Possibly evidenced by

Questions, request for information; statement of misconception
Inaccurate follow-through of instructions, development of preventable complications

Desired Outcomes/Evaluation Criteria—Client Will

Knowledge: Disease Process (NOC)
Verbalize understanding of condition, effects of procedure, and potential complications.

Knowledge: Treatment Regimen (NOC)
Verbalize understanding of therapeutic needs.
Correctly perform necessary procedures and explain reasons for actions.
Initiate necessary lifestyle changes and participate in treatment regimen.

ACTIONS/INTERVENTIONS   **RATIONALE**

Treatment: Disease Process (NIC)
Independent

Review specific surgery or procedure performed and future expectations.

Provides knowledge base from which client can make informed choices.

Review and have client and SO demonstrate dressing change and incision and tube care when indicated. Identify source for supplies.

Promotes competent self-care and enhances independence. *Note:* For incisions closed with a surgical zipper, client should be instructed as to when it is appropriate to peel off the device.

Stress avoidance of environmental risk factors including exposure to crowds or persons with infections.

Reduces potential for acquired infections.

Discuss drug therapy, including use of prescribed and OTC analgesics, and resumption of herbal supplements.

Enhances cooperation with regimen, reduces risk of adverse reactions or untoward effects. *Note:* Herbal preparations such as garlic, ginseng, ginkgo biloba, ginger, and feverfew increase the risk of postoperative bleeding and are contraindicated for several days following surgery.

Identify specific activity limitations.

Prevents undue strain on operative site.

Recommend planned, progressive exercise program.

Promotes return of normal function and enhances feelings of general well-being.

Schedule adequate rest periods.

Prevents fatigue and conserves energy for healing.

Review importance of nutritious diet and adequate fluid intake.

Provides elements necessary for tissue regeneration and healing, and support of tissue perfusion and organ function.

Encourage cessation of smoking.

Smoking increases risk of pulmonary infections, causes vasoconstriction, and reduces oxygen-binding capacity of blood, affecting cellular perfusion and potentially impairing healing.

Identify signs and symptoms requiring medical evaluation, such as nausea or vomiting; difficulty voiding; fever; continued or odoriferous wound drainage; incisional swelling, erythema, or separation of edges; and unresolved pain or changes in characteristics of pain.

Early recognition and treatment of developing complications which may include ileus, urinary retention, infection, and delayed healing, and may prevent progression to more serious or life-threatening situation.

Stress necessity of follow-up visits with providers, including therapists and laboratory.

Monitors progress of healing and evaluates effectiveness of regimen.

Include SO in teaching program and discharge planning. Provide written instructions and teaching materials in client's dominant language. Instruct in use of and arrange for special equipment.

Provides additional resources for reference after discharge. Promotes effective self-care.

ACTIONS/INTERVENTIONS (continued)

Identify available resources, including homecare services, visiting nurse, Meals on Wheels, outpatient therapy, and contact phone number for questions.

RATIONALE (continued)

Enhances support for client during recovery period and provides additional evaluation of ongoing needs or new concerns.

> **POTENTIAL CONSIDERATIONS** following surgical procedure (dependent on client's age, physical condition and presence of complications, personal resources, and life responsibilities)
> • *Fatigue*—increased energy requirements to perform activities of daily living, states of discomfort
> • *risk for Infection*—broken skin, traumatized tissues, stasis of body fluids, presence of pathogens and contaminants, environmental exposure, invasive procedures
> • *Self-Care Deficit/impaired Home Maintenance*—decreased strength and endurance, pain or discomfort, unfamiliarity with neighborhood resources, inadequate support systems
> Refer also to appropriate plans of care regarding underlying condition/specific surgical procedure for additional considerations.

EXTENDED CARE

I. Indications
a. Level of care and needs of the client are frequently the deciding factors in the choice of placement.
b. Short-term rehabilitation—individuals requiring services postdischarge from acute care setting
c. Long-term nursing care—individuals requiring assistance with activities of daily living (ADLs)
  i. Elderly individuals are the primary population requiring assistance with (on average) 4 to 6 ADLs.
  ii. Increasing numbers of younger individuals are requiring care for debilitating conditions when they cannot be managed in the home setting (Family Caregiver Alliance, 2005).

II. Statistics (Family Caregiver Alliance, 2005)
a. Population: In 2002, 1,458,000 people resided in nursing homes nationally, of which almost 75% were women.
b. Cost: In 2002, estimated spending on long-term care services exceeded $103 billion; in 2004, the average daily rate for a private room in a skilled nursing facility was $192, or $70,080 annually; for a semiprivate room, $169, or $61,685 annually.

GLOSSARY

Activities of daily living (ADLs): Basic everyday self-care activities, including bathing, grooming, dressing, feeding, toileting, hygiene, and personal safety.
Instrumental activities of daily living (IADLs): Activities needed to function independently in the home or community, including shopping, meal preparation, housekeeping/home maintenance, laundry, managing medications and health maintenance, use of transportation, and money management.

Long-term or extended care facility: Provision of custodial or personal care services, with ongoing supervision and coordination of care by licensed nurses (RN or LPN/LVN).
Short-term rehabilitation or skilled nursing facility: Provision of registered nursing and rehabilitation services, such as physical, occupational, and/or speech therapies; intravenous (IV) antibiotics or chemotherapy; complicated wound care; and respiratory and nutritional support.

Related Concerns

Acquired immunodeficiency syndrome (AIDS), page 709
Cancer, page 846
Cerebrovascular accident (CVA)/stroke, page 238
Craniocerebral trauma—acute rehabilitative phase, page 220
Dementia of the Alzheimer's type/vascular dementia, page 764
End-of-life care/hospice, page 866
Multiple sclerosis, page 290
Psychosocial aspects of care, page 749
Spinal cord injury, page 271
Surgical intervention, page 782
Ventilatory assistance (mechanical), page 173

Client Assessment Database

Data depend on underlying physical and psychosocial conditions necessitating continuation of structured care.

DIAGNOSTIC DIVISION MAY REPORT	MAY EXHIBIT
TEACHING/LEARNING • *Discharge Plan Considerations:* May require assistance with treatments, self-care activities, health maintenance, and nutritional support ▶ Refer to section at end of plan for postdischarge considerations.	

Diagnostic Studies

Dependent on age, general health, and medical condition. Individuals are often transferred to facility or admitted following an acute care episode where diagnostic studies were previously performed.

TEST WHY IT IS DONE	WHAT IT TELLS ME
BLOOD TESTS • *Complete blood count (CBC):* Battery of screening tests, which typically includes hemoglobin (Hgb); hematocrit (Hct); red blood cell (RBC) count, morphology, indices, and distribution width index; platelet count and size; and white blood cell (WBC) count and differential.	Low Hgb suggests anemia. Elevated Hct may indicate dehydration, whereas decreased Hct suggests fluid overload. An elevated WBC count is indicative of inflammatory process. Decreased WBC count suggests viral processes, requiring further evaluation because immune system may be dysfunctional.
• *Chemistry profile:* Evaluates general organ function and imbalances.	Age-related changes include decreased serum albumin, up to 20% increase in alkaline phosphatase, and decreased urine creatinine clearance.
OTHER DIAGNOSTIC TESTS • *Urinalysis:* Provides information about kidney function.	Determines presence of urinary tract infection (UTI) or diabetes mellitus (DM). *Note:* Bacteria are common in some populations, especially the elderly and bedridden, reflecting urinary stasis.
• *Pulse oximetry:* Determines oxygenation and respiratory function.	Decreased levels indicate need for supplemental oxygen therapy.
• *Communicable disease screens:* Rule out tuberculosis (TB), HIV, venereal disease, and hepatitis.	Testing identifies treatment needs and provides for safety of staff and other residents.
• *Drug screen:* As indicated by usage to identify therapeutic or toxic levels.	Therapeutic drug monitoring aids in establishing individually appropriate drug dosage and frequency to maintain steady state for maximal drug effect and with minimal side effects.
• *Visual acuity testing:* Assesses sight and health of the eyes.	Identifies cataracts or other vision problems.
• *Tonometer test:* Measures intraocular pressure.	Elevation indicates glaucoma.
• *Chest x-rays:* Procedure used to evaluate organs and structures within the chest for symptoms of disease.	Reveals size of heart and lung abnormalities or disease conditions, or changes of the large blood vessels and bony structure of the chest.
• *Electrocardiogram (ECG):* Provides baseline data; detects abnormalities.	ST-segment and T-wave changes, atrial and ventricular dysrhythmias, and various heart blocks are common in the elderly population.

Nursing Priorities

1. Promote physiological and psychological well-being.
2. Provide for security and safety.
3. Prevent complications of disease and/or aging process.
4. Promote effective coping skills and independence.
5. Encourage continuation of healthy habits and participation in plan of care to meet individual needs and wishes.

Discharge Goals

1. Client dealing realistically with current situation.
2. Homeostasis maintained.
3. Injury prevented.
4. Complications prevented or minimized.
5. Client performing ADLs by self or with assistance, as necessary.
6. Plan in place to meet needs after discharge, as appropriate.

NURSING DIAGNOSIS: **risk for Relocation Stress Syndrome**

Risk factors may include
Decreased psychosocial or physical health status
Temporary or permanent move that may be voluntary or involuntary
Past, current, and recent losses
Feelings of powerlessness
Lack of predeparture counseling
Unpredictability of experience

Possibly evidenced by
(Not applicable; presence of signs and symptoms establishes an *actual* diagnosis)

Desired Outcomes/Evaluation Criteria—Client Will

Anxiety Level (NOC)
Demonstrate appropriate range of feelings and appear relaxed.

Psychosocial Adjustment: Life Change (NOC)
Verbalize understanding of reasons for change as able.
Participate in routine and special or social events as capable.
Verbalize acceptance of situation.

ACTIONS/INTERVENTIONS	RATIONALE
Relocation Stress Reduction (NIC)	
Independent	
Provide client and significant other (SO) with a copy of "A Patient's Bill of Rights" and review it with them. Discuss facility's rules about such things as visitors, off-grounds visits, and personal property.	Provides information that can foster confidence that individual rights do continue in this setting and the client is still "his or her own person" and has some control over what happens.
Ascertain if client has completed an advance directive. Provide information, as appropriate.	Assures client/family wishes will be known to provide direction to caregivers.
Determine client's and SO's attitude toward admission to facility and expectations for the future.	If this is expected to be a temporary placement, client's and SO's concerns will be different than if placement is permanent. When client is giving up own home and way of life, feelings of helplessness, loss, and grief are to be expected.
Help family and SO to be honest with client regarding admission. Be clear about actions and events.	Family may have difficulty dealing with decision and reality of permanent placement and may avoid discussing situation with client. Honesty decreases "surprises," assists in maintaining trust, and may enhance coping.
Identify support person(s) important to client and include in care activities, mealtime, and so on, as appropriate.	During adjustment period and times of stress, client may benefit from presence of trusted individual who can provide reassurance and reduce sense of isolation.
Assess level of anxiety and discuss reasons when possible.	Identifying specific problems enables individual to deal more realistically with them and care provider to intervene as necessary, for example, a client who is being neglected or abused or has unrelieved pain may be very anxious and afraid or unable to verbalize.
Develop nurse-client relationship.	Trusting relationships among client, SO, and staff promotes optimal care and support.
Make time to listen to client about concerns, and encourage free expression of feelings including anger, hostility, fear, and loneliness.	Being available in this way allows client to feel accepted and begin to acknowledge and deal with feelings related to circumstances of admission.

(continues on page 804)

ACTIONS/INTERVENTIONS (continued)	RATIONALE (continued)
Acknowledge reality of situation and feelings of client. Accept expressions of anger while limiting aggressive, acting-out behavior.	Permission to express feelings allows for beginning of resolution. Acceptance promotes sense of self-worth. *Note:* Psychosocial and/or physiological disturbances can occur as a result of transfer from one environment to another, especially if the move is unexpected or involuntary.
Assist client to identify strengths and successful coping behaviors and incorporate into problem-solving.	Building on past successes increases likelihood of positive outcome in present situation. Enhances sense of control and management of current deficits.
Orient to physical aspects of facility, schedules, and activities. Introduce to roommate(s) and staff. Give explanation of roles.	Getting acquainted is an important part of admission. Knowledge of where things are and from whom client can expect assistance can be helpful in reducing anxiety.
Determine client's usual schedule and incorporate into facility routine as much as possible.	Consistency provides reassurance and may lessen confusion and enhance cooperation.
Provide above information in written or audiovisual form as well.	Overload of information is difficult to remember. Client can refer to written or audiovisual materials as needed to refresh memory or learn new information.
Give careful thought to room placement. Provide help and encouragement in placing client's own belongings around room. Do not transfer from one room to another without client approval and documentable need.	Location, roommate compatibility, and place for personal belongings are important considerations for helping the client feel "at home." Changes are often met with resistance and can result in emotional upset and decline in physical condition. *Note:* Persons with severe behavioral problems or cognitive dysfunctions may require a private room if similar roommate not available.
Note behavior, presence of suspiciousness or paranoia, irritability, and defensiveness. Compare to SO's description of customary responses.	Increased stress, physical discomfort, and fatigue may temporarily exacerbate mental deterioration and cognitive inaccessibility, and further impair communication and social inaccessibility. This represents a catastrophic episode that can escalate into a panic state and violence.
Be aware of escalating anxiety and presence of delirium. Look for possible causes.	Common causes of delirium include drug toxicity, electrolyte imbalances, withdrawal from alcohol and other drugs, pain, and trauma—especially hip fractures and advanced disease resulting in organ failure.
Collaborative	
Refer to social service or other appropriate agency for assistance. Have case manager or social worker discuss ramifications of Medicare and/or Medicaid if client is eligible for these resources.	Client may not be aware of the resources available, and providing current information about individual coverage and limitations and other possible sources of support will assist with adjustment to new situation.

NURSING DIAGNOSIS: Grieving

May be related to
Perceived, actual, or potential loss of physiopsychosocial well-being, personal possessions, or SO; cultural beliefs about aging and/or debilitation

Possibly evidenced by
Denial of feelings, depression, sorrow, guilt
Alterations in activity level, sleep patterns, eating habits, libido

Desired Outcomes/Evaluation Criteria—Client Will

Grief Resolution (NOC)
Identify and express feelings appropriately.
Progress through the grieving process.
Enjoy the present and plan for the future one day at a time.

ACTIONS/INTERVENTIONS	RATIONALE
Grief Work Facilitation (NIC)	
Independent	
Assess emotional state. Note cultural beliefs and expectations.	Anxiety and depression are common reactions to changes and losses associated with long-term illness or debilitating condition. In addition, changes in neurotransmitter levels, such as increased monoamine oxidase (MAO) and serotonin levels with decreased norepinephrine, may potentiate depression in elderly clients. Personal expectations may affect response to change.

ACTIONS/INTERVENTIONS (continued)	RATIONALE (continued)
Make time to listen to the client. Encourage free expression of hopeless feelings and desire to die.	Allowing these feelings to be expressed, rather than denying or ignoring them, provides a sounding board for the client to hear and reflect on own thoughts, start to deal with the feelings, and consider alternatives.
Assess suicidal potential.	May be related to physical disease, social isolation, and grief. *Note:* Studies indicate women are three times as likely to attempt suicide; however, men are three times as likely to succeed. The elderly are disproportionately likely to die by suicide (National Institute of Mental Health [NIHM], 2008).
Involve SO in discussions and activities to the level of their willingness.	When SOs are involved, there is more potential for successful problem-solving. *Note:* SO may not be available or may choose not to be involved.
Provide liberal touching and hugs as individually accepted.	Conveys sense of concern and closeness to reduce feelings of isolation and enhance sense of self-worth. *Note:* Touch may be viewed as a threat by some clients and escalate feelings of anger or fear.
Identify spiritual concerns. Discuss available resources and encourage participation in religious activities, as appropriate.	Search for meaning is common to those facing changes in life. Participation in religious or spiritual activities can provide sense of direction and peace of mind.
Assist with planning for specifics as necessary, including advance directives to determine code status, living will wishes, making of will, and funeral arrangements, if appropriate.	Having these issues resolved can help client and SO deal with the grieving process and may provide peace of mind.

Collaborative

Refer to other resources as indicated, such as a spiritual advisor, parish nurse, case manager, or social worker.	May need further assistance to resolve some problems.

NURSING DIAGNOSIS: impaired Memory/disturbed Thought Processes

May be related to
Physiological changes of aging, loss of cells or brain atrophy, decreased blood supply, altered sensory input
Pain, effects of medications
Psychological conflicts: disrupted life pattern

Possibly evidenced by
Slower reaction times, gradual memory loss, altered attention span; disorientation; inability to follow
Altered sleep patterns
Personality changes

Desired Outcomes/Evaluation Criteria—Client Will

Cognition (NOC)
Maintain or improve usual reality orientation.

Distorted Thought Self-Control (NOC)
Recognize changes in thinking and behavior.
Identify interventions to deal effectively with situation and deficits.

ACTIONS/INTERVENTIONS	RATIONALE
Cognitive Stimulation (NIC)	
Independent	
Allow adequate time for client to respond to questions or comments and to make decisions.	Reaction time may be slowed with aging due to changes in metabolism and cerebral blood flow or with brain injuries and some neuromuscular conditions.
Discuss happenings of the past. Place familiar objects in room. Encourage the display of photographs and photo albums and frequent visits from SO and friends.	Events of the past may be more readily recalled by the elderly client because long-term memory usually remains intact. Reminiscence or life review and companionship are beneficial to clients.

(continues on page 806)

ACTIONS/INTERVENTIONS (continued)	RATIONALE (continued)
Note presence of short-term memory loss, and provide with such aids as calendars, clocks, room signs, and pictures.	Short-term memory loss presents a challenge for nursing care, especially if the client cannot remember such things as how to use the call bell or how to get to the bathroom. This problem is not in client's control but may be less frustrating if simple reminders are used to assist in providing continual reorientation. It may be helpful for older person and their family to know that short-term memory loss is common and is not necessarily a sign of "senility."
Evaluate individual stress level and deal with it appropriately.	Stress level may be greatly increased because of recent losses, such as poor health, death of spouse or companion, or loss of home. In addition, some conflicts that occur with age come from previously unresolved problems that may need to be dealt with now.
Assess physical status and psychiatric symptoms, especially in presence of recent change in mentation or development of confusion. Institute interventions appropriate to findings.	Not all mental changes are the result of aging, and it is important to rule out physical causes before accepting these as unchangeable. Possibilities include pain that is often unreported and underestimated, metabolic imbalances, adverse toxic medication levels, drug-induced side effects (e.g., anti-Parkinsonian agents, tricyclic antidepressants), or the result of infectious, cardiac, or respiratory disorders (Amella, 2004).
Reorient to person, place, and time, as appropriate.	Helps client maintain focus.
Have client repeat verbal or written instructions.	Verifies hearing and ability to read and comprehend.
Note cyclic changes in mentation or behavior, such as evening confusion, picking at bedclothes, pacing, shouting or angry outbursts, or wandering aimlessly.	"Sundowner syndrome" may occur in response to visual and/or hearing deficits enhanced by declining light or an accumulation of all the sensory stimulation during the day, fatigue, inflexible institution schedules, peak-and-trough drug levels, dehydration, and electrolyte imbalances.
Involve in regular exercise, activity, and diversional programs.	Promotes release of endorphins, enhancing sense of well-being, and can improve thinking abilities.
Schedule at least one rest period per day.	Prevents fatigue; enhances general well-being.
Provide brighter lighting in room and common areas by midafternoon (e.g., 3 p.m.), or earlier on cloudy or winter days.	Maximizes visual perception; may limit evening confusion.
Turn off lights at bedtime. Provide night lights where appropriate.	Reinforces "sleep time" while meeting safety needs.
Support client's involvement in own care. Provide opportunity for choices on a daily basis.	Choice is a necessary component in everyday life. Cognitively impaired clients may respond with aggressive behavior as they lose control in their lives.

Collaborative

Review results of laboratory and diagnostic tests, such as electrolytes, thyroid studies, or full drug screen and computerized tomography (CT) scan.	Aids in establishing cause of changes in mentation and determining treatment options. *Note:* These tests can identify the causes of dementia in 90% of the cases.
Administer medications as indicated, such as donepazil (Aricept), rivastigmine (Exelon), galantamine (Razadyne), and memantine (Namenda).	Aricept, Exelon, and Razadyne are cholinesterase inhibitors used to treat mild to moderate dementia, whereas Namenda, which regulates glutamine activation, is prescribed for the treatment of moderate to severe dementia (NIA, 2008). *Note:* Tacrine (Cognex) is approved for treatment of dementia but is no longer actively marketed and rarely used because of difficulties with dosing, tolerance, and significant hepatotoxicity (Geldmacher, 2007). (Refer to CP: Dementia of the Alzheimer's Type/Vascular Dementia.)

NURSING DIAGNOSIS: compromised family Coping

May be related to
Placement of family member in extended care facility
Temporary family disorganization and role changes
Situational or transitional crises SO may be facing
Client providing little support for SO
Prolonged disease or disability progression that exhausts the supportive capacity of SOs

Possibly evidenced by
SO describes significant preoccupation with personal reactions, such as fear, anticipatory grief, guilt, and anxiety
SO attempts assistive or supportive behaviors with unsatisfactory results
SO withdraws from client
SO displays protective behavior disproportionate—too little or too much—to client's abilities and need for autonomy

NURSING DIAGNOSIS: compromised family Coping (continued)

Desired Outcomes/Evaluation Criteria—Family Will

Family Coping NOC
Identify resources within themselves to deal with the situation.
Interact appropriately with the client and staff, providing support and assistance, as indicated.
Verbalize knowledge and understanding of situation.
Participate in planning for discharge, as appropriate.

ACTIONS/INTERVENTIONS	RATIONALE
Family Support NIC	
Independent	
Introduce staff and provide SO with information about facility and care. Be available for questions. Provide tour of facility.	Helpful to establish beginning relationships. Offers opportunities for enhancing feelings of involvement.
Determine involvement and availability of family and SO.	Clarifies expectations and abilities and identifies needs.
Encourage SO participation in care at level of desire and capability and within limits of safety. Include in social events and celebrations.	Helps family to feel at ease and allows them to feel supportive and a part of the client's life.
Accept choices of SO/family regarding level of involvement in care.	Families may choose to ignore client or may project feelings of guilt regarding placing client in facility by criticizing staff. *Note:* Feelings of dissatisfaction with the staff may be transferred back to the client.
Evaluate SO's and caregiver's level of stress and coping abilities, especially before planning for discharge.	Caring for and about clients with chronic or debilitating conditions places a heavy strain on SO. Recognizing own strengths and areas for improvement provides opportunity for personal growth, enhancing potential for success if client returns home.
Support the caregiver with attention, compassion, time, respect, honesty, advocacy, and understanding.	Nursing interventions need to prepare the caregivers for the challenges they face and meet their needs for compassion and caring.
Identify availability and use of community support systems.	Helps determine areas of need and provides information regarding additional resources to enhance coping.
Be aware of staff's own feelings of anger and frustration about client's and SO's choices and goals that differ from those of staff, and deal with them appropriately.	Group care conferences or individual counseling may be helpful in problem-solving.
Collaborative	
Inform SO of services available to them such as meal tickets, family cooking time or celebrations, group care conference, visiting nurse, caseworker, and other social services.	Promotes feeling of involvement; eases transition in adjustment to client's admission to homecare or facility care.
Advise caregivers of resources available, such as Eldercare Locator, Seniornet, Today's Caregiver, and Caregiver Network, Inc.	Helps nurses, clients, and caregivers feel supported and able to provide more skillful care.
Refer SO and caregivers to stress management classes, as indicated.	Although support groups may be very helpful, learning stress management techniques may be more effective in strengthening individual coping as the focus is on the SO rather than the SO-client relationship.

NURSING DIAGNOSIS: risk for Poisoning, [drug toxicity]

Risk factors may include
Reduced metabolism; impaired circulation; precarious physiological balance, presence of multiple diseases or organ involvement
Use of multiple prescribed and/or over-the-counter (OTC) drugs

Possibly evidenced by
(Not applicable; presence of signs and symptoms establishes an *actual* diagnosis)

Desired Outcomes/Evaluation Criteria—Client Will

Risk Control: Drug Use NOC
Maintain prescribed drug regimen free of untoward side effects.

ACTIONS/INTERVENTIONS	RATIONALE

Medication Management (NIC)

Independent

Determine allergies, medication, and other drug use history.

Review resources such as drug manuals or pharmacist for information about toxic symptoms and side effects. List drug actions and interactions and idiosyncrasies, such as medications that are given with or without foods, as well as those that should not be crushed.

Discuss self-administration of, or access to, OTC products.

Helps avoid repetition or creation of problems.

Provides information about drugs being taken and identifies possible interactions. Toxicity can be increased in the debilitated and older client with symptoms not as apparent. Presence of polypharmacy increases the possibility of drug-drug or drug-food interaction (Amella, 2004).

Limits interference with prescribed regimen, desired drug action, and organ function. May prevent inadvertent overdosing or toxic reactions. *Note:* Appropriate use of OTC products kept at bedside or via free access at nurses' station fosters independence and enhances sense of control and self-esteem.

Identify swallowing problems or reluctance to take tablets or capsules.

Give pills in a spoonful of soft foods, such as applesauce or ice cream; or use liquid form of medication if available.

Open capsules or crush tablets only when appropriate.

May not be able to or want to take medication.

Ensures proper dosage if client is unable, or does not like, to swallow pills.

Should not be done unless absolutely necessary because this may alter absorption of medications; for example, enteric-coated tablets may be absorbed in the stomach when crushed, instead of in the intestines.

Make sure medication has been swallowed.

Observe for changes in condition or behavior.

Ensures effective therapeutic use of medication and prevents pill hoarding.

Behavior may be only indication of drug toxicity, and early identification of problems provides for appropriate intervention. *Note:* Elderly individuals have increased sensitivity to anticholinergic effects of medications; therefore, use of anticholinergics, antiparkinson agents, benzodiazepines, central nervous system (CNS) depressants, and tricyclic antidepressants may cause delirium or confusion.

Use discretion in the administration of sedatives.

A quiet place where the client can pace or be secluded, may be more helpful. If client is destructive or excessively disruptive, pharmacological or mechanical control measures may be required. Convenience of the staff is never a reason for sedating client; however, client safety and rights of other clients need to be taken into consideration.

Collaborative

Review drug regimen routinely with physician and pharmacist.

Provides opportunity to alter therapy by reducing dosage or discontinue medications as client's needs and organ functions change affecting drug absorption, distribution, and renal clearance (Amella, 2004).

Obtain serum drug levels, as indicated.

Determines therapeutic or toxic levels.

NURSING DIAGNOSIS: impaired verbal Communication

May be related to

Degenerative changes—such as reduced cerebral circulation, hearing loss; progressive neurological disease—such as Parkinson's disease, Alzheimer's disease

Laryngectomy or tracheostomy; stroke, traumatic brain injury

Possibly evidenced by

Impaired articulation; difficulty with phonation; inability to modulate speech, find words, name, or identify objects (aphasia, dysarthria)

Diminished hearing ability

Desired Outcomes/Evaluation Criteria—Client Will

Communication (NOC)

Establish method of communication by which needs can be expressed.

Demonstrate congruent verbal and nonverbal communication.

ACTIONS/INTERVENTIONS	RATIONALE
Communication Enhancement: Speech Deficit (NIC)	
Independent	
Assess reason for lack of communication, including CNS and neuromuscular functioning, gag and swallow reflexes, hearing, and teeth and mouth problems.	Identification of the problem is essential to appropriate intervention. Sometimes clients do not want to talk, may think they talk when they do not, may expect others to know what they want, or may not be able to comprehend or be understood.
Determine whether client is bilingual and what language is primary.	With declining cerebral function or diminished thought processes and increased level of stress, client may mix languages or revert to original language.
Investigate how SO communicates with the client.	Provides opportunity to develop or continue effective communication patterns, which have already been established.
Assess client knowledge base and level of comprehension. Treat the client as an adult, avoiding pity and impatience.	Knowing how much to expect of the client can help to avoid frustration and unreasonable demands for performance. However, having an expectation that the client will understand may help raise level of performance.
Establish therapeutic nurse-client relationship through active-listening, being available for problem-solving.	Aids in dealing with communication problems.
Make client aware of presence when entering the room by speaking, turning a light off and on, or touching client or mattress, as appropriate.	Getting attention is the first step in communication.
Make eye contact, place self at or below client's level, and speak face to face.	Conveys interest and promotes contact.
Speak slowly and distinctly, using simple sentences and yes-or-no questions. Avoid speaking loudly or shouting. Supplement with written communication when possible or needed. Allow sufficient time for reply; remain relaxed with client.	Assists in comprehension and overall communication. Client may respond poorly to high-pitched sounds; shouting also obscures consonants and amplifies vowels.
Use other creative measures to assist in communication, such as picture chart or alphabet board, sign language, or lip reading, when appropriate.	Many options are available, depending on individual situation. *Note:* Sign language also may be used effectively with other than hearing-impaired individuals.
Communication Enhancement: Hearing Deficit (NIC)	
Check ears for excess cerumen.	Hardened earwax may decrease hearing acuity and cause tinnitus.
Ascertain if client has or uses hearing aid.	Client may have, but not use, a hearing aid because it may not fit well or it may need batteries.
Be aware that behavioral problems may be associated with hearing loss.	Anger, explosive temper outbursts, frustration, embarrassment, depression, withdrawal, and paranoia may be attempts to deal with communication problems.
Collaborative	
Refer to speech therapists, ear-nose-throat physician, or for audiometry, as needed.	Determines extent of hearing loss and whether a hearing aid is appropriate. May be helpful to a client and staff in improving communication. *Note:* Some sources believe 90% of the clients in extended care facilities have some degree of hearing loss or presbycusis because this is a common age change. Hearing aids are most effective with conductive losses and may help with sensorineural losses.

NURSING DIAGNOSIS: disturbed Sleep Pattern

May be related to
Lack of sleep privacy; sleep partner/roommate
Environmental changes; noise; facility routines

Possibly evidenced by
Change in normal sleep pattern; interrupted sleep
Verbal reports of not feeling well rested; dissatisfaction with sleep
Decreased ability to function

Desired Outcomes/Evaluation Criteria—Client Will

Sleep (NOC)
Report improvement in sleep or rest pattern.
Verbalize increased sense of well-being and feeling rested.

ACTIONS/INTERVENTIONS	RATIONALE

Sleep Enhancement (NIC)
Independent

Ascertain usual sleep habits and changes that are occurring.	Determines need for action and helps identify appropriate interventions.
Provide comfortable bedding and some of own possessions, such as a pillow or an afghan.	Increases comfort for sleep; provides physiological and psychological support.
Establish new sleep routine incorporating old pattern and new environment.	When new routine contains as many aspects of old habits as possible, stress and related anxiety may be reduced, enhancing sleep.
Match with roommate who has similar sleep patterns and nocturnal needs.	Decreases likelihood that "night owl" roommate may delay client's falling asleep or create interruptions that cause awakening.
Encourage some light physical activity during the day. Make sure client stops activity several hours before bedtime, as individually appropriate.	Daytime activity can help client expend energy and be ready for nighttime sleep; however, continuation of activity close to bedtime may act as a stimulant, delaying sleep.
Promote bedtime comfort regimens such as warm bath, massage, a glass of warm milk, or small amount wine or brandy at bedtime.	Promotes a relaxing, soothing effect. *Note:* Milk has soporific qualities, enhancing synthesis of serotonin, a neurotransmitter that helps client fall asleep faster and sleep longer.
Instruct in relaxation measures.	Helps induce sleep.
Reduce noise and light.	Provides atmosphere conducive to sleep.
Encourage position of comfort and assist in turning, if needed.	Repositioning reduces pressure on tissues, enhances muscle relaxation, and promotes rest.
Lower bed and position one side against wall when possible. Avoid use of side rails.	May have fear of falling because of change in size and height of bed. *Note:* Side rails place client at risk for falling when climbing over rails or possible entrapment.
Avoid or limit interruptions such as awakening for medications or therapies.	Uninterrupted sleep is more restful, and client may be unable to return to sleep when wakened.

Collaborative

Administer sedatives and hypnotics with caution, as indicated.	May be given to help client sleep or rest during transition period from home to new setting. *Note:* Avoid habitual use because these drugs decrease REM (rapid eye movement) sleep time.

NURSING DIAGNOSIS: **imbalanced Nutrition: Less [or] More than Body Requirements**

May be related to
Impaired dentition, dulling of senses of smell and taste
Cognitive limitations, depression
Inability to feed self effectively
Sedentary activity level

Possibly evidenced by
Reported or observed dysfunctional eating patterns
Weight under or over ideal for height and frame
Poor muscle tone, pale conjunctiva and mucous membranes
Signs and symptoms of vitamin and protein deficits, electrolyte imbalances

Desired Outcomes/Evaluation Criteria—Client Will

Nutritional Status (NOC)
Maintain normal weight or progress toward weight goal with normalization of laboratory values and be free of signs of malnutrition and obesity.
Demonstrate eating patterns or behaviors to maintain appropriate weight.

ACTIONS/INTERVENTIONS	RATIONALE

Nutrition Management (NIC)
Independent

Perform initial nutritional assessment—admission height, weight, and body mass index (BMI); ability to feed self, chew, and swallow; and eating preferences.	Provides baseline evaluation to help determine dietary needs and formulate dietary plan (Henkel, 2004).
Evaluate activity pattern.	Extremes of exercise, such as sedentary life and continuous pacing, affect caloric needs.

ACTIONS/INTERVENTIONS (continued)

Incorporate favorite foods and maintain as near-normal food consistency as possible, such as soft or finely ground food with gravy or liquid added. Avoid pureed or baby food whenever possible.

Encourage the use of spices, other than sodium, to client's personal taste.

Provide small, frequent feedings, as indicated.

Serve hot foods hot and cold foods cold.

Promote a pleasant environment for eating in dining room or with company, if possible.

Have healthy snack foods, such as cheese, crackers, soup, and fruit available on a 24-hour basis.

Plan for social events and provide for snacks even when working to reduce total calories.

Weigh on a regular basis—preferably, same time of day and in similar clothing.

Assess causes of weight loss or gain, such as dysphagia due to decreased saliva production, neurogenic or psychogenic disturbances, tumors, muscular dysfunction, altered senses of smell and taste, or dysfunctional eating patterns related to depression or dementia.

Review medication regimen for potential effects on food intake.

Check state of client's dental health periodically, including fit and condition of dentures, if present.

Monitor total caloric intake, as indicated.

Observe condition of skin; note muscle wasting; brittle nails; dry, lifeless hair; and signs of poor healing.

Encourage exercise and activity program within individual ability.

Collaborative

Consult with dietitian.

Provide balanced diet with individually appropriate protein, complex carbohydrates, and calories. Include supplements between meals, as indicated.

Administer vitamin and mineral supplements, as appropriate.

Refer to speech therapist for swallowing evaluation, as indicated.

Refer for dental care routinely and as needed.

RATIONALE (continued)

Aids in maintaining intake, especially when mouth and dental problems exist. Baby food is often unpalatable and can decrease appetite and lower self-esteem.

Reduction in number and acuity of taste buds results in food tasting bland and decreases enjoyment of food and desire to eat.

Decreased gastric motility causes client to feel full and reduces intake.

Foods served at the proper temperature are more palatable, and enjoyment may increase appetite.

Eating is, in part, a social event and appetite can improve with increased socialization.

Helps meet individual needs and enhances intake with caloric recommendations.

Eating is part of socialization, and being able to respond to body's needs enhances sense of control and willingness to participate in dietary program.

Monitors nutritional state and effectiveness of interventions.

Aids in adjusting plan of care and choice of interventions. *Note:* In elderly clients, saliva secretion may be decreased by as much as 66%, taste buds atrophy with reduced sensitivity to sweet and salt.

Drug side effects can impact client's intake; for example, corticosteriods may increase intake; angiotensin-converting enzyme (ACE) inhibitors and antihistamines cause change in taste; antidepressants, NSAIDs, and ferrous sulfate can decrease appetite or cause dysphagia; NSAIDs, antibiotics, digoxin, opiates, and chemotherapeutic agents can cause gastrointestinal (GI) distress, nausea, constipation, or mucositis (Henkel, 2004).

Oral infections and dental problems, shrinking gums, reaction of client's oral mucous membranes and saliva (associated with some medications or treatments), loss of teeth or ill-fitting dentures can all decrease client's ability to chew.

If dietary plan is ineffective in meeting individual goals, calorie count or food diary may help identify problem areas.

Reflects lack of adequate nutrition.

Promotes sense of well-being and may improve appetite.

Aids in establishing specific nutritional program to meet individual client needs.

Adjustments may be needed to deal with the body's decreased ability to process protein, as well as decreased metabolic rate and levels of activity. *Note:* Reduced production of salivary ptyalin inhibits digestion of complex carbohydrates in elderly individuals affecting dietary plan. In addition, delayed insulin release by the pancreas and reduced peripheral sensitivity to insulin decrease glucose tolerance.

With age, renal and other regulatory systems cannot compensate as well for errors in intake. Mineral requirements change as hormone levels, metabolism, and GI function change. In addition, absorption can be impaired by medication use and chronic illness.

Information useful in determining diet type or consistency, need for special exercises to strengthen muscles for swallowing, and/or inclusion in a restorative dining program (Henkel, 2004).

Maintenance of oral and dental health and good dentition can enhance intake.

NURSING DIAGNOSIS: Self-Care Deficit: [specify]

May be related to
Depression, discouragement, perceptual or cognitive impairment
Loss of mobility, general debilitation, neuromuscular or musculoskeletal impairment
Pain, discomfort

Possibly evidenced by
Inability to manage ADLs, unkempt appearance

Desired Outcomes/Evaluation Criteria—Client Will

Self-Care: Activities of Daily Living (ADLs) (NOC)
Perform self-care activities within level of own ability.
Demonstrate techniques or lifestyle changes to meet own needs.
Use resources effectively.

ACTIONS/INTERVENTIONS	RATIONALE
Self-Care Assistance (NIC)	
Independent	
Determine current capabilities (using 0–4 scale) and barriers to participation in self-care.	Comprehensive functional assessment includes independent performance of basic ADLs, social activities, sensory abilities, cognition, and ability to ambulate.
Involve client in formulation of plan of care at level of ability.	Enhances sense of control and aids in cooperation and maintenance of independence.
Encourage self-care. Work within present abilities; do not pressure client, but encourage client to reach beyond current capabilities. Provide adequate time for client to complete tasks. Have expectation of improvement and assist as needed.	Doing for oneself enhances feeling of self-worth. Failure can produce discouragement and depression.
Provide and promote privacy, including during bathing or showering.	Modesty may lead to reluctance to participate in care or perform activities in the presence of others.
Use specialized equipment as needed, such as tub transfer seat, grab bars, or raised toilet seat.	Enhances ability to move and perform activities safely.
Give tub bath, using walk-in tub, or two-person or mechanical lift if necessary. Use shower chair and spray attachment, as appropriate. Avoid chilling.	Provides safety for those who cannot get into the tub alone. Shower may be more feasible for some clients, though it may be less beneficial or desirable to the client. Elderly or debilitated clients are more prone to chilling.
Shampoo and style hair, as needed. Provide or assist with manicure.	Aids in maintaining appearance. Shampooing may be required more or less frequently than bathing schedule.
Encourage use of barber or beauty salon if client is able.	Enhances self-image and self-esteem, preserving dignity of the client.
Acquire clothing with modified fasteners, as indicated.	Use of Velcro instead of buttons or shoelaces can facilitate process of dressing, undressing, and toileting.
Encourage and assist with routine mouth and teeth care daily. Promote, or provide, denture care on a regular basis—cleaning, disinfecting, storage, repair, and use of dental adhesive. Use alternate oral hygiene measures as indicated, such as suction toothbrush, backward-bent toothbrush, chlorhexidine and fluoride mouth rinses, and regular suctioning.	Reduces risk of gum disease and tooth loss, enhances oral health, and promotes proper fitting and use of dentures.
Collaborative	
Consult with physical and/or occupational therapists and rehabilitation specialist.	Useful in establishing exercise and activity program, identifying assistive devices to meet individual needs and safety concerns, and facilitating independence.

NURSING DIAGNOSIS: risk for impaired Skin Integrity

Risk factors may include
General debilitation, reduced mobility, changes in skin and muscle mass associated with aging, sensory or motor deficits
Altered circulation, edema, poor nutrition
Excretions and secretions (bladder and bowel incontinence)
Problems with self-care

NURSING DIAGNOSIS: risk for impaired Skin Integrity (continued)

Possibly evidenced by
(Not applicable; presence of signs and symptoms establishes an *actual* diagnosis)

Desired Outcomes/Evaluation Criteria—Client Will

Risk Control (NOC)
Maintain intact skin.
Identify individual risk factors.
Demonstrate behaviors or techniques to prevent skin breakdown or facilitate healing.

ACTIONS/INTERVENTIONS	RATIONALE
Skin Surveillance (NIC)	
Independent	
Inspect skin, tissues, and mucous membranes routinely.	Provides opportunity for early intervention in potential high-risk population, who may have thin, less elastic, and more fragile skin and tissues.
Anticipate and use preventive measures in clients who are at risk for skin breakdown, such as anyone who is thin, obese, aging, or debilitated.	Decubitus ulcers are difficult to heal, and prevention is the best treatment.
Assess nutritional status and initiate corrective measures, as indicated. Provide balanced diet with adequate protein, vitamins, and minerals.	A positive nitrogen balance and improved nutritional state can help prevent skin breakdown and promote ulcer healing. *Note:* May need additional calories and protein if draining ulcer is present.
Encourage adequate fluid intake especially in presence of cognitive impairment or dementia.	Prevention of dehydration is necessary to maintain circulating volume and tissue perfusion, moist mucous membranes, and good skin turgor to reduce risk of ulcer formation.
Maintain strict skin hygiene, using mild, nondetergent soap (if any), drying gently and thoroughly, and lubricating with lotion or emollient.	A daily bath is usually not necessary in elderly clients because there is atrophy of sebaceous and sweat glands, and bathing may create dry skin problems. However, as epidermis thins with age, cleansing and use of lubricants is needed to keep skin soft, pliable, and to protect susceptible skin from breakdown.
Change position frequently in bed and chair. Recommend 10 minutes of exercise each hour and/or perform passive ROM.	Improves circulation, muscle tone, and joint motion and promotes client participation.
Use a rotation schedule in turning client. Use draw or turn sheet. Pay close attention to client's comfort level.	Allows for longer periods free of pressure; prevents shearing or tearing motions that can damage fragile tissues. *Note:* Use of prone position depends on client tolerance and should be maintained for only a short time.
Massage bony prominences gently with lotion or cream.	Enhances circulation to tissues, increases vascular tone, and reduces tissue edema. *Note:* Contraindicated if area is pink or red because cellular damage may occur. Gentle massage around area may stimulate circulation to impaired tissues.
Keep sheets and bedclothes clean, dry, and free from wrinkles, crumbs, and other irritating material.	Avoids friction or abrasion injury of skin.
Use elbow and heel protectors and foam, water, or gel pads for positioning in bed and when up in chair. Avoid use of plastic sheet protectors or incontinent pads.	Reduces risk of tissue abrasions and decreases pressure that can impair cellular blood flow. Promotes circulation of air along skin surface to dissipate heat and moisture. Plastic can actually trap heat and moisture against fragile tissues, increasing risk of tissue irritation and breakdown.
Provide for safety during ambulation, using appropriate adaptive devices, such as a walker or cane.	Loss of muscle strength and flexibility and physical disease process or debilitation may result in impaired coordination.
Limit exposure to temperature extremes and use of heating pad or ice pack.	Decreased sensitivity to pain, heat, or cold increases risk of tissue trauma.
Examine feet and nails routinely and provide foot and nail care as indicated:	Foot problems are common among clients who are elderly, diabetic, bedfast, and/or debilitated.
Keep nails cut short and smooth.	Jagged, rough nails can cause tissue damage and infection.
Use lotion or softening cream on feet.	Prevents drying or cracking of skin; promotes maintenance of healthy skin.
Check for fissures between toes, swab with hydrogen peroxide or dust with antiseptic powder, and place a wisp of cotton between the toes.	Prevents spread of infection and/or tissue injury.
Rub feet with witch hazel or a mentholated preparation and have client wear lightweight cotton socks.	Even though rash may not be present, burning and itching may be a problem. *Note:* Witch hazel may be contraindicated if skin is dry.

(continues on page 814)

ACTIONS/INTERVENTIONS (continued)

Inspect skin surface and folds, especially when incontinence pad or pants are used, and bony prominences routinely. Increase preventive measures when reddened areas are noticed.

Continue regimen for redness and irritation when break in skin occurs.

Observe for decubitus ulcer development, and treat immediately according to protocol.

Collaborative

Provide waterbed, alternating pressure, egg-crate or gel mattress, and pad for chair.

Monitor Hgb and Hct and blood glucose levels.

Refer to podiatrist, as indicated.

Provide whirlpool treatments, as appropriate.

Assist with topical applications, such as hydrogel dressings, skin barrier dressings (Duoderm, Op-Site), collagenase therapy, absorbable gelatin sponges (Gelfoam), and aerosol sprays.

Administer nutritional supplements and vitamins, as indicated.

Prepare for skin grafting. (Refer to CP: Burns, ND: impaired Skin Integrity.)

RATIONALE (continued)

Skin breakdown can occur quickly with potential for infection and necrosis, possibly involving muscle and bone. There is increased risk of redness and irritation around legs due to elastic bands in adult incontinence pads or pants.

Aggressive measures are important because decubitus ulcers can develop in a matter of a few hours.

Timely intervention may prevent extensive damage.

Provides protection and improved circulation by decreasing amount of pressure on tissues.

Anemia, dehydration, and elevated glucose levels are factors in skin breakdown and can impair healing.

May need professional care for such problems as ingrown toenails, corns, bony changes, and skin or tissue ulceration.

Increases circulation and has a débriding action.

Although there are differing opinions about the efficacy of these agents, individual or combination use may enhance healing.

Aids in healing and cellular regeneration.

May be required to close large ulcers.

NURSING DIAGNOSIS: **risk for impaired Urinary Elimination**

Risk factors may include
Changes in fluid or nutritional pattern
Neuromuscular changes
Perceptual or cognitive impairment

Possibly evidenced by
(Not applicable; presence of signs and symptoms establishes an *actual* diagnosis)

Desired Outcomes/Evaluation Criteria—Client Will

Urinary Elimination (NOC)
Maintain or regain effective pattern of elimination.
Initiate necessary lifestyle changes.
Participate in treatment regimen to correct or control situation, such as bladder training program or use of indwelling catheter.

ACTIONS/INTERVENTIONS

RATIONALE

Urinary Elimination Management (NIC)
Independent

Monitor voiding pattern. Identify possible reasons for changes, such as disorientation, neuromuscular impairment, and psychotropic medications.

Palpate bladder. Observe for "overflow" voiding and determine frequency and timing of dribbling or voiding.

Promote fluid intake of 2,000 to 3,000 mL/day within cardiac tolerance; include fruit juices, especially cranberry juice. Schedule fluid intake times appropriately.

Institute bladder program, including scheduled voiding times and Kegel's exercises, involving client and staff in a positive manner.

This information is essential to plan for care and influences choice of individual interventions. Nocturia, frequency, and urgency are common because bladder capacity and/or tone are affected. Bladder pelvic muscles and sphincter tone may also be affected. *Note:* Urinary incontinence occurs more frequently in older adults but is not considered a normal part of aging (Dowling-Castronovo & Bradway, 2008).

Bladder distention indicates urinary retention, which may cause incontinence and infection.

Maintains adequate hydration and promotes kidney function (Dowling-Castronovo & Bradway, 2008). Acid-ash juices act as an internal pH acidifier, retarding bacterial growth. *Note:* Client may decrease fluid intake in an attempt to control incontinence and become dehydrated. Instead, fluids may be scheduled to decrease frequency of incontinence, such as limiting fluids after 6 p.m. to reduce need to void during the night.

Regular toileting times may help control incontinence. Program is more apt to be successful when positive attitudes and cooperation are present.

ACTIONS/INTERVENTIONS (continued)

Assist client to sit upright on bedside commode, or bedpan, if not able to use toilet.

Provide, or encourage, perineal care daily and as needed.

Use adult incontinence pads or pants during day if needed based on individual type and amount of incontinence. Keep client clean and dry. Provide frequent skin care.

Avoid verbal or nonverbal signs of rejection, disgust, or disapproval over failures.

Provide regular catheter care with soap and water, and maintain patency if indwelling catheter is present.

Collaborative

Administer medications as indicated, such as the following:
  Oxybutynin chloride (Ditropan) and tolterodine tartrate (Detrol)
  Vitamin C and methenamine mandelate (Mandelamine)

Maintain condom or indwelling catheter, or provide intermittent catheterization, if needed, using aseptic technique.

Irrigate catheter with acetic acid, if indicated.

RATIONALE (continued)

Provides functional position for voiding.

Reduces risk of contamination and ascending infection.

When training is unsuccessful, this is the preferred method of management (Dowling-Castronovo & Bradway, 2008). *Note:* Avoiding use of incontinence pads during night exposes skin to air, reducing risk of irritation.

Expressions of disapproval lower self-esteem and are not helpful to a successful program.

Prevents infection and/or minimizes reflux (Cravens & Zweig, 2000; Wong & Hooton, 2005).

Promotes bladder sphincter control.

Bladder pH acidifiers retard bacterial growth (Cravens & Zweig, 2000).

May be used if continence cannot be maintained to prevent skin breakdown and resultant problems (Wong & Hooton, 2005). *Note:* A single catheter insertion may lead to bacteriuria in up to 20% of elderly clients, and "chronic indwelling catheterization is not a substitute for good nursing care in the management of incontinence" (Cravens & Zweig, 2000).

May be done to maintain acid pH and retard bacterial growth.

NURSING DIAGNOSIS: risk for Constipation/Diarrhea

Risk factors may include

Changes in, or inadequate, nutrition or fluid intake, poor muscle tone, change in level of activity

Medication side effects

Perceptual or cognitive impairment, depression

Lack of privacy

Possibly evidenced by

(Not applicable; presence of signs and symptoms establishes an *actual* diagnosis)

Desired Outcomes/Evaluation Criteria—Client Will

Bowel Elimination (NOC)

Establish or maintain normal pattern of bowel functioning.

Demonstrate changes in lifestyle as necessitated by risk or contributing factors.

Participate in bowel program as able.

ACTIONS/INTERVENTIONS

Bowel Management (NIC)

Independent

Ascertain usual bowel pattern and aids used, including previous long-term laxative use. Compare with current routine.

Assess reasons for problems, rule out medical causes such as hemorrhoids, drug effect, impaction, bowel obstruction, and cancer.

Determine presence of food and/or drug sensitivities.

Institute individualized program of exercise, rest, diet, and bowel retraining.

Provide diet high in bulk in the form of whole-grain cereals, breads, and fresh fruits—especially prunes and plums.

Decrease or eliminate foods such as dairy products.

Encourage increased fluid intake.

Use adult incontinence pads or pants, if needed. Keep client clean and dry. Provide frequent perineal care. Apply skin protective ointment to anal area.

Keep air freshener in room, at bedside, or in bathroom, as needed.

RATIONALE

Determines extent of problem and indicates type of interventions required. Many clients may already be laxative-dependent, and it is important to reestablish as near-normal functioning as possible.

Identification and treatment of underlying medical condition is necessary to achieve optimal bowel function.

May contribute to diarrhea.

Depends on the needs of the client. Loss of muscular tone reduces peristalsis or may impair control of rectal sphincter.

Improves stool consistency and promotes evacuation.

These foods are known to cause constipation.

Promotes normal stool consistency.

Prevents skin breakdown.

Limits noxious odors and may help reduce client embarrassment and concern.

(continues on page 816)

ACTIONS/INTERVENTIONS (continued)

Give emotional support to client. Avoid "blaming" talk or actions if incontinence occurs.

Collaborative

Administer medications, as indicated, for example:
Bulk-providers and stool softeners such as Metamucil

Camphorated tincture of opium (Paregoric) and diphenoxylate with atropine (Lomotil)

RATIONALE (continued)

Decreases feelings of frustration and embarrassment that can diminish self-esteem.

Promotes regularity by increasing bulk and/or improving stool consistency.
May be needed on a short-term basis when diarrhea persists.

NURSING DIAGNOSIS: impaired physical Mobility/risk for Falls

May be related to
Decreased strength and endurance, neuromuscular impairment
Pain or discomfort
Perceptual or cognitive impairment

Possibly evidenced by
Impaired coordination; limited ROM; decreased muscle mass, strength, control
Reluctance to attempt movement, inability to purposefully move

Desired Outcomes/Evaluation Criteria—Client Will

Mobility (NOC)
Maintain or increase strength and function of affected body parts.
Verbalize willingness to, and participate in, desired activities.
Demonstrate techniques or behaviors that enable continuation or resumption of activities.

ACTIONS/INTERVENTIONS

Environmental Management (NIC)
Independent
Determine functional ability using a scale of 0 to 4 and reasons for impairment.
Note emotional and behavioral responses to altered ability.

Plan activities and visits with adequate rest periods as necessary.

Encourage participation in self-care, occupational, or recreational activities.
Provide chairs with firm, high seats and lifting chairs, when indicated.

Fall Prevention (NIC)
Perform initial and ongoing fall-risk assessment, including fall history, gait and balance assessment, cognition, use of mobility adjuncts, and environmental conditions.

Assist with transfers and ambulation if indicated; show client and SO ways to move safely.

Obtain supportive shoes and well-fitting, nonskid slippers.

Remove clutter, wires or cords, scatter rugs, and extraneous furniture from pathways. Keep floors dry.
Encourage use of hand rails in hallway, stairwells, and bathrooms. Keep bed height in low position.
Review safe use of mobility aids and adjunctive devices such as walker, braces, and prosthetics.
Provide for environmental changes to meet visual deficiencies:

Keep areas well lighted. Accompany and keep close to client when in unfamiliar areas.

RATIONALE

Identifies need for and degree of intervention required.

Physical changes and loss of independence often create feelings of anxiety, anger, frustration, and depression that may be manifested as reluctance to engage in activity.
Can limit or prevent fatigue; conserve energy for continued participation.
Promotes independence and self-esteem; may enhance willingness to participate.
Facilitates rising from seated position.

Information can help determine client's potential for falling and identify which risk factors can be modified such as medications, uncorrected sensory impairments, or poorly fitting shoes.
Prevents accidental falls and injury, especially in the client with altered gait, generalized weakness, orthostatic hypotension, fatigue, and vision disturbances.
Assists client to walk with a firm step, maintains sense of balance and prevents slipping.
Reduces risk of falling and injuring self.

Promotes independence in mobility; reduces risk of falls.

Facilitates activity and reduces risk of injury.

Prevents accidents and reduces sense of sensory deprivation. If client is visually impaired, may need assistance and ongoing orientation to surroundings.
Provides for safety and psychological comfort.

ACTIONS/INTERVENTIONS (continued)

Avoid use of physical restraints.

Speak to client when entering the room, and let client know when leaving.

Encourage client with glasses or contacts to wear them. Be sure glasses are kept clean. Determine reason if glasses are not being worn.

Collaborative

Arrange for regular eye examinations.

Consult with physical and occupational therapists and rehabilitation specialist.

RATIONALE (continued)

Studies show that older adults who are restrained, particularly when visually or cognitively impaired, are more likely to experience a fall than those who are not restrained.

Special actions help client who cannot see to know when someone is there.

Optimal visual acuity facilitates participation in activities and reduces risk of falls and injury. Client may not be wearing glasses because they need adjustment or change in correction.

Identifies development or progression of vision problem such as myopia, hyperopia, presbyopia, astigmatism, cataract, glaucoma, tunnel vision, loss of peripheral fields, and blindness; and specific options for care.

Useful in creating individual exercise and activity program and identifying adjunctive aids. *Note:* Even in the elderly population, inclusion of moderate weight-lifting in the exercise program can improve and maintain the cardiovascular system; decrease obesity and blood pressure; and improve bone density, balance, and muscle tone and strength.

NURSING DIAGNOSIS: deficient Diversional Activity

May be related to
Environmental lack of diversional activity, long-term care requirements
Physical limitations
Depression, cognitive impairment

Possibly evidenced by
Statements of boredom, depression, lack of energy
Disinterest, lethargy, withdrawn behavior, hostility

Desired Outcomes/Evaluation Criteria—Client Will

Leisure Participation (NOC)
Recognize own response and initiate appropriate coping actions.
Engage in satisfying activities within personal limitations.

ACTIONS/INTERVENTIONS

Activity Therapy (NIC)
Independent
Determine avocation and hobbies client previously pursued. Incorporate activities, if appropriate, into present program.

Encourage participation in mix of activities and stimuli, such as music, news program, educational presentations, crafts, and social interactions, as appropriate.

Provide change of scenery when possible, alter personal environment, encourage trips to shop, or participate in local and family events.

Collaborative
Refer to occupational therapist or activity director.

RATIONALE

Encourages involvement and helps to stimulate client mentally and physically to improve overall condition and sense of well-being.

Offering different activities helps client to try out new ideas and develop new interests. Activities need to be personally meaningful for the client to derive the most enjoyment from them such as talking or Braille books for the blind and closed-caption TV broadcasts for the deaf or hearing impaired.

Stimulates energy and provides new outlook for client.

Can introduce and design new programs to provide positive stimuli for the client.

NURSING DIAGNOSIS: risk for Sexual Dysfunction

Risk factors may include
Biopsychosocial alteration of sexuality
Interference in psychological and physical well-being, self-image
Lack of privacy and/or SO

Possibly evidenced by
(Not applicable; presence of signs and symptoms establishes an *actual* diagnosis)

Desired Outcomes/Evaluation Criteria—Client Will

Role Performance (NOC)
Verbalize knowledge and understanding of sexual limitations, difficulties, or changes that have occurred.
Demonstrate improved communication and relationship skills.
Identify appropriate options to meet needs.

ACTIONS/INTERVENTIONS	RATIONALE
Sexual Counseling (NIC)	
Independent	
Note client's and SO's cues regarding sexuality.	May be concerned that condition or environmental restrictions may interfere with sexual function or ability, but is afraid to ask directly.
Determine cultural and religious values and conflicts or other factors that may be present.	Affects client's perception of existing problems and response of others—family, staff, and other residents. Provides starting point for discussion and problem solving.
Assess developmental and lifestyle issues.	Factors such as menopause and aging, adolescence, and young adulthood need to be taken into consideration with regard to sexual concerns about illness and long-term care.
Provide atmosphere in which discussion of sexuality is permitted and encouraged.	When concerns are identified and discussed, problem-solving can begin.
Provide privacy for client and SO.	Demonstrates acceptance of need for intimacy and provides opportunity to continue previous patterns of interaction as much as possible.
Collaborative	
Refer to sex counselor or therapist and family therapy when indicated.	May require additional assistance for resolution of problems.

NURSING DIAGNOSIS: ineffective Health Maintenance

May be related to
Lack of, or significant alteration in, communication skills
Complete or partial lack of gross and/or fine motor skills
Perceptual or cognitive impairment, lack of ability to make deliberate and thoughtful judgments
Lack of material resources

Possibly evidenced by
Demonstrated lack of knowledge regarding basic health practices
Reported or observed inability to take responsibility for meeting basic health needs, impairment of personal support system
Demonstrated lack of behaviors adaptive to internal or external environmental changes

Desired Outcomes/Evaluation Criteria—Client/Caregiver Will

Participation: Health Care Decisions (NOC)
Verbalize understanding of factors contributing to current situation.
Adopt lifestyle changes supporting individual healthcare goals.
Assume responsibility for own healthcare needs when possible.

ACTIONS/INTERVENTIONS	RATIONALE
Health Education (NIC)	
Independent	
Assess level of adaptive behavior, knowledge, and skills about health maintenance, environment, and safety.	Identifies areas of concern or need and aids in choice of interventions.
Provide information about individual healthcare needs.	Provides knowledge base and encourages participation in decision making.

ACTIONS/INTERVENTIONS (continued)

Develop plan with client and SO for self-care incorporating existing disabilities and adapting and organizing care.

Maintain adequate hydration and balanced diet with sufficient protein intake.

Schedule adequate rest with progressive activity program.

Promote good hand washing and personal hygiene. Use aseptic techniques as necessary.

Protect from exposure to infections and avoid extremes of temperature. Recommend the wearing of masks, monitor staff and visitors, and provide other interventions, as indicated.

Encourage cessation of smoking.

Encourage reporting of signs and symptoms as they occur.

Health System Guidance (NIC)

Note client's previous use of professional services, and continue as appropriate. Include in choice of new healthcare providers as able.

Observe for and monitor changes in vital signs such as temperature elevation.

Collaborative

Identify resources for, or administer medications, as indicated, for example:

   Immunizations, such as *Haemophilus influenzae* (flu) and pneumonia

   Antibiotics

Schedule preventive and routine healthcare appointments based on individual needs with cardiologist, podiatrist, ophthalmologist, or dentist.

Refer to support services as indicated, such as home healthcare agency, durable medical equipment company, Senior Resources, social services, national hospice organization, Alzheimer's Disease and Related Disorders Association, American Association of Retired Persons (AARP), Center for Health Care Ethics, Choice in Dying, American Bar Association, Commission on Legal Problems of the Elderly, Internet resources, and Adult Protective Services.

RATIONALE (continued)

Assists client and caregiver to maintain and manage desired level of independence when possible.

Promotes general well-being and aids in disease prevention.

Prevents fatigue and enhances general well-being.

Prevents contamination or cross-contamination, reducing risk of illness or infection.

With age, immune protective responses slow down and physiological reactions to temperature extremes may be impaired. As organ function decreases, especially the thymus gland, and natural antibodies decline, clients are at increased risk for infection. Staff and/or visitors with colds or other infections may expose client to these illnesses. *Note:* Nursing home acquired pneumonia (NHAP) is a common cause of infection in chronic care facilities and is a significant cause of mortality (Cunha, 2008).

Smokers are prone to bronchitis and ineffective clearing of secretions.

Provides opportunity for early recognition of developing complications and timely intervention to prevent serious illness.

Preserves continuity and promotes independence in meeting own healthcare needs.

Early identification of onset of illness allows for timely intervention and may prevent serious complications. *Note:* Elderly persons often display subnormal temperatures, so presence of a low-grade fever may be of serious concern.

Reduces risk of acquiring contagious, potentially life-threatening diseases.

May be used prophylactically, depending on individual disease process or risk factors, and to treat infections.

Promotes optimal recovery and maintenance of health.

Many community resources are available, and often untapped, to make life and care of the individual easier.

POTENTIAL CONSIDERATIONS following discharge from care facility.
Refer to plan of care for diagnosis that required admission.

ALCOHOL: ACUTE WITHDRAWAL

I. Pathophysiology (McKeown & West, 2008)

  a. Alcohol intoxication and withdrawal—complex mechanism

  b. Most clinical effects explained by the interaction of ethanol with various neurotransmitters and neuroreceptors in the brain

  c. Resulting changes in the inhibitory and excitatory neurotransmitters disrupt the neurochemical balance in the brain, causing symptoms of withdrawal.

II. Stages of Withdrawal (Al-Sanouri et al, 2005; Gossman, 2007; McKeown & West, 2008)

  a. Stage I: autonomic hyperactivity

  b. Stage II: hallucinations

  c. Stage III: neuronal excitation

  d. Stage IV: delirium tremens (DTs)

(text continues on page 820)

III. Etiology

a. Individual's desire to repeatedly reach a state of feeling high; numb negative feelings

b. Associated with serious mental health disorders—anxiety, mood disorders, or major depression

c. Personality traits—dependency more common in isolation, loneliness, shyness, depression, dependency, hostile and self-destructive impulsivity, and sexual immaturity

d. Environment—frequently come from a broken home and have a disturbed relationship with their parents

e. Genetics—incidence of alcoholism is higher in biological children of alcoholics, and some people who become alcoholics are less easily intoxicated having a higher threshold for central nervous system (CNS) effects

IV. Statistics

a. Morbidity: The lifetime prevalance of combined alchohol abuse and dependence is approximately 15% (Merck Manuals, 2005); more than 15 million American adults are dependent on alcohol; in 2005, 1.2 million hospital admissions in the United States for problems related to alcohol abuse; (McKeown, 2008); approximately 5% of individuals who have alcohol withdrawal progress to DTs (Gossman, 2007).

b. Mortality: There are more than 100,000 deaths related to health consequences of alcohol abuse annually (Myrick, 2006); dependent on comorbidities, including traumatic injuries (McKeown & West, 2008); with untreated DTs, rate is at 35%, which decreases to less than 5% with early recognition and treatment (Gossman, 2007).

c. Cost: In 2000, there was $185 billion in economic costs related to alcohol abuse in the United States (Myrick, 2006); in 2005, costs are estimated at over $229 billion.

GLOSSARY

Addiction: Dependence on a substance (such as alcohol or other drugs) or an activity, to the point that stopping is very difficult and causes severe physical and mental reactions

Alcohol withdrawal syndrome (AWS): The neurological, psychiatric, and cardiovascular signs and symptoms that result when a person accustomed to consuming large quantities of alcohol suddenly becomes abstinent.

Arcus senilis: White or gray ring-like opacity of the cornea.

Ataxia: Gross incoordination of voluntary muscle movement, reflecting loss of proprioception in chronic alcohol abuse.

Autonomic hyperactivity stage: Usually occurs within 24 hours of the last drink. Symptoms may be mild, characterized by tremulousness, insomnia, anxiety, diaphoresis, mild tachycardia, and gastrointestinal (GI) upset.

Binge: Uninterrupted consumption of a drug for several hours or days.

Blackout: Amnesia for events occurring during the period of alcoholic intoxication, even though consciousness is still maintained during that time.

Delirium tremens (DTs): Potentially fatal form of alcohol withdrawal characterized by disorientation, confusion, impaired attention, pronounced autonomic hyperactivity, and visual and auditory hallucinations. Usually begins at 48 to 72 hours, but can be delayed up to 4 to 5 days. Death is usually due to cardiovascular or respiratory collapse.

Detoxification: Process of removing alcohol or other drugs from the body. This is the initial period addicts must go through to become drug-free. Withdrawal symptoms appear early during this process. Depending on the drug, detoxification lasts for a few days to a week or more.

Gluconeogenesis: Conversion of glycogen to glucose in the liver.

Hallucination stage: Development of false visual (most common), olfactory, or auditory perceptions that have no relation to reality, usually occurring 24 to 36 hours after the cessation of alcohol intake.

Hepatic encephalopathy: Condition used to describe the deleterious effects of liver failure on the central nervous system (CNS). Features include confusion ranging to coma, with alcoholic cirrhosis being the most common cause.

Myelosuppression: Decrease in the production by the bone marrow of red blood cells (RBCs), platelets, and some white blood cells (WBCs).

Neuronal excitation stage: Development of autonomic hyperactivity or seizures occurring within 48 hours after cessation of alcohol consumption.

Nystagmus: An unintentional jittery movement of the eyes. Nystagmus usually involves both eyes and is often exaggerated by looking in a particular direction.

Thrombocytopenia: Low platelet count, which can lead to impaired blood clotting and spontaneous bleeding.

Wernicke's syndrome or Wernicke encephalopathy: Neurological disease characterized by the clinical triad of confusion, inability to coordinate voluntary movement, and eye abnormalities.

Care setting

Client may be inpatient on a behavioral unit, at a substance abuse rehabiltation facility, or outpatient in community programs. Although clients are not generally admitted to the acute care setting with this diagnosis, withdrawal from alcohol may occur secondarily during hospitalization for other illnesses or conditions. A short hospital stay may be required during the acute phase because of severity of general condition or comorbidities, or a delayed discharge from acute care can be the result of alcohol withdrawal beginning within 6 to 48 hours of admission.

Related Concerns

Cirrhosis of the liver, page 445
Heart failure: chronic, page 48
Psychosocial aspects of care, page 749
Substance dependence/abuse rehabilitation, page 835
Upper gastrointestinal/esophageal bleeding, page 306

Client Assessment Database

Data depend on the duration and extent of use of alcohol, concurrent use of other drugs, degree of organ involvement, and presence of other pathology.

DIAGNOSTIC DIVISION MAY REPORT	MAY EXHIBIT
ACTIVITY/REST • Difficulty sleeping, not feeling well rested • Fatigue or weakness	• Abnormal heart rate or blood pressure (BP) in response to activity
CIRCULATION	• Tachycardia common during acute withdrawal • Numerous dysrhythmias may be identified, especially atrial fibrillation • Hypertension common in early withdrawal stage; may become labile or progress to hypotension • Peripheral pulses weak, irregular, or rapid
EGO INTEGRITY • Feelings of guilt, shame; defensiveness about drinking • Denial, rationalization • Multiple stressors or losses— relationships, employment, finances • Use of alcohol to deal with life stressors, boredom	• Anxiety, fear • Irrititability
ELIMINATION • Diarrhea	• Bowel sounds varied (may reflect gastric complications such as hemorrhage)
FOOD/FLUID • Nausea, vomiting; food intolerance	• Gastric distention, ascites, liver and spleen enlargement (seen in cirrhosis) • Muscle wasting; dry, dull hair; swollen salivary glands; inflamed buccal cavity; capillary fragility (malnutrition) • Bowel sounds varied (reflecting malnutrition, electrolyte imbalances, general bowel dysfunction)
NEUROSENSORY • "Internal shakes" • Headache, dizziness, blurred vision • Blackouts	• Psychopathology—paranoia, schizophrenia, major depression (may indicate dual diagnosis) • Level of consciousness (LOC) and orientation varied—confusion, stupor, hyperactivity, distorted thought processes, slurred, incoherent speech • Memory loss, confabulation

(continues on page 822)

DIAGNOSTIC DIVISION MAY REPORT (continued)	MAY EXHIBIT (continued)

	• Affect/mood/behavior—fearful, anxious, easily startled, inappropriate, silly, euphoric, irritable, physically or verbally abusive, depressed, and/or paranoid
	• Hallucinations may be visual, tactile, olfactory, or auditory; for example, client may be picking items out of the air or responding verbally to unseen person or voices
	• *Eye examination:*
	  • Nystagmus—associated with cranial nerve palsy
	  • Pupil constriction (may indicate CNS depression)
	  • Arcus senilis (normal in aging populations, suggests alcohol-related changes in younger individuals)
	• Fine-motor tremors of face, tongue, and hands
	• Seizure—grand mal or partial that is usually brief, generalized, tonic-clonic in nature, and without an aura, occur in a cluster of 1 to 3 seizures with a short postictal period; in 30% to 50% of individuals, the seizures progress to DTs (McKeown & West, 2008)
	• Gait unsteady (ataxia), which may be due to thiamine deficiency or cerebellar degeneration associated with Wernicke's encephalopathy (Merck Manuals, 2005)

PAIN/DISCOMFORT • Constant upper abdominal pain and tenderness radiating to the back (pancreatic inflammation) • Headache (may be "pulsating")	• Guarding affected area • Narrowed focus
RESPIRATION • History of smoking • Chronic respiratory problems	• Tachypnea, hperventilation • Breath sounds diminished, adventitious sounds (suggests pulmonary complications such as respiratory depression or pneumonia)
SAFETY • History of recurrent trauma—falls, fractures, lacerations, burns, or motor vehicle crashes • Violence toward self or others	• Skin—flushed face and palms of hands; scars, ecchymotic areas; fissures at corners of mouth (vitamin deficiency) • Fractures healed or new—signs of recent or recurrent trauma • Temperature elevation, flushing, diaphoresis • Suicidal ideation, suicide attempts—approximately 7% of individuals with alcohol dependence commit suicide (American Foundation for Suicide Prevention [AFSP], 2008)
SEXUALITY • Loss of sexual desire • Not achieving sexual satisfaction, or needing alcohol for satisfying sex • Actual or perceived limitation imposed by disease	• Alteration in relationship with partner
SOCIAL INTERACTION • Frequent sick days off from work or school, fighting with others, arrests for disorderly conduct, or motor vehicle violations such as driving under the influence (DUI) • Denial that alcohol intake has any significant effect on present condition • Dysfunctional family system of origin (generational involvement), problems in current relationships, often alienated from family when problem is chronic • Mood changes affecting interactions with others	• Speech unintelligible or slurred • Family interactions and communications strained and difficult

Client Assessment Database (continued)

DIAGNOSTIC DIVISION MAY REPORT (continued)	MAY EXHIBIT (continued)

TEACHING/LEARNING
- Family history of alcoholism
- History of alcohol and/or other drug use or abuse, tobacco use
- Ignorance and/or denial of addiction to alcohol, or inability to cut down or stop drinking despite repeated efforts, previous periods of abstinence or withdrawal
- History of daily alcohol use for at least 3 months.
- Large amount of alcohol consumed in last 24 to 48 hours ("bingeing")
- Previous hospitalizations for alcoholism or alcohol-related diseases such as cirrhosis and esophageal varices

DISCHARGE PLAN CONSIDERATIONS
- May require assistance to maintain abstinence and begin to participate in rehabilitation program

▸ Refer to section at end of plan for postdischarge considerations.

Diagnostic Studies

TEST WHY IT IS DONE	WHAT IT TELLS ME

BLOOD TESTS
- *Blood alcohol level (BAL):* Measures level of alcohol in the blood.

BAL may or may not be severely elevated, depending on amount consumed, time between consumption and testing, and the degree of tolerance, which varies widely. In the absence of elevated alcohol tolerance, blood levels of 100 mg/dL are associated with loss of control of fine motor movements and confusion when faced with tasks requiring thinking; at 200 mg/dL, very slurred speech, ataxia, and lethargy; at 400 mg/dL, coma and respiratory depression; at 500 mg/dL, death is possible due to respiratory arrest, severe hypotension, and aspiration (Cohen, 2006).

- *Complete blood count (CBC):* Battery of screening tests, which typically includes hemoglobin (Hgb); hematocrit (Hct); RBC count, morphology, indices, and distribution width index; platelet count and size; WBC count and differential.

Blood loss from the GI tract and nutritional deficiencies producing anemia are common in alcohol withdrawal. In addition, alcohol ingestion leads to myelosuppression with a slight reduction in all cell lines. Thrombocytopenia is common. Increased mean corpuscular volume (MCV) suggests anemia based on deficiencies in vitamin B_{12} and folate. WBC count may be increased with infection or decreased if client is immunosuppressed.

- *Glucose and ketones:* Determines ability of liver to manage simple sugars and end-products of sugar metabolism.

Clients with liver disease due to alcoholism have reduced glycogen stores, and alcohol impairs gluconeogenesis. As a consequence, these clients are susceptible to hypoglycemia (McKeown & West, 2008). Ketoacidosis may be present with or without metabolic acidosis. Alcoholic ketoacidosis (AKA) can occur in chronic alcohol abuse with history of recent binge drinking, decreased food intake, and persistent vomiting (O'Brien et al, 2007).

(continues on page 824)

- *Electrolytes:* Substances that dissociate into ions in solution and acquire the capacity to conduct electricity. Common electrolytes include sodium, potassium, chloride, calcium, and phosphate.

Alcoholics with liver disease frequently have abnormal sodium serum concentrations, with hyponatremia (low plasma sodium concentration) as the most common alteration. Decreased serum potassium concentration may be associated with respiratory alkalosis, elevated insulin levels, and elevated epinephrine levels resulting from alcohol withdrawal. Client with chronic alcoholism usually has dietary magnesium deficiency and possibly concurrent alcoholic hepatitis. Alcoholic pancreatitis may cause hypocalcemia.

- *Liver function tests—lactate dehydrogenase (LDH), alanine aminotransferase (ALT), lipase, and amylase:* Determine level of liver and pancreatic dysfunction.

May be elevated, reflecting liver or pancreatic damage.

- *Blood ammonia:* Helps evaluate the cause of the change in consciousness.

Level is elevated if hepatic encephalopathy is present.

- *Nutritional tests—albumin or prealbumin, total protein, carbohydrate-deficient transferrin (CDT), iron, vitamins D and B_{12}, and folate:* Evaluates nutritional status, identifies deficiencies and treatment needs.

Albumin and total protein may be decreased. CDT, a protein molecule involved in iron transport, is a relatively new test that is sometimes used to help identify chronic, heavy drinking. Vitamin deficiencies are usually present, reflecting malnutrition or malabsorption.

OTHER DIAGNOSTIC STUDIES

- *Urinalysis:* Detects and measures various compounds that pass through the urine.

Increased WBCs and/or protein may indicate infection; ketones may be present related to breakdown of fatty acids in malnutrition (pseudodiabetic condition).

- *Chest x-ray:* Procedure used to evaluate organs and structures within the chest for symptoms of disease.

May reveal right lower lobe pneumonia, a common manifestation which may be related to malnutrition, depressed immune system, and aspiration. X-ray may also reveal evidence of chronic lung disorders associated with heavy tobacco use, also common in alcoholics.

- *Electrocardiogram (ECG):* Record of the electrical activity of the heart.

Dysrhythmias, cardiomyopathies, and/or ischemia may be present because of direct effect of alcohol on the cardiac muscle and/or conduction system, as well as effects of electrolyte imbalance. The adrenergic storm produced by alcohol withdrawal increases cardiac demand, which may precipitate infarction in susceptible individuals. Atrial fibrillation is the most common cardiac symptom seen in the alcoholic (Gossman, 2007).

- *Computed tomography (CT) scan of the head:* X-ray procedure that uses a computer to produce a detailed picture of a cross-section of the body.

May be obtained in clients with depressed LOC, in those with multiple seizures or signs of head trauma, and in those with failure to respond to treatment. *Note:* Client with AWS is at risk for intracranial bleeding because of frequent falls, cortical atrophy, and coagulopathy.

- *Clinical Institute Withdrawal Assessment (CIWA):* Clinical rating tool that provides a numerical rating for 10 factors, including nausea and vomiting, tactile disturbances, tremor, auditory and visual disturbances, sweating, anxiety, headache agitation, and orientation (Jennings-Ingle, 2007).

Provides a clinical quantification of the severity of the alcohol withdrawal syndrome and can be rapidly administered at the bedside. Scores of 9 to 15 points correspond with moderate withdrawal, and scores greater than 15 correspond to severe withdrawal symptoms and increased risk of DTs and seizures.

- *Addiction severity index (ASI):* A 161-item multidimensional clinical and research tool that produces a "problem severity profile" of the client, including chemical, medical, psychological, legal, family and social, and employment and support aspects, indicating areas of treatment needs.

Provides basic diagnostic information on a client prior to, during, and after treatment for substance use-related problems as well as for the assessment of change in client status and treatment outcome.

Nursing Priorities

1. Maintain physiological stability during acute withdrawal phase.
2. Promote client safety.
3. Provide appropriate referral and follow-up.
4. Encourage and support significant other (SO) involvement in "intervention" or confrontation process.
5. Provide information about condition, prognosis, and treatment needs.

Discharge Goals

1. Homeostasis achieved.
2. Complications prevented or resolved.
3. Sobriety maintained on a day-to-day basis.
4. Ongoing participation in rehabilitation program or group therapy, such as Alcoholics Anonymous.
5. Condition, prognosis, and therapeutic regimen understood.
6. Plan in place to meet needs after discharge.

This plan of care is to be used in conjunction with CP: Substance Dependence/Abuse Rehabilitation.

NURSING DIAGNOSIS: risk for ineffective Breathing Pattern

Risk factors may include
Direct effect of alcohol toxicity on respiratory center and/or sedative drugs given to decrease alcohol withdrawal symptoms
Tracheobronchial obstruction
Presence of chronic respiratory problems, inflammatory process
Decreased energy, fatigue

Possibly evidenced by
(Not applicable; presence of signs and symptoms establishes an *actual* diagnosis)

Desired Outcomes/Evaluation Criteria—Client Will

Respiratory Status: Ventilation (NOC)
Maintain effective breathing pattern with respiratory rate within normal range, lungs clear, and free of cyanosis or other signs and symptoms of hypoxia.

ACTIONS/INTERVENTIONS	RATIONALE
Respiratory Monitoring (NIC)	
Independent	
Monitor respiratory rate, depth, and pattern as indicated. Note periods of apnea and Cheyne-Stokes respirations.	Frequent assessment is important because toxicity levels may change rapidly. Hyperventilation is common during acute withdrawal phase. Kussmaul's respirations are sometimes present because of acidotic state associated with vomiting and malnutrition. However, marked respiratory depression can occur because of CNS depressant effects of alcohol if acute intoxication is present. This may be compounded by drugs used to control AWS.
Auscultate breath sounds. Note presence of adventitious sounds such as rhonchi, wheezes.	Client is at risk for atelectasis related to hypoventilation and pneumonia.
Airway Management (NIC)	
Elevate head of bed.	Decreases potential for aspiration; lowers diaphragm, enhancing lung inflation.
Encourage coughing, deep-breathing exercises, and frequent position changes.	Facilitates lung expansion and mobilization of secretions to reduce complications from atelectasis or pneumonia.
Have suction equipment and airway adjuncts available.	Sedative effects of alcohol potentiates risk of aspiration, relaxation of oropharyngeal muscles, and respiratory depression, requiring intervention to prevent respiratory arrest.
Collaborative	
Administer supplemental oxygen, if necessary.	Hypoxia may occur with respiratory depression and chronic anemia.
Review serial chest x-rays, arterial blood gases (ABGs), or pulse oximetry, as indicated.	Monitors presence of secondary complications, evaluates effectiveness of respiratory effort, and identifies therapy needs. *Note:* Right lower lobe pneumonia is common in alcohol-debilitated clients and is often due to chronic aspiration. Chronic lung diseases, such as emphysema or bronchitis, are also common.

NURSING DIAGNOSIS: risk for decreased Cardiac Output

Risk factors may include
Direct effect of alcohol on the heart muscle
Altered systemic vascular resistance
Electrical alterations in rate, rhythm, conduction

Possibly evidenced by
(Not applicable; presence of signs and symptoms establishes an *actual* diagnosis)

Desired Outcomes/Evaluation Criteria—Client Will

Circulation Status (NOC)
Display vital signs within client's normal range; absence, or reduced frequency, of dysrhythmias.
Demonstrate an increase in activity tolerance.

ACTIONS/INTERVENTIONS	RATIONALE
Hemodynamic Regulation (NIC)	
Independent	
Monitor vital signs frequently during acute withdrawal.	Hypertension frequently occurs in acute withdrawal phase. Extreme hyperexcitability, accompanied by catecholamine release and increased peripheral vascular resistance, raises BP and heart rate; however, BP may become labile and progress to hypotension. *Note:* Client may have underlying cardiovascular disease, which is compounded by alcohol withdrawal.
Monitor cardiac rate and rhythm. Document irregularities and dysrhythmias.	Long-term alcohol abuse may result in cardiomyopathy and heart failure (HF). Tachycardia is common because of sympathetic response to increased circulating catecholamines. Dysrhythmias may develop with electrolyte imbalance. All of these may have an adverse effect on cardiac output.
Monitor body temperature.	Elevation may occur because of sympathetic stimulation, dehydration, and/or infections, causing vasodilation and compromising venous return and cardiac output.
Monitor intake and output (I&O). Note 24-hour fluid balance.	Preexisting dehydration, vomiting, fever, and diaphoresis may result in decreased circulating volume that can compromise cardiovascular function. *Note:* Hydration is difficult to assess in the alcoholic client because the usual indicators are not reliable, and overhydration is a risk in the presence of compromised cardiac function.
Be prepared for and assist in cardiopulmonary resuscitation.	Causes of death during acute withdrawal stages include cardiac dysrhythmias, respiratory depression and arrest, oversedation, excessive psychomotor activity, severe dehydration or overhydration, and massive infections. Mortality for unrecognized or untreated DTs may be as high as 35% (Gossman, 2007).
Collaborative	
Monitor laboratory studies, such as serum electrolyte levels, RBCs, Hgb and Hct, and platelets.	Potassium and magnesium imbalances potentiate risk of cardiac dysrhythmias. Anemia may be present and platelets can be decreased in late stage alcoholism due to liver dysfunction.
Administer fluids and electrolytes, as indicated.	Severe alcohol withdrawal causes the client to be susceptible to excessive fluid losses associated with fever, diaphoresis, and vomiting; electrolyte imbalances, especially potassium and magnesium; and glucose.
Administer medications, as indicated, for example: Clonidine (Catapres) or atenolol (Tenormin)	Although the use of benzodiazepines is often sufficient to control hypertension during initial withdrawal from alcohol, some clients may require more specific therapy. *Note:* Atenolol and other beta-adrenergic blockers may speed up the withdrawal process and eliminate tremors as well as lower the heart rate, BP, and body temperature.
Potassium	Corrects deficits that can result in life-threatening dysrhythmias.

NURSING DIAGNOSIS: **risk for Injury, [specify]**

Risk factors may include
Cessation of alcohol intake with varied autonomic nervous system responses to the system's suddenly altered state
Involuntary clonic, tonic muscle activity (seizures)
Equilibrium and balancing difficulties, reduced muscle and hand–eye coordination

Possibly evidenced by
(Not applicable; presence of signs and symptoms establishes an *actual* diagnosis.)

Desired Outcomes/Evaluation Criteria—Client Will

Risk Control (NOC)
Demonstrate absence of untoward effects of withdrawal.
Experience no physical injury.

ACTIONS/INTERVENTIONS	RATIONALE
Substance Use Treatment: Alcohol Withdrawal (NIC)	
Independent	
Identify stage of AWS using CIWA. Stage I is associated with signs and symptoms of hyperactivity, such as tremors, sleeplessness, nausea, vomiting, diaphoresis, tachycardia, and hypertension; stage II is manifested by increased hyperactivity plus hallucinations and/or seizure activity; stage III symptoms include DTs and extreme autonomic hyperactivity with profound confusion, anxiety, insomnia, and fever.	AWS usually begins 3 to 36 hours after the last drink. Prompt recognition and intervention may halt progression of symptoms and enhance recovery, improving prognosis. In addition, progression of symptoms indicates need for changes in drug therapy and more intense treatment to prevent death. DTs may not present until 2 to 3 days after last alcohol intake, usually lasting 1 to 5 days.
Monitor and document seizure activity. Maintain patent airway. Provide environmental safety such as padded side rails and bed in low position.	Grand mal seizures are most common and may be related to decreased magnesium levels, hypoglycemia, elevated blood alcohol, or history of head trauma or preexisting seizure disorder. *Note:* In absence of history of seizures or other pathology causing them, they usually stop spontaneously or with magnesium replacement, which reduces CNS excitablilty (Gossman 2007).
Check deep-tendon reflexes. Assess gait, if possible. Palpate upper arm to discern actual withdrawal versus medication-seeking behavior.	Reflexes may be depressed, absent, or hyperactive. Peripheral neuropathies are common, especially in malnourished client. Ataxia is associated with Wernicke's syndrome (thiamine deficiency) and cerebellar degeneration. Three ways to assess whether the client is having actual withdrawal tremors are (1) have the client stick out his or her tongue—it will be tremulous; (2) feel the client's upper arm—withdrawal tremors can be felt bone deep; and (3) have the client visually track a pencil—there will be observable nystagmus.
Assist with ambulation and self-care activities, as needed.	Prevents falls with resultant injury.
Provide for environmental safety when indicated. (Refer to ND: disturbed Sensory Perception [specify], following.)	May be required when equilibrium and hand–eye coordination problems exist.
Collaborative	
Administer medications, as indicated, for example:	
Benzodiazepines (BZDs), such as chlordiazepoxide (Librium), diazepam (Valium), lorazepam (Ativan), oxazemapm (Serax), or clonidine (Catapess)	BZDs are commonly used to control neuronal hyperactivity because of their minimal respiratory and cardiac depression and anticonvulsant properties. Studies have also shown that these drugs can prevent progression to more severe states of withdrawal. Intravneous (IV) or oral (PO) administration is preferred route because intramuscular (IM) absorption is unpredictable. Muscle-relaxant qualities are particularly helpful to client in controlling "the shakes," trembling, and ataxic quality of movements.
Haloperidol (Haldol)	May be used in conjunction with BZDs for clients experiencing agitation and hallucinations, although should be used with caution as it can lower seizure threshold.
Thiamine	Thiamine deficiency may lead to neuritis, Wernecke's syndrome, and/or Korsakoff's psychosis.
Magnesium sulfate	Reduces tremors and seizure activity by decreasing neuromuscular excitability.

NURSING DIAGNOSIS: disturbed Sensory Perception [specify]

May be related to

Chemical alteration: exogenous—alcohol consumption, sudden cessation; endogenous—electrolyte imbalance, elevated ammonia and blood urea nitrogen (BUN)

Sleep deprivation

Psychological stress—anxiety, fear

Possibly evidenced by

Disorientation to time, place, person, or situation

Changes in usual response to stimuli; exaggerated emotional responses, change in behavior

Bizarre thinking

Listlessness, irritability, apprehension, activity associated with visual/auditory hallucinations

Fear and anxiety

Desired Outcomes/Evaluation Criteria—Client Will

Cognition (NOC)

Regain or maintain usual LOC.

Distorted Thought Self-Control (NOC)

Report absence of, or reduced, hallucinations.

Identify external factors that affect sensory-perceptual abilities.

ACTIONS/INTERVENTIONS	RATIONALE
Substance Use Treatment: Alcohol Withdrawal (NIC) *Independent* Assess LOC, ability to speak, and response to stimuli and commands.	Speech may be garbled, confused, or slurred. Response to commands may reveal inability to concentrate, impaired judgment, or muscle coordination deficits.
Observe for behavioral responses such as hyperactivity, disorientation, confusion, sleeplessness, and irritability.	Hyperactivity related to CNS disturbances may escalate rapidly. Sleeplessness is common due to loss of sedative effect gained from alcohol usually consumed before bedtime. Sleep deprivation may aggravate disorientation or confusion. Progression of symptoms may indicate impending hallucinations (stage II) or DTs (stage IV).
Note onset of hallucinations and document as auditory, visual, and/or tactile.	Auditory hallucinations are reported to be more frightening and threatening to client. Visual hallucinations occur more at night and often include insects, animals, or faces of friends or enemies. Clients are frequently observed "picking the air." Yelling may occur if client is calling for help from perceived threat which is usually seen in stage III of AWS.
Provide quiet environment. Speak in calm, quiet voice. Regulate lighting, as indicated. Turn off radio or TV during sleep.	Reduces external stimuli during hyperactive stage. Client may become more delirious when surroundings cannot be seen, but some respond better to quiet, darkened room.
Provide care by same personnel whenever possible.	Promotes recognition of caregivers and a sense of consistency, which may reduce fear.
Encourage SO to stay with client whenever possible.	May have a calming effect, and may provide a reorienting influence.
Reorient frequently to person, place, time, and surrounding environment, as indicated.	May reduce confusion; prevent or limit misinterpretation of external stimuli.
Avoid bedside discussion about client or topics unrelated to the client that do not include the client.	Client may hear and misinterpret conversation, which can aggravate hallucinations.
Provide environmental safety as indicated, for example, place bed in low position, leave doors in full open or closed position, observe frequently, place call light/bell within reach, and remove articles that can harm client.	Client may have distorted sense of reality or be fearful or suicidal, requiring protection from self.
Collaborative Provide seclusion and restraints as necessary, adhering to facility policy regarding restraints.	Clients with excessive psychomotor activity, severe hallucinations, violent behavior, and/or suicidal gestures may respond better to seclusion. Restraints are usually ineffective and add to client's agitation, but occasionally may be required to prevent self-harm.

ACTIONS/INTERVENTIONS (continued)

Monitor laboratory studies such as electrolytes, magnesium levels, liver function studies, ammonia, BUN, glucose, and ABGs.

Administer medications, as indicated, for example:
Anti-anxiety agents as indicated (Refer to ND: Anxiety [severe/panic]/Fear, following.)

Thiamine, vitamins C and B complex, multivitamins, and Stresstabs

RATIONALE (continued)

Changes in organ function may precipitate or potentiate sensory-perceptual deficits. Electrolyte imbalance is common. Liver function is often impaired in the chronic alcoholic, and ammonia intoxication can occur if the liver is unable to convert ammonia to urea. Ketoacidosis is sometimes present without glycosuria; however, hyperglycemia or hypoglycemia may occur, suggesting pancreatitis or impaired gluconeogenesis in the liver. Hypoxemia and hypercarbia are common manifestations in chronic alcoholics who are also heavy smokers.

Reduces hyperactivity, promoting relaxation and sleep. Drugs that have little effect on dreaming may be desired to allow dream recovery or rapid eye movement (REM) rebound to occur, which has previously been suppressed by alcohol use.

Vitamins may be depleted because of insufficient intake and malabsorption. Vitamin deficiency, especially thiamine, is associated with ataxia, loss of eye movement and pupillary response, palpitations, postural hypotension, and exertional dyspnea.

NURSING DIAGNOSIS: Anxiety [severe/panic]/Fear

May be related to
Cessation of alcohol intake, physiological withdrawal
Situational crisis—hospitalization
Threat to self-concept, perceived threat of death

Possibly evidenced by
Feelings of inadequacy, shame, self-disgust, and remorse
Increased helplessness, hopelessness with loss of control of own life
Increased tension, apprehension
Fear of unspecified consequences; identifies object of fear

Desired Outcomes/Evaluation Criteria—Client Will

Anxiety [or] Fear Self-Control (NOC)
Verbalize reduction of fear and anxiety to an acceptable and manageable level.
Express sense of regaining some control of situation and life.
Demonstrate problem-solving skills and use resources effectively.

ACTIONS/INTERVENTIONS

Anxiety Reduction (NIC)
Independent
Identify cause of anxiety, involving client in the process. Explain that alcohol withdrawal increases anxiety and uneasiness. Reassess level of anxiety on an ongoing basis.

Develop a trusting relationship through frequent contact and being honest and nonjudgmental. Project an accepting attitude about alcoholism.
Inform client about what you plan to do and why. Include client in planning process and provide choices when possible.

Reorient frequently. (Refer to ND: disturbed Sensory Perception.)

RATIONALE

Persons in acute phase of withdrawal may be unable to identify and/or accept what is happening. Anxiety may be physiologically or environmentally caused. *Note:* Individuals with alcohol use disorders often also have post-traumatic stress disorder (PTSD) (U.S. Department of Veterans Affairs, 2007).
Provides client with a sense of humanness, helping to decrease paranoia and distrust. Client will be able to detect biased or condescending attitude of caregivers.
Enhances sense of trust, and explanation may increase cooperation and reduce anxiety. Provides sense of control over self in circumstance where loss of control is a significant factor. *Note:* Feelings of self-worth are intensified when one is treated as a worthwhile person.
Client may experience periods of confusion, resulting in increased anxiety.

(continues on page 830)

ACTIONS/INTERVENTIONS (continued)

Collaborative

Administer medications, as indicated, for example:

    Benzodiazepines, such as chlordiazepoxide (Librium), and diazepam (Valium)

    Barbiturates, such as phenobarbital, or possibly secobarbital (Seconal) or pentobarbital (Nembutal)

Arrange "intervention" or confrontation in controlled setting, when client has recovered sufficiently from withdrawal to address addiction issues.

Provide consultation or referral to detoxification or crisis center for ongoing treatment program as soon as medically stable (e.g., oriented to reality).

RATIONALE (continued)

Anti-anxiety agents are given during acute withdrawal to help client relax, be less hyperactive, and feel more in control.

These drugs are sometimes used to treat or prevent alcohol withdrawal seizures, but need to be used with caution because they are respiratory depressants and REM sleep cycle inhibitors.

Process wherein SO and family members, supported by staff, provide information about how client's drinking and behavior have affected each one of them, helps client acknowledge that drinking is a problem and has resulted in current situational crisis.

Client is more likely to contract for treatment while still hurting and experiencing fear and anxiety from last drinking episode. Motivation decreases as well-being increases and person again feels able to control the problem. Direct contact with available treatment resources provides realistic picture of help. Decreases time for client to "think about it," change mind, or restructure and strengthen denial systems.

POTENTIAL CONSIDERATIONS following acute care (dependent on client's age, physical condition and presence of complications, personal resources, and life responsibilities)

Refer to: Substance Abuse/Rehabilitation plan of care, and plans of care for any specific underlying medical condition(s)

Sample clinical pathway follows in Table 15.1.

TABLE 15.1 Sample CP: Alcohol Withdrawal Program. ELOS: 5 Days Behavioral Unit

ND and Categories of Care	Time Dimension	Goals/Actions	Time Dimension	Goals/Actions	Time Dimension	Goals/Actions
Risk for injury R/T varied autonomic and sensory responses	Day 1	Verbalize understanding of safety concerns relative to individual needs Cooperate with therapeutic regimen	Day 3 Day 4	Vital signs stable I&O balanced Display marked decrease in objective symptoms	Day 5	Be free of injury resulting from ETOH withdrawal Display no objective symptoms of withdrawal
Referrals	Day 1	RN-NP or MD If indicated: Internist Cardiologist Neurologist				
Diagnostic studies	Day 1	BA level Drug screen If indicated: CXR Pulse oximetry ECG	Day 2 Serum Mg, amylase	CMP 20 RPR UA	Day 4	Repeat of selected studies as indicated
Additional assessments	Day 1	VS, temp, respiratory status/breath sounds q4h	Day 2–3	VS q8h if stable	Day 4–5	VS qd
	Day 1–4	I&O q8h				
	Ongoing	Motor activity, body language, verbalizations, need for/type of restraint Withdrawal symptoms:				
	Stage I	Tremors, N/V, hypertension, tachycardia, diaphoresis, sleeplessness				
	Stage II	Increased hyperactivity, hallucinations, seizure activity				
	Stage III	Extreme autonomic hyperactivity, profound confusion, anxiety, fever				
Medications Allergies: _____ _____	Day 1	Librium 200 mg PO	Day 3	Librium 120 mg PO	Day 5	Librium 40 mg PO

(continues on page 832)

TABLE 15.1 Sample CP: Alcohol Withdrawal Program. ELOS: 5 Days Behavioral Unit (continued)

ND and Categories of Care	Time Dimension	Goals/Actions	Time Dimension	Goals/Actions	Time Dimension	Goals/Actions
Client education	Day 1–4 Day 2 Day 1	Thiamine 100 mg IM Librium 160 mg PO Orient to room/unit, schedule, procedures	Day 4 Day 3–4	Librium 80 mg PO Need for ongoing therapy Goals/availability of AA program	Day 5	Schedule of follow-up visits if indicated
Additional nursing actions	Day 1 Day 1–2 Ongoing	Bedrest 12 hours if in withdrawal Position change, HOB elevated; C, DB exercises if on bedrest Assist with ambulation, self-care as needed Encourage fluids if free of N/V Provide environmental safety measures, seizure precautions as indicated Reorient as needed	Day 3–5	Activity as tolerated		
Ineffective coping R/T personal vulnerability, situational crisis, inadequate coping methods	Day 1–5 Day 2–5	Participate in development and, evaluation of treatment plan Interact in group sessions	Day 3 Day 4	Verbalize understanding of relationship of ETOH abuse to current situation Identify/make contact with potential resources, support groups	Day 5	Plan on place to meet needs postdischarge
Referrals	Day 1 Day 2–5	Psychiatrist group sessions	Day 4	Community classes: Assertiveness training Stress management		
Additional assessments	Day 1	Understanding of current situation; Drinking pattern, previous withdrawal; other drug use, attitudes toward substance use History of violence	Day 2–3 Day 3–5	Previous coping strategies/consequences Perception of drug use on life, employment, legal issues Congruency of actions based on insight		

Medications	Day 1–2	Relationships with others: personal, work/school; Readiness for group activities	Day 5	Naltrexone 50 mg/day if indicated	Day 5	Medication dose, frequency, side effects; Written instructions for therapeutic program
Client education	Day 1; Day 1–2; Day 2	Physical effects of ETOH abuse; Types/use of relaxation techniques; Consequences of ETOH abuse	Day 3–5; Day 4–5	Human behavior and interactions with others. Community resources for self/family; Identify goals for change		
Additional nursing actions	Day 1–5	Support client's taking responsibility for own recovery; Provide consistent approach/expectations for behavior; Set limits/confront inappropriate behaviors	Day 2–5	Discuss alternative solutions; Provide positive feedback for efforts; Support during confrontation by peer group; Encourage verbalization of feelings, personal reflection		
Imbalanced nutrition: less than body requirements R/T poor intake, effects of ETOH on digestive system, and hypermetabolic response to withdrawal	Day 2–5	Select foods appropriately to meet individual dietary needs	Day 4	Verbalize understandings of effects of ETOH abuse and reduced dietary intake on nutritional status	Day 5	Display stable weight or initial weight gain as appropriate, and laboratory results WNL
Referrals; Diagnostic studies	Day 1 and prn; Day 1	Dietitian; CBC, liver function studies; Serum albumin, transferrin	Day 2–5	Fingerstick glucose prn		
Additional assessments	Day 1; Day 1–2	Weight, skin turgor, condition of mucous membranes, muscle tone; Bowel sounds, characteristics of stools			Day 5	Weight

(continues on page 834)

833

TABLE 15.1 Sample CP: Alcohol Withdrawal Program. ELOS: 5 Days Behavioral Unit (continued)

ND and Categories of Care	Time Dimension	Goals/Actions	Time Dimension	Goals/Actions	Time Dimension	Goals/Actions
	Day 1–5	Appetite, dietary intake				
Medications	Day 1–5	Antacid ac and hs Imodium 2 mg prn	Day 2–5	Multivitamin 1 tab/qd		
Client education	Day 1–2	Individual nutritional needs	Day 4	Principles of nutrition, foods for maintenance of wellness		
Additional nursing actions	Day 1	Liquid/bland diet as tolerated				
	Day 1–5	Encourage small, frequent, nutritious meals/snacks Encourage good oral hygiene pc and hs	Day 2–5	Advance diet as tolerated		

Key: AA, Alcoholics Anonymous; ac, after meals; BA, blood alcohol; C, cough; CBC, complete blood count; CMP, comprehensive metabolic panel; CXR, chext x-ray; DM, diabetes mellitus; ECG, electrocardiogram; ELOS, estimated length of stay; ETOH, ethyl alcohol; HOB, head of bed; hs, hour of sleep; IM, intramuscular; I&O, intake and output; N/V, nausea and vomiting; pc, after meals; PO, by mouth; prn, as needed; q4h, every 4 hours; q8h, every 8 hours; qd, every day; RPR, rapid plasma reagin; R/T, related to; tab, tablet; UA, urinalysis; VS, vital signs; WNL, within normal limits.

SUBSTANCE DEPENDENCE/ABUSE REHABILITATION

I. Pathophysiology

a. Considered a continuum of phases incorporating a cluster of cognitive, behavioral, and physiological symptoms, including loss of control over use of the substance and a continued use of the substance to reach a state of feeling high despite adverse consequences—effects on all body systems, relationship problems, financial difficulties, self- or other-directed violence, exposure to criminal element and activities, legal consequences

b. All commonly abused drugs stimulate the brain's limbic system, elevating dopamine levels and affecting level of alertness, perceptions, emotions, judgment, attention, movement, and sleep (Weekes & Lee, 2008).

c. Commonly misused substances in order of the number of people affected (National Intitute on Drug Abuse [NIDA], 2008a)

  i. Alcohol

  ii. Tobacco products

  iii. Marijuana

  iv. Prescription drugs and pain relievers

  v. Cocaine, crack

  vi. Hallucinogens

  vii. Ecstasy (MDMA)

  viii. Inhalants

  ix. Methamphetamine

  x. Heroin

II. Etiology

a. No single theory developed to date explains condition

b. Multiple predisposing factors implicated in abuse of substances (Merck Manuals, 2005; Townsend, 2006)

  i. Biological—genetic predisposition, chronic pain, illness, trauma

  ii. Biochemical—properties of psychoactive drugs, individual's higher threshold for central nervous system (CNS) effects

  iii. Psychological—depression; personality traits include isolation, low self-esteem, passivity, impulsivity, sexual immaturity

  iv. Sociocultural—unstable home environment, disturbed relationship with parental figures, peer or group pressure, conditioning, availability of substance

  v. Cultural and ethnic influences—attitudes toward alcohol or drug use, expectation that substance can safely relieve distress

III. Statistics

a. Morbidity: Approximately 13% of Americans are alcoholics, another 600,000 to 700,000 are regular cocaine users, and 750,000 are heroine users (Cohagan & Worthington, 2007); in 2004, almost 1.3 million emergency department visits were associated with drug misuse or abuse (Substance Abuse and Mental Health Services Administration [SAMHSA], 2006); in 2006, of the 23.6 million people (aged 12 or older) requiring treatment for substance abuse, only 2.5 million received some form of treatment (NIDA, 2008b).

b. Mortality: In 2005, 33,541 persons died of drug-induced causes in the United States, which includes deaths from use of either legal or illegal drugs and poisoning from medically prescribed and other drugs (Centers for Disease Control and Prevention [CDC], 2005).

c. Cost: In 2002, an estimated $181 billion was spent for illicit drug abuse, with another $185 billion spent for alcohol abuse (NIDA, 2008b).

GLOSSARY

Addiction: Chronic relapsing condition characterized by compulsive drug seeking and abuse and by long-lasting chemical changes in the brain.

Amenorrhea: Absence of menstruation.

CAGE Screening tool: A questionnaire focusing on individual's attempts to Cut down on drinking (or drug use), Annoyance with criticism from others regarding use, Guilt about substance use, and using alcohol (or drug) as an Eye opener or to counter negative effects of withdrawal.

Compulsive: Type of behavior a person exhibits that is overpowering, repeated and, often, irrational.

Craving: Powerful desire for a substance that cannot be ignored.

Detoxification: Medically supervised treatment for alcohol or drug addiction designed to purge the body of intoxicating or addictive substances.

Dual diagnosis: Co-occurring mental illness and substance abuse.

Enabling: Doing for the client what he or she needs to do for self—rescuing. Due to shame and fear, significant others (SOs) and family member(s) often allow the drug or alcohol user to continue disruptive, irrational behavior patterns.

Gynecomastia: Breast enlargement.

Harm-reduction: Program that accepts the reality of drug use while attempting to reduce its harmful consequences to individuals and society. An example could be a "clean-needle program" for intravenous (IV) drug users.

Peer support: Structured relationship in which people meet to provide or exchange emotional support with others facing similar challenges. Peer-to-peer groups are those, such as Alcoholics Anonymous (AA), Narcotics Anonymous (NA), smart recovery, and online forums.

Spider angioma or nevus: Benign growth of dilated capillaries just below the skin surface resembling a spider; often associated with liver disease.

Substance use disorder: Condition that is used to describe a person dependent on or abusing alcohol and/or drugs, including the nonmedical use of prescription drugs.

Care Setting

Client is treated inpatient on behavioral unit or outpatient in a day program or community agency.

Related Concerns

Alcohol: acute withdrawal, page 819
Psychosocial aspects of care, page 749

Client Assessment Database

Data depend on substances involved, duration of use, and organs affected.

MAY REPORT	MAY EXHIBIT
ADDITIONAL DATA REQUIREMENTS • Family issues—discipline, conflict, attitudes • Peer and individual—the individual's delinquency, perception of risk, friends' attitudes and use of substances **TEACHING/LEARNING** • *Discharge Plan Considerations:* May need assistance with long-range plan for recovery ▶ Refer to section at end of plan for postdischarge considerations.	• Family issues—communication • Community—availability of substances, attitudes regarding use • Work or school—attendance, performance or grades

Diagnostic Studies

TEST WHY IT IS DONE	WHAT IT TELLS ME
DRUG SCREENS • *Drug screens:* Serum, urine, saliva, sweat, and/or hair may be tested. • *Screening for use or relapse:* Variety of tools may be used, such as Alcohol Use Disorders Identification Test (AUDIT), CAGE survey, Drug Abuse Screening Test (DAST), and brief Michigan Alcoholism Screening Test (BMAST). • *Addiction Severity Index (ASI) assessment tool:* Produces a "problem severity profile" of the client, including chemical, medical, psychological, legal, family and social, and employment and support aspects. • *Other screening studies (e.g., hepatitis, HIV, tuberculosis [TB]):* Depends on general condition, individual risk factors, and care setting.	Identifies drug(s) being used, including usual drugs of abuse—alcohol, heroin, marijuana, cocaine, and inhalants. Use of a validated tool reveals substance use and dependency. Reveals treatment needs and areas to be addressed. Reveals organ involvement and presence of comorbidities.

Nursing Priorities

1. Provide support for decision to stop substance use and harm reduction.
2. Strengthen individual coping skills.
3. Facilitate learning of new ways to reduce anxiety.
4. Promote family involvement in rehabilitation program.
5. Facilitate family growth and development.
6. Provide information about condition, prognosis, and treatment needs.

Discharge Goals

1. Responsibility for own life and behavior assumed.
2. Plan to maintain substance-free life formulated.
3. Family relationships and enabling issues being addressed.
4. Treatment program successfully begun.
5. Condition, prognosis, and therapeutic regimen understood.
6. Plan in place to meet needs after discharge.

NURSING DIAGNOSIS: **Denial**

May be related to
Personal vulnerability, difficulty handling new situations
Previous ineffective or inadequate coping skills with substitution of drug(s)
Learned response patterns, cultural factors, personal and family value systems

Possibly evidenced by
Delay in seeking or refusal of healthcare attention to the detriment of health and life
No perception of personal relevance of symptoms or danger or denial of impact of condition on life pattern; projection of blame and responsibility for problems
Use of manipulation to avoid responsibility for self

Desired Outcomes/Evaluation Criteria—Client Will

Acceptance: Health Status (NOC)
Verbalize awareness of relationship of substance abuse to current situation.
Engage in therapeutic program.
Verbalize acceptance of responsibility for own behavior.

ACTIONS/INTERVENTIONS	RATIONALE
Behavior Modification (NIC)	
Independent	
Ascertain by what name client would like to be addressed.	Shows courtesy and respect, giving client a sense of orientation and control.
Convey attitude of acceptance, separating individual from unacceptable behavior.	Promotes feelings of dignity and self-worth.
Ascertain reason for beginning abstinence and involvement in therapy.	Provides insight into client's willingness to commit to long-term behavioral change and whether client even believes that he or she can change. *Note:* Denial is one of the strongest and most resistant symptoms of substance abuse. The decision to quit is an important step to success in therapy.
Review definition of drug dependence and abuse with categories of symptoms including patterns of use, impairment caused by use, tolerance to substance.	This information helps client make decisions regarding acceptance of problem and treatment choices.
Answer questions honestly and provide factual information. Keep your word when agreements are made.	Creates trust, which is the basis of the therapeutic relationship.
Provide information about addictive use versus experimental, occasional use; biochemical and genetic disorder theory— genetic predisposition, use activated by environment; and compulsive desire.	Progression of use continuum ranges from experimental or recreational to addictive use. Comprehending this process is important in combating denial. Education may relieve client's guilt and blame and may help awareness of recurring addictive characteristics.
Discuss current life situation and impact of substance use.	First step in decreasing use of denial is for client to see the relationship between substance use and personal problems.
Confront and examine denial and rationalization in peer group. Use confrontation with caring attitude.	Because denial is the major defense mechanism in addictive disease, confrontation by peers can help the client accept the reality of adverse consequences of behaviors and that drug use is a major problem. Caring attitude preserves self-concept and helps decrease defensive response.
Provide information regarding effects of addiction on mood and personality.	Individuals often mistake effects of addiction and use this to justify or excuse drug use.
Remain nonjudgmental. Be alert to changes in behavior such as restlessness and increased tension.	Confrontation can lead to increased agitation, which may compromise safety of client and staff.
Provide positive feedback for expressing awareness of denial in self and others.	Necessary to enhance self-esteem and to reinforce insight into behavior.
Maintain firm expectation that client attend recovery support and therapy groups regularly.	Attendance is related to admitting need for help; to working with denial; and for maintaining long-term, drug-free existence.
Encourage and support client's taking responsibility for own recovery, such as development of alternative behaviors to drug urge and use. Assist client to learn own responsibility for recovering.	Denial can be replaced with positive action when client accepts the reality of own responsibility.
Be aware of own enabling behaviors.	Caregiving lends itself to "taking care" of clients that can backfire in substance abuse treatment.

NURSING DIAGNOSIS: ineffective Coping

May be related to
Personal vulnerability
Negative role modeling, inadequate support systems
Previous ineffective or inadequate coping skills with substitution of drug(s)

Possibly evidenced by
Impaired adaptive behavior and problem-solving skills
Decreased ability to handle stress of illness or hospitalization
Financial affairs in disarray, employment or school difficulties (e.g., losing time on job or not maintaining steady employment; poor work or school performances; on-the-job injuries)
Verbalization of inability to cope or ask for help

Desired Outcomes/Evaluation Criteria—Client Will

Substance Addiction Consequences (NOC)
Identify consequences of using substance as a method of coping.

Coping (NOC)
Identify other ineffective coping behaviors.
Engage in effective coping skills and problem-solving.
Initiate necessary lifestyle changes.

ACTIONS/INTERVENTIONS	RATIONALE
Substance Use Treatment (NIC)	
Independent	
Review program rules and philosophy expectations.	Having information provides opportunity for client to cooperate and function as a member of the group or milieu, enhancing sense of control and sense of success.
Determine understanding of current situation and previous or other methods of coping with life's problems.	Provides information about degree of denial, acceptance of personal responsibility and commitment to change; identifies coping skills that may be used in present situation.
Set limits and confront efforts to get caregiver to grant special privileges, making excuses for not following through on behaviors agreed on, and attempting to continue drug use. Avoid use of labels, such as lying.	Client has learned manipulative behavior throughout life and needs to learn a new way of getting needs met. Following through on consequences of failure to maintain limits can help the client to change ineffective behaviors. Use of labels promotes negative attitudes that can impede therapeutic relationships.
Be aware of staff attitudes, feelings, and enabling behaviors.	Lack of understanding and judgmental or enabling behaviors can result in inaccurate data collection and nontherapeutic approaches.
Encourage verbalization of feelings, fears, and anxiety.	May help client begin to come to terms with long-unresolved issues.
Explore alternative coping strategies.	Client may have little or no knowledge of adaptive responses to stress and needs to learn other options for managing time, feelings, and relationships without drugs.
Assist client to learn and encourage use of relaxation skills, guided imagery, and visualizations.	Helps client relax and develop new ways to deal with stress and to problem-solve.
Structure diversional activity that relates to recovery such as social activity within support group, wherein issues of being chemically free are examined.	Discovery of alternative methods of coping with drug hunger can remind client that addiction is a lifelong process and opportunity for changing patterns is available.
Use peer support to examine ways of coping with drug hunger.	Self-help groups, such as AA, NA, and Crystal Methamphetamine Anonymous, are valuable for learning and promoting abstinence in each member by using understanding and support as well as peer pressure.
Identify possible and actual triggers for relapse. Encourage client to use the acronym HALT—"Am I hungry, angry, lonely, or tired?"	Employment and financial stressors, isolation, unhealthy relationships, being around substance-using friends, hearing certain songs, premenstrual syndrome—the list of possibilities depends on the individual. Being aware of the triggers provides an opportunity to plan for ways to avoid and deal with them.
Encourage involvement in therapeutic writing. Have client begin journaling or writing autobiography.	Therapeutic writing or journaling can enhance participation in treatment; serves as a release for grief, anger, and stress; provides a useful tool for monitoring client's safety; and can be used to evaluate client's progress. Autobiographical activity provides an opportunity for client to remember and identify sequence of events in his or her life that relate to current situation.

ACTIONS/INTERVENTIONS (continued)

Discuss client's plans for living without drugs.

Collaborative
Administer medications, as indicated, for example:
  Disulfiram (Antabuse)

  Metronidazole (Flagyl)

  Acamprosate (Campral EC)

  Buprenorphine (Buprex, Subutex, Suboxone)

  Methadone (Dolophine) and levo-α-acetymethadol (LAAM)

  Naltrexone (Trexan) and nalmefine (Revex)

Encourage involvement with self-help associations such as AA or NA.
Refer to community or social resources such as housing assistance, employment agencies, childcare, food stamps, or alternative schooling.

RATIONALE (continued)

Provides opportunity to develop and refine plans. Devising a comprehensive strategy for avoiding relapses helps client into maintenance phase of behavioral change.

This drug can be helpful in maintaining abstinence from alcohol while other therapy is undertaken. By inhibiting alcohol oxidation, the drug leads to an accumulation of acetaldehyde with a highly unpleasant reaction if alcohol is consumed.

Increasingly used to maintain abstinence from alcohol instead of Antabuse. It has the same gastrointestinal (GI) distress effects but fewer cardiac concerns and lower cost.

Helps prevent relapses in alcoholism by lowering receptors for the excitatory neurotransmitter glutamate. This agent may become drug of choice because it does not make the user sick if alcohol is consumed; it has no sedative, anti-anxiety, muscle relaxant, or antidepressant properties and produces no withdrawal symptoms.

Used in the treatment of opioid addiction. At low doses it produces sufficient agonist effect to enable opioid addicted individuals to discontinue the misuse of opioids without experiencing withdrawal symptoms. This drug carries a lower risk of abuse, dependence, and side effects compared to full opioid agonists (McNicholas, 2004).

Methadone is thought to blunt the craving for or diminish the effects of opioids and is used to assist in withdrawal and long-term maintenance programs. It can allow the individual to maintain daily activities and ultimately withdraw from drug use. LAAM is a long-acting synthetic μ agonist thought to be a safe and effective alternative to methadone maintenance. Harm reduction needs to be considered versus the possibility of exchanging one addiction for another (CDC, 2002).

Used to suppress craving for opioids and may help prevent relapse in the client abusing alcohol. Current research suggests that naltrexone suppresses urge to continue drinking by interfering with alcohol-induced release of endorphins (Leavitt, 2002).

Puts client in direct contact with support system necessary for managing sobriety and drug-free life.

Dealing with life problems in a proactive way enhances coping abilities, reduces sense of isolation and hopelessness, and decreases risk of relapse.

NURSING DIAGNOSIS: Powerlessness

May be related to
Substance addiction with or without periods of abstinence
Episodic compulsive indulgence; attempts at recovery
Lifestyle of helplessness

Possibly evidenced by
Ineffective recovery attempts, statements of inability to stop behavior or requests for help
Constantly thinking about drug and/or obtaining drug
Alteration in personal, occupational, and social life

Desired Outcomes/Evaluation Criteria—Client Will

Health Beliefs: Perceived Control (NOC)
Admit inability to control drug habit and surrender to powerlessness over addiction.
Verbalize acceptance of need for treatment and awareness that willpower alone cannot control abstinence.
Engage in peer support.
Demonstrate active participation in program.
Regain and maintain healthy state with a drug-free lifestyle.

ACTIONS/INTERVENTIONS	RATIONALE

Self-Responsibility Facilitation (NIC)

Independent

Use crisis intervention techniques to initiate behavior changes:

May need to use emergency commitments or other legal holds for the client's safety. Client may be more amenable to acceptance of need for treatment at this time.

Assist client to recognize problem exists. Discuss in a caring, nonjudgmental manner how drug has interfered with life.

In the precontemplation phase, the client has not yet identified that drug use is problematic. While client is hurting, it is easier to admit substance use has created negative consequences.

Involve client in development of treatment plan, using problem-solving process in which client identifies goals for change and agrees to desired outcomes.

During the contemplation phase, the client realizes a problem exists and is thinking about a change of behavior. The client is committed to the outcomes when the decision-making process involves solutions that are promulgated by the individual.

Discuss alternative solutions.

Brainstorming helps creatively identify possibilities and provides sense of control. During the preparation phase, minor action may be taken as individual organizes resources for definitive change.

Assist in selecting most appropriate alternative.

As possibilities are discussed, the most useful solution becomes clear.

Support decision and implementation of selected alternative(s).

Helps the client persevere in process of change. During the action phase, the client engages in a sustained effort to maintain sobriety, and mechanisms are put in place to support abstinence.

Explore support in peer group. Encourage sharing about drug hunger, situations that increase the desire to indulge, and ways that substance has influenced life.

Client may need assistance in expressing self, speaking about powerlessness, and admitting need for help in order to face up to problem and begin resolution.

Assist client to learn ways to enhance health and structure healthy diversion from drug use including maintaining a balanced diet; getting adequate rest; exercise such as walking; slow or long distance running; and acupuncture, biofeedback, or deep meditative techniques.

Learning to empower self in constructive areas can strengthen ability to continue recovery. These activities help restore natural biochemical balance; aid detoxification; and manage stress, anxiety, and use of free time. These diversions can increase self-confidence, thereby improving self-esteem. *Note:* Exercise promotes release of endorphins, creating a feeling of well-being.

Provide information regarding understanding of human behavior and interactions with others, such as transactional analysis.

Understanding these concepts can help the client to begin to deal with past problems and losses, and prevent repeating ineffective coping behaviors and self-fulfilling prophecies.

Assist client in self-examination of spirituality and faith.

Although not mandatory for recovery, surrendering to and faith in a power greater than oneself has been found to be effective for many individuals in substance recovery; may decrease sense of powerlessness.

Instruct in and role-play assertive communication skills.

Effective in helping refrain from use, to stop contact with users and dealers, to build healthy relationships, and to regain control of own life.

Provide treatment information on an ongoing basis.

Helps client know what to expect, and creates opportunity for client to be a part of what is happening and make informed choices about participation and outcomes.

Collaborative

Refer to, or assist with making contact with, programs for ongoing treatment needs—partial hospitalization drug treatment programs, NA, AA, or peer support groups.

Continuing treatment is essential to positive outcome. Follow-through may be easier once initial contact has been made.

NURSING DIAGNOSIS: **imbalanced Nutrition: Less than Body Requirements**

May be related to
Insufficient dietary intake to meet metabolic needs for psychological, physiological, or economic reasons

Possibly evidenced by
Weight loss, weight below norm for height and body build, decreased subcutaneous fat or muscle mass
Reported altered taste sensation, lack of interest in food
Poor muscle tone
Sore, inflamed buccal cavity
Laboratory evidence of protein and vitamin deficiencies

NURSING DIAGNOSIS: **imbalanced Nutrition: Less than Body Requirements** (continued)

Desired Outcomes/Evaluation Criteria—Client Will

Nutritional Status (NOC)
Demonstrate progressive weight gain toward goal with normalization of laboratory values and absence of signs of malnutrition.

Knowledge: Treatment Regimen (NOC)
Verbalize understanding of effects of substance abuse and reduced dietary intake on nutritional status.
Demonstrate behaviors or lifestyle changes to regain and maintain appropriate weight.

ACTIONS/INTERVENTIONS	RATIONALE
Nutrition Therapy (NIC)	
Independent	
Assess height, weight, age, body build, strength, and activity and rest levels. Note condition of oral cavity.	Provides information on which to base individual caloric needs and dietary plan. Type of foods may be affected by condition of mucous membranes and teeth.
Take anthropometric measurements, such as midarm muscle circumference, triceps skinfold, and percentage of body fat, when available.	Calculates subcutaneous fat and muscle mass to aid in determining dietary needs.
Note total daily calorie intake. Recommend client maintain a diary of intake, as well as times and patterns of eating.	Information will help identify nutritional deficiencies.
Evaluate energy expenditure (e.g., pacing or sedentary), and establish an individualized exercise program.	Activity level affects nutritional needs. Exercise enhances muscle tone and may stimulate appetite.
Provide opportunity to choose foods and snacks to meet dietary plan.	Enhances sense of control, may promote resolution of nutritional deficiencies, and helps evaluate client's understanding of dietary teaching.
Recommend monitoring weight weekly.	Provides information regarding effectiveness of dietary plan.
Collaborative	
Consult with dietitian.	Useful in establishing individual dietary needs and plan, and provides additional resource for learning.
Review laboratory studies as indicated, such as glucose, serum albumin or prealbumin, and electrolytes.	Identifies anemias, electrolyte imbalances, and other abnormalities that may be present, requiring specific therapy.
Refer for dental consultation as necessary.	Teeth are essential to good nutritional intake, and oral hygiene and dental care are often a neglected area in this population.

NURSING DIAGNOSIS: **chronic low Self-Esteem**

May be related to
Social stigma attached to substance abuse, expectation that one controls behavior
Negative role models, abuse, neglect, dysfunctional family system
Life choices perpetuating failure, situational crisis with loss of control over life events
Biochemical body change—withdrawal from alcohol and/or other drugs

Possibly evidenced by
Self-negating verbalization, expressions of shame and guilt
Evaluation of self as unable to deal with events, confusion about self, purpose, or direction in life
Rationalizing away and rejecting positive feedback about self

Desired Outcomes/Evaluation Criteria—Client Will

Self-Esteem (NOC)
Identify feelings and underlying dynamics for negative perception of self.
Verbalize acceptance of self as is and an increased sense of self-worth.
Set goals and participate in realistic planning for lifestyle changes necessary to live without drugs.

ACTIONS/INTERVENTIONS	RATIONALE
Self-Esteem Enhancement (NIC)	
Independent	
Provide opportunity for and encourage verbalization and discussion of individual situation.	Client often has difficulty expressing self, even more difficulty accepting the degree of importance substance has assumed in life and its relationship to present situation.

(continues on page 842)

ACTIONS/INTERVENTIONS (continued)	RATIONALE (continued)
Assess mental status. Note presence of other psychiatric disorders.	Many clients use substances in an attempt to obtain relief from depression or anxiety, which may predate use and/or be the result of substance use. Approximately 60% of substance-dependent clients have underlying psychological problems or a dual diagnosis, and treatment for both is imperative to achieve and maintain abstinence.
Spend time with client. Discuss client's behavior and use of substance in a nonjudgmental way.	The nurse's presence conveys acceptance of the individual as a worthwhile person.
Provide grief counseling, as indicated.	Discussion provides opportunity for insight into the problems abuse has created for the client. Life losses secondary to alcohol or other drug abuse problems need to be addressed to enable client to move forward with rehabilitation.
Provide reinforcement for positive actions and encourage client to accept this input.	Failure and lack of self-esteem have been problems for this client, who needs to learn to accept self as an individual with positive attributes.
Observe family interactions and SO dynamics and level of support.	Substance abuse is a family disease, and how the members act and react to the client's behavior affects the course of the disease and how client sees self. Many unconsciously become "enablers," helping the individual to cover up the consequences of the abuse. (Refer to ND: dysfunctional Family Processes, following.)
Encourage expression of feelings of guilt, shame, and anger.	The client often has lost respect for self and believes that the situation is hopeless. Expression of these feelings helps client begin to accept responsibility for self and take steps to make changes.
Help client acknowledge that substance use is the problem and that problems can be dealt with without the use of drugs. Confront the use of defenses—denial, projection, and rationalization.	When drugs can no longer be blamed for the problems that exist, client can begin to deal with the problems and live without substance use. Confrontation helps client accept the reality of the problems as they exist.
Ask client to list and review past accomplishments and positive happenings.	There are things in everyone's life that have been successful. Often when self-esteem is low, it is difficult to remember these successes or to view them as successes.
Use techniques of role rehearsal.	Assists client to practice developing skills to cope with new role as a person who no longer uses or needs drugs to handle life's problems.
Collaborative	
Involve client in group therapy.	Group sharing helps encourage verbalization because other members of the group are in various stages of abstinence from drugs and can address the client's concerns or denial. The client can gain new skills, hope, and a sense of family or community from group participation.
Formulate plan to treat other mental illness problems.	Clients who seek relief for other mental health problems through drugs will continue to do so once discharged. Both the substance use and the mental health problems need to be treated together to maximize abstinence potential. Treatment may be difficult because of difficulty of taking initiative, thinking realistically, and problem-solving. Behavioral methods seem to be most helpful.
Administer antipsychotic medications, such as quetiapine (Seroquel) or olanzapine (Zyprexa or Zydis), as necessary.	Prolonged or profound psychosis following lysergic acid diethylamide (LSD) or phencyclidine (PCP) use can be treated with these drugs because it is probably the result of an underlying functional psychosis that has now emerged. Methamphetamine psychosis often does not reverse. *Note:* Avoid the use of phenothiazines because they may decrease seizure threshold and cause hypotension in the presence of LSD or PCP use.
Monitor for diabetes, weight gain, and dyslipidemia.	Atypical antipsychotics (e.g., Zyprexa) are associated with these effects and should be monitored closely for changes in glucose control. Measurement of fasting blood glucose at the beginning of therapy and periodical monitoring during therapy are recommended.

NURSING DIAGNOSIS: dysfunctional Family Processes

May be related to
Abuse of substance(s), resistance to treatment
Family history of substance abuse
Addictive personality
Inadequate coping skills, lack of problem-solving skills

Possibly evidenced by
Anxiety, anger or suppressed rage, shame, and embarrassment
Emotional isolation, loneliness, vulnerability, repressed emotions
Disturbed family dynamics, closed communication systems, ineffective spousal communication and marital problems
Altered role function, disruption of family roles
Manipulation, dependency, criticizing, rationalization or denial of problems
Enabling to maintain drinking or substance abuse, refusal to get help or inability to accept and receive help appropriately

Desired Outcomes/Evaluation Criteria—Family Will

Family Coping (NOC)
Verbalize understanding of dynamics of enabling behaviors.
Participate in individual family programs.
Identify ineffective coping behaviors and consequences.
Initiate and plan for necessary lifestyle changes.
Take action to change self-destructive behaviors and alter behaviors that contribute to partner's/SO's addiction.

ACTIONS/INTERVENTIONS	RATIONALE
Substance Use Treatment (NIC)	
Independent	
Review family history and explore roles of family members, circumstances involving drug use, strengths, and areas for growth.	Determines areas for focus and potential for change.
Explore how the SO has coped with the client's habit—use of denial, repression, rationalization, projection, feelings of hurt, and loneliness.	The person who enables also suffers from the same feelings as the client and uses ineffective methods for dealing with the situation, necessitating help in learning new, more effective coping skills.
Determine understanding of current situation and previous methods of coping with life's problems.	Provides information on which to base present plan of care.
Assess current level of functioning of family members.	Affects individual's ability to cope with situation.
Determine extent of enabling behaviors being evidenced by family members and explore with each individual and client.	People want to be helpful and do not want to feel powerless to help their loved one stop substance use and change the behavior that is so destructive. However, the substance abuser often relies on others to rescue them by covering up own inability to cope with daily responsibilities.
Provide information about enabling behavior, addictive disease characteristics for both user and nonuser.	Awareness and knowledge of behaviors such as avoiding and shielding, taking over responsibilities, rationalizing, and subserving, provide opportunity for individuals to begin the process of change.
Identify and discuss sabotage behaviors of family members.	Even though family member(s) may verbalize a desire for the individual to become substance free, the reality of interactive dynamics is that they may unconsciously not want the individual to recover because this would affect their own role in the relationship. Additionally, they may receive sympathy and attention from others—secondary gain.
Encourage participation in therapeutic writing, such as journaling (narrative) or guided or focused writing.	Serves as a release for feelings such as anger, grief, and stress, and helps move individuals forward in treatment process.
Provide factual information to client and family about the effects of addictive behaviors on the family and what to expect after discharge.	Many clients and SOs are not aware of the nature of addiction. If client is using legally obtained drugs, he or she may believe this does not constitute abuse.
Encourage family members to be aware of their own feelings and look at the situation with perspective and objectivity. They can ask themselves: "Am I being conned? Am I acting out of fear, shame, guilt, or anger? Do I have a need to control?"	When the enabling family members become aware of their own actions that perpetuate the addict's problems, they need to decide to change themselves. If they change, the client can then face the consequences of his or her own actions and may choose to get well.
Provide support for enabling partner(s). Encourage group work.	Families and SOs need support to produce change as much as the person who is addicted.

(continues on page 844)

ACTIONS/INTERVENTIONS (continued)

Assist the client's partner to become aware that client's abstinence and drug use are not the partner's responsibility.

Help the recovering partner who is enabling to distinguish
between destructive aspects of behavior and genuine
motivation to aid the user.

Note how partner relates to the treatment team.

Explore conflicting feelings the enabling partner may have
about treatment such as feelings similar to those of
abuser—blend of anger, guilt, fear, exhaustion, embarrassment, loneliness, distrust, grief, and possibly relief.

Involve family in discharge referral plans.

Be aware of staff's enabling behaviors and feelings about
client and enabling partners.

Collaborative

Involve in substance abuse treatment plan.

Encourage involvement with self-help associations, AA or NA,
Al-Anon, Alateen, and professional family therapy.

RATIONALE (continued)

Partners need to learn that user's habit may or may not
change despite partner's involvement in treatment.

Enabling behavior can be partner's attempts at personal
survival.

Determines enabling style. A parallel exists between how partner relates to user and to staff, based on partner's feelings
about self and situation.

Useful in establishing the need for therapy for the partner. This
individual's own identity may have been lost, she or he
may fear self-disclosure to staff, and may have difficulty
giving up the dependent relationship.

Drug abuse is a family illness. Because the family has been so
involved in dealing with the substance abuse behavior,
family members need help adjusting to the new behavior
of sobriety and abstinence. Incidence of recovery is almost
doubled when the family is treated along with the client.

Lack of understanding of enabling can result in nontherapeutic
approaches to clients and their families.

Can be voluntary, court ordered, or via the Department of
Human Services involvement.

Puts client and family in direct contact with support systems
necessary for continued sobriety and to assist with problem
resolution.

NURSING DIAGNOSIS: Sexual Dysfunction

May be related to

Altered body function—neurological damage and debilitating effects of drug use (particularly alcohol and opiates)

Possibly evidenced by

Progressive interference with sexual functioning

For men, a significant degree of testicular atrophy is noted with testes smaller and softer than normal, gynecomastia,
impotence, and decreased sperm counts

For women, loss of body hair, thin soft skin, and spider angioma (elevated estrogen); amenorrhea; increase in miscarriages

Desired Outcomes/Evaluation Criteria—Client Will

Substance Addiction Consequences (NOC)
Verbally acknowledge effects of drug use on sexual functioning and reproduction.

Sexual Functioning (NOC)
Identify interventions to correct and overcome individual situation.

ACTIONS/INTERVENTIONS

Sexual Counseling (NIC)
Independent

Ascertain client's beliefs and expectations. Have client describe
problem in own words.

Encourage and accept individual expressions of concern.

Provide educational opportunities such as pamphlets or consultation with appropriate persons regarding effects of drug
on sexual functioning.

Provide information about individual's condition.

Assess drinking and drug history of pregnant client. Provide
information about effects of substance abuse on the reproductive system and fetus including increased risk of premature birth, brain damage, and fetal malformation.

RATIONALE

Determines level of knowledge, identifies misperceptions,
level of concern regarding sexually transmitted diseases
(STDs), level of risk reduction, and specific learning needs.

Most people find it difficult to talk about this sensitive subject
and may not ask directly for information.

Much of denial and hesitancy to seek treatment may be reduced
as a result of sufficient and appropriate information.

Sexual functioning may have been affected by the drug itself,
and/or by psychological factors, such as stress or depression. Information can assist client to understand own
situation and identify actions to be taken.

Awareness of the negative effects of alcohol and other drugs
on reproduction may motivate client to stop using substance. When client is pregnant, identification of potential
problems aids in identifying concerns and planning for
future fetal needs.

ACTIONS/INTERVENTIONS (continued)	RATIONALE (continued)
Discuss prognosis for sexual dysfunction, such as impotence or low sexual desire.	Impotence may be reversed with abstinence from drug(s) for many individuals; however, for some erectile dysfunction will be permanent.
Collaborative Refer for sexual counseling, if indicated.	Couple may need additional assistance to resolve more severe problems or situations. Client may have difficulty adjusting if drug has improved sexual experience such as heroin, which decreases dyspareunia in women and premature ejaculation in men. Furthermore, the client may have engaged enjoyably in bizarre, erotic sexual behavior under influence of the stimulant drug; client may have found no substitute for the drug, may have driven a partner away, and may have no motivation to adjust to sexual experience without drugs.
Review results of sonogram if pregnant.	Assesses fetal growth and development to identify possibility of fetal alcohol syndrome or other harmful drug effects and future needs. There are concerns about placental abruption with the use of methamphetamine and cocaine.

NURSING DIAGNOSIS: deficient Knowledge [Learning Need] regarding condition, prognosis, treatment, self-care, and discharge needs

May be related to
Lack of information, information misinterpretation, lack of recall
Cognitive limitations or interference with learning—other mental illness problems or organic brain syndrome

Possibly evidenced by
Statements of concern, questions, misconceptions
Inaccurate follow-through of instructions, development of preventable complications
Continued use in spite of complications or adverse consequences

Desired Outcomes/Evaluation Criteria—Client Will

Knowledge: Substance Abuse Control (NOC)
Verbalize understanding of own condition or disease process, prognosis, and potential complications.
Verbalize understanding of therapeutic needs.
Identify and initiate necessary lifestyle changes to remain drug free.
Participate in treatment program including plan for follow-up and long-term care.

ACTIONS/INTERVENTIONS	RATIONALE
Learning Facilitation (NIC) *Independent* Be aware of and deal with anxiety of client and family members.	Anxiety can interfere with ability to hear and assimilate information.
Provide an active role for the client and SO in the learning process using discussions, group participation, and role-playing.	Learning is enhanced when persons are actively involved.
Provide written and verbal information as indicated. Include list of articles, books, Internet resources, and special TV programs related to client and family needs and encourage reading and discussing what they learn.	Helps client and SO make informed choices about future and can be a useful addition to other therapeutic approaches.
Assess client's knowledge of own situation including disease process, prognosis, complications, and needed changes in lifestyle.	Assists in planning for long-range changes necessary for maintaining sobriety and drug-free status. Client may have street knowledge of the drug but be ignorant of medical facts.
Pace learning activities to individual needs.	Facilitates learning because information is more readily assimilated when timing is considered.
Teaching: Disease Process (NIC) Review condition, prognosis, and future expectations.	Provides knowledge base from which client can make informed choices.
Discuss relationship of drug use to current situation.	Often client has misperception or denial of real reason for admission to the medical or psychiatric care setting.

(continues on page 846)

Educate about effects of specific drug(s) used; for example, PCP is deposited in body fat and may reactivate, causing flashbacks even after long interval of abstinence; alcohol use may result in mental deterioration and liver involvement or damage; cocaine can damage postcapillary vessels and increase platelet aggregation, promoting thromboses and infarction of skin or internal organs, causing localized atrophie blanche or sclerodermatous lesions.

Information will help client understand possible long-term effects of drug use.

Discuss potential for reemergence of withdrawal symptoms in stimulant abuse as early as 3 months or as late as 9 to 12 months after discontinuing use.

Even though intoxication may have passed, client may manifest denial, drug hunger, and periods of "flare-up," wherein there is a delayed recurrence of withdrawal symptoms such as anxiety, depression, irritability, sleep disturbance, or compulsiveness with food, especially sugars.

Inform client of effects of disulfiram (Antabuse) in combination with alcohol intake and importance of avoiding use of alcohol-containing products such as cough syrups, foods, candy, mouthwash, aftershave, and cologne.

Interaction of alcohol and Antabuse results in nausea and hypotension, which may produce fatal shock. Individuals on Antabuse are sensitive to alcohol on a continuum, with some being able to drink while taking the drug and others having a reaction with only slight exposure. Reactions also appear to be dose related.

Review specific aftercare needs; for example, PCP user should drink cranberry juice and continue use of ascorbic acid; alcohol abuser with liver damage should refrain from drugs, anesthetics, or use of household cleaning products that are detoxified in the liver.

Promotes individualized care related to specific situation. Cranberry juice and ascorbic acid enhance clearance of PCP from the system. Substances that have the potential for liver damage are more dangerous in the presence of an already damaged liver.

Discuss variety of helpful organizations and programs that are available for assistance or referral such as AA, Dual Recovery Anonymous (DRA), or NA.

Long-term support is necessary to maintain optimal recovery. Psychosocial needs and other issues may need to be addressed.

POTENTIAL CONSIDERATIONS following acute care (dependent on client's age, physical condition and presence of complications, personal resources, and life responsibilities)
- *ineffective self Health Management/ineffective family Therapeutic Regimen Management*—decisional conflicts, excessive demands made on individual or family, family conflict, perceived seriousness/benefits
- *ineffective Coping*—vulnerability, situational crises, multiple life changes, inadequate relaxation, inadequate/loss of support systems
- *readiness for enhanced family Coping*—needs sufficiently gratified and adaptive tasks effectively addressed to enable goals of self-actualization to surface

Physical needs depend on substance effect on organ systems—refer to appropriate medical plans of care for additional considerations.

CANCER

I. Pathophysiology
  a. General term describing a disturbance of cellular growth and referring to a group of 150 different known diseases or types
  b. The metastatic behavior or "natural history" of cancer varies according to the primary site of diagnosis—metastatic pattern for primary breast cancer may be from the breast to the bone, lung, liver, and/or brain.

II. Classification
  a. Four main classifications of cancer according to tissue type
    i. Lymphomas: cancers originating in infection-fighting organs
    ii. Leukemias: cancers originating in blood-forming organs
    iii. Sarcomas: cancers originating in bones, muscle, or connective tissue
    iv. Carcinomas: cancers originating in epithelial cells
  b. Within these broad categories, a cancer is classified by histology, stage, and grade.

III. Etiology
  a. Cellular disease that can arise from any body tissue with manifestations that result from failure to control the proliferation and maturation of cells.
  b. Multiple risk factors or cancer-causing agents
    i. Chemicals
    ii. Radiation
    iii. Viruses
    iv. Human behaviors and lifestyles that affect cancer risk
    v. Tobacco use
    vi. Poor nutrition
    vii. Inactivity, obesity
    viii. Sun exposure
    ix. Workplace or occupational exposure
    x. Pollution—air, water, soil

c. Biological factors that may increase or reduce risk
  i. Inflammation
  ii. DNA repair mechanisms
  iii. Immunologic responses
  iv. Heredity

IV. Statistics (American Cancer Society [ACS], 2007)
  a. Morbidity: In 2007, 1,444,920 new cancer cases were projected in the United States.
  b. Mortality: In 2007, there were an estimated 559,650 deaths from all types of cancer in the United States.
  c. Cost: In 2006, there were aproximately $206.3 billion in direct and indirect costs for cancer.

GLOSSARY

Adenocarcinoma: Cancer arising in gland-forming tissue. An example is breast cancer.

Adjuvant therapy: Treatment given in addition to the primary treatment.

Alopecia: Hair loss.

Biotherapy: Treatment to boost or restore the ability of the immune system to fight cancer. Also used to lessen certain side effects that may be caused by some cancer treatments. Agents used in biotherapy include monoclonal antibodies, growth factors, and vaccines.

Cachexia: Loss of body weight and muscle mass as a result of anorexia, nausea and vomiting, or hypermetabolism.

Cancer-related fatigue (CRF): Persistent and subjective sense of tiredness that can occur with cancer or cancer treatment, which interferes with usual functioning and can drastically affect the client's quality of life.

Carcinogen: Any substance that causes cancer.

Carcinoma: Cancer that begins in the lining or covering of an organ.

Desquamation: Shedding of the skin as a reaction to radiotherapy. In its mildest form, it is "dry" when the skin flakes in a powdery form. In a more severe form ("wet"), the deeper layers of the skin are exposed.

Metastasis: Spread of cancer to another organ, usually through the bloodstream.

Mucositis: A complication of some cancer therapies in which the lining of the digestive system becomes inflamed; often seen as sores in the mouth.

Nadir: Period of time following chemotherapy treatment when blood counts generally are at their lowest levels and client is at greatest risk of developing infection and other blood-related side effects.

Peripheral progenitor cell (stem cell) transplant: Method of replacing blood-forming cells destroyed by cancer treatment. Immature blood cells (stem cells) in the circulating blood that are similar to those in the bone marrow are given to the client after treatment.

Radiation dermatitis: Skin condition that is a common side effect of radiation therapy. The affected skin becomes painful, red, itchy, and blistered.

Staging: Classification of the primary tumor (T), lymph node involvement (N), combined with tests to see if the cancer has metastasized (M).

Stomatitis: Inflammation of the mucous membranes of the mouth.

Superior vena cava syndrome (SVCS): Condition in which a tumor presses against the superior vena cava—the large vein that carries blood from the head, neck, arms, and chest to the heart. This pressure blocks blood flow to the heart and may cause coughing; difficulty in breathing; and swelling of the face, neck, and upper arms.

Tumor: An abnormal mass of tissue, either benign (noncancerous) or malignant (cancerous).

Tumor marker: Substance detectable in the blood or urine that suggests the presence of cancer.

Vein flare: Painless local allergic reaction identified by redness along the vein used to infuse chemotherapeutic agent; urticaria or hives may also be present. Usually subsides within 30 to 60 minutes without treatment.

Care Setting

Cancer centers may focus on staging and major treatment modalities for complex cancers. Treatment for managing adverse effects, such as malnutrition and infection, may take place in short-stay, ambulatory, or community setting. More cancer clients are receiving care at home because of personal choice and healthcare costs.

Related Concerns

End-of-life care/hospice, page 866

Hysterectomy, page 611

Adult leukemias, page 516

Lung cancer: postoperative care, page 144

Lymphomas, page 525

Mastectomy, page 619

Prostatectomy, page 596

Psychosocial aspects of care, page 749

Radical neck surgery: laryngectomy (postoperative care), page 160

Sepsis/septicemia, page 686

Total nutritional support: parenteral/enteral feeding, page 469

Urinary diversions/urostomy (postoperative care), page 578

Data depend on organs or tissues involved and stage of disease. Refer to appropriate plans of care for additional assessment information.

DIAGNOSTIC DIVISION MAY REPORT	MAY EXHIBIT
ACTIVITY/REST • Weakness • Fatigue • Changes in rest pattern and usual hours of sleep per night • Presence of factors affecting sleep, such as pain, anxiety, night sweats, more frequent elimination needs • Limitations of participation in hobbies, exercise, usual activities	• Inability to maintain usual routines or desired level of activity or work • Lack of energy • Disinterest in surroundings • Compromised concentration
CIRCULATION • Palpitations • Chest pain on exertion	• Changes in blood pressure (BP) • Fluctuations in heart rate
EGO INTEGRITY • Stress factors—financial, job, role changes • Ways of handling stress—smoking, drinking, delay in seeking treatment, religious or spiritual crisis • Concern about changes in appearance such as alopecia, disfiguring lesions, surgery, profound weight loss, edema, weight gain, or rash • Denial of diagnosis • Feelings of powerlessness, hopelessness, helplessness, worthlessness, guilt, loss of control	• Denial, withdrawal, anger • Depression
ELIMINATION • Changes in bowel pattern—blood in stools, pain with defecation, constipation, or diarrhea • Changes in urinary elimination—pain or burning on urination, hematuria, frequent urination or nocturia	• Changes in bowel sounds • Abdominal distention • Diarrhea • Dysuria, frequency, incontinence
FOOD/FLUID • Poor dietary habits, such as low-fiber, high-fat, additives, preservatives • Anorexia, altered taste • Nausea and vomiting • Difficulty swallowing, mouth sores • Food intolerances	• Changes in weight, severe weight loss, cachexia • Wasting of muscle mass • Changes in skin moisture or turgor • Edema • Ulcerations of oral mucosa
NEUROSENSORY • Dizziness, syncope • Lack of coordination, unstable balance • Numbness or tingling of extremities • Sensation of coldness • Difficulty performing fine motor skills such as buttoning shirt	

PAIN/DISCOMFORT
• Varying degrees of pain from mild discomfort to severe pain
• Pain localized in a specific area
• Quality or description
  • Stabbing, throbbing, dull, aching (somatic pain often present with surgery or metastases in bone)
  • Pressure-like, cramping, gnawing, squeezing—visceral pain that may be referred from one site to another
  • Sharp, burning, shooting pain, may be accompanied by numbness and tingling in extremities—neuropathic pain caused from damage to nervous system
	• Guarding behaviors, positioning to avoid pain
	• Facial mask
	• Sleep disturbance
	• Restlessness, moaning, crying, irritability, lethargy
	• Self-focusing; narrowed focus
	• Reduced interaction with others
	• Depression

DIAGNOSTIC DIVISION MAY REPORT (continued)	MAY EXHIBIT (continued)

RESPIRATION
- Dyspnea with exertion
- History of chronic respiratory disease
- Smoking—tobacco, marijuana
- Living with someone who smokes
- Asbestos or dust exposure—coal, sandstone, silica, and the like

SAFETY
- Occupational, professional or environmental exposure to toxic chemicals, carcinogens
- Excessive or prolonged sun exposure

(MAY EXHIBIT)
- Skin rashes, ulcerations
- Dry, leather-like skin

SEXUALITY
- Sexual concerns such as impact on relationship, change in level of satisfaction, impotence, menopausal symptoms
- Nulligravida greater than 30 years of age, multigravida
- Multiple sex partners, early sexual activity, genital herpes
- Exposure to human papillomavirus (HPV)

SOCIAL INTERACTION
- Inadequate or weak support system
- Marital history regarding in-home satisfaction, support, or help
- Concerns about role function and responsibility

TEACHING/LEARNING
- Family history of cancer, for example multiple family members—mother, grandmother, aunt, or sister—with breast cancer
- Primary site, date discovered or diagnosed
- Metastatic disease—additional sites involved (if none, natural history of primary will provide important information for looking for metastasis)
- Treatment history—previous treatment for cancer—place and treatments given

DISCHARGE PLAN CONSIDERATIONS
- May require assistance with finances, medications, treatments, wound care and supplies, transportation, food shopping and preparation, self-care, homemaker or maintenance tasks, provision for childcare, changes in living facilities, or hospice

▶ Refer to section at end of plan for postdischarge considerations.

Test selection depends on history, clinical manifestations, and index of suspicion for a particular cancer.

TEST WHY IT IS DONE	WHAT IT TELLS ME
BLOOD TESTS • *Tumor markers:* Substances produced and secreted by tumor cells and found in serum; for example, carcinoembryonic antigen (CEA), prostate-specific antigen (PSA), α-fetoprotein (AFP), human chorionic gonadotropin (hCG), CA15-3, CA19-9, and CA125.	Helpful in diagnosing cancer but more useful as prognostic indicator and/or therapeutic monitor. For example, CA125 levels are monitored in ovarian cancer with levels often high prior to surgery, but should be lower after surgery or with a response to chemotherapy. If the cancer begins to grow, the CA125 level will usually begin to increase before any other signs or symptoms are evident.
• *Hormone receptors:* Estrogen and progesterone receptor assay done on breast tissue.	Provides information about whether or not hormonal manipulation can be therapeutic in breast cancer treatment.
• *Her-2/neu amplification:* Cellular proto-oncogene that stimulates cell growth.	Amplification (a large number of these receptors found on the cell surface) results in more aggressive breast cancers and, usually, a worse prognosis with earlier appearance of metastatic disease.
• *Gene mutations:* BRCA-1 and BRCA-2 function as tumor suppressor genes.	If these genes are mutated, there may be an increased lifetime risk of acquiring breast, ovarian, prostatic, and possibly other cancers.
• *Complete blood count (CBC):* Battery of screening tests, which typically includes hemoglobin (Hgb); hematocrit (Hct); red blood cell (RBC) count, morphology, indices, and distribution width index; platelet count and size; and white blood cell (WBC) count and differential.	May reveal anemia; changes in RBCs and WBCs; and reduced or increased platelets.
OTHER DIAGNOSTIC STUDIES • *Scans—magnetic resonance imaging (MRI), computed tomography (CT), positron emission tomography (PET), or ultrasound:* May be done for diagnostic purposes, identification of metastasis, and evaluation of response to treatment.	Knowledge of the etiology and natural history or pattern of metastasis of a cancer type is important in planning the client's care and in evaluating the client's progress, prognosis, and physical complaints.
• *Biopsy—fine-needle aspiration (FNA), needle core, incisional or excisional:* May be taken from various sites, such as bone marrow (e.g., leukemia), skin, or organ.	Differentiates diagnosis and delineates treatment options.

Nursing Priorities

1. Support adaptation and independence.
2. Promote comfort.
3. Maintain optimal physiological functioning.
4. Prevent complications.
5. Provide information about disease process, condition, prognosis, and treatment needs.

Discharge Goals

1. Dealing with current situation realistically.
2. Pain alleviated or controlled.
3. Homeostasis achieved.
4. Complications prevented or minimized.
5. Disease process, condition, prognosis, and therapeutic choices and regimen understood.
6. Plan in place to meet needs after discharge.

NURSING DIAGNOSIS: **Fear/Anxiety [specify level]**

May be related to
Situational crisis—cancer
Threat to, or change in, health, socioeconomic status, role functioning, interaction patterns
Threat of death
Separation from family—hospitalization, treatments
Interpersonal transmission or contagion of feelings

NURSING DIAGNOSIS: Fear/Anxiety [specify level] (continued)

Possibly evidenced by

Increased tension, shakiness, apprehension, restlessness, insomnia

Expressed concerns regarding changes in life events

Feelings of helplessness, hopelessness, inadequacy

Sympathetic stimulation, somatic complaints

Desired Outcomes/Evaluation Criteria—Client Will

Fear [or] Anxiety Self-Control (NOC)

Display appropriate range of feelings and lessened fear.

Appear relaxed and report anxiety is reduced to a manageable level.

Demonstrate use of effective coping mechanisms and active participation in treatment regimen.

ACTIONS/INTERVENTIONS	RATIONALE
Anxiety Reduction (NIC)	
Independent	
Review client's and significant other's (SO's) previous experience with cancer. Determine what the doctor has told client and what conclusion client has reached.	Clarifies client's perceptions; assists in identification of fear(s) and misconceptions based on diagnosis and experience with cancer.
Encourage client to share thoughts and feelings.	Provides opportunity to examine realistic fears and misconceptions about diagnosis.
Provide open environment in which client feels safe to discuss feelings or to refrain from talking.	Helps client feel accepted in present condition without feeling judged and promotes sense of dignity and control.
Maintain frequent contact with client. Talk with and touch client, as appropriate.	Provides assurance that the client is not alone or rejected; conveys respect for and acceptance of the person, fostering trust.
Be aware of effects of isolation on client when required by immunosuppression or radiation implant. Limit use of isolation clothing, as possible.	Sensory deprivation may result when sufficient stimulation is not available and may intensify feelings of anxiety, fear, and alienation.
Assist client and SO in recognizing and clarifying fears to begin developing coping strategies for dealing with these fears.	Coping skills are often stressed after diagnosis and during different phases of treatment. Support and counseling are often necessary to enable individual to recognize and deal with fear and to realize that control and coping strategies are available.
Provide accurate, consistent information regarding diagnosis and prognosis. Avoid arguing about client's perceptions of situation.	Can reduce anxiety and enable client to make decisions and choices based on realities.
Permit expressions of anger, fear, and despair without confrontation. Give information that feelings are normal and are to be appropriately expressed.	Acceptance of feelings allows client to begin to deal with situation.
Explain the recommended treatment, its purpose, and potential side effects. Help client prepare for treatments.	The goal of cancer treatment is to destroy malignant cells while minimizing damage to normal ones. Treatment may include curative, preventive, or palliative surgery as well as chemotherapy, internal or external radiation, or newer, organ-specific treatments such as whole-body hyperthermia or biotherapy. Bone marrow or peripheral progenitor cell transplant may be recommended for some types of cancer.
Explain procedures, providing opportunity for questions and honest answers. Stay with client during anxiety-producing procedures and consultations.	Accurate information allows client to deal more effectively with reality of situation, thereby reducing anxiety and fear of the unknown.
Provide primary and consistent caregivers whenever possible.	May help reduce anxiety by fostering therapeutic relationship and facilitating continuity of care.
Provide calm, quiet environment.	Facilitates rest, conserves energy, and may enhance coping abilities.
Identify stage and degree of grief client and SO are currently experiencing. (Refer to ND: Grieving, following.)	Choice of interventions is dictated by stage of grief and negative coping behaviors, such as anger, withdrawal, and denial.
Note ineffective coping such as poor social interactions, helplessness, giving up everyday functions, and usual sources of gratification.	Identifies individual problems and provides support for client and SO in using effective coping skills.
Be alert to signs of denial or depression, such as withdrawal and anger, or making inappropriate remarks. Determine presence of suicidal ideation and assess potential on a scale of 1 to 10.	Client may use defense mechanism of denial and express hope that diagnosis is inaccurate. Feelings of guilt, spiritual distress, physical symptoms, or lack of cure may cause the client to become withdrawn and believe that suicide is a viable alternative.

(continues on page 852)

Encourage and foster client interaction with support systems, including counselors, spiritual leader, and local cancer resources.

Reduces feelings of isolation. If family support systems are not available, outside sources may be needed immediately.

Provide reliable and consistent information and support for SO.

Allows for better interpersonal interaction and reduction of anxiety and fear.

Include SO as indicated and client desires when major decisions are to be made.

Provides a support system for the client and allows the SO to be involved appropriately.

Collaborative

Administer anti-anxiety medications, such as lorazepam (Ativan) or alprazolam (Xanax), as indicated.

May be useful for brief periods of time to help client handle feelings of anxiety related to diagnosis or situation during periods of high stress, to assist client with diagnostic procedures, such as lying still during scan, and/or to minimize nausea.

Refer to additional resources for counseling and support as needed.

May be useful from time to time to assist client and SO in dealing with anxiety.

NURSING DIAGNOSIS: Grieving

May be related to

Anticipated loss of physiological well-being—loss of body part, change in body function; change in lifestyle
Perceived potential death of client

Possibly evidenced by

Changes in eating habits, sleep patterns, activity level, libido, and communication patterns
Denial of potential loss, choked feelings, anger

Desired Outcomes/Evaluation Criteria—Client Will

Grief Resolution (NOC)
Identify and express feelings appropriately.
Continue normal life activities, looking toward and planning for the future, one day at a time.
Verbalize reality and acceptance of situation.

ACTIONS/INTERVENTIONS

RATIONALE

Grief Work Facilitation (NIC)
Independent

Expect initial shock and disbelief following diagnosis of cancer and/or traumatizing procedures such as disfiguring surgery, colostomy, and amputation.

Few clients are fully prepared for the reality of the changes that can occur.

Assess client and SO for stage of grief currently being experienced. Explain process, as appropriate.

Knowledge about the grieving process reinforces the normalcy of feelings and reactions being experienced, helping client deal more effectively with them.

Provide open, nonjudgmental environment. Use therapeutic communication skills of active-listening, acknowledgment, and so on.

Promotes and encourages realistic dialogue about feelings and concerns.

Encourage verbalization of thoughts and concerns, accepting expressions of sadness, anger, and rejection. Acknowledge normalcy of these feelings.

Client may feel supported in expression of feelings by the understanding that deep and often conflicting emotions are normal and experienced by others in this difficult situation.

Be aware of mood swings, evidence of conflict, expressions of anger or hostility, and other acting-out behavior. Set limits on inappropriate behavior and redirect negative thinking.

May be client's way of expressing or dealing with feelings of despair and spiritual distress reflecting ineffective coping and need for additional interventions. Preventing destructive actions enables client to maintain control and sense of self-esteem.

Note signs of debilitating depression. Ask client direct questions about state of mind. Listen for statements of despair, guilt, and hopelessness, such as "There's nothing to live for."

Studies show that many cancer clients are at higher risk for suicide (Miller et al, 2008; Misono et al, 2008). They are especially vulnerable when recently diagnosed and/or discharged from hospital.

Reinforce teaching regarding disease process and treatments. Be honest; do not give false hope while providing emotional support.

Client and SO benefit from factual information. Honest answers promote trust and provide reassurance that correct information will be given.

Review past life experiences, role changes, and coping skills.

Opportunity to identify skills that may help individuals cope with grief of current situation more effectively.

ACTIONS/INTERVENTIONS (continued)	RATIONALE (continued)

Hope Instillation (NIC)

Identify positive aspects of the situation.

Possibility of remission and slow progression of disease and/or new therapies can offer hope for the future.

Discuss ways client and SO can plan together for the future. Encourage setting of realistic goals.

Having a part in problem-solving and planning can provide a sense of control over anticipated events.

Assist client and SO to identify strengths in self, situation, and support systems.

Recognizing these resources provides opportunity to work through feelings of grief.

Encourage participation in care and treatment decisions.

Allows client to retain some control over life.

Refer to appropriate counselor as needed, such as psychiatric clinical nurse specialist, social worker, hospice counselor, psychologist, and clergy.

Can help alleviate distress or palliate feelings of grief to facilitate coping and foster growth.

Collaborative

Refer to visiting nurse, home health agency as needed, or hospice program, if appropriate.

Provides support in meeting physical and emotional needs of client and SO, and can supplement the care family and friends are able to give.

Refer to CP: End of Life/Hospice Care, ND: anticipatory Grieving/death Anxiety, for additional interventions.

NURSING DIAGNOSIS: **situational low Self-Esteem**

May be related to

Biophysical—disfiguring surgery and chemotherapy or radiotherapy side effects, such as loss of hair, nausea, vomiting, weight loss, anorexia, impotence, sterility, overwhelming fatigue, and uncontrolled pain

Psychosocial—threat of death, feelings of lack of control, doubt regarding acceptance by others, and fear and anxiety

Possibly evidenced by

Verbalization of change in lifestyle, fear of rejection or reaction of others, negative feelings about body, feelings of helplessness, hopelessness, powerlessness

Preoccupation with change or loss

Not taking responsibility for self-care, lack of follow-through

Change in self-perception and other's perception of role

Desired Outcomes/Evaluation Criteria—Client Will

Self-Esteem (NOC)

Verbalize understanding of body changes, acceptance of self in situation.

Begin to develop coping mechanisms to deal effectively with problems.

Demonstrate adaptation to changes and events that have occurred as evidenced by setting of realistic goals and active participation in work, play, and personal relationships, as appropriate.

ACTIONS/INTERVENTIONS	RATIONALE

Chemotherapy [or] Radiation Therapy Management (NIC)

Independent

Discuss with client and SO how the diagnosis and treatment are affecting the client's personal life and home and work activities.

Aids in defining concerns to begin problem-solving process.

Review anticipated side effects associated with a particular treatment, such as alopecia or disfiguring surgery, including possible effects on sexual activity and sense of attractiveness or desirability. Tell client that not all side effects occur and that others may be minimized.

Anticipatory guidance can help client and SO begin the process of adaptation to new state and to prepare for some side effects such as buying a wig before radiation and scheduling time off from work, as indicated. (Refer to ND: risk for Sexual Dysfunction.)

Encourage discussion of and problem-solve concerns about effects of cancer or cancer treatments on role as homemaker, wage earner, or parent.

May help reduce problems that interfere with acceptance of treatment or aggravate progression of disease.

Acknowledge difficulties client may be experiencing. Give information that counseling is often necessary and important in the adaptation process.

Validates reality of client's feelings and gives permission to take whatever measures are necessary to cope with what is happening.

Evaluate support structures available to and used by client and SO.

Helps with planning for care while hospitalized and after discharge.

Provide emotional support for client and SO during diagnostic tests and treatment phase.

Although some clients adjust to cancer effects or side effects of therapy, many need additional support during this period.

(continues on page 854)

ACTIONS/INTERVENTIONS (continued)

Use touch during interactions, if acceptable to client, and maintain eye contact.

Collaborative

Refer client and SO to supportive group programs, such as I Can Cope, Reach to Recovery, Man to Man Prostate Cancer Group, or Leukemia/Lymphoma Society.

Refer for professional counseling as indicated.

RATIONALE (continued)

Affirmation of individuality and acceptance is important in reducing client's feelings of insecurity and self-doubt.

Group support is usually very beneficial for both client and SO, providing contact with other clients with cancer at various levels of treatment and/or recovery, validating feelings, and assisting with problem-solving.

May be necessary to regain and maintain a positive psychosocial structure if client and SO support systems are deteriorating.

NURSING DIAGNOSIS: acute/chronic Pain

May be related to
Disease process—compression or destruction of nerve tissue, infiltration of nerves or their vascular supply, obstruction of a nerve pathway, inflammation, metastasis to bones
Side effects of various cancer therapy agents

Possibly evidenced by
Reports of pain
Self-focusing, narrowed focus
Alteration in muscle tone; facial mask of pain
Distraction/guarding behaviors
Autonomic responses, restlessness (acute pain)

Desired Outcomes/Evaluation Criteria—Client Will

Pain Level (NOC)
Report maximal pain relief or control with minimal interference with activities of daily living (ADLs).

Pain Control (NOC)
Follow prescribed pharmacological regimen.
Demonstrate use of relaxation skills and diversional activities as indicated for individual situation.

ACTIONS/INTERVENTIONS

Pain Management (NIC)
Independent

Determine pain history, for example, location of pain, frequency, duration, and intensity using a rating scale (scale of 0–10), or verbal rating scale—"no pain" to "excruciating pain"; and relief measures used. Believe client's report.

Determine timing and precipitants of "breakthrough" pain when using around-the-clock agents, whether oral, intravenous (IV), topical, transmucosal, epidural, or patch medications.

Evaluate painful effects of particular therapies, such as surgery, radiation, chemotherapy, or biotherapy. Provide information to client and SO about what to expect.

Provide nonpharmacological comfort measures such as massage, repositioning, and back rub; as well as diversional activities, such as music, reading, and TV.

Encourage use of stress management skills and complementary therapies such as relaxation techniques, visualization, guided imagery, biofeedback, laughter, music, aromatherapy, and Therapeutic Touch.

Provide cutaneous stimulation, such as heat and cold packs, or massage.

RATIONALE

Information provides baseline data to evaluate need for, and effectiveness of, interventions. Pain of more than 6 months' duration constitutes chronic pain, which may affect therapeutic choices. Recurrent episodes of acute pain can occur within chronic pain, requiring increased level of intervention. *Note:* The pain experience is an individualized one composed of both physical and emotional responses.

Pain may occur near the end of the dose interval, indicating need for higher dose or shorter dose interval. Pain may be precipitated by identifiable triggers, or occur spontaneously, requiring use of short half-life agents for rescue or supplemental doses.

A wide range of discomforts are common such as incisional pain, burning skin, low back pain, mouth sores, or headaches, depending on the procedure or agent being used. Pain is also associated with invasive procedures to diagnose or treat cancer.

Promotes relaxation and helps refocus attention.

Enables client to participate actively in nondrug treatment of pain and enhances sense of control. Pain produces stress and, in conjunction with muscle tension and internal stressors, increases client's focus on self, which in turn increases the level of pain.

May decrease inflammation, muscle spasms, reducing associated pain.

ACTIONS/INTERVENTIONS (continued)

Be aware of barriers to cancer pain management related to client, as well as the healthcare system.

Evaluate pain relief at regular intervals. Adjust medication regimen as necessary.
Inform client and SO of the expected therapeutic effects and discuss management of side effects.

Collaborative
Discuss use of alternative or complementary therapies, such as acupuncture, if client desires.
Develop individualized pain management plan with the client and physician. Provide written copy of plan to client, family and SO, and care providers.

Administer analgesics, as indicated, for example:

Opioids such as codeine, morphine (MSContin, Kadian), oxycodone (oxycontin), hydrocodone (Vicodin), hydromorphone (Dilaudid), methadone (Dolophine), fentanyl (Duragesic, Actiq, Fentora), or oxymorphone (Numorphan, Opana)

Acetaminophen (Tylenol) and nonsteroidal anti-inflammatory drugs (NSAIDs), including aspirin, ibuprofen (Motrin, Advil), peroxicam (Feldene), or indomethacin (Indocin)
Corticosteroids, such as dexamethasone (Decadron) or prednisone

Anticonvulsants, such as phenytoin (Dilantin), valproic acid (Depakote), clonazepam (Klonopin), gabapentin (Neurontin), or pregabalin (Lyrica)
Antidepressants, such as amitriptyline (Elavil), imipramine (Tofranil), doxepin (Sinequan), trazodone (Desyrel), or duloxetine (Cymbalta)
Antihistamines, such as hydroxyzine (Atarax, Vistaril)

Radioisotopes, such as strontium-89 (Metastron) or Samarium SM 153 lexidronam (Quadramet)

Bisphosphonates, such as Pamidronate (Aredia) or zoledronic acid (Zometa)

Provide and instruct in use of PCA, as appropriate.

Instruct in use of electrical stimulation (e.g., transcutaneous electrical nerve stimulation [TENS]) unit.

RATIONALE (continued)

Clients may be reluctant to report pain for reasons such as fear that disease is worse; worry about unmanageable side effects of pain medications; belief that pain has meaning, such as "God wills it," they should overcome it; or that pain is merited or deserved for some reason. Healthcare system problems include factors such as inadequate assessment of pain, concern about controlled substances or client addiction, inadequate reimbursement, and cost of treatment modalities.
Goal is maximum pain control with minimum interference with ADLs.
This information helps establish realistic expectations and confidence in own ability to handle what happens.

May provide reduction or relief of pain without drug-related side effects.
An organized plan beginning with the simplest dosage schedules and least invasive modalities improves chance for pain control. Particularly with chronic pain, client and SO must be active participant in pain management and all care providers need to be consistent.
A wide range of analgesics and associated agents may be employed around the clock to manage pain. *Note:* Addiction to or dependency on drug is not a concern.
Effective for localized and generalized moderate to severe pain, with long-acting or controlled-release forms available. Routes of administration include oral; transmucosal; transdermal; nasal; rectal; and subcutaneous, IV, epidural, and intrathecal infusions, which may be delivered via patient-controlled analgesia (PCA). Fentanyl citrate (Oralet) is available as a transmucosal agent that is absorbed through the mucosa of the inner cheek. *Note:* Intramuscular (IM) route is not recommended for pain medications because absorption is not reliable, in addition to being painful and inconvenient.
Adjuvant drugs are useful for mild to moderate pain and can be combined with opioid and other modalities.

May be effective in controlling pain associated with inflammatory process including metastatic bone pain, acute spinal cord compression, and neuropathic pain.
Useful for peripheral pain syndromes associated with neuropathic pain, especially shooting pain, postherpetic neuralgia.

Effective for neuropathic pain (e.g., tingling, burning pain) and pain resulting from surgery, chemotherapy, or nerve infiltration.
Mild anxiolytic agent with sedative and analgesic properties. May produce additive analgesia with therapeutic doses of opioids and may be beneficial in limiting opioid-induced nausea or vomiting.
Effective in treating pain resulting from osteoblastic metastatic bone lesions. Drug onset is about 1 week with duration of 2 to 4 months. May help reduce dosage of opioid analgesics. *Note:* Bone marrow, WBC, and platelet counts may be suppressed for up to 8 weeks after administration of the drug.
Specific inhibitors of osteoclastic activity that treat hypercalcemia and reduce bone pain and fractures especially in multiple myeloma, breast, and prostate cancers.
Provides for timely drug administration, preventing fluctuations in intensity of pain, often at lower total dosage than would be given by conventional methods.
TENS blocks nerve transmission of pain stimulus, providing reduction and relief of pain without drug-related side effects. Can be used in combination with other modalities.

(continues on page 856)

Prepare for and assist with procedures such as nerve blocks, cordotomy, commissural myelotomy, or radiation therapy.

May be used in severe, intractable pain unresponsive to other measures. *Note:* Radiation is especially useful for bone metastasis and may provide fast onset of pain relief even with only one treatment.

Refer to structured support group, psychiatric clinical nurse specialist, psychologist, or spiritual advisor for counseling, as indicated.

May be necessary to reduce anxiety and enhance client's coping skills, decreasing level of pain. *Note:* Hypnosis can heighten awareness and help to focus concentration to decrease perception of pain.

NURSING DIAGNOSIS: imbalanced Nutrition: Less than Body Requirements

May be related to
Hypermetabolic state associated with cancer
Consequences of chemotherapy, radiation, surgery—anorexia, gastric irritation, taste distortions, nausea
Emotional distress, fatigue, poorly controlled pain

Possibly evidenced by
Reported inadequate food intake, altered taste sensation, loss of interest in food, perceived or actual inability to ingest food, vomiting
Body weight 20% or more under ideal for height and frame, decreased subcutaneous fat and muscle mass
Sore, inflamed buccal cavity
Diarrhea and/or constipation, abdominal cramping

Desired Outcomes/Evaluation Criteria—Client Will

Nutritional Status (NOC)
Demonstrate stable weight or progressive weight gain toward goal with normalization of laboratory values and be free of signs of malnutrition.

Knowledge: Diet (NOC)
Verbalize understanding of individual interferences to adequate intake.
Participate in specific interventions to stimulate appetite and increase dietary intake.

ACTIONS/INTERVENTIONS

RATIONALE

Nutrition Therapy (NIC)
Independent
Monitor daily food intake and have client keep food diary, as indicated.

Identifies nutritional strengths and deficiencies.

Measure height, weight, and skinfold thickness, or other anthropometric measurements, as appropriate. Ascertain amount of recent weight loss. Weigh daily or as indicated.

If these measurements fall below minimum standards, client's chief source of stored energy, fat tissue, is depleted.

Assess skin and mucous membranes for pallor, delayed wound healing, and enlarged parotid glands.

Helps in identification of protein-calorie malnutrition, especially when weight and anthropometric measurements are less than normal.

Encourage client to eat high-calorie, nutrient-rich diet, with adequate fluid intake. Encourage use of supplements and frequent, smaller meals spaced throughout the day.

Metabolic tissue and needs are increased as to eliminate waste products. Supplements can play an important role in maintaining adequate caloric and protein intake.

Create pleasant dining atmosphere; encourage client to share meals with family and friends.

Makes mealtime more enjoyable, which may enhance intake.

Encourage open communication regarding anorexia.

Often a source of emotional distress, especially for SO who wants to feed client frequently. When client refuses, SO may feel rejected or frustrated.

Chemotherapy Management (NIC)
Adjust diet before and immediately after treatment such as clear, cool liquids; light or bland foods; candied ginger; dry crackers; toast; and carbonated drinks. Give liquids 1 hour before or 1 hour after meals.

The effectiveness of diet adjustment is very individualized in relief of post-therapy nausea. Clients must experiment to find best solution and combinations. Avoiding fluids during meals minimizes becoming "full" too quickly.

Control environmental factors, such as strong or noxious odors and noise. Avoid overly sweet, fatty, or spicy foods.

Can trigger nausea and vomiting response.

Encourage use of relaxation techniques, visualization, guided imagery, and moderate exercise before meals.

May prevent onset or reduce severity of nausea, decrease anorexia, and enable client to increase oral intake.

ACTIONS/INTERVENTIONS (continued)	RATIONALE (continued)

Identify the client who experiences anticipatory nausea or vomiting, and take appropriate measures.

Psychogenic nausea and vomiting occurring before chemotherapy generally does not respond to antiemetic drugs. Change of treatment environment or client routine on treatment day may be effective.

Evaluate effectiveness of antiemetic agents.

Individuals respond differently to all medications. First-line antiemetics may not work, requiring alteration in or use of combination drug therapy.

Hematest stools and gastric secretions.

Certain therapies, such as antimetabolites, inhibit renewal of epithelial cells lining the gastrointestinal (GI) tract, which may cause changes ranging from mild erythema to severe ulceration with bleeding.

Collaborative

Review laboratory studies, as indicated, such as total lymphocyte count, serum transferrin, and albumin or prealbumin.

Helps identify the degree of biochemical imbalance or malnutrition and influences choice of dietary interventions. *Note:* Anticancer treatments can also alter nutrition studies, so all results must be correlated with the client's clinical status.

Administer medications, as indicated, for example:

5-HT3 receptor antagonists, such as ondansetron (Zofran), granisetron (Kytril), dolasetron (Anzemet), and palonosetron (Aloxi); NK-1 receptor antagonist aprepitant (Emend); phenothiazines, such as prochlorperazine (Compazine) and thiethylperazine (Torecan); antidopaminergics such as metoclopramide (Reglan); antihistamines, such as diphenhydramine (Benadryl); and cannabinoids such as dronabinol (Marinol)

Most antiemetics act to interfere with stimulation of true vomiting center, and chemoreceptor trigger zone agents also act peripherally to inhibit reverse peristalsis. These medications are often prescribed routinely before, during, and after chemotherapy to prevent nausea and vomiting.

Corticosteroids such as dexamethasone (Decadron); benzodiazepines such as lorazepam (Ativan); and butyrophenones, such as haloperidol (Haldol) or droperidol (Inapsine)

Combination therapy such as Compazine with Decadron and/or Ativan is often more effective than single agents.

Vitamins, especially A, D, and B_6

Prevents deficit related to decreased absorption of fat-soluble vitamins. Deficiency of B_6 can contribute to or exacerbate depression, irritability, and neuropathy. *Note:* Some medical providers recommend avoiding such antioxidants as E and C because they may interfere with chemotherapy and radiation.

Antacids and/or proton pump inhibitors such as esomeprazole (Nexium), lansoprazole (Prevacid), or pantoprazole (Protonix)

Minimizes gastric irritation, decreases nausea, and reduces risk of mucosal ulceration.

Administer antiemetic on a regular schedule before or during and after administration of antineoplastic agent and radiation, as appropriate.

Nausea and vomiting are frequently the most disabling and psychologically stressful side effects of chemotherapy.

Nutrition Therapy (NIC)

Refer to dietitian or nutritional support team.

Provides for specific dietary plan to meet individual needs and reduce problems associated with protein or calorie malnutrition and micronutrient deficiencies.

Insert and maintain nasogastric (NG) or feeding tube for enteric feedings, or central line for total parenteral nutrition (TPN), if indicated.

In the presence of severe malnutrition (e.g., loss of 25%–30% body weight) or if client has been nothing-by-mouth status (NPO) for 5 days and is unlikely to be able to eat for another week, tube feeding or TPN may be necessary to meet nutritional needs.

NURSING DIAGNOSIS: risk for deficient Fluid Volume

Risk factors may include
Excessive losses through normal routes—vomiting, diarrhea; and/or abnormal routes—indwelling tubes, wounds, fistulas
Hypermetabolic state
Impaired intake of fluids

Possibly evidenced by
(Not applicable; presence of signs and symptoms establishes an *actual* diagnosis)

Desired Outcomes/Evaluation Criteria—Client Will

Hydration (NOC)
Display adequate fluid balance as evidenced by stable vital signs, moist mucous membranes, good skin turgor, prompt capillary refill, and individually adequate urinary output.

ACTIONS/INTERVENTIONS	RATIONALE

Fluid/Electrolyte Management (NIC)

Independent

Monitor intake and output (I&O) and specific gravity. Include all output sources, such as emesis, diarrhea, or draining wounds. Calculate 24-hour balance.	Continued negative fluid balance, decreasing renal output, and concentration of urine suggest developing dehydration and need for increased fluid replacement.
Weigh, as indicated.	Sensitive measurement of fluctuations in fluid balance.
Monitor vital signs. Evaluate peripheral pulses and capillary refill.	Reflects adequacy of circulating volume.
Assess skin turgor and moisture of mucous membranes. Note reports of thirst.	Indirect indicators of hydration status and degree of deficit.
Encourage increased fluid intake as individually appropriate and tolerated.	Assists in maintenance of fluid requirements and reduces risk of harmful side effects such as hemorrhagic cystitis in client receiving cyclophosphamide (Cytoxan).
Observe for bleeding tendencies, such as oozing from mucous membranes or puncture sites and presence of ecchymosis or petechiae.	Early identification of problems that may occur as a result of cancer and/or therapies, allows for prompt intervention.
Minimize venipunctures such as combining IV starts with blood draws. Encourage client to consider central or peripheral venous catheter placement.	Reduces potential for hemorrhage and infection associated with repeated venous puncture.
Avoid trauma and apply pressure to puncture sites.	Reduces potential for bleeding and hematoma formation.

Collaborative

Provide IV fluids as indicated.	Given for general hydration and to dilute antineoplastic drugs and reduce adverse side effects—nausea, vomiting, or nephrotoxicity.
Administer antiemetic therapy. (Refer to ND: imbalanced Nutrition: Less than Body Requirements.)	Alleviation of nausea and vomiting decreases gastric losses and allows for increased oral intake.
Monitor laboratory studies, such as CBC, electrolytes, and serum albumin.	Provides information about level of hydration and corresponding deficits. *Note:* Malnutrition and effects of decreased albumin levels potentiates fluid shifts or edema formation.
Administer transfusions, as indicated:	
RBCs	May be needed to restore blood count and prevent manifestations of anemia often present in cancer clients, such as tachycardia, tachypnea, dizziness, and weakness.
Platelets	Thrombocytopenia may occur as a side effect of chemotherapy, radiation, or cancer process increasing the risk of bleeding from mucous membranes and other body sites. Spontaneous bleeding may occur with platelet count of 5,000.
Avoid use of aspirin, gastric irritants, platelet inhibitors, or herbs such as ginseng, green tea, garlic, ginger, ginkgo, or willow bark.	These substances can negatively affect clotting mechanism and/or potentiate risk of bleeding.

NURSING DIAGNOSIS: **Fatigue**

May be related to

Decreased metabolic energy production, increased energy requirements— hypermetabolic state, effects of treatment
Overwhelming psychological and emotional demands
Altered body chemistry—side effects of pain and other medications, chemotherapy, radiation therapy, biotherapy

Possibly evidenced by

Unremitting, overwhelming lack of energy; inability to maintain usual routines, decreased performance, impaired ability to concentrate, lethargy, listlessness
Disinterest in surroundings

Desired Outcomes/Evaluation Criteria—Client Will

Endurance (NOC)
Report improved sense of energy.
Perform ADLs and participate in desired activities at level of ability.

ACTIONS/INTERVENTIONS	RATIONALE

Energy Management (NIC)

Independent

Have client rate fatigue, using a numeric scale, if possible, and the time of day when it is most severe.	Helps in developing a plan for managing CRF to improve client's quality of life (de Nijs et al, 2008).

ACTIONS/INTERVENTIONS (continued)

Plan care to allow for rest and uninterupted sleep periods. Schedule activities for periods when client has most energy. Involve client and SO in schedule planning.

Establish realistic activity goals with client.

Assist with self-care needs when indicated; keep bed in low position and pathways clear of furniture; and assist with ambulation.

Encourage client to do whatever possible, such as self-bathing, sitting up in chair, and walking. Increase activity level as individual is able.

Encourage aerobic exercise, as client is able, with goal of 30 minutes per day.

Monitor physiological response to activity, such as changes in BP or heart and respiratory rate.

Perform pain assessment and provide pain management.

Encourage nutritional intake. (Refer to ND: imbalanced Nutrition: Less than Body Requirements.)

Encourage adequate fluid intake. (Refer to ND: risk for deficient Fluid Volume.)

Collaborative

Provide supplemental oxygen, as indicated.

Refer to physical and occupational therapy.

RATIONALE (continued)

Frequent rest periods and/or naps are needed to conserve and restore energy. Planning will allow client to be active during times when energy level is higher, which may restore a feeling of well-being and a sense of control.

Provides for a sense of control and feelings of accomplishment.

Weakness may make ADLs difficult to complete or place the client at risk for injury during activities.

Enhances strength and stamina and enables client to become more active without undue fatigue.

Aerobic exercise minimizes fatigue, increases strength and stamina, and stimulates release of natural endorphins, which promotes sense of well-being.

Tolerance varies greatly depending on the stage of the disease process, nutrition state, fluid balance, and reaction to therapeutic regimen.

Poorly managed cancer pain can contribute to fatigue.

Adequate intake and use of nutrients is necessary to meet energy needs and build energy reserves for activity.

Prevents dehydration, which increases fatigue.

Presence of anemia or hypoxemia reduces O_2 available for cellular uptake and contributes to fatigue.

Programmed daily exercises and activities help client maintain or increase strength and muscle tone and enhance sense of well-being. Use of adaptive devices may help conserve energy.

NURSING DIAGNOSIS: risk for Infection

Risk factors may include

Inadequate secondary defenses and immunosuppression such as bone marrow suppression—dose-limiting side effect of both chemotherapy and radiation

Malnutrition; chronic disease process

Invasive procedures

Possibly evidenced by

(Not applicable; presence of signs and symptoms establishes an *actual* diagnosis)

Desired Outcomes/Evaluation Criteria—Client Will

Immune Status (NOC)

Remain afebrile.

Achieve timely healing, as appropriate.

Knowledge: Infection Control (NOC)

Identify and participate in interventions to prevent and reduce risk of infection.

ACTIONS/INTERVENTIONS

RATIONALE

Infection Protection (NIC)
Independent

Promote good hand-washing procedures by staff and visitors. Screen and limit visitors who may have infections.

Emphasize personal hygiene.

Monitor temperature.

Encourage fluids. (Refer to ND: risk for deficient Fluid Volume.)

Protects client from sources of infection, such as visitors and staff who may have an upper respiratory infection (URI).

Limits potential sources of infection.

Temperature elevation may occur, if not masked by corticosteroids or anti-inflammatory drugs, because of various factors including chemotherapy side effects, disease process, or infection. Early identification of infectious process enables appropriate therapy to be started promptly.

Adequate fluid intake enhances immune system and aids natural defense mechanisms.

(continues on page 860)

Assess all systems (e.g., skin, respiratory, genitourinary) for signs and symptoms of infection on a continual basis.

Reposition frequently; keep linens dry and wrinkle free.

Promote adequate rest and exercise periods.

Stress importance of good oral hygiene.

Avoid or limit invasive procedures, as possible. Adhere to aseptic techniques.

Collaborative

Monitor CBC with differential WBC and granulocyte count and platelets, as indicated.

Obtain cultures, as indicated.

Administer antibiotics, as indicated.

Early recognition and intervention may prevent progression to more serious situation such as sepsis.

Reduces pressure and irritation to tissues and may prevent skin breakdown.

Limits fatigue, yet encourages sufficient movement to prevent stasis complications—pneumonia, decubitus ulcers, or thrombus formation.

Development of stomatitis increases risk of infection and secondary overgrowth.

Reduces risk of contamination and limits portal of entry for infectious agents.

Bone marrow activity may be inhibited by effects of chemotherapy, the disease state, or radiation therapy. Monitoring status of myelosuppression is important for preventing further complications, such as infection, anemia, or hemorrhage, and scheduling drug delivery. *Note:* The nadir is usually seen 7 to 10 days after administration of chemotherapy.

Identifies causative organism(s) and appropriate therapy.

May be used to treat identified infection or given prophylactically in immunocompromised client.

NURSING DIAGNOSIS: risk for impaired Oral Mucous Membrane

Risk factors may include

Side effect of some chemotherapeutic agents (e.g., antimetabolites) and radiation

Dehydration, malnutrition, NPO restrictions for more than 24 hours

Possibly evidenced by

(Not applicable; presence of signs and symptoms establishes an *actual* diagnosis)

Desired Outcomes/Evaluation Criteria—Client Will

Oral Hygiene (NOC)

Display intact mucous membranes, which are pink, moist, and free of inflammation or ulcerations.

Self-Care Oral Hygiene (NOC)

Verbalize understanding of causative factors.

Demonstrate techniques to maintain or restore integrity of oral mucosa.

ACTIONS/INTERVENTIONS

RATIONALE

Oral Health Maintenance (NIC)

Independent

Assess dental health and oral hygiene periodically.

Encourage client to assess oral cavity daily, noting changes in mucous membrane integrity. Note reports of burning in the mouth, changes in voice quality, ability to swallow, sense of taste, development of thick saliva, or blood-tinged emesis.

Discuss with client areas needing improvement and demonstrate methods for good oral care.

Initiate and recommend oral hygiene program to include the following:

Avoidance of commercial mouthwashes and lemon or glycerine swabs

Use of mouthwash made from warm water with salt and baking soda; dilute solution of hydrogen peroxide may be used for bleeding or infected tissue

Identifies prophylactic treatment needs before initiation of chemotherapy or radiation and provides baseline data of current oral hygiene for future comparison.

Stomatitis generally occurs 7 to 14 days after treatment begins, but signs may be seen as early as day 3 or 4, especially if there are any preexisting oral problems. The range of response extends from mild erythema to severe ulceration and may extend the length of the GI tract, which can be very painful, can inhibit oral intake, and is potentially life threatening. Early identification enables prompt treatment.

Good care is critical during treatment to control stomatitis complications.

Products containing alcohol or phenol may exacerbate mucous membrane dryness or irritation.

May be soothing to the membranes. Rinsing before meals may improve the client's sense of taste. Rinsing after meals and at bedtime dilutes oral acids and relieves xerostomia.

ACTIONS/INTERVENTIONS (continued)

Brushing with soft toothbrush or foam swab

Flossing gently or use WaterPik cautiously

Keeping lips moist with lip gloss or balm, K-Y Jelly, Chapstick
Use of mints, other hard candy or artificial saliva (Ora-Lube, Salivart), as indicated

Instruct regarding dietary changes such as avoiding hot or spicy foods and acidic juices; suggest use of straw; ingest soft or blenderized foods, popsicles, and ice cream, as tolerated.
Encourage fluid intake as individually tolerated.

Discuss effects of smoking and alcohol intake, if indicated, and address concerns.
Monitor for, and explain to client, signs of oral superinfection such as thrush.

Collaborative
Refer to dentist before initiating chemotherapy or head and neck radiation.
Culture suspicious oral lesions.

Administer medications, as indicated, for example:
Analgesic rinses, such as GelClair, mixture of Koatin, pectin, diphenhydramine [Benadryl], and topical lidocaine [Xylocaine]

Antifungal mouthwash preparation, such as nystatin (Mycostatin) and antibacterial Biotane
Antinausea agents

Opioid analgesics, such as hydromophone (Dilaudid) or morphine

RATIONALE (continued)

Prevents trauma to delicate, fragile tissues. *Note:* Toothbrush should be changed every month.
Removes food particles that can promote bacterial growth. *Note:* Water under pressure has the potential to injure gums and force bacteria under gum line.
Promotes comfort and prevents drying and cracking of tissues.
Stimulates secretions and provides moisture to maintain integrity of mucous membranes, especially in presence of dehydration and reduced saliva production.
Severe stomatitis may interfere with nutritional and fluid intake leading to negative nitrogen balance or dehydration. Dietary modifications may make foods easier to swallow and may feel soothing.
Adequate hydration helps keep mucous membranes moist, preventing drying and cracking.
May cause further irritation and dryness of mucous membranes.
Early recognition provides opportunity for prompt treatment.

Prophylactic examination and repair work before therapy reduce risk of infection.
Identifies organism(s) responsible for oral infections and suggests appropriate drug therapy.

Aggressive analgesia program may be required to relieve intense pain. *Note:* Rinse should be used as a swish-and-spit rather than a gargle, which could anesthetize client's gag reflex.
May be needed to treat or prevent secondary oral infections, such as *Candida, Pseudomonas,* and herpes simplex.
When given before beginning mouth care regimen, may prevent nausea associated with oral stimulation.
May be required for acute episodes of moderate to severe oral pain.

NURSING DIAGNOSIS: **risk for impaired Skin/Tissue Integrity**

Risk factors may include
Effects of radiation and chemotherapy
Immunological deficit
Altered nutritional state; anemia

Possibly evidenced by
(Not applicable; presence of signs and symptoms establishes an *actual* diagnosis)

Desired Outcomes/Evaluation Criteria—Client Will

Risk Control (NOC)
Identify interventions appropriate for specific condition.
Participate in techniques to prevent complications and promote healing, as appropriate.

ACTIONS/INTERVENTIONS

RATIONALE

Chemotherapy [or] Radiation Therapy Management (NIC)
Independent
Assess skin frequently for side effects of cancer therapy; note breakdown and delayed wound healing. Emphasize importance of reporting open areas to caregiver.

A reddening and/or tanning effect called radiation dermatitis may develop within the field of radiation. Dry desquamation with dryness and pruritus, moist desquamation with blistering, ulceration, hair loss, and loss of dermis and sweat glands may also be noted. In addition, skin reactions—allergic rashes, hyperpigmentation, pruritus, increased risk of sunburn, acne-like skin eruptions, and alopecia—may occur with some chemotherapy agents.

(continues on page 862)

ACTIONS/INTERVENTIONS (continued)	RATIONALE (continued)
Bathe with lukewarm water and mild soap.	Maintains cleanliness without irritating the skin.
Encourage client to avoid vigorous rubbing and scratching and to pat skin dry instead of rubbing.	Helps prevent skin friction or trauma to sensitive tissues.
Turn or reposition frequently.	Promotes circulation and prevents undue pressure on skin and tissues.
Review skin care protocol for client receiving radiation therapy:	Designed to minimize trauma to area of radiation therapy.
Avoid rubbing or use of soap, lotions, creams, ointments, powders, or deodorants on area; avoid applying heat or attempting to wash off marks or tattoos placed on skin to pinpoint location for radiation therapy.	These factors can potentiate or otherwise interfere with radiation delivery and may actually increase reaction.
Recommend wearing soft, loose cotton clothing; have female client avoid wearing bra if it creates pressure.	Skin is very sensitive during and after treatment, and all irritation should be avoided to prevent dermal injury.
Apply cornstarch, Aquaphor, Lubriderm, Eucerin, or other water-soluble moisturizing gel to area twice daily or more frequently, as needed.	Helps control dampness or pruritus. Maintenance care is required until skin and tissues have regenerated and are back to normal.
Encourage liberal use of sunblock and breathable, protective clothing.	Protects skin from ultraviolet rays and reduces risk of recall reactions.
Review skin care protocol for client receiving chemotherapy:	
Use appropriate peripheral or central venous catheter, dilute anticancer drug per protocol, and ascertain that IV is infusing well.	Reduces risk of tissue irritation or extravasation of agent into tissues.
Instruct client to notify caregiver promptly of discomfort at IV insertion site.	Development of irritation indicates need for alteration of rate or dilution of chemotherapy and/or change of IV site to prevent more serious reaction.
Assess skin, IV site, and vein for erythema, edema, tenderness, weltlike patches, itching, burning, swelling, soreness, and blisters progressing to ulceration or tissue necrosis.	Presence of phlebitis or extravasation requires immediate discontinuation of antineoplastic agent and medical intervention. *Note:* Vein flare, a localized reaction, may resolve without intervention based on individual reaction.
Wash skin immediately with soap and water if antineoplastic agents are spilled on unprotected skin of client or caregiver.	Dilutes drug to reduce risk of skin irritation and chemical burn.
Advise clients receiving 5-fluorouracil (5-FU) and methotrexate to avoid sun exposure. Withhold methotrexate if sunburn is present.	Sun can cause exacerbation of burn spotting, a side effect of 5-FU, or can cause a red "flash" area with methotrexate, which can exacerbate drug's effect.
Review expected dermatological side effects seen with chemotherapy such as rash, hyperpigmentation, acne-like eruptions, and peeling of skin on palms.	Anticipatory guidance helps decrease concern if side effects do occur.
Inform client that if alopecia occurs, hair could grow back after completion of chemotherapy, but may or may not grow back after radiation therapy.	Anticipatory guidance may help adjustment to, or preparation for, baldness. Men are often as sensitive to hair loss as women. Radiation's effect on hair follicles may be permanent, depending on radiation dosage.
Collaborative	
Administer appropriate antidote if extravasation of IV should occur, for example:	Reduces local tissue damage.
Dimethyl sulfoxide (DMSO)	Some studies suggest benefit with topical DMSO for mitomycin and doxorubicin (Adriamycin). *Note:* Injection of diphenhydramine (Benadryl) may relieve urticaria of vein flare.
Hyaluronidase (Wydase)	Injected subcutaneously for vincristine (Oncovin), vinblastine (Velban), etoposide (VP16), vindesine (Eldisine), vinorelbine (Navelbine), teniposide (Vm26), or paclitaxel (Taxol) infiltration.
Thiosulfate	Injected subcutaneously for nitrogen mustard and large amounts, greater than 20 mL, of concentrated cisplatin.
Apply ice pack or warm compresses per protocol.	Controversial intervention depends on type of agent used. Ice restricts blood flow, keeping drug localized, whereas heat enhances dispersion of neoplastic drug or antidote, minimizing tissue damage.

NURSING DIAGNOSIS: **risk for Constipation/Diarrhea**

Risk factors may include
Irritation of the GI mucosa from either chemotherapy or radiation therapy, malabsorption of fat
Hormone-secreting tumor, carcinoma of colon
Poor fluid intake, low-bulk diet, lack of exercise, use of opioids and antiemetics

Possibly evidenced by
(Not applicable; presence of signs and symptoms establishes an *actual* diagnosis)

Desired Outcomes/Evaluation Criteria—Client Will

Bowel Elimination (NOC)
Maintain usual bowel consistency and pattern.
Verbalize understanding of factors and appropriate interventions or solutions related to individual situation.

ACTIONS/INTERVENTIONS	RATIONALE
Bowel Management (NIC)	
Independent	
Ascertain usual elimination habits.	Data required as baseline for future evaluation of therapeutic needs and effectiveness.
Assess bowel sounds and monitor and record bowel movements (BMs) including frequency and consistency—particularly during first 3 to 5 days of vinca alkaloid therapy, and when on pain and/or nausea medications.	Defines problem—diarrhea or constipation. *Note:* Constipation is one of the earliest manifestations of neurotoxicity.
Monitor I&O and weight.	Dehydration, weight loss, and electrolyte imbalance are complications of diarrhea. Inadequate fluid intake may potentiate constipation.
Encourage adequate fluid intake, increased fiber in diet, and regular exercise.	May reduce potential for constipation by improving stool consistency and stimulating peristalsis; can prevent dehydration associated with diarrhea.
Provide small, frequent meals of foods low in residue if not contraindicated, maintaining needed protein and carbohydrates, such as eggs, cooked cereal (oatmeal), or bland cooked vegetables.	Reduces gastric irritation. Use of low-fiber foods can decrease irritability and provide bowel rest when diarrhea present.
Adjust diet as appropriate—avoid foods high in fat, such as butter, fried foods, and nuts; foods with high-fiber content and those known to cause diarrhea or gas including cabbage, baked beans, and chili; food or fluids high in caffeine; or extremely hot or cold food and fluids.	GI stimulants that may increase gastric motility and frequency of stools.
Check for impaction if client has not had BM in 3 days, or if abdominal distention, cramping, and headache are present.	Further interventions and alternative bowel care may be needed.
Collaborative	
Monitor laboratory studies, such as electrolytes, as indicated.	Electrolyte imbalances may be the result of, or contribute to, altered GI function.
Administer the following, as indicated:	
IV fluids	Prevents dehydration and dilutes chemotherapy agents to diminish side effects.
Antidiarrheal agents	May be indicated to control severe diarrhea.
Stool softeners and laxatives	Prophylactic use may prevent further complications in some clients, such as those who will receive vinca alkaloid, have poor bowel pattern before treatment, or have decreased motility. *Note:* Enemas and suppositories are to be avoided when possible as they increase the potential for infection and are uncomfortable and unpleasant for the client.

Risk factors may include
Knowledge or skill deficit about alternative responses to health-related transitions, altered body function or structure, illness, and medical treatment
Overwhelming fatigue
Fear, anxiety
Lack of privacy and SO

Possibly evidenced by
(Not applicable; presence of signs and symptoms establishes an *actual* diagnosis)

Desired Outcomes/Evaluation Criteria—Client Will

Role Performance (NOC)
Verbalize understanding of effects of cancer and therapeutic regimen on sexuality and measures to correct or deal with problems.
Maintain sexual activity at a desired level as possible.

ACTIONS/INTERVENTIONS

RATIONALE

Sexual Counseling (NIC)
Independent

Discuss with client and SO the nature of sexuality and reactions when it is altered or threatened. Provide information about normality of these problems and that many people find it helpful to seek assistance with adaptation process.

Advise client of side effects of prescribed cancer treatment that are known to affect sexuality.

Provide private time for hospitalized client. Knock on door and receive permission from client and SO before entering.

Acknowledges legitimacy of the problem. Sexuality encompasses the way men and women view themselves as individuals and how they relate between and among themselves in every area of life.

Anticipatory guidance can help client and SO begin the process of adaptation to new state.

Sexual needs do not end because the client is hospitalized. Intimacy needs continue and an open and accepting attiude for the expression of those needs is essential.

Collaborative

Refer to sex therapist, as indicated.

May require additional assistance in dealing with situation.

NURSING DIAGNOSIS: risk for interrupted Family Processes

Risk factors may include
Situational or transitional crises—long-term illness, change in roles or economic status
Developmental—anticipated loss of a family member

Possibly evidenced by
(Not applicable; presence of signs and symptoms establishes an *actual* diagnosis)

Desired Outcomes/Evaluation Criteria—Family Will

Family Coping (NOC)
Express feelings freely.
Demonstrate individual involvement in problem-solving process directed at appropriate solutions for the situation.
Encourage and allow member who is ill to handle situation in own way.

ACTIONS/INTERVENTIONS

RATIONALE

Family Process Maintenance (NIC)
Independent

Note components of family, presence of extended family, and others including friends and neighbors.

Identify patterns of communication in family and patterns of interaction between family members.

Assess role expectations of family members and encourage discussion about them.

Assess energy direction: Are efforts at resolution or problem-solving purposeful or scattered?

Note cultural and religious beliefs.

Listen for expressions of helplessness.

Deal with family members in a warm, caring, respectful way. Provide verbal and written information and reinforce, as necessary.

Encourage appropriate expressions of anger without reacting negatively to them.

Acknowledge difficulties of the situation, such as the diagnosis and treatment of cancer, or possibility of death.

Identify and encourage use of previously successful coping behaviors.

Stress importance of continuous open dialogue between family members.

Helps client and caregiver know who is available to assist with care and provide respite and support.

Provides information about effectiveness of communication and identifies problems that may interfere with family's ability to assist client and adjust positively to diagnosis and treatment of cancer.

Each person may see the situation in own individual manner, and clear identification and sharing of these expectations promote understanding.

Provides clues about interventions that may be appropriate to assist client and family in directing energies in a more effective manner.

Affects client and SO reaction and adjustment to diagnosis, treatment, and outcome of cancer.

Helpless feelings may contribute to difficulty adjusting to diagnosis of cancer and cooperating with treatment regimen.

Provides feelings of empathy and promotes individual's sense of worth and competence in ability to handle current situation.

Feelings of anger are to be expected when individuals are dealing with the difficult, potentially fatal illness of cancer. Appropriate expression enables progress toward resolution of the stages of the grieving process.

Communicates acceptance of the reality the client and family are facing.

Most people have developed effective coping skills that can be useful in dealing with current situation.

Promotes understanding and assists family members to maintain clear communication and resolve problems effectively.

ACTIONS/INTERVENTIONS (continued)

RATIONALE (continued)

Collaborative

Refer to support groups, clergy, and family therapy, as indicated.

May need additional assistance to resolve problems of disorganization that may accompany diagnosis of potentially terminal illness.

NURSING DIAGNOSIS: deficient Knowledge [Learning Need] regarding illness, prognosis, treatment, self-care, and discharge needs

May be related to
Lack of exposure or recall; information misinterpretation, myths
Unfamiliarity with information resources
Cognitive limitation

Possibly evidenced by
Questions, request for information; verbalization of problem
Statement of misconception
Inaccurate follow-through of instructions; development of preventable complications

Desired Outcomes/Evaluation Criteria—Client Will

Knowledge: Disease Process (NOC)
Verbalize accurate information about diagnosis, prognosis, and potential complications at own level of readiness.

Knowledge: Treatment Regimen (NOC)
Verbalize understanding of therapeutic needs.
Correctly perform necessary procedures and explain reasons for the actions.
Initiate necessary lifestyle changes and participate in treatment regimen.
Identify and use available resources appropriately.

ACTIONS/INTERVENTIONS

RATIONALE

Teaching: Disease Process (NIC)
Independent

Review with client and SO understanding of specific diagnosis, treatment alternatives, and future expectations.

Determine client's perception of cancer and cancer treatment(s). Ask about client's own or previous experience or experience with other people who have, or had, cancer.

Provide clear, accurate information in a factual but sensitive manner. Answer questions specifically, but do not bombard with nonessential details.

Provide anticipatory guidance with client and SO regarding treatment protocol, length of therapy, expected results, and possible side effects. Be honest with client.

Provide written materials about cancer, treatment, and available support systems.

Ask client for verbal feedback, and correct misconceptions about individual's type of cancer and treatment choices.
Review specific medication regimen and use of over-the-counter (OTC) drugs.
Outline normally expected limitations, if any, on ADLs including difficulty cooking meals when nauseated or fatigued and loss of work time because of effects of treatments.
Address specific home care needs such as ability to live alone, perform necessary treatments or procedures, and acquire supplies.
Do predischarge home evaluation, as indicated.

Validates current level of understanding, identifies learning needs, and provides knowledge base from which client can make informed decisions.
Aids in identification of ideas, attitudes, fears, misconceptions, and gaps in knowledge about cancer.

Helps with adjustment to the diagnosis of cancer by providing needed information along with time to absorb it. *Note:* Rate and method of giving information may need to be altered to decrease client's anxiety and enhance ability to assimilate information.
Client has the "right to know" and participate in decisions. Accurate and concise information helps to dispel fears and anxiety, helps clarify the expected routine, and enables client to maintain some degree of control.
Anxiety and preoccupation with thoughts about life and death often interfere with client's ability to assimilate adequate information. Written materials provide reinforcement and clarification about information as client needs it.
Misconceptions about cancer may be more disturbing than facts and can interfere with treatments or delay healing.
Enhances ability to manage self-care and avoid potential complications and drug reactions or interactions.
Enables client and SO to begin to put limitations into perspective and plan for, or adapt, as indicated.

Provides information regarding changes that may be needed in current plan of care to meet therapeutic needs.

Aids in transition to home setting by providing information about needed changes in physical layout and the acquisition of needed supplies.

(continues on page 866)

ACTIONS/INTERVENTIONS (continued)	RATIONALE (continued)
Refer to community resources, as indicated, such as social services, home health agencies, Meals on Wheels, local chapter of American Cancer Society, respite care, hospice center, or other services.	Promotes competent self-care and optimal independence. Maintains client in home or desired setting.
Review with client and SO the importance of maintaining optimal nutritional status.	Promotes well-being, facilitates recovery, and is critical in enabling the client to tolerate treatments.
Encourage diet variations and experimentation in meal planning and food preparation such as cooking with sweet juices or wine and serving foods cold or at room temperature, as appropriate.	Creativity may enhance flavor and intake, especially when protein foods taste bitter.
Recommend cookbooks that are designed for cancer clients.	Helps provide specific menu and recipe ideas.
Recommend increased fluid intake and fiber in diet, as well as routine exercise.	Improves consistency of stool and stimulates peristalsis.
Instruct client to assess oral mucous membranes routinely, noting erythema or ulceration.	Early recognition of problems promotes early intervention, minimizing complications that may impair oral intake and provide avenue for systemic infection.
Initiate medical and support referrals for smoking or alcohol cessation program if client desires.	Decreases irritation to mucous membranes, enhances healing, and promotes general well-being.
Advise client concerning skin and hair care: avoid harsh shampoos, hair dyes, permanents, salt water, and chlorinated water; avoid exposure to strong wind and extreme heat or cold; avoid sun exposure to target area for 1 year after end of radiation treatments; and regularly apply sunblock (SPF 15 or greater).	Prevents additional hair damage and skin irritation and may prevent recall reactions.
Review signs and symptoms requiring medical evaluation such as infection, delayed healing, drug reactions, and increased pain; or swelling of face or hands and arms that may worsen when lying down, dyspnea, cough, headache, and visual disturbances suggestive of SVCS.	Early identification and treatment may limit severity of complications. *Note:* The use of central venous access devices for various therapies—chemotherapy, TPN, or antibiotic administration—may cause local vein trauma leading to SVCS days, months, or even years after catheter insertion.
Stress importance of continuing medical follow-up.	Provides ongoing monitoring of progression or resolution of disease process and opportunity for timely diagnosis and treatment of complications and early detection of second malignancies. *Note:* Some complications can develop long after therapy is completed such as pathological fractures, radiation cystitis, or pneumonitis. Periodic thyroid function tests are indicated for clients with radiation to the neck and upper chest because hypothyroidism may develop.
Encourage periodic review of advance directives. Promote inclusion of family and SO in decision-making process.	Client, family, and SO need to reevaluate choices as condition changes and treatment options become available or are exhausted.

POTENTIAL CONSIDERATIONS following acute hospitalization (dependent on client's age, physical condition and presence of complications, personal resources, and life responsibilities)

In addition to Potential Considerations in specific plans of care such as leukemia, mastectomy:
- *ineffective Coping*—situational crises, vulnerability
- *Self-Care Deficit/impaired Home Maintenance*—decreased strength and endurance, pain or discomfort, depression, insufficient finances, unfamiliarity with neighborhood resources, inadequate support systems
- *risk for Caregiver Role Strain*—illness severity of care receiver, significant home care needs, situational stressors, complexity or amount of caregiving tasks
- *acute/chronic Pain*—disease process—compression or destruction of nerve tissue, infiltration of nerves, or their vascular supply, obstruction of a nerve pathway, inflammation
- *ineffective self Health Management*—complexity of therapeutic regimen, economic difficulties, decisional conflict, perceived barriers, powerlessness, social support deficits

---

END-OF-LIFE CARE/HOSPICE

I. Purpose—provides care and support to the client and family in the client's final stage of a terminal illness when a return to health is not possible

II. Indications
    a. Criteria (Allen, 2008)
        i. Physician certification of terminal illness
        ii. Life expectancy of 6 months or less

iii. Presence of a family member or other caregiver continuously in the home when the client is no longer able to safely care for self

  b. Care of the dying person encompasses several dimensions (Malloy et al, 2008).

  i. Management of pain and other physical symptoms—nausea, vomiting, fatigue, anorexia, functional decline

  ii. Psychological and spiritual support

  1. Provide client and family the opportunity to consider the meaning of their lives.

  2. Encourage participation in making plans and shaping the course of their living while preparing for death.

  iii. Bereavement support after death for family

III. Trajectories of Death Appropriate for Hospice Care (Glaser & Strauss, 1968; Lunney, 2007)

  a. Steady decline, short terminal phase, as may occur with certain cancers

  b. Slow decline with periodic crises and then death, as may occur with chronic obstructive pulmonary disease (COPD), heart or kidney failure

  c. Lingering, expected death as expected in frail elderly, dementias, stroke, Parkinson's disease

IV. Barriers to Using Hospice Services (Malloy et al, 2008)

  a. Influence of managed care on end-of-life care

  i. Lack of understanding of hospice goals and services provided

  ii. Delay in referral to services

  b. Client's or family member's denial or avoidance of death; negative perception of hospice

  c. Access to care

  i. Limitations of insurance coverage

  ii. Medicare payment source requires care be provided by a Medicare-certified hospice program.

  d. Lack of continuity of care across care settings

  e. Caregiver fatigue (psychological and physical) that can compromise the care provided in the home

V. Statistics

  a. Availability: There were 4,100 Medicare-certified programs serving 1.2 million clients in 2005 (Lunney, 2007).

  b. Mortality: There are 2.4 million deaths in the United States each year, of which approximately 44% occur in hospitals, 25% in nursing homes, and 25% in the home setting (Ferrell, 2007).

  c. Cost: In 2001, Medicare expenditures for hospice services were $3.6 billion (Hospice Association of America [HAA], 2002).

GLOSSARY

Advance directives: Used to give other people, including healthcare providers, information about client's wishes for medical care, at a time when client is not physically or mentally able to speak for self. The most common types of advance directives are the living will and the durable power of attorney for healthcare.

End-of-life care: General term that refers to the comprehensive care given in the advanced or terminal stages of illness.

Hospice care: Type of care designed to help clients and their families during the final stages of a terminal illness. Hospice treatment is concentrated primarily on maintaining comfort.

Locus of control: The site of control in an individual—internal or external.

Mindfulness: Method of staying in the moment.

Palliative care: Philosophy of care with the goal of improving the quality of life of clients and their families facing life-threatening illness, through the prevention and relief from suffering. This type of care can encompass treatment of disease processes; provides more than comfort care.

Care Setting

Although much of the care of the dying is still provided by nurses in hospitals (primarily in oncology and critical care areas), other care settings are becoming more common including the home, assisted living or extended care facilities, or hospice inpatient units.

Related Concerns

Cancer, page 846

Extended care, page 801

Psychosocial aspects of care, page 749

Client Assessment Database

Data depend on underlying terminal condition, involvement of other body systems, and stage of dying process. Refer to care plan(s) reflecting underlying pathology of terminal condition for specific assessements related to that condition.

DIAGNOSTIC DIVISION MAY REPORT	MAY EXHIBIT
ACTIVITY/REST • Fatigue • General weakness • Sleep disturbances	• Deep sadness • Apathy, withdrawal

(continues on page 868)

DIAGNOSTIC DIVISION MAY REPORT (continued)	MAY EXHIBIT (continued)

ELIMINATION
• Abdominal discomfort
	• *End Stage:*
	  • Constipation (effect of opioids, decreased fluids)
	  • Dark urine, oliguria

EGO INTEGRITY • Inability to care for self and decision to accept hospice services • Feelings of helplessness, hopelessness, sorrow, anger; choked feelings • Fear of the dying process, loss of physical and/or mental abilities • Concern about impact of death on significant other (SO) and family; difficulty coping—client and/or family • Inner conflict about beliefs, meaning of life and death; moral distress • Financial concerns, lack of preparation (e.g., will, power of attorney, funeral)	• Deep sadness, crying, anxiety • Apathy, social isolation, withdrawal • Grieving • Spiritual distress
FOOD/FLUID • Decreasing appetite • Nausea • Anorexia	• Weight loss • Decreased muscle mass, subcutaneous fat • Poor skin turgor, dry mucous membranes • Difficulty swallowing

NEUROLOGICAL	• *End Stage:*
	  • Decreasing level of consciouness (LOC)
	  • Agitation, restlessness
	  • Terminal delirium

PAIN/DISCOMFORT • Acute or chronic pain	• Muscle tension, restlessness • Facial grimacing

RESPIRATION	• *End Stage:*
	  • Adventitious breath sounds—rhonchi, wheezes
	  • Abnormal breathing patterns

SAFETY	• Erythemia over body prominences • Skin breakdown, pressure ulcers • Perineal infection—candidiasis
SOCIAL INTERACTION • Apprehension about caregiver's ability to provide care • Changes in family roles and usual patterns of responsibility • Loneliness	• Altered communication pattern • Difficulty adapting to changes imposed by condition and dying process • Family coping concerns

Nursing Priorities

1. Control pain.
2. Prevent or manage complications.
3. Maintain quality of life as possible.

4. Plans in place to meet client's and family's last wishes such as care setting, advance directives, will, and funeral.

NURSING DIAGNOSIS: acute/chronic Pain

May be related to
Injuring agents—biological, chemical, physical, psychological
Chronic physical disability

Possibly evidenced by
Verbal or coded report, preoccupation with pain
Changes in appetite, eating, weight, sleep patterns, altered ability to continue desired activities; fatigue
Guarded or protective behavior, distraction behavior—pacing, repetitive activities, reduced interaction with others
Facial mask, expressive behavior—restlessness, moaning, crying, irritability
Self-focusing, narrowed focus—altered time perception, impaired thought processes
Alteration in muscle tone—varies from flaccid to rigid
Autonomic responses—diaphoresis, changes in blood pressure (BP), respiration, pulse
Sympathetic mediated responses—temperature, cold, changes of body position, hypersensitivity

Desired Outcomes/Evaluation Criteria—Client Will

Pain Control (NOC)
Report pain is relieved or controlled.
Verbalize methods that provide relief.
Follow prescribed pharmacological regimen.
Demonstrate use of relaxation skills and diversional activities, as indicated.

Family/SO(s) Will

Cooperate in pain management program.

ACTIONS/INTERVENTIONS	RATIONALE
Pain Management (NIC)	
Independent	
Perform a comprehensive pain evaluation, including location, characteristics, onset, duration, frequency, quality, severity using a scale of 0 to 10 or a similar scale, and precipitating or aggravating factors. Note cultural issues impacting reporting and expression of pain. Determine client's acceptable level of pain.	Provides baseline information from which a realistic plan can be developed, keeping in mind that verbal and behavioral cues may have little direct relationship to the degree of pain perceived. *Note:* Often client does not feel the need to be completely pain free but is able to be more functional when pain is at lower level on the pain scale.
Determine possible pathophysiological and psychological causes of pain, such as may be caused by inflammation, fractures, cancer process, surgery, grief, fear, anxiety, or delirium.	Pain is associated with many factors that may be interactive and increase the degree of pain experienced.
Assess client's perception of pain, being aware of client's cognitive status along with behavioral and psychological responses. Determine client's attitude toward, and use of, pain medications and locus of control—internal or external.	Helps identify client's needs, ability to adequately express self, and pain control methods found to be helpful or not helpful in the past. *Note:* Individuals with external locus of control may take little or no responsibility for pain management.
Encourage client and family to express feelings and concerns about opioid use.	Inaccurate information regarding drug use, fear of addiction, or oversedation could impair pain management efforts.
Verify current and past analgesic and drug use, including alcohol.	May provide insight into what has or has not worked in the past or may impact therapy plan.
Assess degree of personal adjustment to diagnosis, such as anger, irritability, withdrawal, and acceptance.	These factors are variable and often affect the perception of pain, ability to cope, and pain management.
Discuss with SO(s) ways in which they can assist client and reduce precipitating factors.	Promotes involvement in care and belief that there are things they can do to help.
Identify specific signs and symptoms and changes in pain requiring notification of healthcare provider and medical intervention.	Unrelieved pain may be associated with progression of terminal disease process or with complications that require medical management.
Involve caregivers in identifying effective comfort measures for client, such as use of nonacidic fluids, oral swabs, lip salve, and suctioning; skin and perineal care; and use of laxatives. Instruct in use of any needed equipment, such as suction and oxygen.	Managing troubling symptoms, such as nausea, dry mouth, dyspnea, and constipation, can reduce client's suffering and family anxiety, thus improving quality of life and allowing client and family to focus on other issues.
Demonstrate and encourage use of relaxation techniques such as guided imagery, music, and meditation.	Can supplement analgesic therapy, especially during periods when client desires to minimize sedative effects of medication.
Monitor for, and discuss possibility of, changes in mental status such as agitation, confusion, and restlessness.	Although causes of deterioration are numerous in terminal stages, early recognition and management of the psychological component are integral parts of pain management.

(continues on page 870)

ACTIONS/INTERVENTIONS (continued)

Collaborative

Establish pain management plan with client, family, and healthcare providers, including options for management of breakthrough pain.

Schedule and administer analgesics, as indicated, to maximal dosage. Use various modalties such as patch, lollipop, sublingal, or combinations of medications, as indicated.

Plan for aggressive pain managament, as indicated. Notify physician if regimen is inadequate to meet pain control goal.

Instruct client, family, and caregiver in use of sustained-release formulations, around-the-clock dosing, and breakthrough pain management and technology such as pump or patient-controlled analgesia (PCA) for pain control.

Review medicinal options to treat constipation.

RATIONALE (continued)

Inadequate pain management remains one of the most significant deficiencies in the care of the dying client. A stepwise plan or analgesic ladder developed in advance increases client's level of trust that comfort will be maintained, reducing anxiety.

Helps maintain "acceptable" level of pain. Various drugs, dosages, and combinations allow for smaller doses and fewer side effects.

Primary goal is for client to be comfortable. Sometimes frequent alterations are required in achieving this, but medications and comfort measures must be sufficient to ensure that client is not suffering.

By understanding and managing these factors, pain relief can be enhanced and quality of life improved.

Various "cocktails" are available to manage constipation associated with use of opioid pain medications, reduced peristalsis, and lack of food intake. This is a frequent problem that must be managed to reduce client discomfort.

Refer to CP: Cancer, ND: acute/chronic Pain for additional interventions.

NURSING DIAGNOSIS: Activity Intolerance/Fatigue

May be related to

Generalized weakness

Bedrest or immobility, progressive disease state or debilitating condition

Imbalance between oxygen supply and demand

Cognitive deficits, emotional status secondary to underlying disease process or depression

Pain, extreme stress

Possibly evidenced by

Report of lack of energy, inability to maintain usual routines

Verbalizes no desire and/or lack of interest in activity

Lethargic, drowsy; decreased performance

Disinterested in surroundings; introspection

Desired Outcomes/Evaluation Criteria—Client Will

Energy Conservation (NOC)

Identify negative factors affecting performance and eliminate or reduce their effects when possible.

Adapt lifestyle to energy level.

Verbalize understanding of potential loss of ability in relation to existing condition.

Endurance (NOC)

Maintain or achieve slight increase in activity tolerance evidenced by manageable level of fatigue or weakness.

Remain free of preventable discomfort and/or complications.

ACTIONS/INTERVENTIONS

Energy Management (NIC)

Independent

Assess sleep patterns and note changes in thought processes and behaviors.

Recommend scheduling activities for periods when client has most energy. Adjust activities as necessary, reducing intensity level or discontinuing activities, as indicated.

Encourage client to do whatever possible, for example, self-care, sit in chair, or visit with family and friends. Plan for shorter activites.

Instruct client, family, and caregiver in energy conservation techniques. Stress necessity of allowing for frequent rest periods following activities.

RATIONALE

Multiple factors can aggravate fatigue, including sleep deprivation, emotional distress, side effects of medication, and progression of disease process.

Prevents overexertion and allows for some activity within client's ability.

Provides for sense of control and feeling of accomplishment.

Enhances performance while conserving limited energy and preventing increase in level of fatigue.

ACTIONS/INTERVENTIONS (continued)	RATIONALE (continued)
Plan family and friend visits around client's increased sleep time and shorter periods of alertness.	Client may become tired easily and will sleep more. In addition, client may have periods of unresponsiveness or confusion, or seem to be in a dream state. This may be distressing to some visitors.
Demonstrate proper performance of activities of daily living (ADLs), ambulation, and position changes. Identify safety issues such as use of assistive devices, temperature of bath water, and keeping pathways clear of furniture.	Protects client and caregiver from injury during activities.
Encourage nutritional intake and use of supplements, as appropriate.	Client may or may not want to eat, but food can be offered, if client is able to eat. Easy-to-digest foods that client enjoys may help meet energy needs for activity.
Discuss future plans regarding food and fluid, as indicated. Help client's family understand that forced eating and drinking may harm instead of help.	As the body starts the natural process of dying, the need for food and fluids decreases due to the shut down of body systems. At this point, dehydration associated with the dying process actually causes analgesic effects (Allen, 2008). Intravenous (IV) fluids and enteral feedings do not prolong life of the dying person. In fact, they may increase discomfort and hasten death. For example, IV fluids can cause edema, increased pain from inflammation, and fluid overload, whereas enteral feedings can cause pulmonary congestion and pneumonia (Suter et al, 2008).
Document cardiopulmonary response to activity—weakness, fatigue, dyspnea, arrhythmias, and diaphoresis.	Can provide guidelines for participation in activities and changes in the plan of care and level of assistance required.
Monitor breath sounds. Note feelings of panic or air hunger.	Hypoxemia increases sense of fatigue and impairs ability to function.

Collaborative

Provide supplemental oxygen as indicated and monitor response.	Increases oxygenation, reducing anxious feelings. Evaluates effectiveness of therapy.

NURSING DIAGNOSIS: Grieving/death Anxiety

May be related to
Anticipated loss of physiological well-being, change in body function
Perceived death of client

Possibly evidenced by
Changes in eating habits, sleep pattern, activity level, libido, and communication pattern
Denial of potential loss, choked feelings, anger
Fear of the process of dying, loss of physical and/or mental abilities
Negative death images or unpleasant thoughts about any event related to death or dying, anticipated pain related to dying
Powerlessness over issues related to dying, total loss of control over any aspect of one's own death, inability to problem-solve
Worrying about impact of one's own death on SO(s), being the cause of others' grief and suffering, concerns of overworking the caregiver as terminal illness incapacitates

Desired Outcomes/Evaluation Criteria—Client Will

Grief Resolution (NOC)
Identify and express feelings appropriately.
Continue normal life activities, looking toward and planning for the future, one day at a time.
Verbalize understanding of the dying process and feelings of being supported in grief work.

Dignified Life Closure (NOC)
Experience personal empowerment in spiritual strength and resources to find meaning and purpose in grief and loss.

Family Will

Grief Resolution (NOC)
Verbalize understanding of the stages of grief and loss.
Ventilate conflicts and feelings related to illness and death.

ACTIONS/INTERVENTIONS	RATIONALE

Grief Work Facilitation (NIC)

Independent

Facilitate development of a trusting relationship with client and family.

Trust is necessary before client and family can feel free to open personal lines of communication with the hospice team and address sensitive issues.

Assess client and SO for stage of grief currently being experienced. Explain process, as appropriate.

Knowledge about the grieving process reinforces the normalcy of feelings and reactions being experienced and can help client deal more effectively with them.

Provide open, nonjudgmental environment. Use therapeutic communication skills of active-listening, acknowledgment, and so on.

Promotes and encourages realistic dialogue about feelings and concerns.

Encourage verbalization of thoughts and concerns. Accept expressions of sadness, anger, and rejection. Acknowledge normalcy of these feelings.

Client may feel supported in expression of feelings by the understanding that deep and often conflicting emotions are normal and experienced by others in this difficult situation (Otis-Green, 2008b).

Be aware of mood swings, hostility, and other acting-out behavior. Set limits on inappropriate behavior and redirect negative thinking.

Indicators of ineffective coping and need for additional interventions. Preventing destructive actions enables client to maintain control and sense of self-esteem.

Monitor for signs of debilitating depression such as statements of hopelessness, desire to "end it now." Ask client direct questions about state of mind.

Client may be especially vulnerable when recently diagnosed with end-stage disease process and/or when discharged from hospital. Fear of loss of control or concerns about managing pain effectively may cause client to consider suicide.

Reinforce teaching regarding disease process and provide information as requested and appropriate about dying. Be honest; do not give false hope while providing emotional support.

Client and SO benefit from factual information. Individuals may ask direct questions about death, and honest answers promote trust and provide reassurance that correct information will be given.

Review past life experiences, role changes, sexuality concerns, and coping skills. Promote an environment conducive to talking about things that interest client.

This is an opportunity to identify skills that may help individuals cope with grief of current situation more effectively. *Note:* Issues of sexuality remain important at this stage, such as feelings of masculinity or femininity, giving up caretaker or provider role within family, and ability to maintain sexual activity or closeness, if desired.

Investigate evidence of conflict; expressions of anger; and statements of despair, guilt, hopelessness, and inability to grieve.

Interpersonal conflicts and angry behavior may be client's and SO's way of expressing or dealing with feelings of despair or spiritual distress, necessitating further evaluation and support.

Determine way that client and SO understand and respond to death—cultural expectations; learned behaviors; experience with death of close family members or friends; and beliefs about life after death, spirituality, or faith in a higher power.

These factors affect how each individual faces death and influences how he or she may respond and interact.

Assist client and SO to identify strengths in self or situation and support systems.

Recognizing these resources provides opportunity to work through feelings of grief.

Be aware of own feelings about death. Accept whatever methods client and SO have chosen to help each other through the process.

Caregiver's anxiety and unwillingness to accept reality of possibility of own death may block ability to be helpful to client and SO, necessitating enlisting the aid of others to provide needed support.

Dying Care (NIC)

Provide open environment for discussion with client and SO, when appropriate, about desires and plans pertaining to death including making a will, burial arrangements, tissue donation, death benefits, insurance, time for family gatherings, and how to spend remaining time.

If client and SO are mutually aware of impending death, they may more easily deal with unfinished business or desired activities. Having a part in problem-solving and planning can provide a sense of control over anticipated events.

Encourage participation in care decisions.

Allows client to retain some control over life.

Visit frequently and provide physical contact as appropriate and desired, or provide frequent phone support as appropriate for setting. Arrange for care provider or support person to stay with client, as needed.

Helps reduce feelings of isolation and abandonment. Provides respite and time for SO and family to meet own needs and complete required activities.

Provide time for acceptance, final farewell, and arrangements for memorial or funeral service according to individual spiritual, cultural, and ethnic needs.

Accommodation of personal and family wishes helps reduce anxiety and may promote sense of peace.

Collaborative

Determine spiritual needs and/or conflicts and refer to appropriate team members including clergy or spiritual advisor and parish nurse.

Providing for spiritual needs, forgiveness, prayer, devotional materials, or sacraments as requested can relieve spiritual pain and provide a sense of peace. (Refer to ND: risk for Spiritual Distress.)

ACTIONS/INTERVENTIONS (continued)	RATIONALE (continued)
Refer to appropriate counselor, as needed, such as psychiatric clinical nurse specialist, social worker, psychologist, and pastoral support.	Compassion and support can help alleviate distress or palliate feelings of grief to facilitate coping and foster growth.
Refer to visiting nurse or home health agency if hospice services not available.	Provides support in meeting physical and emotional needs of client and SO, and can supplement the care family and friends are able to give.
Identify need for and appropriate timing of antidepressants or anti-anxiety medications.	May alleviate distress and enhance coping, especially for clients not requiring analgesics.

NURSING DIAGNOSIS: compromised [or] disabled family Coping/Caregiver Role Strain

May be related to
Inadequate or incorrect information or understanding by a primary person, unrealistic expectations

Temporary preoccupation by significant person who is trying to manage emotional conflicts and personal suffering; client providing little support in turn for the primary person

Significant person with chronically unexpressed feelings of guilt, anxiety, hostility, despair

Temporary family disorganization and role changes, highly ambivalent family relationships

Prolonged disease or disability progression that exhausts the supportive capacity of significant persons, increasing care needs, dependency

Possibly evidenced by
Client expressing despair about family reactions or lack of involvement, history of poor relationship between caregiver and care receiver

Inability to complete caregiving tasks, altered caregiver health status

SO describing preoccupation about personal reactions; displaying intolerance, abandonment, rejection

SO attempting assistive or supportive behaviors with less than satisfactory results

Family behaviors that are detrimental to well-being

Apprehension about future regarding caregiver's ability to provide care

Desired Outcomes/Evaluation Criteria—Family/Caregiver Will

Caregiver Performance: Direct [or] Indirect Care (NOC)
Identify resources within themselves to deal with situation.
Participate positively in care of client, within limits of abilities.
Engage in problem-solving with direct care providers to meet client's individual needs.

Caregiver-Patient Relationship (NOC)
Express realistic understanding of situation and expectations of client.
Provide opportunity for client to deal with situation in own way.

ACTIONS/INTERVENTIONS	RATIONALE
Family Involvement Promotion (NIC) *Independent* Assess level of anxiety present in family and SO.	Anxiety level needs to be dealt with before problem-solving can begin. Individuals may be so preoccupied with own reactions to situation that they are unable to respond to another's needs.
Establish rapport and acknowledge difficulty of the situation for the family.	May assist SO to accept what is happening and be willing to share problems with healthcare providers.
Determine level of coping impairment. Evaluate current behaviors that may be interfering with the care of client.	Information about family problems such as divorce or separation, alcoholism, other drug abuse, or abusive situation will be helpful in determining options and developing an appropriate plan of care.
Note client's emotional and behavioral responses resulting from increasing weakness and dependency such as depression, withdrawal, hostility, hallucinations, and delusions.	Approaching death is most stressful when client and family coping responses are strained, resulting in increased frustration, guilt, and anguish.
Discuss underlying reasons for client behaviors with family.	When family members know why client is behaving differently, it may help them understand, accept, and deal with unusual behaviors.
Assist family and client to understand "who owns the problem" and who is responsible for resolution. Avoid placing blame or guilt.	When these boundaries are defined, each individual can begin to take care of own self and stop taking care of others in inappropriate ways.

(continues on page 874)

873

ACTIONS/INTERVENTIONS (continued)	RATIONALE (continued)
Determine current knowledge and perceptions of the situation.	Provides information on which to begin planning care and make informed decisions. Lack of information or unrealistic perceptions can interfere with individual's responses to illness situation.
Assess current actions of SO and how they are received by client.	SO may be trying to be helpful, but actions are not perceived as such by client. SO may be withdrawn or too protective.
Facilitate family conference, include all family members, as appropriate. Provide and reinforce information about terminal illness, death, and future family needs.	Knowledge can help the family prepare for eventualities and deal with the actual death process. Increases understanding of necessary activities and steps to be taken to deal with funeral preparations, legal and financial concerns, and survivor issues.

Caregiver Support (NIC)

ACTIONS/INTERVENTIONS	RATIONALE
Determine caregiver's health, level of commitment, responsibility, and involvement in care. Use assessment tool, such as Burden Interview, to further clarify caregiver's abilities, when appropriate.	Terminal care taxes caregiver and may alter ability to meet client's and own needs (Otis-Green, 2008a).
Ascertain caregiver's understanding and acceptance of client's wishes and advance directives.	If caregiver is not in total agreement with client's wishes, role strain may be intensified as specific decisions are made regarding care and termination of therapies.
Involve SO in information giving, problem-solving, and care of client, as appropriate. Instruct in medication administration techniques, needed treatments, and appropriate complementary and alternative therapies, such as massage, herbs, aromatherapy, and relaxation techniques. Ascertain adeptness with required equipment.	Information can reduce feelings of helplessness and uselessness. Helping a client and family find comfort is often more important than adhering to strict routines. However, family caregivers need to feel confident with specific care activities and equipment. *Note:* Use of complementary and alternative medicine is increasing for pain and symptom relief with lessened side effects.
Provide positive feedback for efforts.	Helps caregiver recognize and feel valued for contribution to care.
Stress importance of self-nurturing, personal needs, and social contacts.	Taking time for self can help lessen risk of being overwhelmed by situation.
Identify and schedule alternative care resources, such as family, friends, sitter, and respite services, as needed.	As client's condition worsens, primary caregiver will require additional help from other sources to maintain client at home as desired while still meeting own needs for rest and personal time.

Collaborative

ACTIONS/INTERVENTIONS	RATIONALE
Refer to appropriate resources for assistance, as indicated, including counseling, psychotherapy, financial, spiritual, and respite care.	May need additional assistance in resolving family issues, making peace, and maintaining personal well-being.
Arrange for appropriate prescriptions for SO (e.g., sedative and hypnotic).	Mild medication may be beneficial in reducing anxiety and promoting sleep, which, in turn, can enhance coping ability.

NURSING DIAGNOSIS: risk for Spiritual Distress

Risk factors may include
Physical or psychological stress, energy-consuming anxiety
Situational losses
Blocks to self-love, low self-esteem, inability to forgive

Possibly evidenced by
(Not applicable; presence of signs and symptoms establishes an *actual* diagnosis)

Desired Outcomes/Evaluation Criteria—Client and SO Will

Dignified Life Closure (NOC)
Identify meaning and purpose in one's life that reinforces hope, peace, and contentment.
Verbalize acceptance of self as being worthy, not deserving of illness or death.
Identify and use resources appropriately.

ACTIONS/INTERVENTIONS	RATIONALE

Spiritual Support (NIC)

Independent

Listen to client's and SO's reports and expressions of anger or concern.

Determine client's religious or spiritual orientation, current involvement, and presence of conflicts in current circumstances.

Assess sense of self-concept, worth, and ability to enter into or maintain loving relationships.

Explore interpretation and relationship of spirituality, concept of life, and death and illness to client's spiritual centeredness.

Explore ways that spirituality or religious practices, such as music, prayer, meditation, and rituals, have affected client's life.

Determine support systems available to and used by client and SO.

Encourage client to be introspective in search for peace and harmony.

Establish environment that promotes free expression of feelings and concerns.

Have client and SO identify and prioritize current and immediate needs regarding faith, influence, and community.

Make time for nonjudgmental discussion of cultural and philosophical issues and questions about spiritual impact of illness and/or impending death.

Discuss difference between grief and guilt and help client to identify and deal with each, assuming responsibility for own actions.

Use therapeutic communication skills of gentle stillness, reflection, conveying respect through tone of voice and body language, and active-listening.

Review coping skills used and their effectiveness in current situation.

Suggest use of story telling, journaling, or taping thoughts.

Determine how involved in physical care the family members want to be. Establish with client and SO wishes for the moment of death.

Collaborative

Encourage participation in desired religious activities, prayer, meditation, contact with minister, spiritual advisor, or grief counselor.

May reveal many conflicting thoughts and beliefs, for example, that illness or situation is a punishment for wrongdoing or that death is desirable or feared. Dying client faces momentous losses of physical control and function, of independence, of relationships, of possibilities, and ultimately of life itself. To family members and friends, the loss of a loved one causes great stress and temporarily impairs concentration, decision making, and work performance.

Provides insight as to where client currently is and what hopes for the future may be. *Note:* Individuals reporting high spirituality were less hopeless, had less desire to hasten their deaths, and had less suicidal ideation.

Necessary to provide firm foundation for growth and guiding client and family through life closure and completion tasks.

Identifying the meaning of these issues may be helpful in forming or stating a belief system that enables client to move forward. Comfort can be gained when family and friends share client's beliefs and support search for spiritual knowledge.

Allows client to explore spiritual needs and decide what fits own view, and provides support for dealing with current situation.

May help identify strengths and weaknesses in relationship dynamics that the client and SOs may want to address such as expressing love, forgiveness, and support.

Finding peace within will carry over to relationships with others and one's outlook on life and death.

May help identify the real need of the day. For example, the dying person may not hope for cure or postponement of death, but rather that on the next day he or she will feel better with fewer physical and emotional discomforts.

Helps client and SO focus on what needs to be done and identify manageable steps to take.

Spiritual or religious practices, customs, and rituals often play important roles, especially at a time of such significant transition in life.

Identifies persons at risk for complicated grief and bereavement and its associated depression and complications. May provide opportunities for resolution.

Encourages client and SO to identify and express end-of-life concerns, hopes, fears, and expectations openly and honestly in a caring milieu.

Helps client and SO remember and call upon strengths that have been helpful in other situations. May free the client to be "more" creative, loving, and into the experience of well-being.

Helps client explore and find own solutions to concerns. Identifies strengths to incorporate into plan and techniques needing revision.

Clarification of specific wishes can be helpful in reducing stress and allow for needed differences in response.

May prove beneficial to both client and family members in reflecting on life and death issues. Can assist in clarifying values and ideas, recognizing and resolving feelings, and promoting comfort. Validating one's beliefs in an external way can support and strengthen the inner self.

Refer to CP: Psychosocial Aspects of Care, ND: risk for impaired Religiosity for additional interventions.

DISASTER CONSIDERATIONS

I. Problem

a. The bigger the disaster or catastrophe, the greater the number of people involved and the wider the effect

b. Physical effects of a catastrophic event can vary depending on the type of disaster.

   i. Explosive devices, transportation accidents, hurricanes, or floods—burns and brain and crush injuries

   ii. Release of chemical agents—burns, pulmonary or other organ damage, neurological impairment

   iii. Biological weapons or reemerging infections (avian flu or pandemic influenza)—mass infections

   iv. Radioactive contamination or exposure—burns, radiation sickness, cancer

II. Consequences

a. Following any disaster, those involved—victims, rescuers, and the surrounding community—suffer from a variety of responses.

b. Disaster or extreme events can have indirect health-related effects.

   i. Exacerbation of chronic condition, such as heart or lung problems

   ii. Precipitation of emergent conditions such as premature births, seizures, or psychiatric conditions

c. Psychological ramifications

   i. Immediate stressors may cause anxiety or panic disorders.

   ii. The playing and replaying of the events in one's mind may lead to suicidal thoughts and post-traumatic stress disorder (PTSD).

   iii. Repeated media coverage can magnify the effects; people far removed from the scene may also suffer.

GLOSSARY

Biological agents: Viruses (smallpox), bacteria (anthrax, *Salmonella*), other agents including toxins (botulism) that can cause illness or death.

Chemical agents: Poisonous gases, liquids, or solids including nerve agents (sarin), biotoxins (ricine), choking or pulmonary agents (chlorine, ammonia), blood agents (cyanide), caustics (hydrofluoric acid), visicants or blister agents (lewisite, mustard gas), or long-acting anticoagulants (super warfarin) that can cause serious injury or death.

Disaster: Generally refers to a catastrophic natural or man-made event affecting a large population resulting in injury, death, and destruction of property that overwhelms local resources.

Eye movement desensitization and reprocessing (EMDR): Information processing psychotherapy technique integrating elements of psychodynamic, cognitive behavioral, interpersonal, experiential, and body-centered therapies to assist individuals to deal with anxious feelings and stress associated with traumatic memories.

Post-traumatic stress disorder (PTSD): Intense physical and psychological distress that ensues following a traumatic event, manifested by horrifying memories, reexperiencing the event or flashbacks, recurring fears, and feelings of helplessness. May be acute—beginning within 6 months and not lasting longer than 6 months; chronic—lasting longer than 6 months; or delayed—period of latency of 6 months or more.

Care Setting

Wherever disaster occurs, to include triage areas, aid stations, clinics, hospital and emergency centers, and shelters.

Related Concerns

Burns: thermal, chemical, and electrical—acute and convalescent phases, page 667

Craniocerebral trauma, page 220

Fractures, page 632

Pneumonia, page 131

Sepsis/septicemia, page 686

Psychosocial aspects of care, page 749

Client Assessment Database

Data depend on specific injuries incurred and presence of chronic conditions (refer to specific plans of care for appropriate data, such as burns, multiple trauma, cardiac and respiratory conditions, and so forth) and timing of presentation for care.

DIAGNOSTIC DIVISION MAY REPORT	MAY EXHIBIT
ACTIVITY/REST • Sleep disturbances—recurrent intrusive dreams of the event, nightmares, difficulty in falling or staying asleep; hypersomnia with intrusive thoughts, flashbacks • Fatigue	• Listlessness

Client Assessment Database (continued)

DIAGNOSTIC DIVISION MAY REPORT (continued)	MAY EXHIBIT (continued)
CIRCULATION • Palpitations • Hot flashes or chills	• Tachycardia • Sweating • Cold, clammy hands • Elevated blood pressure (BP) (anxiety) • Decreased BP (dehydration, hypovolemia)
EGO INTEGRITY • Excessive worry about event • Avoidance of circumstances or locations associated with incident • Sense of inner turmoil • Dry mouth, upset stomach, lump in throat • Perceived threat to physical integrity or self-concept • Questioning of God's purpose, abandonment	• Facial expression in keeping with level of anxiety—furrowed brow, strained face, eyelid twitch • Labile emotions • Inappropriate humor
ELIMINATION • Frequent urination • Diarrhea	
FOOD/FLUID • Lack of interest in food, dysfunctional eating pattern—decreased or increased intake • Nausea, vomiting, gastric distress	
NEUROSENSORY • Lightheadedness, dizziness • Anticipation of misfortune to self or others • Feeling stuck • Absence of other mental disorder	• Confusion, memory loss • Motor tension, shakiness, jitteriness, trembling, easily startled • Apprehensive expectation, rumination • Excessive vigilance, hyperattentiveness • Distractibility, difficulty concentrating or making decisions, shortened attention span • Irritability, impatience • Psychic numbing
PAIN/DISCOMFORT • Muscle aches, tension headaches, chest pain • Pain related to physical injuries or comorbid conditions	• Guarding or distraction behaviors
RESPIRATORY • Shortness of breath • Smothering sensation	• Increased respiratory rate
SAFETY • Increased smoking, substance use or abuse • Fear of harm to self or others	
SEXUALITY • Decreased libido	
SOCIAL INTERACTIONS • Concern for well-being of others • Questioning own actions, survival • Difficulty participating in social settings • Reluctance to engage in usual activities, work	• Withdrawal

(continues on page 878)

DIAGNOSTIC DIVISION MAY REPORT (continued)	MAY EXHIBIT (continued)
TEACHING/LEARNING • *Discharge plan considerations:* Dependent on individual situation, level of support, and available resources	

Diagnostic Studies

Dependent on injuring agent and exposure and availability of resources for testing and procedures.

Nursing Priorities

1. Prevent or treat life-threatening conditions.
2. Prevent further injury and spread of infection.
3. Support efforts to cope with situation.
4. Facilitate integration of event.
5. Assist community in preparing for future occurrences.

Discharge Goals

1. Free of preventable complications.
2. Anxiety or fear reduced to a manageable level.
3. Beginning to cope effectively with situation.
4. Plan in place to meet needs after discharge.
5. Community preparedness enhanced.

NURSING DIAGNOSIS: risk for[/or actual] Injury—Trauma, Suffocation, or Poisoning

Risk factors may include
Biological—immunization level of community, presence of microorganism
Contact with chemical pollutants, poisonous agents
Exposure to open flame or flammable material
Acceleration and deceleration forces
Contamination of food or water

Possibly evidenced by
(Not applicable; presence of signs and symptoms establishes an *actual* diagnosis)

Desired Outcomes/Evaluation Criteria—Client/Caregivers Will

Physical Injury Severity (NOC)
Minimize degree of and prevent further injury.

Personal Safety Behavior (NOC)
Verbalize understanding of condition and specific needs.
Identify interventions appropriate to situation.
Demonstrate behaviors necessary to protect self from further injury.
Accept responsibility for own care and follow up as individually able.

ACTIONS/INTERVENTIONS	RATIONALE
Triage: Disaster (NIC) *Independent* Acquire information about nature of emergency, accident, or disaster.	Identifies basic resource needs and helps to prepare staff for appropriate level of response based on customary injuries and healthcare needs usually associated with specific event.
Prepare area and equipment; check and restock supplies.	Assists in providing safe medical and nursing care in anticipation of emergency need.
Assist in prioritizing (triaging) clients for treatment. Monitor for and treat life-threatening injuries.	Promotes efficient care of those who can be medically treated and maximizes use of resources. *Note:* In routine emergency situations, the goal is to do the best for each individual. However, in a disaster, the focus of treatment shifts to do the greatest good for the greatest number.

ACTIONS/INTERVENTIONS (continued)	RATIONALE (continued)
Determine primary needs and specific complaints of client. Check for medical alert tag.	Information necessary for triaging to appropriate services. *Note:* Pediatric clients are better able to compensate during early hypovolemic shock than adults, creating a false impression of normalcy (American Academy of Pediatrics [AAP], 2006).
Obtain additional medical information including preexisting conditions, allergies, and current medication. Perform more in-depth assessment as time allows and condition warrants.	Provides for assessment and treatment of conditions that might not be evident initially.
Determine client's developmental level, decision-making ability, level of cognition, and competence.	Affects treatment plan regarding issues of informed consent, self-care, client teaching, and discharge.
Evaluate individual's response to event, mood, coping abilities, and personal vulnerability.	People react to traumatic situations in many ways and may exhibit a wide range of responses—from no visible response to wild emotions. This may result in carelessness or increased risk taking without considerations of consequences, or inability to act on own behalf, including protecting self.
Ascertain knowledge of needs and injury prevention and motivation to prevent further injury.	Indicator of need for information and assistance with making positive changes, promoting safety and sense of security.
Discuss importance of self-monitoring of conditions and emotions that can contribute to occurrence of injury—shock state, ignoring basic needs, fatigue, anger, and irritability.	Recognizing these factors and dealing with them appropriately, including seeking support and assistance, can reduce individual risks.
Note socioeconomic status and availability and use of resources.	May determine ability to access help for identified problems.

Collaborative

Work with other agencies, such as law enforcement, fire department, Red Cross, and ambulance and EMTs, as indicated. Follow prearranged roles when participating in a community disaster plan.	During a disaster, many people are involved with care of victims. Most communities have disaster plans in which nurses will participate.
Identify and manage life-threatening situations—airway problems, bleeding, and diminished consciousness.	Stabilization of medical condition is necessary before proceeding with additional therapies.

Triage: Emergency Care (NIC)

Obtain and assist with diagnostic studies, as indicated.	Choice of studies is dependent on individual situation and availability of resources.
Provide therapeutic interventions as individually appropriate. (Refer to specific CPs; e.g., Burns, Fractures, Crainocerebral Trauma, Myocardial Infarction, Chronic Obstructive Pulmonary Disease [COPD], Ventilatory Assistance [mechanical].)	Specific needs of client and the level of care available at a particular site determine response.
Provide written instructions and list of resources for later review.	Client and significant other(s) (SO[s]) are generally not able to assimilate information at time of crisis and may need reinforcement or want additional information.
Identify community resources including shelter, neighbors, friends, and government agencies available for assistance.	May need assistance or ongoing monitoring postdischarge to deal with self-care needs as well as safe housing and other life requirements. *Note:* Release of client without active support increases personal risk because of possibility of unrecognized or subacute injury or delayed psychological response.
Refer to other resources, as indicated, such as counseling and psychotherapy.	Immediate "debriefing" or counseling is beneficial for dealing with crisis to enhance ability to meet own needs.

NURSING DIAGNOSIS: risk for Infection

Risk factors may include
Environmental exposure, inadequate acquired immunity
Trauma, tissue destruction, invasive procedures
Chronic disease, malnutrition
Insufficient knowledge to avoid exposure to pathogens

Possibly evidenced by
(Not applicable; presence of signs and symptoms establishes an *actual* diagnosis)

(continues on page 880)

Desired Outcomes/Evaluation Criteria—Client Will

Risk Control (NOC)
Verbalize understanding of individual exposure and risk factor(s).
Identify interventions to prevent and reduce risk of infection.

Infection Severity (NOC)
Be free and demonstrate resolution of infection.

ACTIONS/INTERVENTIONS	RATIONALE
Infection Control (NIC)	
Independent	
Note risk factors for occurrence of infection—environmental exposure, compromised host, traumatic injury, loss of skin integrity. Determine client's proximity to incident. Be aware of incubation period for various diseases.	Understanding nature and properties of infectious agents and individual's exposure determines choice of therapeutic intervention. *Note:* Those upwind of an aerosol release of a biological agent may have little or no exposure to the agent. (Refer to Table 15.2, at the end of plan of care, for pertinent information.)
Observe for signs and symptoms of infective agent and systemic infection—fever, chills, diaphoresis, altered level of consciousness (LOC), and positive blood cultures. Investigate presence of rash.	Initial symptoms of some agents include fever, fatigue, joint aches, and headache similar to influenza. The infection may even be misdiagnosed as an influenza-like infection (ILI), unless healthcare providers maintain an index of suspicion and obtain additional diagnostic studies. *Note:* The immature immunological system of children places them at higher risk for developing infections (AAP, 2006).
Practice and demonstrate proper hand-washing technique.	First-line defense to limit spread of infections.
Provide for infection precautions or isolation, as indicated—standard precautions of gown, gloves, face shield or goggles, respiratory mask or filter, and reverse or negative pressure room.	Reduces risk of cross-contamination to staff, visitors, and other clients.
Group or cohort individuals with same diagnosis or exposure as resources require.	Limited resources may dictate open wardlike environment, but need to control spread of infection still exists.
Monitor visitors and caregivers for infectious diseases.	Prevents exposure of client to further infection and may reveal additional cases.
Review individual nutritional needs, appropriate exercise program, and need for rest.	Essential for well-being and recovery.
Instruct client/SO(s) in techniques to prevent spread of infection, protect the integrity of skin, and care for wounds or lesions.	Self-care activities that may provide protection for client and others.
Emphasize necessity of taking antibiotics as directed, especially dosage and length of therapy.	Premature discontinuation of treatment when client begins to feel well may result in return of infection. However, unnecessary use of antibiotics may result in development of secondary infections or resistant organisms.
Involve community in education programs geared to increasing awareness of spread and prevention of communicable diseases.	Helps to reduce incidence of disease in the community as well as manage the dissemination of information.
Collaborative	
Obtain appropriate specimens for observation and culture and sensitivities testing—nose and throat swabs, sputum, blood, urine, or feces.	Provides information to diagnose infection and determine appropriate therapeutic interventions.
Assist with medical procedures, such as incision and drainage of abscess, bronchoscopy, or wound care, as indicated.	Helps determine causative factors for appropriate treatment and facilitates recovery.
Administer and monitor medication regimen (e.g., antimicrobials, topical antibiotics) and note client's response.	Determines effectiveness of therapy and presence of side effects.
Provide passive protection such as immune globulin, active protection (e.g., vaccination), or chemoprophylaxis, as appropriate.	May prevent development of infection following exposure or reduce the likelihood of acquiring disease in the future. (Refer to Table 15.3 at the end of plan of care.)
Alert proper authorities to presence of specific infectious agent and number of cases.	Diseases that could be caused by biological releases or that spread rapidly through populations have reporting requirements to local, state, and national agencies, such as the state health department or the Centers for Disease Control and Prevention (CDC). These agencies, in turn, have responsibilities for the public safety and welfare.

Anxiety (severe/panic)/Fear

May be related to
Situational crisis, exposure to toxins
Real or perceived threat to physical well-being, threat of death
Interpersonal transmission of concerns or fears
Unconscious conflict about essential values, beliefs
Unmet needs

Possibly evidenced by
Persistent feelings of apprehension and uneasiness, sense of impending doom
Scanning and vigilance or lack of awareness of surroundings
Sympathetic stimulation, extraneous movements—restlessness, foot shuffling, hand/arm fidgeting, rocking movements
Focus on self, overexcited
Impaired functioning; verbal expressions of having no control or influence over situation, outcome, or self-care

Desired Outcomes/Evaluation Criteria—Client Will

Anxiety [or] Fear Self-Control (NOC)
Acknowledge and discuss feelings.
Verbalize accurate knowledge of current situation and potential outcomes.
Identify healthy ways to successfully deal with stress.
Report anxiety is reduced to a manageable level.
Demonstrate problem-solving skills appropriate for individual situation.
Use resources and support systems effectively.

ACTIONS/INTERVENTIONS	RATIONALE
Crisis Intervention (NIC)	
Independent	
Determine degree of anxiety or fear present; associated behaviors, such as laughter, crying, calm or agitation, excited or hysterical behavior; expressions of disbelief and/or self-blame; and reality of perceived threat.	Clearly understanding client's perception is pivotal to providing appropriate assistance in overcoming the fear. Individual may be agitated or totally overwhelmed. Severe anxiety increases risk for client's own safety as well as the safety of others in the environment. *Note:* Children are affected by their own reaction to the event as well as the transmission of anxiety or fear being experienced by parents and care providers, thus magnifying the psychological impact on the child (AAP, 2006).
Note degree of disorganization.	Client may be unable to handle activities of daily living (ADLs) or work requirements and may need more intensive evaluation and intervention. Children may regress—girls may express anxiety and sadness, whereas boys are more likely to display behavioral problems (AAP, 2006).
Maintain and respect client's personal space boundaries—approximately 4-foot circle around client.	Entering client's personal space without permission or invitation could result in an overwhelming anxiety response and, possibly, an overt act of violence.
Create quiet area as able. Maintain a calm, confident manner. Speak in even tone using short simple sentences.	Decreases sense of confusion, overstimulation, and enhances sense of safety. Helps client focus on what is said and reduces transmission of anxiety.
Develop trusting relationship with client.	Trust is the basis of a therapeutic nurse-client relationship and enables them to work together effectively.
Identify whether incident has reactivated preexisting or coexisting situations—physical or psychological.	Concerns or psychological issues will be recycled every time trauma is reexperienced and affect how the client views the current situation.
Determine presence of physical symptoms, such as numbness, headache, tightness in chest, nausea, and pounding heart.	Physical problems need to be differentiated from anxiety symptoms so that appropriate treatment can be given.
Identify psychological responses—anger, shock, acute anxiety, panic, confusion, and denial. Record emotional changes.	Although these are normal responses at the time of the trauma, they will recycle again and again until they are dealt with adequately.
Discuss with client perception of what is causing anxiety or panic.	Increases ability to connect symptoms to subjective feeling of anxiety, providing opportunity to gain insight and control, and make desired changes.
Assist client to correct any distortions being experienced. Share perceptions with client.	Perceptions based on reality will help to decrease fearfulness. How the nurse views the situation may help client to see it differently.
Explore with client and SO the manner in which the client has coped with anxiety-producing events before the trauma.	May help client regain sense of control and recognize significance of trauma.

(continues on page 882)

Engage client in learning new coping behaviors, such as progressive muscle relaxation and thought stopping.

Demonstrate and encourage use of techniques to reduce or manage stress, and vent emotions such as anger and hostility.

Give positive feedback when client demonstrates better ways to manage anxiety and is able to calmly and/or realistically appraise own situation.

Collaborative

Administer medications, as indicated, for example:

   Anti-anxiety agents, such as Diazepam (Valium), buspirone (BuSpar), alprazolam (Xanax), and oxazepam (Serax)

   Antidepressants, such as Fluoxetine (Prozac), paroxetine (Paxil), and bupropion (Wellbutrin)

Refer for additional therapies such as hypnosis, EMDR, or Thought Reprocessing Therapy, as appropriate.

Coordinate release or discharge to family, friend, or emergency services, as indicated.

Educate victims and public about risks and steps being taken to deal with problem. Include other members of healthcare teams, stressing risks to themselves. Refer to such resources as the CDC or specific Web sites.

Replacing maladaptive behaviors can enhance ability to manage and deal with stress. Interrupting obsessive thinking allows client to use energy to address underlying anxiety, while continued rumination about the incident can actually retard recovery.

Reduces likelihood of eruptions that can result in abusive behavior.

Provides acknowledgment and reinforcement, encouraging use of new coping strategies. Enhances ability to deal with fearful feelings and gain control over situation, promoting future successes.

Provides temporary relief of anxiety symptoms, enhancing client's ability to cope with situation. Also useful for alleviating feelings of panic and intrusive nightmares.

Used to decrease anxiety, lift mood, aid in management of behavior, and ensure rest until client regains control of own self. Helpful in suppressing intrusive thoughts and explosive anger.

When used by trained therapist, these short-term therapies are particularly effective with individuals who have been traumatized or who have problems with anxiety and depression. Systematic desensitization, reframing, and reinterpretation of memories may be achieved through hypnosis.

Triaging and maximum use of resources may limit time allotted for care, and client may not be ready to meet own needs or assume full responsibility for self.

Nurses have a role in community education because they are close to the individuals affected. Providing accurate information and credible resources helps limit level of concern and transmission of anxiety. Current, timely information regarding biological concerns and healthcare needs can be accessed through such Web sites as www.cdc.gov, www.hhs.gov, and www.fbi.gov.

NURSING DIAGNOSIS: Spiritual Distress

May be related to

Physical and psychological stress; energy-consuming anxiety

Situation, loss(es), intense suffering

Separation from religious or cultural ties

Challenged belief and value system

Possibly evidenced by

Expressions of concern about disaster; the meaning of life, death and/or belief systems

Inner conflict about current loss of normalcy and effects of the disaster, anger directed at deity, engaging in self-blame

Seeking spiritual assistance or chooses not to participate

Reports of somatic symptoms

Desired Outcomes/Evaluation Criteria—Client Will

Spiritual Health (NOC)

Verbalize increased sense of self-concept and hope for future.

Discuss beliefs and values about spiritual issues.

Verbalize acceptance of self as being worthy.

ACTIONS/INTERVENTIONS

RATIONALE

Spiritual Support (NIC)

Independent

Determine client's religious or spiritual orientation, current involvement, and presence of conflicts.

Provides baseline for planning care and accessing appropriate resources.

ACTIONS/INTERVENTIONS (continued)

Establish environment that promotes free expression of feelings and concerns. Provide calm, peaceful setting when possible.

Listen to client's and SO's reports or expressions of anger, concern, alienation from God, belief that situation is a punishment for wrongdoing, and so forth.

Note sense of futility, feelings of hopelessness and helplessness, and lack of motivation to help self.

Listen to expressions of inability to find meaning in life or reason for living. Evaluate for suicidal ideation.

Determine support systems available to client and SO(s).

Ask how you can be most helpful. Convey acceptance of client's spiritual beliefs and concerns.

Make time for nonjudgmental discussion of philosophical issues or questions about spiritual impact of events and current situation.

Discuss difference between grief and guilt and help client to identify and deal with each, assuming responsibility for own actions and expressing awareness of the consequences of acting out of false guilt.

Use therapeutic communication skills of reflection and active-listening.

Discuss use of, and provide opportunities for client and SO to experience meditation, prayer, and forgiveness. Provide information that anger with God is a normal part of the grieving process.

Assist client to develop goals for dealing with life situation.

Collaborative

Identify and refer to resources that can be helpful such as pastoral or parish nurse, religious counselor, crisis counselor, psychotherapy, and Alcoholics or Narcotics Anonymous.

Encourage participation in support groups.

RATIONALE (continued)

Promotes awareness and identification of feelings so they can be dealt with.

Helpful to understand client's and SO's point of view and how they are questioning their faith in the face of tragedy.

These thoughts and feelings can result in the client feeling paralyzed and unable to move forward to resolve the situation.

May indicate need for further intervention to prevent suicide attempt.

Presence or lack of support systems can affect client's recovery.

Promotes trust and comfort, encouraging client to be open about sensitive matters.

Helps client to begin to look at basis for spiritual confusion. *Note:* There is a potential for care provider's belief system to interfere with client finding own way. Therefore it is most beneficial to remain neutral and not espouse own beliefs.

Blaming self for what has happened impedes dealing with the grief process and needs to be discussed and dealt with.

Helps client find own solutions to concerns.

Can help to heal past and present pain.

Enhances commitment to goal, optimizing outcomes and promoting sense of hope.

Specific assistance to resolve life stressors such as relationship problems, substance abuse, or suicidal ideation are important to advance recovery process.

Discussing concerns and questions with others can help client resolve feelings.

NURSING DIAGNOSIS: risk for Post-Trauma Syndrome

Risk factors may include
Events outside the range of usual human experience
Serious threat or injury to self or loved ones, witnessing violent death or tragic events
Disasters; destruction of one's home or community; epidemics
Exaggerated sense of responsibility and survivor's role in the event

Possibly evidenced by
(Not applicable; presence of signs and symptoms establishes an *actual* diagnosis)

Desired Outcomes/Evaluation Criteria—Client/Caregivers Will

Anxiety [or] Fear Self-Control (NOC)
Express own feelings and reactions openly, avoiding projection.
Demonstrate ability to deal with emotional reactions in an individually appropriate manner.
Report absence of physical manifestations such as pain, nightmares, flashbacks, or fatigue associated with the event.

ACTIONS/INTERVENTIONS

Crisis Intervention (NIC)
Independent
Determine involvement in event— survivor, SO, and family, rescue or aid worker, healthcare provider, or family member of responder.

RATIONALE

All those concerned with a traumatic event are at risk for emotional trauma and have needs related to their situation and involvement in the event. *Note:* Close involvement with victims or survivors affects individual responses and may prolong emotional suffering.

(continues on page 884)

ACTIONS/INTERVENTIONS	RATIONALE
Evaluate life factors and stressors currently or recently occurring, such as displacement from home due to catastrophic event—illness, injury, natural disaster, or terrorist attack. Identify how client's past experiences may affect current situation.	Affects client's reaction to current event and is basis for planning care and identifying appropriate supports and resources.
Listen for comments of taking on responsibility such as "I should have been more careful . . . or gone back to get her."	Indicators of "survivor's guilt" and blaming self for actions that can delay recovery and impair general well-being.
Identify client's current coping mechanisms.	Noting positive or negative skills provides direction for care.
Determine availability and usefulness of client's support systems—family, social, community, and so forth.	Family and others close to the client may also be at risk and require assistance to cope with the trauma.
Provide information about signs and symptoms of post-trauma response, especially if individual is involved in a high-risk occupation.	Awareness of these factors helps individual identify need for assistance when they occur.
Identify and discuss client's strengths as well as vulnerabilities.	Provides information to build on for coping with traumatic experience.
Evaluate individual's perceptions of events and personal significance, for example, a rescue worker trained to provide lifesaving assistance but recovering only dead bodies.	Events that trigger feelings of despair and hopelessness may be more difficult to deal with, and require long-term interventions.
Provide emotional and physical presence by sitting with client and SO and offering solace.	Strengthens coping abilities.
Encourage expression of feelings. Note whether feelings expressed appear congruent with events experienced.	It is important to talk about the incident repeatedly. Incongruencies may indicate deeper conflict and can impede resolution.
Note presence of nightmares, reliving the incident, loss of appetite, irritability, numbness and crying, and family or relationship disruption.	These responses are normal in the early post-incident time frame. If prolonged and persistent, they may indicate need for more intensive therapy.
Provide a calm, safe environment.	Helps client deal with the disruption in personal life.
Encourage and assist client in learning stress-management techniques.	Promotes relaxation and helps individual exercise control over self and what has happened.
Collaborative	
Recommend participation in debriefing sessions that may be provided following major disaster events.	Dealing with the stresses promptly may facilitate recovery from event and prevent exacerbation.
Identify employment and community resource groups.	Provides opportunity for ongoing support to deal with recurrent feelings related to the trauma.
Administer medications, as indicated, such as the following: Antipsychotics, for example, phenothiazines such as chlorpromazine (Thorazine) and haloperidol (Haldol)	Low doses may be used for reduction of psychotic symptoms when loss of contact with reality occurs, usually for clients with especially disturbing flashbacks.
Carbamazepine (Tegretol)	Used to alleviate intrusive recollections and flashbacks, impulsivity, and violent behavior.

NURSING DIAGNOSIS: ineffective community Coping

May be related to
Natural or human-made disasters—earthquakes, floods, reemerging infectious agents, terrorist activity
Deficits in social support services and resources
Ineffective or nonexistent community systems such as lack of, or inadequate emergency medical system, transportation system, or disaster planning systems

Possibly evidenced by
Deficits of community participation, community does not meet its own expectations
Expressed vulnerability, community powerlessness
Stressors perceived as excessive
Excessive community conflicts
High illness rates

Desired Outcomes/Evaluation Criteria—Community Will

Community Competence (NOC)
Recognize negative and positive factors affecting community's ability to meet its own demands or needs.
Identify alternatives to inappropriate activities for adaptation and problem-solving.
Report a measurable increase in necessary or desired activities to improve community functioning.

ACTIONS/INTERVENTIONS	RATIONALE

Community Disaster Preparedness (NIC)
Independent

Evaluate community activities as related to meeting collective needs within the community itself and between the community and the larger society. Note immediate needs including healthcare, food, shelter, and funds.

Note community reports of functioning, including areas of weakness or conflict.

Identify effects of related factors on community activities.

Determine availability and use of resources. Identify unmet demands or needs of the community.

Determine community strengths.

Encourage community members and groups to engage in problem-solving activities.

Develop a plan jointly with the members of the community to address immediate needs.

Create plans managing interactions within the community itself and between the community and the larger society.

Make information accessible to the public. Provide channels for dissemination of information to the community as a whole including print media, radio and television, reports and community bulletin boards, Internet resources, speaker's bureau, reports to committees, councils, or advisory boards.

Make information available in different modalities and geared to differing educational levels and cultures within the community.

Seek out and evaluate needs of underserved populations.

RATIONALE column:

Provides a baseline to determine community needs in relation to current concerns or threats.

Provides a view of how the community itself sees these areas.

In the face of a current threat, local or national, community resources need to be evaluated, updated, and given priority to meet the identified need.

Information necessary to identify what else is needed to meet the current situation.

Promotes understanding of the ways in which the community is already meeting the identified needs.

Promotes a sense of working together to meet the needs.

Deals with deficits in support of identified goals.

Meets collective needs when the concerns or threats are shared beyond a local community.

Readily available accurate information can help citizens make informed decisions to deal with the situation.

Using languages other than English and making written materials accessible to all members of the community will promote understanding.

The homeless and those residing in lower income areas may have special needs requiring additional resources.

NURSING DIAGNOSIS: readiness for enhanced community Coping

May be related to
Social support available
Resources available for problem-solving
Community has a sense of power to manage stressors

Possibly evidenced by
Active planning by community for predicted stressors
Active problem-solving by community when faced with issues
Positive communication among community members and between community and aggregates and larger community
Resources sufficient for managing stressors

Desired Outcomes/Evaluation Criteria—Community Will

Community Competence (NOC)
Identify positive and negative factors affecting management of current and future problems or stressors.
Have an established plan in place to deal with various contingencies.
Report a measurable increase in ability to deal with potential events.

ACTIONS/INTERVENTIONS	RATIONALE

Program Development (NIC)
Independent

Review community plans to monitor for and deal with untoward events.

Assess effects of related factors on management of problems or stressors.

Determine community strengths and weaknesses. Identify limitations in current pattern of community activities that can be improved through adaptation and problem-solving.

RATIONALE:

Provides a baseline for comparison of preparedness with other communities and developing plan to address concerns.

Identifies areas that need to be addressed to enhance community coping.

Plan can be built on strengths, and areas of weakness can be addressed.

(continues on page 886)

ACTIONS/INTERVENTIONS (continued)

Evaluate community activities as related to management of problems or stressors within the community itself and between the community and the larger society.

Define and discuss current needs and anticipated or projected concerns.

Identify and prioritize community goals.

Promote community awareness about the problems of design of buildings, equipment, transportation systems, and workplace practices that may compound disaster or impact disaster response.

Identify available resources—persons, groups, financial, governmental, as well as other communities.

Seek out and involve underserved and at-risk groups within the community.

Assist the community to form partnerships within the community and between the community and the larger society.

Establish mechanism for self-monitoring of community needs and evaluation of efforts.

Participate in exercises and activities to test preparedness.

Use multiple formats—TV, radio, print media, billboards, computer bulletin boards, speaker's bureau, and reports to community leaders and groups on file that are accessible to the public.

RATIONALE (continued)

Disasters occurring in the community or the country affect the local community and need to be recognized and addressed.

Agreement on scope and parameters of needs is essential for effective planning.

Helps to bring the community together to meet a common concern or threat. Helps maintain focus and facilitates accomplishment.

Provides opportunity for making changes that promote safety.

Important to work together to meet goals. Major catastrophes affect more than local community, and communities need to work together to deal with and accomplish growth.

Supports communication and commitment of community as a whole.

Promotes long-term developmental growth of the community.

Facilitates proactive rather than reactive responses by the community.

Provides opportunities to verify appropriateness of plans and problem-solve deficiencies.

Keeps the community informed and involved regarding plans, needs, and outcomes of tests of the plans.

TABLE 15.2 Clinical Characteristics of Critical Biological Agents—7/1/00

Disease	Signs and Symptoms	Physical Exam	Clinical Test	Key Differential Diagnosis	Incubation Period	Duration of Illness	Case Fatality	U.S. Epidemiology
Inhalational Anthrax	Fever, malaise, cough, mild chest discomfort, possible short recovery phase then onset of dyspnea, diaphoresis, stridor, cyanosis, shock. Death 24–36 hours after onset of severe symptoms. Hemorrhagic meningitis in up to 50%.	Nonspecific physical findings.	Serology, gram stain, culture, polymerase chain reaction (PCR); chest x-ray (CXR)—widened mediastinum. Rarely pneumonia.	Hantavirus pulmonary syndrome (HPS), dissecting aortic aneurysm (no fever)	1–6 days (up to 45 days)	3–5 days	~100% if untreated	None
Pneumonic plague	High fever, chills, headache, hemoptysis and toxemia, rapid progression to dyspnea, stridor, and cyanosis. Death from respiratory failure, shock, and bleeding.	Rales, hemoptysis, purpura	Gram stain, culture, serum immunoassay for capsular antigen, PCR, immunohistochemical stains (IHC)	HPS, tuberculosis (TB), community acquired pneumonia (CAP), meningococcemia, rickettsioses	2–3 days	1–6 days	Usually fatal unless treated in 12–24 hours	2–3 cases/yr, mainly in SW U.S.
Tularemia	Typhoidal—aerosol, gastrointestinal, and intradermal challenge. Fever, headache, malaise, chest discomfort, anorexia, nonproductive cough. Pneumonia in 30–80%. Oculoglandular from inoculation of conjunctiva with periorbital edema.	No adenopathy with typhoidal illness	Serology, culture, PCR, IHC; CXR—pneumonia, mediastinal lymphadenopathy, or pleural effusion.	Atypical CAP, Q fever, brucellosis	1–10 days (average 3–5 days)	>2 wks	10–35% untreated	150 case/yr, transmitted by ticks/deer flies or contact with infected animals
Smallpox	Fever, back pain, vomiting, malaise, headache, rigors. Papules 2–3 days later, progressing to pustular vesicles. Abundant on face and extremities initially.	Papules, pustules, or scabs of similar stage, many on face/extremities, palms/soles	Guamierl bodies on Glemsa or modified silver stain, virions on electron microscopy, PCR, viral isolation, IHC	Varicella, vaccinia, monkeypox, cowpox, disseminated herpes zoster	7–17days (average 12 days)	4 wks	Up to 30% higher in flat-type or hemorrhagic disease	None

(continues on page 888)

TABLE 15.2   Clinical Characteristics of Critical Biological Agents—7/1/00 (continued)

Disease	Signs and Symptoms	Physical Exam	Clinical Test	Key Differential Diagnosis	Incubation Period	Duration of Illness	Case Fatality	U.S. Epidemiology
Botulism	Ptosis, blurred vision, diplopia, generalized weakness, dizziness, dysarthria, dysphonia, dysphagia, followed by symmetrical descending flaccid paralysis and respiratory failure.	No fever, client alert, postural hypotension, pupils unreactive, normal sensation, variable muscle weaknesss	Serology, toxin assays/anaerobic cultures of blood/stool; electromyography studies	Guillain Barré, myasthenia gravis, tick paralysis, Mg^{++} intoxication, organophosphate poisoning, polio	1–5 days	Death 24–72 hours or respiratory support for months	High mortality without respiratory support	30 cases/yr; food intoxication, wound infections, or honey ingestion (infants)
Filoviruses (Marburg, Ebola)	Fever, severe headache, malaise, myalgia, maculo-papular rash day 5; progression to pharyngitis, hematemasis, melena, uncontrolled bleeding; shock/death 6–9 days.	Petechia, ecchymoses, conjunctivitis, uncontrolled bleeding	Serology, PCR, IHC, electron microscopy (EM); elevated liver enzymes, thrombocytopenia	Meningococcemia, malaria, typhus, leptospirosis, borreliosis, thrombotic thrombocytopenic purpura (TTP), rickettsiosis, hemolytic uremic syndrome (HUS), arenaviruses	2–19 days (average 4–10 days)	Days to weeks	>80%	None
Arenaviruses (Lassa, Junin, Sabia, Machupo, Guanarito)	Fever, malaise, headache, N/V, pharyngitis, cough, retro-intestinal pain, bleeding, tremors of tongue and hands (Junin), shock, aspetic meningitis, coma, hearing loss in some.	Conjunctivitis, petechia, ecchymoses, flushing over head and upper torso	Serology, viral isolation, PCR, IHC; leukopenia, thrombocytopenia, proteinuria	Leptospirosis, meningococcemia, malaria, typhus, borreliosis, rickettsiosis, TTP, HUS, filoviruses	5–21 days Lassa; 7–16 days Sabia, Junin, Machapo, Guanarito	7–15 days	15–30%	None

Source: Biological Warfare and Terrorism: Medical Issues and Response—Student Material Booklet. U.S. Army Medical Research Institute of Infectious Diseases, September 2000.

TABLE 15.3 BW Agents: Vaccine, Therapeutics, and Prophylaxis

Disease	Vaccine	Chemotherapy	Chemoprophylaxis (PX)	Comments
Anthrax	Bioport vaccine (licensed) 0.5 mL SC at 0, 2, 4 wk; 6, 12, 18 mo then annually	Ciprofloxacin 400 mg IV q 8–12 h Doxycycline 200 mg IV, then 100 mg IV q 8–12 h Penicillin 2 million units IV q2h	Ciprofloxacin 500 mg PO bid × 4 wk if unvaccinated, begin initial doses of vaccine Doxycycline 100 mg PO bid × 4 wk plus vaccination	Potential alternates for Rx: gentamicin, erythromycin, and chloramphenicol PCN for sensitive organisms only
Cholera	Wyeth–Ayerst Vaccine 2 doses 0.5 mL IM or SC at 0, 7–30 days, then boosters q6 mo	Oral rehydration therapy during period or high fluid loss Tetracycline 500 mg q6h × 3 d Doxycycline 300 mg once, or 100 mg q12h × 3 d Ciprofloxacin 500 mg q12h × 3 d		Vaccine not recommended for routine protection in endemic areas (50% efficacy, short term) Alternates for Rx: erythromycin, trimethoprim and sulfamethoxazole, and furazolidone Quinolones for tetra/doxy resistant strains
Q Fever	IND 610—inactivated whole cell vaccine given as single 0.5 mL SC injection	Tetracycline 500 mg PO q6h × 5–7 d Doxycycline 100 mg PO q12h × 5–7 d	Tetracycline start 8–12 d post-exposure × 5 d Doxycycline start 8–12 d post-exposure × 5 d	Currently testing vaccine to determine the necessity of skin testing prior to use.
Glanders	No vaccine available.	Antibiotic regimens vary depending on localization and severity of disease—refer to text.	Post-exposure prophyaxsis may be tried with TMP-SMX	No large therapeutic human trials have been conducted owing to the rarity of naturally occurring disease.
Plague	Greer inactivated vaccine (FDA licensed) is no longer available: 1.0 mL, IM; 0.2 mL, IM 1–3 mo later; 6.2 mL 5–6 mo after dose 2; 0.2 mL boosters at 6, 12, 18 mo after dose 3 then q 1–2 years	Streptomycin 30 mg/kg/d IM in 2 divided doses × 10 d (or gentamicin) Doxycycline 200 mg IV then 100 mg IV bid × 10–14 d Chloramphenicol 1 g IV qid × 10–14 d	Doxycycline 100 mg PO bid × 7 or duration of exposure Ciprofloxacin 500 mg PO bid × 7 d Doxycycline 100 mg PO bid × 7 d Tetracycline 500 mg PO qid × 7 d	Plague vaccine not protective against aerosol challenge in animal studies. Alternate Rx: trimethoprim-sulfamethoxazole Chloramphenicol for plague meningitis
Tularemia	IND—live attenuated vaccine: one dose by scarification	Streptomycin 30 mg/kg IM divided bid × 10–14 d Gentamicin 3–5 mg/kg/d IV × 10–14 d	Doxycycline 100 mg PO bid × 14 d Tetracycline 500 mg PO qid × 14 d	
Brucellosis	No human vaccine available	Doxycycline 200 mg/d PO plus rifampin 600–900 mg/d PO × wk Ofloxacin 400/rifampin 600 mg/d PO × 6 wks	Doxycycline and rifampin × 3 wk	Trimethoprim-sulfamethoxazole (TMP-SMX) may be substituted for rifampin; however, relapse may reach 30%
Viral encephalitides	VEE DOD TC-3 live attenuated vaccine (IND): 0.5 mL SC × 1 dose VEE DOD C-84 (formalin inactivated TC-83) (IND): 0.5 mL SC for up to 3 h EEE inactivated (IND): 0.5 mL SC at 0 & 28 d WEE inactivated (IND): 0.5 mL SC at 0, 7, and 28 d	Supportive therapy: analgesics and anticonvulsants prn	NA	TC-83 rectogenic in 20%. No seroconversion in 20%. Only effective against subtypes IA, IB, and IC. C-84 vaccine used for nonresponders to TC-83. EEE and WEE inactivated vaccines are poorly immunogenic; multiple immunizations are required.

(continues on page 890)

TABLE 15.3 BW Agents: Vaccine, Therapeutics, and Prophylaxis (continued)

Disease	Vaccine	Chemotherapy	Chemoprophylaxis (PX)	Comments
Viral hemorrhagic fevers	AHF Candid #1 vaccine (x-protective for BHF) (IND) RVF inactivated vaccine (IND)	Ribavarin (CCHF/ arenaviruses) 30 mg/kg IV initial dose 15 mg/kg IV q6h × 4 d 7.5 mg/kg IV q8h × 6 d Passive antibody for AHF, BHF, Lassa fever, and CCHF	NA	Aggressive supportive care and management of hypotension very important.
Smallpox	Wyeth calf lymph vaccinia vaccine (licensed): 1 dose by scarification	Cidofovir (effective in vitro); animal studies ongoing	Vaccinia immune globulin 0.6 mL/kg IM (within 3 d of exposure, best within 24 h)	Pre- and postexposure vaccination recommended if >3 years since last vaccine.
Botulism	DOD pentavaient toxoid for serotypes A-E (IND): 0.5 mL deep SC at 0, 2, 12 wk, then yearly boosters	DOD heptavalent equine despeciated antitoxin for serotypes A-G (IND): 1 vial (10 mL) IV CDC trivaient equine antitoxin for serotypes A, B, E (licensed)		Skin test for hypersensitivity before equine antitoxin administration
Straphylococcus enterotoxin B	No vaccine available.	Ventilatory support for inhalation exposure		
Ricin	No vaccine available.	Inhalation: supportive therapy G-1: gastric lavage, superactivated charcoal, cathartics		
T-2 Mycotoxins	No vaccine available.		Decontamination of clothing and skin	

Key: AHF, Argentine hemorrhagic fever; BHF, Bovine hemorrhagic fever; bid, twice a day; CCHF, Crimean-Congo hemorrhagic fever; CDC, Centers for Disease Control and Prevention; DOD, U.S. Department of Defense; EEE, Eastern equine encephalitis; FDA, Food and Drug Administration; IM, intramuscular; IND, investigational new drug; IV, intravenous; NA, not applicable; PCN, penicillin; PO, by mouth; q, every; Rx, prescription; SC, subcutaneous; VEE, Venezuelan equine encephalitis; WEE, Western equine encephalitis.
Source: Biological Warfare and Terrorism: Medical Issues and Response—Student Material Booklet. U.S. Army Medical Research Institute of Infectious Diseases, September 2000.

PEDIATRIC CONSIDERATIONS

I. Challenges
a. Undergoing medical treatment can be emotionally and psychologically difficult for the child (infant through adolesent) and his or her family.
b. Children are not "small adults" and require child-friendly care with adaptation of interventions dependent on maturation of body systems and organ function and the child's age and developmental level (London et al, 2007).
   i. Growth—generally follows a predictable pattern influenced by gender, heredity, environmental factors (such as nutrition), and cultural practices
   ii. Development—each child's maturational pattern is unique; however, the sequence for acquisition of skills is uniform in children, essentially proceeding from the head down and from the center of the body out to the extremities.
c. Special approaches are required to meet the physical, emotional, social, spiritual, and cultural needs of the hospitalized child and his or her family.

   i. Child-sized equipment
   ii. Diversional activities—age-appropriate play rooms, games, arts, recreation
   iii. Learning opportunities—age-appropriate print and visual teaching tools, tutoring during prolonged hospitalization
   iv. Family-centered care—inclusion of all members, as appropriate, with consideration of sociocultural and spiritual factors

II. Developmental Factors Relating to Hospitalization
(Morgan Stanley Children's Hospital of New York, n.d.; The Children's Hospital of Philadelphia, n.d.)
a. Infant—birth to 12 months
   i. Just learning to make sense of the world; child can become very unsettled when cared for by multiple or different providers.
   ii. Cannot understand how various procedures and treatments that he or she perceives to "hurt" can actually produce recovery or make them well
   iii. From about age 6 months and older, child can become very afraid if parents leave him or her.

b. Toddler—12 to 36 months

    i. Issues of separation, rather than being ill, can be the major stress for child if required to stay in hospital without parent or familiar caregiver.

    ii. Has no concept or understanding of what is happening when they are ill

    iii. Does not understand time and space so all this can be very frightening for them

c. Preschool—3 to 5 years

    i. Fear of the unknown and being left alone are major concerns.

    ii. Have limited ability to distinguish fantasy from reality

    iii. Tend to misunderstand words they hear, leading to misconceptions

    iv. May view hospitalization as a punishment—fearing needles, body mutilation, or loss of function

d. School-age child—6 to 11 years

    i. Almost all school-age children will have seen and heard about illness and hospitals on TV.

    ii. May have seen people "die" in hospital and know about cancer and other illnesses that can cause children to die

    iii. Need to know what will happen to them, and that they will not die from this illness—may be too frightened to ask about this themselves

    iv. Often misunderstand what they overhear; require opportunities to ask questions

e. Adolescent—12 to 18 years

    i. Understands what causes illness and how it affects the body

    ii. Fears separation from peers and group activities

    iii. Hospitalization represents a loss of control over almost all areas of life, even the most basic aspects—when the teen eats, sleeps, or uses the bathroom, coupled with a loss of privacy at a time when self-consciousness is peaking.

    iv. May express anger or indifference to mask feelings of fear

    v. May feel bothered by frequent examinations by different professionals

    vi. Hospitalization represents a challenge to all teens, especially teens from ethnic, religious, or cultural minority groups.

III. Statistics

a. More than 3 million children in the United States are hospitalized annually (Schmidt et al, 2007).

GLOSSARY

Development: The qualitative increase in a child's capabilities or function, attainment or mastery of skills.

Growth: Increase in physical size and internal development as measured by multiple factors, such as height, weight, blood pressure, and sexual maturation, as well as the number of words in vocabulary.

Major Theories of Development (London, 2007):

Behaviorism: The research of animal behaviorists was applied to children and demonstrated that behaviors can be elicited by positive reinforcement or extinguished by negative reinforcement. Application of theory to hospitalization—repetition of desired behaviors can be encouraged by providing positive reinforcement for child's efforts.

Ecologic theory: Although controversy exists about heredity (nature) versus environment (nurture) and which one has more influence in human development, this theory recognizes the effect of both through mutual interactions between the child and the various levels of the environment (from close to remote) in all of life's settings. Application of theory to hospitalization—use of tool based on this theory to assess child's interface with varied levels of the environment identifies areas of strength that can help with addressing individual challenges or areas that are nonsupportive.

Erikson's Theory of Psychosexual Development: Describes psychosocial stages during eight periods of human life with a particular challenge that is needed for healthy development to occur. Application of theory to hospitalization—interrupts usual support provided by family and peers and adds a situational crisis to the normal developmental crisis experienced by the child.

Freud's Theory of Psychosexual Development: Early childhood experiences form the unconscious motivation for actions in later life. Application of theory to hospitalization—defensive mechanisms, such as regression and repression, may be used by the child to cope with excess anxiety, and the crisis of illness can interfere with normal developmental processes.

Kohlberg's Theory of Moral Development: Using Piaget's cognitive theory as a basis for moral development, three levels of moral reasoning—preconventional, conventional, and postconventional—were identified with associated age ranges. Application of theory to hospitalization—based on stage of development, decisions made by the child may reflect a desire to avoid punishment, to please others, or to present a sense of social responsibility. This provides some direction to care providers as they present information to the child to assist them in the decision-making process.

Piaget's Theory of Cognitive Development: The child's view of the world is influenced largely by age and maturational ability and matures naturally. Application of theory to hospitalization—level of cognitive development and thought processes affects choice of approaches when providing appropriate stimulation and creating teaching plans for the child.

(text continues on page 892)

Social Learning Theory: Children learn attitudes, beliefs, customs, and values through their social contacts with adults and other children, and they model the behavior they see. Application of theory to hospitalization—the provision of positive role model, such as a peer experiencing a similar situation, facilitates learning and child's cooperation with interventions.

Temperament Theory: The child both influences, and is influenced by, the enviroment and has innate qualities of personality or certain patterns of temperament that he or she brings to daily life. Application of theory to hospitalization—understanding the child's temperament provides opportunities to alter or manipulate the environment to meet the child's needs and maximize the experience.

Resiliency Theory: A child's characteristics and how these traits interact with the environment determines his or her resiliency or ability to use healthy responses even in adverse situations. In the face of a crisis, the child and the family have protective characteristics that provide strength and risk factors or characteristics that magnify challenges. Application of theory to hospitalization—providing positive reinforcement for protective characteristics encourages continuation of desired behaviors that can be used to support the period of adjustment and facilitate adaptation to change. Identification of risk factors provides an opportunity to target interventions and teaching activities to assist family and child to deal more effectively with the challenge and increase their resiliency.

Care Setting

Any setting in which nursing contact with children occurs and care is provided.

Client Assessment Database

Data depend on the specific pathology necessitating therapeutic interventions.

Assessment Factors—in addition to routine assessment of current condition or comorbidities

SUBJECTIVE	OBJECTIVE
INDIVIDUAL	
• Perception of body and its functions in health, illness, and in this situation	• Age, developmental level, gender
• Emotional reactions in feeling or sensory terms; for example, client states, "I feel scared"	• Personality, temperament
• Food and eating concerns	• Patterns of communication with significant others (SOs)
• Sleep patterns	• Behavior when anxious, afraid, impatient, withdrawn, or angry
• Lifestyle differences requiring considerarion—dietary, spiritual, sexual identity, other community (e.g., religious order, commune, homeless)	• Emotional response to current treatment or hospitalization
	• How child experiences illness versus reality of situation
SIGNIFICANT OTHERS	
• Nuclear family, extended family; peer group, friends	• Interaction processes within the family
• Family developmental cycle	
• Child's role in family tasks and functions	
• How are SOs affected by the illness and prognosis?	
SOCIOECONOMIC	
	• Social class, value system
	• Social acceptability of current situation
CULTURAL	
• Ethnic background, heritage, and residence	
• Family beliefs regarding caring and curing	
• Family health-seeking behaviors, illness referral system	
• Family values related to health and treatment	
• Cultural factors related to illness in general and to pain response	

Client Assessment Database (continued)

SUBJECTIVE (continued)	OBJECTIVE (continued)
DISEASE/CONDITION • Past experience with illness, hospitalization, healthcare systems and providers • Family and child expectations if illness is terminal	• Response of child and family to situation or condition requiring treatment • Nature of condition—acute, chronic, recurrent • Emotional response to current treatments • Availability and use of resources

Nursing Priorities

1. Enhance level of comfort and minimize pain.
2. Reduce anxiety and fear.
3. Provide growth-promoting environment for child and parent(s).
4. Prevent or minimize complications.

Discharge Goals

1. Pain relieved or controlled.
2. Child and family dealing appropriately with current situation.
3. Safe environment maintained.
4. Plan in place to meet needs after discharge.

NURSING DIAGNOSIS: acute/chronic Pain

May be related to
Injuring agents—biological, chemical, physical, psychological

Possibly evidenced by
Verbal cues
Changes in appetite and eating, sleep pattern
Guarding, protective behavior; restlessness, moaning, crying, irritability
Autonomic responses

Desired Outcomes/Evaluation Criteria—Child Will

Pain Level (NOC)
Report or indicate pain is relieved or controlled.
Manifest decreased restlessness and irritability.
Demonstrate age-appropriate blood pressure (BP), pulse, and respiratory rates.

Pain Disruptive Effects (NOC)
Participate in usual activities within level of ability.

ACTIONS/INTERVENTIONS	RATIONALE
Pain Management (NIC) *Independent* Perform routine comprehensive pain assessment, including location, characteristics, onset, duration, frequency, quality, and severity using some type of rating scale, such as numbers or visual analog, facial expressions, or color scale. Accept child's description of pain, noting precipitating, exacerbating, and relieving factors. Investigate changes in frequency or description of pain. Observe for guarding, rigidity, crying, and restlessness. Monitor heart rate, BP using correctly sized cuff, and respiratory rate, noting age-appropriate normals and variations. Note location and type of surgical incisions or trauma.	Assessment of children involves observational skills and may require enlisting the aid of parent or caregiver to clarify cues and verbalizations. Choice of rating scale is dependent on age and developmental level (Suresh, 2002). Pain is subjective and cannot be experienced by others. *Note:* In presence of chronic pain situation, use of a pain diary may be appropriate for adolescents (Suresh, 2002). May signal worsening of condition or development of complications. Nonverbal expressions, body movement, and behavioral state may signal pain or changes in pain severity, especially in infants and younger children (Suresh, 2002). Changes in autonomic responses may indicate increased pain before child verbalizes. *Note:* Autonomic responses change with acute pain, not chronic pain. BP may be lower than normal or higher than normal. Influences degree and severity of pain manifestations.

(continues on page 894)

ACTIONS/INTERVENTIONS (continued)

Provide comfort measures, such as holding, repositioning, back rub, and use of breathing or guided visualization relaxation techniques, as indicated.

Identify ways to avoid or minimize pain, such as splinting surgical incisions during coughing, sleeping on a firm mattress, or wearing brace on sprains.

Encourage sleep and rest periods.

Encourage diversional activities such as TV, music, reading, playing quiet games, and texting friends.

Review procedures and expectations and tell child when it will hurt. Provide distraction during painful procedures, such as deep breathing or counting, or looking at something that interests child.

Encourage expression of feelings about pain.

Suggest parent and caregiver be with child during procedures, as possible.

Collaborative

Collaborate in treatment of underlying conditions or disease process.

Administer medications, such as opioid and nonsteroidal analgesics, as indicated. Use multiple routes to deliver analgesia, such as oral, nebulized, transdermal, or patient-controlled analgesia (PCA), as indicated by current situation.

RATIONALE (continued)

Nonpharmacological pain management promotes relaxation; may reduce level of pain and enhance coping.

Many factors may reduce pain intensity based on specific situation. Child can quickly learn and use such pain management techniques, enhancing sense of control as well as comfort.

Helps reduce fatigue and enhances coping ability.

Helps distract child's attention from pain and reduces tension.

Although the procedure may still be stressful, child will find it easier to handle if he or she knows what to expect and has developed coping strategies.

Can relieve anxiety and help reduce intensity of pain.

Provides comforting presence.

Treating cause, when possible, can eliminate pain.

Depending on the cause and type of pain, as well as its chronicity, various means of pain management may be needed to overcome or control pain.

NURSING DIAGNOSIS: Anxiety/Fear; ineffective Coping

May be related to

Situational and maturational crises; interpersonal transmission or contagion

Threat to, or change in, health status

Natural or innate origin—pain, loss of physical support

Separation from support system in potentially stressful situation—hospitalization, hospital procedures

Learned response—conditioning, modeling from or identification with others

Possibly evidenced by

Excessive psychomotor activity, restlessness, crying, lack of eye contact, withdrawal, sleep disturbances, nightmares

Avoidance or attack behaviors, reports of being scared, expressed concerns about changes

Social inhibition, shy, withdrawn demeanor

Desired Outcomes/Evaluation Criteria—Child Will

Anxiety Level (NOC)

Appear relaxed and report or demonstrate relief from somatic manifestations of anxiety.

Demonstrate a decrease in somatic complaints and physical symptoms when faced with stressful situations such as impending separation from SO.

Anxiety Self-Control (NOC)

Engage in age-appropriate activities in absence of parent or primary caregiver without fear or distress noted.

ACTIONS/INTERVENTIONS

Anxiety Reduction (NIC)

Independent

Establish an atmosphere of calmness, trust, and genuine positive regard.

Prepare child for activites and procedures. Provide explanations in language appropriate for age. Use terms familiar to child, such as for care activities—"walk" instead of "ambulate"—or procedures—"take a picture" instead of "fluoroscope." Provide opportunity for client to ask questions, observe or touch equipment as appropriate.

RATIONALE

Trust and unconditional acceptance are necessary for satisfactory therapeutic relationship. Calmness is important because anxiety is easily transmitted from one person to another, and children are often adept at sensing changes in the moods of adults around them.

Accurate and age-appropriate communication promotes trust and creates an atmosphere where child feels free to ask questions. Based on child's developmental level, tour of facility or surgical suite and observation of "machinery" in action may help reduce concerns regarding the unknown. *Note:* Children may become frightened of things they cannot articulate.

ACTIONS/INTERVENTIONS (continued)	RATIONALE (continued)
Ensure child of his or her safety and security—listen to child, identify needs, and be available for support.	Strange people and surroundings, changes in routine, and loss of control in situation create anxiety and can be very frightening. Children may believe that situation is punishment for some wrongdoing—imagined or real—on their part. Providing information and being available can be reassuring.
Be honest with child and parents by saying, "Yes, this will hurt and I will help you manage it."	Promotes trust and belief that child will not be left alone to deal with situation.
Refrain from conversations unrelated to child in his or her presence or failing to include child in conversations regarding him or her.	Ignoring the child or talking about, instead of to, the child or allowing child to overhear partial or unrelated conversations may be very stressful and result in child imagining things that are incorrect.
Maintain home routines whenever possible. Encourage child and parents to bring transitional object from home, such as familiar toys, handheld computer games or digital music player, special pillow or blanket, some favorite pictures, or posters, if hospitalized.	Use of age-appropriate object enhances sense of security when child or adolescent is hospitalized or in treatment setting.
Provide consistency of caregivers.	Becoming acquainted with caregiver enhances sense of security, facilitates communication, and lessens anxiety.
Promote child and family contact and interaction. Encourage parents to participate in care planning and care provision.	Family involvement in activities promotes continuity of family unit, provides opportunity to learn and practice new skills, and enhances coping skills.
Emphasize importance of staff and family giving verbal prompts in anticipation of absences. Provide honest information about leaving and returning.	Avoidance of these issues increases the likelihood of anxiety responses when separation occurs.
Help family support child emotionally by being available and active-listening.	Conveys acceptance of child and confidence in ability to cope with situation.
Encourage contact with peers via phone, texting, online chats, or visits, as appropriate.	Helps child stay connected with friends and life outside hospital (Merck Manuals, 2005b). *Note:* Computer access requires monitoring, or blocking of, inappropriate Web sites for client's safety.
Provide child with age-appropriate choices, when possible.	Promotes sense of control, demonstrates regard for individual.
Schedule ample time for play and age-appropriate diversions. Use play materials, such as puppets, doll house, doctor/nurse kits, fairy tale stories, clay, coloring book, and so on.	Promotes normalcy and helps divert attention from situation. Play therapy enables child to explore conflicts, express fears, and release tension.
Engage in exercise program as appropriate to situation.	Provides physical outlet for energy, releasing tension. May stimulate release of endorphins, decreasing anxiety and enhancing child's ability to deal with illness and situation.
Collaborative	
Administer medications, as indicated.	Mild sedation can be effective in ameliorating symptoms of anxiety and enhancing child's receptiveness to therapeutic regimen.

NURSING DIAGNOSIS: Activity Intolerance [specify level]/Fatigue

May be related to
Generalized weakness, bedrest or immobility
Imbalance between oxygen supply and demand
Pain, extreme stress

Possibly evidenced by
Report of fatigue or weakness, lack of energy, exertional discomfort or dyspnea, inability to maintain usual routine
Listless, lethargic; abnormal heart rate or BP response to activity

Desired Outcomes/Evaluation Criteria—Child Will

Endurance (NOC)
Participate in customary activities at desired level.
Report display or absence of fatigue.

ACTIONS/INTERVENTIONS	RATIONALE
Activity Therapy (NIC)	
Independent	
Ascertain child's usual level of activity, taking into account age and developmental level.	Establishes baseline in order to determine needed interventions and to assess progress of recovery.

(continues on page 896)

ACTIONS/INTERVENTIONS (continued)

Note how present situation is affecting level of activity—immobilization, use of restraints, casts or traction, presence of heart or respiratory impairment, cancer, and treatments.

Determine usual sleep and rest routine and any bedtime rituals or security objects. Plan care with adequate rest periods.

Adjust activities, reducing intensity level or discontinuing activities, as needed. Assist with activities of daily living (ADLs) and promote exercise, as indicated.

Promote participation in individually appropriate recreational and diversional activities.

Promote optimal mobility, providing safe transport such as wagon, child-size wheelchair, or walker.

Monitor response to activity, including BP, pulse, respiratory rate, skin color, and behavior.

Collaborative

Provide and monitor response to oxygen administration via appropriate route and effects of medication.

Refer to physical and occupational therapists.

RATIONALE (continued)

Presence of certain disease processes, trauma, or treatment modalities have potential for interfering with child's usual and desired level of activity.

Attempting to maintain usual sleep routines promotes rest and maximizes energy and endurance.

Protects child from injury and enhances ability to participate in activity to improve strength.

Enhances sense of well-being and expectation of return to usual activities.

Provides normalcy to child, who is not accustomed to inactivity, and will help reduce complications associated with immobility.

Helps identify and monitor degree of fatigue and potential for complications. *Note:* Charts list different respiratory rates for different ages. However, a quick method to use as a guide is this: If you feel out of breath watching a child breathe, the rate is abnormally fast; if you feel the need to help a child breathe, the rate is probably too slow.

Oxygen may be needed to improve tolerance to activity and treat underlying cause for fatigue. High-flow oxygen via non-rebreather mask is ideal if child can tolerate it. Blow-by oxygen can provide some benefit if child refuses to wear mask.

Helpful to develop activity and exercise programs to meet individual and family needs.

NURSING DIAGNOSIS: **risk for delayed Growth and Development**

Risk factors may include
Separation from parents and family, peer group
Environmental and stimulation deficiencies, effects of physical disability or confinement
Inadequate care; multiple caretakers; prolonged, painful treatments

Possibly evidenced by
(Not applicable, presence of signs and symptoms establishes an *actual* diagnosis)

Desired Outcomes/Evaluation Criteria—Child Will

Child Development: [specify age group] (NOC)
Perform motor, social, and/or expressive skills typical of age group within scope of present capabilities.
Demonstrate weight and growth-stabilization or progress toward age-appropriate size.

ACTIONS/INTERVENTIONS

Development Enhancement: Child [or] Adolescent (NIC)
Independent

Determine existing factors or condition(s) that could contribute to growth or development deviation, such as chronic illness, substance use or abuse, familial history of pituitary tumors, Marfan's syndrome, and genetic anomalies.

Determine child's birth weight and length and compare present growth with norms.

Note chronological age and familial factors, such as body build and stature. Review expectations for current height and weight percentiles and degree of deviation.

Measure developmental level using age-appropriate tests, such as the Denver Developmental Screening Test. Note reported losses or alterations in functional level.

Determine child's cognitive and perceptual level, such as grade level in school. Note behavioral reaction to environment and stimuli, such as withdrawal or aggression.

RATIONALE

Plan of care will be based on individual factors present, immediacy of threat, and potential long-term complications. *Note:* Tobacco, alcohol, or other drug use are major health-care concerns for children.

Identifies the child's status compared with other children of the same age.

Aids in determining growth expectations (Sutter Health, n.d.).

Provides comparative baseline and basis for choosing developmentally appropriate interventions.

Illness or injury can lead to a temporary increase in level of dependency and a decline in functional level. Although this may not be of major concern for the short term, chronic and recurrent conditions may delay acquisition of important developmental milestones.

ACTIONS/INTERVENTIONS (continued)

Note severity and pervasiveness of situation. For example, is the child showing effects of long-term physical or emotional abuse or neglect versus experiencing recent onset situational disruption or inadequate resources during period of crisis or transition?

Determine occurrence and frequency of significant stressful events in the child's life, including losses, separation, and environmental changes, such as abandonment, divorce, death of parent or sibling, and relocation.

Discuss nature and effectiveness of parenting and caregiving activities, noting inadequate, inconsistent, unrealistic, or insufficient expectations as well as lack of stimulation, limit setting, or responsiveness.

Provide parents with information regarding normal growth and development, as appropriate, including pertinent reference materials.

Identify realistic goals with child and parents. Discuss actions to take to avoid or minimize preventable complications.

Encourage self-care activities, as appropriate, such as feeding, grooming, and playing. Provide privacy when desired and when privacy is safe for child.

Collaborative

Assist with therapy to treat or correct underlying conditions, such as Crohn's disease, cardiac problems, or renal disease; endocrine problems, such as hypothyroidism, type 1 diabetes mellitus, or growth hormone abnormalities; and genetic or intrauterine growth retardation, infant feeding problems, or nutritional deficits.

Include family, nutritionist, physical and occupational therapists, and other specialists in developing plan of care.

Refer to available community resources as appropriate such as public health programs, medical equipment suppliers, nutritionist, substance abuse program, and specialist in endocrine conditions or genetics.

Contact client's school for educational resource or tutor and learning plan, as indicated.

RATIONALE (continued)

Problems existing over a long period may have more severe effects and require longer course of treatment to reverse.

Lack of resolution or repetition of stressor can have a cumulative effect over time and result in regression in, or deterioration of, functional level.

Assessment of parenting and potential for conflict and negative interaction between parent or caregiver and child identifies interventions needed to maximize care.

Helps parents understand potential changes in relation to current illness or problem.

Provides anticipatory guidance (Sutter Health, n.d.). Increases probability of reaching goals and managing situation more effectively. Can enhance sense of control and independence.

Promotes independence and maintenance of self-esteem.

Illness, hospitalization, treatments, and separation from parents and family have a negative effect on physical and psychological growth and development.

Multidisciplinary team involvement increases likelihood of a well-rounded plan of care that meets child's special and varied needs.

Although acute situations may be readily resolved with limited support and few ill effects, chronic or recurrent conditions require many resources to maximize growth potential of child and family.

Prevents child from falling behind in studies and provides sense of normalcy during prolonged illness or hospitalization (Merck Manuals, 2005b).

NURSING DIAGNOSIS: risk for imbalanced Nutrition: Less than Body Requirements

Risk factors may include

Inability to ingest or digest food or absorb nutrients because of biological, psychological, or economic factors

Increased metabolic demands

Possibly evidenced by

(Not applicable, presence of signs and symptoms establishes an *actual* diagnosis)

Desired Outcomes/Evaluation Criteria—Child Will

Nutritional Status (NOC)

Ingest nutritionally adequate diet for age, activity level, and metabolic demands.

Demonstrate stable weight or progressive weight gain toward goal.

ACTIONS/INTERVENTIONS

Nutrition Management (NIC)

Independent

Identify child at risk for malnutrition, such as with intestinal surgery, hypermetabolic states, restricted intake, and/or prior nutritional deficiencies.

RATIONALE

Provides opportunity for timely intervention.

(continues on page 898)

ACTIONS/INTERVENTIONS (continued)	RATIONALE (continued)
Determine ability to chew, swallow, and taste. Note presence of conditions affecting food intake, such as lactose intolerance, cystic fibrosis, diabetes, inflammatory bowel diseases, or eating disorders.	These factors can affect specific dietary choices, desire to eat and/or ingestion and digestion of nutrients.
Determine child's current nutritional status using age-appropriate measurements, including weight and body build, strength, activity level, and sleep and rest cycles.	Identifies individual nutritional needs and provides comparative baseline.
Auscultate bowel sounds. Note characteristics of stool, including color, amount, and frequency of bowel movements.	Provides information about digestion and bowel function and may affect choice and timing of feeding.
Elicit information from child/parent regarding typical daily food intake, determining foods and beverages normally consumed. Note types of snacks. Discuss eating habits and food preferences—likes and dislikes.	Baseline information to determine adequacy of intake. Knowledge of child's specific likes and dislikes may be helpful in meeting child's nutritional needs during a time when appetite is suppressed or child has no interest in food.
Determine psychological factors and cultural or religious desires or influences on dietary choices.	Dietary beliefs, such as vegetarianism, can affect nutritional intake. Usual ethnic food choices can improve a child's intake when appetite is poor.
Review drug regimen, noting potential side effects, and possible interactions with other medications, over-the-counter (OTC) drugs, and herbs.	Timing of medication doses and interaction with certain foods can alter effect of medication or digestion and absorption of nutrients.
Determine whether infant is breast-fed or formula-fed, and note typical pattern of feedings during a 24-hour period. Note type and amounts of solid foods infant or toddler eats.	Providing usual and typical feedings is important to infant well-being and early growth.
Discuss with parent what types of candy, other sweets, snacks, and beverages child eats or drinks.	Identifies what child eats in a typical day. Provides opportunity for identifying teaching needs and providing healthy snacks.
Emphasize importance of well-balanced, nutritious intake. Provide information regarding individual nutritional needs and ways to meet these needs within financial constraints. Avoid arguing over food intake. Provide food without comment.	Although nutritious intake is important, arguing over food is counterproductive. Providing age-appropriate guidelines to children as well as to parents or care provider may help them in making healthy choices. *Note:* Childhood obesity with associated long-term physical and psychological effects is also a potential concern regardless of current weight.
Clarify caregiver access to and use of resources, such as food stamps, budget counseling, Women, Infants, and Children (WIC) program, community food bank, and/or other appropriate assistance programs.	May be necessary to improve child's intake and/or availability of food to meet nutritional needs.
Collaborative	
Establish a nutritional plan that meets individual needs incorporating specific food restrictions and special dietary needs.	Corrects or controls underlying causative factors, such as with diabetes, cancer, malabsorption syndrome, and anorexia.
Consult dietitian or nutritional team, as indicated.	Helps determine individual nutritional needs and therapeutic diet.
Review laboratory studies, such as serum albumin or prealbumin, transferrin, amino acid profile, iron, blood urea nitrogen (BUN), nitrogen balance studies, glucose, liver function, electrolytes, and total lymphocyte count.	Indicators of nutritional health and effects of nutrients in organ function.
Refer for dental hygiene care, nutritional counseling, or psychiatric or family therapy, as indicated.	May be needed to provide assistance, support, and direction for meeting nutritional needs not only in the present but for achieving long-term goals as well.
Refer to home care resources when indicated by specific condition or illness.	Assists with initiation and supervision of home nutrition therapy when used.

NURSING DIAGNOSIS: risk for Injury (specify: Trauma, Suffocation, Poisoning)

Risk factors may include

Developmental age; cognitive or emotional difficulties

Disease or injury process; use of restraining device

Use of pharmaceutical agents, narrow therapeutic margin of safety of some drugs, exposure to substances—tobacco, alcohol, street drugs

Lack of safety or drug education or precautions

Immune or autoimmune dysfunction; malnutrition; exposure to nosocomial agents

Possibly evidenced by

(Not applicable, presence of signs and symptoms establishes an *actual* diagnosis)

NURSING DIAGNOSIS: risk for Injury (specify: Trauma, Suffocation, Poisoning) (continued)

Desired Outcomes/Evaluation Criteria—Child Will

Risk Control (NOC)
Be free of injury.

Caregiver/Parent—Will

Verbalize understanding of individual risk factors that contribute to possibility of injury.
Take steps to correct identified risks and protect child from hazards.

ACTIONS/INTERVENTIONS	RATIONALE
Risk Surveillance (NIC)	
Independent	
Identify individual risk factors, such as airway patency, therapeutic use of potentially toxic medications, invasive lines or procedures, exposure to latex products, impaired neurological status, seizure activity, exposure to safety hazards, immobility, use of restraints, presence of fractures, malnutrition, and fluid deficit or excess.	Provides opportunity to modify environment and eliminate factors that place child at risk.
Handle infant and child gently. Limit use of restraints, and when used, release restraints periodically per protocol.	Skin and tissues are fragile and are at risk for damage.
Provide appropriate level of supervision.	Permits monitoring of child's well-being and allows for timely intervention.
Initiate safety precautions as individually appropriate, such as bed in low position, padded side rails, infection precautions, and medications in childproof containers.	Preventing injuries and complications is a prime responsibility of parents and caregivers.
Have age-appropriate equipment available including properly sized BP cuff, intravenous (IV) catheters, airway adjuncts, and oxygen mask or hood; suction equipment, ventilator bag, low-flow IV pump, or warming devices.	Prevents treatment-related injuries and ensures availability of age- or size-appropriate life-saving equipment.
Monitor medication administration closely, especially dosage measurements and conversions. Use pediatric concentrations of medications when available.	Provides for effective therapeutic management, prevents overdose, and reduces risk for toxic reactions.
Ascertain recurrent exposure to latex products including gloves, catheters, and tubing. Note history of allergies or eczema.	Repeat exposure increases risk of developing sensitivity or adverse reaction to latex products.
Review home situation for safety hazards. Ascertain parent or caregiver knowledge of safety needs and injury prevention in home setting.	Promotes a safe environment. *Note:* Specific attention needs to be focused on childhood recreational and sports injuries, including impact of repeated concussions which is often underestimated.
Provide written resources for parent or caregiver and child, including information about safety issues, such as immunizations, obesity, smoking, substance use, and safer sex practices.	Provides information for later review and self-paced learning.
Encourage parent or caregiver to learn cardiopulmonary resuscitation (CPR) and individually appropriate procedures or emergency interventions and responses, such as carrying an EpiPen.	Being prepared for emergencies promotes confidence for adults and children in their own ability to deal with their situation.
Collaborative	
Refer to community education programs and resources, such as Family Effectiveness Training, as indicated.	Can provide additional opportunities for improving parenting skills and obtaining necessary equipment.

NURSING DIAGNOSIS: risk for imbalanced Fluid Volume

Risk factors may include
Lack of adequate intake, increase in fluid needs such as with fever
Rapid or sustained loss—hemorrhage, burns, vomiting, diarrhea, fistulas
Rapid or excessive fluid replacement

Possibly evidenced by
(Not applicable; presence of signs and symptoms establishes an *actual* diagnosis)

(continues on page 900)

NURSING DIAGNOSIS: risk for imbalanced Fluid Volume (continued)

Desired Outcomes/Evaluation Criteria—Child Will

Hydration (NOC)
Demonstrate adequate fluid balance as evidenced by stable vital signs, palpable pulses of good quality, normal skin turgor, moist mucous membranes; individual appropriate urinary output; lack of excessive weight fluctuation—loss or gain; and absence of edema.

Parent/Caregiver Will

Verbalize understanding of child's fluid needs.
Promote adequate age-appropriate fluid intake.

ACTIONS/INTERVENTIONS	RATIONALE
Fluid Management (NIC)	
Independent	
Note potential sources of fluid loss and intake, presence of conditions such as diabetes or burns, and use of total parenteral nutrition (TPN).	Causative and contributing factors for fluid imbalances.
Note child's age, size, weight, and cognitive abilities.	Affects ability to tolerate fluctuations in fluid level and ability to respond to fluid needs.
Monitor vital signs; color of palms, soles of feet, and mucous membranes; weight; skin turgor; breath sounds; urinary and gastric output; amount of blood draws; and hemodynamic measurements.	Indicators of hydration status. *Note:* Hypotension indicative of developing shock may not be readily observed in child until very late in the clinical course because of vasoconstriction.
Review child's intake of fluids.	Children often do not take in enough oral fluids to meet hydration needs.
Determine child's normal pattern of elimination and whether child is toilet trained.	Provides information for baseline and comparison. If child is in diapers, output may be determined by weighing diapers.
Determine whether child has problems with urination, such as urine retention, bed-wetting, burning, or holding.	Evaluation of these issues is important for determining cause and treatment of underlying problem.
Note use of drainage devices such as nasogastric (NG) tube or wound drain and use of laxatives, enemas, and suppositories.	May increase fluid and electrolyte losses.
Collaborative	
Administer IV fluids via control device.	Because smaller volumes are administered, close monitoring and regulation is required to prevent fluid overload while correcting fluid balance.
Replace electrolytes, as indicated, by oral route whenever possible.	Replacement solutions formulated for children are often safer and better tolerated when given orally if time and condition allows. *Note:* Child with mild dehydration not caused by trauma may respond well to oral rehydration starting with 5 to 10 mL by mouth every 15 to 20 minutes and increasing according to tolerance.
Monitor laboratory results, such as hemoglobin/hematocrit (Hgb/Hct), BUN, urine osmolality, and specific gravity.	Indicators of adequacy of hydration and effectiveness of therapeutic interventions.
Arrange with laboratory to combine common tests and draw smallest amount of blood that is necessary to perform required studies.	Excessive or repetitive blood draws may markedly reduce Hgb and Hct levels in pediatric client.

NURSING DIAGNOSIS: interrupted Family Processes/impaired Parenting

May be related to
Situational transition and/or crises—illness, trauma, disabling and/or expensive treatments; shift in health status of a family member; modification in family finances or social status
Lack of or ineffective role model; lack of support between or from SO(s)
Separation from parent; interruption in bonding process; lack of appropriate response of child to parent or parent to child
Lack of knowledge; unrealistic expectation for self, child, partner

Possibly evidenced by
Changes in communication patterns, participation in decision making
Expressions of conflict within family
Frequent verbalization of disappointment in child, resentment toward child, inability to care for or discipline child
Lack of parental attachment behaviors
Growth and/or developmental lag in child

NURSING DIAGNOSIS: **interrupted Family Processes/impaired Parenting** (continued)

Desired Outcomes/Evaluation Criteria—Parent/Caregiver Will

Family Functioning (NOC)
Verbalize positive feelings about parenting abilities.
Be involved in problem-solving solutions for current situation.
Develop skills to deal with present situation.
Strengthen parenting skills.

ACTIONS/INTERVENTIONS	RATIONALE
Family Support (NIC) *Independent*	
Determine existing situation and parental perception of the problems, noting presence of specific factors such as psychiatric or physical illness, and disabilities of child or parent.	Identification of the individual factors will aid in focusing interventions and establishing a realistic plan of care.
Identify developmental stage of the family—first child, new infant, school-age or adolescent children, or stepfamily.	These factors affect how family members view current problems and choices of solutions.
Determine cultural and religious influences on parenting and expectations of self and child.	This information is crucial to helping the family identify and develop a treatment plan that meets its specific needs, enhancing likelihood of success.
Assess parenting skill level, considering intellectual, emotional, and physical strengths and limitations.	Identifies areas of need for further education, skill training, and factors that might interfere with ability to assimilate new information.
Note attachment behaviors between parent and child(ren), recognizing cultural background. Encourage parent(s) to hold and spend time with child, particularly newborn or infant.	Lack of eye contact and touching may indicate bonding problems. Failure to bond effectively with newborn is thought to affect subsequent parent-child interaction.
Observe interactions between parent(s) and child(ren).	Identifies relationships, communication skills, and feelings about one another.
Note presence and effectiveness of extended family support systems.	Provides role models for parent(s) to help them develop own style of parenting. *Note:* Role models may be negative and/or controlling.
Emphasize positive aspects of situation, maintaining a positive attitude toward parent's capabilities and potential for improving.	Helping parent(s) to feel accepting about self and individual capabilities will promote growth.
Involve all members of the family in learning activities.	Learning new skills is enhanced when everyone is participating and interacting.
Encourage parent(s) to identify positive outlets for meeting own needs, such as going to a movie or out to dinner. Discuss use of home care and respite services, as appropriate.	Parent often believes it is "selfish" to do things for own self, that children are primary. However, parents are important, children are important, and the family is important. As a rule, when parents take care of themselves, their coping abilities are enhanced and they are better parents. *Note:* Siblings also require time with parents to attend to their needs, and to have positive interactions.
Discuss issues of stepparenting and ways to achieve positive relationships in a blended family.	Blending two families can be a very demanding task, and preconceived ideas can be counterproductive.
Collaborative	
Refer to resources such as books, classes, and support groups.	Providing information and/or role models can help people learn to negotiate and develop skills for parenting and living together.

NURSING DIAGNOSIS: **risk for imbalanced Body Temperature**

Risk factors may include
Extremes of age or weight; dehydration, exposure to cold or hot environments, illness or trauma affecting temperature regulation

Possibly evidenced by
(Not applicable; presence of signs and symptoms establishes an *actual* diagnosis)

Desired Outcomes/Evaluation Criteria—Child Will

Thermoregulation (NOC)
Regain or maintain appropriate body temperature for age and size.

Parent/Caregiver Will

Risk Control (NOC)
Provide proper environmental controls and safeguards.

ACTIONS/INTERVENTIONS	RATIONALE

Temperature Regulation (NIC)
Independent

Note conditions promoting fevers—infection, inflammation, hot environment, and dehydration.	Determines choice of interventions.
Measure and monitor child's temperature, using properly functioning thermometer.	Inaccurate measurement can result in inappropriate treatment.
Discuss variables in temperature measurements for age of child and where temperature is measured.	Knowledge of normal ranges for age of child—newborn through adolescent—is critical to knowing when a fever requires treatment. Temperature may be measured orally, rectally, and at the axillary space, with rectal measurement being on average approximately 1 degree higher than oral, and axillary being 1 degree lower than oral. *Note:* Temperature of 100.4°F (38°C) or greater in newborns and infants needs immediate attention. For toddlers and older children, temperatures up to 104°F (40°C) may be tolerated unless accompanied by other signs, such as poor color, breathing problems, severe lethargy, headache, or stiff neck (Cincinnati Children's Hospital Medical Center [CCHMC], 2006).
Be aware of heat loss related to age and body mass.	Newborn is more vulnerable to heat loss than older child because of body surface area, higher metabolic rate, and sensitivity to environmental conditions.
Observe for seizure activity. Provide safety precautions, as indicated.	Higher fevers may trigger febrile seizures in susceptible children.
Adjust bedclothes, linens, and environment. Apply cool cloth to head and bathe in lukewarm bath.	Limiting linens and use of room fan can help lower body temperature. *Note:* Use of alcohol sponge bath is contraindicated as fumes are inhaled by infant.

Collaborative

Administer antipyretics, for example, acetaminophen (Tylenol), 10 to 15 mg/kg every 4 hours or ibuprofen (Motrin), 10 to 15 mg/kg every 6 hours, as indicated. Avoid use of aspirin.	Some degree of fever may be useful for fighting infection; however, excessive levels may have adverse effects and require intervention. Aspirin is believed to be associated with the onset of Reye's syndrome (London et al, 2007).

NURSING DIAGNOSIS: risk for ineffective Health Maintenance

Risk factors may include
Unachieved developmental tasks
Perceptual or cognitive impairment
Ineffective individual or family coping
Lack of material resources, psychosocial supports

Possibly evidenced by
(Not applicable; presence of signs and symptoms establishes an *actual* diagnosis)

Desired Outcomes/Evaluation Criteria—Parent Or Caregiver Will

Health Seeking Behavior (NOC)
Identify necessary health maintenance activities.
Verbalize understanding of factors contributing to current situation.
Develop plan to meet specific needs.

ACTIONS/INTERVENTIONS	RATIONALE

Health System Guidance (NIC)
Independent

Explore with parents how child's health status is maintained—nutrition, exercise, sleep and rest, immunization status, and environmental issues such as childcare setting and homelessness.	Identifies strengths; may reveal problems requiring immediate intervention.
Discuss mother's health status when pregnant such as exposure to toxic agents, substance use, and complications of pregnancy or birth.	Helps identify issues, such as fetal alcohol syndrome, that may arise in child's future health status.

ACTIONS/INTERVENTIONS (continued)

Ascertain frequency of routine health exams, including eye and dental care, monitoring by primary care provider, and immunizations. Note availability and use of resources. Problem-solve barriers to meeting healthcare needs.

Note desire and level of ability to meet health maintenance needs, as well as self-care ADLs.

Develop plan with parent or caregiver for child's care.

Provide time to listen to concerns of parent or caregiver.

Provide anticipatory guidance for periods of wellness, and identify ways parent can adapt when progressive illness or long-term health problems occur.

Provide for communication and coordination between the healthcare facility team and community healthcare providers.

Monitor adherence to prescribed medical regimen. Determine causes for deviations.

Provide information about individual healthcare needs. Identify signs and symptoms requiring further evaluation and follow-up.

Collaborative

Make referral as needed for community support services such as homemaker, skilled nursing care, well-baby clinic, and respite care.

Refer to social services, as indicated.

Arrange for palliative or hospice services, if needed.

RATIONALE (continued)

Identifies areas of child's healthcare that may be lacking, and provides parents with information about areas that need to be monitored and care provided to promote optimum health. *Note:* Financial issues, such as being under- or uninsured, having high insurance co-pays, or a lack of transportation may restrict ability to follow through on needed or routine care.

Care providers and children who can provide much of their own care may have areas of need, either because of illness or other stressors.

Allows for incorporating existing strengths or limitations and assistance in adapting and organizing care, as necessary.

Long-term care for chronically ill child or acute care for a child can be very challenging to parent's physical, emotional, and financial resources.

Information and support is vital for maintaining and managing effective health practices.

Promotes continuity of care and continuation of goals.

Additional education or problem-solving may be required for success of therapeutic plan.

Provides for prevention of complications and early intervention in times of illness.

Provides for childcare and parental support in home setting to enhance coping with therapeutic regimen.

May need assistance with financial, housing, or legal concerns.

May be indicated when illness is prolonged or terminal.

POTENTIAL CONSIDERATIONS following acute hospitalization (dependent on client's age, physical condition and presence of complications, and family resources)
Refer to primary diagnosis for specific concerns.
- *ineffective self Health Management*—perceived seriousness, economic difficulties, complexity of regimen and excessive demands made on family, family patterns of healthcare
- *delayed Growth and Development*—effects of physical disability, prescribed dependence, environmental and stimulation deficiencies

FLUID AND ELECTROLYTE IMBALANCES

I. Homeostasis
   a. The body is equipped with homeostatic mechanisms to keep the composition and volume of body fluids within narrow limits.
   b. Organs involved in this mechanism are kidneys, lungs, heart, blood vessels, adrenal glands, parathyroid glands, and pituitary gland.

II. Composition
   a. Body fluid is composed primarily of water and electrolytes and is divided into two types.
   i. Intracellular—within the cells
   ii. Extracellular—interstitial or tissue fluid, intravascular or plasma, and transcellular, such as cerebrospinal or synovial fluids

Related Concerns

All plans of care specific to underlying health condition causing imbalance, such as diabetes mellitus (DM), heart failure (HF), upper gastrointestinal (GI) bleeding, renal failure, and dialysis.

Metabolic acidosis—primary base bicarbonate deficiency, page 483

Metabolic alkalosis—primary base bicarbonate excess, page 488

Respiratory acidosis (primary carbonic acid excess), page 195

Respiratory alkalosis (primary carbonic acid deficit), page 200

Nursing Priorities

1. Restore homeostasis.
2. Prevent or minimize complications.
3. Provide information about condition, prognosis, and treatment needs, as appropriate.

Discharge Goals

1. Homeostasis restored.
2. Free of complications.
3. Condition, prognosis, and treatment needs understood.
4. Plan in place to meet needs after discharge.

Fluid Balance

Note: Because fluid and electrolyte imbalances usually occur in conjunction with other medical conditions, the following information is offered as a reference. The interventions are presented in a general format for inclusion in the primary plan of care.

GLOSSARY

Dehydration: Loss of too much body water, which can affect cellular and organ function.

Fluid balance: State in which the volume of body water and its solutes (electrolytes and nonelectrolytes) are within normal limits and there is normal distribution of fluids within the intracellular and extracellular compartments.

Fluid volume deficit: Imbalance in fluid volume in which there is loss of fluid from the body not compensated for by an adequate intake of water. The major causes are (1) insufficient fluid intake and (2) excessive fluid loss from vomiting; diarrhea; suctioning of gastric contents; or drainage through operative wounds, burns, or fistulae.

Fluid volume excess: Overabundance of water in the interstitial fluid spaces or body cavities (edema) or an excess of fluid within the blood vessels (hypervolemia). Factors that contribute to the accumulation of excess fluid are (1) dilatation of the arteries, as occurs in inflammatory process; (2) reduced effective osmotic pressure, as in hypoproteinemia, lymphatic obstruction, and increased capillary permeability; (3) increased venous pressure, as in congestive heart failure, thrombophlebitis, and cirrhosis of the liver; and (4) retention of sodium due to increased reabsorption of sodium by the renal tubules.

Hypervolemia: Increase in the volume of circulating blood; also known as fluid overload or fluid excess. Excess fluid can accumulate in the intravascular space and/or the interstitial space.

Hypovolemia: Decreased, circulating volume in the intravascular compartment; also known as fluid deficit, or dehydration. Relative and absolute hypovolemic states can commonly coexist in certain clinical conditions as well. A client who is relatively hypovolemic may have adequate volume; however, it does not remain or exist in the intravascular space. In other words, it is not effective circulating volume. Absolute hypovolemia is considered to be measurable fluid (greater than 500 mL/day).

Interstitial fluid: Extracellular fluid bathing most tissues, excluding the fluid within the lymph and blood vessels.

Intracellular fluid: Portion of total body water with its dissolved solutes within the cell membranes.

Orthopnea: Labored breathing occurring when laying flat.

Osmotic pressure: Pressure produced by a solution in a space divided by a semipermeable membrane due to a differential in the concentrations of solute. The colloid osmotic pressure is influenced by proteins. This is due to the proteins being the only dissolved substance in the plasma and interstitial fluid that do not diffuse readily through the capillary membrane.

Positive fluid balance: Fluid gain is greater than fluid loss, which might suggest a problem with either the renal or cardiovascular system.

Tachypnea: Abnormally rapid respirations.

HYPERVOLEMIA (EXTRACELLULAR FLUID VOLUME EXCESS)

I. Predisposing or Contributing Factors

a. Excess sodium intake: sodium-containing foods, medications, or fluids (orally/intravenously); excessive or rapid administration of hypertonic or, possibly, isotonic parenteral fluids

b. Hormone imbalance: increased release of antidiuretic hormone (ADH), excessive adrenocorticotropic hormone (ACTH) production, hyperaldosteronism

c. Decreased plasma proteins: chronic liver disease with ascites, major abdominal surgery, malnutrition or protein depletion

d. Chronic kidney disease, acute renal failure (ARF)

e. HF

Client Assessment Database

DIAGNOSTIC DIVISION MAY REPORT	MAY EXHIBIT
ACTIVITY/REST • Fatigue • Generalized weakness	
CIRCULATION	• Hypertension, elevated central venous pressure (CVP) • Pulse full and bounding • Tachycardia usually present; bradycardia—late sign of cardiac decompensation • Extra heart sounds (S_3) • Edema variable from dependent to generalized • Neck and peripheral vein distention
ELIMINATION • Decreased urinary output, polyuria if renal function is normal • Diarrhea	
FOOD/FLUID • Anorexia; nausea, vomiting • Thirst—may be absent, especially in elderly	• Abdominal girth increased with visible fluid wave on palpation (ascites) • Sudden weight gain, often in excess of 5% of total body weight • Edema initially dependent, pitting may progress to facial or periorbital, general or anasarca
NEUROSENSORY	• Changes in level of consciousness from lethargy, disorientation, confusion to coma • Aphasia • Muscle twitching, tremors, seizure activity • Hyperreflexia, rigid paralysis—severe hypernatremia
PAIN/DISCOMFORT • Headache • Abdominal cramps	
RESPIRATION • Shortness of breath • Productive cough	• Tachypnea with or without dyspnea, orthopnea • Crackles
SAFETY	• Fever • Skin changes in color, temperature, and turgor, such as taut and cool where edematous

(continues on page 906)

DIAGNOSTIC DIVISION MAY REPORT (continued)	MAY EXHIBIT (continued)
TEACHING/LEARNING • Refer to predisposing or contributing factors **DISCHARGE PLAN CONSIDERATIONS** • May require assistance with changes in therapeutic regimen, dietary management ▶ Refer to plan of care concerning underlying medical or surgical condition for possible postdischarge considerations.	

Diagnostic Studies

TEST WHY IT IS DONE	WHAT IT TELLS ME
BLOOD TESTS • *Hematocrit (Hct):* Measures the proportion of blood that is made up of red blood cells. Normal adult female range is 37% to 47%;normal adult male range is 40% to 54%.	Elevated in dehydration due to hemoconcentration; decreased with fluid overload.
• *Serum sodium (Na+):* Sodium is the body's most abundant extracellular ion. It plays a key role in maintaining fluid balance—where sodium goes, water will follow. Normal adult range is 135 to 146 mEq/L.	Serum sodium may be high, low, or normal, depending on cause for fluid excess and balance of other electrolytes, including intracellular potassium. Because sodium is the only cation to exert significant osmotic pressure, sodium levels are closely linked to both blood volume and blood.
• *Serum potassium (K+):* An essential intracellular ion needed to regulate water balance, levels of acidity, and blood pressure (BP). Normal range is 3.5 to 5.5 mEq/L.	Normal or decreased in fluid overload unless renal damage present. Potassium deficit may occur with kidney dysfunction or diuretic therapy.
• *Blood urea nitrogen (BUN):* Measures the amount of urea nitrogen in blood; used primarily to evaluate kidney function. Normal range is 7 to 25 mg/dL.	Normal or decreased in fluid overload unless renal damage present.
• *Plasma proteins:* Plasma proteins (such as albumin) help to transport substances and water throughout the body. Albumin helps maintain intravascular pressure. More than half of the protein in blood serum is albumin. Normal albumin range is 3.5 to 5.5 U/L.	May be decreased. The most common cause of decreased plasma albumin levels is related to inflammatory processes, including hemodilution, loss of extravascular space, increased consumption by cells locally, and decreased synthesis. Approximately 75% of the total colloid osmotic pressure is related to albumin (Hankins, 2006).
• *Serum glucose:* Type of sugar found in blood. Normal adult fasting range is 70 to 99 mg/dL.	May be elevated if dehydration is result of osmotic diuresis associated with metabolic acidosis.
• *Serum osmolality:* An indirect measurement of the number of particles—sodium, glucose, and urea—in plasma, reflecting fluid balance. Normal range is 275 to 295 mOsm/kg.	Usually unchanged, although hypo-osmolality may occur with hyponatremia.
OTHER DIAGNOSTIC STUDIES • *Urine sodium:* Measures the amount of sodium in urine and must be evaluated in association with blood levels. Concentrations may mirror blood levels or be the opposite. Normal values (generally) are 15 to 250 mEq/L/day.	The body normally excretes excess sodium; so, the concentration in the urine may be elevated because it is elevated in the blood. It may also be elevated in the urine when the body is losing too much sodium. If blood sodium levels are low due to insufficient intake, then urine concentrations will also be low.
• *Urine specific gravity:* Measures the concentration of particles in urine such as glucose, sodium, and urea. Normal range is 1.002 to 1.028.	Decreased levels can be associated with fluid excess and such conditions as diabetes insipidus.

NURSING DIAGNOSIS: excess Fluid Volume

May be related to
Excess fluid or sodium intake
Compromised regulatory mechanism

Possibly evidenced by
Signs and symptoms noted in database

Desired Outcomes/Evaluation Criteria—Client Will

Fluid Overload Severity (NOC)
Demonstrate stabilized fluid volume as evidenced by balanced intake and output (I&O), vital signs within client's normal range, stable weight, and absence of signs of edema.

Knowledge: Treatment Regimen (NOC)
Verbalize understanding of individual dietary and fluid restrictions.
Demonstrate behaviors to monitor fluid status and prevent or limit recurrence.

ACTIONS/INTERVENTIONS	RATIONALE
Hypervolemia Management (NIC)	
Independent	
Monitor vital signs as well as CVP, if available.	Tachycardia and hypertension are common manifestations. Tachypnea usually present with or without dyspnea. Elevated CVP may be noted before dyspnea and adventitious breath sounds occur. Hypertension may be a primary disorder or occur secondary to other associated conditions such as HF.
Auscultate lung and heart sounds.	Adventitious sounds (crackles) and extra heart sounds (S_3) are indicative of fluid excess, possibly resulting in rapid development of pulmonary edema.
Assess for presence and location of edema formation.	Edema can be either a cause or a result of various pathological conditions reflecting four competing forces: blood hydrostatic and osmotic pressures and interstitial fluid hydrostatic and osmotic pressures. The dynamic interaction of these four forces allows fluid to shift from one body compartment to another. Edema may be generalized or localized in dependent areas. Elderly clients may develop dependent edema with relatively little excess fluid.
Note presence of neck and peripheral vein distention, along with pitting edema, and dyspnea.	Signs of cardiac decompensation and HF.
Maintain accurate I&O. Note decreased urinary output and positive fluid balance on 24-hour calculations.	Decreased renal perfusion, cardiac insufficiency, and fluid shifts may cause decreased urinary output and edema formation.
Weigh, as indicated. Be alert for acute or sudden weight gain.	One liter of fluid retention equals a weight gain of 1 kilogram (2.2 pounds).
Give oral fluids with caution. If fluids are restricted, set up a 24-hour schedule for fluid intake.	Fluid restrictions, as well as extracellular shifts, can aggravate drying of mucous membranes, and client may desire more fluids than are prudent.
Monitor infusion rate of parenteral fluids closely; administer via control device, as necessary.	Rapid fluid bolus or prolonged excessive administration potentiates volume overload and risk of cardiac decompensation.
Encourage coughing and deep-breathing exercises.	Pulmonary fluid shifts potentiate respiratory complications.
Maintain semi-Fowler's position if dyspnea or ascites is present.	Gravity improves lung expansion by lowering diaphragm and shifting fluid to lower abdominal cavity.
Turn or reposition, and provide skin care at regular intervals.	Reduces pressure and friction on edematous tissue, which is more prone to breakdown than normal tissue.
Encourage bedrest. Schedule care to provide frequent rest periods.	Limited cardiac reserves result in fatigue and activity intolerance. Rest, particularly lying down, favors diuresis and reduction of edema.
Provide safety precautions as indicated, such as use of side rails, bed in low position, frequent observation, and soft restraints, if required.	Fluid shifts may cause cerebral edema and changes in mentation, especially in the geriatric population. *Note:* Use of restraints may increase agitation and can pose a safety threat.
Collaborative	
Assist with identification and treatment of underlying cause.	Refer to listing of predisposing and contributing factors to determine treatment needs.

(continues on page 908)

ACTIONS/INTERVENTIONS (continued)	RATIONALE (continued)
Monitor laboratory studies, such as sodium, potassium, BUN, and arterial blood gases (ABGs), as indicated.	Extracellular fluid shifts, sodium and water restriction, and renal function all affect serum sodium levels. Potassium deficit may occur with kidney disfunction or diuretic therapy. BUN may be increased as a result of renal dysfunction. ABGs may reflect metabolic acidosis.
Provide balanced protein, low-sodium diet. Restrict fluids, as indicated.	If serum proteins are low because of malnutrition or gastrointestinal (GI) losses, intake of dietary proteins can enhance colloidal osmotic gradients and promote return of fluid to the vascular space. Restriction of sodium or water decreases extracellular fluid retention.
Administer diuretics: loop diuretic such as furosemide (Lasix), thiazide diuretic such as hydrochlorothiazide (Esidrix), or potassium-sparing diuretic such as spironolactone (Aldactone).	To achieve excretion of excess fluid, either a single thiazide diuretic or a combination of agents may be selected, such as thiazide and spironolactone. The combination can be particularly helpful when two drugs have different sites of action, allowing more effective control of fluid excess.
Replace potassium losses, as indicated.	Potassium deficit may occur, especially if client is receiving potassium-wasting diuretic. This can cause lethal cardiac dysrhythmias if untreated.
Prepare for and assist with dialysis or ultrafiltration, if indicated	May be done to rapidly reduce fluid overload, especially in the presence of severe cardiac or renal failure.

HYPOVOLEMIA (EXTRACELLULAR FLUID VOLUME DEFICIT)

I. Classification (Stevens, 2008)
   a. Absolute: measurable intravascular loss or hemorrhage
   b. Relative: secondary to internal fluid shifts or insensible losses

II. Predisposing or Contributing Factors
   a. Excessive fluid losses: vomiting, gastric suctioning, diarrhea, polyuria, diaphoresis, wounds or burns, intraoperative fluid loss, hemorrhage

   b. Insufficient or decreased fluid intake: preoperative and postoperative nothing-by-mouth (NPO) status
   c. Systemic infections, fever
   d. Intestinal obstruction or fistulas
   e. Pancreatitis, peritonitis, cirrhosis, ascites, adrenal insufficiency
   f. Kidney disease, diabetic ketoacidosis, hyperglycemic hyperosmotic nonketotic coma (HHNC), diabetes insipidus, syndrome of inappropriate antidiuretic hormone (SIADH)

Client Assessment Database

DIAGNOSTIC DIVISION MAY REPORT	MAY EXHIBIT
ACTIVITY/REST • Fatigue • Generalized weakness	
CIRCULATION	• Hypotension, including postural changes • Pulse weak or thready • Tachycardia • Neck veins flattened • Central venous pressure (CVP) decreased
ELIMINATION • Constipation or, occasionally, diarrhea • Abdominal cramps	• Urine volume decreased; oliguria • Dark, concentrated color

Client Assessment Database (continued)

DIAGNOSTIC DIVISION MAY REPORT (continued)	MAY EXHIBIT (continued)
FOOD/FLUID • Thirst • Loss of appetite • Nausea and vomiting • Complete, sudden cessation of intake; or prolonged diminished intake of fluids	• Weight loss often exceeding 2% to 8% of total body weight • Abdominal distention • Mucous membranes dry, furrows on tongue, decreased tearing and salivation • Skin dry with poor turgor or pale, moist, clammy (shock)
NEUROSENSORY • Tingling of the extremities • Vertigo, syncope	• Behavior change such as apathy, restlessness, confusion
RESPIRATION	
SAFETY	• Tachypnea • Temperature usually subnormal, although fever may occur
TEACHING/LEARNING • Refer to predisposing or contributing factors • Use, misuse of diuretics	
DISCHARGE PLAN CONSIDERATIONS • May require assistance with changes in therapeutic regimen, dietary management ◗ Refer to plan of care concerning underlying medical or surgical condition for possible considerations after discharge.	

Diagnostic Studies

TEST WHY IT IS DONE	WHAT IT TELLS ME

BLOOD TESTS
• *Complete blood count (CBC):* Battery of screening tests, which typically includes hemoglobin (Hgb); hematocrit (Hct); red blood cell (RBC) count, morphology, indices, and distribution width index; platelet count and size; and white blood cell (WBC) count and differential.
  • *Hgb:* Normal adult female range, 12 to 16 g/dL; normal adult male range, 14 to 18 g/dL.
  • *Hct:* Normal adult female range, 37% to 47%; normal adult male range, 40% to 54%.
	Hgb, Hct, and RBC count may be increased because of hemoconcentration. These factors will be decreased with hemorrhage.

• *Serum sodium:* Sodium is the body's most abundant extracellular ion. Normal range is 135 to 145 mEq/L.	May be normal, high, or low.
• *Plasma proteins:* Plasma proteins, such as albumin, help to transport substances and water throughout the body. Albumin helps maintain intravascular pressure. More than half of the protein in blood serum is albumin. Normal albumin range is 3.5 to 5.5 U/L.	Levels are increased.
• *Blood urea nitrogen (BUN)/creatinine (Cr):* Measurement of ratio of two serum laboratory values—BUN and serum Cr. Normal BUN/Cr ratio is 10 to 20:1. • *Serum lactate:* Measures lactic acid to help detect and evaluate the severity of hypoxia and metabolic acidosis.	BUN out of proportion to Cr level is associated with hypovolemia or other causes of dimished renal blood flow. Ratio greater than 20:1 confirms diagnosis of dehydration (Mentes, 2006). Elevated lactate levels may be present with hypoperfusion, as may occur with hypovolemic shock, and signifies ongoing oxygen debt at the tissue and cellular level (Stevens, 2008).

(continues on page 910)

TEST **WHY IT IS DONE** (continued)	**WHAT IT TELLS ME** (continued)
OTHER DIAGNOSTIC STUDIES • *Urine sodium:* Measures the amount of sodium in urine and must be evaluated in association with blood levels. Concentrations may mirror blood levels or be the opposite. Normal values (generally) are 15 to 250 mEq/L/day.	Usually decreased when losses are from diarrhea and fluid loss or kidney failure. Levels may be higher than normal if sodium intake is excessive or kidneys are not reabsorbing sodium.
• *Urine specific gravity:* Measures concentration of particles to water. Normal range is 1.002 to 1.028.	Increased with dehydration, water restriction, and conditions causing water loss, such as vomiting, diarrhea, and certain types of kidney failure.

NURSING DIAGNOSIS: deficient Fluid Volume

May be related to
Active fluid loss—hemorrhage, vomiting, gastric intubation, diarrhea, burns, wounds, fistulas
Regulatory failure—adrenal disease, recovery phase of acute renal failure (ARF); diabetic ketoacidosis (DKA), HHNC; diabetes insipidus, systemic infections

Possibly evidenced by
Signs and symptoms noted in client database

Desired Outcomes/Evaluation Criteria—Client Will

Fluid Balance (NOC)
Maintain fluid volume at a functional level as evidenced by individually adequate urinary output with normal specific gravity, stable vital signs, moist mucous membranes, good skin turgor, and prompt capillary refill.

Knowledge: Treatment Regimen (NOC)
Verbalize understanding of causative factors and purpose of therapeutic interventions.
Demonstrate behaviors to monitor and correct deficit, as appropriate.

ACTIONS/INTERVENTIONS	**RATIONALE**
Hypovolemia Management (NIC) *Independent*	
Monitor vital signs and CVP. Note presence and degree of postural blood pressure (BP) changes. Observe for temperature elevations or fever.	Tachycardia is present along with a varying degree of hypotension, depending on degree of fluid deficit. CVP measurements are useful in determining degree of fluid deficit and response to replacement therapy. Fever increases metabolism and exacerbates fluid loss.
Palpate peripheral pulses; note capillary refill and skin color and temperature. Assess mentation.	Conditions that contribute to extracellular fluid deficit can result in inadequate organ perfusion to all areas and may cause circulatory collapse and shock.
Monitor urinary output. Measure or estimate fluid losses from all sources such as gastric losses, wound drainage, and diaphoresis.	Fluid replacement needs are based on correction of current deficits and ongoing losses. A decreased urinary output may indicate insufficient renal perfusion or hypovolemia, or polyuria can be present, requiring more aggressive fluid replacement.
Weigh daily and compare with 24-hour fluid balance. Measure edematous areas such as abdomen and limbs.	Although weight gain and fluid intake greater than output may not accurately reflect intravascular volume, these measurements provide useful data for comparison.
Evaluate client's ability to manage own hydration.	Impaired gag and swallow reflexes, anorexia, nausea, oral discomfort, and changes in level of consciousness (LOC) are among the factors that affect client's ability to replace fluids orally.
Ascertain client's beverage preferences, and set up a 24-hour schedule for fluid intake. Encourage foods with high fluid content.	Relieves thirst and discomfort of dry mucous membranes and augments parenteral replacement. *Note:* Sense of thirst is often diminished in the older adult.
Turn frequently, gently massage skin, and protect bony prominences.	Tissues are susceptible to breakdown because of vasoconstriction and increased cellular fragility.

ACTIONS/INTERVENTIONS (continued)

Provide skin and mouth care. Bathe every other day using mild soap. Apply lotion, as indicated.

Provide safety precautions, as indicated, such as use of side rails where appropriate, bed in low position, frequent observation, and soft restraints if required.

Investigate reports of sudden or sharp chest pain, dyspnea, cyanosis, increased anxiety, and restlessness.

Monitor for sudden or marked elevation of BP, restlessness, moist cough, dyspnea, basilar crackles, and frothy sputum.

Collaborative

Assist with identification and treatment of underlying cause.

Monitor laboratory studies, as indicated

Administer IV solutions, as indicated, for example:
   Isotonic solutions such as 0.9% NaCl (normal saline) and 5% dextrose/water

   0.45% NaCl (half-normal saline) and lactated Ringer's (LR) solution

   Colloids such as dextran, Plasmanate or albumin, or hetastarch (Hespan)

   Whole blood or packed RBC transfusion and autologous collection of blood

Provide tube feedings, including free water, as appropriate.

RATIONALE (continued)

Skin and mucous membranes are dry with decreased elasticity because of vasoconstriction and reduced intracellular water. Daily bathing may increase dryness.

Decreased cerebral perfusion frequently results in changes in mentation or altered thought processes, requiring protective measures to prevent client injury. *Note:* The use of restraints may increase agitation and can pose a safety risk.

Hemoconcentration and increased platelet aggregation may result in systemic emboli formation.

Too rapid a correction of fluid deficit may compromise the cardiopulmonary system, especially if colloids are used in general fluid replacement.

Refer to listing of predisposing or contributing factors to determine treatment needs. *Note:* Dehydration is the most common fluid and electrolyte imbalance in older adults.

Depending on the avenue of fluid loss, differing electrolyte and metabolic imbalances may be present and require correction. For example, use of glucose solutions in clients with underlying glucose intolerance may result in serum glucose elevation and increased urinary water losses.

Crystalloids provide prompt circulatory improvement, although the benefit may be transient because of increased renal clearance.

As soon as the client is normotensive, a hypotonic solution (0.45% NaCl) may be used to provide both electrolytes and free water for renal excretion of metabolic wastes. *Note:* Buffered crystalloids (LR) are used with caution because they may potentiate the risk of metabolic acidosis.

Corrects plasma protein concentration deficits, thereby increasing intravascular osmotic pressure and facilitating return of fluid into vascular compartment.

Indicated when hypovolemia is related to active blood loss.

Enteral replacement can provide proteins and other needed elements in addition to meeting general fluid requirements when swallowing is impaired.

SODIUM

I. Function
   a. Primarily responsible for osmotic pressure in that compartment
   b. Enhances neuromuscular conduction or transmission of impulses and is essential for maintaining acid–base balance
   c. Chloride is carried by sodium and will display the same imbalances.

II. Normal Laboratory Values
   a. Serum sodium range: 135 to 145 mEq/L
   b. Intracellular sodium: 10 mEq/L
   c. Serum chloride range: 95 to 105 mEq/L

Hyponatremia (Sodium Deficit)

III. Predisposing or Contributing Factors
   a. Primary hyponatremia—loss of sodium
      i. Heavy sweating (e.g., heat exhaustion), wounds or trauma (hemorrhage), burns, gastric suctioning, vomiting, diarrhea, small-bowel obstruction, peritonitis, salt-wasting renal dysfunction, adrenal insufficiency (Addison's disease)
      ii. Lack of sufficient dietary sodium, severe malnutrition, infusion of sodium-free solutions
   b. Dilutional hyponatremia—water gains
      i. Excessive water intake
      ii. Electrolyte-free intravenous (IV) infusion
      iii. Water intoxication—psychiatric illness, too aggressive hypotonic IV therapy, tap-water enemas
      iv. Gastric irrigations with electrolyte-free solutions
      v. Presence of tumors or central nervous system (CNS) disorders predisposing to syndrome of inappropriate antidiuretic hormone (SIADH), heart failure (HF), renal failure, nephrotic syndrome, hepatic cirrhosis, diabetes mellitus (DM), or hyperglycemia
      vi. Freshwater near-drowning
      vii. Use of certain drugs—hypoglycemia medications, barbiturates, antipsychotics, aminophylline, morphine (may stimulate pituitary gland to secrete excessive amounts of antidiuretic hormone [ADH]), anticonvulsants, some antineoplastic agents, or nonsteroidal anti-inflammatory drugs (NSAIDs)

Client may be asymptomatic until serum sodium level is less than 125 mEq/L, depending on rapidity of onset.

General

DIAGNOSTIC DIVISION MAY REPORT	MAY EXHIBIT
ACTIVITY/REST • Malaise • Generalized weakness, faintness • Muscle cramps	
EGO INTEGRITY • Anxiety	• Restlessness, apprehension
FOOD/FLUID • Nausea, anorexia • Thirst • Low-sodium diet • Diuretic use	
NEUROSENSORY • Headache • Blurred vision • Vertigo	• Loss of coordination • Personality changes • Stupor
TEACHING/LEARNING • Refer to predisposing or contributing factors • Use of oral hypoglycemic agent, potent diuretics, NSAIDs, other drugs that impair renal water excretion	
DISCHARGE PLAN CONSIDERATIONS • May require assistance with changes in therapeutic regimen, dietary management ▶ Refer to plan of care concerning underlying medical or surgical condition for possible considerations after discharge.	

Sodium/Water Deficit

Sodium less than 135 mEq/L, urine specific gravity elevated, and serum osmolality normal.

DIAGNOSTIC DIVISION MAY REPORT	MAY EXHIBIT
CIRCULATION	• Hypotension • Tachycardia • Peripheral pulses diminished • Pallid, clammy skin

DIAGNOSTIC DIVISION MAY REPORT (continued)	MAY EXHIBIT (continued)
ELIMINATION • Abnormal cramping • Diarrhea	• Urinary output decreased
FOOD/FLUID • Anorexia • Nausea, vomiting	• Poor skin turgor • Mucous membranes dry, decreased saliva and perspiration • Soft, sunken eyeballs
NEUROSENSORY • Dizziness	• Muscle twitching • Lethargy, restlessness, confusion, stupor
RESPIRATION	• Tachypnea
SAFETY	• Skin flushed, dry, hot • Fever

Sodium Deficit/Water Excess

Sodium less than 135 mEq/L, urine specific gravity low, serum osmolality decreased.

Client Assessment Database

DIAGNOSTIC DIVISION MAY REPORT	MAY EXHIBIT
CIRCULATION	• Hypertension • Generalized edema **When Na+ less than 120 mEq/L:** • Hypotension with vasomotor collapse • Rapid, thready pulse • Cold, clammy skin; fingerprinting on sternum • Cyanosis
ELIMINATION	• Urinary output increased
NEUROSENSORY	• Muscle twitching • Restlessness • Changes in mentation—more severe when problem is acute, develops rapidly **When Na+ less than 120 mEq/L:** • Hyporeflexia • Convulsions • Coma
PAIN/DISCOMFORT • Headache • Abdominal cramps	

Diagnostic Studies (depend on associated fluid level)

TEST — WHY IT IS DONE	WHAT IT TELLS ME
BLOOD TESTS	
• *Serum sodium:* Sodium is the body's most abundant extracellular ion. It plays a key role in maintaining fluid balance—where sodium goes, water will follow. Normal adult range is 135 to 146 mEq/L.	Decreased, less than 135 mEq/L. However, signs and symptoms may not occur until level is less than 120 mEq/L.
• *Serum potassium:* An essential intracellular ion needed to regulate water balance, levels of acidity, and blood pressure (BP). Normal range is 3.5 to 5.5 mEq/L.	May be decreased as the kidneys attempt to conserve sodium at the expense of potassium.
• *Serum chloride/bicarbonate ($HCO_3{}^-$):* Normal range for chloride is 95 to 107 mEq/L, whereas normal range for $HCO_3{}^-$ is 18 to 23 mmol/L.	Levels are decreased depending on which ion is lost with the sodium.
• *Serum osmolality:* An indirect measurement of the number of particles (sodium, glucose, and urea) in plasma, reflecting fluid balance. Normal range is 275 to 295 mOsm/kg.	Commonly low, but may be normal as in pseudohyponatremia, or high as in hyperglycemic hyperosmotic nonketotic coma (HHNC).
• *Hematocrit (Hct):* Volume percentage of red blood cells (RBCs) in whole blood. Normal range for adult female is 37% to 47%; normal range for adult male is 40% to 54%.	Depends on fluid balance—fluid excess versus dehydration.
OTHER DIAGNOSTIC STUDIES	
• *Urine sodium:* Measures the amount of sodium in urine and must be evaluated in association with blood levels. Concentrations may mirror blood levels or be the opposite. Normal values (generally) are 15 to 250 mEq/L/day.	Less than 15 mEq/L indicates renal conservation of sodium due to sodium loss from a nonrenal source, unless sodium-wasting nephropathy is present. Urine sodium greater than 20 mEq/L indicates syndrome of inappropriate antidiuretic hormone (SIADH).
• *Urine osmolality:* Measures concentration of particles to water in urine. Normal range for random specimen is 50 to 1,400 mOsm/kg.	Usually low unless SIADH present; in which case, it will exceed serum osmolality.
• *Urine specific gravity:* Measures the concentration of particles in urine such as glucose, sodium, and urea. Normal values range from 1.002 to 1.028.	May be decreased or increased if SIADH is present.

NURSING DIAGNOSIS: risk for Electrolyte Imbalance

Risk factors may include
Vomiting, diarrhea
Renal dysfunction
Treatment-related side effects such as gastric suctioning, electrolyte free intravenous (IV) solutions, medications
Water intoxication

Possibly evidenced by
(Not applicable, presence of signs and symptoms establishes an *actual* diagnosis)

Desired Outcomes/Evaluation Criteria—Client Will

Electrolyte & Acid/Base Balance (NOC)
Display heart rate, BP, and laboratory results within normal limits (WNL) for client; absence of muscle weakness; and neurological irritability.

ACTIONS/INTERVENTIONS	RATIONALE
Electrolyte Management: Hyponatremia (NIC) *Independent*	
Identify client at risk for hyponatremia and the specific cause such as sodium loss or fluid excess.	Provides clues for early intervention. Hyponatremia is a common imbalance, especially in the elderly, and may range from mild to severe. Severe hyponatremia can cause neurological damage or death if not treated promptly.
Monitor intake and output (I&O). Calculate fluid balance. Weigh daily.	Indicators of fluid balance are important because either fluid excess or deficit may occur with hyponatremia.

ACTIONS/INTERVENTIONS (continued)	**RATIONALE** (continued)
Assess level of consciousness (LOC) and neuromuscular response.	Sodium deficit may result in decreased mentation to the point of coma, as well as generalized muscle weakness, cramps, or convulsions.
Maintain quiet environment; provide safety and seizure precautions.	Reduces CNS stimulation and risk of injury from neurological complications such as seizures.
Note respiratory rate and depth.	Co-occurring hypochloremia may produce slow and shallow respirations as the body compensates for metabolic alkalosis.
Encourage foods and fluids high in sodium such as milk, meat, eggs, carrots, beets, and celery. Use fruit juices and bouillon instead of plain water.	Unless sodium deficit causes serious symptoms requiring immediate IV replacement, the client may benefit from slower replacement by oral method or removal of previous salt restriction.
Irrigate nasogastric (NG) tube (when used) with normal saline instead of water.	Isotonic irrigation will minimize loss of gastrointestinal (GI) electrolytes.
Observe for signs of circulatory overload, as indicated.	Administration of sodium-containing IV fluids in presence of HF increases risk.
Collaborative	
Assist with treatment of underlying cause.	Refer to listing of predisposing or contributing factors to determine treatment needs.
Monitor serum and urine electrolytes and osmolality.	Evaluates therapy needs and effectiveness.
Provide or restrict fluids, depending on fluid volume status.	In presence of hypovolemia, volume losses are replaced with isotonic saline (e.g., normal saline), or, on occasion, hypertonic solution (3% NaCl) when hyponatremia is life threatening. In the presence of fluid volume excess, or SIADH, fluid restriction is indicated. *Note:* Too rapid or excessive administration of hypertonic solutions can be lethal.
Administer medications, as indicated, for example: Furosemide (Lasix)	Effective in reducing fluid excess to correct sodium and water balance.
Sodium chloride	Used to replace deficits in the presence of chronic or ongoing losses.
Potassium chloride	Corrects potassium deficit, especially when diuretic is used.
Demeclocycline (Declomycin)	Useful in treating chronic SIADH, or when severe water restriction may not be tolerated. *Note:* May be contraindicated in clients with liver disease because nephrotoxicity may occur.
Captopril (Capoten)	May be used in combination with a loop diuretic (e.g., Lasix) to correct fluid volume excess, especially in the presence of HF.
Prepare for/assist with dialysis as indicated.	May be done to restore sodium balance without increasing fluid level when hyponatremia is severe or response to diuretic therapy is inadequate.

SODIUM (continued)

Hypernatremia (Sodium Excess)

IV. Predisposing or Contributing Factors

a. Excessive water losses: polyuria (as may occur with diabetes insipidus); use of osmotic diuretics (such as mannitol); presence of fever, profuse sweating, vomiting, diarrhea

b. Extracellular fluid volume excesses: renal disease, HF, primary aldosteronism, excessive steroids, Cushing's disease; excessive ingestion or infusion of sodium; saltwater near-drowning

c. Insufficient water intake: administration of tube feedings or high-protein diets with minimal fluid intake, self-medication, "ulcer diet" primarily using half and half or whole milk

Sodium Excess/Water Deficit

Sodium greater than 145 mEq/L and elevated urine specific gravity.

DIAGNOSTIC DIVISION MAY REPORT	MAY EXHIBIT
ACTIVITY/REST • Weakness	• Muscle rigidity, tremors • Generalized weakness
CIRCULATION	• Decreased BP, postural hypotension • Tachycardia **If sodium/water excess—Na+ greater than 145 mEq/L, urine specific gravity decreased:** • Elevated BP, hypertension
ELIMINATION	• Decreased urinary output **If sodium/water excess:** • Polyuria
FOOD/FLUID • Thirst	• Mucous membranes dry, sticky • Tongue dry, swollen, rough **If sodium/water excess:** • Skin pale, moist, taut with pitting edema • Weight gain
NEUROSENSORY	• Irritability, lethargy, coma—depending on rapidness of onset rather than actual serum sodium level • Delusions, hallucinations • Muscle irritability, seizure activity
RESPIRATION	• Dyspnea
TEACHING/LEARNING • Refer to predisposing or contributing factors	
DISCHARGE PLAN CONSIDERATIONS • May require assistance with changes in therapeutic regimen, dietary management ▶ Refer to plan of care concerning underlying medical or surgical condition for possible considerations after discharge.	

TEST WHY IT IS DONE	WHAT IT TELLS ME
BLOOD TESTS • *Serum sodium:* Sodium is the body's most abundant extracellular ion. It plays a key role in maintaining fluid balance—where sodium goes, water will follow. Normal adult range is 135 to 146 mEq/L.	Levels are increased. Serum levels greater than 160 mEq/L may be accompanied by severe neurological signs.

Diagnostic Studies (continued)

TEST WHY IT IS DONE (continued)	WHAT IT TELLS ME (continued)
• *Serum chloride:* Measures the amount of chloride in fluid portion of blood. It works with other electrolytes to maintain fluid and acid–base balance. Normal adult range is 95 to 105 mEq/L.	Increased with dehydration and metabolic acidosis. May be lower than normal if SIADH is present.
• *Serum potassium:* An essential intracellular ion needed to regulate water balance, levels of acidity, and BP. Normal range is 3.5 to 5.5 mEq/L.	Levels are decreased.
• *Serum osmolality:* An indirect measurement of the number of particles (sodium, glucose, and urea) in plasma, reflecting fluid balance. Normal range is 275 to 295 mOsm/kg.	Greater than 295 mOsm/L with dehydration. Is reduced in presence of extracellular fluid excess and less than 200 mOsm/L with excessive polyuria.
• *Hct:* Volume percentage of RBCs in whole blood. Normal range for adult female is 37% to 47%; normal range for adult male is 40% to 54%.	May be normal or elevated depending on fluid status.

OTHER DIAGNOSTIC STUDIES

• *Urine sodium:* Measures the amount of sodium in urine and must be evaluated in association with blood levels. Concentrations may mirror blood levels or be the opposite. Normal values (generally) are 15 to 250 mEq/L/day.	Levels are decreased.
• *Urine osmolality:* Measures concentration of particles to water in urine. Normal range for random specimen is 50 to 1,400 mOsm/kg.	Levels are elevated.
• *Urine specific gravity:* Measures the concentration of particles in urine, such as glucose, sodium, and urea. Normal values range from 1.002 to 1.028.	Increased with water deficit; decreased when hypernatremia is due to polyuria.

NURSING DIAGNOSIS: risk for Electrolyte Imbalance

Risk factors may include
Vomiting, diarrhea
Renal disease, diabetes insipidus
Fever, profuse sweating
Treatment-related side effects such as osmotic diuretics
High-protein diet

Possibly evidenced by
(Not applicable, presence of signs and symptoms establishes an *actual* diagnosis)

Desired Outcomes/Evaluation Criteria—Client Will

Electrolyte & Acid/Base Balance (NOC)
Display BP, heart rate, and laboratory results WNL for client and absence of neuromuscular irritability and cognitive impairment.

ACTIONS/INTERVENTIONS	RATIONALE
Electrolyte Management: Hypernatremia (NIC)	
Independent	
Monitor BP.	Either hypertension or hypotension may be present depending on the fluid status. Presence of postural hypotension may affect activity tolerance.
Identify client at risk for hypernatremia and likely cause such as water deficit or sodium excess.	Early identification and intervention prevents serious complications associated with this problem.
Note respiratory rate and depth.	Deep, labored respirations with air hunger suggest metabolic acidosis due to hyperchloremia, which can lead to cardiopulmonary arrest if not corrected.
Monitor I&O and urine specific gravity. Weigh daily. Assess presence and location of edema.	These parameters are variable, depending on fluid status, and are indicators of therapy needs and effectiveness.

(continues on page 918)

Evaluate LOC and muscular strength, tone, and movement.	Sodium imbalance may cause changes that vary from confusion and irritability to seizures and coma. In presence of water deficit, rapid rehydration may cause cerebral edema.
Maintain safety and seizure precautions, as indicated, such as bed in low position and use of padded side rails.	Sodium excess and cerebral edema increase risk of convulsions.
Assess skin turgor, color, and temperature and mucous membrane moisture.	Water-deficit hyponatremia manifests by signs of dehydration.
Provide and encourage meticulous skin care and frequent repositioning.	Maintains skin integrity.
Provide frequent oral care. Avoid use of mouthwash that contains alcohol.	Promotes comfort and prevents further drying of mucous membranes.
Offer debilitated client fluids at regular intervals. Give free water to client receiving enteral feedings.	May prevent hypernatremia in client who is unable to perceive or respond to thirst.
Recommend avoidance of foods high in sodium such as canned soups and vegetables, processed foods, snack foods, and condiments.	Reduces risk of sodium-associated complications.

Collaborative

Assist with identification and treatment of underlying cause.	Refer to listing of predisposing or contributing factors to determine treatment needs.
Monitor serum electrolytes, osmolality, and arterial blood gases (ABGs), as indicated.	Evaluates therapy needs and effectiveness. *Note:* Co-occurring hyperchloremia may cause metabolic acidosis, requiring further intervention.
Increase oral (PO) and IV fluid intake.	Replacement of total body water deficit will gradually restore sodium and water balance.
Restrict sodium intake and administer diuretics as indicated.	Restriction of sodium intake while promoting renal clearance lowers serum sodium levels in the presence of extracellular fluid excess.

POTASSIUM

I. Function
   a. Major cation of the intracellular fluid
   b. Responsible for maintaining intracellular osmotic pressure
   c. Also regulates neuromuscular excitability, aids in maintenance of acid–base balance, synthesis of protein, and metabolism of carbohydrates
II. Normal laboratory values
   a. Serum range: 3.5 to 5.0 mEq/L
   b. Total body: 42 mEq/L

Hypokalemia (Potassium Deficit)

III. Predisposing or Contributing Factors
   a. Renal loss: use of potassium-wasting diuretics, diuretic phase of acute tubular necrosis (ATN), healing phase of burns, diabetic acidosis, Cushing's syndrome, nephritis, hypomagnesemia; use of sodium penicillins, amphotericin B, carbenicillin, steroids; licorice abuse

   b. Gastrointestinal (GI) loss: profuse vomiting, excessive diarrhea, laxative abuse, prolonged gastric suction, inflammatory bowel disease, fistulas
   c. Inadequate dietary intake: anorexia nervosa, starvation, high-sodium diet
   d. Shift into cells: total parenteral nutrition (TPN), alkalosis, or excessive secretion or administration of insulin
   e. Other: sweat losses (heavily perspiring person acclimated to heat); liver disease

Client Assessment Database

DIAGNOSTIC DIVISION MAY REPORT	MAY EXHIBIT
ACTIVITY/REST • Generalized weakness • Lethargy, fatigue	

DIAGNOSTIC DIVISION MAY REPORT (continued)	MAY EXHIBIT (continued)
CIRCULATION	• Hypotension • Pulses weak or diminished, irregular • Heart sounds distant • Dysrhythmias—premature ventricular contractions (PVCs), ventricular tachycardia, fibrillation
ELIMINATION	• Nocturia, polyuria if factors contributing to hypokalemia include heart failure (HF) or diabetes mellitus (DM) • Bowel sounds diminished, decreased bowel motility, paralytic ileus • Abdominal distention
FOOD/FLUID • Anorexia, nausea, vomiting • Thirst	
NEUROSENSORY • Paresthesias	• Depressed mental state, confusion, apathy, drowsiness, irritability, coma • Hyporeflexia, tetany, paralysis—flaccid quadriparesis
PAIN/DISCOMFORT • Muscle pain, cramps	
RESPIRATION	• Hypoventilation, decreased respiratory depth due to muscle weakness, paralysis of diaphragm • Apnea • Cyanosis
TEACHING/LEARNING • Refer to predisposing or contributing factors • May use or misuse herbal supplements that can cause or exacerbate hypokalemia—aloe, caraway, castor oil, dandelion, elder flower, flaxseed, glycerol, licorice, peppermint oil, psyllium, yarrow	
DISCHARGE PLAN CONSIDERATIONS • May require assistance with changes in therapeutic regimen, dietary management ▶ Refer to plan of care concerning underlying medical or surgical condition for possible considerations after discharge.	

Diagnostic Studies

TEST WHY IT IS DONE	WHAT IT TELLS ME
BLOOD TESTS • *Serum potassium:* An essential intracellular ion needed to regulate water balance, levels of acidity, and blood pressure (BP). Normal range is 3.5 to 5.5 mEq/L.	Levels are decreased. Hypokalemia can result from two general causes: either from an overall depletion in the body's potassium or from excessive uptake of potassium by muscle from surrounding fluids.

(continues on page 920)

TEST WHY IT IS DONE (continued)	WHAT IT TELLS ME (continued)
• *Serum chloride:* Measures the amount of chloride in the fluid portion of the blood. It works with other electrolytes, such as potassium, sodium, and carbon dioxide, to help keep the proper balance of body fluids and maintain the body's acid–base balance. Normal adult range is 95 to 105 mEq/L.	Levels are often decreased. *Note:* Use of diuretics may cause chloride (as well as potassium) depletion.
• *Serum magnesium:* An essential intracellular ion needed to regulate water balance, levels of acidity, and BP. Normal range is 3.5 to 5.5 mEq/L.	Hypomagnesemia occurs and exacerbates potassium loss and sodium retention.
• *Arterial blood gases (ABGs):* Measures blood acidity and levels of oxygen and carbon dioxide in the blood. Used to determine how well lungs are able to move oxygen into the blood and remove carbon dioxide from the blood.	Imbalances may be noted in pH and bicarbonate.
OTHER DIAGNOSTIC STUDIES • *Electrocardiogram (ECG):* Record of the electrical activity of the heart.	The following changes can be associated with hypokalemia: low voltage, flat or inverted T wave; appearance of U wave; depressed ST segment; peaked P waves; prolonged QT interval; and ventricular dysrhythmias.

NURSING DIAGNOSIS: risk for Electrolyte Imbalance

Risk factors may include
Vomiting, diarrhea, profuse sweating
Renal dysfunction; diabetic acidosis
Treatment-related side effects such as diuretics, some antibiotics, TPN
Starvation, high-sodium diet

Possibly evidenced by
(Not applicable, presence of signs and symptoms establishes an *actual* diagnosis)

Desired Outcomes/Evaluation Criteria—Client Will

Electrolyte & Acid/Base Balance (NOC)
Display heart rhythm and laboratory results within normal limit (WNL) for client and absence of muscle weakness, paresthesias, and cognitive impairment.

ACTIONS/INTERVENTIONS	RATIONALE
Electrolyte Management: Hypokalemia (NIC) *Independent* Monitor heart rate and rhythm.	Changes associated with hypokalemia include abnormalities in both conduction and contractility. Tachycardia may develop as well as potentially life-threatening atrial and ventricular dysrhythmias—PVCs, sinus bradycardia, atrioventricular (AV) blocks, AV dissociation, and ventricular tachycardia.
Monitor respiratory rate, depth, and effort. Encourage cough and deep-breathing exercises; reposition frequently.	Respiratory muscle weakness may proceed to paralysis and eventual respiratory arrest.
Assess level of consciousness (LOC) and neuromuscular function, noting strength, sensation, and movement.	Apathy, drowsiness, irritability, tetany, paresthesias, and coma may occur.
Auscultate bowel sounds, noting absence or change.	Paralytic ileus commonly follows gastric losses through vomiting, gastric suction, or protracted diarrhea.
Maintain accurate record of urinary, gastric, and wound losses.	Guide for calculating fluid and potassium replacement needs.
Monitor rate of intravenous (IV) potassium administration using microdrop or pump infusion devices. Check for side effects. Provide ice pack, as indicated.	Ensures controlled delivery of medication to prevent bolus effect and reduce associated discomfort such as burning sensation at IV site. When solution cannot be administered via central vein and slowing rate is not possible or effective, applying ice pack to infusion site may help relieve discomfort.

ACTIONS/INTERVENTIONS (continued)	RATIONALE (continued)
Encourage intake of foods and fluids high in potassium such as bananas, oranges, dried fruits, red meat, turkey, salmon, leafy vegetables, peas, baked potatoes, tomatoes, winter squash, coffee, colas, and tea. Discuss use of potassium chloride salt substitutes for client receiving long-term diuretics.	Potassium may be replaced and level maintained through the diet when the client is allowed oral food and fluids. Dietary replacement of 40 to 60 mEq/L/day is typically sufficient if no abnormal losses are occurring.
Review drug regimen for potassium-wasting drugs, such as furosemide (Lasix), hydrochlorothiazide (Diamox), IV catecholamines, gentamicin (Garamycin), carbenicillin (Geocillin), and amphotericin B (Fungizone).	If alternate agents (e.g., potassium-sparing diuretics such as spirinolactone [Aldactone], triamterene [Dyrenium], amiloride [Midamor]) cannot be administered or when high-dose sodium drugs are administered (e.g., carbenicillin), close monitoring and replacement of potassium are necessary.
Discuss preventable causes of condition such as nutritional choices and the proper use of laxatives.	Provides opportunity for client to prevent recurrence. Also, dietary control is more palatable than oral replacement medications.
Watch for signs of digoxin toxicity when used: reports of nausea, vomiting, blurred vision, increasing atrial dysrhythmias, and heart block.	Low potassium enhances effect of digoxin, slowing cardiac conduction. *Note:* Combined effects of digoxin, diuretics, and hypokalemia may produce lethal dysrhythmias.
Observe for signs of metabolic alkalosis such as hypoventilation, tachycardia, dysrhythmias, tetany, and changes in mentation.	Frequently associated with hypokalemia.
Collaborative	
Assist with treatment of underlying cause.	Refer to listing of predisposing or contributing factors to determine treatment needs. *Note:* Hypokalemia is life threatening, therefore early detection is crucial.
Monitor laboratory studies, such as the following: Serum potassium	Levels should be checked frequently during replacement therapy, especially in the presence of insufficient renal function.
ABGs	Correction of metabolic alkalosis raises serum potassium level and reduces replacement needs. Correction of acidosis drives potassium back into cells, resulting in decreased serum levels and increased replacement needs.
Administer oral and/or IV potassium.	May be required to correct deficiencies when changes in medication, therapy, and/or dietary intake are insufficient. *Note:* Even in severe deficit, parenteral replacement should not exceed 40 mEq every 2 hours. Dietary supplementation may also be used to produce a gradual equilibration if client is able to take oral food and fluids.

POTASSIUM (continued)

Hyperkalemia (Potassium Excess)

IV. Predisposing or Contributing Factors

a. Potassium retention: decreased renal excretion (e.g., renal disease, acute failure, hypoaldosteronism, Addison's disease), hypovolemia, use of potassium-conserving diuretics—especially when associated with potassium supplements, use of nonsteroidal anti-inflammatory drugs (NSAIDs)

b. Excessive potassium intake: salt substitutes, drugs containing potassium, improper use of oral potassium supplements, too-rapid IV administration of potassium, massive transfusion of banked blood

c. Shift or release of potassium out of cells: severe catabolism, burns, crush injuries, myocardial infarction (MI), severe hemolysis, rhabdomyolysis, chemotherapy with cytotoxic drugs, respiratory or metabolic acidosis, anoxia, hyperglycemia with insulin deficiency, use of some beta-adrenergic blockers, profound digoxin toxicity

d. Other: use of certain medications such as captopril, heparin, cyclosporine

Client Assessment Database

Data depend on degree of elevation and length of time condition has existed.

DIAGNOSTIC DIVISION MAY REPORT	MAY EXHIBIT
ACTIVITY/REST • Vague muscular weakness	• Restlessness, irritability

(continues on page 922)

DIAGNOSTIC DIVISION MAY REPORT (continued)	MAY EXHIBIT (continued)
CIRCULATION	• Irregular pulse, bradycardia, heart block, asystole
EGO INTEGRITY • Apprehension	
ELIMINATION • Intermittent abdominal cramps • Diarrhea	• Urine volume decreased • Hyperactive bowel sounds
FOOD/FLUID • Nausea, vomiting	
NEUROSENSORY • Paresthesias—often of face, tongue, hands, feet • Slurred speech	• Decreased deep-tendon reflexes • Progressive, ascending flaccid paralysis • Twitching, seizure activity • Apathy, confusion
PAIN/DISCOMFORT • Muscle cramps, pain	
TEACHING/LEARNING • Refer to predisposing or contributing factors	
DISCHARGE PLAN CONSIDERATIONS • May require assistance with changes in therapeutic regimen, dietary management	
▶ Refer to plan of care concerning underlying medical or surgical condition for possible considerations after discharge.	

Diagnostic Studies

TEST WHY IT IS DONE	WHAT IT TELLS ME
BLOOD TESTS • *Serum potassium:* An essential intracellular ion needed to regulate water balance, levels of acidity, and BP. Normal range is 3.5 to 5.5 mEq/L.	Levels are increased.
• *Serum magnesium:* An essential intracellular ion needed to regulate water balance, levels of acidity, and BP. Normal range is 3.5 to 5.5 mEq/L.	Levels may be elevated if renal failure is present.
OTHER DIAGNOSTIC STUDIES • *ECG:* Record of the electrical activity of the heart	In the presence of hyperkalemia, these changes may be seen: T waves tall and peaked or tented; prolonged PR interval; loss of P waves; widening of QRS complex; shortened QT interval and ST segment depression; atrial or ventricular dysrhythmias—bradycardia, atrial arrest, complete heart block, ventricular fibrillation, and cardiac arrest.

NURSING DIAGNOSIS: risk for Electrolyte Imbalance

Risk factors may include
Renal disease
Treatment-related side effects such as diuretics, NSAIDs, cytotoxic drugs, medications containing potassium, massive transfusion with banked blood

Possibly evidenced by
(Not applicable, presence of signs and symptoms establishes an *actual* diagnosis)

Desired Outcomes/Evaluation Criteria—Client Will

Electrolyte & Acid/Base Balance (NOC)
Display heart rate/rhythm and laboratory results WNL for client and absence of muscle weakness, paresthesias, and cognitive impairment.

ACTIONS/INTERVENTIONS	RATIONALE
Electrolyte Management: Hyperkalemia (NIC)	
Independent	
Identify client at risk or the cause of the hyperkalemia, such as excessive intake of potassium or decreased excretion.	Influences choice of interventions. Early identification and treatment can prevent complication. *Note:* A major cause of hypokalemia is decreased renal excretion.
Instruct client in use of potassium-containing salts or salt substitutes, taking potassium supplements safely.	The client is often able to prevent hyperkalemia through management of supplements, diet, and other medications.
Monitor respiratory rate and depth. Elevate head of bed. Encourage coughing and deep-breathing exercises.	Clients may hypoventilate and retain CO_2, leading to respiratory acidosis. Muscular weakness can affect respiratory muscles and lead to respiratory complications.
Monitor heart rate and rhythm. Be aware that cardiac arrest can occur.	Excess potassium depresses myocardial conduction. Bradycardia can progress to cardiac fibrillation and arrest.
Monitor urinary output.	In kidney failure, potassium is retained because of improper excretion. Potassium should not be given if oliguria or anuria is present.
Assess LOC and neuromuscular function, including movement, strength, and sensation.	Client is usually awake and alert; however, muscular paresthesia, weakness, and flaccid paralysis may occur.
Encourage and assist with range-of-motion (ROM) exercises, as tolerated.	Improves muscular tone and reduces muscle cramps and pain.
Encourage frequent rest periods; assist with care activities, as indicated.	General muscle weakness decreases activity tolerance.
Review drug regimen for medications containing potassium or affecting potassium excretion such as penicillin G, spironolactone (Aldactone), amiloride (Midamor), and hydrochlorothiazide (Dyazide, Maxzide).	Requires regular monitoring of potassium levels and may require alternate drug choices or changes in dosage or frequency.
Identify and discontinue dietary sources of potassium, such as tomatoes, broccoli, orange juice, bananas, bran, chocolate, coffee, tea, eggs, dairy products, and dried fruits, if indicated.	Facilitates reduction of potassium level and may prevent recurrence of hyperkalemia.
Recommend an increase in carbohydrates and fats and foods low in potassium such as canned fruits, refined cereals, and apple or cranberry juice.	Reduces exogenous sources of potassium and prevents catabolic tissue breakdown with release of cellular potassium.
Stress importance of client's notifying future caregivers when chronic condition potentiates development of hyperkalemia, such as oliguric renal failure.	May help prevent recurrence of hyperkalemia.
Collaborative	
Assist with treatment of underlying cause.	Refer to listing of predisposing and contributing factors to determine treatment needs.
Monitor laboratory results, such as serum potassium and ABGs, as indicated.	Evaluates therapy needs and effectiveness. *Note:* Hypoventilation may result in respiratory acidosis, thereby increasing serum potassium levels.
Administer medications, as indicated, for example: Diuretics such as furosemide (Lasix)	Loop or thiazide diuretics promote renal clearance and excretion of potassium.
IV glucose with insulin and sodium bicarbonate	Short-term emergency measure to move potassium into the cell, thus reducing toxic serum level. *Note:* Use with caution in presence of HF or hypernatremia.

(continues on page 924)

Calcium chloride or calcium gluconate	Temporary stopgap measure that antagonizes toxic potassium depressant effects on heart and stimulates cardiac contractility. *Note:* Calcium is contraindicated in clients on digoxin because it increases the cardiotonic effects of the drug and may cause dysrhythmias.
Sodium polystyrene sulfonate (Kayexalate, SPS suspension), administered orally, per nasogastric (NG) tube, or rectally	Resin removes potassium by exchanging potassium for sodium or calcium in the GI tract. Sorbitol enhances evacuation. *Note:* Use cautiously in clients with HF and/or edema, and in the elderly because it increases sodium level. In addition, Kayexalate may cause hyperchloremia.
Beta-adrenergic agonist such as albuterol (Proventil)	Nebulizer administration has been effective in clients receiving hemodialysis and may also attenuate the hypoglycemic effect of insulin administration.
Infuse potassium-based medication or solutions slowly.	Prevents administration of concentrated bolus, allows time for kidneys to clear excess free potassium.
Provide fresh blood or washed red blood cells (RBCs), if transfusions required.	Fresh blood has less potassium than banked blood because breakdown of older RBCs releases potassium.
Prepare for and assist with dialysis.	May be required when more conservative methods fail or are contraindicated such as severe HF.

CALCIUM

I. Function
a. Bone formation and reabsorption
b. Neural transmission and muscle contraction
c. Regulation of enzyme systems
d. Coenzyme in blood coagulation

II. Normal laboratory values
a. Serum: 4.5 to 5.3 mEq/L
b. Total body: 8.5 to 10.5 mg/dL—directly related to the serum albumin, calcium is bound to the protein, and must be considered if only total serum readings are available
c. Ionized: 2.1 to 2.6 mEq/L—physiologically active and clinically important, especially in critically ill clients; altered by changes in pH (affects how much calcium is bound to protein) or increased serum levels of fatty acids, lactate, and bicarbonate

Hypocalcemia (Calcium Deficit)

III. Predisposing or Contributing factors
a. Primary or surgical hypoparathyroidism, transient hypocalcemia following thyroidectomy; hyperphosphatemia, hypomagnesemia

b. Massive subcutaneous tissue infections, acute pancreatitis, burns, peritonitis, malignancies
c. Excessive gastrointestinal (GI) losses: draining fistula, diarrhea, fat malabsorption syndromes, chronic laxative use (particularly phosphate-containing laxatives and enemas)
d. Extreme stress situations with mobilization and excretion of calcium
e. Diuretic and terminal phase of renal failure
f. Inadequate dietary intake, lack of milk or vitamin D, excessive protein diet
g. Alcoholism: primary effect of ethanol, plus intestinal malabsorption, hypomagnesemia, hypoalbuminemia, and pancreatitis
h. Use of anticonvulsants, antibiotics, corticosteroids; loop diuretics, drugs that lower serum magnesium (e.g., cisplatin, gentamycin)
i. Infusion of citrated blood, calcium-free infusions; rapid infusion of Plasmanate
j. Malignant neoplasms with bone metastases
k. Alkalotic states
l. Decreased ultraviolet exposure

> **Client Assessment Database**

Data depend on duration, severity, and rate of onset of hypocalcemia.

DIAGNOSTIC DIVISION MAY REPORT	MAY EXHIBIT
CIRCULATION	• Hypotension • Pulses weak or decreased, irregular— weak cardiac contraction or premature dysrhythmias
ELIMINATION • Abdominal pain • Diarrhea	• Abdominal distention—paralytic ileus

Client Assessment Database (continued)

DIAGNOSTIC DIVISION MAY REPORT (continued)	MAY EXHIBIT (continued)
FOOD/FLUID • Nausea, vomiting	• Difficulty swallowing
HYGIENE	• Coarse, dry skin; alopecia (chronic)
NEUROSENSORY • Numbness and tingling of fingers and toes • Muscle cramps	• Anxiety, confusion, irritability, alteration in mood • Memory impaired • Depression • Hallucinations, psychoses • Muscle spasms—carpopedal and laryngeal • Increased deep-tendon reflexes, tetany • Tonic, clonic seizure activity • Positive Trousseau's and Chvostek's signs
RESPIRATION	• Labored shallow breathing, stridor—spasm of laryngeal muscles
SAFETY	• Bleeding with no, or minimal, trauma
TEACHING/LEARNING • Refer to predisposing or contributing factors	
DISCHARGE PLAN CONSIDERATIONS • May require assistance with changes in therapeutic regimen, dietary management ▶ Refer to plan of care concerning underlying medical or surgical condition for possible considerations after discharge.	

Diagnostic Studies

TEST WHY IT IS DONE	WHAT IT TELLS ME
BLOOD TESTS • *Serum calcium:* Essential mineral for proper functioning of muscles, nerves, and heart. Is required in blood clotting and in formation of bones. Only about 1% of calcium circulates in blood. Normal total calcium ranges from 8.4 to 10.2 mg/dL.	Total calcium is decreased in conditions of low albumin levels, extreme deficiency of dietary calcium caused by malnutrition, and disorders of the kidney.
• *Serum magnesium:* An essential intracellular ion needed to regulate water balance, levels of acidity, and blood pressure (BP). Normal range is 3.5 to 5.5 mEq/L.	May be decreased—follows calcium.
• *Serum albumin:* A transport protein, one of the total proteins in blood. More than half of the protein in blood serum is albumin. Normal albumin range is 3.5 to 5.5 U/L.	A low albumin level causes a deceptively low calcium level due to protein binding.
• *Bleeding/clotting studies, such as protime (PT) and platelets:* Calcium is an essential part of the clotting mechanism.	Deficit may lead to excessive bleeding.
• *Arterial blood gases (ABGs):* Measures blood acidity and levels of oxygen and carbon dioxide in the blood.	Alkalosis causes surplus bicarbonate to bind with free calcium, impairing function. Acidosis frees calcium, potentiating hypercalcemia.

(continues on page 926)

TEST **WHY IT IS DONE** (continued)	**WHAT IT TELLS ME** (continued)
OTHER DIAGNOSTIC STUDIES • *Electrocardiogram (ECG):* Record of the electrical activity of the heart.	Changes that may be seen with hypocalcemia: prolonged QT interval—characteristic but not necessarily diagnostic. In severe deficiency, T waves may flatten or invert, giving appearance of hypokalemia or myocardial ischemia; ventricular tachycardia may develop.

NURSING DIAGNOSIS: risk for Electrolyte Imbalance

Risk factors may include
Diarrhea, chronic laxative abuse
Renal failure
Treatment-related side effects of medications such as anticonvulsants, antibiotics, corticosteroids, diuretics

Possibly evidenced by
(Not applicable, presence of signs and symptoms establishes an *actual* diagnosis)

Desired Outcomes/Evaluation Criteria—Client Will

Electrolyte & Acid/Base Balance (NOC)
Display heart rhythm and laboratory results within normal limits (WNL) for client and absence of neuromuscular irritability and respiratory impairment.

ACTIONS/INTERVENTIONS	RATIONALE
Electrolyte Management: Hypocalcemia (NIC) *Independent* Monitor heart rate and rhythm.	Calcium deficit along with associated hypomagnesemia weakens cardiac muscle contractility.
Assess respiratory rate, rhythm, and effort. Have tracheostomy equipment available.	Laryngeal stridor may develop and result in respiratory arrest.
Observe for neuromuscular irritability, including tetany, or seizure activity. Assess for presence of Chvostek's and Trousseau's signs.	Calcium deficit causes repetitive and uncontrolled nerve transmission, leading to muscle spasms and hyperirritability.
Provide quiet environment and seizure precautions, as appropriate.	Reduces central nervous system (CNS) stimulation and protects client from potential injury.
Encourage relaxation and stress reduction techniques including deep-breathing exercises, guided imagery, and visualization.	Tetany can be potentiated by hyperventilation and stress. *Note:* Direct pressure on the nerves, such as tightening BP cuff, may trigger tetany.
Check for bleeding from any source, such as mucous membranes, puncture sites, wounds, or incisions. Note presence of ecchymosis and petechiae.	Alterations in coagulation can occur as a result of calcium deficiency.
Review client's drug regimen such as use of insulin, mithramycin (Mithracin), parathyroid injection, and digoxin.	Some drugs can lower magnesium levels, affecting calcium level. The effect of digoxin is enhanced by calcium, and, in clients receiving calcium, digoxin intoxication may develop.
Discuss use of laxatives and antacids.	Those containing phosphate may negatively affect calcium metabolism.
Review dietary intake of vitamins and fat.	Insufficient ingestion of vitamin D and fat impairs absorption of calcium.
Identify sources to increase calcium and vitamin D in diet such as dairy products, beans, cauliflower, eggs, oranges, pineapples, sardines, and shellfish. Restrict intake of phosphorus such as foods containing barley, bran, whole wheat, rye, liver, nuts, and chocolate.	Vitamin D aids in absorption of calcium from intestinal tract. Phosphorus competes with calcium for intestinal absorption.
Encourage use of calcium-containing antacids if needed, such as Titralac, Dicarbosil, and Tums.	Possible sources for oral replacement to help maintain calcium levels, especially in clients at risk for osteoporosis.
Stress importance of meeting calcium needs.	Adverse effects of long-term deficiency include tooth decay, eczema, cataracts, and osteoporosis.

ACTIONS/INTERVENTIONS (continued)

Collaborative

Assist with identification and treatment of underlying cause.

Monitor laboratory studies.
Administer the following:
  Calcium gluconate, gluceptate, or chloride intravenously (IV)

Oral preparations, such as calcium lactate/carbonate
Magnesium sulfate IV or orally (PO), if indicated
Vitamin D supplement

RATIONALE (continued)

Refer to listing of predisposing and contributing factors to determine treatment needs.
Evaluates therapy needs and effectiveness

Provides rapid treatment in acute calcium deficit, especially in presence of tetany or convulsions. *Note:* Calcium chloride is not used as often because it is irritating to the vein and can cause tissue sloughing if it leaks into tissues.
Oral preparations are useful in correcting subacute deficiencies.
Hypomagnesemia is a precipitating factor in calcium deficit.
May be used in combination with calcium therapy to enhance calcium absorption once concomitant phosphate deficiency is corrected.

CALCIUM (continued)

Hypercalcemia (Calcium Excess)

IV. Predisposing or Contributing Factors

  a. Hyperparathyroidism, hyperthyroidism, multiple myeloma or other malignancies (e.g., cancer of breast, lung), renal disease, skeletal muscle paralysis, parathyroid tumor, sarcoidosis, adrenal insufficiency, tuberculosis (TB)
  b. Excessive or prolonged use of vitamins A and D and calcium-containing antacids; prolonged use of thiazide diuretics, theophylline, lithium
  c. Multiple fractures, bone tumors, osteoporosis, osteomalacia, prolonged immobilization causing imbalance between the rate of bone formation and resorption
  d. Milk-alkali syndrome as a side effect of prolonged milk and antacid self-medication for gastric pain or ulcer
  e. Hypophosphatasia, hyperproteinemia
  f. Anticancer drugs: tamoxifen, androgens, estrogens

Client Assessment Database

DIAGNOSTIC DIVISION MAY REPORT	MAY EXHIBIT
ACTIVITY/REST • General malaise, fatigue, weakness • Lethargy	• Incoordination, ataxia
CIRCULATION	• Hypertension • Irregular pulse, dysrhythmias, bradycardia
ELIMINATION • Constipation or diarrhea	• Polyuria, nocturia • Kidney stones or calculi
FOOD/FLUID • Anorexia, nausea, vomiting • Thirst • Abdominal pain	• Poor skin turgor • Dry mucous membranes
NEUROSENSORY • Headache	• Hypotonicity, muscular relaxation, flaccid paralysis • Depressed or absent deep-tendon reflexes • Drowsiness, apathy, confusion, stupor, coma • Paranoia, personality change, inappropriate or bizarre behaviors, psychosis • Decreased attention span, memory loss • Depression • Slurred speech

(continues on page 928)

DIAGNOSTIC DIVISION MAY REPORT (continued)	MAY EXHIBIT (continued)
PAIN/DISCOMFORT • Epigastric, abdominal, deep flank pain • Bone or joint pain **TEACHING/LEARNING** • Refer to predisposing or contributing factors **DISCHARGE PLAN CONSIDERATIONS** • May require assistance with changes in therapeutic regimen, dietary management ▶ Refer to plan of care concerning underlying medical or surgical condition for possible considerations after discharge.	

Diagnostic Studies

TEST WHY IT IS DONE	WHAT IT TELLS ME
BLOOD TESTS • *Serum calcium:* Essential mineral for proper functioning of muscles, nerves, and heart. It is required in blood clotting and in formation of bones. Only about 1% of calcium circulates in blood. Normal total calcium levels range from 8.4 to 10.2 mg/dL.	Levels are increased.
• *Blood urea nitrogen (BUN):* Measures the amount of urea nitrogen in blood; used primarily to evaluate kidney function. Normal range is 7 to 25 mg/dL.	Increased if kidney stones calculi have caused kidney damage.
• *Serum phosphate:* Test of trace metal used to help diagnose and evaluate the severity of conditions that affect the GI tract, interfering with the absorption of calcium and magnesium.	Phosphate levels may be low when parathyroid hormone inversely promotes calcium uptake and calcium competes with phosphate for absorption and transport with vitamin D.
OTHER DIAGNOSTIC STUDIES • *Urine calcium:* Measures amount of calcium passed in urine over 24-hour period.	Levels are increased. Test may be done to determine whether a kidney stone has developed because of high amounts of calcium in the urine. May also be done to check for problems with the parathyroid glands.
• *X-rays, computed tomography (CT) scan, or magnetic resonance imaging (MRI):* Helps identify contributing factors or effects of elevated calcium level.	May reveal evidence of bone cavitation, pathological fracture, or osteoporosis, reflecting an imbalance between bone formation and resoption; or urinary calculi associated with hypercalcemia.
• *ECG:* Record of the electrical activity of the heart.	Changes seen with hypercalcemia include shortened QT interval and inverted T waves. In severe deficit, QRS may widen, PR interval lengthens, and ventricular prematurities develop.

NURSING DIAGNOSIS: risk for Electrolyte Imbalance

Risk factors may include
Renal disease
Treatment-related side effects of medications such as thiazide diuretics, theophylline, lithium, anticancer drugs
Hyperthyroidism; hyperparathyroidism

Possibly evidenced by
(Not applicable, presence of signs and symptoms establishes an *actual* diagnosis)

NURSING DIAGNOSIS: **risk for Electrolyte Imbalance** (continued)

Desired Outcomes/Evaluation Criteria—Client Will

Electrolyte & Acid/Base Balance (NOC)
Display heart rhythm, muscle strength, cognitive status, and laboratory results WNL for client.

ACTIONS/INTERVENTIONS	RATIONALE
Electrolyte Management: Hypercalcemia (NIC)	
Independent	
Monitor cardiac rate and rhythm. Be aware that cardiac arrest can occur in hypercalcemic crisis.	Overstimulation of cardiac muscle occurs with resultant dysrhythmias and ineffective cardiac contraction. Sinus bradycardia, sinus dysrhythmias, wandering pacemaker, and atrioventricular (AV) block may be noted. Hypercalcemia creates a predisposition to cardiac arrest.
Assess level of consciousness and neuromuscular status, including muscle movement, strength, and tone.	Nerve and muscle activity is depressed. Lethargy and fatigue can progress to convulsions or coma.
Monitor intake and output (I&O); calculate fluid balance.	Efforts to correct original condition may result in secondary imbalances and complications.
Encourage fluid intake of 3 to 4 L/day, including sodium-containing fluids (within cardiac tolerance) and use of acid-ash juices, such as cranberry and prune, if kidney stones present or suspected.	Reduces dehydration, encourages urinary flow and clearance of calcium, and reduces risk of stone formation. *Note:* Sodium favors calcium excretion and can be used if not contraindicated by other conditions.
Strain urine if flank pain occurs.	Large amount of calcium present in kidney parenchyma may lead to stone formation.
Auscultate bowel sounds.	Hypotonicity leads to constipation when the smooth muscle tone is inadequate to produce peristalsis.
Maintain bulk in diet.	Constipation may be a problem because of decreased GI tone.
Encourage frequent repositioning and range-of-motion (ROM) and/or muscle-setting exercises with caution. Promote ambulation if client is able.	Muscle activity may reduce calcium shifting from the bones that occurs during immobilization. *Note:* Increased risk for pathological fractures exists because of calcium shifts out of the bones.
Provide safety measures, including gentle handling when moving client.	Reduces risk of injury and pathological fractures.
Review drug regimen, noting use of calcium-elevating drugs, such as heparin, tetracyclines, methicillin, and phenytoin.	May affect drug choice or require reduction in oral sources of calcium.
Identify and restrict sources of calcium intake such as dairy products, eggs, and spinach and calcium-containing antacids such as Titralac, Dicarbosil, and Tums, if indicated.	Foods or drugs containing calcium may need to be limited in chronic conditions causing hypercalcemia.
Collaborative	
Assist with treatment of underlying cause.	Refer to listing of predisposing or contributing factors to determine treatment needs.
Monitor laboratory studies such as calcium, magnesium, and phosphate.	Monitors therapy needs and effectiveness.
Administer isotonic saline and sodium sulfate IV or PO.	Emergency measures in severe hypercalcemia used to dilute extracellular calcium concentration and inhibit tubular reabsorption of calcium, thereby increasing urinary excretion.
Administer medications, as indicated, for example:	
Diuretics, such as furosemide (Lasix)	Diuresis promotes renal excretion of calcium and reduces risks of fluid excess from isotonic saline infusion.
Sodium bicarbonate	Induces alkalosis, thereby reducing the ionized calcium fraction.
Phosphate	Rapid-acting agent that induces calcium excretion and inhibits resorption of bone.
Glucocorticoid therapy	Inhibits intestinal absorption of calcium and reduces inflammation and associated stress response that mobilizes calcium from the bone.
Mithramycin (Mithracin)	Cytotoxic antibiotic that lowers serum calcium by inhibiting inappropriate bone resorption, typically seen in malignancies or hyperparathyroidism.
Disodium edetate (EDTA)	Chelating action lowers serum calcium level.
Calcitonin	Promotes movement of serum calcium into bones, temporarily reducing serum calcium levels, especially in the presence of increased parathyroid hormone.
Neutra-Phos and Fleet Phospho-Soda	These drugs bind calcium in the GI tract, promoting excretion.
Prepare for and assist with hemodialysis.	Rapid reduction of serum calcium may be necessary to correct life-threatening situation.

MAGNESIUM

I. Function
a. Influences carbohydrate metabolism, secretion of parathyroid hormone, sodium and potassium transport across the cell membrane, and synthesis of protein and nucleic acid
b. Activates adenosine triphosphate (ATP) and mediates neural transmission within the central nervous system (CNS)
c. Deficit often associated with hypokalemia and promotes intracellular potassium loss and sodium accumulation, altering and exacerbating membrane excitability
d. Normal laboratory value—serum range 1.5 to 2.5 mEq/L or 1.8 to 3.0 mg/dL

Hypomagnesemia (Magnesium Deficit)

II. Predisposing or Contributing Factors
a. Gastrointestinal (GI) losses: biliary or intestinal fistula, surgery (bowel resection, small-bowel bypass); severe, protracted diarrhea, laxative abuse; impaired GI absorption or malabsorption syndrome, gastric or colon cancer, prolonged gastric suction
b. Protein or calorie malnutrition, enteral or parenteral feeding without adequate magnesium replacement
c. Prolonged intravenous (IV) infusion of magnesium-free solutions, multiple transfusions with citrated blood products
d. Chronic alcoholism, alcohol withdrawal, pancreatitis
e. Hyperaldosteronism: primary or secondary (e.g., cirrhosis or heart failure [HF])
f. Toxemia of pregnancy
g. Renal losses: severe renal disease, diuretic phase of acute renal failure (ARF), vigorous and/or prolonged diuresis with mercurial thiazides or loop diuretics, syndrome of inappropriate antidiuretic hormone (SIADH)
h. Drugs that affect magnesium balance: aminoglycosides (gentamicin, tobramycin), antifungals (amphotericin B), chemotherapy agents (cisplatin), antirejection agents (cyclosporine), excessive doses of calcium or vitamin D supplements
i. Diabetic ketoacidosis, malignancies causing hypercalcemic states, severe burns, sepsis, hypothermia, hypoparathyroidism, hypercalcemia, hyperthyroidism

Client Assessment Database

DIAGNOSTIC DIVISION MAY REPORT	MAY EXHIBIT
ACTIVITY/REST	
• Generalized weakness	• Ataxia
• Insomnia	
• Vertigo	
CIRCULATION	
	• Tachycardia, dysrhythmias
	• Hypotension (vasodilation), occasional hypertension
FOOD/FLUID	
• Anorexia, nausea	
• Diarrhea	
NEUROSENSORY	
• Paresthesia (legs, feet)	• Nystagmus
• Vertigo	• Musculoskeletal fasciculations or tremors, neuromuscular irritability or spasticity, spontaneous carpopedal spasms, hyperactive deep tendon reflexes, clonus
	• Seizure activity, convulsions
	• Tetany; positive Babinski's, Chvostek's, and Trousseau's signs
	• Disorientation, apathy, depression, irritability, agitation, hallucinations, psychoses, coma
TEACHING/LEARNING	
• Refer to predisposing or contributing factors	
DISCHARGE PLAN CONSIDERATIONS	
• May require assistance with changes in therapeutic regimen, dietary management	
⬩ Refer to plan of care concerning underlying medical or surgical condition for possible postdischarge considerations.	

Diagnostic Studies

TEST WHY IT IS DONE	WHAT IT TELLS ME
BLOOD TESTS • *Serum magnesium:* An essential intracellular ion needed to regulate water balance, levels of acidity, and blood pressure (BP). Normal range is 3.5 to 5.5 mEq/L.	Decreased, less than 1.5 mEq/L or 1.8 mg/dL. Usually symptoms do not appear until level is less than 1 mEq/L.
• *Calcium:* Essential mineral for proper functioning of muscles, nerves, and heart. It is required in blood clotting and in formation of bones. Only about 1% of calcium circulates in blood. Normal total calcium ranges from 8.4 to 10.2 mg/dL.	May be decreased unless there is a hypercalcemic condition causing the magnesium deficit.
• *Potassium:* An essential intracellular ion needed to regulate water balance, levels of acidity, and BP. Normal range is 3.5 to 5.5 mEq/L.	Decrease associated with severe hypomagnesemia.
OTHER DIAGNOSTIC STUDIES • *Electrocardiogram (ECG):* Record of the electrical activity of the heart.	Changes associated with hypomagnesemia include prolonged PR and QT intervals, widened QRS complex, ST-segment depression, and T-wave inversion.

NURSING DIAGNOSIS: risk for Electrolyte Imbalance

Risk factors may include
Excessive losses
Renal disease
Diabetic ketoacidosis, hyperaldosteronism
Treatment-related side effects of medications such as diuretics, aminoglycosides, antifungals, chemotherapy agents
Malnutrition

Possibly evidenced by
(Not applicable, presence of signs and symptoms establishes an *actual* diagnosis)

Desired Outcomes/Evaluation Criteria—Client Will

Electrolyte & Acid/Base Balance (NOC)
Display heart rate and rhythm, muscle strength, cognitive status, and laboratory results within normal limits (WNL) for client and absence of neuromuscular irritability.

ACTIONS/INTERVENTIONS	RATIONALE
Electrolyte Management: Hypomagnesemia (NIC) *Independent* Monitor cardiac rate and rhythm, noting tachydysrhythmias and characteristic ECG changes.	Magnesium influences sodium and potassium transport across the cell membrane and affects excitability of cardiac tissue.
Monitor for signs of digoxin intoxication when used, including reports of nausea or vomiting and blurred vision; increasing atrial dysrhythmias and heart block.	Magnesium deficit may precipitate digoxin toxicity.
Assess level of consciousness (LOC) and neuromuscular status, noting movement, strength, and reflexes and tone; note presence of Chvostek's and Trousseau's signs.	Confusion, irritability, and psychosis may occur. However, more common manifestations are muscular including hyperactive deep tendon reflexes, muscle tremors, spasticity, or generalized tetany.
Monitor status of airway and swallowing.	Laryngeal stridor and dysphagia can occur when depletion is moderate to severe.
Take seizure or safety precautions, such as padded side rails, bed in low position, and frequent observation, as indicated.	Changes in mentation or the development of seizure activity in severe hypomagnesemia increases the risk of client injury.
Provide quiet environment and subdued lighting.	Reduces extraneous stimuli; promotes rest.
Encourage range-of-motion (ROM) exercises, as tolerated.	Reduces deleterious effects of muscle weakness and spasticity.
Place footboard or cradle on bed.	Elevation of linens may reduce spasms.
Auscultate bowel sounds.	Muscle weakness or spasticity may reduce peristalsis and bowel function.

(continues on page 932)

ACTIONS/INTERVENTIONS (continued)	RATIONALE (continued)
Encourage intake of dairy products, whole grains, green leafy vegetables, meat, and fish.	Provides oral replacement for mild magnesium deficits; may prevent recurrence.
Instruct client in proper use of laxatives and diuretics.	Deficit may be the result of abuse of these drugs.
Observe for signs of magnesium toxicity during replacement therapy—thirst, feeling hot and flushed, diaphoresis, anxiety, drowsiness, hypotension, increased muscular and nervous system irritability, or loss of patellar reflex.	Rapid, excessive IV replacement may lead to toxicity and life-threatening complications.
Collaborative	
Assist with treatment of underlying cause.	Refer to listing of predisposing or contributing factors. *Note:* Studies have shown that chronic alcoholism with malnutrition is the most common cause of hypomagnesemia in the United States.
Monitor laboratory studies such as serum magnesium, calcium, and potassium levels.	Evaluates therapy needs and effectiveness. *Note:* These electrolytes are interrelated, symptoms may be similar, and deficits of more than one may be present.
Administer medications, as indicated, for example:	
Magnesium sulfate or magnesium chloride IV, monitoring administration closely	IV replacement is preferred in severe deficit because absorption of magnesium from intestinal tract varies inversely with calcium absorption. However, potential for drug interaction with digitalis preparations may lead to increased cardiac dysrhythmias or heart block. *Note:* Calcium gluconate is the antidote should hypermagnesemia be evidenced by depressed deep tendon reflexes or respiratory depression and hypotension (late sign).
Magnesium sulfate intramuscularly (IM) or magnesium hydroxide orally (PO) (Amphojel and milk of magnesia)	May be given for mild deficit or in nonemergent situations. Injections should be deep IM to decrease local tissue reaction.
Magnesium-based antacids such as Mylanta, Maalox, Gelusil, and Riopan	Can supplement dietary replacement. *Note:* Use of these products may cause diarrhea, which can be alleviated by concurrent use of aluminum-containing products such as Amphojel and Basaljel.

MAGNESIUM (continued)

Hypermagnesemia (Magnesium Excess)

III. Predisposing or Contributing Factors

a. Reduced renal function (e.g., acute processes or age), chronic renal disease or failure, or dialysis with hard water

b. Excessive intake or absorption—too-rapid replacement of magnesium (as in pregnancy-induced hypertension or premature labor), excessive use of magnesium-containing drugs or products, such as Maalox, milk of magnesia, and Epsom salts

c. Untreated diabetic ketoacidosis

d. Hyperparathyroidism, aldosterone deficiency, adrenal insufficiency

e. Extracellular fluid volume depletion (e.g., after diuretic abuse)

f. Saltwater near-drowning, hypothermia, shock

g. Chronic diarrhea; diseases that interfere with gastric absorption

Client Assessment Database

DIAGNOSTIC DIVISION MAY REPORT	MAY EXHIBIT
ACTIVITY/REST	
• Generalized weakness	• Drowsiness, lethargy, stupor
• Fatigue	
CIRCULATION	
	• Hypotension (mild to severe)
	• Pulses weak, irregular, bradycardia (12–15 mEq/L), cardiac arrest (greater than 25 mEq/L)

DIAGNOSTIC DIVISION MAY REPORT (continued)	MAY EXHIBIT (continued)
FOOD/FLUID • Nausea	
NEUROSENSORY	• Depressed deep tendon reflexes (7–10 mEq/L) progressing to flaccid paralysis • Decreased LOC, lethargy progressing to coma • Slurred speech
RESPIRATION	• Hypoventilation progressing to apnea (12–15 mEq/L)
SAFETY	• Skin flushing, sweating
TEACHING/LEARNING • Refer to predisposing or contributing factors	
DISCHARGE PLAN CONSIDERATIONS • May require assistance with changes in therapeutic regimen, dietary management ▶ Refer to plan of care concerning underlying medical or surgical condition for possible considerations after discharge.	

Diagnostic Studies

TEST WHY IT IS DONE	WHAT IT TELLS ME
BLOOD TESTS • *Serum magnesium:* An essential intracellular ion needed to regulate water balance, levels of acidity, and BP. Normal range is 3.5 to 5.5 mEq/L.	Client is symptomatic when levels are greater than 3 mEq/L. High levels (10–20 mEq/L) result in respiratory depression, coma, and cardiac arrest.
OTHER DIAGNOSTIC STUDIES • *ECG:* Record of the electrical activity of the heart.	Changes associated with hypermagnesemia include prolonged PR and QT intervals, widened QRS, elevated T waves, development of heart block, and cardiac arrest.

NURSING DIAGNOSIS: risk for Electrolyte Imbalance

Risk factors may include
Chronic diarrhea
Renal dysfunction
Treatment-related side effects of such as medications containing magnesium, diuretic abuse, dialysis with hard water
Diabetic ketoacidosis

Possibly evidenced by
(Not applicable, presence of signs and symptoms establishes an *actual* diagnosis)

Desired Outcomes/Evaluation Criteria—Client Will

Electrolyte & Acid/Base Balance (NOC)
Display heart rhythm, muscular strength, cognitive status and laboratory results WNL for client and absence of respiratory impairment.

ACTIONS/INTERVENTIONS	RATIONALE
Electrolyte Management: Hypermagnesemia (NIC)	
Independent	
Monitor cardiac rate and rhythm.	Bradycardia and heart block may develop, progressing to cardiac arrest as a direct result of hypermagnesemia on cardiac muscle.
Monitor BP.	Hypotension unexplained by other causes is an early sign of toxicity.
Assess LOC and neuromuscular status, including reflexes, muscle tone, movement, and strength.	CNS and neuromuscular depression can cause decreasing level of alertness, progressing to coma, and depressed muscular responses, progressing to flaccid paralysis.
Monitor respiratory rate, depth, and rhythm. Encourage coughing and deep-breathing exercises. Elevate head of bed, as indicated.	Neuromuscular transmissions are blocked by magnesium excess, resulting in respiratory muscular weakness and hypoventilation, which may progress to apnea.
Check patellar reflexes periodically.	Absence of these reflexes suggests magnesium levels about 7 mEq/L or greater. If untreated, cardiac and respiratory arrest can occur.
Encourage increased fluid intake, if appropriate.	Increased hydration enhances magnesium excretion, but fluid intake must be cautious in event of renal or cardiac failure.
Monitor urinary output and 24-hour fluid balance.	Renal failure is the primary contributing factor in hypermagnesemia, and, if it is present, fluid excess can easily occur.
Promote bedrest; assist with personal care activities, as needed.	Flaccid paralysis, lethargy, and decreased mentation can reduce activity tolerance and ability.
Recommend avoidance of magnesium-containing antacids, such as Maalox, Mylanta, Gelusil, and Riopan, in client with renal disease. Caution clients with renal disease to avoid over-the-counter (OTC) drug use without discussing with healthcare provider.	Limits oral intake to help prevent hypermagnesemia.
Collaborative	
Assist with treatment of underlying cause.	Refer to listing of predisposing and contributing factors to determine treatment needs. *Note:* Most frequently occurs in clients with advanced renal failure.
Monitor laboratory studies, as indicated	Evaluates therapy needs and effectiveness.
Administer IV fluids and thiazide diuretics, as indicated.	Promotes renal clearance of magnesium if kidney function is normal.
Administer 10% calcium chloride or gluconate IV.	Antagonizes action and reverses symptoms of magnesium toxicity to improve neuromuscular function.
Assist with dialysis, as needed.	In the presence of renal disease or failure, dialysis may be needed to lower serum levels.

BIBLIOGRAPHY

CHAPTER 1

Books

American Nurses Association: Code of ethics for nurses. American Nurses Association, Silver Spring, MD, 2001.

American Nurses Association: Nursing scope and standards of practice. American Nurses Association, Silver Spring, MD, 2004.

National Center for Health Statistics. (2007). Health, United States, 2007, with chartbook on trends in the health of Americans. National Center for Health Statistics, Hyattsville, MD, 2007.

Articles

Aiken, LH, et al: Hospital nurse staffing and patient mortality, nurse burnout, and job dissatisfaction. JAMA 288(16):1987–1993, 2002.

Blegen, MA, Goode, CJ, and Reed, L: Nursing staffing and patient outcomes. Nurs Res 47(1):43–50, 1998.

Buerhaus, PJ: Is a nursing shortage on the way? Nursing98 28(8): 34–35, 1998.

Dunton, N, et al: Nurse staffing and patient falls on acute care hospital units. Nurs Outlook 52(1):53–59, 2004.

Keenan, G, Tschannen, D, and Wesley, M: Standardized nursing terminologies can transform practice. JONA 38(3):103–106, 2008.

Keenan, GM, et al: The HANDS project: Studying and refining the automated collection of a cross-setting clinical data set. Comp Inform Nurs 20(3):89–100, 2002.

Kohl, BA, et al: Effect of telemedicine on mortality and length of stay in a university ICU. Crit Care Med 35(12):A22, 2007.

Leape, LL, and Berwick, DM: Five years after to err is human: What have we learned? JAMA 293(19):2384–2390, 2005.

Mark, BA, Harless, D, and Berman, WF: Nurse staffing and adverse events in hospitalized children. Policy Polit Nurs Pract 8(2): 83–92, 2007.

Matthews, JT: The nursebot project: Developing a personal robotic assistant for frail older adults in the community. Home Health Care Management & Practice 14(5):403–405, 2002.

Needleman, J, et al: Nurse staffing levels and the quality of care in hospitals. New Eng J Med 346(22):1715–1722, 2002.

Pineau, J, et al: Towards robotic assistants in nursing homes: Challenges and results. Rob Auton Syst 42(3-4):271–281, 2003.

Rivera, D, and Halvorson, G: We're in it together. Modern Healthcare 38(11):22, 2008.

Solovy, A, Hoppszallern, S, and Brown, S: Ten lessons from the top 100; Healthcare most wired. Hosp Health Network 81(7):40–53, 2007.

Yang, KP: Relationships between nurse staffing and client outcomes. J Nurs Res 11(3):149–158, 2003.

Electronic Resources

American Nurses' Association Health Care Agenda 2005. Retrieved March 2008 from **http://nursingworld.org/MainMenuCategories/ HealthcareandPolicyIssues/Reports/HealthCareAgenda.aspx**

Center for American Nurses: Restructuring and redesigning nurses' work environments, 2007 revised. Retrieved March 2008 from **http://www.centerforamericannurses.org/positions/ finalworkenviron.pdf**

HHS Secretary Leavitt: 500-Day Plan for improving the health, safety, and well-being of America. Retrieved March 2008 from **www.hhs.gov/500DayPlan**

Park, HK, et al: A nursing robot system for the elderly and the disabled. Int J of Human-friendly Welfare Robotic Systems 2(4):11–16, 2001. Retrieved April 2008 from **http://web.cecs.pdx.edu/~mperkows/ Rehabilitation_Robots/nursing-robot.pdf**

Pollack, ME, et al: Pearl: A mobile robotic assistant for the elderly, 2002. Retrieved May 2008 from **http://www.eecs.umich.edu/~pollackm/ distrib/aaai02wkshp.pdf**

State Health Access Data Assistance Center: The coverage gap: A state-by-state report on access to care. Prepared by University of Minnesota, 2006a. Retrieved March 2008 from **http://www.sph .umn.edu/img/assets/18528/CTUW2006_TheCoverageGap.pdf**

State Health Access Data Assistance Center: Shifting ground: Changes in employer-sponsored health insurance. Prepared by University of Minnesota, 2006b. Retrieved March 2008 from **http://www.sph .umn.edu/img/assets/18528/CTUW2006_ShiftingGround.pdf**

CHAPTER 2

Books

American Nurses Association: Nursing's social policy statement. American Nurses Association, Kansas City, MO, 1980.

American Nurses Association. Standards of clinical nursing practice. American Nurses Association, Kansas City, MO, 1991.

American Nurses Association: Nursing's social policy statement. American Nurses Association, Washington, DC, 1995.

American Nurses Association: Nursing: Scope and Standards of Practice. American Nurses Association, Silver Spring, MD, 2004.

NANDA-I: Nursing diagnoses: Definitions and classification. NANDA International, Philadelphia, 2007.

Pesut, DJ, and Herman, J: Clinical reasoning, the art and science of critical and creative thinking. Delmar, Albany, NY, 1999.

Shore, LS: Nursing Diagnosis: What It Is and How To Do It, A Programmed Text. Medical College of Virginia Hospitals, Redmond, VA, 1988.

Articles

Aquilino, ML, and Keenan, G: Having our say: Nursing's standardized nomenclature. AJN 100(7):33–38, 2000.

Delaney, C, and Maas, M: Reliability of nursing diagnoses documented in a computerized nursing information system. Nurs Diagn 11(3): 121–134, 2000.

CHAPTER 3

Books

Pesut, DJ, and Herman, J: Clinical reasoning, the art and science of critical and creative thinking. Delmar, Albany, NY, 1999.

Articles

Hickman, JS: A critical assessment of critical thinking in nursing education. Holistic Nurse Practitioner 7(3):36–47, 1993.

Electronic Resources

Scriven, M, and Paul, R: Critical thinking as defined by the National Council for Excellence in Critical Thinking. Presented at the 8th Annual International Conference on Critical Thinking and Education Reform, Summer 1987. Retrieved February 2009 from **http:// www.criticalthinking.org/aboutCT/define_critical_thinking.cfm**

CHAPTER 4

Books

Abraham, WT: The expanding role of natruiretic peptide treatment in management of heart failure. CME Offering. University of Minnesota, Minneapolis, MN, 2004.

American College of Cardiology/American Heart Association Task Force: Practice guidelines for the management of patients with AMI. Elsevier Science, New York, 1999.

Bezruchka, S: Altitude illness prevention and treatment. The Mountaineers, Seattle, WA, 1998.

The Criteria Committee of the New York Heart Association: Nomenclature and criteria for diagnosis of diseases of the heart and great vessels, ed 9. Little, Brown & Co, Boston, 1994, pp 253–256.

Deglin, JH, and Vallerand, AH: Davis's drug guide for nurses, ed 10. FA Davis, Philadelphia, 2007.

LeFever Kee, J: Laboratory and diagnostic tests with nursing implications, ed 7. Pearson Prentice Hall, Upper Saddle River, NJ, 2005.

Smeltzer, S, et al: Brunner and Suddarth's textbook of medical-surgical nursing, ed 11. Lippincott, Williams & Wilkins, Philadelphia, 2008.

Van Leeuwen, AM, Kranpitz, TR, and Smith, L: Davis's comprehensive handbook of laboratory and diagnostic tests with nursing implications, ed 2. FA Davis, Philadelphia, 2006.

Wilson, BA, et al: Prentice Hall nurse's drug guide 2008. Pearson Prentice Hall, Upper Saddle River, NJ, 2008.

Articles

Abbott, AV: Diagnostic approach to palpitations. Am Fam Physician 71(4):743–755, 2005.

Adams, JE, and Miracle, VA: Cardiac biomarkers: Past, present, and future. Am J Crit Care 7(6):418–423, 1998.

Albert, N: Heart failure: The physiologic basis for current therapeutic concepts. Crit Care Nurse June (suppl):2–13, 1999.

Alpert, JS, et al: Myocardial infarction redefined—A consensus document of The Joint European Society of Cardiology/American College of Cardiology Committee for the Redefinition of Myocardial Infarction. JACC 36(3):959–969, 2000.

Artinian, MT: The psychosocial aspects of heart failure. AJN 103(12):32–42, 2003.

Artinian, MT: Innovations in blood presssure monitoring. AJN 104(8):53–60, 2004.

Balser, JR: Managing arrhythmias after cardiac surgery. AACN News 17(2):10–11, 2000.

Berger R, et al: B-type natriuretic peptide predicts sudden death in clients with chronic heart failure. Circulation (105):2328–2331, 2002.

Bond, EA, et al: The left ventricular assist device. AJN 103(1): 33–41, 2003.

Braun, LT: Cardiovascular disease: Strategies for risk assessment and modification. J Cardiovas Nurs 21(6)(suppl):S20–S42, 2006.

Braun, LT, and Davidson, MH: Cholesterol-lowering drugs bring benefits to high-risk populations even when LDL is normal. J Cardiovas Nurs 18(1):44–49, 2003.

Bridges, EJ, and Woods, SL: Cardiovascular chronobiology: Implications for critical care nursing. Crit Care Nurse 18(4):49–64, 1998.

Cheek, D, and Cesan, A: What's different about heart disease in women? Nursing2003 33(8):36–42, 2003.

Chobanian, AV, et al: Seventh report of Joint National Committee (JNC) on detection, evaluation, and treatment of high blood pressure. Hypertension 42(6):1206–1252, 2003.

Church, V: Staying on guard for DVT and PE. Nursing 2000 30(2): 34, 2000.

Church, V: Managing the risk of DVT and PE. Nursing 2001 31(12): 1–10, 2001.

Colwell, CW, and Hardwick, ME: Natural history of venous thromboembolism. Tech Orthop 19:236–239, 2004.

Coughlin, RM: Recognizing ventricular arrhythmias and preventing sudden cardiac death: Be prepared to stop these dangerous arrhythmias. Am Nurse Today 2(5):38–43, 2007.

Coviello, JS, and Nystrom, KV: Obesity and heart failure. J Cardiovasc Nurs 18(5):360–368, 2003.

Craft, J: Eplerenone (Inspra), a new aldosterone antagonist for the treatment of systemic hypertension and heart failure. Proc (Bayl Univ Med Cent) 17(2):217–220, 2004.

Crowther, M, and McCourt, K: Get the edge on deep vein thrombosis. Nurs Manage 35(1):21–29, 2004.

Crowther, M, and McCourt, K: Venous thromboembolism: A guide to prevention and treatment. Nurse Pract 30(8):26–43, 2005.

Crumlish, CM, et al: When time is muscle. AJ, 100(1):26, 2000.

Cucinelli, C: Minimally invasive coronary artery bypass surgery. Crit Care Nurse 23(1):54, 2000.

Cunningham, C: Managing hospitalized client with heart failure: What you need to know about the new practice guidelines for evaluation, care, and treatment of heart failure clients in the hospital. Am Nurse Today 1(1):44–50, 2006.

Curtis, A: Prophylactic defibrillators for the prevention of sudden cardiac death: The SCD-HeFT Trial. American College of Cardiology Presentation. March 7–10, New Orleans, LA, 2004.

D'Arcy, Y: Controlling pain: Managing postoperative CABG pain. Nursing99 29(9):17, 1999.

Daly, J, et al: Health status, perceptions of coping and social support immediately after discharge of survivors of acute myocardial infarct. Am J Crit Care 9(1):62–69, 2000.

Day, MW: Recognizing and managing deep vein thrombosis. Nursing2003 33(5):36–41, 2003.

De Jong, MJ, and Morton, PG: Predictors of atrial dysrhythmias for patients undergoing coronary artery bypass grafting. Am J Crit Care 9(6):388–396, 2000.

de Lissovoy, G: Economic issues in the treatment and prevention of deep vein thrombosis from a managed care perspective. Am J Manag Care 7(17)(suppl):S535–S538; (discussion) S538–S544, 2001.

Dracup, KA, and Cannon, C: Combination treatment strategies for management of acute myocardial infarction: New directions with current therapies. Crit Care Nurse April (suppl):3–15, 1999.

Edgar, WF, Ebersole, N, and Mayfield, MG: MIDCAB. AJN 99(7):40, 1999.

Elmer, PJ, et al: Effects of comprehensive lifestyle modification on diet, weight, physical fitness, and blood pressure control: 18-month results of a randomized trial. Ann Intern Med 144(7):485–495, 2006.

Fareed, M, Suri, K, and Qureshi, AI: Prehypertension as a risk factor for cardiovascular diseases. J Cardiovasc Nurs 21(6):478–482, 2006.

Fort, CW: Can you solve this mystery? The patient might have DVT . . . or is it FES? Nursing Made Incredibly Easy! 1(2):10, 2003.

Freeman, JJ, and Hedges, C: Cardiac arrest: The effect on the brain. AJN 103(6):51–55, 2003.

Futterman, LG, and Lemberg, L: Encephalopathies following cardiac surgery. Am J Crit Care 7(6):450–453, 1998.

Futterman, LG, and Lemberg, L: Low-molecular-weight heparin: Antithrombotic agent whose time has come. Am J Crit Care 8(1):520–523, 1999.

Futterman, LG, and Lemberg, L: Update on management of acute myocardial infarction: Facilitated percutaneous coronary intervention. Am J Crit Care 9(1):70–76, 2000.

Geerts, WH, et al: Prevention of venous thromboembolism. Chest (126):338S–400S, 2004.

Gibbon-Clements, T, et al: The challenge of warfarin therapy. AJN 100(3):38, 2000.

Goldsborough, MA, et al: Prevalence of leg wound complications after coronary artery bypass grafting: Determination of risk factors. Am J Crit Care 8(3):149–153, 1999.

Gylys, K, and Gold, M: Acute coronary syndromes—New developments in pharmacological treatment strategies. Crit Care Nurse April (suppl):3–14, 2000.

Heart Failure Society of America: Evaluation of clients for ventricular dysfunction and heart failure. J Card Fail 12(1):e16–e25, 2006.

Heidenreich, PA, et al: Cost effectiveness of screening with B-type natriuretic peptide to identify patients with reduced left ventricular ejection fraction. J Am Coll Cardiol 17 43(6):1019–1026, 2004.

Heller, GA: Atrial fibrillation: Soothing the savage beat. Nursing99 29(2):26, 1999.

Hill, MN, et al: Hypertension care and control in underserved urban African American men: Behavioral and physiologic outcomes at 36 months. Am J Hypertens 16:906–913, 2003.

Hu, A, et al: Factors influencing patient knowledge of warfarin therapy after mechanical heart valve replacement. J Cardiovasc Nurs 21(3):169–175, 2006.

Hunt, S, et al: ACC/AHA 2005 guideline update for the diagnosis and management of chronic heart failure in the adult. American College of Cardiology/American Heart Association Practice Guidelines. Circulation 112:1–82, 2005.

Hussar, DA: New drugs. Part II. Nursing99 29(2):45, 1999.

Kanbay, M, et al: Relation between serum thyroid hormone and "nondipper" circadian blood pressure variability. Kidney Blood Press Res 30(6):416–420, 2007.

Kark, VA: The future of minimally invasive cardiac surgery. OR Nurse 2(1):25–30, 2008.

Karmath, B, and Thornton, W: Auscultation of the heart. Hosp Phys Sept:39–43, 2002.

Kearney, K: Digitalis toxicity. AJN 100(6):51–52, 2000.

Kehl-Pruett, W: Deep vein thrombosis in hospitalized patients: A review of evidence-based guidelines for prevention. Dimens Crit Care Nurs 25(2):53–59, 2006.

Keib, CN: Mediastinitis following coronary artery bypass graft surgery: Pathogenesis, clinical presentation, risks, and management. J Cardiovasc Nurs 21(6):493–499, 2006.

Khan, NA, et al: The Canadian recommendations for management of hypertension. Can J Cardiol 20(1):41–54, 2004.

Kline-Rogers, E, Marlin, JS, and Smith, DD: New era of reperfusion in acute myocardial infarction. Crit Care Nurse 19(1):21–31, 1999.

Kozuk, JL: NSAIDs and anti-hypertensives: An unhappy union. AJN 100(6):40, 2000.

Kuncl, N, and Nelson, KM: Getting the skinny on lipid-lowering drugs. Nursing2000 30(7):52, 2000.

Lackey, SA: Suppressing the scourge of AMI. Nurs 36(5):36–41, 2006.

Lewis, AM: Cardiovascular emergency. Nursing99 29(6):51, 1999.

Livorsi-Moore, J, Gulanick, M, and Rosko, PH: Port access: Another advance in cardiovascular surgery. AJN 99(7):52, 1999.

Logan, P, and Moore, J:. Hypertension: Getting back to the basics. Nursing 2004 May (suppl):1–7, 2004.

MacCallum, EM, Hanlon, SJ, and Byrne, KH: Beyond aspirin: How glycoprotein inhibitors ease acute coronary syndromes. Nursing99 29(12):34, 1999.

Mair, M: Monophasic and biphasic defibrillators. AJN 103(8): 58–60, 2003.

Marchigiano, G, Riendeau, D, and Morse, CJ: New technology applications: Thrombolysis of acute deep vein thrombosis. Crit Care Nurs Quart 29(4):312–323, 2006.

McKinney, BC: Solving the puzzle of heart failure. Nursing99 29(5):33, 1999.

Metules, TJ: Cardiac tamponade. RN 62(12):26, 1999.

Miller, DD, and Shaw, LJ: Coronary artery disease: Diagnostic and prognostic models for reducing patient risk. J Cardiovas Nurs 21(6) (suppl): S2–S16, 2006.

Mosca, L, et al: Evidence-based guidelines for cardiovascular disease prevention in women. J Am Coll Cardiol 43(5):900–921, 2004.

Murphy, MJ, and Berding, CB: Use of measurements of myoglobin and cardiac troponins in acute myocardial infarction. Crit Care Nurse 19(1):58–65, 1999.

No author listed: Angioplasty vs clot busters. Harv Health Lett 24(11): 7, 1999.

No author listed: Chest pain in women—in the head or in the heart? Harv Heart Lett 10(12):2, 2000.

No author listed: Heart attacks without chest pain: The danger is greater. Harv Heart Lett 11(1):5, 2000.

No author listed: New techniques for preventing strokes. Focus on Healthy Aging 3(8):1, 2000.

No author listed: Triglycerides and heart disease. Harv Heart Lett 11(1): 5, 2000.

Owens, SG: Nursing management of arrhythmias after cardiac surgery. AACN News 17(2):11–12, 2000.

Pantilat, SZ, and Steimle, AE: Palliative care for clients with heart failure. JAMA 291:2476–2482, 2004.

Platek, UN, and Atzori, M: PTMR. AJN 99(7):64, 1999.

Ridker, PM: Clinical application of C-reactive protein for cardiovascular disease detection and prevention. Circulation 107:363–369, 2003.

Rochett, JL: Endothelial dysfunction and the promise of ACE inhibitors. AJN 99(10):44, 1999.

Rosmund, W, et al: Heart disease and stroke statistics—2007 update: A report from the American Heart Association Statistics Committee and Stroke Statistics Subcommittee. Circulation 115:e69–e171, 2007.

Sakallaris, BR, et al: Same-day transfer of patients to the cardiac telemetry unit after surgery: The rapid after bypass back into telemetry (RABBIT) program. Crit Care Nurse 20(2):50–68, 2000.

Savage, LS, and Grap, MJ: Telephone monitoring after early discharge for cardiac surgery patients. Am J Crit Care 8(3):154–159, 1999.

Sesso, HD, et al: C-reactive protein and the risk of developing hypertension JAMA. 290:2945–2951, 2003.

Shapiro, D, Goldstein, IB, and Jamner, LD: Effects of anger/hostility, defensiveness, gender, and family history of hypertension on cardiovascular reactivity. Psychophysiology 32(5):425–435, 1995.

Sims, JM, and Miracle, VA: Easy ECG series. Part II. Using the ECG to detect myocardial infarction. Nursing99 29(8):41, 1999.

Siomko, AX: Demystifying cardiac markers. AJN 100(1):36, 2000.

Smith, SC, et al: AHA/ACC guidelines for secondary prevention for patients with coronary and other atherosclerotic vascular disease: 2006 update. Circulation 113:2363–2372, 2006.

Sorensen, ER, Lorme, TB, and Heath, D: Improve cardiac outcomes with TEG. Nurs 2008 Crit Care 1(2):18–24, 2006.

Steinke, EE: Sexual counseling after myocardial infarction. AJN 100(12):38–43, 2000.

Stockman, J: In too deep: Understanding deep vein thrombosis. Nursing Made Incredibly Easy! 6(2):29–38, 2008.

Tasota, FJ, and Tate, J: Eye on diagnostics: Assessing digoxin levels. Nurs 2000 30(3):24, 2000.

Tenenbaum, A, et al: Functional capacity impairment in patients with coronary artery disease: Prevalence, risk factors and prognosis. Cardiol 100(4):207–215, 2003.

Walke, LM, et al: The burden of symptoms among community-dwelling older persons with advanced chronic disease. Arch Int Med 164(21):2321–2324, 2004.

Whitman, GR: Nursing-sensitive outcomes in cardiac surgery patients. J Cardiovasc Nurs 19(5):293–298, 2004.

Wingate, S: Caring for persons with advanced heart failure. Home Healthc Nurse 25(8):511–520, 2007.

Woods, A: Managing the silent killer. Nursing Made Incredibly Easy! 2(2):12–25, 2004.

Woods, A, and Moshang, J: Lowering risks of diabetes, hypertension, and heart disease. Holist Nurs Pract 20(1):5–9, 2006.

Woods, AD: Managing hypertension: Help your patient keep the lid on high BP. Nursing99 29(3):41, 1999.

Yee, CA: Atrial fibrillation: The ruthless irregular rhythm. Nurs 2008 Crit Care 1(5):30–37, 2006.

Yutsis, P: High blood pressure: Prescription drugs causing more problems than they solve? J Longev 6(1):21, 2000.

Zevola, DR, and Maier, B: Improving the care of cardiothoracic surgery patients through advanced nursing skills. Crit Care Nurse 19(1): 34–44, 1999.

Electronic Resources

Alaeddini, J, and Shriani, J: Angina pectoris, 2007. Retrieved March 2008 from **http://www.emedicine.com/med/topic133.htm**

American Association for Clinical Chemistry: Lab tests online, n.d. Retrieved March 2008 from **http://www.labtestsonline.org/**

American Heart Association: Cholesterol levels. Retrieved February 2009 from **http://www.americanheart.org/presenter.jhtml?identifier=4500**

American Heart Association: Heart disease and stroke statistics—2004 update, 2004. Retrieved May 2008 from **http://www.americanheart .org/downloadable/heart/1079736729696HDSStats2004UpdateRE V3-19-04.pdf**

American Heart Association: Heart disease and stroke statistics—2007 update, 2007. Retrieved January 2008 from **http://circ.ahajournals .org/cgi/content/full/CIRCULATIONAHA.106.179918**

Breen, P: DVT: What every nurse should know. RN2000 63(4):58–62, 2000. Retrieved May 2008 from **http://rn.modernmedicine.com/ rnweb/data/articlestandard//rnweb/342004/114305/article.pdf**

Bussey, HI: Deep vein thrombosis and pulmonary embolus estimates are substantially higher than previously thought, 2007. Retrieved January 2008, from **http://www.clotcare.com/clotcare/ deepveinthrombosispulmonaryembolismstats.aspx**

Centers for Disease Control and Prevention: Heart failure fact sheet, 2006a. Retrieved March 2008 from **http://www.cdc.gov/DHDSP/ library/fs_heart_failure.htm**

Centers for Disease Control and Prevention: High blood pressure fact sheet, 2006b. Retrieved March 2008 from **http://www.cdc.gov/ DHDSP/library/fs_bloodpressure.htm**

Centers for Disease Control and Prevention: Health, United States, 2007, p 280, 2007a. Retrieved January 2008 from **http://www.cdc.gov/ nchs/data/hus/hus07.pdf**

Centers for Disease Control and Prevention: Heart disease fact sheet, 2007b. Retrieved March 2008 from **http://www.cdc.gov/heartdisease/**

Cleveland Clinic: Cleveland Clinic Heart and Vascular Guide, 2007. Various articles concerning current and future practice in heart surgery procedures. Retrieved May 2008 from **http://www.clevelandclinic .org/heartcenter/pub/guide/disease/cad/treatment_heartsurg.htm**

The Criteria Committee of the New York Heart Association: 1994 Revisions to Classification of Functional Capacity and Objective Assessment of Patients with Diseases of the Heart. From Nomenclature and criteria for diagnosis of diseases of the heart and great vessels, ed 9. Little, Brown & Co, Boston, Mass, 1994, pp 253–256. Retrieved January 2008 from **http://americanheart.org/ presenter.jhtml?identifier=1712**

Earhart, A, and Tomlinson, M: Deep vein thrombosis: Prevention, diagnosis, and treatment, 2007. Retrieved May 2008 from **http://rn .modernmedicine.com/rnweb/article/articleDetail.jsp?id=405276**

Garcia, M: Heart disease: Diagnosing heart disease: Cardiac computed tomography (CT), 2006. Retrieved February 2008 from **http://www. webmd.com/heart-disease/guide/ct-heart-scan?ecd=wnl_nal_112907**

Griffin, RM: Heart-failure treatment by device, 2003. Retrieved November 2004 from **http://www.mywebmd.com**

HeartCenterOnline: Ablation. Retrieved November 2004 from **http://www.heartcenteronline.com**

HeartCenterOnline: Coronary artery bypass surgery. Retrieved November 2004 from **http://www.heartcenteronline.com**

HeartCenterOnline: Electrophysiology study. Retrieved November 2004 from **http://www.heartcenteronline.com**

HeartCenterOnline: Inflammation reduced with "beating heart" surgery: Study, 2003. Retrieved November 2004 from **http://yourtotalhealth. ivillage.com/inflammation-reduced-with-beating-heart-surgery- study.html**

HeartCenterOnline: Maze procedure. Retrieved November 2004 from **http://www.heartcenteronline.com**

HeartCenterOnline: Minimally invasive bypass surgery. Retrieved November 2004 from **http://heart centeronline.com**

HeartCenterOnline: Pacemaker. Retrieved November 2004 from **http://www.heartcenteronline.com**

High blood pressure and ED: When medicine is the problem. Retrieved December 2007 from **http://www.webmd.com/solutions/ hbp-and-sex/medications-and-ed**

Hix, JK, and Vidt, DG: Initial evaluation. Thyroid dysfunction and hypertension: What's the connection? The Cleveland Clinic Disease Management Project, 2004. Retrieved January 2008 from **http://www.clevelenadclinicmed.com**

Hobbs, R, and Boyle, A: Heart failure: Definition. Cleveland Clinic, 2004. Retrieved April 2008 from **http://www.clevelandclinicmeded.com/ medicalpubs/diseasemanagement/cardiology/heartfailure/ heartfailure.htm#ref2**

McKhann, GM, et al: Stroke and encephalopathy after cardiac surgery: An update. Stroke 37:562–571, 2006. Retrieved May 2008, from **http://stroke.ahajournals.org/cgi/content/full/strokeaha;37/2/562**

McKhann, GM, et al: Encephalophy and stroke after coronary artery bypass grafting. Arch Neurol 59(9):1422–1428, 2002. Retrieved May 2008 from **http://archneur.ama-assn.org/cgi/content/full/ 59/9/1422?ck=nck**

National Center for Health Statistics: Heart disease. Retrieved January 2008 from **http://www.cdc.gov/nchs/data/nvsr/nvsr55/ nvsr55_19.pdf**

National Heart, Lung and Blood Institute: NHLBI Issues New High Blood Pressure Clinical Practice Guidelines, 2003. Article for U.S. Department of Health and Human Services National Institutes of Health (NIH) News website. Retrieved November 2004 from **http://wwwl.nih.gov/news/pr/may2003/nhlbi-14.htm**

National Heart, Lung and Blood Institute: NHLBI Factbook, 2007. Retrieved January 2008 from **http://www.nhlbi.nih.gov/about/ factbook/chapter4.htm**

National Heart, Lung and Blood Institute: Disease statistics. Retrieved January 2008, from **http://www.nhlbi.nih.gov/about/factbook/ chapter4.htm#4_2**

National Heart, Lung and Blood Institute: Morbidity and Mortality: 2007 Chart Book on Cardiovascular, Lung and Blood Diseases. Retrieved March 2008 from **http://www.nhlbi.nih.gov/resources/docs/ 07-chtbk.pdf**

No author listed: Advances for patients: Drug-eluting stents. Presentation of the 2004 Transcatheter Cardiovascular Therapeutics Symposium. Washington, DC. Retrieved November 2004 from **http://www.ptca .org/articles/tct2004_summary.html**

Parks, R: Tips for following the Dietary Approaches to Stop Hypertension (DASH) diet, 2007. Retrieved December 2007 from **http://www .cigna.com/healthinfo/zp3284.html#zp3285**

Schreiber, D: Deep vein thrombosis and thrombophlebitis, 2007. Retrieved May 2008 from **http://www.emedicine.com/emerg/topic122.htm**

Warner, J, and Nazario, B: New heart failure drug approved by FDA: Inspra reduces risk of death after heart attack, 2003. Retrieved November 2004 from **http://aolsvc.health.webmd**

Wedro, BC: Heart rhythm disorders, 2007. Retrieved May 2008 from **http://www.medicinenet.com**

Zarra, N, and Asani, S: Cardiac care: Managing postoperative bleeding, 2008. Retrieved April 2008 from **http://rn.modernmedicine.com/ rnweb/article/articleDetail.jsp?id=502761**

CHAPTER 5

Books

Blair, KA: The aging pulmonary system. In Stanley, M, Blair, KA, and Beare, PG (eds): Gerontological nursing: Promoting successful aging with older adults, ed 3. FA Davis, Philadelphia, 2005.

Clochesy, JM: Interventions for critically ill clients with respiratory problems. In Ignatavicius, DD, and Workman, ML (eds): Medical-surgical nursing: Critical thinking for collaborative care, ed 5. Elsevier Saunders, St. Louis, MO, 2006.

DeConti, RC: Carcinomas of the head and neck. In Skeel, RT (ed): Handbook of cancer chemotherapy, ed 6. Lippincott, Williams & Wilkins, Philadelphia, 2003.

Deglin, JH, and Vallerand, AH: Davis's drug guide for nurses, ed 10. FA Davis, Philadelphia, 2007.

Felver, L: Acid-base homeiostasis and imbalances. In Copstead, LEC, and Banasik, JL (eds): Pathophysiology, ed 3. Elsevier Saunders, St. Louis, MO, 2005.

Fink, JG, and Hess, DR: Secretion clearance techniques. In Hess, DR, et al (eds): Respiratory care: Principles and practices. Saunders, Philadelphia, 2002.

Ginsberg, RJ, Vokes, EE, and Rosenzweig, K: Non–small cell lung cancer. In DeVita, VT, Hellman, S, and Rosenberg, SA (eds): Cancer principles and practice of oncology, ed 6. Lippincott-Raven, Philadelphia, 2001.

Hoang, T, and Schiller, J: Carcinoma of the lung. In Skee, R (ed): Handbook of cancer chemotherapy, ed 6. Lippincott, Williams & Wilkins, Philadelphia, 2003.

Pagana, KD, and Pagana, TJ: Mosby's manual of diagnostic and laboratory tests, ed 3. Mosby, St. Louis, MO, 2006.

Schumann, L: Respiratory function and alterations in gas exchange. In Copstead, LEC, and Banasik, JL (eds): Pathophysiology, ed 3. Elsevier Saunders, St. Louis, MO, 2005

Springhouse, PA (ed): When acids and bases tip the balance. In Fluids & electrolytes made incredibly easy! Lippincott, Williams & Wilkins, Philadelphia, 1997.

Springhouse, PA (ed): Pathophysiology made incredibly easy!, ed 3. Lippincott, Williams & Wilkins, Philadelphia, 2006.

Articles

Anderson, KL: Change in quality of life after lung volume reduction surgery. Am J Crit Care 8(6):389–396, 1999.

Banning, M: Chronic obstructive pulmonary disease: Clinical signs and infections. Br J Nurs 15(16):874–880, 2006.

Barry, RM: Trauma nursing penetrating chest wounds. RN 67(5):36–41, 2004.

Baumann, M, and Noppen, M: Pneumothorax. Respirology 9:157–164, 2004.

Benninger, M, and Segreti, J: Is it bacterial or viral? Criteria for distinguishing bacterial and viral infections. Suppl J Fam Prac 3: S5–S11, 2008.

Boutotte, JM: Keeping TB in check. Nursing99 29(3):34, 1999.

Boyle, AH, and Locke, DC: Update on chronic obstructive pulmonary disease. Medsurg Nurs 13(1):42–48, 2004.

Braman, SS: Asthma and chronic obstructive pulmonary disease in later life. Generations Fall:33–38, 2006.

Burman, ME, and Wright, WL: Diagnosis and management of community-acquired pneumonia: Evidence-based practice. J Nurse Pract 10: 633–649, 2007.

Burns, SM: Pharmacological and ventilatory management of acute asthma exacerbations. Crit Care Nurse 19(4):39–54, 1999.

Byers, JF, and Sole, ML: Analysis of factors related to the development of ventilator-associated pneumonia: Use of existing databases. Am J Crit Care 9(5):344–349, 2000.

Carroll, P: Evolutions/revolutions: Respiratory monitoring. RN 62(5):69, 1999.

Centers for Disease Control and Prevention: Guidelines for the investigation of contacts of persons with infectious tuberculosis and Guidelines for using the QuantiFERON®-TB Gold test for detecting *Mycobacterium tuberculosis* infection, United States. MMWR 54:RR-15, 2005.

Chrisp, DR: Action stat: Tension pneumothorax. Nursing2000 30(5):33, 2000.

Coleman, PR: Pneumonia in the long-term care setting: Etiology, management, and prevention. J Gerontol Nurs 4:14–23, 2004.

Coughlin, AM, and Parchinsky, C: Go with the flow of chest tube therapy. Nursing2006 36(3):36–41, 2006.

Covey, ML, and Larson, JL: Beats and breaths: Exercise and COPD. AJN 104(5):40–43, 2004.

Cross, S: Managing exacerbations of chronic obstructive pulmonary disease. Br J Nurs 14(11):607–609, 2005.

Dasta, JF, et al: Daily cost of an intensive care unit day: The contribution of mechanical ventilation. Crit Care Med 33(6):1266–1271, 2005.

DeVito Dabbs, A, et al: Pattern and predictors of early rejection after lung transplantation. Am J Crit Care 12:497–507, 2003.

Donnelly, LE, and Duncan, FR: Therapy for chronic obstructive pulmonary disease in the 21st century. Drugs 63(19):1973–98, 2003.

Endicott, L, et al: Operating a sustainable disease management program for chronic obstructive pulmonary disease. Lippincotts Case Manag 8(6):282, 2003.

Esteban, A, et al: Characteristics and outcomes in adult patients receiving mechanical ventilation. JAMA 287:345–355, 2002.

Fahlman MM, et al: Salivary s-IgA response to training in functionally limited elders. J Aging Phys Act 11:502–515, 2003.

Faul, JL, et al: Quality of life and lung volume reduction surgery. Am J Crit Care 8(6):359–360, 1999.

Fay, S, and Narayan, MC: Diagnosis: Tuberculosis. Home Healthc Nurse 24(4):236–46, 2006.

Forastiere, A, et al: Head and neck cancer. N Engl J Med 345: 1890–1900, 2001.

Frakes, MA, Evans, T: TB—Your vigilance is vital. RN 67(11): 30–35, 2004.

Girard, TD, and Bernard, GR: Mechanical ventilation in ARDS. Chest 131:921–29, 2007.

Gronkiewicz, C, and Brokgren-Okonek, M: Acute exacerbation of COPD. Nursing application of evidence-based guidelines. Crit Care Nurs Q 27(4):336–352, 2004.

Holcomb, S: Asthma update. Dimen Crit Care Nurs 23(3):101–107, 2004.

Horne, C, and Derrico, D: Mastering ABGs. AJN 99(8):26, 1999.

Jacavone, J, and Young, J: Use of pulmonary rehabilitation strategies to wean a difficult-to-wean patient: Case study. Crit Care Nurse 18(6):29–37, 1998.

Jemal, A, et al: Cancer statistics. CA Cancer J Clin 55:10–50, 2005

Kinloch, D: Instillation of normal saline during endotracheal suctioning: Effects on mixed venous oxygen saturation. Am J Crit Care 8(4):231–240, 1999.

Kowalski, SD, and Rayfield, CA: A post hoc descriptive study of patients receiving propofol. Am J Crit Care 8(1):507–513, 1999.

Kreamer, KM: Getting the lowdown on lung cancer. Nursing2003 33(11):36–42, 2003.

Legon, K: Teaching incentive spirometry. Nursing99 29(11):60, 1999.

Lewis, AM: Respiratory emergency. Nursing99 29(8):62, 1999.

Lutfiyya, MN, et al: Diagnosis and treatment of community-acquired pneumonia. Am Fam Physician 73:442–50, 2006.

Mason, DJ: Put this in your pipe and smoke it. AJN 99(11):7, 1999.

McEnroe-Ayers, DM, and Lappin, JS: Act fast when your patient has dyspnea. Nursing2004 34(7):36–41, 2004.

McGann, E: Medication compliance in adults with asthma. AJN 99(3): 45, 1999.

Murphy, KR, Cecil, B, and Sarver, NL: Asthma: Helping patients breathe easier. Nurse Pract 29(10):38–55, 2004.

Myrianthefs, PM, et al: Nosocomial pneumonia. Crit Care Nurs Q 27(3):241–257, 2004.

Niederman, MS: Cost effectiveness in treating VAP. Crit Care 5:243–244, 2001.

No author listed: Bronchial hygiene therapy: From traditional hands-on techniques to modern technological advances. AJN 102(1):37, 2002.

No author listed: Understanding pneumothorax. Nursing2002 32(11):74–76, 2002.

Olmos, RAV, et al: Thallium-201 SPECT in the diagnosis of head and neck cancer. J Nucl Med 38(6):873–879, 1997.

Orgill, R, Krempl, GA, and Medina, JE: Acute pain management following laryngectomy. Arch Otolaryngol Head Neck Surg 128:829–832, 2002.

Owens, CL: New directions in asthma management. AJN 99(3):26, 1999.

Pierce, LNB: Protocols for practice: Applying research at the bedside—traditional and nontraditional modes of mechanical ventilation. Crit Care Nurse 20(1):81–86, 2000.

Pieterman, RM, et al: Preoperative staging of non–small-cell lung cancer with positron-emission tomography. N Engl J Med 343: 254–261, 2000.

Polomano, RC, and Farrar, JT: Pain and neuropathy in cancer survivors: Surgery, radiation, and chemotherapy can cause pain; research could improve its detection and treatment. AJN 106(3, suppl): 39–47, 2006.

Powers, J, and Bennett, SJ: Measurement of dyspnea in patients treated with mechanical ventilation. Am J Crit Care 8(4):254–261, 1999.

Pruitt, B and Jacobs, M: Best-practice interventions: How can you prevent ventilator-assisted pneumonia? Nursing2006 36(2):36–41, 2006.

Roman, M, Weinstein, A, and Macaluso, S: Primary spontaneous pneumothorax. Medsurg Nurs 12(3):161–169, 2000.

Rose-Ped, AM, et al: Complications of radiation therapy for head and neck cancers: The patient's perspective. Cancer Nurs 25(6): 461–467, 2002.

Ruppert, RA: The last smoke. AJN 99(11):26, 1999.

Schleder, B: Taking charge of hospital-acquired pneumonia. Nurse Pract 29(3):50–53, 2004.

Schmelz, JO, et al: Effects of position of chest drainage tube on volume drained and pressure. Am J Crit Care 8(5):319–323, 1999.

Schouchoff, B, and Rodriguez, A: Blunt chest trauma. Top Emerg Med 23(1):1–11, 2001.

Schultz, TR: Community-acquired pneumonia: Hunting the elusive respiratory infection. Nursing Made Incredibly Easy! 1(1):29–34, 2003a.

Schultz, TR: On the trail of community-acquired pneumonia. Nurs Manage 34(2):27–31, 2003b.

Seneff, MG, et al: The impact of long-term acute-care facilities on the outcome and cost of care for patients undergoing prolonged mechanical ventilation. Crit Care Med 28(2):342–350, 2000.

Shortall, SP, and Perkins, LA: Interpreting the ins and outs of pulmonary function tests. Nursing99 29(12):41, 1999.

Silverman, PM, et al: Carcinoma of the larynx and hypopharynx: Computed tomographic-histopathologic correlations. Radiology 151:697–702, 1984.

St. John, RE: Protocols for practice: Applying research at the bedside—airway management. Crit Care Nurse 19(4):79–83, 1999.

Sud, S, et al: Effect of mechanical ventilation in the prone position on clinical outcomes in patients with acute hypoxemic respiratory failure: a systematic review and meta-analysis. Can Med Assoc J 178(9):1153–1161, 2008.

Tomioka, H: Development of new antituberculous agents based on new drug targets and structure—activity relationships. Expert Opinion on Drugs 3(1):21–49, 2008.

Trudeau, ME, and Solano-McGuire, SM: Evaluating the quality of COPD care. AJN 99(3):47, 1999.

Wong, F: A new approach to ABG interpretation. AJN 99(8):34, 1999.

Woodruff, DW: How to ward off complications of mechanical ventilation. Nursing99 29(11):34, 1999.

Yantis, MA, and Nieman, W: Resting easy with PAP therapy. Nursing2000 30(4):62, 2000.

Electronic Resources

Allen, J: Mechanical ventilation, 2001. Retrieved May 2008 from **http://home.columbus.rr.com/allen/mechanical ventilation.htm**

American Association for Cancer Research: Lung cancer fact sheet, no date. Retrieved May 2008 from **http://www.aacr.org/home/public--media/for-the-media/fact-sheets/organ-site-fact-sheets/lung-cancer.aspx**

American Association for Cancer Research: Organ-site fact sheets, 2008. Retrieved August 2008 from **http://www.aacr.org/home/public--media/for-the-media/fact-sheets/organ-site-fact-sheets.aspx**

American Association for Respiratory Care (AARC): Exercise testing for evaluation of hypoxemia and/or desaturation, 2001 revision and update. Retrieved February 2004 from **http://www.guideline.gov**

American Cancer Society (ACS): Detailed guide: Laryngeal and hypopharyngeal cancer, 2007. Retrieved May 2008 from **http://documents.cancer.org/148.00/148.00.pdf**

American Cancer Society (ACS): What causes non-small cell lung cancer?, updated 2008. Retrieved May 2008 from **http://www.cancer.org/docroot/CRI/content/CRI_2_2_2x_What_Causes_Non-small_Cell_Lung_Cancer.asp?sitearea=**

American Head and Neck Society: Management of cancer of the head and neck imaging: General guidelines, n.d. Retrieved February 2008 from **http://www.ahns.info/clinicalresources/guidelines.php**

American Lung Association: Spontaneous pneumothorax fact sheet, 2005. Retrieved May 2008 from **http://www.lungusa.org/site**

American Lung Association: Search LungUSA. Chronic bronchitis and emphysema, 2006. Retrieved March 2008 from **http://www.lungusa.org**

American Lung Association: Asthma and children fact sheet, 2007a. Retrieved March 2008 from **http://www.lungusa.org**

American Lung Association: Asthma in adults fact sheet, 2007b. Retrieved March 2008 from **http://www.lungusa.org**

American Lung Association: Search LungUSA, Pneumonia, 2007c. Retrieved May 2008 from **http://www.lungusa.org**

Atrium Medical Corporation: Managing chest drainage, 2007a. Retrieved May 2008 from **http://www.atriummed.com/PDF/bluehandbook.pdf**

Atrium Medical Corporation: Managing dry suction chest drainage, 2007b. Retrieved May 2008 from **http://www.atriummed.com/PDF/greenhandbook.pdf**

Byrd, RP, et al: Ventilation, mechanical, 2006. Retrieved May 2008 from **http://www.emedicine.com/med/TOPIC3370.HTM**

Campbell, WJ, and de la Torre, JI: Head and neck cancer: Squamous cell carcinoma, updated 2008. Retrieved February 2008 from **http://www.emedicine.com/plastic/topic376.htm**

Carroll, P: Chest drainage. Continuing Education Program. Atrium Medical Corporation, 2004. Retrieved April 2008 from **http://www.antriummed.com**

Chang, AK, and Mukherji, P: Pneumothorax, iatrogenic, spontaneous and pneumomediastinum, 2007. Retrieved May 2008 from **http://www.emedicine.com/emerg/TOPIC469.HTM**

Centers for Disease Control and Prevention: Reported tuberculosis in the United States, 2007. Retrieved September 2008 from **http://www.cdc.gov/tb/surv/2007/default.htm**

Cunha, BA: Nosocomial pneumonia, 2006. Retrieved May 2008 from **http://www.emedicine.com/med/TOPIC3229.HTM**

Dewar, M, and Curry, RW: Chronic obstructive pulmonary disease: Diagnostic considerations, 2006. Am Fam Physician 73(4):669–676. Retrieved March 2008 from **http://www.aafp.org/afp**.

Elias, A and Baldini, EH: Patient information: Treatment of small cell lung cancer, 2008. Retrieved May 2008 from **http://www.uptodate.com/patients/content/topic.do?topicKey=~nn88VFHbEjbw**

Global Initiative for Chronic Obstructive Lung Disease (GOLD): Global strategy for the diagnosis, management, and prevention of COPD, 2007. Retrieved March 2008 from **http://www.goldcopd.org**

Grogano, AW: Acid-base tutorial, 2008. Retrieved April 2008 from **http://www.acid-base.com/index.php**

Herchline, T, and Amorosa, JK: Tuberculosis, 2007. Retrieved April 2008 from **http://www.emedicine.com/med/TOPIC2324.HTM**

Lee, JM, et al: Health-related quality of life burden of head and neck cancer. Retrieved May 2008 from **http://www.abtassociates.com/posters/ISPOR2003-quality.pdf**

Lombard, LE: Laryngectomy rehabilitation, 2003. Retrieved December 2004 from **http://www.emedicine.com**

Memorial Sloan-Kettering Cancer Center: Lung cancer: Overview, 2008. Retrieved May 2008 from **http://www.mskcc.org/mskcc/print/12163.cfm**

Mouth Cancer Foundation: Home page—Statistics, 2008. Retrieved May 2008 from **http://www.rdoc.org.uk/**

National Cancer Institute (NCI): A snapshot of head and neck cancers, updated 2007a. Retrieved May 2008 from **http://planning.cancer.gov/disease/Head_and_Neck-Snapshot.pdf**

National Cancer Institute: SEER fact sheet—Cancer: Larynex, 2007b. Retrieved Mary 2008 from **http://seer.cancer.gov/statfacts/html/laryn.html**

National Cancer Institute: What you need to know about lung cancer, 2008. Retrieved May 2008 from **http://www.cancer.gov/cancertopics/wyntk/lung/allpages**

National Center for Health Statistics (NCHS): Pneumonia, 2007. Retrieved May 2008 from **http://www.cdc.gov/nchs.FASTATS/pneumonia.htm**

National Heart, Lung and Blood Institute (NHLBI): COPD Learn more breathe better, 2008a. Retrieved March 2008 from **http://www.nhlbi.nih.gov/health/public/lung/copd/index.htm**

National Heart Lung and Blood Institute (NHLBI): What are pleurisy and other disorders of the pleura?, 2008b. Retrieved May 2008 from **http://www.nih.gov/health/dci/Diseases/pleurisy/pleurisy_all.html**

National Heart Lung and Blood Institute: What is pneumonia?, 2008c, March. Retrieved May 2008 from **http://www.nhlbi.nih.gov/health/dci/Diseases/pnu/pnu_all.html**

National Institute for Clinical Excellence: Chronic obstructive pulmonary disease. Management of COPD in adults in primary and secondary care. Clinical Guideline 12. Developed by the National Collaborating Centre for Chronic Conditions, 2004. Retrieved March 2008 from **http://www.nice.org/uk/CG012quickrefguide**

NIH Senior Health: Lung cancer treatments and research—Standard treatments, reviewed November 13, 2008. Retrieved May 2008 from **http://nihseniorhealth.gov/lungcancer/standardtreatments/06.html**

No author listed: Collapsed lung (Pneumothorax), 2008. Retrieved May 2008 from **http://www.webmd.com/a-to-zguides/collapsed-lung-pneumothorax-topic-overview**

No author listed: Facts about coronary angioplasty (PTCA), n.d. Article for North Suburban Cardiology Group, Ltd. Retrieved November 2004 from **http://www.nscardiology.com**

No author listed: Lung cancer: Various fact sheets from oncologychannel website, n.d. Retrieved April 2008 from **http://www.oncologychannel.com/lungcancer/index.shtml**

No author listed: Mechanical ventilation, n.d. Retrieved May 2008 from http://en.wikipedia.org/wiki/Mechanical_ventilation

No author listed: Pneumonia, 2007. Retrieved May 2008 from **http://www.webmd.com/a-to-zguides/pneumonia-topic-overview?page=2**

Oral Cancer Foundation: Oral cancer facts, 2008. Retrieved February 2008 from **http://www.oralcancerfoundation.org/facts/index.htm**

Payne, K, and Rhoads, C: Cardiac calcium scoring, 2003. Retrieved November 2004 from **http://my.webmd.com**

Petrossian, GA: Angiojet, 2000. Retrieved November 2004 from **http://www. heartcenteronline.com**

Sharma, S: Pneumonia, bacterial, 2007. Retrieved May 2008 from **http://www.emedicine.com/med/topic1852.htm**

U.S. Cancer Statistics Working Group: United States Cancer Statistics: 2004 Incidence and Mortality. Department of Health and Human Services, Centers for Disease Control and Prevention, and National Cancer Institute, 2007. Retrieved April 2008 from **http://www.cdc.gov/cancer/lung/statistics/**

World Health Organization: Report: Global tuberculosis control—Surveillance, planning, financing, 2008. Retrieved April 2008 from **http://www.who.int/tb/publications/global_report/2008/summary/en/index.html**

CHAPTER 6

Books

Abrams, AC, Pennington, SS, and Lammon, CB: Clinical drug therapy: Rationales for nursing practice, ed 8. Lippincott, Williams and Wilkins, Philadelphia, 2007.

Deglin, JH, and Vallerand, AH: Davis's drug guide for nurses, ed 10. FA Davis, Philadelphia, 2007.

Finkelstein EA, Corso, PS, and Miller, TR: The incidence and economic burden of injuries in the United States. Oxford University Press, New York, 2006.

Granacher, RP Jr: Traumatic brain injury: Methods for clinical and forensic neuropsychiatric assessment. CRC Press, Boca Raton, FL, 2003.

Halper, J, et al: Multiple sclerosis: Best practices in nursing care. Medicallance, Columbia, MD, 2000.

Hausman, KA: Interventions for clients with problems of the central nervous system. In Ignatavicius, DD, and Workman, ML (eds): Medical-surgical nursing: Critical thinking for collaborative care, ed 5. Elsevier Saunders, St. Louis, MO, 2006.

Nettina, SM: Lippincott manual of nursing practice, ed 8. Lippincott, Williams and Wilkins, Philadelphia, 2006.

Smeltzer, SS, et al: Brunner and Suddarth's textbook of medical-surgical nursing, ed 11. Lippincott, Williams and Wilkins, Philadelphia, 2008.

Springhouse, PA: Handbook of diseases, ed 3. Lippincott, Williams & Wilkins, Philadelphia, 2003.

Van Leeuwen, AM, Kranpitz, TR, and Smith, L: Davis's comprehensive handbook of laboratory tests with nursing implications, ed 2. FA Davis, Philadelphia, 2006.

Articles

Abour, R: Aggressive management of intracranial dynamics. Crit Care Nurse 18(3):30–40, 1998.

Aref, AA, and Schmitt, BP: Open-angle glaucoma: Tips for earlier detection and treatment selection. J Fam Pract 54(2):117–125, 2005.

Black, T, Soltis, T, and Bartlett, C: Using the functional independence measure instrument to predict stroke rehabilitation outcomes. Rehab Nurs 24(3):109–114/121, 1999.

Bonner, SM: My aching back: Relieving the pain of herniated disk. Nursing Made Incredibly Easy! 6(1):19–30, 2008.

Brook, IM, et al: Expenditures and health status among adults with back and neck problems. JAMA 299(6):656–64, 2008.

Chotikul, L: Spinal implants. RN 63(5):28–31, 2000.

Crimlisk, JT, and Grande, MM: Neurologic assessment for the acute medical surgical nurse. Orthop Nurs 23(1):3–9, 2004.

Cross, C: Seizures: Regaining control. RN 67(12): 44–51, 2004.

Dryden, T, Baskwill, A, and Preyde, M: Massage therapy for the orthopaedic patient: A review. Orthop Nurs 23(5):327–332, 2004.

Eck, M: Through the labyrinth: The twists and turns of brain injury. AJN 100(9):25, 2000.

Edwards, RR, et al: Ethnic differences in pain tolerance: Clinical implications in a chronic pain population. Psychosom Med 63: 316–323, 2001.

Fagley, MU: Taking charge of seizure activity. Nursing2007 37(9): 42–47, 2007.

Fonte, N, and Moore, KN: Urological care of the spinal cord-injured patient. J Wound Ostomy and Continence Nurs 35(3):323–331, 2008.

Franges, EZ: A sudden storm: Caring for seizure patients. LPN2008 2(2):28–36, 2006.

Galvin, T.J: Dysphagia: Going down and staying down. AJN 101(1):37–42, 2001.

Gambrell, M, and Flynn, N: Seizures 101. Nursing2004, 34(8): 36–41, 2004.

Gordon, MO, et al: The ocular hypertension treatment study: Baseline factors that predict the onset of primary open-angle glaucoma. Arch Ophthalmol 120(6):714–720, 2002.

Gray, M: Urinary retention: Management in the acute care setting. AJN 100(8):36–43, 2000.

Harvey, J: Countering "brain attacks." Nurs Manage 35(8):27–32, 2004.

Hazard, RG: Movement brings relief: Using lumbar CPM as a postrehab strategy for patients with recurring low back pain. Rehab Manage 13(7):40–42, 2000.

Hilton, L: We've got your back: Recovery from spinal cord injuries starts with the first hours of critical care. NurseWeek Mountain West, January 10, 2005, p 12, 2005.

Kavchak-Keyes, MA: Autonomic hyperreflexia. Rehab Nurs 25(1): 31–35, 2000.

Keating, DJ, et al: Postacute brain injury rehab: Where do we go from here? Rehab Manage 13(7):36–38, 2000.

Kennedy, MS: News: Growing older, seeing less: Blindness and visual impairment are on the rise in older Americans. AJN 104 (7):21, 2004.

Kowing, D, and Kester, E: Keep an eye out for glaucoma. Nurse Pract 32(7):18–23, 2007.

Lathbury, K: The road ahead—Managing a spinal cord injury. Case Manager 11(3):55–57, 2000.

Lee, S, et al: Anterior minimally invasive approaches for the cervical spine. Orthop Clin North Am, 38(3):327–337, 2007.

Lemke, DM: Sympathetic storming after severe traumatic brain injury. Crit Care Nurse 27(1):30-37, 2007.

Lewis, AM: Neurologic emergency! Nursing99 29(10):54, 1999.

Lublin, FD, and Reingold, SC: Defining the clinical course of multiple sclerosis: Results of an international survey. National Multiple Sclerosis Society (USA) Advisory Committee on Clinical Trials of New Agents in Multiple Sclerosis. Neurology 46(4):907–911, 1996.

Manchikanti, L, et al: Evidence-based practice guidelines for interventional techniques in the management of chronic spinal pain. Pain Physician 6:3–81, 2003.

Martin, L: Computer-assisted management of primary open-angle glaucoma. Comp Inform Nurs 14(5):267, 1996.

Modlin, SJ: Service dogs as interventions: State of the science. Rehab Nurs 25(6):212–219, 2000.

Morrison, K: Improving the care of stroke patients. Using an evidence-based quality improvement initiative enhances outcomes for stroke patients. Am Nurse Today 38–43, 2007.

Nickolaus, MJ: Diabetes insipidus: A current perspective. Crit Care Nurse 19(6):18–30, 1999.

O'Leary, JM, and Sarkarati, M: Aging with SCI. Rehab Manage 13(5):66–70, 2000.

Offenbacher, H, et al: Assessment of MRI criteria for a diagnosis of MS. Neurology 43:905–909, 1993.

Phillips, RA: Treating carotid artery stenosis to prevent stroke. Nursing Made Incredibly Easy! 5(1):40–48, 2007.

Pohl, PS, and Richards, LG: Decreasing stroke deficits. Rehab Manage 13(3):32–35, 2000.

Posser, CM, et al: New diagnostic criteria for multiple sclerosis: Guidelines for research protocols. Ann Neurol 13:227–231, 1983.

Reddy, L, and Santoni, C: Heads up on cerebral bleeds. Nursing2006 36(5, ED Insider):4-9, 2006.

Reeves, K, and Barash, S: Managing intrathecal baclofen pump implantation. Rehab Rep 10(10):28–29, 1999.

Rigby, D: Underactive bladder syndrome. Nurs Stand 19:57–64, 2005.

Rothke, SE, and Michael, E: Integrating the head injury team. Rehab Manage 13(2):38–40, 96, 2000.

Santoni-Reddy, LC: Heads up on cerebral bleeds. Nursing Made Incredibly Easy! 2(3):8–16, 2004.

Sauerbeck, LR: Primary stroke prevention. AJN 106(11):40–49, 2006.

Schappert, SM: Office visits for glaucoma: United States, 1991–92. Vital and Health Statistics of the Centers for Disease Control and Prevention (CDC) Division of Health Care Statistics, 1995.

Secrest, JA: Transformation of the relationship: The experience of primary support persons of stroke survivors. Rehab Nurs 25(3):93–99, 2000.

Secrest, JA, and Thomas, SP: Continuity and discontinuity: The quality of life following stroke. Rehab Nurs 24(6):240–246, 1999.

Stockert, PA: Getting UTI patients back on track. RN 62(3):49–52, 1999.

Stuifbergen AK, and Harrison, TC: Complementary and alternative therapy use in persons with multiple sclerosis. Rehab Nurs 28:141–147, 158, 2003.

Sullivan, MP, and Sharts-Hopko, NC: Preventing the downward spiral: Osteoporosis and MS. AJN 100(8):26–32, 2000.

Teasell, RW, et al: Cardiovascular consequences of loss of supraspinal control of the sympathetic nervous system after spinal cord injury. Arch Phys Med Rehab 4:81, 2000.

Thurman D, et al: Traumatic brain injury in the United States: A public health perspective. J of Head Trauma and Rehab, 14(6):602–615, 1999.

Travers, PL: Autonomic dysreflexia: A clinical rehabilitation problem. Rehab Nurs 24(1):19–23, 1999.

Turner, JA, et al: Chronic pain associated with spinal cord injuries: A community survey. Arch Phys Med Rehabil (82):501–508, 2001.

Weeks, SK, Hubbartt, E, and Michaels, TK: Keys to bowel success. Rehab Nurs 25(2):66–69, 2000.

Weir, NU: An update on cardioembolic stroke. Postgraduate Med J 84: 133–142, 2008.

Winkelman, C: Effect of backrest position on intracranial and cerebral perfusion pressure in traumatically brain-injured adults. Am J Crit Care 9(6):373–380, 2000.

Wong, FW: Prevention of secondary brain injury. Crit Care Nurse 20(5):18–27, 2000.

Zink, EK, and McQuillan, K: Managing traumatic brain injury. Nursing2005 35(9):36–43, 2005.

Electronic Resources

American Academy of Orthopaedic Surgeons (AAOS): Clinical guideline on low back pain/sciatica (acute) (phases I and II), 2002. Retrieved January 2005 from **http://www.guide line.gov**

American Heart Association and American Stroke Association: Heart disease and stroke statistics. Update at-a-glance, 2008. Retrieved May 2008 from **http://www.americanheart.org/presenter.jhtml ?identifier=3037327**

American Optometric Association (AOA) Consensus Panel: Care of the patient with primary angle closure glaucoma: Reference guide for clinicians, 1994. Retrieved February 2008 from **http://www.aoa.org/ documents/CPG-5.pdf**

Barrett, AM, and John, ST: Spatial neglect, 2007. Retrieved May 2008 from **www.emedicine.com/neuro/topic719.htm**

Bilkovski, RN: Transient ischemic attack (mini-stroke), 2003. Retrieved January 2005 from **http://www.emedicinehealth.com**

Bitan, FD: Motion preservation: An overview, 2008. Retrieved April 2008 from **http://www.bitanmd.com/procedures/disc.php**

Brandt, JD, Gordon, MO, and Kass, MA: Central corneal thickness in the ocular hypertension treatment study (OHTS), n.d. Retrieved February 2008 from **https://vrcc.wustl.edu/OHTS%20Central %20Corneal%20Thickness%2010-01.pdf**

Brown University: Glaucoma, n.d. Retrieved May 2008 from **http:// biomed.brown.edu/Courses/BI108/2006-108websites/ group02glaucoma/glaucoma.html**

Campagnolo, DI: Autonomic dysreflexia in spinal cord injury, 2006. Retrieved June 2008 from **http://www.emedicine.com/pmr/ TOPIC217.HTM**

Cavazos, JE, and Lum, F: Seizures and epilepsy: Overview and classification, 2007. Retrieved March 2008 from **http://www.emedicine.com/ neuro/TOPIC415.HTM**

Centers for Disease Control and Prevention: Facts about traumatic brain injury, 2006. Retrieved March 2008 from **http://www.cdc.gov/ncipc/ tbi/FactSheets/Facts_About_TBI.pdf**

Charite, SB: Get artificial disc replacement (ADR) surgery at Stenum Hospital. Public information materials from Get ADR.com website, updated 2006. Retrieved January 2005 from **http://www.getadr.com**

Centre for Neuro Skills: TBI resource guide: Glasgow coma scale, 2006. Retrieved May 2008 from **http://www.neuroskills.com/ glasgow.shtml**

Defense and Veterans Brain Injury Center: Blast injury FAQs, 2005. Retrieved May 2008 from **http://www.dvbic.org/cms.php?p =Blast_injury**

Devinsky, O (ed): Complex partial seizures, 2004. Retrieved May 2008 from **http://www.epilepsy.com/epilepsy/seizure_complexpartial**

Eidelson, SG: Minimally invasive and open surgical procedures. Excerpt from: Save your aching back and neck: Patient information, ed 2, 2002. Retrieved May 2008 from **http://www.spineuniverse.com/ displayarticle.php/article2002.html**

Epilepsy Foundation: 1995–2005: Statistics, n.d. Retrieved March 2008 from **http://www.epilepsyfoundation.org/about/statistics.cfm**

Food and Drug Administration, Center for Devices and Radiological Health: New humanitarian device approval: OP-1 Putty - H020008, updated 2004. Retrieved May 2008 from **http://www.fda.gov/cdrh/ MDA/DOCS/h020008.html**

Gale Encyclopedia of Surgery: Laminectomy, 2007. Retrieved May 2008 from **http://www.surgeryencyclopedia.com/Fi-La/ Laminectomy.html**

Geisser, B: Communicating the diagnosis of multiple sclerosis, 2005. National Multiple Sclerosis Society. Retrieved June 2008 from **http://www.nationalmssociety.org/for-professionals/ healthcare-professionals/publications/index.aspx**

Glaucoma Foundation: About glaucoma, 2009. Retrieved March 2009 from **http://www.glaucoma-foundation.org/education_content .php?i=7**

Glaucoma Research Foundation: Treating glaucoma, n.d. Retrieved February 2008 from **http://www.glaucoma.org/treating/index.php**

Huff, JS, Huff, M, and Plantz, SH: Epilepsy, 2003. Retrieved December 2004 from **http://www.emedicine.com**

Langlois JA, Rutland-Brown W, and Thomas KE: Traumatic brain injury in the United States: Emergency department visits, hospitalizations, and deaths. Centers for Disease Control and Prevention, National Center for Injury Prevention and Control, 2006. Retrieved May 2008 from **http://www.ninds.nih.gov/disorders/tbi/detail_tbi.htm**

Lazoff, M: Multiple sclerosis, 2008. Retrieved June 2008 from **http://www.emedicine.com/emerg/topic321.htm**

Lehmkuhl, LD (ed): Brain injury glossary. HDI Publishers, 1992. Retrieved May 2008 from **http://www.neuroskills.com/glossary.shtml**

Lynch, DM: Cranberry for prevention of urinary tract infections. Am Fam Physician, 70:2175–2177, 2004. Retrieved May 2008 from **http://www.aafp.org/afp/20041201/2175.html**

Medline Plus: Herniated nucleus pulposus (slipped disk). Medical Encyclopedia, 2006. Retrieved March 2008 from **http://www.nlm.nih.gov/medlineplus/ency/article/000442.htm**

de Menezes, MS: Status epilepticus, 2004. Retrieved December 2004 from **http://www.emedicine.com**

Nassisi, D: Stroke, hemorrhagic, 2008. Retrieved May 2008 from **http://www.emedicine.com/emerg/topic557.htm**

National Ambulatory Medical Care Survey (NAMCS): Office visits for glaucoma: United States, 1991–1992. Advance report #262, updated 2007. Retrieved February 2008 from **http://www.cdc.gov/nchs/data/ahcd/publist12-03-07.pdf**

National Center for Health Statistics: Health, United States, 2006 (with chartbook on trends in the health of Americans). Hyattsville, MD, 2006. Retrieved May 2008 from **http://www.cdc.gov/nchs/data/hus/hus06.pdf**

National Heart, Lung and Blood Institute: Morbidity and mortality: 2007 Chartbook on cardiovascular, lung, and blood Diseases, 2007. Retrieved May 2008 from **http://www.nhlbi.nih.gov/resources/docs/cht-book.htm**

National Institute for Neurological Disorders and Stroke (NINDS): Multiple sclerosis: Hope through research, 1996, updated 2008. Retrieved June 2008 from **http://www.ninds.nih.gov/disorders/multiple_sclerosis/detail_multiple_sclerosis.htm**

National Institutes of Health: Stroke scale, 2003. Retrieved March 2009 from **http://www.ninds.nih.gov/doctors/NIH_Stroke_Scale.pdf**

National Institutes of Neurological Disorders and Stroke: Traumatic brain injury: Hope through research, 2002. Retrieved May 2008 from **http://www.ninds.nih.gov/disorders/tbi/detail_tbi.htm**

National Institutes of Neurological Disorders and Stroke: Spinal cord injury: Hope through research, 2003. Retrieved June 2008 from **http://www.ninds.nih.gov/disorders/sci/detail_sci.htm**

National Institutes of Neurological Disorders and Stroke: Seizures and epilepsy: Hope through research, updated 2008. Retrieved March 2009 from **http://www.ninds.nih.gov/disorders/epilepsy/detail_epilepsy.htm#79193109**

The National Society for Epilepsy: Information on epilepsy: Anti-epileptic drugs used in adults, 2007. Retrieved March 2008 from **http://www.epilepsynse.org.uk/pages/info/leaflets/AED.cfm**

National Spinal Cord Injury Statistical Center (NSCISC): Facts and figures at a glance, updated 2008. Retrieved May 2008 from **http://www.spinalcord.uab.edu/show.asp?durki=116979&site=1021&return=19775**

North American Spine Society: Herniated disc. In North American Spine Society phase III clinical guidelines for multidisciplinary spine care specialists, n.d. Retrieved January 2005 from **http://guideline.gov**

Pascotto, A, and Soreca, E: Glaucoma, complications and management of glaucoma filtering, 2004. Retrieved January 2005 from **http://www.emedicine.com**

Sahrakar, K, and Melicharek, M: Lumbar disc disease, 2006. Retrieved April 2008 from **http://www.emedicine.com/med/TOPIC2902.HTM**

Santillo, VM, and Lowe, FC: Cranberry juice for the prevention and treatment of urinary tract infections. Drugs Today 43(1):47, 2008. Retrieved May 2008 from **http://journals.prous.com/journals/servlet/xmlxsl/pk_journals.xml_summary_pr?p_JournalId=4&p_RefId=1032055&p_IsPs=N**

Schachter, SC (ed): Simple partial seizures, 2006. Retrieved May 2008 from **http://www.epilepsy.com/epilepsy/seizure_simplepartial**

Schiffer, S: Procedures: Spine and neck surgical procedures. Retrieved March 2008 from **http://www.drschiffer.com/**

Schwanke, J: Gene putty helps body grow new bone, 2001. Retrieved January 2005 from **http://webmdpractice.health**

Scott, DD, and Williamson, SF: Multiple sclerosis, 2004. Retrieved January 2005 from **http://www.emedicine.com**

Silver, B: Medical treatment of stroke, 2004. Retrieved January 2005 from **http://www.emedicine.com**

Stowkoski, LA: Stroke and stroke nursing: Safeguarding the brain. Article for Medscape Nurses, 2007. Retrieved May 2008 from **http://www.medscape.com/viewarticle/558615**

Texas Tech University Managed Health Care Network Pharmacy and Therapeutics Committee: Acute seizures and seizure disorder: Guideline from bibliographic source, n.d. Retrieved December 2004 from **http://www.guideline.gov**

University of Utah: Multiple sclerosis. Physical Medicine and Rehabilitation website, 2001. Retrieved June 2008 from **http://healthcare.utah.edu/healthinfo/adult/rehab/multscle.htm**

CHAPTER 7

Books

Boehmke, MM: Interventions for clients with inflammatory intestinal disorders. In Ignatavicius, DD, and Workman, ML (eds): Medical-surgical nursing: Critical thinking for collaborative care. Elsevier Saunders, St. Louis, MO, 2006.

Gibbs, JR: Interventions for clients with stomach disorders. In Copstead, LEC, and Banasik, JL (eds): Pathophysiology, ed 3. Elsevier Saunders, St. Louis, MO, 2005.

Mettina, S: Manual of nursing practice, ed 8. Lippincott, Williams & Wilkins, Philadelphia, 2006.

National Women's Health Information Center. U.S. Department of Health and Human Services, Office on Women's Health: Inflammatory bowel disease, 2005.

Sartin, JS: Alterations in function of the gallbladder and exocrine pancreas. In Copstead, LEC, and Banasik, JL (eds): Pathophysiology, ed 3. Elsevier Saunders, St. Louis, MO, 2005a.

Sartin, JS: Gastrointestinal disorders. In Copstead, LEC, and Banasik, JL (eds): Pathophysiology, ed 3. Elsevier Saunders, St. Louis, MO, 2005b.

Swearingen, P: Manual of medical-surgical nursing care: Nursing interventions and collaborative management. Mosby, St. Louis, MO, 2003.

Articles

Cullen, DJE, et al: Peptic ulcer bleeding in the elderly: Relative roles of helicobacter pylori and non-steroidal anti-inflammatory drugs. Gut 41:459–462, 1997.

DeBartoli, N, et al: *Helicobacter pylori* eradication: A randomized prospective study of triple therapy versus triple therapy plus lactoferrin and probiotics. Am J Gastroenterol 102:951–956, 2007.

Dorn, SD, and Sandler, RS: Inflammatory bowel disease is not a risk factor for cardiovascular disease mortality: Results from a systematic review and meta-analysis. Am J Gastroenterol 102(3):662667, 2007.

Gignoux, BM, et al: Three-luminal nasojejunal tube in digestive surgery: Preliminary feasibility study. Ann Circ 127(8):629–630, 2002.

Hanauer, SB: Inflammatory bowel disease: Epidemiology, pathogenisis, and therapeutic opportunities. Inflamm Bowel Dis (12):Suppl 1:S3–S9, 2006.

Kane, SV: Systematic review: Adherence issues in the treatment of ulcerative colitis. Aliment Pharmacol Ther 23(5):577–585, 2006.

Krumberger, JM: How to manage an upper GI bleed. RN 68(5):29–33, 2005.

Loftus, EV: Mortality in inflammatory bowel disease: Peril and promise. Gastroenterology 125(6):1881–1883, 2003.

Loftus, EV: Clinical epidemiology of inflammatory bowel disease: Incidence, prevalence, and environmental influences. Gastroenterology 126:1504–1517, 2004.

Movius, M: What's causing the gut pain? RN 69(7):25–30, 2006.

Ringhofer, J: Meeting the needs of your ostomy patient. RN 68(8):37–41, 2005.

Smith, GD: The management of acute upper gastrointestinal bleeding. Nurs Times 100(26):40, 2004.

Turnbull, GB: The ostomy files: Ostomy statistics: The $64,000 question. Ostomy Wound Manage 49(6):22–23, 2003.

Electronic Resources

A.D.A.M. Encyclopedia: Crohn's disease, 2007. Retrieved June 2008 from **http://www.drugs.com/enc/crohn-s-disease.html**

Ansari, P: Appendicitis, 2007. Merck Manuals Online Medical Library. Retrieved March 2008 from **http://www.merck.com/mmpe/sec02/ch011/ch011e.html**

Azer, SA: Intestinal perforation, 2006. Retrieved June 2008 from **http://www.emedicine.com/med/TOPIC2822.HTM**

Brett, A: Capsule endoscopy in obsure GI bleeding, 2007. Journal Watch. Retrieved March 2008 from **http://www.medscape.com/viewarticle/552205**

Clark, J: Ileostomy guide, 2005. Retrieved June 2008 from **http://www.uoaa.org/ostomy_info/**

Clark, J, and Grover, P: Colostomy guide, 2004. Retrieved June 2008 from **http://www.uoaa.org/ostomy_info/**

Crohn's and Colitis Foundation of America: About Crohn's disease and ulcerative colitis. Retrieved June 2008 from **http://www.ccfa.org/about/press/ibdfacts**

DeCaestecker, J, and Straus, J: Upper gastrointestinal bleeding: Surgical perspective, updated 2006. Retrieved June 2008 from **http://www.emedicine.com/med/topic3566.htm**

Gladden, D, and Migala, AF: Cholecystitis, 2007. Retrieved June 2008 from **http://www.emedicine.com/MED/topic346.htm**

Helwick, CA: Essay for Gale encyclopedia of medicine, 2002. Retrieved June 2008 from **http://www.healthatoz.com/**

Heuman, DM, et al: Cholelithiasis, 2006. Retrieved June 2008 from **http://www.emedicine.com/med/TOPIC836.HTM**

Kean, WF, et al: Adult peritoneal dialysis-related peritonitis treatment recommendations: 2000 update, 2000. Retrieved June 2008 from **http://www.ispd.org/guidelines/articles/update/index.html**

Lab Tests Online. Retrieved March 2008 from **http://www.labtestsonline.org**

Layke, JC, and Lopez, PP: Gastric cancer: Diagnosis and treatment, 2004. Am Fam Phys 69(5):1133–1140. Retrieved June 2008 from **http://www.aafp.org/afp/20040301/1133.html**

Leung, Y, Devlin, S, and Meddings, J: Duodenal ulcers, 2007. Retrieved March 2008 from **http://www.emedicine.com/med/TOPIC591.HTM**

National Cancer Institute: Stomach (gastric) cancer screening, updated 2008. Retrieved June 2008 from **http://www.cancer.gov/cancertopics/pdq/screening/gastric/healthprofessional/allpages/print**

National Digestive Diseases Information Clearinghouse (NDDIC): Irritable bowel syndrome. NIH publication 07-693, September 2007. Retrieved June 2008 from **http://www.digestive.niddk.nih.gov/ddiseases/pubs/ibs/**

National Vital Statistics and Records (NVSR): Deaths: Preliminary data for 2003, 2005. Retrieved March 2008 from **http://www.cdc.gov/nchs/data/nvsr/nvsr53/nvsr53_15.pdf**

Peralta, R, Napalitano, LM, and Guzofski, S: Peritonitis and abdominal sepsis, 2006. Retrieved June 2008 from **http://www.emedicine.com/med/TOPIC2737.HTM**

Salles, N, and Megraud, R: Current management of *H. pylori* infections in the elderly, 2007. Expert Rev Anti Infect Ther 5(5):845–856. Retrieved March 2008 from **http://www.medscape.com/viewarticle/565635**

Santacroce, L, and Ochoa, JB: Appendicitis, 2006. Retrieved March 2008 from **http://www.emedicine.com/med/TOPIC3430.HTM**

Varma, MK, and Allen, AW: Gastrointestinal bleed, upper, 2005. Retrieved June 2008 from **http://www.emedicine.com/Radio/topic302.htm**

CHAPTER 8

Books

Bernal-Mizrachi, E, and Bernal-Mizrachi, C: Diabetes mellitus and related disorders. In Green, GB, et al (eds): The Washington manual of medical therapeutics, ed 31. Lippincott, Williams & Wilkins, St. Louis, 2004.

Clutter, WE: Endocrine diseases: Hyperthyroidism. In Green, GB et al (eds): The Washington manual of medical therapeutics, ed. 31. Lippincott, Williams & Wilkins, St. Louis, 2004.

Felver, L: Acid-base homeostasis and imbalances. In Copstead, LEC, and Banasik, JL (eds): Pathophysiology, ed 3. Elsevier Saunders, St. Louis, MO, 2005.

Ignatavicius, DD: Interventions with clients with problems of the binary system and pancreas. In Ignatavicius, DD, and Workman, ML (eds): Medical-surgical nursing: Critical thinking for collaborative care, ed 5. Elsevier Saunders, St. Louis, MO, 2006.

Joint Commission on Accreditation of Healthcare Organizations (JCAHO): Comprehensive accreditation manual for hospitals. The official handbook. JCAHO, Oakbrook Terrace, IL, 1997.

Klein, S: Nutrition support. In Green, GB, et al (eds): The Washington manual of medical therapeutics, ed 31. Lippincott, Williams & Wilkins, St. Louis, 2004.

LeFever Kee, J: Laboratory and diagnostic tests with nursing implications, ed 7. Prentice Hall, Upper Saddle River, NJ, 2005.

Lemone, P, and Burke, K: Medical surgical nursing: Critical thinking in client care, ed 4. Prentice Hall, Upper Saddle River, NJ, 2008.

Lewis, SL, et al: Medical surgical nursing: Assessment and management of clinical problems, ed 7. Mosby Elsevier, St. Louis, 2007.

Mehler, PS, and Anderson, AE: Eating disorders: A guide to medical care and complications. The John Hopkins University Press, Baltimore, 1999.

Murphy, MB: Interventions for clients with liver problems. In Ignatavicius, DD, and Workman, ML (eds): Medical-surgical nursing: Critical thinking for collaborative care, ed 5. Elsevier Saunders, St. Louis, 2006.

Springhouse (ed): Pathophysiology made incredibly easy!, ed 3. Lippincott, Williams & Wilkins, Philadelphia, 2005.

Springhouse (ed): Fluids & electrolytes made incredibly easy! Lippincott, Williams & Wilkins, Philadelphia, 2007.

Townsend, M: Psychiatric mental health nursing, concepts of care in evidence-based practice, ed 5. FA Davis, Philadelphia, 2006.

Venes, D, Biderman, A, and Taber, CW (eds): Taber's cyclopedic medical dictionary, ed 20. FA Davis, Philadelphia, 2005.

Articles

American Diabetes Association: American Diabetes Association's 2004 position statement: Diagnosis and classification of diabetes mellitus. Diabetes Care 27(Suppl 1):S5–S10, 2004a.

American Diabetes Association: Summary of revisions for the 2004 clinical practice recommendations. Diabetes Care 27(Suppl 1):S3, 2004b.

American Diabetes Association: Standards of medical care in diabetes—2007. Diabetes Care 30(Suppl 1):S4–S41, 2007.

Apfell, SC, et al: New option for diabetic neuropathy. AJN 99(2):20, 1999.

Astle, SM: Restoring electrolyte balance. RN 68(5):34–39, 2005.

Beauchamp-Johnson, BM: Scale down bariatric surgery's risks. Men in Nurs 1(3):20–26, 2006.

Birn, CS: CE 355: Endoscopic ultrasound reveals GI tract secrets. NurseWeek Mountain West 1(17), 2005.

Blackwood, HS: Obesity: A rapidly expanding challenge. Nurs Manage 35(5):27–35, 2004.

Bockhold, KM: Who's afraid of hepatitis C? AJN 100(5):26, 2000.

Booker, KJ, et al: Comparison of 2 methods of managing gastric residual volumes from feeding tubes. Am J Crit Care 9(5):318–324, 2000.

Bouldin, M, et al: The effect of obesity surgery and obesity comorbidity. Am J Med Sci 331(4):183–193, 2006.

Bowers, S: All about tubes: Your guide to enteral feeding devices. Nursing2000 30(12):41, 1999.

Brettler, SJ: Defenses gone awry: Primary biliary cirrhosis. RN 66(9):38–43, 2003.

Cammon, SA, and Hackshaw, HS: Are we starving our patients? AJN 100(5):43–46, 2000.

Cheever, KH: Early enteral feeding of patients with multiple trauma. Crit Care Nurse 19(6):40–51, 1999.

Cole, L: Unraveling the mystery of acute pancreatitis. Dimen Crit Care Nurs 21(3):86–89, 2002.

Corbell, CF, and Cook, D: Diabetes ABCs: Do you know them, get them, improve them? Home Healthc Nurse 22(7):452–459, 2004.

Davidson, JE, et al: Critical care of the morbidly obese. Crit Care Nurse Q 26(2):105–116, 2003.

Dudek, SG: Malnutrition in hospitals: Who's assessing what patients eat? AJN 100(4):36, 2000.

Durston, S: The ABCs—and more—of hepatitis. Nursing Made Incredibly Easy! 2(4):22–32, 2004.

Fagenholz, PJ, et al: Direct medical costs of acute pancreatitis hospitalizations in the United States. Pancreas, 35(4):302–307, 2007.

Farooqi, IS, and O'Rahilly, S: Genetic factors in human obesity. Obesity Reviews 2007 8(Suppl 1):37–40, 2007.

Fisher, JN: Management of thyrotoxicosis. South Med J 95(5): 493–505, 2002.

Fleming, DR: Challenging traditional insulin injection practices. AJN 99(2):72, 1999.

Funnell, MM, and Barlage, DL: Saying a mouthful about oral diabetes drugs. Nursing2000 30(11):34, 2000.

Funnell, MM, and Kruger, DF: Type 2 diabetes: Treat to target. Nurs Pract 29(1):11–13, 2004.

Gallagher, S: Taking the weight off with bariatric surgery. Nursing2004 34(3):58–64, 2004.

Gallagher, S: Tailoring care for obese patients. RN 62(5):43, 1999.

Gopalan, S, and Khanna, S: Enteral nutrition delivery technique. Curr Opin Clin Nutr Metab Care 6(3):313–317, 2003.

Halmi, KA, et al: Comorbidity of psychiatric diagnosis in anorexia. Arch Gen Psychiatry 48:712–718, 1991.

Halpin-Landry, JE, and Goldsmith, S: Feet first: Diabetes care. AJN 99(2):26, 1999.

Heathcote, EJ: Management of primary biliary cirrhosis. Hepatology 31(4):1005–1022, 2000.

Heidelbaugh, JJ, and Bruderly, M: Cirrhosis and chronic liver failure: Part I. Diagnosis and evaluation. Am Fam Physician 74:765–774, 2006.

Holleman, CB: Monitoring CSII therapy. AJN 100(3):86, 2000.

Hussar, DA: New drugs 2003, part III. Nursing2003 33(8):55–61, 2003.

Iscoe, KE, et al: Efficacy of continuous real-time blood glucose monitoring during and after prolonged high-intensity cycling exercise: Spinning with a continuous glucose monitoring system. Diabetes Technol Ther, 8(6):627–635, 2006.

Jorgensen, RA: Nonalcoholic fatty liver disease. Gastroenterol Nurs 26(4):150–154, 2003.

Klainberg, M: (1999). Primary biliary cirrhosis. AJN 99(12):38, 1999.

Kohn-Keeth, C: How to keep feeding tubes flowing freely. Nursing2000 30(3):58, 2000.

Konick-McMahan, J: Riding out a diabetic emergency. Nursing99 29(9):34, 1999.

Lambright, JA: Preventing hepatitis. Nursing99 29(8):66, 1999.

Leininger, SM: The role of nutrition in wound healing. Crit Care Nurse 25(1):13–21, 2002.

McConnel, EA: Clincal do's and don'ts: Administering an insulin injection. Nursing99 29(12):18, 1999.

McInnis, KJ: Diet, exercise, and the challenge of combating obesity in primary care. J Cardiovas Nurs 18(2):93–100, 2003.

Metheny, NA, Aud, MA, and Wunderlich, RJ: A survey of bedside methods used to detect pulmonary aspiration of enteral formula in intubated tube-fed patients. Am J Crit Care 8(3):160–167, 1999.

Murphy, K: The skinny on eating disorders. Nursing Made Incredibly Easy! 5(3):40–48, 2007.

No author listed: Comparing psychotherapies for bulimia. Harv Ment Health Lett 17(99):8, 2001.

Noble, KA: Name that tube. Nursing2003 33(3):56–62, 2003.

O'Brien, B, Davis, S, and Erwin-Toth, P: G-tube site care: A practical guide. RN 62(2):52, 1999.

O'Neil, KM: Thyrotoxic hypokalemic paralysis: A case study. Crit Care Nurse 19(6):31–34, 1999.

Olohan, K, and Zappitelli, D: The insulin pump. AJN 103(4):48–56, 2003.

Olson, RS: An update in diabetes management. Rehab Nurs 25(5): 177–184, 2000.

Orbanic, S: Understanding bulimia, signs, symptoms and the human experience. AJN 101(3):35, 2001.

Padula, CA, et al: Enteral feedings: What the evidence says. AJN 104(7):62–69, 2004.

Parini, S: Hepatitis C: Update your knowledge of this silent stalker. Nursing2003 22(4): 57–63, 2003.

Peeples, M, and Seley, JJ: Diabetes care: The need for change. AJN 107(6Suppl):13–19, 2007.

Perkins, H.K: Where is bariatric rehab on the safety scale? Rehab Rep 10(6):19–23, 1999.

Powers, J, et al: Beside placement of small-bowel feeding tubes in the intensive care unit. Crit Care Nurse 23(1):1624, 2003.

Racette, SB, Deusinger, SS, and Deusinger, RH: Obesity: Overview of prevalence, etiology and treatment. Phys Ther 83:276–288, 2003.

Rose, C: The role of nurses in caring for the eating disordered patient. HealthReach [newsletter], Denver Health Medical Center, 2001.

Salemeh, JR: Bariatric surgery: Past and present. Am J Med Sci 331(4):194–200, 2006.

Scemons, D: Are you up-to-date on diabetes medications? Nursing2007 37(7):45–49, 2007.

Schantz, S: Child and adolescent obesity, BMI and the school nurses role. NASN Newsletter 7:22–24, 2007.

Scherer, MJ: Breaking barriers—Important factors to consider when advising bariatric clients on home modification and assistive technology. Rehab Manage 12(6):74–77, 1999.

Shovein, JT, Damozo, RJ, and Hyams, I: Hepatitis A: How benign is it? AJN 100(3):43, 2000.

Simmons-Holcomb, S: An update on hepatitis. Dimen Crit Care Nurs 21(5):170–177, 2002.

Speranza, M, et al: Predictive value of alexithymia in patients with eating disorders: A 3-year prospective study, 2007. J Psychosom Res 63(4):365–371.

Trujillo, EB, Robinson, MK, and Jacobs, DO: Nutritional assessment in the critically ill. Crit Care Nurse 19(1):67–78, 1999.

Trus, TL, Pope, GD, and Finlayson, SR: National trends in utilization and outcomes of bariatric surgery. Surg Endosc 19(5):616–620, 2005.

Vink, T, et al: Association between an agouti-related protein gene polymorphism and anorexia nervosa. Mol Psychiatry 6(3):325–328, 2001.

Winfield, M: Bariatric rehab: What you should know about the new drug therapies. Rehab Rep 10(10):13–17, 1999.

Young, J: Action stat! Myxedema coma. Nursing99 29(1):64, 1999a.

Young, J: Action stat! Thyroid storm. Nursing99 29(8):33, 1999b.

Electronic Resources

American Association for Clinical Chemistry: T3, T4, TSH, n.d. Public resource on clinical lab testing. Retrieved January 2005 from **http://www.labtestsonline.org**

American Association of Clinical Endocrinologists (AACE): Medical guidelines for clinical practice for the evaluation and treatment of hyperthyroidism and hypothyroidism, amended 2006. Retrieved June 2008 from **http://www.aace.com/pub/pdf/guidelines/hypo _hyper.pdf**

American Diabetes Association (ADA): Direct and indirect costs of diabetes in the Untited States, n.d. Retrieved June 2008 from **http://www .diabetes.org/diabetes-statistics/cost-of-diabetes-in-us.jsp**

American Liver Foundation: Hepatitis B and C fact sheet and hepatitis and liver disease in the United States, n.d. Retrieved February 2005 from **http://www.liverfoundation.org**

Baker, R: Treatment of patients with HIV/HCV coinfection: An overview. Article for HIV and Hepatitis.com website, 2007. Retrieved June 2008 from **http://www.hivandhepatitis.com/hiv_hcv_co_inf/2007/101907 _a.html**

Balentine, JR: Pancreatitis, reviewed July 2007. Retrieved February 2005 from **http://www.emedicinehealth.com/pancreatitis/article_em.htm**

Bernstein, BE: Eating disorder: Anorexia, 2008. Retrieved June 2008 from **http://www.emedicine.com/ped/TOPIC115.HTM#ref5**

Brandis, K: Acid-base tutorial. Chapters 5 and 7, 2006. Retrieved June 2008 from **http://www.anaesthesiamcq.com/AcidBaseBook/ ABindex.php**

Buggs, AM, and Kim, JK: Hepatitis, 2006. Retrieved April 2008 from **http://www.emedicine.com/emerg/TOPIC244.HTM**

Centers for Disease Control and Prevention: Fact sheet: CDC efforts to reduce or prevent obesity, 2005a. Retrieved July 2008 from **http://www.cdc.gov/od/oc/media/pressrel/fs050419.htm**

Centers for Disease Control and Prevention: National hospital discharge survey: 2005 annual summary, 2005b. Retrieved June 2008 from **http://www.cdc.gov/nchs/data/series/sr_13/sr13_165.pdf**

Centers for Disease Control and Prevention: National diabetes fact sheet: General information and national estimates on diabetes in the United States, 2005c. Retrieved June 2008 from **http://www.cdc.gov/diabetes/pubs/factsheet05.htm**

Centers for Disease Control and Prevention: Obesity among adults in the United States—No statistically significant change since 2003–2004. Data Brief Number 1, 2007. National Center for Health Statisitcs. Retrieved June 2008 from **http://www.cdc.gov/nchs/pressroom/07newsreleases/obesity.htm**

Christenson, JL: Essentials of promoting healthy sexuality in the treatment of eating disorders, 2008. HealthReach. Retrieved June 2008 from **http://www.empoweringchange.com/pdf/health.pdf**

Da Liburd, J: Eating disorder: Anorexia, 2004. Retrieved January 2005 from **http://www.emdicine.com**

Encinosa, WE, et al: Use and cost of bariatric surgery and prescription weight-loss medications, 2005. Retrieved June 2008 from **http://www.medscape.com/viewarticle/508412**

Fallon, LF: Thyroidectomy. Encyclopedia of surgery: A guide for patients and caregivers, 2003. Retrieved June 2008 from **http://www.surgeryencyclopedia.com/St-Wr/Thyroidectomy.html**

Farkas, TA, and Waldrop, R: Anorexia nervosa, 2006. Retrieved June 2008 from **http://www.emedicine.com/EMERG/topic34.htm**

Foster, R, and Smith-Coggins, R: Bulimia, 2004. Retrieved January 2005 from **http://www. emedicine.com**

Gardner, TB, Berk BS, and Yakshe, P: Pancreatitis, acute, 2008. Retrieved June 2008 from **http://www.emedicine.com/med/topic1720.htm**

Gilroy, RK, and Mukherjee, S: Hepatitis A, 2006. Retrieved June 2008 from **http://www.emedicine.com/med/topic991.htm**

Gorham, E: Working with families of eating disordered patients to create an environment for recovery, 2005. HealthReach. Retrieved June 2008 from **http://healthwithinreach.com/HealthReach/HealthReach%20%20FEB%2005.pdf**

Haines, C: Diabetes: Treating diabetes with insulin, 2006. Retrieved January 2008 from **http://www.webmd.com/content/Article/46/1667_50931.htm**

Hepatitis Foundation International (HFI): Herbs and nutritional supplements, n.d. Retrieved February 2005 from **http://www.hepatitisresources-calif.org**

Hepatitis Foundation International: The ABCs of hepatitis, 2003. Retrieved June 2008 from **http://www.hepfi.org/living/liv_abc.html?gclid=CJL_8MnxnpQCFRdinAodlUx8fQ**

Hepatitis-Central: Some herbal remedies should not be taken because they can trigger serious side effects, 1998. Retrieved January 2005 from **http://www.hepatitis-central.com/hcv/herbs/donotuse.html**

Hsiang-Ching, K, et al: Deaths: Final data for 2005. National vital statistics reports 56(10), 2008. Hyattsville, MD, National Center for Health Statistics. Retrieved June 2008 from **http://www.cdc.gov/nchs/data/nvsr/nvsr56/nvsr56_10.pdf**

Huang, LH, and Priestley, MA: Alkalosis, metabolic, 2007. Retrieved June 2008 from **http://www.emedicine.com/ped/TOPIC69.HTM**

Joint Commission on Accreditation of Healthcare Organizations (JCAHO): Standards: Environment of care list of standards TX.4, updated April 2002. Retrieved March 2008 from **http://nyspi.org/JCHO/jcahotx4.htm**

Kalapatapu, RK, et al: Bulimia, 2008. Retrieved June 2008 from **http://www.emedicine.com/MED/topic255.htm**

Kaplan, EL, and Angelos, P: Surgery of the thyroid gland, updated 2006. Thyroid Disease Manager. Retrieved June 2008 from **http://www.thyroidmanager.org/Chapter21/21-frame.htm**

Kaye, WH: Atypicals in the treatment of anorexia nervosa. Broadening the horizon of atypical antipsychotic applications. CME article for Medscape, pp 65–67, 2004. Retrieved January 2005 from **http://www.medscape.com**

Kumrow, D, and Dahlen, R: Thyroidectomy: Understanding the potential for complications. Medsurg Nurs 11(5):228–235, 2002. Retrieved June 2008 from **http://findarticles.com/p/articles/mi_m0FSS/is_5_11/ai_n18614288/pg_1?tag=artBody;col1**

Lie, D: Recommendations for acute pancreatitis. CME article for Medscape Nurses, 2007. Retrieved June 2008 from **http://www.medscape.com/viewarticle/557675?src=mp**

Mears, E: Nutritional assessment: An opportunity for laboratorians to improve health care. Clinical Laboratory News, 2005. Retrieved March 2008 from **http://www.nutritionperspectives.com/content/NutritionalAssessment.cfm**

Medical encyclopedia: Overweight, 2007. Retrieved June 2008 from **http://www.nih.gov/medlineplus/ency/article/003101.htm**

Moreno, MA, and Judd, R: Eating disorder: Bulimia, 2008. Retrieved June 2008 from **http://www.emedicine.com/ped/TOPIC298.HTM**

Mukherjee, S: Hepatitis B, 2005. Retrieved June 2008 from **http://www.emedicinehealth.com/hepatitis_b/article_em.htm**

National Diabetes Information Clearinghouse: National diabetes statistics, 2007. Retrieved June 2008 from **http://diabetes.niddk.nih.gov/dm/pubs/statistics/#12**

National Heart, Lung and Blood Institute: What are overweight and obesity?, 2008. Diseases and Conditions Index. Retrieved July 2008 from **http://www.nhlbi.nih.gov/health/dci/Diseases/obe/obe_whatare.html**

National Institute of Diabetes and Digestive and Kidney Disorders (NIDDK): Chronic hepatitis C: Current disease management, 2006. NIH publication 07-4230. Retrieved July 2007 from **http://digestive.niddk.nih.gov/ddiseases/pubs/chronichepc/**

National Institute of Mental Health: National Comorbidity Survey and National Comorbidity Survey Replication: Collaborative psychiatric epidemiology surveys, 2007. Retrieved June 2008 from **http://www.icpsr.umich.edu/CPES/**

No author listed: Hepatitis, A, B, and C: Learn the differences, n.d. Retrieved March 2009 from **http://www.immunize.org/catg.d/p4075abc.pdf**

No author listed: Cirrhosis, last updated March 2009. Retrieved March 2009 from **http://www.nlm.nih.gov/medlineplus/cirrhosis.html**

No author listed: Pancreatic diseases, updated March 2009. Retrieved February 2005 from **http://www.nlm.nih.gov/medlineplus/pancreaticdiseases.html**

Obideen, L, and Yashke, P: Pancreatitis, chronic, 2008. Retrieved June 2008 from **http://www.emedicine.com/med/topic1721.htm**

Pancreas Foundation: Diseases of the pancreas: FAQ, n.d. Retrieved February 2005 from **http://www.pancreasfoundation.org**

Payne, K: Thyroid hormone tests and hyperthyroidism treatment overview. Two articles for WebMD with AOL website, 2004. Retrieved January 2005 from **http://aolsvc. health.webmd.aol.com**

Priestley, MA: Acidosis, metabolic, 2006. Retrieved June 2008 from **http://www.emedicine.com/PED/topic15.htm**

Pryor, T: Eating disorders at middle age, the desperate housewives effect. Eating Disorder Center of Denver, 2007. Retrieved June 2008 from **http://www.empoweringchange.com/pdf/EDCD-Midlife-study.pdf**

PsychCentral: Eating disorders cost millions of dollars for many U.S. businesses, 2004. Retrieved June 2008 from **http://psychcentral.com/blog/archives/2004/08/17/eating-disorders-cost-millions-of-dollars-for-many-us-businesses/**

Ross, DS: Patient information: Antithyroid drugs, 2004. Retrieved January 2005 from **http://patients.uptodate.com**

Schraga, ED: Hyperthyroidism, thyroid storm, and Graves' disease, 2008. Retrieved June 2008 from **http://www.emedicine.com/EMERG/topic269.htm**

Schwartz, JM, Ingram, K, and Flora, KD: Hepatitis E, 2006. Retrieved June 2008 from **http://63.240.86.189/med/topic995.htm**

Scientific Registry of Transplant Recipients: Fast facts about transplants, Jan 1, 2006–Dec 31, 2007. Retrieved June 2008 from **http://www.ustransplant.org/csr/current/fastfacts.aspx**

South Carolina Dept of Mental Health: Eating disorder statistics, 2006. Retrieved June 2008 from **http://www.state.sc.us/dmh/anorexia/statistics.htm**

Spengler, R: Thyroid scan and radioactive iodine uptake test, n.d. Retrieved January 2005 from **http://aolsvc.health.webmd.aol.com**

Taylor, CR: Cirrhosis, 2008. Retrieved June 2008 from **http://www .emedicine.com/radio/TOPIC175.HTM**

Thomas, CP, and Hamwai, K: Metabolic acidosis, 2007. Retrieved June 2008 from **http://www.emedicine.com/med/topic1458.htm**

University of Michigan: Patient information sheet: Thyroid and parathyroid surgery. Department of Surgery, Division of Endocrine Surgery, University of Michigan Health System Website, n.d. Retrieved January 2005 from **http://www.um-edocrine-surgery.org**

U.S. Department of Health and Human Services: Health, United States, 2006. DHHS publication 2006-1232. Retrieved June 2008 from **http://www.cdc.gov/nchs/data/hus/hus06.pdf**

U.S. Deptartment of Health and Human Services, National Institutes of Health: Classification of overweight and obesity by BMI, waist circumference, and associated disease risks, n.d. Retrieved July 2008 from **http://www.nhlbi.nih.gov/health/public/heart/obesity/ lose_wt/risk.htm**

Uwaifo, GI, and Arioglu, E: Obesity, 2006. Retrieved July 2008 from **http://www.emedicine.com/med/TOPIC1653.HTM**

Weight-control Information Network: Bariatric surgery for severe obesity, updated 2008. Retrieved June 2008 from **http://win.niddk.nih.gov/ publications/gastric.htm**

Wolf, DC: Cirrhosis, 2007. Retrieved June 2008 from **http://www .emedicine.com/med/TOPIC3183.HTM**

Wright, S: Patient information on minimally invasive thyroidectomy, n.d. Retrieved June 2008 from **http://www.thyroidectomy.com/ minimally-invasive-thyroidectomy-thyroid-graves.htm**

Yakshe, P: Pancreatitis, acute, 2005. Retrieved January 2005 from **http://www.emedicine.com**

Yaseen, S, and Thomas, C: Metabolic acidosis, 2007. Retrieved June 2008 from **http://www.emedicine.com/med/TOPIC1459.HTM**

Youngerman-Cole, S: Thyroidectomy: Surgery overview, 2004. Retrieved January 2005 from **http://aolsvc.health.webmd.aol.com**

CHAPTER 9

Books

Beers, MK (ed): The Merck manual of diagnosis and therapy, ed 11. Merck Research Laboratories, West Point, PA, 2006.

Evens, A, and Tallman, M: Acute leukemias. In Skeel, RT (ed): Handbook of cancer chemotherapy, ed 6. Lippincott, Williams & Wilkins, Philadelphia, 2003.

Iltano, JK, et al: ONS core curriculum for oncology nursing, ed 4. Elsevier Saunders, Philadelphia, 2005.

Katz, A: Breaking the silence on cancer and sexuality: A handbook for healthcare providers. Oncology Nursing Society, Philadelphia, 2006.

National Institutes of Health: The management of sickle cell disease, ed 4. NIH Pub #02–2117, Bethesda, MD, 2002.

Pui CH, Heslop HE, and Hoelzer, D: Advances in pediatric and adult acute lymphoblastic leukemia. In Oncology 2002: The American Society of Clinical Oncology 2002 Education Book. American Society of Clinical Oncology, Alexandria, VA, 2002, pp 32–57.

Stein, R, Morgan, D, and Greer, J: Hodgkin's disease and non-Hodgkin's lymphoma. In Skeel, RT (ed): Handbook of cancer chemotherapy, ed 6. Lippincott, Williams & Wilkins, Philadelphia, 2003.

Visovsky, C: Interventions for clients with hematologic problems. In Ignatavicius, DD and Workman, ML (eds): Medical-surgical nursing: Critical thinking for collaborative care, ed 5. Elsevier Saunders, St. Louis, MO, 2006.

Articles

Basile, J: Clinical considerations and practical recommendations for the primary care practitioner in the management of anemia of chronic kidney disease. South Med J 100(12):1200–1207, 2007.

Cerrato, PL: Complementary therapies: Diet and herbs for BPH? RN 63(2):63–64, 2000.

Corwin, H, and Krantz, S: Anemia of the critically ill: Acute anemia of chronic disease. Crit Care Med 29(9):S199–S200, 2001.

Day, SW, and Wynn, LW: Sickle cell pain and hydroxyurea. AJN 100(11):34–38, 2000.

Gorman, K: Sickle cell disease: Do you doubt your patient's pain? AJN 99(3):38–43, 1999.

Gutaj, DA: Oncology today: Lymphoma. RN 63(8):32–37, 2000.

Hays, K, and McCartney, S: Nursing care of the patient with chronic lymphocytic leukemia. Semin Oncol Nurs 25(1):75, 1998.

Hebbar, AK, and Gibson, MV: Recognizing and managing anemia of chronic disease. Patient Care 40(11):36–40, 2006.

Kanarek, R: Facing the challenge of childhood leukemia. AJN 98(7): 42, 1998.

Kosits, C, and Callaghan, M: Rituximab: A new monoclonal antibody therapy for non-Hodgkin's lymphoma. Oncol Nurs Forum 27(1): 51, 2000.

Krantz, SB: Pathogenesis and treatment of the anemia of chronic disease. Am J Med Sci 307(5):353–359, 1994.

Mackey, H, and Klemm, P: Leukemia: Aggressive therapies predispose patients to a host of side effects. AJN (4)Suppl:27–31, 2000.

Medoff, E: Oncology today: Leukemia. RN 63(9):42–49, 2000.

Mitchell, R: Sickle cell anemia. AJN 99(5):36–37, 1999.

Mohanty, D, Mukherjee, MB, and Colah, RB: Iron deficiency anaemia in sickle cell disorders in India. Indian J Med Res 127: 366–369, 2008.

Montoya, V, Wink, D, and Sole, M: Adult anemia: Determine clinical significance. Nurse Pract 27(3):38–53, 2002.

Mullen, E: Hodgkin lymphoma: An update. J Nurse Pract 3(6):393–403, 2007.

Rogers, B: Looking at lymphoma and leukemia. Nursing2005 35(7):56–63, 2005.

Roy, C, Weinstein, D, and Andrews, N: 2002 E. Mead Johnson award for research in pediatrics lecture: The molecular biology of the anemia of chronic disease: A hypothesis. Pediat Res 53(3):507–512, 2003.

Stremick, K, and Gallagher, E: Malignant lymphomas. AJN (4)Suppl:18–22, 2000.

Thompson, KA: Detecting Hodgkin's disease. AJN 99(5):61–64, 1999.

Electronic Resources

American Cancer Society (ACS): What happens after treatment for Hodgkin Disease?, 2007. Retrieved July 2008 from **http://www .cancer.org/docroot/CRI/content/CRI_2_4_5x_What_Happens _After_Treatment_for_Hodgkin_Disease.asp?sitearea=**

CureResearch.com: Statistics about anemia, updated 2003. Retrieved June 2008 from **http://www.cureresearch.com/a/anemia/stats.htm**

Distenfeld, A, and Woermann, U: Sickle Cell Anemia, 2007. Retrieved July 2008 from **http://www.emedicine.com/MED/topic2126.htm**

Dunleavy, KM, Kass, E, and Wilson, W: Lymphoma of the head and neck, 2007. Retrieved July 2008 from **http://www.emedicine.com/ ent/TOPIC742.HTM**

Gajra, A, Vajpayee, N, and Grethlein, S: Lymphoma, B-cell, 2007. Retrieved July 2008 from **http://www.emedicine.com/med/ topic1358.htm**

Hu, W, and Hale, KL: Lymphoma, 2005. Retrieved July 2008 from **http://www.emedicinehealth.com/lymphoma/article_em.htm**

Iron Disorders Institute: Sickle cell anemia and complicated iron, 2006. Retrieved July 2008 from **http://www.irondisorders.org/Disorders/ ComplicatedIron.asp**

Leukemia & Lymphoma Society: Facts 2007–2008. The National Cancer Institute's Surveillance, Epidemiology and End Results Program, Cancer Statistics Review (SEER), 1975–2004. Published online by SEER. Retrieved July 2008 from **http://seer.cancer.gov/**

Luekemia & Lymphoma Society: The Lymphomas, 2006. Retrieved July 2008 from **http://www.leukemia-lymphoma.org/hm_lls**

McIntyre, J, Moral, MA, and Bozzo, J: Combination therapies with valproic acid in cancer: Initial clinical approach. Drugs of the Future 32(1):45, 2007. Retrieved July 2008 from **http://journals.prous.com/ journals/servlet/xmlxsl/pk_journals.xml_summary_pr?p _JournalId=2&p_RefId=1052960&p_IsPs=N**

National Cancer Institute: Cancer trends progress report—2007 update: Costs of cancer care, updated November 2007. Retrieved July 2008 from **http://progressreport.cancer.gov/doc_detail.asp?pid=1&did =2007&chid=75&coid=726&mid**

National Heart, Lung and Blood Institute: Anemia: Who is at risk?, updated 2007. Diseases and Conditions Index. Retrieved June 2008 from **http://www.nhlbi.nih.gov/health/dci/Diseases/anemia/anemia_whoisatrisk.html**

National Heart, Lung and Blood Institute: Sickle cell anemia, 2008. Retrieved September 2008 from **http://www.nhlbi.nih.gov/health/dci/Diseases/Sca/SCA_All.html**

National Institute of Diabetes and Digestive and Kidney Diseases: Anemia in kidney disease and dialysis, 2005. Retrieved June 2008 from **http://kidney.niddk.nih.gov/kudiseases/pubs/anemia/#treatment**

Perry, M, and Rasool, H: Chronic lymphocytic leukemia, 2005. Retrieved July 2008 from **http://www.emedicine.com/med/topic370.htm**

Phillips, K: Response to EPO for anemia, 2002. Retrieved June 2008 from **http://www.medscape.com/viewarticle/436160**

Seiter, K: Acute myelogenous leukemia, 2006. Retrieved July 2008 from **http://www.emedicine.com/med/TOPIC34.HTM**

Steiner, CA, and Miller, JL: Statistical briefing #21: Sickle cell disease patients in U.S. hospitals 2004, 2006. Agency for Healthcare Research and Quality. Retrieved July 2008 from **http://www.hcup-us.ahrq.gov/reports/statbriefs/sb21.pdf**

Swierzewski, SJ: Leukemia treatments, 2007. Retrieved July 2008 from **http://www.oncologychannel.com/leukemias/chemotherapy.shtml**

Taher, A, and Kazzi, ZN: Anemia, sickle cell, 2007. Retrieved July 2008 from **http://www.emedicine.com/emerg/TOPIC26.HTM**

CHAPTER 10

Books

Caputi, LJ: Interventions for male clients with reproductive problems. In Ignatavicius, DD, and Workman, ML: Medical-surgical nursing: Critical thinking for collaborative care, ed 5. Elsevier Saunders, St. Louis, MO, 2006.

Centers for Disease Control and Prevention, National Center for Health Statistics: National hospital discharge survey: 2004 annual summary with detailed diagnosis and procedure data. Department of Health and Human Services publication 2006-1733, GPO, Hyattsville, MD, 2006.

Choka, KP: Renal failure. In Copstead, LEC, and Banasik, JL: Pathophysiology, ed 3. Elsevier Saunders, St. Louis, MO, 2005.

Doenges, ME, Moorhouse, MF, and Murr, AC: Nurse's pocket guide diagnoses, prioritized interventions, and rationales, ed 11. FA Davis, Philadelphia, 2008.

Karch, AM: Lippincott's nursing drug guide. Lippincott, Williams & Wilkins, Ambler, PA, 2008.

Lacharity, LA: Interventions for clients with acute and chronic renal failure. In Ignatavicius, DD, and Workman, ML. Medical-surgical nursing: Critical thinking for collaborative care, ed 5. Elsevier Saunders, St. Louis, MO, 2006.

National Institutes of Health (NIH): Urostomy and Continent Urinary Diversion. Publication no. 06–5629, Washington DC, May 2006.

Porth, CM: Essentials of pathophysiology: Concepts of altered health states, ed 2. Lippincott, Williams & Wilkins, Philadelphia, 2007.

Springhouse, A (ed): Pathophysiology made incredibly easy! Lippincott, Williams & Wilkins, Philadelphia, 2005.

Springhouse, A (ed): Emergency nursing made incredibly easy! Lippincott, Williams & Wilkins, Ambler, PA, 2007.

U.S. Renal Data System: USRDS 2007 Annual data report. National Institutes of Health, Department of Health and Human Services, Washington DC, 2007.

Wei, JT, Calhoun, EA, and Jacobsen, SJ: Benign prostatic hyperplasia. In Litwin, MS, and Saigal, CS (eds): Urologic diseases in America. National Institutes for Health. NIH publication 07-5512:43–67, Washington, DC, 2007.

Winkleman, C: Interventions for clients with urinary problems. In Ignatavicius, DD, and Workman, ML (eds): Medical-surgical nursing: Critical thinking for collaborative care, ed 5. Elsevier Saunders, St. Louis, MO, 2006.

Wolfson, AB, et al: Clinical practice of emergency medicine, ed 4. Lippincott, Williams & Wilkins, Philadelphia, 2005.

Articles

Arkouche, W, et al: Twenty-five years of experience with out-center hemodialysis. Kidney Int 56(6):2269–2275, 1999.

Bak, GP: Teaching ostomy patients to regain their independence. Am Nurse Today 3(3):30-34, 2008.

Bent, S, et al: Saw palmetto for benign prostatic hyperplasia. N Engl J Med 354(6): 557–566, 2006.

Burrows-Hudson, S: Chronic kidney disease: An overview. AJN 105(2):40–49, 2005.

Calabrese, DA: Prostate cancer in older men. Urol Nurs 24(4): 258–264, 2004.

Campbell, D: How acute renal failure puts the brakes on kidney function. Nursing2003 33(1):59–63, 2003.

Chan, CT, et al: Regression of left ventricular hypertrophy after conversion to nocturnal hemodialysis. Kidney Int 61(6):2235–2239, 2002.

Chertow, GM, et al: The association of intradialytic parenteral nutrition with survival in hemodialysis patients. Am J Kidney Dis 24: 921, 1994.

Colwell, JC, Goldberg, M, and Carmel, J: The state of the standard diversion. J Wound Ostomy Continence Nurs 28(1):6–17, 2001.

Cook, L: The value of lab values. AJN 99(5):66–75, 1999.

Davison, BJ, et al: Client evaluation of a discharge program following a radical prostatectomy. Urol Nurs 24(6):483–489, 2004.

Finkielstein, VA, and Goldfarb, DS: Strategies for preventing calcium oxalate stones. CMAJ 174(10):1407–1409, 2006.

Gilchrist, K: Benign prostatic hyperplasia: Is it a precursor to prostatic cancer? Nurse Pract 29(6):30–37, 2004.

Goodman, ED, and Ballou, MB: Perceived barriers and motivators to exercise in hemodialysis patients. Nephrol Nurs J 31(1):23–29, 2004.

Gray, M: Urinary retention: Management in the acute care setting, part 1. AJN 100(7):40–47, 2000.

Greifzu, SP: Oncology today: Prostate cancer. RN 63(6):26–31, 2000.

Held-Warmkessel, J: How to care for men with prostate cancer. Nursing99, 29(11):51–53, 1999.

Holcolm, SS: Keeping kidney function flowing. Nursing Made Incredibly Easy! 2(5):30–40, 2004.

Holcomb, SS: Evaluating chronic kidney disease risk. Nurse Pract 30(4):12–25, 2005.

Kaplow, R, and Barry, R: Continuous renal replacement therapies. AJN 102(11):26–33, 2002.

Kearney, K: Dialysis disequilibrium syndrome. AJN 100(2):53–54, 2000.

King, B: Meds and the dialysis patient. RN 63(7):54–59, 2000.

Leydig, EJ: Are you endangering your patients? RN 68(2):29–31, 2005.

Little, C: Renovascular hypertension. AJN 100(2):46–51, 2000.

McGlynn, B, et al: Management of urinary incontinence following radical prostatectomy. Urol Nurs 24(6):475–482, 2004.

No author listed: Research News Item: Don't give your kidneys a jolt! Nutr Today 39(5):213, 2004.

Osborne, D: Managing patients with a distended bladder. Clin J Oncol Nurs 4(2):103, 2000.

Parsons, JK, et al: Lower urinary tract symptoms and the risk of falls in older men. J Urol 179(suppl):140; Abstract 394, 2008.

Paton, M: CRRT: Help for acute renal failure. Nursing Made Incredibly Easy! 5(5):28–38, 2007.

Pieper, B, et al: Discharge information needs of patients after surgery. J Wound Ostomy Continence Nurs 33(3):281–290, 2006.

Polzien, G: Chronic kidney disease and kidney failure important numbers to know. Home Health Nurs, 25(10):655–660, 2007.

Pupim, LB, Flakoll, PJ, and Brouillette, JR: Intradialytic parenteral nutrition improves protein and energy homeostasis in chronic hemodialysis patients. J Clin Invest 110(4):483–492, 2002.

Saigal, C, and Joyce, G: Economic costs of benign prostatic hyperplasia in the private sector. J Urol 173(4):1309–1313, 2005.

Shiller, J: Greenlight laser: BPH treatment shows promise. RN 70(11):28–32, 2007.

Sienty, MK, and Dawson, N: Preventing urosepsis from indwelling urinary catheters. AJN 99(1):24C–24H, 1999.

Wojcik, M, and Dennison, D: Photoselective vaporization of the prostate in ambulatory surgery. AORN J 83(2):330, 2006.

Young, J: Kidney stone. Nursing2000 30(7):33, 2000.

Zellner, KM: Acute tubular necrosis. RN 62(10): 42–45, 1999.

Electronic Resources

Agency for Healthcare Research and Quality (AHRQ): Clinical summary guide: Treatments for clinically localized prostate cancer, 2008. Retrieved July 2008 from **http://effectivehealthcare.ahrq.gov/healthInfo .cfm?infotype=sg&DocID=99&ProcessID=9**

Agraharkar, M, and Gupta, R: Acute renal failure, updated 2007. Retrieved July 2008 from **http://emedicine.medscape.com/article/ 243492-overview**

Alper, AB, and Young, BA: Uremia, 2008. Retrieved July 2008 from **http://www.emedicine.com/MED/topic2341.htm**

American Cancer Society (ACS): Urostomy: A guide, revised 2007. Retrieved July 2008 from **http://www.cancer.org/docroot/CRI/ content/CRI_2_6x_Urostomy.asp**

American Urological Association Education and Research, Inc.: AUA guideline on the management of benign prostatic hyperplasia: Diagnosis and treatment recommendations, updated 2003. Retrieved March 2008 from **http://www.guideline.gov/summary/summary .aspx?ss=15&doc_id=3740&nbr=2966**

American Urological Association Foundation: Continent urinary diversion, n.d. Public information fact sheet. Retrieved February 2005 from **http://www.urologyhealth.org**

American Urological Association Foundation: Kidney (renal) failure, n.d. Public information fact sheet. Retrieved February 2005 from **http://www.urologyhealth.org**

Bargman, G: Mechanical and other noninfectious complications of PD. Power point presentation for Medscape Nephrology, 2007. Retrieved July 2008 from **http://www.medscape.com/viewarticle/559642**

Centers for Disease Control and Prevention, National Center for Health Statistics: 2005 National hospital discharge survey. Advance data from vital and health statistics, No. 385, July 12, 2007. Retrieved July 2008 from **http://www.cdc.gov/nchs/data/ad/ad385.pdf**

Clark, J, and DuBois, H: Urostomy guide.United Ostomy Associations of America, 2005. Retrieved July 2008 from **http://www.uoaa.org/ ostomy_info/pubs/uoa_urostomy_en.pdf**

Costa, JA, and Kreder, K: Urinary diversions and neobladders, 2006. Retrieved July 2008 from **http://www.emedicine.com/MED/ topic3083.htm**

Craig, S: Renal calculi, 2006. Retrieved July 2008 from **http://www .emedicine.com/emerg/TOPIC499.HTM**

Diagnostic Center For Disease: Robotic prostatectomy—A race to failure?, 2008. Retrieved July 2008 from **http://www .medicalnewstoday.com/articles/112626.php**

Guilli, LF, et al: Open prostatectomy. Surgery encyclopedia: A guide for patients and caregivers, n.d. Retrieved July 2008 from **http:// www.surgeryencyclopedia.com/La-Pa/Open-Prostatectomy.html**

How, PP, and Lau, AH: Malnutrition in patients undergoing hemodialysis: Is intradialytic parenteral nutrition the answer?, 2005. Retrieved July 2008 from **http://www.medscape.com/viewarticle/496192**

Korman, HJ, and Harris, M: Prostate cancer: Radical perineal resection, 2007. Retrieved July 2008 from **http://www.emedicine.com/med/ topic3053.htm**

Krause, RS: Renal failure, chronic and renal dialysis, 2006. Retrieved July 2008 from **http://www.emedicine.com/emerg/topic501.htm**

Leslie, SW: Nephrolithiasis: Acute renal colic, 2007. Retrieved July 2008 from **http://www.emedicine.com/med/topic3437.htm**

Leveillee, RJ, Patel, VR, and Bird, VG: Prostate hyperplasia, benign, updated 2006. Retrieved March 2008 from **http://www.emedicine .com/MED/topic1919.htm**

Lohr, JT, and Sherk, SD: Cystectomy. Gale encyclopedia of surgery: A guide for patients and caregivers, 2004. Retrieved July 2008 from **http://www.surgeryencyclopedia.com/Ce-Fi/Cystectomy.html**

Mayo Clinic Staff: Bladder cancer, 2004. Retrieved February 2005 from **http://mayoclinic.com**

Milenkovic, M, Russo, A, and Elixhauser, A: Hospital stays for prostate cancer, 2004. AHRQ Healthcare cost and utilization project. Statistical brief #30, 2007. Retrieved July 2008 from **http://www.hcup -us.ahrq.gov/reports/statbriefs/sb30.pdf**

Morbidity and Mortality Weekly Report: Prevalence of chronic kidney disease and associated risk factors—United States 1999–2004, 2007. Retrieved July 2008 from **http://www.cdc.gov/mmwr/preview/ mmwrhtml/mm5608a2.htm**

National Cancer Institute: Surveillance epidemiology and end results (SEER), 2008. Retrieved July 2008 from **http://seer.cancer.gov/ statfacts/html/urinb.html?statfacts_page=urinb.html&x=12&y=16**

National Institute of Diabetes and Digestive and Kidney Diseases: Treatment methods for kidney failure: peritoneal dialysis, 2001. Retrieved July 2008 from **http://findarticles.com/p/articles/ mi_m0652/is_2001_April_15/ai_82877258**

National Institute of Diabetes and Digestive and Kidney Diseases: Medical therapy of prostatic symptoms, 2003. Retrieved July 2008 from **http://www.niddk.nih.gov/patient/mtops/mtops-q&a.htm**

National Institutes of Health (NIH): Eat right to feel right on hemodialysis. NIH publication 03-4274, 2003. Retrieved February 2005 from the National Kidney and Urologic Diseases Information Clearinghouse, **http://www.kidney.niddk.nih.gov**

National Institutes of Health: Fact sheet: Chronic kidney disease and kidney failure, 2007. Retrieved July 2008 from **http://www.nih.gov/ about/researchresultsforthepublic/kidney.pdf**

National Institutes of Health: Kidney failure: Choosing a treatment that's right for you. NIH publication 03-2412, 2003. Retrieved February 2005 from **http://www.kidney.niddk.nih.gov**

National Institutes of Health: Kidney stones in adults. NIH Public information fact sheet, publication 05-2495, 2004. Retrieved February 2005 from **http://www.kidney.niddk.nih.gov**

National Institutes of Health: Hemodialysis dose and adequacy. Patient information fact sheet. National Institute of Diabetes and Digestive and Kidney Diseases. NIH publication 03-4556, n.d. Retrieved February 2005 from **http://www.kidneyniddk.nih.gov**

National Kidney Foundation: Clinical practice guidelines, 2000. Retrieved February 2005 from **http://www.kidney.org/professionals/kdoqi/ guidelines.cfm**

National Kidney Foundation: End-stage renal disease in the United States, 2008. Retrieved July 2008 from **http://www.kidney.org/news/ newsroom/fsitem.cfm?id=38**

National Kidney and Urologic Diseases Information Clearinghouse (NKUDIC): Hemodialysis dose and adequacy, 2005. Retrieved July 2008 from **http://kidney.niddk.nih.gov/Kudiseases/pubs/ hemodialysisdose/**

National Kidney and Urologic Diseases Information Clearinghouse (NKUDIC): Treatment methods for kidney failure: Hemodialysis. NIH publication 07-4666, 2006. Retrieved July 2008 from **http:// kidney.niddk.nih.gov/kudiseases/pubs/hemodialysis/index.htm**

National Kidney and Urologic Diseases Information Clearinghouse: Treatment methods for kidney failure: Peritoneal dialysis. NIH publication 06-4688, 2006. Retrieved July 2008 from **http://kidney .niddk.nih.gov/kudiseases/pubs/peritoneal/index.htm**

National Kidney and Urologic Disease Information Clearinghouse: Kidney and urologic disease statistics for the United States. NIH publication 08-3895, 2008. Retrieved July 2008 from **http://kidney.niddk.nih.gov/kudiseases/pubs/kustats/**

National Kidney and Urologic Diseases Information Clearinghouse: Vascular access for hemodialysis. NIH Publication 08-4554, 2008. Retrieved July 2008 from **http://kidney.niddk.nih.gov/Kudiseases/ pubs/vascularaccess/**

Nazario, B: Enlarged prostate: Is it time for surgery?, 2006. Retrieved July 2008 from **http://www.webmd.com/solutions/enlarged _prostate/surgery**

No author listed: Benign prostatic hyperplasia (BPH). How is it treated?, updated January 2009. Retrieved July 2008 from **http://www .drugdigest.org/DD/HC/Treatment/0,4047,550246,00.html**

Pearle, MS, Calhoun, E, and Curhan, GC: Urolithiasis. In Litwin, MS, and Saigal, CS, eds: Urologic Diseases in America. U.S. Department of Health and Human Services, National Institutes of Health, National Institute of Diabetes and Digestive and Kidney Diseases. Washington,

DC: U.S. Government Printing Office publication 07-5512, pp 281–319, 2007. Retrieved July 2008 from **http://kidney .niddk.nih.gov/statistics/uda/Urolithiasis-Chapter08.pdf**

Perl, J, and Chan, CT: Sleep apnea in peritoneal dialysis: Nocturnal versus continuous ambulatory treatment. Nat Clin Pract Nephrol 3:72–73, 2007. Retrieved July 2008 from **http://www.nature.com/ncpneph/ journal/v3/n2/full/ncpneph0392.html**

Poit, CA: The ins and outs of continent urinary diversions, 2003. Nursing Spectrum Education/CE Self-Modules. Retrieved February 2005 from **http://nsweb.nursingspectrum.com**

Rhodes, M: Kidney stones, 2007. Retrieved July 2008 from **http://www .webmd.com/kidney-stones/kidney-stones-adults**

Rubenstein, J, and McVary, KT: Transurethral microwave thermotherapy of the prostate (TUMT), 2004. Retrieved February 2005 from **http://www.emedicine.com**

Sinert, R, and Peacock, PR: Renal failure, acute, 2006. Retrieved July, 2008 from **http://www.emedicine.com/emerg/topic500.htm**

Sofocleous, CT, et al: Dialysis fistula, 2008. Retrieved July 2008 from **http://www.emedicine.com/Radio/topic759.htm**

U.S. Renal Data System: Annual data report. Economic costs of ESRD. Reference section K, 2004. Retrieved July 2008 from **http://www .usrds.org/2004/ref/K_tables_04.pdf**

Verrelli, M: Chronic renal failure, 2006. Retrieved July 2008 from **http://www.emedicine.com/med/topic374.htm**

Wedro, BC: Kidney stones: Symptoms, causes, and treatment, 2007. Retrieved July 2008 from **http://www.emedicinehealth.com/ kidney_stones/article_em.htm**

Wolf, JS: Nephrolithiasis, 2004. Retrieved February 2005 from **http://www.emedicine.com**

CHAPTER 11

Books

American Cancer Society: Cancer facts and figures 2004. American Cancer Society, Atlanta, 2004.

Mohamed, I, and Skeel, RT: Carcinoma of the breast. In Skeel RT, (ed): Handbook for cancer chemotherapy, ed 6. Lippincott Williams & Wilkins, Philadelphia, 2003.

Winer EP, et al: Malignant tumors of the breast. In DeVita, VT, Hellman, S, and Rosenberg, SA (eds): Cancer: Principles and practice of oncology. Lippincott Williams & Wilkins, Philadelphia, 2001.

Articles

Augustus, CE: Beliefs and perspectives of African American women who have had hysterectomies. J Transcul Nurs 13(4):296–302, 2002.

Bunde, M, et al: On-line hysterectomy support: Characteristics of website experience. Cyberpsychol Behav 10(1):80–85, 2007.

Buren, JM, and Linton, C: The role of exercise in treating lymphedema. Rehab Manage 13(6):26–31, 2000.

Curry H: Menorrhagia and hysterectomy. AJN 102(1):14–19, 2002.

DiPalma, AM, and DiPalma, JA: Women's colonic digestive health. Gastroenterol Nurs 25(1):3–8, 2002.

Ely, S, and Vioral, AN: Breast cancer overview. Plast Surg Nurs 27(3):128–133, 2007.

Katz, A: Sexuality after hysterectomy: A review of the literature and discussion of nursing roles. J Adv Nurs 42(3):297–303, 2003.

Klingman, L: Assessing the female reproductive system. AJN 99(8):37–43, 1999.

Ligibel, JA, et al: Impact of a mixed strength and endurance exercise intervention on insulin levels in breast cancer survivors. J Clin Oncol 26(6):907–912, 2008.

Mazmanian, CM: Hysterectomy: Holistic care is key. RN 62(6):32–35, 1999.

Moreria, V: Hysterectomy: Nursing the physical and emotional wounds. Nurs Times 96(20):41–42, 2000.

Oetker-Black, SL: Preoperative teaching and hysterectomy outcomes. AORN J 77(6):1215–1218, 1221–1231; 2003.

Risser, N, and Murphy, M: Literature review: Women's health care: Sexual function after hysterectomy. Nurs Pract 29(2):49, 2004.

Ruth-Sahd, LA, and Zulkosky, KD: Cervical cancer: Caring for patients undergoing total pelvic exenteration. Crit Care Nurse 19(1):46–57, 1999.

Sharts-Hopko, NC: Hysterectomy for nonmalignant conditions. AJN 101(9):32–36, 2001.

Thomas, S, and Greifzu, SP: Oncology today: Breast cancer. RN 63(4):40–45, 2000a.

Thomas, S, and Greifzu, SP: Oncology today: Breast reconstruction. RN 63(4):45–47, 2000b.

Warren, A, et al: Lymphedema: A comprehensive review. Ann Plast Surg 59(4):464–472, 2007.

Electronic Resources

American Cancer Society: Lymphedema: What every woman with breast cancer should know, 2007. Retrieved July 2008 from **http://www .cancer.org/docroot/MIT/content/MIT_7_2x_Lymphedema_and _Breast_Cancer.asp**

American College of Obstetricians and Gynecologists: Hysterectomy, 2008. Retrieved June 2008 from **http://www.acog.org/publications/ patient_education/bp008.cfm**

Bachmann, G, and Patel, S: Hysterectomy, 2004. Retrieved February 2005 from **http://www.emedicine.com**

Brown, ML, et al: Estimating health care costs related to cancer treatment from SEER-Medicare data. Med Care 40(8 Suppl):IV-104–IV-117, 2002. Retrieved July 2008 from **http://progressreport.cancer.gov/ graphs-excel/tabl2costsofcancercarebycancer.xls**

Forchuk, C, et al: Postoperative arm massage: A support for women with lymph node dissection. Cancer Nurs 27(1):25–32, 2004. Retrieved February 2005 from **http://www.medscape.com**

Gor, HB, Bachmann, G, and Patel, S: Hysterectomy, 2006. Retrieved June 2008 from **http://www.emedicine.com/med/TOPIC3315.HTM**

Institute for Clinical Systems Improvement: Cervical cancer screening, 2003. Retrieved February 2005 from National Guideline Clearinghouse. **http://www.guideline.gov**

Institute for Clinical Systems Improvement: Menopause and hormone therapy (HT): Collaborative decision-making and management, 2006. Retrieved June 2008 from National Guideline Clearing House. **http://www.guideline.gov**

Mayo Clinic: Abdominal hysterectomy, 2008. Retrieved June 2008. **http://www.mayoclinic.com/health/hysterectomy/HQ00905**

Mayo Clinic: Mastectomy, 2007. Retrieved July 2008 from **http:// www.mayoclinic.com/health/mastectomy-lumpectomy/ BC99999/PAGE=BC00015**

Medline Plus: Estrogen and progestin (hormone replacement therapy), reviewed 2007. Retrieved June 2008 from **http://www.nlm.nih.gov/ medlineplus/druginfo/medmaster/a601041.html**

National Cancer Institute: Breast Cancer, various articles, including statistics, n.d. Retrieved July 2008 from **http://www.cancer.gov/ cancertopics/types/breast**

National Cancer Institute: Pain control-support for people with cancer. NIH publication 07-6287, 2008. Retrieved July 2008 from **http:// www.cancer.gov/cancertopics/paincontrol.pdf**

National Comprehensive Cancer Network (NCCN): Breast cancer treatment guidelines for patients, 2007. Retrieved July 2008 from **http://www .nccn.org/patients/patient_gls/_english/_breast/contents.asp**

National Guideline Clearinghouse: Management of breast cancer in women: A national clinical guideline, 1998. Retrieved July 2008 from **http://www.guideline.gov/summary/summary.aspx?ss=15&doc_id =8510&nbr=4745**

National Guideline Clearinghouse: Surgical alternatives to hysterectomy in the management of leiomyomas, 2000. American College of Obstetricians and Gynecologists (ACOG). Retrieved from **http://www.guideline.gov**

National Uterine Fibroids Foundation: Statistics, 2004. Retrieved June 2008 from **http://www.nuff.org/health_statistics.htm**

National Women's Health Information Center, U.S. Department of Health and Human Services: Hysterectomy, updated July 1, 2006. Retrieved June 2008 from **http://womenshealth.gov/faq/hysterectomy.htm**

Parker, WH: About hysterectomy, n.d. Retrieved June 2008 from **http://www.parkermd.com/about-hysterectomy.htm**

Parker, WH, and Parker, RL: If you absolutely need a hysterectomy. In A gynecologist's second opinion, ed 2. Plume, New York, 2003. Retrieved June 2008 from **http://www.gynsecondopinion.com/hysterectomy.htm**

Walling, AD: Laparoscopic vs. abdominal hysterectomy: A comparison. Am Family Phys 70(8), 2006. Retrieved June 2008 from **http://www.aafp.org/afp/20041015/tips/19.html**

WebMD: Women's health: Hysterectomy—Recovery, 2006a. Retrieved June 2008 from **http://women.webmd.com/tc/hysterectomy-recovery**

WebMD: Women's health: Hysterectomy—Comparison of hysterectomy procedures, 2006b. Retrieved June 2008 from **http://women.webmd.com/tc/hysterectomy-comparison-of-hysterectomy-procedures**

CHAPTER 12

Books

No author listed: Zimmer traction manual. Zimmer Orthopaedic Surgical Products, Inc., 2005–2006.

Articles

Aulivola, B, et al: Major lower extremity amputation. Arch Surg 139(4): 395–399, 2004.

Bailey, J: Getting a fix on orthopedic care. Nursing2003 33(6):58–63, 2003.

Bryant, G: Stump care. AJN 101(2):67–71, 2001.

Fort, CW: Getting a fix on long-bone fractures. Nursing2002 32(6):321–326, 2002.

Frakes, M, and Evans, T: Major pelvic fractures. Crit Care Nurse 24(2):24–30, 2004.

Kurtz, SM, et al: Future clinical and economic impact of revision total hip and knee arthroplasty. J Bone Joint Surg Am 89 (Suppl 3): 144–151, 2007.

Pasero, C: Using superficial cooling for pain control. AJN 99(3): 24, 1999.

Prehoden, ME: Crush injury: Compromised circulation can threaten limb survival. AJN, 99(3):35, 1999.

Wilson, T: Advanced prosthetic devices aid amputees. Disabled Am Veterans (DAV) Magazine, November/December, 2004.

Electronic Resources

Barclay, L: National Osteoporosis Foundation issues guidelines for osteoporosis management. CE article, 2008. Retrieved July 2008 from **http://www.medscape.com/viewarticle/570594**

Clontz, AS, Annonio, D, and Walker, L: Trauma nursing: Amputation, 2004. Retrieved February 2005 from **http://rnweb.com**

DiGioia, AM: Total joint replacement educational series part 6: Surprising statistics about knee and hip replacement surgery. J Bone and Joint Surg 89-A(12), 2007. Retrieved July 2008 from **http://www.amd3.org/ROblog/2008/01/total-joint-replacement-educat-2.html**

Ellis, W, Kishner, S, and Laborde, JM: Gait analysis after amputation, 2007. Retrieved July 2008 from **http://www.emedicine.com/orthoped/topic633.htm**

Ertl, JP, and Ertl, W: Amputations of the lower extremity, 2005. Retrieved February 2005 from **http://www.emedicine.com**

Liu, SS, et al: Trends in mortality, complications, and demographics for primary hip arthroplasty in the United States. International Orthopaedics, 2008. Retrieved July 2008 from **http://www.ncbi.nlm.nih.gov/pubmed/18461326**

Martines, K, Mipro, RC, and Bodeau, VS: Upper limb prosthetics, 2006. Retrieved July 2008 from **http://www.jackgoldsurgical.com/PRODUCTS/eMedicine%20-%20Upper%20Limb%20Prosthetics%20%20Article%20by%20Kevin%20Martinez,%20MD.htm**

National Guideline Clearinghouse: Skeletal pin site care, 2005. Retrieved July 2008 from **http://www.guideline.gov/summary/summary.aspx?ss=15&doc_id=7420&nbr=004379&string=pin+AND+care#s25**

National Institute of Arthritis and Musculoskeletal and Skin Diseases: Osteoporosis, 2007. Retrieved July 2008 from **http://www.niams.nih.gov/Health_Info/Bone/Osteoporosis/default.asp**

National Limb Loss Information Center (NLLIC) Staff: Wound care: Preventing infection. Amputee Coalition of America Fact Sheet, revised 2009. Retrieved April 2009 from **http://www.amputee-coalition.org/fact_sheets/woundcare.html**

National Osteoporosis Foundation (NOF): Fast facts on osteoporosis, n.d. Retrieved July 2008 from **http://www.nof.org/osteoporosis/diseasefacts.htm**

No author listed: ON-Q PainBuster® Patient Guidelines, n.d. Retrieved July 2008 from **www.surgicalspecialties.com.au/download_file.asp?file=downloads/onq/brochures/onq_pain_patientguide.pdf**

Partners Against Pain and NLLIC Staff: Pain management and the amputee. National Limb Loss Information Center (NLLIC) Fact Sheet, updated September 18, 2008. Retrieved April 2009 from **http://www.amputee-coalition.org/fact_sheets/painmgmt.html**

Rasul, AT, and Wright, J: Total joint replacement rehabilitation, 2007. Retrieved July 2008 from **http://www.emedicine.com/pmr/topic221.htm**

Rhodes, LA: Phantom limb pain. In Malawer, MM, and Sugarbaker, PH (eds): Musculoskeletal cancer surgery. Springer, New York, 2001. Retrieved February 2005 from **http://www.sarcoma.org/publications/mcs/ch24.pdf**

Richeimer, S: Phantom limb pain. The Richeimer Pain Report, July 2000. Retrieved February 2005 from **http://www.helpfor pain.com/arch2000jul.htm**

Schuch, CM: Consumer guide for amputees: A guide to lower limb prosthetics: Part 1—Prosthetic designs: Basic concepts. inMotion: a Publication of the Amputee Coalition of America 8(2), 1998, updated 2004. Retrieved February 2005 from **http://www.amputee-coalition.org**

Shonski, C: Pain management: A discussion of the various techniques and types of drugs currently available for pain control with medicines. inMotion: A Publication of the Amputee Coalition of America 8(5), 1998. Retrieved February 2005 from **http://www.amputee-coalition.org/inmotion/sep_oct_98/painmgt.html**

Swain, R, and Ross, D: Lower extremity compartment syndrome: When to suspect acute or chronic pressure buildup, 1999. Retrieved February 2005 from **http://www.postgradmed.com**

U.S. Bone and Joint Decade: The burden of musculoskeletal diseases. American Academy of Orthopaedic Surgeons, Rosemont, IL, 2008. Retrieved July 2008 from **http://www.boneandjointburden.org/**

Wheeless, CR: Compartment syndrome pressure monitoring in Wheeless textbook of orthapeadics. Retrieved July 2008 from **http://www.wheelessonline.com/ortho/12584**

CHAPTER 13

Books

Van Leeuwen, AM, Kranptiz, TR, and Smith, L: Davis's comprehensive handbook of laboratory and diagnostic tests with nursing implications, ed 2. FA Davis, Philadelphia, 2006.

Articles

Demling, RH, and DeSanti, L: Management of partial thickness facial burns (comparison of topical antibiotics and bio-engineered skin substitutes). Burns, 25:256–261, 1999.

DeSanti, L: Pathophysiology and current management of burn injury. Adv Skin Wound Care, 18(6):323–332, 2005.

Hettiaratchy, S, and Dziewulski, P: Pathophysiology and types of burns. BMJ 328:1427–1429, 2004.

Johnson, RM, and Richard, R: Partial-thickness burns: Identification and management. Adv Skin Wound Care 16(4):178–186, 2003.

Morgan, ED, Bledsoe, SC, and Barker, J: Ambulatory management of burns. Am Fam Physician 62(9):2015–2026, 2000.

No author listed: Complementary therapy—Massage therapy and burn debridement. AJN 99(1):15, 1999.

Sheridan, RL: Evaluating and managing burn wounds. Dermatol Nurs 12(1):17–18, 21–28, 2000.

Wiebelhaus, P, and Hansen, SL: Burns: Handle with care. RN 62(11):
52–57, 1999.

Wiebelhaus, P, and Hansen, SL: What you should know about managing
burn emergencies. Nursing2001 31(1):36–41, 2001.

Electronic Resources

American Burn Association: Burn incidence and fact sheet, 2007.
Retrieved March 2008 from **http://www.ameriburn.org/resources
_factsheet.php**

Centers for Disease Control and Prevention: Fire deaths and injuries: Fact
sheet, 2007. Retrieved May 2008 from **http://www.cdc.gov/ncipc/
factsheets/fire.htm**

EAST Practice Management Guidelines Work Group: Practice management guidelines for nutritional support of the trauma patient, n.d.
Eastern Association for the Surgery of Trauma (EAST). Available at
National Guideline Clearinghouse. Retrieved February 2005 from
http//:www.guidelines.gov

Edlich, RF, Drake, DB, and Long, WB: Burns, thermal, 2006. Retrieved
March 2008 from **http://www.emedicine.com/plastic/topic518.htm**

Serebrisky, D, and Nazarian, EB: Inhalation injury, 2006. Retrieved
March 2008 from **http://www.emedicine.com/ped/topic1189.htm**

World Health Organization, International Society for Burn Injuries: Facts
about injuries: Burns. Retrieved May 2008 from **http://www
.ameriburn.org/WHO-ISBIBurnFactsheet.pdf**

CHAPTER 14

Books

Abrams, AC, Pennington, SS, and Lammon, CB: Clinical drug therapy:
Rationales for nursing practice, ed 8. Lippincott, Williams and
Wilkins, Philadelphia, 2007.

Deglin, JD, and Vallerand, AH: Davis's drug guide for nurses, ed 10.
FA Davis, Philadelphia, 2007.

Flynn, JA, and Johnson, T: The Johns Hopkins White Papers: Arthritis.
Stuart Jordon, Baltimore, 2008.

Nettina, SM: Lippincott manual of nursing practice, ed 8. Lippincott,
Williams and Wilkins, Ambler, PA, 2006.

Sampson, JG: Interventions for clients with HIV/AIDS and other
immunodeficiencies. In Ignatavicius, DD, and Workman, ML:
Medical-surgical nursing: Critical thinking for collaborative care,
ed 5. Elsevier Saunders, St. Louis, MO, 2006.

Smeltzer, SS, et al: Brunner and Suddarth's textbook of medical-surgical
nursing, ed 11. Lippincott, Williams and Wilkins, Philadelphia, 2008.

Van Leeuwen, AM, Kranptiz, TR, and Smith, L: Davis's comprehensive
handbook of laboratory and diagnostic tests with nursing implications,
ed 2. FA Davis, Philadelphia, 2006.

Workman, ML: Concepts of inflammation and the immune response.
In Ignatavicius, DD, and Workman, ML: Medical-surgical nursing:
Critical thinking for collaborative care, ed 5. Elsevier Saunders,
St. Louis, MO, 2006.

Articles

Abuedo, MA: Regulations, technology guide multivisceral transplant
success. OR Nurse 1(7):24–29, 2007.

Angus DC, et al: Epidemiology of severe sepsis in the United States:
Analysis of incidence, outcome, and associated costs of care.
Crit Care Med 29:1303–1310, 2001.

Arhens, T: Sepsis: Stopping an insidious killer. Am Nurse Today
2(1):36–39, 2007.

Bruce, ML, and Peck, B: New rheumatoid arthritis treatments. Holistic
Nurs Pract 19(5):197–204, 2005.

Carroll, P: Monitoring the gut to prevent MODS. RN 62(10):34–37, 1999.

Cavanaugh, JC: A qualitative study of stress and coping strategies used by
well spouses of lung transplant candidates. Fam Syst Health/J
Cardiovasc Nurs 10(2):58–70, 2001.

Centers for Disease Control and Prevention: Estimated numbers of persons living with HIV/AIDS, by year and selected characteristics,
2001–2005—33 states and U.S. dependent areas with confidential
name-based HIV infection reporting. Washington, DC, revised 2007.

Coe, PF: Managing pulmonary hypertension in heart transplantation:
Meeting the challenge. Crit Care Nurse 20(2):22–28, 2000.

Cook, L: The value of lab values. AJN 99(5):66–75, 1999.

Crone, CC, and Wise, TN: Psychiatric aspects of transplantation, II:
Preoperative issues. Crit Care Nurse 19(3):51–63, 1999.

Crone, CC, and Wise, TN: Psychiatric aspects of transplantation, III:
Postoperative issues. Crit Care Nurse 19(4):28–38, 1999.

Garcia-Jones, S: A step-by-step approach to HIV/AIDS. Nurse Pract
31(6):26–39, 2006.

Good, EW: Caring for patients with donor organs. Nursing2000 30(6):34,
2000.

Grady, KL: When to transplant: Recipient selection for heart transplantation. J Cardiovasc Nurs 10(2):58–70, 1996.

Greenwald, JL, et al: A rapid review of Rapid HIV Antibody Tests. Curr
Infect Dis Rep 8:125–131, 2006.

Hoffman, RL, and Reeder, SJ: Mycophenolate mofetil (CellCept): The
newest immunosuppressant. Crit Care Nurse 18(3):50–57, 1998.

Jones, SG: A step-by-step approach to HIV/AIDS. Nurse Pract
31(6):26–39, 2006.

Kleinpell, RM: Stop severe sepsis in its tracks. Nursing2008 1(1):
20–26, 2006.

Kurz, JM, and Cavanaugh, JC: A qualitative study of stress and coping
strategies used by well spouses of lung transplant candidates.
Families, Systems, & Health 19(2)181–197, 2001.

Mallard, VJ, et al: Increasing knowledge of sexually transmitted infection
risk. Nurse Pract 32(2):26–32, 2007.

Martin, SA: Posttransplant lymphoproliferative disease in a pediatric
multivisceral transplant recipient. Crit Care Nurse 18(3):74–80, 1998.

Moons, P: Post-transplant immunosuppression. Heart Lung 27:34, 1998.

No author listed: AIDS File: Achieving medication adherence. AJN
99(1):17, 1999.

No author listed: AIDS File: Return to unsafe sexual behaviors. AJN
99(9):17, 1999.

Pressly, KB, and Quattlebaum, LS: Infection control: Vibrio vulnificus
sepsis. Crit Care Nurse 20(5):78–83, 2000.

Ramsburg, KL: Rheumatoid arthritis. AJN 100(11):40–43, 2000.

Rayl, J: Home care of the cancer patient. Adv Nurses 2(14):23–33, 2000.

Rayl, J: Home health care of the post-transplant patient. Adv Nurses
2(12):25–35, 2000.

Ress, B: AIDS/HIV—Caring for patients with HIV disease in the millen-
nium. Crit Care Nurse, 21(1):69–76, 2001.

Schmelzer, M, and Stam, MA: A hidden menace: Hemolytic uremic syndrome. AJN 100(11):26–32, 2000.

Sears, JR, and Ganger, PM: Antibiotics to treat RA. RN 63(1):41–42,
2000.

Sheff, B: Reining in a runaway infection. Nursing99 29(10):60–61, 1999.

Sullivan, DM, and Schoonover-Shoffner, K: Sorting through the stem cell
hype. J Christian Nurs 24(4):182–189, 2007.

Swam, A, Daley, AM, and Crowley, A: Contraceptive counseling for adolescents with HIV. Nurse Pract 32(5):38–45, 2007.

Tahan, HA: Patients waiting for heart transplantion: An analysis of vulnerability. Crit Care Nurse 18(4):40–48, 1998.

Veitz, A: Managing the side effects of chemotherapy. Adv Nurses
2(14):11–13, 2000.

Webb, A, and Norton, M: Clinical assessment of symptom-focused health
related quality of life in HIV/AIDS. JANAC 15(2):67–81, 2004.

Wood, S, and Lavieri, MC: What you need to know about sepsis.
Nursing2007 37(3):46–51, 2007.

Electronic Resources

United Nations Programme on HIV/AIDS and World Health
Organization: AIDS epidemic update, December 2007. Retrieved
August 2008 from **http://data.unaids.org/pub/EPISlides/2007/
2007_epiupdate_en.pdf**

American College of Rheumatology: Guidelines for the management of
rheumatoid arthritis, updated 2002. Retrieved March 2008 from
http://www.rheumatology.org/publications/guidelines/index.asp

Armington, K: How to recognize and prevent HIV infections. Clin
Advisor (December):36–42, 2007. Retrieved August 2008 from

http://www.clinicaladvisor.com/content/Issue_Story.26.0.html?&no_cache=1&tx_cortlandtmagissue_pi1%5Bpointer%5D=0&tx_cortlandtmagissue_pi1%5Bmode%5D=1&tx_cortlandtmagissue_pi1%5BshowUid%5D=2005

Arthritis Foundation: Rheumatoid arthritis: What is it?, 2007. Retrieved March 2008 from **http://www.arthritis.org/disease-center.php?disease_id=31**

Arthritis Foundation and National Pharmaceutical Council: A closer look at arthritis, 2002. Retrieved July 2008 from **http://www.npcnow.org/resources/PDFs/CL_Arthritis.pdf**

Burdette, SD, and Parilo, M: Systemic inflammatory response syndrome, 2007. Retrieved August, 2008 from **http://www.emedicine.com/med/topic2227.htm**

Centers for Disease Control and Prevention: HIV/AIDS surveillance report: Cases of HIV infection and AIDS in the United States and dependent areas, 2005. Vol. 17, revised 2007. Retrieved August 2008 from **http://www.cdc.gov/hiv/topics/surveillance/resources/reports/2005report/pdf/2005SurveillanceReport.pdf**

Cunha, BA: Sepsis, bacterial, 2008. Retrieved August 2008 from **http://www.emedicine.com/MED/topic3163.htm**

Dubin, J: HIV infection and AIDS, 2008. Retrieved July 2008 from **http://www.emedicine.com/EMERG/topic253.htm**

Glynn, M, and Rhodes, P: Estimated HIV prevalence in the United States at the end of 2003. National HIV Conference, Atlanta, 2005. Abstract T1-B1101. Retrieved March 2008 from **http://www.aegis.com/conferences/NHIVPC/2005/T1-B1101.html**

Gupta, K, and Bhagia, SM: Rheumatoid arthritis, updated 2006. Retrieved July 2008 from **http://www.emedicine.com/pmr/TOPIC124.HTM**

Hauboldt, RH: 2007 U.S. organ and tissue transplant cost estimate, 2007. Retrieved August 2008 from **http://www.milliman.com/expertise/healthcare/publications/rr/pdfs/2007-US-Organ-Transplant-RR11-01-07.pdf**

Health24: Symptoms and phases of HIV infection & Aids, updated July 20, 2004. Retrieved March 2008 from **http://www.health24.com/medical/Condition_centres/777-792-814-1756,22216.asp**

Highleyman, L: The stages of HIV disease. San Francisco AIDS Foundation, 2005. Retrieved July 2008 from **http://www.thebody.com/content/treat/art2506.html**

Hutchinson, AB, et al: The economic burden of HIV in the United States in the era of highly active antiretroviral therapy: Evidence of continuing racial and ethnic differences. J Acquir Immune Defic Syndr 43(4):451–457, 2006. Retrieved July 2008 from **http://www.ncbi.nlm.nih.gov/pubmed/16980906NAM**

Joint United Nations Programme on HIV/AIDS: 2006 Report on the global AIDS epidemic, 2006. Retrieved March 2008 from **http://www.unaids.org/en/KnowledgeCentre/HIVData/GlobalReport/**

Khamsi, R: Drug-resistant HIV battled in a new way. HIV Drug Resistance Database, 2007. Retrieved August 2008 from **http://www.newscientist.com/article.ns?id=dn10893**

King, RD, and Worthington, R: Arthritis, rheumatoid, updated 2006. Retrieved July 2008 from **http://www.emedicine.com/EMERG/topic48.htm**

Matsumoto, AK, Bathon, J, and Bingham, CO: Rheumatoid arthritis treatment, n.d. Retrieved March 2008 from **http://www.hopkins-arthritis.org/arthritis-info/rheumatoid-arthritis/rheum_treat.html**

National Institute of Arthritis and Musculoskeletal and Skin Disease: Rheumatoid arthritis, updated 2004. Retrieved March 2008 from **http://www.niams.nih.gov/Health_Info/Rheumatic_Disease/default.asp**

New York Times: Rheumatoid arthritis in-depth report, 2007. Retrieved March 2008 from **http://health.nytimes.com/health/guides/disease/rheumatoid-arthritis/print.html**

No author listed: Stages of HIV, updated 2004. Retrieved March 2008 from **http://www.aidsmap.com/en/docs/6DF087FA-BF76-4957-8E6E-637D4840AE34.asp**

No author listed: Currently approved drugs for HIV: A comparative chart, revised 2008. Retrieved March 2008 from **http://www.aidsmeds.com/articles/DrugChart_10632.shtml**

No author listed: AIDSinfo, n.d. Retrieved August 2008 from **http://aidsinfo.nih.gov/guidelines**

Noble, R: Introduction to HIV types, groups and subtypes, 2008. Retrieved August 2008 from **http://www.avert.org/hivtypes.htm**

Ojo, AO, et al: Chronic renal failure after transplantation of a nonrenal organ. N Engl J Med, 349(10):931–940, 2003. Retrieved August 2008 from **http://www.ncbi.nlm.nih.gov/pubmed/12954741**

Parimon, T, et al: Pretransplant lung function, respiratory failure, and mortality after stem cell transplant. Am J Respir and Crit Care Med 172(3):384–390, 2005. Retrieved August 2008 from **http://ajrccm.atsjournals.org/cgi/content/full/172/3/384**

Pellegrino, B, and Schmidt, RJ: Immunosuppression, 2007. Retrieved August 2008 from **http://www.emedicine.com/med/topic3558.htm**

Powderly, WG: Opportunistic infections, 1999. Retrieved August 2008 from **http://doctor.medscape.com/viewarticle/412669**

Saag, M: Annual U.S. health care costs per AIDS patient, 2002. Retrieved August 2008 from **http://www.kaisernetwork.org/daily_reports/rep_index.cfm?DR_ID=12268**

Sharma, S, and Mink, S: Septic shock, 2007. Retrieved August 2008 from **http://www.emedicine.com/med/topic2101.htm**

Sharma, S, and Unruh, H: History of adult transplantation, 2006. Retrieved August 2008 from **http://www.emedicine.com/med/TOPIC3497.HTM**

Twyman, T: Tissue matching for transplants, 2004. Retrieved August 2008 from **http://genome.wellcome.ac.uk/doc_WTD020937.html**

U.S. Department of Health and Human Services: OPTN/SRTR annual report: Survival rate data tables, 2007. Retrieved August 2008 from **http://www.ustransplant.org/annual_reports/current/113_surv-new_dh.htm**

U.S. Food and Drug Administration: Information on COX-2, updated July 18, 2005. Retrieved March 2008 from **http://www.fda.gov/cder/drug/infopage/cox2/**

U.S. Organ and Procurement Network and the Scientific Registry of Transplant Recipients: Annual report: Transplant data 1997–2006, 2007. Retrieved August 2008 from **http://www.ustransplant.org/annual_reports/current/**

CHAPTER 15

Books

American Psychiatric Association: DSM-IV-TR, diagnostic and statistical manual of mental disorders, ed 4, text revision. Washington, DC, 2000, pp 583–595.

Deglin, JH, and Valler, AH: Davis's drug guide for nurses, ed 9. FA Davis, Philadelphia, 2005.

Doenges, M, Townsend, M, and Moorhouse, M: Psychiatric nursing care plans, ed 3. FA Davis, Philadelphia, 1998.

Erickson, E: Childhood and society, ed 2. WW Norton, New York, 1963.

Feldman, D, and Lasher, SA: The end-of-life handbook: A compassionate guide to connecting with and caring for a dying loved one. New Harbinger Publications, Oakland, CA, 2008.

Glaser, BG, and Strauss, AL: Time for dying. Aldine, Chicago, 1968.

Hartung, J, and Galvin, M: Energy psychology and EMDR: Combining forces to optimize treatment. WW Norton, New York, 2003.

Hausman, KA: Interventions for clients with problems of the central nervous system. In Ignatavicius, DD, and Workman, ML. Medical-surgical nursing: Critical thinking for collaborative care, ed 5. Elsevier Saunders, St. Louis, MO, 2006.

Kowalak, J, et al: Handbook of signs and symptoms, ed 2. Lippincott Williams & Wilkins, Springhouse, PA, 2002.

London, ML, et al: Maternal & child nursing care, ed 2. Pearson Prentice Hall, Upper Saddle River, NJ, 2007.

Nelson-Marsh, JD: Chronic disorders of neurologic function. In Copstead, LEC, and Banasik, JL (eds): Pathophysiology, ed 3. Elsevier Saunders, St. Louis, MO, 2005.

Skeel, R (ed): Handbook of cancer chemotherapy, ed 6. Lippincott Williams & Wilkins, Philadelphia, 2003.

Theander, S: Outcome and prognosis in anorexia nervosa and bulimia. In Szmukler, GI, et al (eds): Anorexia nervosa and bulimic disorders. Pergamon, London, 1985.

Townsend, MC: Psychiatric mental health nursing concepts of care in evidence-based practice, ed 5. FA Davis, Philadelphia, 2006.

University of Missouri: Handbook of disabilities, substance abuse. Product of RECP7 and Curators of the University of Missouri, Columbia, 2006.

U.S. Department of Health and Human Services: Results from the 2006 national survey on drug use and Health: National findings. DHHS publication (SMA) 07-4293. U.S. Department of Health and Human Services, Substance Abuse and Mental Health Services Administration. Office of Applied Studies, Rockville, MD, September 2007, p 69.

Venes, D (ed): Taber's cyclopedic medical dictionary, ed 20. FA Davis, Philadelphia, 2005.

Young, B, Flamm, JA, and Graham RM: Improved options for better care: The role of new HIV-1 protease inhibitors. A continuing education monograph, 3/2004.

Articles

Allen, CH: Providing compassionate end-of-life care. Nursing Made Incredibly Easy! 6(4):46–53, 2008.

Amella, EJ: Presentation of illness in older adults. Am J of Nurs 104(10):40–51, 2004.

Barry, M: How growth factors help chronic wounds heal. Nursing2000 30(5):52–53, 2000.

Bayard, M, et al: Alcohol withdrawal syndrome. Am Fam Physician 69(6):1443–1450, 2004.

Brenner, ZR: Preventing postoperative complications: What's old, what's new, what's tried-and-true. Nursing99 29(10):34–39, 1999.

Bridges, KJ, Trujillo, EB, and Jacobs, DO: Nutrition: Alcohol-related thiamine deficiency and malnutrition. Crit Care Nurse 19(6):80–85, 1999.

Brown, MK, and Worobec, F: Hypodermoclysis: Another way to replace fluids. Nursing2000 30(5):58–59, 2000.

Chau Patel, CT, et al: Vacuum-assisted wound closure. AJN, 100(12):45–48, 2000.

Clinical rounds: Wound closure. Nursing2000 30(5):62, 2000.

Creechan, T: Combining mechanical ventilation with hospice care in the home: Death with dignity. Crit Care Nurse 20(3):49, 2000.

Criddle, L: Critical Care Extra: A pinch of salt: Therapy should be on slow restoration of the serum sodium level. AJN 106(10): 72CC–72DD, 2006.

Daniels, SM: Improved care for surgical patients. OR Nurse 2008 1(7):18–22, 2008.

Daus, C: Maintaining mobility: Assistive equipment helps the geriatric population stay active and independent. Rehab Manage 12(5):58–61, 1999.

Deering, CG, and Jennings, D: Communicating with children and adolescents. AJN 102 (3):34, 2002.

Derby, SA: Opioid conversion guidelines for managing adult cancer pain. AJN 99(10):62–65, 1999.

Dest, VM: Oncology today: New horizons—Colorectal cancer. RN 63(3):54–59, 2000.

DiMaria-Ghalili, RA, and Amella, E: Nutrition in older adults. AJN 105(3):50, 2005.

Egan, KA, and Arnold, RL: Grief and bereavement care. AJN 103(9):42–52, 2003.

Ewing, JA: Detecting alcoholism: The CAGE questionnaire. JAMA 252:1905–1907, 1984.

Ferrell, B, Coyne, P, and Uman, G: End-of-life care: Nurses speak out. Nursing2000 30(7):54–57, 2000.

Furman, J: Taking a holistic approach to the dying time. Nursing2000 30(6):46, 2000.

Gaguski, ME: A private place: Consolation for grieving families. AJN 99(4):18, 1999.

Giarelli, E, Pisano, R, and McCorkle, R: Stable and able. AJN 100(12):26, 2000.

Ginther, C: Schuckit addresses state-of-the-art addiction treatments. Psychiatr Times 16(4):55–57, 1999.

Granholm, E, et al: Tropicamide effects on pupil size and pupillary light reflexes in Alzheimer's and Parkinson's disease. Int J Psychophysiol 47:95–115, 2003.

Gray-Vickery, P: Combating abuse, part 1: Protecting the older adult. Nursing2000 30(7):34–38, 2000.

Grogan, TA: Bringing bloodless surgery into the mainstream. Nursing99 29(11):58–61, 1999.

Halmi, KA, et al: Comorbidity of psychiatric diagnoses in anorexia nervosa. Arch Gen Psychiatry 48:712–718, 1991.

Hankins, J: The role of albumin in fluid and electrolyte balance. J Infusion Nursing 29(5):260–265, 2006.

Henderson-Martin, B: No more surprises: Screening patients for alcohol abuse. AJN 100(9):26–32, 2000.

Hess, CT: Wound care: When to use hydrocolloid dressings. Nursing99 29(11):20, 1999.

Hess, CT: Wound care: When to use composite dressings. Nursing2000 30(5):26, 2000.

Horn, LB: Reducing the risk of falls in the elderly. Rehab Manage 13(5):36–38/96, 2000.

Jennings-Ingle, S: The sobering facts about alcohol withdrawal syndrome. Nursing Made Incredibly Easy! 5(1):50–60, 2007.

Kearney, K: Hyperkalemia. AJN 100(1):55–56, 2000.

Kirckhoff, KT, et al: Intensive care nurses' experiences with end-of-life care. Am J Crit Care 9(1):36, 2000.

Kleinbeck, S: Development of the perioperative nursing data set. AORN J 70(1):15–28, 1999.

Komurcu, S, et al: Common symptoms in advanced cancer. Semin Oncol 27(1):24–33, 2000.

Lussier-Cushing, et al: Is your medical/surgical patient withdrawing from alcohol? Nursing2007 37(10):50–55, 2007.

Mazanec, P, and Tyler, MK: Cultural considerations in end-of-life care. AJN 103(3):50–57, 2003.

McKee, RJ: Clarifying advance directives. Nursing99 29(5):52, 1999.

Mentes, J: Oral hydration in older adults: Greater awareness is needed in preventing, recognizing, and treating dehydration. AJN 106(6): 40–49, 2006.

Miller, J: Potassium in the balance: Understanding hyperkalemia and hypokalemia. LPN2007 2(5):42–49, 2006.

Munoz, C, and Hilgenberg, C: Ethnopharmacology. AJN 105(8): 40–48, 2005.

Nelson, K, et al: Common complications of advanced cancer. Semin Oncol 27(1):34–44, 2000.

Nevius, KS, and D'Arcy, Y: Decrease recovery time with proper pain management. OR Nurse 2008 2(4):34–39, 2008.

de Nijs, EJM, Ros, W, and Gripdonck, MH: Nursing intervention for fatigue during the treatment for cancer. Cancer Nursing 31(3): 191–206, 2008.

No author listed: Treatment of alcoholism—Part II. Harvard Mental Health Lett 16(12):1, 2000.

No author listed: Disaster and trauma. Harvard Mental Health Lett 18(7):1–5, 2002.

Ott, BB: Advance directives: The emerging body of research. Am J Crit Care 8(1):514–519, 1999.

Panke, JT: Difficulties in managing pain at the end of life. AJN 102(7):26–33, 2002.

Pasero, C, and McCaffery, M: Pain control: Using agonist-antagonist opioids and antagonist drugs. AJN 99(1):20–23, 1999.

Pitorak, EF: Care at the time of death. AJN 103(7):42–52, 2003.

Rentz, CA: Alzheimer's disease: An elusive thief. Nurs Manage 39(6):33–37, 2008.

Sachse, DS: Emergency: Delirium tremens. AJN 100(5):41–42, 2000.

Salati, DS: Caring for a sick child in a nonpediatric setting. Nursing2004 34(4):54–61, 2004.

Scanlon, C: Ethical concerns in end-of-life care. AJN 103(1):48–53, 2003.

Schiffman, RF: Drug and substance use in adolescents. MCN, Am J Maternal/Child Nurs 29(1):21–27, 2004.

Schmidt, C, et al: Hospitalized children's perceptions of nurses and nurse behaviors. MCN, Am J of Maternal/Child Nurs, 32(6):336–342, 2007.

Schmidt, TC: New eye on diagnostics: Assessing a sodium and fluid imbalance. Nursing2000 30(1):18, 2000.

Schutzius, P: Update on wound care. Rehab Manage 12(6):30–34, 1999.

Sharer, J: Tackling sundowning in a patient with Alzheimer's disease. MedSurg Nurs 17(1):27–30, 2008.

Sheehan, DK, and Schirm, V: End-of-life care of older adults. AJN 103 (11):48–57, 2003.

Skokal, W: How to spot this catheter complication. RN 62(10):26–28, 1999.

Smith, R: Increasing independence: Advancements in rolling walkers get clients back into the outside world. Rehab Manage 12(5):62, 1999.

Snow, D: Addiction: Working with relapse. AJN 99(7):69, 1999.

Solomon, PR, et al: A 7 minute neurocognitive screening battery highly sensitive to Alzheimer's disease. Arch Neurol 56(1):123–124, 1999.

Sprigle, S: Prescribing pressure ulcer treatment. Rehab Manage 13(5):72–77, 2000.

Springer, R: The Surgical Care Improvement Project—Focusing on infection control. Plast Surg Nurs 27(3):163–167, 2007.

Star, JH: Radiation is lonely. RN 63(8):40–42, 2000.

Stewart, KB, and Richards, AB: Recognizing and managing your patient's alcohol abuse. Nursing2000 30(2):56–59, 2000.

Stevens, WJ: Fluid balance and resuscitation: Critical aspects of ICU care. Nursing2008 Critical Care 3(2):12–21, 2008.

Stockdell, R, and Amella, EJ: How to try this: The Edinburgh Feeding Evaluation in Dementia Scale. AJN 108(8):46–54, 2008.

Stuppaeck, CH, et al: Assessment of the alcohol withdrawal syndrome: Validity and reliability for the translated and modified Clinical Institute Withdrawal Assessment for Alcohol scale (CIWA-A). Addiction 89(10):1287–1202, 1994.

Suter, PM, Rogers, J, and Strack, C: Hospice & palliative pare: Artificial nutrition for the terminally ill: A reasoned approach. Home Healthcare Nurse 26(1):23–29, 2008.

Tesselaar, H: Joe wanted to die alone . . . or so he said. Nursing99 29(5):54, 1999.

Thompson, J: A practical guide to wound care. RN 63(1):48–52, 2000.

Tilden, VP: Advance directives. AJN 100(12):48, 2000.

Vassallo, BM: The spiritual aspects of dying at home. Holistic Nurs Pract 15(2):19–29, 2001.

Virani, R, and Sofer, D: Improving the quality of end-of-life care. AJN 103 (5):52–60, 2003.

Wolfe, S: Are you ready for bloodless medicine? RN 63(5):42–46, 2000.

Zambroski, CH: Hospice as an alternative model of care for older patients with end-stage heart failure. J Cardiovasc Nurs 19(1):76–85, 2004.

Pamphlets

Forest Pharmaceuticals: Understanding and living with Alzheimer's Disease, your guide to treatment and help. Treatment options and expectations. In it Together series, 2007.

The Mayo Clinic: Pain-pill addiction: What's the risk? Mayo Foundation for Medical Education and Research, June 2006.

No author listed: The family matters: Substance abuse and the American family. New York: The National Center on Addiction and Substance Abuse at Columbia University, New York, 2005.

No author listed: What does America think about addiction prevention and treatment? Robert Wood Johnson Foundation, Princeton, NJ, 2007.

Electronic Resources

Al-Sanouri, I, Dikin, M, and Soubani, AO: Critical care aspects of alcohol abuse, 2005. Retrieved August 2008 from **http://www.medscape .com/viewarticle/501977_2**

Alvarez, N: Alzheimer disease in individuals with Down syndrome, 2008. Retrieved August 2008 from **http://www.emedicine.com/neuro/ TOPIC552.HTM**

Alzheimer's Association: FDA-approved treatments for Alzheimer's, 2007. Retrieved August 2008 from **http://www.alz.org/national/ documents/topicsheet_treatments.pdf**

Alzheimer's Association: 2008 Alzheimer's disease facts and figures. Alzheimer's & Dementia 4(2), 2008. Retrieved March 2008 from **http://www.alz.org/national/documents/report_alzfactsfigures2008.pdf**

Alzheimer's Disease Education and Referral Center: Treatment, 2008. Retrieved August 2008 from **http://www.nia.nih.gov/Alzheimers/ AlzheimersInformation/Treatment/**

American Academy of Pediatrics (AAP): Pediatric terrorism and disaster preparedness: A resource for pediatricians. Foltin, GL, Schonfeld, DJ, and Shannon, MW (eds): AHRQ publication 06(07)-0056. Agency for Healthcare Research and Quality, Rockville, MD, 2006. Retrieved August 2008 from **http://www.ahrq.gov/research/pedprep/ pedresource.pdf**

American Cancer Society: Cancer facts & figures 2007. Retrieved August 2008 from **http://www.cancer.org/downloads/STT/ CAFF2007PWSecured.pdf**

American Cancer Society: Cancer facts & figures 2007—Special section: Cancer-related pain, 2007, pp 22–31. Retrieved August 2008 from **http://www.cancer.org/downloads/STT/CAFF2007PWSecured.pdf**

American Council for Drug Education (ACDE): Basic facts about drugs: Alcohol. Retrieved August 2008 from **http://www.acde.org/parent/ Research.htm**

American Foundation for Suicide Prevention (AFSP): Facts and figures: Alcohol and suicide, 2008. Retrieved August 2008 from **http:// www.afsp.org/index.cfm?fuseaction=home.viewpage&page_id= 050fea9f-b064-4092-b1135c3a70de1fda**

Anandarajah, G, and Hight, E: Spirituality and medical practice: Using the HOPE questions as a practical tool for spiritual assessment. Am Fam Physician 63(1):81–89, 2001. Retrieved August 2008 from **http://www.aafp.org/afp/20010101/81.html**

Association of periOperative Registered Nurses (AORN): Correct site surgery tool kit: Building a safer tomorrow, 2009. Available from **http://www.aorn.org/PracticeResources/ToolKits/ CorrectSiteSurgeryToolKit/**

Barklay, L: CSF markers predict Alzheimer's in patients with mild cognitive impairment, 2002. Retrieved August 2008 from **http://www .medscape.com/viewarticle/444954**

Burns, MJ, Price, JB, and Lekawa, ME: Delirium tremens, updated July 24, 2008. Retrieved April 2009 from **http://emedicine .medscape.com/article/166032-overview**

Centers for Disease Control and Prevention: Methadone maintenance treatment, 2002. Retrieved August 2008 from **http://www.cdc.gov/ idu/facts/Methadone.htm**

Centers for Disease Control and Prevention: Coping with a traumatic event: Information for health professionals, reviewed 2005. Retrieved August 2008 from **http://www.bt.cdc.gov/masscasualties/ copingpro.asp**

Centers for Disease Control and Precention: Deaths: Final data for 2005. National Vital Statistics Report 56(10), 2008. Retrieved August 2008 from **http://www.cdc.gov/nchs/data/nvsr/nvsr56/nvsr56_10.pdf**

Centers for Disease Control and Prevention: National Vital Statistics Reports 56(16), June 11, 2008. Retrieved August 2008 from **http://www.cdc.gov/nchs/data/nvsr/nvsr56/nvsr56_16.pdf**

The Children's Hospital of Philadelphia: Preparing your child for hospitalization and medical procedures, n.d. [Portal to age-specific sites] Retrieved August 2008 from **http://www.chop.edu/consumer/jsp/ division/generic.jsp?id=82125**

Cincinnati Children's Hospital Medical Center: Evidenced based clinical practice guidelines for fever of uncertain source in children 2 to 36 months of age, reviewed 2006. Retrieved August 2008 from **http://www.guideline.gov/summary/summary.aspx?doc_id=5613& nbr=003783&string=child+AND+fever+AND+treatment**

Cohagan, A, and Worthington, R: Alcohol and substance abuse evaluation, 2007. Retrieved August 2008 from **http://www.emedicine.com/ EMERG/topic20.htm**

Cohen, JS: Alcohol intoxication: Signs and symptoms, reviewed 2006. Retrieved August 2008 from **http://www.emedicinehealth.com/ alcohol_intoxication/page2_em.htm**

Cravens, DD, and Zweig, S: Urinary catheter management. Am Fam Physician, 61(2):369–76, 2000. Retrieved August 2008 from **http://www.aafp.org/afp/20000115/369.html**

Cunha, BA: Nursing home acquired pneumonia, updated 2008. Retrieved August 2008 from **http://www.emedicine.com/med/topic3230.htm**

Dowling-Castronovo, A, and Bradway, C: Urinary incontinence—Nursing standards of practice protocol, updated 2008. Retrieved August 2008 from **http://consultgerirn.org/topics/urinary_incontinence/want _to_know_more**

Emanuel, L, et al: The last hours of living: Practical advice for clinicians, 2006. Retrieved August 2008 from **http://www.medscape.com/ viewprogram/5808?src=nursecenl**

EMDR Institute Inc: A brief description of EMDR, 2004. Retrieved August 2008 from **http://www.emdr.com/briefdes.htm**

Ericson, N: Substance abuse: The nations' number one health problem. U.S. Department of Justice, Office of Justice Programs, Office of Juvenile Justice and Delinquency Prevention, May 2001. Retrieved August 2008 from **http://www.ncjrs.gov/pdffiles1/ojjdp/ fs200117.pdf**

Family Caregiver Alliance: Selected long-term care statistics, 2005. Retrieved August 2008 from **http://www.caregiver.org/caregiver/jsp/ content_node.jsp?nodeid=440**

Ferrell, B: End-of-life eduation for nurses, 2007. Retrieved August 2008 from **http://www.medscape.com/viewarticle/559790?src=mp**

Geldmacher, DS: Treatment guidelines for Alzheimer's disease: Redefining perceptions in primary care. Prim Care Companion J Clin Psychiatry 9(2):113–121, 2007. Retrieved August 2008 from **http:// www.pubmedcentral.nih.gov/articlerender.fcgi?artid=1896294**

Gossman, WG: Delirium tremens, 2007. Retrieved August 2008 from **http://www.emedicine.com/emerg/TOPIC123.HTM**

Henkel, GE: Nutrition basics for LTC. Caring for the Ages 5(1):12–22, 2004. Retrieved August 2008 from **http://www.amda.com/ publications/caring/january2004/nutrition.cfm**

Hospice Association of America: Hospice facts & statistics, updated 2002. Retrieved August 2008 from **http://www.nahc.org/consumer/ hpcstats.html**

Joint Commission on Accreditation of Healthcare Organizations: Universal protocol for preventing wrong site, wrong procedure, wrong person surgery(tm), 2003. Retrieved January 2005 from **http:// www.jcaho.org/index.htm**

Joint Commission on Accreditation of Healthcare Organizations: 2008 Hospital National Patient Safety Goals. "Prevent Errors in Surgery" section. Retrieved August 2008 from **http://www.jointcommission.org/**

Joint Commission on Accreditation of Healthcare Organizations: Office-Based Surgery National Patient Safety Goals, 2008. Retrieved August 2008 from **http://www.jointcommission.org/**

Joint Commission on Accreditation of Healthcare Organizations: 2008 Ambulatory National Patient Safety Goals. Retrieved August 2008 from **http://www.jointcommission.org/**

Kaplan, RJ: Cancer and rehabilitation, updated 2006. Retrieved August 2008. **http://www.emedicine.com/pmr/topic226.htm**

Kids Health for Parents: Fever and taking your child's temperature, reviewed 2007. Retrieved August 2008 from **http://kidshealth.org/ parent/general/aches/fever.html**

Kiecolt-Glaser, JK, et al: Psychosocial modifiers of immunocompetence in medical students. Psychosom Med 46(1):7–14, 1984. Retrieved August 2008 from **http://www.ncbi.nlm.nih.gov/pubmed/6701256**

Kiecolt-Glaser, JK, et al: Emotions, morbidity, and mortality: New perspectives from psychoneuroimmunology. Annu Rev Psychol 53:83–107, 2002. Retrieved August 2008 from **http://arjournals .annualreviews.org/doi/abs/10.1146/annurev.psych.53.100901.135217**

Kresevic, DM, and Mezey, M: Asssessment of function of critical importance in acute care of older adults. Geriatric guideline. National Guideline Clearinghouse, 2003. Available from **http://www .guideline.gov**

Kuljis, RO: Alzheimer's disease, 2007. Retrieved August 2008 from **http://www.emedicine.com/neuro/TOPIC13.HTM**

Leavitt, SB: Evidence for the efficacy of Naltrexone in the treatment of alcohol dependence (alcoholism), 2002. Retrieved August 2008 from **http://www.dpt.samhsa.gov/pdf/NTXWPFinalPDF.pdf**

Lunney, J: Trajectories of dying: There's more than one way to go. Science and Theology Seminar, Oak Ridge, TN, 2007. Retrieved August 2008 from **http://fumcor.org/clientimages/33585/ science_theology/lunneytn21007.pdf**

Lyons, SS: Fall prevention for older adults, 2004. University of Iowa Gerontological Interventions Research Center. National Guideline Clearinghouse. Available from **http://www.guideline.gov**

Malloy, P, et al: End-of-life care: Improving communication skills to enhance palliative care. Top Adv Nurs Pract eJournal, 2008. Retrieved August 2008 from **http://www.medscape.com/viewarticle/574420**

McKeown, NJ, and West, PL: Withdrawal syndromes, 2008. Retrieved August 2008 from **http://www.emedicine.com/EMERG/ topic643.htm**

McNicholas, L: Clinical guidelines for the use of Buprenorphine in the treatment of opioid addiction: A treatment improvement protocol (TIP 40), 2004. Retrieved August 2008 from **http://buprenorphine .samhsa.gov/Bup_Guidelines.pdf**

Medical College of Georgia: Antibody detection in Alzheimer's may improve diagnosis, treatment. ScienceDaily, 2004. Retrieved August 2008 from **http://www.sciencedaily.com/releases/2004/06/ 040603064539.htm**

Merck Manuals Alcohol: Wernicke's encephalopathy, 2005a. Retrieved August 2008 from **http://www.merck.com/mmpe/sec15/ch198/ ch198b.hrml#sec15-ch198b-234**

Merck Manuals: Children with chronic health conditions, 2005b. Retrieved August 2008 from **http://www.merck.com/mmpe/ sec19/ch268/ch268c.html**

Miller, M, et al: Cancer and the risk of suicide in older Americans. J Clin Oncol 26(29):4720–4724, 2008. Retrieved August 2008 from **http://www.ncbi.nlm.nih.gov/sites/entrez/18695256?dopt=Abstract &holding=f1000,f1000m,isrctn**

Misono, S, et al: Incidence of suicide in persons with cancer. J Clin Oncol 26(29):4731–4738, 2008. Retrieved August 2008 from **http://www .ncbi.nlm.nih.gov/pubmed/18695257?ordinalpos=1&itool =EntrezSystem2.PEntrez.Pubmed.Pubmed_ResultsPanel.Pubmed _RVDocSum**

Morgan Stanley Children's Hospital of New York Presbyterian: Preparing a child for surgery, n.d. [Portal to age-specific sites.] Retrieved August 2008 from **http://www.childrensnyp.org/mschony/P03032.html**

Munetz, MR, and Benjamin, S: How to examine patients using the Abnormal Involuntary Movement Scale. Hosp Commun Psychiatry 39(11):1172–1177, 1988. Reference courtesy of the Virtual En-psychlopedia by Dr. Bob, **http://www.dr-bob.org/tips/aims.html**

Myrick, H: Diagnosis of alcohol dependence. Medscape Psychiatry & Ment Health 11(2), 2006. Retrieved August 2008 from **http://www .medscape.com/viewarticle/543758**

National Institute on Aging: Alzheimer's disease medications fact sheet, updated 2008. Retrieved August 2008 from **http://www.nia.nih.gov/ Alzheimers/Publications/medicationsfs.htm**

National Institute on Alcohol Abuse and Alcoholism: Twelve-month prevalence and population estimates of DSM-IV alcohol abuse by age, sex, and race-ethnicity: United States, 2001–2002. Retrieved August 2008 from **http://www.niaaa.nih.gov/Resources/DatabaseResources/ QuickFacts/AlcoholDependence/abusdep1.htm**

National Institute on Drug Abuse: Principles of drug addiction treatment: A research based guide, 2000. Retrieved August 2008 from **http://www.nida.nih.gov/PODAT/PODATindex.html**

National Institute on Drug Abuse: Commonly abused drugs, updated 2008a. Retrieved August 2008 from **http://www.drugabuse.gov/ DrugPages/DrugsofAbuse.html**

National Institute on Drug Abuse: NIDA InfoFacts: Treatment approaches for drug addiction, revised 2008b. Retrieved August 2008 from **http://www.drugabuse.gov/infofacts/Treatmeth.html**

National Institute of Mental Health (NIMH): Suicides in the U.S.: Statistics and prevention, reviewed 2008. NIH Publication 06-4594. Retrieved August 2008 from **http://www.nimh.nih.gov/health/ publications/suicide-in-the-us-statistics-and-prevention.shtml**

The Nemours Foundation: 10 Kids' Health Issues to watch in 2007. Retrieved August 2008 from **http://kidshealth.org/parent/positive/ family/issues_2007.html**

No author listed: Blood test results—Normal ranges, updated August 11, 2007. Retrieved August 2008 from **http://www.bloodbook.com/ ranges.html**

O'Brien, MC, Alson, R, and Jobe, D: Alcoholic ketoacidosis, updated 2007. Retrieved August 2008 from **http://www.emedicine.com/ emerg/topic21.htm**

Office of National Drug Control Policy (ONDC): Teens and prescription drugs: An analysis of recent trends on the emerging threat, 2007. Retrieved August 2008 from **http://www.mediacampaign.org/teens/ brochure.pdf**

Robins, JL, et al: Research on psychoneuroimmunology: Tai chi as a stress management approach for individuals with HIV disease. Appl Nurs Res 19(1):2–9, 2006. Retrieved August 2008 from **http:// www.ncbi.nlm.nih.gov/pubmed/16455435**

Robinson, RG, and Krishnan, KR: Depression and the medically ill. In Davis, KL, Charney, D, Coyle, JT, and Nemeroff, C (eds.): Neuropsychopharmacology: The fifth generation of progress. American College of Pharmacology, 2002. Retrieved August 2008 from **http://www.acnp.org/Docs/G5/CH81_1179-1186.pdf**

Schaffer Library of Drug Policy: Handbook for medical practitioners and other health care workers on alcohol and drug problems, updated June 19, 2003. Retrieved August 2008 from **http://www.druglibrary .org/schaffer/Other/ALC_INT.HTM**

Schneider Institute for Health Policy, Brandeis University: Substance abuse: The nation's number one health problem, 2001. Retrieved August 2008 from **http://www.ncjrs.gov/pdffiles1/ojjdp/fs200117.pdf**

Substance Abuse and Mental Health Services Administration: Data on drug-related emergency room visits, 2006. Retrieved August 2008 from **http://www.samhsa.gov/news/newsreleases/060510 _dawn2.htm**

Sucholeik, R, and Caselli, RJ: Dementia: Overview of pharmacotherapy, updated July 16, 2007. Retrieved April 2009 from **http://emedicine .medscape.com/article/1136306-overview**

Suresh, S: Chronic pain management in children and adolescents, 2002. Retrieved August 2008 from **http://www.childsdoc.org/spring2002/ chronicpain.asp**

Surgical Care Improvement Project: Various articles, n.d. Available from **http://www.ihi.org/IHI/Topics/PatientSafety/SurgicalSiteInfections/ Resources/SurgicalCareImprovementProject.htm**

Sutter Health: Monographs on child growth and development, n.d. Retrieved August 2008 from **http://www.kids.sutterhealth.org/ health/development.html**

Thomas, A: Depression and physical illness, 2005. Retrieved August 2008 from **http://www.netdoctor.co.uk/diseases/depression/ depressionandphysicalillness_000601.htm**

University of Iowa Gerontological Interventions Research Center: Oral hygiene care for functionally dependent and cognitively impaired older adults. National Guideline Clearinghouse, 2002. Available from **http://www.guideline.gov**

University of Texas at Austin, School of Nursing, Family Nurse Practitioner Program: Initiating exercise in adults with chronic illness. National Guideline Clearinghouse, 2004. Available from **http://www.guideline.gov**

University of Washington: Specific strategies for coping with physical and behavioral problems, 2002. Retrieved March 2008 from **http:// depts.washington.edu/adrcweb/UnderstandingAD/Strategies.shtml**

U.S. Department of Veterans Affairs: National Center for PTSD fact sheet: PTSD and problems with alcohol use, updated 2007. Retrieved August 2008 from **http://www.ncptsd.va.gov/ncmain/ncdocs/ fact_shts/fs_alcohol.html**

Weekes, AJ, and Lee, DS: Substance abuse: Cocaine, updated 2008. Retrieved August 2008 from **http://www.emedicine.com/PED/ topic2666.htm**

Wong, ES, and Hooton, TM: Guidelines for prevention of catheter-associated urinary tract infections. Centers for Disease Control and Prevention, updated 2005. Retrieved August 2008 from **http://www.cdc.gov/ncidod/dhqp/gl_catheter_assoc.html**

Presentations

Lewis, MM: End of life care in long term care settings. Presentation: End of Life Care and Bereavement, National Geropsychology Conference, University of Colorado at Colorado Springs, 2008.

Otis-Green, S: Building your legacy: Making moments matter. Presentation: End of Life Care and Bereavement, National Geropsychology Conference, University of Colorado at Colorado Springs, 2008a.

Otis-Green, S: Grief and bereavement care. Presentation: End of Life Care and Bereavement, National Geropsychology Conference, University of Colorado at Colorado Springs, 2008b.

INDEX OF NURSING DIAGNOSES

A

Activity intolerance: anemias—iron deficiency, pernicious, aplastic, hemolytic and, 498; end-of-life care/hospice and, 870; heart failure: chronic and, 56; hypertension: severe and, 43; leukemias and, 524; myocardial infarction and, 81; pediatric considerations and, 895; pneumonia and, 138

Airway clearance, ineffective: burns: thermal, chemical, electrical and, risk for, 672; COPD and asthma, 124; disc surgery and, risk for, 265; lung cancer (postoperative care) and, 149; pneumonia and, 135; pulmonary tuberculosis and, 191; radical neck surgery: laryngectomy (postoperative care) and, 164; seizure disorders and, risk for, 217; thyroidectomy and, risk for, 430; ventilatory assistance (mechanical) and, 178

Anxiety: alcohol: acute withdrawal and, 829; angina (coronary artery disease, acute coronary syndrome) and, 72; benign prostatic hyperplasia and, 594; burns: thermal, chemical, electrical and, 682; cancer and, 850; disaster considerations and, 881; glaucoma and, 208; herniated nucleus pulposus (ruptured intervertebral disc) and, 259; hyperthyroidism: Graves' disease, thyrotoxicosis and, 426; inflammatory bowel disease: ulcerative colitis, Crohn's disease and, 330; lung cancer (postoperative care) and, 151; mastectomy and, 623; myocardial infarction and, 82; pediatric considerations and, 894; peritonitis and, 356; psychosocial aspects of care and, 754; renal dialysis and, 566; surgical intervention and, 787; transplantation considerations and, 753; upper gastrointestinal/esophageal bleeding and, 313; ventilatory assistance (mechanical) and, 180

Anxiety, death: AIDS and, 735; end-of-life care/hospice and, 871; mastectomy and, 623

Aspiration, risk for: total nutritional support: parenteral/enteral feeding and, 479

Autonomic dysreflexia, risk for: spinal cord injury (acute rehabilitative phase) and, 286

B

Bleeding, risk for: AIDS and, 728; cirrhosis of the liver and, 454; hepatitis and, 441; prostatectomy and, 598; upper gastrointestinal/esophageal bleeding and, 310

Body image, disturbed: burns: thermal/chemical/electrical and, 683; cirrhosis of the liver and, 456; eating disorders: anorexia nervosa/bulimia nervosa and, 378; eating disorders: obesity and, 393; fecal diversions: postoperative care of ileostomy and colostomy and, 336; radical neck surgery: laryngectomy (postoperative care) and, 170; renal dialysis and, 567; rheumatoid arthritis and, 745; urinary diversions/urostomy (postoperative care) and, 582

Body temperature, risk for imbalanced: pediatric considerations and, 901; surgical intervention and, 792

Bowel incontinence: dementia of the Alzheimer's type/vascular dementia and, 777; spinal cord injury (acute rehabilitative phase) and, 283

Breathing pattern, ineffective: AIDS and, 727; alcohol: acute withdrawal and, 825; cardiac surgery: postoperative care and, 107; cholecystectomy and, 365; cirrhosis of the liver and, 453; craniocerebral trauma and, risk for, 229; disc surgery and, 265; obesity: bariatric surgery and, 399; pancreatitis and, 468; peritoneal dialysis and, 574; pneumothorax/hemothorax and, 156; seizure disorders and, 217; spinal cord injury (acute rehabilitative phase) and, 275; surgical intervention and, 793; ventilatory assistance (mechanical) and, 175

C

Cardiac output, decreased: alcohol: acute withdrawal and, 826; angina (coronary artery disease, acute coronary syndrome) and, 70; cardiac surgery: postoperative care and, 104; dysrhythmias and, 93; heart failure: chronic and, 53; hypertension: severe and, 41; hyperthyroidism (Graves' disease, thyrotoxicosis) and, 422; myocardial infarction and, 83; renal failure: acute and, 543; renal failure: chronic and, 553

Caregiver role strain, risk for: dementia of the Alzheimer's type/vascular dementia and, 781; end-of-life care/hospice and, 873; multiple sclerosis and, 302

Comfort, impaired: cardiac surgery: postoperative care and, 106; thrombophlebitis: deep vein thrombosis and, 116

Communication, impaired verbal: cerebrovascular accident/stroke and, 246; extended care and, 808; radical neck surgery: laryngectomy (postoperative care) and, 165; thyroidectomy and, 341; ventilatory assistance (mechanical) and, 179

Conflict, decisional: psychosocial aspects of care and, 751

Confusion, acute: cirrhosis of the liver and, risk for, 455

Confusion, chronic: dementia of the Alzheimer's type/vascular dementia and, 770

Constipation: anemias (iron deficiency, anemia of chronic disease, pernicious, aplastic, hemolytic) and, 500; cancer and, 862; dementia of the Alzheimer's type/vascular dementia and, 777; disc surgery and, 267; extended care and, 805; fecal diversions: postoperative care of ileostomy and colostomy and, 341; hysterectomy and, 614; spinal cord injury (acute rehabilitative phase) and, 283

Constipation, risk for: renal dialysis and, 565; total joint replacement and, 661

Coping, ineffective: cerebrovascular accident/stroke and, 249; herniated nucleus pulposus (ruptured intervertebral disc) and, 259; hypertension: severe and, 45; inflammatory bowel disease: ulcerative colitis, Crohn's disease and, 332; multiple sclerosis and, risk for, 299; pediatric considerations and, 894; psychosocial aspects of care and, 751; substance dependence/abuse rehabilitation and, 838; transplantation considerations (postoperative and lifelong) and, 744

Coping, ineffective community: disaster considerations and, 884

Coping, readiness for enhanced community: disaster considerations and, 885

Coping, compromised family: dementia of the Alzheimer's type/vascular dementia and, 779; end-of-life care/hospice and, 873; extended care and, 806; multiple sclerosis and, 300; psychosocial aspects of care and, risk for, 752

Coping, readiness for enhanced family: psychosocial aspects of care and, risk for, 753

D

Denial, ineffective: substance dependence/abuse rehabilitation and, 837

Development, risk for delayed: pediatric considerations and, 896

Diarrhea: anemias—iron deficiency, anemia of chronic disease, pernicious, aplastic hemolytic and, 500; cancer and, risk for, 863; extended care and, risk for, 815; fecal diversions: postoperative care of ileostomy and colostomy and, risk for, 341; hysterectomy and, risk for, 614; inflammatory bowel disease: ulcerative colitis, Crohn's disease and, 327; obesity: bariatric surgery and, 403

Diversional activity, deficient: extended care and, 817

E

Electrolyte imbalance, risk for: hypercalcemia (calcium excess) and, 928; hyperkalemia (potassium excess) and, 923; hypermagnesemia (magnesium excess) and, 933; hypernatremia (sodium excess) and, 917; hypocalcemia (calcium deficit) and, 926; hypokalemia (potassium deficit) and, 920; hypomagnesemia (magnesium deficit) and, 931; hyponatremia (sodium deficit) and, 914

F

Falls, risk for: extended care and, 816

Family processes, dysfunctional: substance dependence/abuse rehabilitation and, 843

Family processes, interrupted: cancer and, risk for, 864; craniocerebral trauma (acute rehabilitative phase) and, 236; pediatric consideration and, 900

Fatigue: diabetes mellitus/diabetic ketoacidosis and, 415; hepatitis and, 439; HIV-positive client and, 701; hyperthyroidism (Graves' disease, thyrotoxicosis) and, 425; multiple sclerosis and, 294; total nutritional support: parenteral/enteral feeding and, 481

Fear: alcohol: acute withdrawal and, 829; benign prostatic hyperplasia and, 594; burns: thermal, chemical, electrical and, 682; cancer and, 850; dementia of the Alzheimer's type/vascular dementia and, 773; disaster considerations and, 881; lung cancer (postoperative care) and, 151; myocardial infarction and, 82; pediatric considerations, 894; peritonitis and, 356; psychosocial aspects of care and, 754; renal dialysis and, 566; surgical intervention and, 787; transplantation considerations (postoperative and lifelong) and, 743; upper gastrointestinal/esophageal bleeding and, 313; ventilatory assistance (mechanical) and, 180

Fluid volume, deficient: diabetes mellitus/diabetic ketoacidosis and, 410; hypovolemia and, 910

Fluid volume, excess: cirrhosis of the liver and, 451; heart failure: chronic and, 57; hemodialysis and, risk for, 578; hypervolemia and, 907; myocardial infarction and, risk for, 86; peritoneal dialysis and, risk for, 570; renal failure: acute and, 541

Fluid volume, risk for deficient: adult leukemias and, 521; AIDS and, 715; appendectomy and, 347; benign prostatic hyperplasia and, 593; burns: thermal, chemical, electrical and, 673; cancer, 857; cholecystectomy and, 366; cholecystitis with cholelithiasis and, 361; eating disorders: anorexia nervosa/bulimia nervosa and, 377; fecal diversions: postoperative care of ileostomy and colostomy and, 338; hemodialysis and, 577; hepatitis and, 441; inflammatory bowel disease: ulcerative colitis, Crohn's disease and, 328; obesity: bariatric surgery and, 400; pancreatitis and, 464; peritoneal dialysis and, 571; peritonitis and, 353; pneumonia and, 140; prostatectomy and, 598; renal failure: acute and, 546; sepsis/septicemia and, 694; sickle cell crisis and, 511; surgical intervention and, 795; urolithiasis (renal calculi) and, 609

Fluid volume, risk for imbalanced: pediatric considerations and, 899; total nutritional support: parenteral/enteral feeding, 480

G

Gas exchange, impaired: AIDS and, risk for, 717; COPD and asthma and, 126; fractures and, risk for, 639; heart failure: chronic and, risk for, 58; lung cancer (postoperative care) and, 148; lymphomas and, risk for, 530; pancreatitis and, 468; pneumonia and, 136; pulmonary tuberculosis and, risk for, 192; respiratory acidosis (primary carbonic acid excess) and, 199; respiratory alkalosis (primary carbonic acid deficit) and, 202; sepsis/septicemia and, risk for, 695; sickle cell crisis and, 507; thrombophlebitis: deep vein thrombosis and, 117

Glucose level, risk for unstable blood: diabetes mellitus/diabetic ketoacidosis and, 411; pancreatitis and, 466

Grieving: cancer and, 852; dementia of the Alzheimer's type/vascular dementia and, 774; end-of-life care/hospice and, 871; extended care and, 804; hysterectomy and, risk for, 616; psychosocial aspects of care and, 757; spinal cord injury (acute rehabilitative phase) and, 281

Growth and development, delayed: pediatric considerations and, risk for, 896

H

Health maintenance, ineffective: dementia of the Alzheimer's type/vascular dementia and, 780; extended care and, 818; pediatric considerations and, risk for, 902

Home maintenance, impaired: dementia of the Alzheimer's type/vascular dementia and, 780

Hopelessness: multiple sclerosis and, 298

I

Infection, risk for: adult leukemias and, 520; anemias (iron deficiency, anemia of chronic disease, pernicious, aplastic, hemolytic) and, 501; appendectomy and, 346; craniocerebral trauma (acute rehabilitative phase) and, 234; diabetes mellitus/diabetic ketoacidosis and, 413; hepatitis and, 442; obesity: bariatric surgery and, 403; pancreatitis and, 467; peritoneal dialysis and, 573; peritonitis and, 352; pneumonia and, 137; pulmonary tuberculosis and, 186; renal failure: acute and, 546; sickle cell crisis and, 513; total nutritional support: parenteral/enteral feeding and, 477; ventilatory assistance (mechanical) and, 182

Injury, risk for: alcohol: acute withdrawal and, 827; dementia of the Alzheimer's type/vascular dementia and, 768; disaster considerations and, risk for, 878; hemodialysis and, 575; pediatric considerations and, 898; surgical intervention and, 789; thryoidectomy and, 431; total nutritional support: parenteral/enteral feeding and, 478

Injury, risk for perioperative positioning: surgical intervention and, 788

K

Knowledge, deficient: adult leukemias and, 524; AIDS and, 727; amputation and, 653; anemias—iron deficiency, pernicious, aplastic, hemolytic and 501; angina (coronary artery disease, acute coronary syndrome) and, 73; appendectomy and, 348; benign prostatic hyperplasia and, 594; burns: thermal/chemical/electric and, 684; cancer and, 865; cardiac surgery: postoperative care and, 109; cerebrovascular accident (CVA)/stroke and, 252; cholecystectomy and, 368; cholecystitis with cholelithiasis and, 363; cirrhosis of the liver and, 457; COPD and asthma and, 129; craniocerebral trauma (acute rehabilitative phase) and, 237; diabetes mellitus/diabetic ketoacidosis and, 416; disc surgery and, 268; dysrhythmias and, 98; eating disorders: anorexia nervosa/bulimia nervosa and, 381; eating disorders: obesity and, 395; fecal diversions: postoperative care of ileostomy and colostomy and, 342; fractures and, 644; gastrectomy/gastric resection and, 319; glaucoma, 209; heart failure: chronic and, 60; herniated nucleus pulposus (ruptured intervertebral disc) and, 260; hepatitis and, 444; HIV-positive client and, 703; hypertension: severe and, 46; hyperthyroidism (Graves' disease, thyrotoxicosis) and, 428; hysterectomy and, 617; inflammatory bowel disease: ulcerative colitis, Crohn's disease and, 333; lymphomas and, 534; lung cancer (postoperative care) and, 152; mastectomy and, 627; multiple sclerosis and, 303; myocardial infarction and, 87; obesity: bariatric surgery and, 404; pancreatitis and, 468; peritonitis and, 356; pneumonia and, 141; pneumothorax/hemothorax and, 160; prostatectomy and, 601; pulmonary tuberculosis and, 194; radical neck surgery: laryngectomy (postoperative care) and, 171; renal dialysis and, 568; renal failure: acute and, 547; renal failure: chronic and, 558; rheumatoid arthritis and, 737; seizure disorders and, 219; sepsis/septicemia and, 696; sickle cell crisis and, 514; spinal cord injury (acute rehabilitative phase) and, 288; substance dependence/abuse rehabilitation and, 845; surgical intervention and, 786, 800; total nutritional support: parenteral/enteral feeding and, 482; thrombophlebitis: deep vein thrombosis and, 118; thyroidectomy and, 433; total joint replacement and, 662; transplantation considerations (postoperative and lifelong) and, 745; upper gastrointestinal/esophageal bleeding and, 315; urinary diversions/urostomy (postoperative care) and, 587; urolithiasis (renal calculi) and, 609; ventilatory assistance (mechanical) and, 185

L

Lifestyle, sedentary: eating disorders: obesity and, 392

Liver function, risk for impaired: hepatitis and, 437

M

Memory, impaired: extended care and, 805

Mobility, impaired physical: amputation and, 652; burns: thermal, chemical, electric and, 680; cerebrovascular accident (CVA)/stroke and, 244; craniocerebral trauma (acute rehabilitative phase) and, 233; disc surgery and, 266; extended care and, 816; fractures and, 640; herniated nucleus pulposus (ruptured intervertebral disc) and, 259; mastectomy and, 626; renal dialysis and, 563; rheumatoid arthritis and, 734; sickle cell crisis and, 512; spinal cord injury (acute rehabilitative phase) and, 277; total joint replacement and, 660

N

Nausea: lymphomas and, 532

Neglect, unilateral: cerebrovascular accident (CVA)/stroke and, 253

Nutrition: less than body requirements, imbalanced: AIDS and, 718; anemias—iron deficiency, anemia of chronic disease, pernicious, aplastic, hemolytic and, 499; burns: thermal, chemical, electric and, 679; cancer and, 856; cholecystitis with cholelithiasis and, risk for, 362; cirrhosis of the liver and, 449; COPD and asthma and, 128; craniocerebral trauma (acute rehabilitative phase) and, risk for, 235; dementia of the Alzheimer's type/vascular dementia and, risk for, 776; eating disorders: anorexia nervosa/bulimia nervosa, 374; eating disorders: obesity and, 390; extended care and, 810; fecal diversions: postoperative care of ileostomy and colostomy and, risk for, 339; gastrectomy/gastric resection and, risk for, 318; hepatitis and, 440; HIV-positive client and, 702; hyperthyroidism (Graves' disease, thyrotoxicosis) and, risk for, 425; inflammatory bowel disease: ulcerative colitis, Crohn's disease and, risk for, 328; obesity: bariatric surgery and, risk for, 401; pancreatitis and, 465; pediatric considerations and, risk for, 897; peritonitis and, risk for, 355; pneumonia and, risk for, 139; pulmonary tuberculosis and, 193; radical neck surgery: laryngectomy (postoperative care) and, 169; renal dialysis and, 562; renal failure: acute and, risk for, 545; substance dependence/abuse rehabilitation and, 840; total nutritional support: parenteral/enteral feeding and, 474; ventilatory assistance (mechanical) and, 181

Nutrition: more than body requirements, imbalanced: dementia of the Alzheimer's type/vascular dementia and, risk for, 776; extended care and, 810; hypertension: severe and, 44

O

Oral mucous membrane, impaired: AIDS and, 722; cancer and, risk for, 860; radical neck surgery: laryngectomy (postoperative care) and, 169; renal failure: chronic and, risk for, 557; ventilatory assistance (mechanical) and, 181

P

Pain, acute: adult leukemias and, 523; AIDS and, 720; amputation and, 649; angina (coronary artery disease, acute coronary syndrome) and, 68; appendectomy and, 348; benign prostatic hyperplasia and, 593; burns: thermal, chemical, electrical and, 675; cancer and, 854; cardiac surgery: postoperative care and, 106; cholecystitis with cholelithiasis and, 360; disc surgery and, 265; end-of-life care/hospice and, 869; fecal diversions: postoperative care of ileostomy and colostomy and, 337; fractures and, 636; herniated nucleus pulposus (ruptured intervertebral disc) and, 257; hypertension: severe and, 43; inflammatory bowel disease: ulcerative colitis, Crohn's disease and, 331; lung cancer (postoperative care) and, 150; mastectomy and, 624; myocardial infarction and, 79; pancreatitis and, 463; peritoneal dialysis and, 572; pediatric considerations and, 893; peritonitis and, 354; pneumonia and, 138; prostatectomy and, 600; radical neck surgery: laryngectomy (postoperative care) and, 168; rheumatoid arthritis and, 732; sickle cell crisis and, 509; spinal cord injury (acute rehabilitative phase) and, 280; surgical intervention and, 796; total joint replacement and, 657; thrombophlebitis: deep vein thrombosis and, 116; thyroidectomy and, 432; upper gastrointestinal/esophageal bleeding and, 314; urinary diversions/urostomy (postoperative care) and, 583; urolithiasis (renal calculi) and, 606

Pain, chronic: AIDS and, 720; cancer and, 854; end-of-life care/hospice and, 869; heart failure: chronic and, risk for, 59; herniated nucleus pulposus (ruptured intervertebral disc) and, 257; pediatric considerations and, 893; rheumatoid arthritis and, 732; sickle cell crisis and, 509; upper gastrointestinal/esophageal bleeding and, 314

Parenting, impaired: eating disorders: anorexia nervosa/bulimia nervosa and, 380; pediatric considerations and, 900

Perfusion, ineffective tissue: burns: thermal, chemical, electrical and, 678; disc surgery and, 263; hysterectomy and, risk for, 615; myocardial infarction and, 84; obesity: bariatric surgery and, risk for, 400; sickle cell crisis and, 510; thrombophlebitis: deep vein thrombosis and, 114; tissue perfusion and, risk for, 799

Perfusion, ineffective peripheral tissue: amputation and, 650

Perfusion, risk for ineffective cerebral tissue: cerebrovascular accident (CVA)/stroke and, 242; craniocerebral trauma (acute rehabilitative phase) and, 226

Poisoning, risk for: dysrhythmias (including digoxin toxicity) and, 97; extended care and, 807

Post-trauma syndrome, risk for: disaster considerations and, 883; psychosocial aspects of care and, 762

Powerlessness: AIDS and, 727; diabetes mellitus/diabetic ketoacidosis and, 415; multiple sclerosis and, 298; substance dependence/abuse rehabilitation and, 839

Protection, ineffective: renal failure: chronic and, risk for, 555

R

Religiosity, risk for impaired: psychosocial aspects of care and, 759

Relocation stress syndrome, risk for: dementia of the Alzheimer's type/vascular dementia and, 782; extended care and, 803

Role performance, ineffective: burns: thermal, chemical, electrical and, 683; radical neck surgery: laryngectomy (postoperative care) and, 170; rheumatoid arthritis and, 735

S

Self-care deficit: cerebrovascular accident (CVA)/stroke and, 248; dementia of the Alzheimer's type/vascular dementia and, 775; extended care and, 812; multiple sclerosis and, 296; renal dialysis and, 564; rheumatoid arthritis and, 736

Self-esteem: cirrhosis of the liver and, 456

Self-esteem, chronic low: eating disorders: anorexia nervosa/bulimia nervosa and, 378; eating disorders: obesity and, 393; multiple sclerosis and, 297; seizure disorders and, 218; substance dependence/abuse rehabilitation and, 841

Self-esteem, situational low: amputation and, 648; cancer and, 853; hepatitis and, 442; hysterectomy and, 613; mastectomy and, 625; multiple sclerosis and, 297; psychosocial aspects of care and, 756; renal dialysis and, 567; seizure disorders and, 218; spinal cord injury (acute rehabilitative phase) and, 282

Sensory Perception, disturbed: alcohol: acute withdrawal and, 828; cerebrovascular accident (CVA)/stroke and, 247; craniocerebral trauma (acute rehabilitative phase) and, 230; dementia of the Alzheimer's type/vascular dementia and, 772; diabetes mellitus/diabetic ketoacidosis and, risk for, 414; glaucoma and, 207; spinal cord injury (acute rehabilitative phase) and, 279; surgical intervention and, 794

Sexual dysfunction: cancer and, risk for, 863; dementia of the Alzheimer's type/vascular dementia and, risk for, 778; extended care and, risk for, 818; fecal diversions: postoperative care of ileostomy and colostomy and, risk for, 341; hysterectomy and, risk for, 616; lymphomas and, 533; prostatectomy and, risk for, 600; substance dependence/abuse rehabilitation and, 844; urinary diversions/urostomy (postoperative care) and, risk for, 586

Shock, risk for: sepsis/septicemia and, 692; upper gastrointestinal/esophageal bleeding and, 313;

Skin integrity, impaired: burns: thermal, chemical, electrical and, 681; cardiac surgery: postoperative care and, 108; cholecystectomy and, 367; fecal diversions: postoperative care of ileostomy and colostomy and, 338; mastectomy and, 624; radical neck surgery: laryngectomy (postoperative care) and, 166; surgical intervention and, 798

Skin integrity, risk for impaired: AIDS and, 721; cancer and, 861; cirrhosis of the liver and, 452; heart failure: chronic and, 60; eating disorders: anorexia nervosa/bulimia nervosa and, 381; extended care and, 812; fecal diversions: postoperative care of ileostomy and colostomy and, 335; fractures and, 641; hepatitis and, 443; obesity: bariatric surgery and, 402; renal failure: chronic and, 557; sickle cell crisis and, 513; spinal cord injury (acute rehabilitative phase) and, 287; urinary diversions/urostomy (postoperative care) and, 580

Sleep deprivation: dementia of the Alzheimer's type/vascular dementia and, 774; fecal diversions: postoperative care of ileostomy and colostomy and, 340;

Sleep pattern, disturbed: extended care and, 809

Social interaction, impaired: eating disorders: obesity and, 394

Social isolation: AIDS and, 726; HIV-positive client and, risk for, 706

Spiritual distress: disaster considerations and, 882; end-of-life care/hospice and, risk for, 874

Suffocation, risk for: pneumothorax/hemothorax and, 159; seizure disorders and, 215

Swallowing, impaired: cerebrovascular accident (CVA)/stroke and, risk for, 250

T

Therapeutic regimen management, family: HIV-positive client and, 707

Tissue integrity, impaired: cancer and, risk for, 861; cholecystectomy and, 367; fecal diversions: postoperative care of ileostomy and colostomy and, 338 (risk for, 335); fractures and, risk for, 641; hepatitis and, risk for, 443; hyperthyroidism (Graves' disease, thyrotoxicosis) and, risk for, 427; mastectomy and, 624; radical neck surgery: laryngectomy (postoperative care) and, 166; spinal cord injury (acute rehabilitative phase) and, risk for, 287; surgical intervention and, 798

Trauma, risk for: dementia of the Alzheimer's type/vascular dementia and, 768; disc surgery (spinal) and, 264; fractures and, 635; peritoneal dialysis and, 572; pneumothorax/hemothorax and, 159; seizure disorders and, 215; spinal cord injury (acute rehabilitative phase) and, 277

U

Urinary elimination, impaired: dementia of the Alzheimer's type/vascular dementia and, 777; extended care and, risk for, 814; hysterectomy and, 613; multiple sclerosis and, 301; prostatectomy and, 597; spinal cord injury (acute rehabilitative phase) and, 284; urinary diversions/urostomy (postoperative care) and, 585; urolithiasis (renal calculi) and, 607

Urinary retention: benign prostatic hyperplasia and, 591; disc surgery and, risk for, 268; hysterectomy and, 613

V

Ventilation, impaired spontaneous: ventilatory assistance (mechanical) and, 175

Ventilatory weaning response, dysfunctional: ventilatory assistance (mechanical) and, risk for, 183

Violence, risk for other-directed: psychosocial aspects of care and, 761

Violence, risk for self-directed: psychosocial aspects of care and, 761

W

Walking, impaired: rheumatoid arthritis and, 734